Other books by members of
the Boston Women's Health Book Collective

Changing Bodies, Changing Lives
The New Ourselves, Growing Older
Ourselves and Our Children

OUR BODIES, OURSELVES

for the New Century

A BOOK BY AND FOR WOMEN

The Boston Women's Health

Book Collective

A TOUCHSTONE BOOK

Published by
SIMON & SCHUSTER

TOUCHSTONE
Rockefeller Center
1230 Avenue of the Americas
New York, NY 10020

Copyright © 1984, 1992, 1998 by the Boston Women's Health Book Collective
All rights reserved,
including the right of reproduction
in whole or in part in any form.

TOUCHSTONE and colophon are registered trademarks
of Simon & Schuster Inc.

Designed by Barbara Bachman

Manufactured in the United States of America

3   5   7   9   10   8   6   4

Library of Congress Cataloging-in-Publication Data
Our bodies, ourselves for the new century : a book by and for women /
the Boston Women's Health Book Collective.
    p.   cm. — (A Touchstone book.)
Originally published in 1984 under the title: Our bodies, ourselves.
Includes bibliographical references and index.
1. Women—Health and hygiene.   2. Women—Diseases.   3. Women—
Psychology.   I. Boston Women's Health Book Collective.
II. Our bodies, ourselves.
RA778.N49   1998
613'.04244—dc21   98-12725
CIP
ISBN 0-684-84231-9

We dedicate this book to three beloved women's health activists
whose passionate, inventive dedication to women's health,
and willingness to ask the difficult questions,
shaped a movement.

| Esther Rome (1945–1995) | Rachel Fruchter (1940–1997) | Mary Catherine Raugust Howell (1932–1998) |

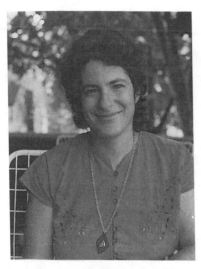

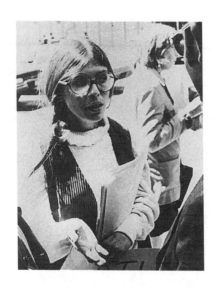

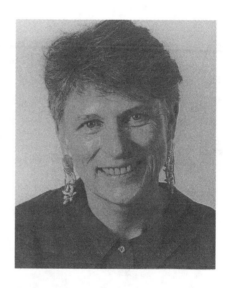

A founder of the Boston Women's Health Book Collective in 1969, Esther Rome co-authored every edition of *Our Bodies, Ourselves* as well as the recent *Sacrificing Our Selves for Love.* An irrepressible activist, Esther organized groundbreaking consumer input at the national level on key women's health issues such as breast implants and tampon safety. / *Nathan Rome*

A founder of HealthRight in New York City in the early 1970s, Rachel Fruchter significantly improved the quality and accessibility of health care for immigrant women in the New York area and nationwide through her tireless research, writing, and advocacy, especially in the area of cervical cancer.

Pediatrician, psychotherapist, lawyer, writer, and activist, Mary Howell was the very first woman dean at Harvard Medical School (Associate Dean for Student Affairs, 1972–1975), where she courageously documented and publicized the pervasive discrimination against women in the medical field. She co-founded the National Women's Health Network; contributed to many editions of *Our Bodies, Ourselves;* and spent her last years helping lesbian and gay families adopt children.

Acknowledgments

THE PRODUCTION CREW FOR *OUR BODIES, OURSELVES FOR THE NEW CENTURY*

1998 Update/Revision Committee: Paula Brown Doress-Worters, Linda King, Judith Lennett, Judy Norsigian, Wendy C. Sanford, and Jennifer Yanco
Senior Editor: Wendy C. Sanford
Coordinator and Junior Editor: Linda King
Graphics Team: Joan Ditzion, Linda King, Judith Lennett, and Sally Whelan
Editor for Tone and Voice: Carolivia Herron
Text Editors: Denise Bergman, Karen Kahn, Jacqueline Lapidus, Jane Pincus, and Kiki Zeldes
Librarians: Jamie Penney and Cindy Irvine
Electronic Resources Coordinator: Kiki Zeldes
Liaison to the Spanish-language Adaptation Project: Mayra Canetti
Final Manuscript Review: Judy Norsigian, Wendy C. Sanford, and April Taylor
Volunteers and Interns *(thank you!):* Trisha Brown, Elizabeth Butler, AnneMarie Clattenburg, Tanya Goldsmith, Regina Graham, Rebecca Herzig, Cecil Lyon Sanford, Laura Tandara, and Jennifer Young
Technical Support: Jamie Penney and Suzanne Nam

SPECIAL THANKS

We want to express special thanks to the following:

- **to our families and friends,** who loved and supported us through this long project and frequently contributed ideas, time, and energy to the book itself.

Polly Attwood	Judy Lapidus
Gerry and Artis Bergman	Kimo Lindon
Amanda Canetti	Elisabeth Morrison
Patricia Cooper	Amanda Mosola
Jesse Decker	Kyra Zola Norsigian
Anneka Shorai Dickson-King	Agnes Norsigian
	Gene Papa
Bruce, Rob, and Sam Ditzion	Anna Yanco Papa
	Ed Pincus
Pat Gozemba	Matthew Sanford
Georgia J. Herron	Helen Sheingold

Helen Horigan	Allen J. Worters
Kate Hogan	Jeanne Yanco
Eyvonne King	Amy Zeldes
Sasha Scot-Paul King	

- to our hard-working **friends at Simon & Schuster:** Sarah Baker, Francine Kass, and Patricia Bozza
- to the active members of the **BWHBC Board of Directors** during the revisions project: Cassandra Clay, June Cooper, Joan Ditzion, Paula Doress-Worters, Diane Hamer, Mirza Lugardo, Judy Norsigian, Michele Russell, Wendy C. Sanford, Ruth Seidman, Ester Shapiro, and Sally Whelan
- to the **Founders of the BWHBC:** Ruth Bell Alexander, Pamela Berger, Joan Ditzion, Vilunya Diskin, Paula Doress-Worters, Nancy Miriam Hawley, Elizabeth MacMahon-Herrera, Pamela Morgan, Judy Norsigian, Jane Pincus, Esther Rome (1945–1995), Wendy C. Sanford, Norma Swenson, and Sally Whelan
- to the women of the **BWHBC staff** during the very challenging revisions project: Maria Baez, Alba Bonilla, Mayra Canetti, Cindy Irvine, Judith Lennett, Judy Norsigian, Jamie Penney, Norma Swenson, April Taylor, Sally Whelan, and Jennifer Yanco

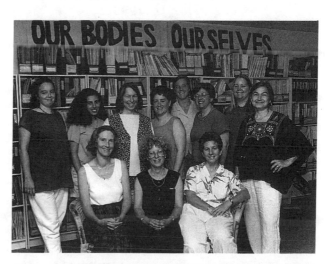

Some staff of the 1998 revisions project/Ellen Shub

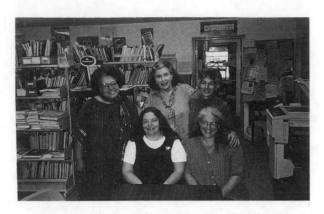

More staff of the 1998 revisions project/Judith Lennett

GENERAL THANKS—1998 Edition

The success of this book depends on many hours of volunteer labor on the part of the Production Crew (listed above) and writers, and a vast array of women and men who comment on drafts, send resources, put us in touch with activists and experts, type manuscripts, and tell us their stories. Most of the people who contributed to particular chapters of *Our Bodies, Ourselves for the New Century* are thanked on the chapter title pages. Thank you, too, to the following: Deborah Adams, Mikki Ansin, Byllye Avery, Dana Chesnulovitch, Donna R. Cooper, Ann Duerr, Sally Edwards and Sally Thompson, Maureen Ferrera, Mary Fillmore, Elana Freedom, Norm Fruchter, Cheryl Giles, Peggy Gillespie, Maryann Gontarz, Hilary and Julie Goodridge, Monique Harriton, Gerry Howard, Jenny Jones, Anne Kahn, Jane Kirk, Jill Kneerim, Judith Kurland, Carolyn Lejustc, Ilene Lerner, Christine McGoldrick, Susie Meikle, Rosie Muñoz-Lopez, Joann Neuroth, Magda Pedraza, Stanley Pillemer, Joanna Rankin, Nathan Rome, Miloslava Růžková, Maryellen Schroeder, Meghan-Morgan Shannon, Laurie Sheridan, Nina Solomita, Margaret Wheeler.

GENERAL THANKS—All Editions Prior to 1998

Thank you to Bonnie Acker; Sue Ade; Lois Alix; Amy Alpern; Carol Altobelli; Majeeda Amadadeen; Davida Andelman; Vicky Anderson; Beth Andrews; George Annas; Naomi Armon; Hilde Armour; Harriet Arnoldi; Connie Arsenault; Arthritis and Health Resource Center; Gisela Ashley; Diane Austras; Byllye Avery; Tricia Axsom; Diane Balser; Kim Bancroft; David Banta; Faith Nobuko Barcus; Phoebe Barnes; Kathleen Barry; Pauline Bart; Margaret Belbin; Ruth Bell; Alan, Noah, and Laurel Berger; Riva Berkovitz; Davi Birnbaum; Alice Bonis; Bea Bookchin; Shafia Bossman; Ursula Bowring-Trenn; Pam Boyle; Almont Bracy; Etta Breit; Belle Brett; Jan Brin; Linda Brion-Meisels; Steven Brion-Meisels; Abraham and Ethel Brown; Kathy Brownback; Agnes Butcher; Norma Canner; Barbara Carmen; Casa Myrna Vasquez; Robin Casarjian; Mary Rae Cate; Susie Chancey; Wendy Chavkin; Donna

Cherniac; Cindy Chin; Aram Chobanian; Ann Chronis; Peggy Clark; Savitri Clarke; Yarrow Anne Cleaves; Connie Clement; Cindy Cohen; Deborah Catherine Cohen; Nancy Cohen; Robert S. Cohen; Tom Conry; Liz Coolidge; Betty Corpt; Maria Corsaro; Mary Costanza; Terry Courtney; Olivia Cousins; Belita Cowan; Trudy Cox; Frannye Crocker; Megan Crowe-Rothstein; Emily Culpepper; John Cutler; Lynne Dahlborg; William Darrow; Martha Davis-Perry; Caro Dellenbaugh; Catherine DeLorey; Debby DeVaughn; Andrew Dibner; Annette Dickinson; Martin, Leah, and Aaron Diskin; Loretta Dixson; Rose Dobosz; Jan Dodds; Hannah and Benjamin Doress; Karen Dorman; Barbara Dow; Hugh Drummond; Kim Ducharme; Buffy Dunker; Wendy Dunning; Jane Dwinell; Sally Edwards; Susan Eisenberg; Helen Eisenstein; Carol Englander; Judy English; Carol Epple; Samuel S. Epstein; Wendy Roberts Epstein; Kitty Ernst; Tish Fabens; Martha Farrar; Lee Farris; Carolyn Fawcett; Richard Feinbloom; Geri Ferber; Fertility Consciousness Group; Cynthia Fertman; Ron Fichtner; JoAnne Fischer; Alice Fisher; Dan and Caitlin Fisher; Maureen Flammer; Mary Flinders; Becky Fowler; Cary Fowler; Dorothy Frauenhofer; Nancy Friedman; Stella Friml; Rose Frisch; Dana Gallagher; Paula Garbarino; Jean Gardelia; Linda Gardner; Linda Gaynor; Carole Geddis-Dlugasch; Tobin Gerhardt; Lois Gibbs; Paige Gidney; Cheryl Giles; Betty Gittes; Evelyn Gladu of Omega, Somerville, Mass.; Leonard Glantz; Ann Godoff; Pat Gold; Meg Goldman; Arnold A. Goldstein; Sharon Golub; Mary Moore Goodlett; Jennifer Gordon; Jocelyn Gordon; Ruth Gore and the Goldennaires; Freedom House, Roxbury, Mass.; Benina Gould; Gray Panthers; Meryl Green; Tova Green; Miriam Greenspan; Betsy Grob; Ione Gunnerson; Joan Gussow; Cynthia Hales; Diana Long Hall; Eleanor Hamilton; Jalna Hanmer; Sandie Harris; Michelle Harrison; Philip Hart; Pat Haseltine; Robert Hatcher; Josh and Gina Hawley; Marie Hayes; Lester Hazell; Muriel Heiberger; Lori Heise; Ingeborg Helling; Susan Helmrich; Judy Herman; Curdina Hill; Ruth Hill, Black Women's Oral History Project, Radcliffe Institute; Hella Hoffman; Kate Hoffman; Beryl-Elise Hoffstein; Joanne Holt; Bar-

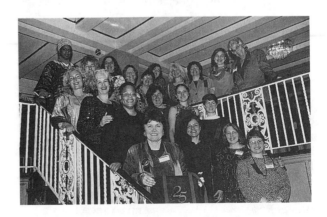

Some board, staff, and friends of the Boston Women's Health Book Collective/Ellen Shub

bara Homan; Barbara Horgan; Mary Howell; Ruth Hubbard; Jeanne Hubbuch; Maile Hulihan; Vilma Hunt; Suzanne Ingrao; Rick Ingrasci; Jeanne Jackson; Sandy Jaffe; Mary Jane Jarrett; Pat Jerabek; Kathryn Jewell; Gail Johnson; Leila Joseph; Myla Kabat-Zinn; Alexandra Kaplan; Peg Kapron; Amy Kasanjian; Linda Katzman; Augusta Kaufman; David Kaufman; Jay Kaufman; Peggy Hershenson Kaufman; Patrice Keegan; Lorrie Kendler; Cheryl Kennedy and Julia Perez; Jamie Keshet; Edith Kessler; Nina Kimche; Joanne Klys; Jenny Knaus; Joan Knight; Thurmond Knight; Pat Kraepelian-Bartels; Philip Kraft; Helen Kramer; Mark Kramer; Karen Kruskal; Ruth Kundsin; Ann LaCasse; Eben LaCasse; Kirsten LaCasse; Marianne LaLuz; Hildegarde Lambrom; Rachel Lanzerotti; Nan Lassin; Nancy Lastoff; Tesair Lauve; Nancy Lessin; Stephen Lester; Maggie Lettvin; Debbie LeVan; Jane Levin; Mitch Levine; Myrna Lewis; Heidi Lewitt; Rinchen Lhamo; Frederick Li; Ricky Lieberman; Bonnie Liebman; Dottie Limont; Lee Lindbert; Liz Linderman; Jessica Lipnak; Judy Lipshutz; Mary Logan; Dylan Loman; Carin Layne Loman; Susan Love; Barbara Low; Ruth Lubic; Brinton Lykes; Peggy Lynch; Ana Machado de Oliveira; P'nina Macher; Howie Machtinger; Catherine MacKinnon; Una MacLean; Brian MacMahon; Elizabeth MacMahon; Carol Mamber; Elizabeth Markson; Lisa Marlin; Irene Marotta; Caroline Marvin; Eliot Masters; Raquel Matas; Lourdes Mattei; Elizabeth Matz; Charlotte Mayerson; Art Mazer; Katie Mazer; William M. Mazer; Renee Mazon; Maggie McCarthy-Herzig; Bill McCormack; Jeffrey and Noah McIntyre; Patty McLean; Martha P. Megee; Jeanne Melvin; Mary Beth Menaker; Barbara Menning; Halford and Nellie Meras; Irma Meridy; Donald Miller; Jean Baker Miller; Miriam Miller; William Minniciello; Denise Minter; Nora Mitchell; Ramona Monteverde, Montreal Health Press; Helen Boulware Moore; Susanne Morgan; Beth Morrison; Marilyn Morrissey; Sonia Muchnick; Charlotte Muller; J. B. Mulligan, Multinational Monitor Staff; Sister Angela Murdaugh; Maryann Napoli; Ruth Nelson, Network of Women in Trade and Technical Jobs; Holly Newman; Marjorie Newman; Louise Newton; Nancy Nichols; Steve Nickerson, Nine-to-Five Health and Safety Committee; Barbara Norfleet; Roy Norsigian; Abigail November; Older Women's League; Oral History Project of the Cambridge Arts Council; Pat O'Reilly; Julie Snow Osherson; Patricia Papernow; Jane Patterson; Cynthia Pearson; Donald Pedicini; Jamie Penney; Jackie Petrillo; Robbie Pfeufer; Connie Phillips; Ed, Sami, and Ben Pincus; Beatrice Pitcher; Jackie Pitullo; Jo Polk-Matthews; Sara Poli; Jane Porcino; Ruth Porham; Clare Potter; Terri Powell; Gina Prenowitz; Abraham Press;

Helane Press; Janet Press; Rosellen Primrose; Susan Quass; Kathleen Quinlan; Minrose Quinn; Pat Rackowski; Jill Rakusen; Carolyn Ramsey; Eloise Rathbone-McCuan; Brenda Reeb; Elsie Reethof; Mira Reicher; Margaret Reid; C. J. Reilly; Erica Reitmayer; Susan Rennie; Ulrike Rettig; Susan Reverby; Naomi Ribner; Marcie Richardson; Claudia Richter; Pat Ricker; Virginia Robison; Lisa Rofel; Nathan, Judah, and Micah Rome; Eva Rooks; Alan Rosen; Lynn Rosenberg; Anita Rossien; Alice Rothchild; Natalie and Peter Rothstein; Donna Roux; Alice Ryerson; Alma Sabatini; Pat Sacry; Carol Sakala; Stephen, Daniel, and Nikki Salk; Jackie Samson; Toni Sandmaier; Linda Sanford; Frank Santora; Cheryl Schaffer; Nancy Schlick; Miriam Schocken; Cyprienne Schroeppel; Allyson Schwartz; Janet Schwartz; Jeremy Schwartz; Helen Scott; Mary Scully; Barbara Seaman; Eli Shapiro; Catherine Shaw; Rene Shaw; Susan Shaw; Beth Shearer; Helen Sheingold; Karen Sheingold; Sayre Sheldon; Laurie Shields; Andrea Siani; Sergio Siani; Ben Siegel; Jane Siegel; Diane Siegelman; Sandra Signor; Marge Silver; Phyllis Silverman; Yehudit Silverman; Jane Simmons-Nashinoff; Barbara Sindriglis; Joan Sing; Dan Sipe; Susan Siroty; Peggy Sloane; Seymour Small; Annette Smith; Barbara Smith; Beverly Smith; Lee Smith; Mary Smith; Leni Sollinger; Tish Sommers; Ethel Sondik; Heidi Spoerle; Selma Squires; Karen Stamm; Cecilia Stanley; Karen Starr; Judith Stein; Susan Steiner; Sheila Stillman; John Stoeckle; Carol A. Stollar; Sheera Strick; Suzanne Stuart; Jana Suchankova; Edith Bjornson Sunley; Carol Sussman; Judy Sutphen; Kate Swan; Chris Sweeney; John and Sarah Swenson; Cheryl Tabb; Linda Tate; Claire Taylor; Rosemary Taylor; Marsha Tennis; Bernice Thomas; Winnie Thomas; Helen Thornton; Peggy Thurston; Jean Tock; Sally Tom; Barbara Tomaskovic-Devey; Donald Tomaskovic-Devey; Melinda Tuhus; Trude Turnquist; Kathy Ullman; Stephanie Urdang; Carol Doyle Van Valkenburgh; Martha H. Verbrugge; Gretchen Von Mering; Margo Wallach; Lila Wallis; Susan Wanger; Gail Washor-Liebhaver; Barbara Waxman; David, Jesse, and Marya Wegman; Laura Weil; Michelle Weiner; Joan Caplan Weizer; Phoebe Wells; Laura Wexler; Sally Whelan; Beatrice Whiting; Lillian Whitney; Paul Wiesner; Valerie Wilk; Diane Willow Williams; Laurie Williams; Fran Wiltsie; Susan Winick; Ann Withorn; Glorianne Wittes; Simon Wittes, Will Wittington; Karen Wolf; Tom, Alexi, and Lea Wolf; Alice Wolfson; Jean Wolhandler; Women of the Boston-Area Socialist-Feminist Group; WOOSH (Women Organizing for Occupational Safety and Health); Lisa Yost; Geraldine Zetzel; Irv, Warren, and Amanda Zola; and Jane Sprague Zones.

Contents

....

Preface to the 25th Anniversary Edition

One of my introductions to the women's health movement came in 1971, from two women—Carol Downer and Lorraine Rothman—in Gainesville, Florida. They came to talk to us about claiming our bodies. After much sharing, we learned for the first time about the demystification of medicine and why it's important for women to understand and be in control of their own bodies. We were intrigued and excited by the thought of taking charge of our reproduction, of having the power to change our lives. We were told that women all over the country were beginning to question their medical care and that people were starting to develop women-specific health information. The Boston Women's Health Book Collective was just such a group, and with their first publication of *Our Bodies, Ourselves,* they showed us an example of women taking health care into their own hands.

This meeting occurred at a turning point in my life. My husband, at age thirty-three, had just suffered a massive heart attack and died. The trauma of this event made me question everything, particluarly the medical system and how health information was disseminated. In the early seventies, an awareness of the dangers of high blood pressure was not common knowledge. Although my husband and I were both educated, I with a master's degree and Wesley just four months away from his doctorate, in the end it didn't matter how much education we had. If you don't know how to take care of yourself, you are basically ignorant. I also realized that health information had to be shared within the context of one's life in order for it to produce lifestyle changes.

It was easy for me to be receptive to the words of these women as they talked about the *right* to have medical information and the importance, or even necessity, of active patient participation. Their words were so inspiring that five of us (Judy Levy, Margaret Parrish, Joan Edelson, Betsy Randall-David, and I) opened the doors of the Gainesville Women's Health Center (GWHC) in May 1974. This center provided first-trimester abortions and well-woman gynecological services.

The political climate of the seventies encouraged the continual growth of the women's health movement. And at the heart of this activism was the Boston Women's Health Book Collective, which convened the historic conference of 1975 in Boston, with five of us from the GWHC attending. The impact of that conference still resonates today in the hearts and souls of many of us, as it taught us to question the status quo and create a sensitive health care delivery system. In fact, it confirmed my commitment to the women's health movement. In 1978, I cofounded an alternative birthing center, Birthplace, and founded the National Black Women's Health Project in 1981.

Our Bodies, Ourselves is the bible for women's health. Countless women have told me that they consult it before physician visits and after diagnosis and are always comforted by its straightforward, honest approach. I have given away hundreds of copies to all kinds of women, those who can read it openly as well as those who are embarrassed and need to read it privately.

Our Bodies, Ourselves modeled for us the importance of talking about health problems with other women. Most of us participated in the conspiracy of silence. We felt ashamed about our illnesses, and this isolation contributed to further ill health. The truth of the matter is, *Our illness is our business.* Over the years, many of us have learned that we don't need to suffer in silence anymore. We now know that sharing helps us make knowledgeable decsions about our health and our lives.

The women's health movement started health care reform in the seventies. Women spoke out about the lack of health information given, the abuse of medical procedures and the unavailability of safe contraceptives. They said no to the disease approach to natural female processes such as birth and menopause and established the rationale for outpatient surgical procedures. Over the years, we have seen many of the demands of the women's health movement incorporated into standard health care procedure. Since the U.S. sees itself as the best health care system in the world, we are justified in making sure it lives up to its reputation.

Our Bodies, Ourselves has served as a way for women, across ethnic, racial, religious and geographical boundaries, to start examining their health from a perspective that will bring about change. The change begins with the individual, who then brings about effective community change. The struggle continues. *La lucha continua.*

—Byllye Avery

In 1970, a young woman training to become a pediatrician gave me a copy of a book by women and about women, printed on newspaper stock and cheaply bound. I was forty-one and just beginning to heal from a traumatic few years of a disastrous marriage. I had just arrived from Puerto Rico and was struggling to find my identity as a Puerto Rican professional and a single mother in New York City. When I read that first edition, titled *Women and Their Bodies,* I felt a surge of joy. The authors spoke to me as if I had been part of the discussion group.

This incredibly talented group of women, initially meeting about their frustration with doctors, had decided to empower themselves. They learned about their bodies, discussed their feelings and shared their knowledge with other women. Their individual and collective strength shone from the pages, giving me strength to grow as well. Their book validated my own nascent perceptions of our need for a different kind of medicine, one that respected and valued people's wisdom and autonomy. The courage and clarity of the women in valuing themselves and one another, in drawing the political lessons from their personal experiences, helped me start what became my lifelong work. I joined other advocates for our right to health. I joined the women's health movement. I became a charter member of the National Women's Health Network, a strong voice for women on health issues.

In the early seventies, my staff at Lincoln Hospital, a beleaguered city hospital in the South Bronx, included a group of pediatricians-in-training who were activists striving to change social inequities. As part of a group of doctors, nurses, and other hospital workers known as the Lincoln Collective, they were not always in harmony with hospital rules and regulations or other staff. The Lincoln Collective's goal was to improve health care for disfranchised communities. As a result, our library copies of the various editions of *Our Bodies, Ourselves* were dogeared and worn. Their contents were used for classes, discussions, and teaching materials for community groups.

I believe those readings, discussions and organizing efforts that the Book Collective sparked sensitized doctors and nurses to listen to and respect women as partners in seeking health. I hope it also led them to question accepted health care practices for women that women were questioning. I know that women who used the book challenged the young professionals into new ways of communicating with their patients.

Through the years, the Book Collective has undertaken difficult revisions, additions and expansions. New knowledge and changing needs, political realities and points of view compelled the authors to renew each edition. What has made each generation of women rejoice in discovering themselves in *Our Bodies, Ourselves* is that it still emanates from women's experiences as faithfully as ever. The idea that women's self-knowledge is the source of our knowledge of health, health promotion and health care is as valid now as it was twenty-five years ago.

Women now constitute an unprecedentedly high proportion of health care professionals and administrators. Although underrepresented in the higher ranks of pay and power, they exert a growing influence on the way women are treated by the health care system. But health care is undergoing radical changes, from a system controlled by doctors to large corporate entities controlled by managers far removed from patients and doctors. This calls for greater vigilance. In the world of "managed care," cost control rules, not quality or quantity of care.

Now, more than ever, we women must empower ourselves and our communities to participate knowingly in mounting health efforts. Promotion of health and prevention of illness must become paramount on our agenda. Women must lead the struggles to reverse the trend toward denying health care access to growing numbers of women—women of low income, of color, immigrant, with disabilities or who are aging are particularly vulnerable. The majority of the over 40 million people without health care coverage in this country are women and children—a national disgrace.

The new *Our Bodies, Ourselves* speaks to us, helping us understand and take better care of ourselves, and of one another. As the Book Collective has done for a quarter of a century, it challenges us and equips us to organize and fight for our rights to health. The women of the Collective make it clear that we cannot achieve a healthier us without achieving a healthier, more equitable health care system and ultimately a more equitable society.

—Helen Rodriguez-Trias

When the group that was to become the Boston Women's Health Book Collective first met in 1969, I was working as a political columnist for *New York* magazine. I was also white and thirty-five years old and had become middle-class courtesy of going to college. In other words, I was part of that small demographic slice of people most likely to get the best health care information. As a journalist, I was even in a position to research what I didn't know.

Yet what "best" meant in those largely prefeminist days was whatever limited information the medical establishment considered appropriate—for patients in general and for women in particular. As a result, I assumed that my body needed attention only when it didn't work, and that the large portions of animal fat, refined sugar, hormones and chemicals in our recommended diets couldn't be too dangerous or they wouldn't be there. Like the third or so of American women who had abortions even when they were illegal, I believed that if I needed an abortion, I had no choice but to risk my life and safety in a criminal underworld. After having one abortion and to avoid taking this risk a second time, I followed the "best" medical advice and took the high-dose contraceptive pill for a decade. In addition to such self-destructive acts, I had many habits based on unchallenged beliefs: for instance, that bingeing on sugar was okay as long as my weight was normal, that only heart attack–prone men had to worry about cholesterol or cardiovascular fitness, and that male violence was inevitable and could only be avoided by female caution.

All these conditions of life seemed to be the price

for being female. So did submitting our female bodies to doctors who were over 90% male (though childbearing meant that women used the health care system about 30% more than men did), and lying feet up like a dying bug in the common gynecological position (a horizontal pose so uniform that even women giving birth were forced to do so against gravity).

I often tell these personal observations because trusting, comparing and compiling our own experience is the revolutionary act taught to us by the Boston Women's Health Book Collective—as it is by feminism in all areas of life. Only remembering a prefeminist time of even greater disempowerment will allow us to see how revolutionary and prescient the message of twenty-five years ago really was. If women with the most resources had to endure ignorance, humiliation and a lack of empathy for female bodies (plus such special punishments as the mysteriously high rate of hysterectomies among women who could afford them), then those with fewer resources risked punishments that were far more lethal (for instance, higher mortality rates for breast cancer due to late discovery among poor women).

Much has changed in this past quarter century of a forceful and populist women's health movement, from increased mental health and life expectancy among women to the increased confidence and influence of women health consumers. Though there are still unacceptable differentials by race, class, age, sexuality and ability, the lives of the female half of America have been touched in a way that shows us how lifesaving a raised consciousness and collective activism can be. Indeed, the lives of men, too, have been improved and perhaps lengthened by such female-led reforms as labeling drugs with information about side effects (a cause advanced by protests against the contraceptive pill) and counselors who accompany a patient through procedures (an innovation pioneered by abortion clinics).

Nonetheless, there are still life-threatening reasons to keep learning from one another's experience, and to increase our activism. A medical and sexual double standard still tries to convince us that males, whether as doctors or lovers, know more about women's bodies than women do. Everyone from profiteering polluters to the beauty police still sends us to the medical establishment for unnecessary fixing. Drug companies still have more profit motive and government support for discovering expensive "cures" than for instituting already known, inexpensive preventions. The few still get better health care than the many. And there are newer areas where information and self-authority are crucial—from birth, fertility, and transplant technologies to fetal cell therapy that is promising for many diseases, yet is being withheld by threats from anti-abortion forces.

But we now know that we can topple hierarchies by starting with our bodies. After all, male-dominant, racist and other unjust systems must control female bodies as the most basic means of production, the means of reproduction, in order to "own" children through systems of legitimacy, to decide how many workers and soldiers the nation needs, and to maintain the degree of race (and class) "purity" that keeps hierarchical systems going.

Whether we are insisting on safe pregnancies or safe abortions, exposing male violence as a major health problem or exposing carcinogens in the environment, exercising our rights as sexual beings or as health consumers, we're taking control of our own bodies. Indeed, women are providing a model of empowerment and activism for male health consumers, too.

Now, this movement is worldwide—as is *Our Bodies, Ourselves*. It has been adapted and adopted in many different countries and cultures, and is available in many languages—and still growing.

Within these pages, you will find wisdom that can only come from shared experience. Listen to it—and add your own.

—Gloria Steinem

Overleaf: Some of the many contributors to the 1998 edition

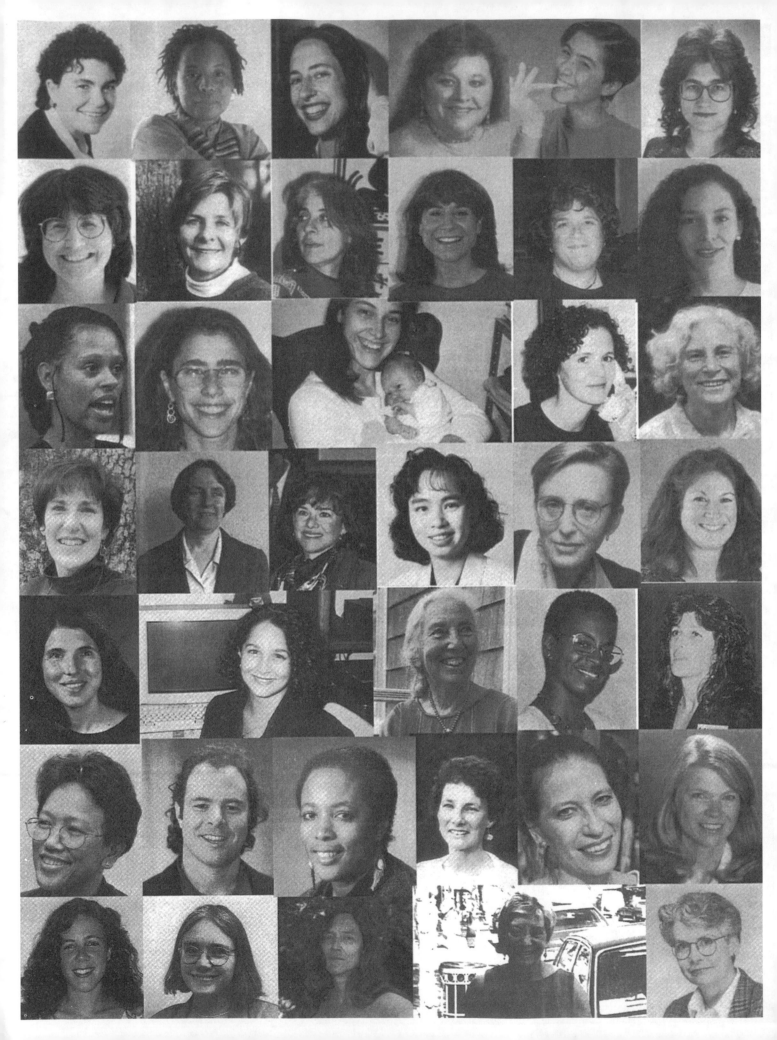

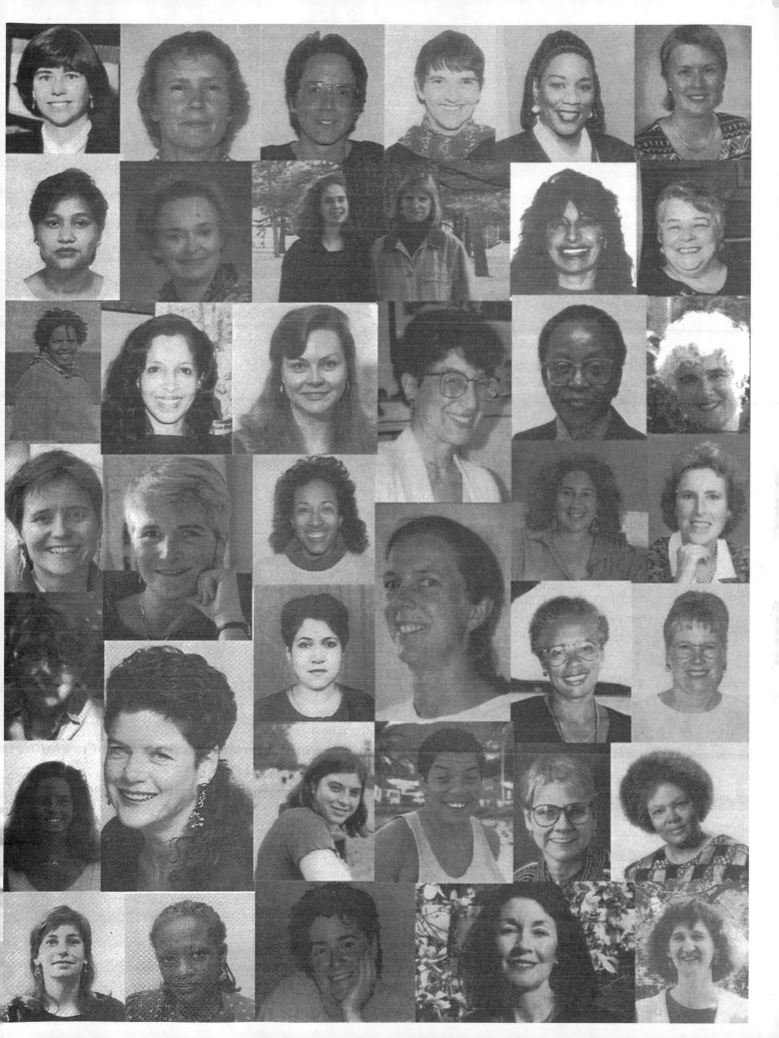

Introduction

....

By Jane Pincus

WITH SPECIAL THANKS TO Ruth Bell
Alexander, Joan Ditzion, Vilunya Diskin,
Paula Doress-Worters, Linda King, Elizabeth
MacMahon-Hererra, Judy Luce, Judy
Norsigian, Jamie Penney, Wendy C. Sanford,
Norma Swenson, Sally Whelan, Jennifer
Yanco, and Kiki Zeldes

Welcome to *Our Bodies, Ourselves for the New Century*! We offer first-time readers and old friends a greatly updated and expanded book that remains true to its beginnings. First published in 1970, the book grew out of a course by and for women about health, sexuality, and child-bearing. The original contributors began meeting weekly in Boston at the end of the dynamic 1960s, when women throughout the U.S. and the world were getting together to share experiences and expose the injustices in women's lives. In recounting our life stories and health care experiences, we discovered with surprise and elation that the "personal is political"—that we were not alone in what happened to us. By pooling all we knew about ourselves, we could create a useful body of knowledge. We soon realized that forces much larger than ourselves determined the availability and quality of health and medical care, and that by working in unison and sharing our knowledge and clout, we could become a force to alter the system to meet our needs. The resulting book became a road map for women and helped to launch and sustain the national and international women's health movement, selling more than four million copies in many languages throughout the world.

Unlike most health books on the market, *Our Bodies, Ourselves for the New Century* is unique in many respects: It is based on, and has grown out of, hundreds of women's experiences. It questions the medicalization of women's bodies and lives, and highlights holistic knowledge along with conventional biomedical information. It places women's experiences within the social, political, and economic forces that determine all of our lives, thus going beyond individualistic, narrow, "self-care" and self-help approaches, and views health in the context of the sexist, racist, and financial pressures that affect far too many girls, women, and families adversely. It condemns medical corporate misbehavior driven by "bottom-line" management philosophy and the profit motive. Most of all, *Our Bodies, Ourselves* encourages you to value and share your own insights and experiences, and to use its information to question the assumptions underlying the care we all receive so that we can deal effectively with the medical system and organize for better care.

This newest *Our Bodies, Ourselves* has been thor-

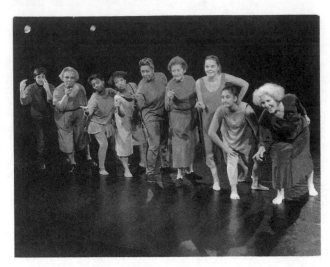

Members of the Intergenerational Troop, Back Porch Dance Company/Eric Levinson

oughly revised, and every chapter contains new and updated information. We have listed and critiqued on-line health resources for women. The chapters "Body Image" and "Sexuality" deal for the first time with issues of racism. We emphasize overwork, violence, and girls' increasing use of tobacco as major threats to women's health, and we highlight more than ever the importance of good food and exercise. We explore the new issues that arise as more lesbians choose to have children. We include transgender and transsexual issues, and discuss women living with HIV as well as the most recent safer sex advice. We explore more extensively the connections between race, class, and gender-based oppressions as they affect the health of women. We offer tools for negotiating the complex and often unregulated "managed care" system, which affects women's lives much more profoundly than men's, and discuss its advantages and disadvantages. Most important, we advocate for an equitable, single-payer national health care system.

Over these past three decades, *Our Bodies, Ourselves* has grown in scope and depth. From the start, the original authors have involved more and more women in its creation, adding new perspectives to each edition, expanding the "we" that appears so frequently throughout the book. This expansion has been a vital process, as the many contributing communities—lesbians, women of color, women with disabilities, older and younger women, to mention several—have changed in self-definition and focus.

While it is exciting that this book stays alive, growing and changing, the process of becoming more inclusive has been difficult and painful at times. For example, like many groups initially formed by white women, we have struggled against society's, and our own, internalized presumption that middle-class white women are representative of all women and thus have the right to define women's health issues and set priorities. This assumption does a great injustice by ignoring and silencing the voices of women of color,

depriving us all of hard-won wisdom and crucial, life-saving information. This time around, many more women of color have been involved in creating this book, writing some of the chapters, and editing and critically reading every chapter. During this process, tensions sometimes arose about what to include or leave out and how to frame certain issues. The resulting vigorous discussions have greatly enriched the book's content. But as in any organic process, some conflicts still remain to be resolved.

Those of us who worked on the original edition are now in our 50s or older. Some of us have made the politics of women's health our lives' work. To continue the book's long history and to ensure that it remains up-to-date, hundreds of women—including "ordinary" women, community organizers, social scientists, student interns, friends, health activists, and medical professionals—have contributed to this edition. Many women who were not yet born when the first edition of *Our Bodies, Ourselves* was published—including some daughters of Health Book Collective members—have shaped the book significantly with their voices and experiences. More than ever before, the staff of the Women's Health Information Center has anchored our research efforts, responding to readers, gathering and documenting health information, participating in national and international women's health endeavors, and strengthening the women's and documentation center movements.

Despite the achievements of the larger women's health movement, it is clear that the same forces that created the need for *Our Bodies, Ourselves* twenty-nine years ago exist today. Disparities in health continue to grow. Determinants of poor health, such as poverty, homelessness, and hunger have worsened, disproportionately affecting communities of color, non-English-speaking women, and women with low incomes in this country and throughout the world. The medical system remains a vast business more tightly connected than ever to drug and medical supply corporations, and increasingly controlled by larger national and international profit-making industries. As "consumers" we must still fight for control and accountability in health plans. Industries continue to pollute water, land, and air. Our increasingly conservative national government embraces the wishes and demands of business interests while seriously reducing or eliminating crucial federal funds for programs dedicated to maintaining and improving our health and lives. Welfare "reform" is causing even more anguish for immigrants and mothers with low incomes.

Thus, as the millennium approaches, our original goals for this book remain as important to us as ever: to fit as much information about women's health between the covers of this book as we can, providing women with tools to enable all of us to take charge of our health and lives; to support women and men who work for progressive change; and to work to create a just society in which good health is not a luxury or a privilege but a human right.

One of the most valuable things we did in our early

While the information contained in *Our Bodies, Ourselves* will hopefully empower you and give you useful tools and ideas, this book is not intended to replace professional health and medical care.

years together was to talk in small groups about our lives. In doing so, we were reclaiming an important part of our common heritage as women who have always, in traditional communities, achieved wisdom by exchanging experiences with one another. We encourage you to meet together, to speak out and listen to one another, and to learn from one another. We recognize that in these times, more women must work harder than ever before and have very little time left over, even for our families. See what you can do close to home, in your living rooms, in your communities. Seek each other out at church, synagogue, or mosque; at the YWCA; at a nearby women's center; and at informal gatherings. Find ways to support the work of nonprofit groups whose efforts you value. Talk together and organize around crucial issues. Fighting back can be good for you and can feel good, too!

We gain political strength by identifying what we have in common, respecting the special needs of each group, and standing in unity. Despite everyone's efforts, this unity remains fragile. We are still evolving ways to form communities that will stand in solidarity with one another. Too often, differences in race, class, ethnicity, financial circumstance, sexual orientation, values, strategies, and degrees of power make it difficult to listen to one another, and these differences divide us. By telling the truth about our lives, women with dissimilar backgrounds and experiences make it more possible for every woman's voice to be heard and for every woman's life to be nurtured. To transform the world into a healthy place we need the energy of *all* women.

The Boston Women's Health Book Collective is a nonprofit organization devoted to education about women and health. Our many projects and services include a Women's Health Information Center; extensive distribution of free materials to women and organizations in the United States and other countries; several midwifery and reproductive health projects; assistance for women in other countries to develop their own translation/adaptions of *Our Bodies, Ourselves;* and a speakers bureau. Royalties income from the sale of *Our Bodies, Ourselves* is not sufficient to support our work. Therefore, the Collective continually needs additional funding from contributions and grants. Tax-deductible donations (made payable to BWHBC) are welcome. Send to Box 192, West Somerville, MA 02144. Thank you.

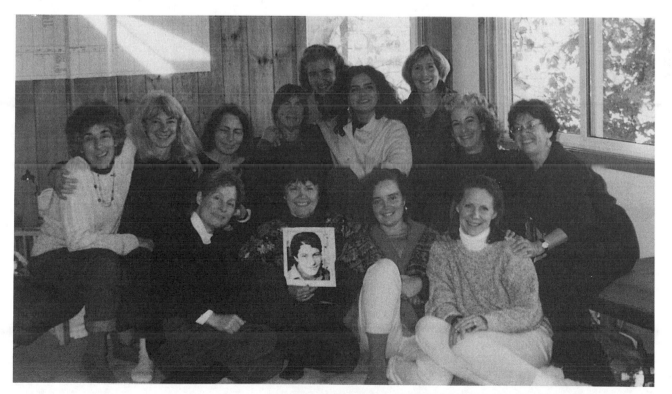

Founders of the Boston Women's Health Book Collective 1996/Judith Lennett

An Introduction to Online Women's Health Resources

By Kiki Zeldes

WITH SPECIAL THANKS TO Carol Sakala and
Norma Meras Swenson

....

The Internet—a vast network of interconnected computers—offers a wealth of free information and resources on many different aspects of women's health. This can be a great boon to women seeking informaton or support on virtually any topic: medical care, preventive care, research, disabilities, sexuality, feminist politics. Through a computer with Internet access, a woman entering menopause can research hormone treatments or self-help approaches; a pregnant lesbian can discuss parenting issues with other lesbian moms; a woman on welfare can find organizations that may help her advocate for the assistance she needs. Because the Internet has become hugely popular and widely available in the years since we last updated *Our Bodies, Ourselves,* we decided to include a brief introduction and a listing of some of the most useful resources currently available.

The first thing you need is a computer that has access to the Internet. (If you don't have a computer at work, school, or home, see box below.) If you have a computer but aren't online, many different commercial companies or local Internet Service Providers (ISPs) will sell you online access. As of the beginning of 1998,

the usual cost for unlimited access is about $20 a month, but both technology and access fees change rapidly. If you need more information on how to get online or how to do things once you get there, check out a book such as *Internet for Dummies* or *Health Online.**

The World Wide Web, the most commonly used and most visible part of the Internet, consists of page-like computer files, identified by an address (called a URL), that contain all sorts of multimedia information, including text, photographs, video images, and sound. The magic of the Web is that files (also known as sites or pages) are "linked" to other files, so that after reading an online newspaper article by a woman with breast cancer who chose a lumpectomy instead of a mastectomy, you can click your mouse and read a medical journal article stored on a computer halfway around the world about the success rates of each procedure. Three other Internet resources—newsgroups, mailing lists, and chat rooms—are more interactive

* Tom Ferguson. *Health Online.* Reading, MA: Addison-Wesley, 1996; and John Levine et al. *Internet for Dummies.* Foster City, CA: IDG Books Worldwide, 1997.

IF YOU DON'T HAVE A COMPUTER (OR HAVE NEVER USED ONE) . . .

Don't turn this page! You may still be able to take advantage of the great resources on the Internet. Some libraries and community centers such as community colleges, Y's, job-training centers, settlement houses, and cable television public access stations offer free or low-cost Internet access and instruction. To find out whether this is available in your community, try calling your local public library; it may have free access or may know where you can get it. Also, the Community Technology Centers Network (CTC) maintains a list of over 250 community centers in the U.S. (most in or around large cities) that offer free or low-cost access to computers and computer-related technology such as the Internet. You can contact it at:

Community Technology Centers Network
55 Chapel Street; Newton, MA 02158; (617) 969-7100, ext. 2727
E-mail: ctcnet@edc.org
Web site: http://www.ctcnet.org

and allow you to communicate with other people about a specific topic. For example, on the alt.support.depression newsgroup and in the *depress* mailing list, people discuss the experience of depression and share information on coping and treatment.

Although the Internet has tremendous potential as a resource for health and medical information, the quality of the information currently available varies greatly. Remember to consider the source and critically view any material you find, just as you would newspapers, magazines, and television shows (see box below). Anyone can create a Web site and put up any information he or she wants. Some sites push dubious medicine, both Western and alternative; some are concerned only with selling you their products; and some sites (as well as some research studies) are biased by the drug companies, professional societies, and other advertisers who support them. For more information on being a critical consumer of health information, see "Where to Find the Information We Need," chapter 25, The Politic of Women's Health and Medical Care, p. 707. The U.S. Food and Drug Administration Web site has some helpful articles specifically geared toward online users; to read them go to http://www.fda.gov/fdac/features/596_info.html.

Because there are so many Internet sites relevant to women's health, we've chosen general sites that are excellent places to begin searching for the information you want. At the end of each chapter, in the Resources listings, we also list a sampling of sites specifically related to each chapter topic. As you look through these listings, remember that changes in the online world are occurring so rapidly it's impossible for any written publication to stay up to date. This means that some sites may have changed or disappeared by the time you read this, and that we don't necessarily endorse all of the sites' contents.

FEMINIST AND/OR CONSUMER-ORIENTED HEALTH SITES

THE FEMINIST MAJORITY FOUNDATION ONLINE
http://www.feminist.org

Has a wide variety of resources for women, including the Feminist Internet Gateway, which lists the "Best on the Net on Feminism." Includes extensive information on women and work, violence against women, lesbian issues, and global feminism, and gives an inclusive list of resources on physical health, with a focus on reproduction and breast health.

NOAH: NEW YORK ONLINE ACCESS TO HEALTH
http://www.noah.cuny.edu

This outstanding site, a collaborative project of four New York organizations including the City University of New York and the New York Public Library, is committed to providing relevant, unbiased, and accurate consumer health information to an underserved population. Currently available in both Spanish and English, the site has information on topics ranging from aging to diabetes to patient rights.

WELLNESS WEB
http://www.wellweb.com

Created collaboratively by consumers and health care professionals, this site is designed to help people find the best and most appropriate medical information and support. Very easy to use; provides evenhanded treatment of both Western and alternative medicine.

WOMEN'S HEALTH RESOURCES ONLINE
http://cwhn.ca/resource/resource.html

Sponsored by the Canadian Women's Health Network, this site contains information and links on growing older, controlling fertility, and the medical system and women. Information is available in both French and English.

WOMEN'S RESOURCES AND LINKS
http://feminist.com

An excellent site put together by women whose goals are to promote awareness, education, activism, and empowerment. Has a nationwide database of thousands of women's resources that allow you to locate a women's service—including adoption agencies, battered women's shelters, and AIDS organizations—near you. The inclusive health section has links to many sites on general women's health, reproductive health, cancer, and AIDS.

WWW VIRTUAL LIBRARY FOR WOMEN
http://www.nwrc.org/vlwomen.htm

Put together by the National Women's Resource Center, this site has an excellent guide to health information for women in all different stages of the life cycle.

GOVERNMENT SITES

CENTERS FOR DISEASE CONTROL AND PREVENTION
http://www.cdc.gov

The CDC Web site offers practical information on diseases, health risks, and prevention guidelines and strategies. It also provides access to CDC databases and summaries of hundreds of CDC publications. The Office of Women's Health pages provide basic information on violence and injury, STDs, HIV/AIDS, AIDS in the later years, tobacco use, reproductive health, and breast and cervical cancer.

HEALTHFINDER
http://www.healthfinder.gov

Created in the spring of 1997 by the U.S. Department of Health and Human Services (DHSS), this is a centralized site where you can search for online information from many different federal agencies, including the Centers for Disease Control and Prevention (CDC), the National Institutes of Health (NIH), and the Food and Drug Administration (FDA). DHSS has also created the National Women's Health Information Clearinghouse, which is located at http://www.4women.org

OFFICE OF MINORITY HEALTH RESOURCE CENTER
http://www.omhrc.gov/welcome.htm

Maintained by the U.S. Department of Health and Human Services, this site holds a database of materials on specific health concerns of African Americans, Asians, Hispanics/Latinos, Native Americans, and Native Hawaiians/Pacific Islanders.

GENERAL HEALTH INFORMATION SITES

THE COCHRANE COLLABORATION
http://som.flinders.edu.au/fusa/cochrane/default.html

The Cochrane Collaboration is an international network of individuals and institutions committed to preparing, maintaining, and disseminating high-quality systematic reviews of health care information on a wide array of topics ranging from childbirth to breast cancer to strokes. Its work includes a Database of Systematic Reviews (CDSR) whose aim is to help people make well-informed decisions about health care by assessing

---

HOW TO KNOW WHERE YOU ARE ON THE WEB

When you're online and jumping from Web site to Web site, it's not always easy to determine who is providing the information you're currently looking at. For clues, look on the site for an icon or symbol called "Who We Are" or "About_____." Also look at the site's URL (which is usually listed in a box labeled "location" near the top part of your screen): the name or initials of the organization are often part of the URL, as is a two- or three-letter "root domain" designation that tells you the nature of the organization. For example, the designation *edu* stands for educational institution, *org* for nonprofit organization, *gov* for government agency, *com* for commercial company, *net* for network, *ca* for Canada, and *uk* for Great Britain. By looking at the URL http://www.cdc.gov, you can figure out that you are at a site created by a government agency (gov) whose initials are probably cdc (they are—the Centers for Disease Control).

---

the quality of existing research. Some of the abstracts of these unique and immensely useful reviews are available online (other Cochrane information is available only through subscription or medical libraries); for more information see "Evidence-Based Practice and the Cochrane Collaboration," chapter 25, The Politics of Women's Health and Medical Care, p. 710.

MEDICINE NET
http://www.medicinet.com

An easy-to-use site with plenty of practical medical information, including a medical dictionary and inclusive sections on first aid, pharmacy information, and diseases and treatments.

MEDSCAPE
http://www.medscape.com

A more technical site with a wide range of patient informaton. Offers access to Medline, an index with summaries of thousands of medical journal articles. The service is free, but you have to sign up.

NETHEALTH'S GUIDE TO THE INTERNET
http://www.nethealth.com/intro.html

Billed as "Your Gateway to Health Information," this site has an ever-expanding list of links on a wide range of health topics, from addictions to back pain to computers in medicine and disability resources.

SEARCH ENGINES

Search engines are Web sites that allow you to use keywords to search for what you want on the Internet. No search engine includes all the information on the Internet, so try a few to get the information you want. Some excellent beginnings:

METACRAWLER
http://www.metacrawler.com

Searches multiple search engines.

SELF-HELP RESOURCES
http://www.cmhc.com/selfhelp.htm

A comprehensive guide to online resources. You can type in your particular topic of interest (anything from addictions to repetitive strain injuries) and find an inclusive list of online resources, including Web sites and mailing lists.

STARTING POINT, HEALTH ONLINE
http://www.stpt.com/health/health.html

WWWOMEN ONLINE
http:///www.wwwomen.com

Bills itself as "The Premier Search Directory for Women Online!"

YAHOO!-HEALTH
http://www.yahoo.com/health

Excellent and comprehensive overall search tool. Lists of different indexes to health, live events, and new health headlines. A great place to begin a search.

To search for a newsgroup or mailing list on a specific topic, go to the Web site Liszt Select (http://www.liszt.com) or Deja News (http://www.dejanews.com) and enter keywords on your selected topic.

PART ONE:

Taking Care of Ourselves

Introduction

By Wendy Sanford, with Nancy Miriam Hawley and Jane Pincus

Revised by Jennifer Yanco and Judy Norsigian for the 1998 edition

This first section of *Our Bodies, Ourselves for the New Century* offers basic information we as women need to take care of our health at home and in the workplace. Conventional medical care, with its heavy emphasis on drugs, surgery, and crisis intervention, sometimes helps us when we are sick, but it does not always keep us healthy. To a great extent, what makes us healthy or unhealthy is how we are able to live our daily lives: the quality of the food we eat and the air we breathe; access to health care; how we exercise; how much rest we get; how much stress we live with; how much we use alcohol, tobacco, or other drugs; how safe or hazardous our workplaces are; whether we experience the threat or reality of sexual violence. Some of these things are under our control as individuals. Many, however, are not; we can influence them only by working with others to bring changes: pressuring an employer to remove hazards, forming a co-op for cheaper high-quality food, protesting the pollution from a nearby chemical plant, starting a network of "safe houses" for women who may be experiencing domestic abuse.

The resources available to us, especially our financial resources, greatly influence our daily health. In an unjust society, some people can afford to take better care of their health than others. It is a major aim of the feminist movement to make the crucial tools for health and survival available to everyone.

All through this book we emphasize wherever possible *what women can do*—for ourselves, for each other—in staying healthy, healing ourselves, and working for change.

HEALTHISM *

Healthism, simply put, is an overemphasis on keeping healthy. Many persons today (particularly the more affluent) have become preoccupied with staying healthy. We may become preoccupied with controlling the more manageable health factors like diet and exercise because we feel powerless to change major factors like the health care system, contaminated water supplies, and toxins in our food and the air we breathe. When we are overly focused on fitness or a "healthy lifestyle" as goals to strive for (or as the measure of a "healthy" society), we deflect attention from the more important goals of social justice and peace.

* One of the first social critics to introduce the concept of healthism was Robert J. Crawford, in his article "Healthism and the Medicalization of Everyday Life," which appeared in the *International Journal of Health Services* (vol. 10, no. 3, 1980).

Even though prevention is crucial, and is dangerously glossed over by conventional medicine, it, too, can be overemphasized. In expanding the concept of prevention ever further, we risk defining more and more aspects of life in terms of health and illness—that is, according to a medical model. We may end up seeing exercise, eating, meditation, fresh air, or dance, for example—all pleasures in their own right—simply as measures of our potential health or nonhealth. In this way, ironically, we further medicalize our lives.

Keeping healthy can also become a moral issue. Individuals are made to feel guilty for getting sick. People shake their heads disapprovingly over those who "don't take care of themselves." In many cases, this amounts to blaming the victim; it shows a failure to recognize both the social and economic influences on health habits and the complexity of illness. With personal habits, too, a certain tendency to judge creeps in: "She *should* have more control over her smoking" or "She *should* get more exercise, stop eating so much sugar." Even when these are matters of personal choice, a moralistic healthism is inappropriate. And it doesn't help people change, even when they may want to.

STRESS

Common to most of the chapters in this unit is an appreciation of stress as a major health factor. Humans, like all animals, have innate stress-alarm systems originally designed to help us fight or run away when faced with danger. In earlier, simpler times, this fight-or-flight response was appropriate. In today's world, however, the dangers are no longer so obvious or so simple. We experience multiple, prolonged, often ambiguous stresses (see box at right) for which immediate action is often impossible. We squelch the fight-or-flight response over and over again in the course of a single day. One commonly expressed theory is that years of failing to discharge the body's stress response can damage the body's immune (disease-fighting) system and may contribute to different kinds of ill health.

Body image pressures are a huge source of stress for women; unrealistic internalized notions of how we should look often lead us to try to alter our appearance by doing things that compromise our health. The stress of living under the constant onslaught of racism has serious health consequences that are finally beginning to be seriously examined by the scientific community. As women, we bear the stress of living under the threat of sexual violence—on the streets, in our workplaces, and in our homes. Job stress continues to increase as more and more of us are heads of households and have to work longer hours to make ends meet. This, combined with cutbacks in social services, is an enormous source of stress. Food can be one of the greatest sources of stress: Do we have enough to feed ourselves and our families? Do we have access to good, wholesome, uncontaminated food? The extent to

CAUSES AND SYMPTOMS OF STRESS

In our culture today, stress is often defined in a simplistic way: stress is working too hard or having a "type A" personality. But the causes of stress are complex and often beyond our personal control.

Some Causes of Stress

- Financial insecurity
- Job loss
- Death of somebody we love and/or need
- Ending or beginning a relationship
- Job changes or a new job
- Having a baby
- Moving
- Being discriminated against because of race, class, age, looks, sexual orientation, religion, or physical disability
- An illness for which we can find no appropriate care
- A diet low in fresh foods and high in sugar, white flour, caffeine, additives, and salt
- Environmental pollution
- The threat of nuclear war

Stresses Specific to Women

- A majority of women now combine outside jobs with full responsibility for home and children. In addition, we may feel—from others, from ourselves—the pressure to be "perfect" at each of these.
- Most jobs pay women little and don't allow us to use our abilities.
- Many women are single parents; many have low incomes.
- Some of us are at home all day with small children.
- We face sexual harassment and abuse on the street, in workplaces, at home.

Symptoms of Excessive Stress

- Headaches
- Neck, back, and shoulder pains
- Nervous twitches, "tics"
- Insomnia
- Skin rashes
- Greater susceptibility to colds, influenza, or other illnesses
- Worsening of existing conditions or illnesses
- Depression, anxiety, irritability, nervousness, despair
- Jaw pains and toothaches (from grinding teeth)
- Cankers, cold sores
- Stomachaches, diarrhea, loss of or increase in appetite
- Increased frequency of herpes episodes

which we are able to eat well influences our ability to deal with stress. At the same time, increasing numbers of women and girls suffer from eating problems—some of them life-threatening, like anorexia and bulimia. Some of us turn to alcohol, tobacco, and other drugs to help us deal with stress; these solutions frequently make matters worse for us.

There are many ways to minimize the effects of stress in our lives by taking care of ourselves—eating well, exercising, and exploring such things as meditation, holistic approaches to health, psychotherapy, and other approaches to caring for our psychological and emotional health—and by enjoying simple pleasures like foot rubs, long hot baths, and time to ourselves. It helps us to complain when we need to, ask our friends for encouragement, to laugh often, and to cry when we need to. But it is important, too, to try to identify the *causes* of negative or excessive stress in our lives, and to change as many as we can.*

This isn't always easy or possible, especially by ourselves. The following chapters attempt to distinguish carefully between what we can do as individuals and the social factors that we must change by working together. In many cases, the fact of joining together with others to bring about needed change can provide us with the energy and hope that are important sources of health and well-being in and of themselves.†

---

* Many businesses have introduced "stress-reduction" programs for employees. These programs, however, emphasize only what *individuals* can do and rarely address the *sources* of stress in the workplace, because to do so would mean expensive changes such as reducing the workload or eliminating safety hazards.

† Please see chapter 27, Organizing for Change, which outlines the kind of work that serves to help us as individuals and as a society.

Chapter 1

Body Image

By Demetria Iazzetto, Linda King, and Jennifer Yanco, based on earlier work by Wendy Sanford, with the women of Boston Self-Help

WITH SPECIAL THANKS TO Allison Abner, Debbie Levine, Marsha Saxton, Judith Stein, Becky Thompson, Linda Villarosa, Kiki Zeldes, and the 6th grade girls *

*T*ake *a moment* to close your eyes and visualize your body. How do you feel about what you see?

Are your breasts too big or too small? Your butt too big or too flat? What about your stomach or thighs—too fat? Is your nose too broad? Do you wish you were taller or more petite? Is your body too hairy or your skin too dark?

If you're like most women, you answered yes to some of these questions. Almost every woman judges some part of her body—sometimes all of it—as not quite right.[1]

Think about the tremendous diversity of female bodies: we are tall, short, thin, fat, large-boned and hefty, tiny and frail; our eyes vary in color and shape; our skin color ranges from blue-black or ebony to deep browns to copper to olive to pink; our hair is many-colored and has an almost infinite range of tex-

tures. Yet, we are all measured against unrealistic standards promoted by the advertising and beauty industries and grounded in fantasies about how a woman should look and behave. A woman who recently quit her job, after a manager told her to change her braided hairstyle or leave, reflects:

Everybody talks about diversity, but if everybody has to fit a certain mold, well, that's not wanting diversity. It's asking people to change who they really are.[2]

What are the forces that lead us to believe we're not okay the way we are? What do we think would change in our lives if we could change our bodies and our looks? What would being more "attractive" give us? More friends? More self-confidence? A better job? How can we learn to feel better about our bodies and more loving toward ourselves and other women despite the onslaught of messages about how we "should" look? Just imagine what would happen if we were to take all the energy we expend trying to conform to society's standards of beauty and direct it elsewhere. What else

* Over the years since 1969, the following women have contributed to the many versions of this chapter: Frances Deloatch, Mary Fitzgerald, Jean Gillespie, Nancy Miriam Hawley, Janna Zwerner Jacobs, Joan Lastovica, Oce, Rosemarie Ouilette, Jane Pincus, Esther Rome, Marsha Saxton, Judith Stein, Jill Wolhandler.

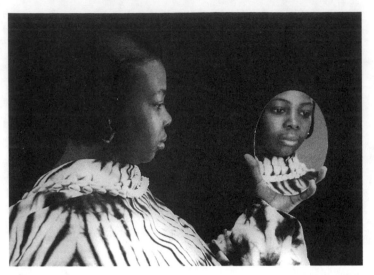

Robin Melavalin

could we be doing with our time? Our money? Our energy?

We generally begin our lives feeling comfortable in our bodies. As infants and children we learn about and explore ourselves and the world through our bodies. As we grow up we may become less at home in our skin. We may find that as girls we are often valued more for our bodies than for our minds, and as we reach adolescence we may feel that to fit in and be popular we need to look and act in a certain way. If we don't look and act that way, we may find ourselves harassed and isolated. The teenage years can be hard on all young women, but these years are particularly difficult for those whose appearance is further from the ideal promoted in the media. If we look more masculine than other girls, if our hair is nappy, if our skin is dark, if we have a disability or have problems with our skin, if we are fat, or if we develop too soon or too late, we may begin to shrink from taking up the space we deserve. We may feel pressured to change our bodies rather than enjoy them as they are.

How we feel about our looks and how at home we feel in our bodies is complex and develops in response to the many and often contradictory messages we get from society at large and in response to our actual experiences living in our bodies. Some of the pressure to be different from the way we are comes from outside ourselves, from the media images that constantly bombard us, and from the reactions we get from others; some of the pressure comes from deep inside ourselves, from how we internalize our experiences as females in this culture.

Too often our experiences living in our bodies make it difficult for us to accept ourselves. Many of us have experienced violence and abuse that make us feel unsafe in our bodies. One in four women will be raped in her lifetime;[3] one in three girls is sexually abused by age 18.[4] Virtually all of us have experienced unwanted attention from men, whether in the form of compliments, derisive comments, or unsolicited touching. Every woman of color will experience racism. If our culture has different ideals of female beauty from those of the dominant Euro-American culture, the messages we receive from parents and relatives may contradict those of our peers and the media and may cause us additional pain and confusion.

As a result of these violations, many of us have come to feel that our bodies—as they are—are not safe places to be. We may respond by wanting to look like the woman on the cover of a glossy beauty magazine, thinking that if we had the perfect body, we would be shielded from insults to our sense of self and from discrimination. Or we may respond by rejecting our female bodies, feeding our hunger for acceptance with bags of junk food or starving ourselves so that our bodies take on the shapes of preadolescent girls.

We are wounded when a physical characteristic or set of characteristics is loaded with negative expectations. If we have black skin and African features, or olive skin and Asian features, or dark curly hair and a prominent nose as do many Jews and Arabs, or if we have a visible disability, or if we are perceived as "overweight," our experiences from an early age may be marked by other people's negative reactions to our physical selves. We may have come to dislike, mistrust, or even hate our bodies as a result, feeling that they, rather than the society we live in, have betrayed us.

Many of us are painfully aware that how we look is directly related to how others treat us, to our romantic prospects, to where we can live, to our employment possibilities. Recently, in a major settlement against the Publix supermarket chain, one of the plaintiffs reported being refused a promotion and actually demoted because she was "overweight."[5] Black women, especially those in service jobs, encounter reactions to our hair on a daily basis, including policies banning braids or other African hairstyles from the workplace.[6]

Every society throughout history has had standards of beauty, but at no other time has there been such an intense media blitz telling us what we should look like. Magazine covers, films, TV shows, and billboards surround us with images that constantly reinforce the idea that "beauty" is everything. But what is "beauty" and what does it mean to strive to be "beautiful"? The current ideal woman portrayed in the dominant American culture is white, thin, able-bodied, shapely, muscular, tall, blond, smooth-skinned, and young.[7] The list of what a woman must do to achieve the perfect look is endless, yet paradoxically, it is absolutely essential that in the end she look totally natural! Despite changes in fashion and in attitudes toward women, today's ideal woman is in fact not so different from the original blond Barbie doll. We may find Barbie's distorted body amusing, but as a caricature of the state-of-the-art white ideal of female beauty, Barbie is the standard that millions of little girls learn to desire at an early age. The fact that she has been joined by numerous ethnic variations doesn't minimize her power as a popular icon. This state-of-the-art white model puts a particular burden on women of color who are under "stress to conform to an ideal that is genetically impossible for most of us to achieve."[8]

Never before have there been so many businesses dedicated to selling "beauty" and so many women willing to buy their products. We are sold an infinite array of products and programs to alter our appearance. Almost everywhere we look we receive similar messages: without these jeans (and the skinny body in them), you'll never find a man; without straight, bright, white teeth you'll never find success. The pressure to conform is promoted by a market whose success depends on convincing us that we don't look good enough and is reinforced by employers and others who have control over where we work, where we live, and our opportunities to enjoy good health.

Many of us spend precious time, money, and emotional energy trying to make our bodies conform to standards that have little to do with who we are or what our bodies actually look like. The cost, both economical and psychological, is enormous. We may expose ourselves to serious health hazards: dangerous chemicals in cosmetics,[9] hair products, depilatories, and vaginal deodorants; malnourishment caused by low-calorie diets; skin disorders caused by skin lighteners and suntanning. We may wear clothes and shoes that severely hamper our freedom of movement, making it difficult for us to defend ourselves if threatened; have tattoos or piercings done in nonsterile environments, putting ourselves at risk of contracting hepatitis or HIV; or undergo highly risky cosmetic surgery to radically change the shape of our eyes, our noses, our faces, our breasts, or our thighs.

We all participate in maintaining the popular myths and fantasies of how we should look. Not only do most of us try in one way or another to conform, but we have learned to judge others by the same standards we use to judge ourselves. We look at each other in school, on the street, at work, at the gym and compare: we want to know how well we are doing in the competition for female perfection. Sometimes we reject the dominant fantasies about how we should look only to create an alternative ideal, wanting ourselves and our friends to fit other, equally oppressive stereotypes like the Amazon or Earth Mother.

The choices we make about our appearances can affect how we feel about other women. Think about it. When we constantly diet and exercise to be thin, how do we view women who are fat? When white women go to great lengths to emulate the state-of-the-art model, how does this affect their relationships with women of color? If we remove the hair on our legs, under our arms, on our faces, or other parts of our bodies, how do we feel about women who don't? None of these actions are good or bad in and of themselves. We all make choices based on what we think is best for us. We don't often think, however, of how these choices affect our relationships with other women. Sometimes our efforts to alter our bodies to emulate some ideal may distance us from women who are, through choice or not, further from that ideal. We might term these women who are different from ourselves "other," "uncool," or "minority" and keep them at the margins of our consciousness. But when we do this, when we constantly judge ourselves and others by standards that are narrowly defined and inevitably out of reach, we drive a wedge between ourselves and other women.

Most of us will, at times in our lives, make some concessions to the dominant ideals for reasons of economic and social survival. If we can recognize, however, when we are reshaping our bodies to fit someone else's demands, we can begin to develop a different relationship to ourselves. As we become conscious of the model body image and the forces that push us to emulate that image, we can learn to know the differences between our authentic selves and the compromises we make with the outside world. We can start feeling freer to make our own choices.

There are many ways to begin this journey. We can explore ways to feel attractive and appreciated that nurture us and respect our integrity as persons. We can find ways of ornamenting our bodies that do not expose us to health risks. We can take the time to learn to appreciate the sheer pleasures of being in our bodies. We can explore ways to enjoy the sensuality of our bodies, through being outdoors, walking, swimming, dancing, taking a hot bath, or getting a massage. We can focus more of our energy on developing other aspects of ourselves through involvement in our communities and through learning and sharing what we know with those around us. We can talk with other women about body image and begin to name the deadly assumptions underlying the standards of female beauty. We can recognize how we've accepted these ideals and how our buying into them reinforces their power.

Thankfully, growing numbers of women question our need to change our bodies to fit the ideals. Many of us are finding power in defining our own standards of beauty. As more of us learn to love and value ourselves and each other just as we are, and as we begin dismantling the stereotypes that equate physical characteristics with our value as persons, media images and social messages will have a lesser impact on our sense of self. Finding new and positive ways of thinking about our bodies allows us to extend the same accepting attitudes to other women and also affects how others perceive us. No matter what our size, shape, color, or physical ability, if we love ourselves and believe in our own beauty, we are more likely to find that others see that beauty, too. And if they don't, believing in ourselves gives others less power over us.

RACISM AND BODY IMAGE

WE LATINA WOMEN

We Latina Women
Fit perfectly
into Rape Culture
because we're so Hot
We can be Raped

We're such dancing,
slick, dark skinned,
inherently sexy,
Hot oily little things
Screaming for Domination.
Oh Mira!
We Want
A Boss!

We are told to forget we are Human
My Black Sisters
Fit so perfect
Because they're such exotic
animal—jungle—Beast-like
Tiger women
that want nothing but sex
and to be Fucked
with
that they are they, less Human

While My Asian Sisters
are so perfectly submissive, slave giving, oriental,
kiss your toes, serve you tea,
24/7 Mistress
with that subordinate-passive

Childlike behavior is considered the non the not
*   really yet Human*
The perfect Rape Culture
is a continuum
taking every Woman
every Man

every Human being
turning, twisting, forming, re-molding, breaking,
*   shaking, silencing,*
slicing, denying us to the death
which is not Human
not soul, heart, mind, voice
which is just
where they want us.

— T I N A   D ' E L I A

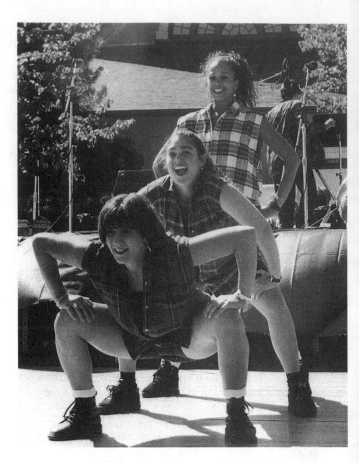

Gerard Evans

The impact of racial discrimination on women of color means that no matter how good we may feel about ourselves, we still have to go through our lives fighting off negative assumptions about our very qualities as human beings. For women of color, the path to womanhood is punctuated with assaults on our self-esteem. Growing up, we may notice that the closer a girl approximates the "ideal" the more she is valued. The closer a girl is to looking like a full-blooded African, the more likely it is that she will be called upon to prove that she is honest, reliable, intelligent—all the qualities assumed to adhere to her white and lighter-skinned black girlfriends. This sets girls against each other at a time when they need each other most. When others mistrust you and call into question your very personhood solely on the basis of the color of your skin or the shape of your eyes or the texture of your hair, this can drive a wedge between you and your friends, whose skin color shields them from such mistreatment. They may be hurt and shocked by others' treatment of you; they don't want to believe that it's truly based on your appearance. They may get little support from parents, teachers, or other adults who greet their concerns with little interest ("It's not your problem, dear"), with silence ("Oh, is that so?"), or with outright denial ("That couldn't be; she must have been doing something to irritate the teacher"). Adults engaged in active antiracism efforts may be more able to provide the kind of support needed to break the cycle of racism.

Racism is deeply embedded in our culture and encoded in our relations with one another. Every one of us is affected by it; all of us are hurt by it. As women we need to have strategies for how to break the silences that reinforce this system, which privileges white-skinned Euro-Americans over people of color, and those with lighter skin over those with darker.[10] Women of color are less likely to be valued for who we are or what we are capable of than our white sisters, who, unless proved otherwise, are assumed to embody those qualities that we must constantly prove we have. It is sobering to realize that a perfectly good woman may have to go through her entire life battling mistreatment and confronting false assumptions about her person because of other people's racism. Those of us who are white women need to see how our silent acceptance of privileges based on race serves to perpetuate the discrimination that wastes the energy and drains the spirits of women of color. It can be frightening to look seriously at this issue; what will we see? And once it is seen, what will we have to do about it? Women of color are always aware of their color; they have no choice but to be. If white women had to be as aware of their whiteness, how would that shape our relationships with each other? Recognizing and naming the way skin privilege operates can open up the possibility for us to see how racism divides us not only from other women but from our own authentic selves.

At first, I didn't want to hear about the power and privilege inherent in my white skin. I wanted simply to identify with women of color—it was easier, and I didn't have to feel guilty or ashamed. Now, after years of anti-racism work, I understand I can do both: I do identify with the women of color in my life, but I also see that our experiences will always be different because we live in a country dominated by people with white skin—skin like mine. I can work to change that reality, but not until I accept that it is the reality.

PHYSICAL DISABILITY AND THE PRESSURE TO BE PHYSICALLY PERFECT

While coming to love and accept our bodies is a difficult process for almost all women in this society, it is especially hard for those of us with physical disabilities. More than 20 million women in this country walk with a limp; move in a wheelchair or with crutches; have impaired sight, speech, or hearing; live with a chronic illness; have lost a limb to fire or accident or disease; need special assistance with simple bodily functions; or wear the scars of some damaging event. Many of these millions of women are silent and invisible—many of us who are able choose to hide our differences in order to avoid the pain of being objectified or stigmatized. Women of color with disabilities experience triple jeopardy: they face daily discrimination based on color, gender, and disability. Because of racial discrimination, a woman of color suffering an asthma attack, for example, may be less likely to get the immediate aid she needs from bystanders; this can sometimes mean the difference between life and death for her.

With a body that doesn't "measure up," we learn pretty quickly what our culture really wants from women.

Having a disability made me very aware at an early age of the messages I was receiving from the larger society about how I was supposed to look and how you're supposed to be. Also, as the doctors poked and studied me endlessly, I learned more quickly than some nondisabled women that I'm seen as an object.

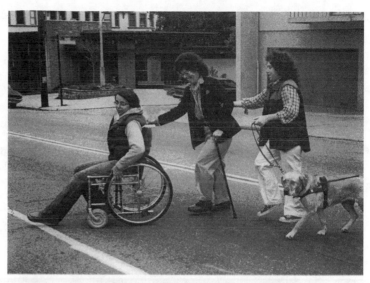

Lesbians with Disability Support Group, originally appearing in *The Lesbian Photo Album* **(1981)/**Cathy Cade

My family's thing was that girls dated in order to find a prospective mate. Since I had cerebral palsy, they assumed I was never going to marry. So why should I date? And I've only just begun to wear a dress this year, because I was always encouraged to wear pants. There was no reason for me to dress like a woman because I wasn't one. That wasn't part of my identity.

If we are white, the more our bodies vary from the able-bodied norm, the less families, friends, and physicians expect or allow us to be sexual (see "Sex and Disability," chapter 11, Sexuality, p. 251). If we can't have children, we are pitied for not being "real" women. As women of color we find that sometimes other stereotypes apply. We may want to have children and be discouraged from doing so because white people don't want to see us reproduce. Even as women with disabilities we are often sexualized and may be more vulnerable to sexual violence.

As women who may not be "pleasing" to look at we are expected to compensate, and we come to expect it of ourselves: we learn to smile a lot and be sweet, or clown around, so people won't feel so uncomfortable around us. Or, believing in our own unworthiness, we fall into the background, trying to make ourselves as invisible as possible.

Other "female" stereotypes surface quickly—we are weak, less intelligent, need protection. If we can't control our movements or bodily functions, people think we are mentally incompetent.

My family thinks of epilepsy as a mental illness.

People see my body and don't expect me to be smart.

Like many women, only more so, we are treated like children far into our adult lives.

People will pinch me on the cheek and use words that you would use to a first- or second-grader.

The doctors still talk to my parents or to the person with me instead of directly to me, as though I'm a child, and I'm sick of it.

As women with physical disabilities, like women with emotional or cognitive disabilities, we find it difficult but important to assert our adulthood, our legal rights, our power, our individuality, and our intelligence. This process is crucial for all women.

Until 1990, severe job discrimination penalized us for having unacceptable bodies and created strong economic incentive for "fitting in" and minimizing differences. As one woman said, "We are not disabled; it is society that disables us by being so unsupportive." With the passage of the 1990 Americans with Disabilities Act, we now have legal protections enabling us to participate more fully in society. The act specifically prohibits discrimination against people with disabilities in employment, transportation, public accommodations, state and city government, and communications.

Sooner or later, if we're lucky, we realize how angry we are at always having had to hide our true feelings and the realities of our lives.

After I got my braces removed at age 12, I did everything I could to hide my skinny, scarred legs, including wearing knee socks or long pants in the hottest weather. Slowly my anger grew at the restrictions I was accepting. Partly with the help of other disabled women, I came to see my underlying feeling that if people saw my legs they'd not only reject me for being ugly, but they'd somehow see the years in the hospital or how dependent and scared I'd been. I began to reevaluate these experiences as simply things that had happened, not who I am. I wear shorts when I want to now, and I like my legs the way they are.

Finally I like my body, and because of my disability that statement has added significance. There is something "WRONG" with my body, so how can I possibly feel good about it or enjoy life in it? Simple answers are: I have no choice and I want to. The more complex answer is that there is nothing wrong with my body. It falls within the wide range of human experience and is therefore both natural and normal. I've been in this body all my life, I was born with it and I'll die with it. It's part of who I am, and I'd be someone else without this body just the way it is.

Dialogue between disabled and nondisabled women reveals that we have much in common. A woman with a brittle bone condition wrote:

I can't quite pinpoint when I began to listen to the experiences of able-bodied women and relate them to my own. It may have been when someone said that she couldn't go out of the house because her skin was so spotty, or when a beautiful black woman told me how all her life she had wanted to be white like her friend at school, or it could have been when a friend of mine who had always been my envy for being followed around by drooling men said that she was so lonely because people only reacted to her stunning body and never to the person inside it. . . . It may have been none of this that made the turning point for me, but instead it could have been the way some of the women put their arms around me and called me their beautiful sister that made me begin to see that we are not so different after all.[11]

BODY IMAGE, WEIGHT, AND SIZE

In many cultures and historical periods women have been proud to be large—being fat was a sign of fertility, of prosperity, of the ability to survive. Even in the U.S. today, where fear of fat reigns in most sectors of the culture, some racial and ethnic groups love and enjoy large women. For example, Hawaiians often consider very large women quite beautiful, and studies show that some black women experience more body satisfaction and are less concerned with dieting, fatness, and weight fluctuations than are white women.[12] However, the weight loss, medical, and advertising industries have an enormous impact on women across racial and ethnic boundaries. These industries all insist that white and thin is beautiful and that fatness is always a dangerous problem in need of correction. The popular notion that some communities are less influenced than others has meant that women of color in particular have a hard time being taken seriously when they have eating disorders. A black woman suffering from an eating disorder says:

After all, don't black people prize wide hips and fleshy bodies? Isn't obesity so prevalent in our communities because it is actually accepted? Don't black women have very positive body images? . . . Anorexia and its kin supposedly strike only adolescent, middle- and upper-middle-class white girls . . . Women like me are winging it, seeking out other sisters with the same concerns, wondering if we are alone on this journey.[13]

Fat women daily encounter hostility and discrimination. If we are fat, health practitioners often attribute our health problems to "obesity," postpone treatment until we lose weight, accuse us of cheating if we don't, make us so ashamed of our size that we don't go for help, and make all kinds of assumptions about our emotional and psychological state ("She must have emotional problems to be so fat"). Yet, as many of us have long suspected, it is now being acknowledged that it is cardiovascular fitness and not fatness we need to look at if we are concerned about health. Some of our ill health as fat women results from the stress of living with fat-hatred—social ridicule and hostility, isolation, financial pressures resulting from job discrimination,

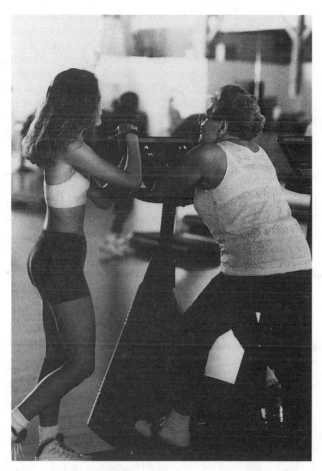

Charles Daniels

We need a widespread rebellion of women who are tired of worrying about their weight, who understand that weight is not a matter of health or discipline but a weapon our culture uses against us to keep us in our place and feeling small. We need to quietly say no to ridiculous weight standards, reassuring ourselves that we're good and worthwhile human beings even if we aren't a size 6, and further, to protest those standards more demonstrably, on behalf of others as well. Both decisions require a change in attitude which, while not necessarily impolite, is rather less tolerant of the everyday demeaning comments about body size that women now accept as their due. In other words, we need to begin to throw our weight around.

—Laura Fraser[14]

AGING AND BODY IMAGE

As we grow older we may experience painful feelings of loss when we notice the signs of aging that change our appearance and eventually require us to develop a new body image. Though many cultures value the wisdom and beauty of their elders (American Indian, Asian, and Polynesian cultures are some examples), the dominant Euro-American culture in the U.S. is highly youth-oriented. Though old men are sometimes given respect for their power and authority, old women are the most marginalized members of our society. As we age in this culture we cannot help but be painfully aware of how the forces of sexism and ageism intersect and severely impinge on the lives of old women. Old women who also face discrimination based on race, sexual orientation, or physical ability have an even more difficult time.

As we age we often become keenly aware of how others respond to us differently. Recognizing that our society values women who most closely resemble the dominant ideals of female "beauty," we may feel hurt by the loss of our youthful looks.

When I walk down the street with my daughter now, I notice that when male heads turn in our direction they are looking at her. My pride in her blossoming young womanhood is bittersweet, because I miss getting that attention myself.

Employers may unfairly dismiss us as incompetent and useless if we don't present a contemporary (read "youthful") image. We may be denied opportunities for promotion if we "look our age" or have "let ourselves go" by refusing to diet or dye our hair. There are times, though, when our experience is valued, particularly if we value ourselves. As one woman explained,

I've found that walking "big" may indeed pay the rent . . . at least I'm having more luck on the job mar-

lack of exercise because of harassment, and, perhaps most important, the hazards of repeated dieting.

Low-calorie dieting has become a national obsession. Many of us are convinced that making women afraid to be fat is a form of social control. Fear of fat keeps women preoccupied, robs us of our pride and energy, keeps us from taking up space.

I don't like myself heavy, I want to feel thin, streamlined and spare, and not like a toad. I have taken antifat thinking into myself so deeply that I hate myself when I am even ten pounds "overweight," whatever that means.

We can be more relaxed about our weight

- By experimenting with what weight feels comfortable to us rather than trying primarily to be thin.
- By being more accepting of weight variations through the life cycle.
- By developing a clearer understanding of which health problems are truly associated with weight (See chapter 2, Food).
- By exercising and eating nutritious food to feel healthy, and letting our body weight set itself accordingly.

ket since perceiving myself as a strong gentle African queen instead of an old black woman without a job.

Youthful appearance may be overvalued in our social groups and relationships as well. As a result, some of us feel more confident when we can delay the outward signs of aging by using makeup and hair dyes. Some cosmetics can have negative health effects. For example, commercial hair dyes may contain cancer-causing chemicals. One woman noted:

Most lesbians' culture is youth-oriented, and I feel better with my hair brown rather than gray. People don't look at me as though I'm old.

Yet, a growing number of us believe that our years and experience entitle us to wear our graying hair, wrinkles, and extra pounds—badges of mature womanliness—with pride. Being older provides a time for us to experiment with different colors, unconventional styles, and new ways of presenting ourselves.

I look in the mirror and am always a little surprised that with my graying hair and some new wrinkles, I don't feel what I'm "supposed" to be feeling. If I were not constantly bombarded from reading, media, and society in general with reminders that now I'm supposed to be in crisis, withdrawing, feeling depressed, isolated, incapable, or ashamed, these ideas wouldn't occur to me. I am simply building on what was before, seeking out new opportunities. I am, as always, energetic and involved.

I don't want to deny my experiences and I feel that if I dislike my aging looks I'm denying all the wonderful parts of my life. I don't want to do that.

WORKING TOGETHER FOR CHANGE

A better self-image doesn't pay the rent or cook supper or prevent nuclear war. Feeling better about ourselves doesn't change the world by itself, but it can give us energy to do what we want and to work for change.

Learning to accept and love our bodies and ourselves is an important and difficult ongoing struggle. But to change the societal values underlying body image, we need to do more than love ourselves. We need to focus our attention on the forces that drive wedges between us as women: racism, sexism, ableism, ageism, and our national obsession with size and shape. To truly create change, to create a world in which all women can make choices about our appearances for ourselves and not others, we must incorporate all women into the heart of how we see ourselves. From this expanded horizon of sisterhood, we may begin to value the lives of women who previously meant nothing to us. We may begin to realize that

understanding their lives is essential to understanding our own lives and realizing our full potential as women.

If we can begin to eliminate the hatred and ridicule levied against women who don't fit the "state-of-the-art" ideal, we can lessen the stress of "not fitting in." We also open the possibility of building a social-change movement that links all women who seek a world where each of us can celebrate and delight in our physical bodies. Working together to change the attitudes and conditions that restrict us, we feel proud and more able to take control of our lives.

We need each others' help to change the deeply entrenched attitudes that make us dislike our own bodies and that interfere with our relationships with other women. Here are some things groups of women can do together:

- Find ways to diversify our circle of friends—learn about the concerns of older women through the Grey Panthers; attend a meeting of a disability rights group; find out if there is a Fat Liberation group in your area and see what it is doing.
- Find women who are exploring ways to combat racism, and form or join an antiracist group.
- Support magazines that show women of all colors, sizes, shapes, and abilities—real women as we know them, not airbrushed, white-looking, thin models (see Resource section).
- Take a course or attend a lecture on race and gender studies, disability issues, women's body image, or the psychology of women to understand the complex dynamics of body image in our culture.
- Write a letter to a TV station or magazine or clothing store that shows positive (or negative) images of women of color, and let them know what you think.
- Read whatever you can find on race and body size issues that support self-acceptance instead of trying to make your body conform to any "ideal." Discuss with others these ideas and how to put them into daily practice in your own life.
- Plan together how to challenge ourselves and others when we judge women on the basis of skin color and appearance.
- Form or join a group or organization that promotes self-acceptance and self-love for all our sizes and in all our diversity.
- Learn more about how our bodies work, through self-help sessions and/or discussion.

Shifting to a body perspective in which every woman matters in a public sense takes a major shift in consciousness. Breaking the silent hold of state-of-the-art body image on female self-esteem, relationships, and social and economic opportunities requires us to adopt a conception of womanhood that is informed by physical, emotional, and spiritual diversity. Valuing this diversity is critical to dismantling the insidious and toxic effect of discrimination based on how we look. Finding ways to change the societal forces that make accepting ourselves so difficult is a process that can begin at any point in our lives and can continue as long as we live. This mission, if taken on, will lead us toward a future in which every woman can experience the joy of being valued completely for who she is.

NOTES

1. An informal survey conducted by the authors at the magazine rack of a local drugstore revealed the way we compartmentalize our bodies. Of the 12 women's magazines on display, ten had cover articles on some body part and how to alter it: "The Ultimate Butt Workout" *(Glamour),* "20 Kissable Lips" *(Cosmopolitan),* "Bad Hair Day" *(Ladies' Home Journal),* "Your Breasts" *(Marie Claire),* "Shrink Your Stomach" *(Good Housekeeping),* "Butt, Abs and Thighs" *(Redbook),* "Frizzy Hair" *(Seventeen),* "Sunproof Skin" and "Wiltproof Hair" *(Mirabella),* "Better Butt" *(Shape).* Imagine a men's magazine with a similar headline: "10 Steps to a Perkier Penis."
2. LaToya Rivers, quoted in "No-braiding policies have some firms in a twist," by Diane E. Lewis, *Boston Globe,* May 6, 1997, C-6.
3. Diana Russell, *Sexual Exploitation: Rape, Child Sexual Abuse, and Sexual Harassment* (Beverly Hills, CA: Sage Publications, 1984).
4. ———, *The Secret Trauma: Incest in the Lives of Girls and Women* (New York: Basic Books, 1986), 61.
5. *Boston Globe,* February 16, 1997.
6. Lewis, "No-braiding policies."
7. "A recent perusal of an issue of a top fashion magazine revealed that 80 of the 83 models were white. Seventy-four were blonde. All were tall and slim, far removed from the average American woman's height and weight —5'4," 145 lbs." From Charlice Hurst, "Sizing up the problem: The politics of body image for women of color," in *Third Force* (May/June 1997): 17.
8. Hurst, "Sizing up the problem."
9. See, for example, "Alpha Hydroxy Acids in Cosmetics," in *FDA Backgrounder: Current and Useful Information from the Food and Drug Administration* (BG-97-4, February 19, 1997).
10. Motivated by the impact of colorism on our relationships as people of color, and as a step toward healing those relationships, the organizers of the conference "Skin Trade: Women, Complexion and Caste" (at Brandeis University, March 1997) provided a forum for the exploration of intra- and interracial/ethnic expressions of skin color preferences for women of various racial and ethnic groups. The organizers also offer workshops and discussion groups that focus on the role of skin color, facial features, and body type in the lives of women (see Resources).
11. Jo Campling, ed., *Images of Ourselves: Women with Disabilities Talking* (London: Routledge and Kegan Paul, 1981), 26–27.
12. Andrea D. Powell and Arnold S. Kahn, "Racial differences in women's desires to be thin," *International Journal of Eating Disorders* 17, no. 2 (March 1995): 191–95.
13. Hurst, "Sizing up the problem."
14. Laura Fraser, *Losing It: America's Obsession with Weight and the Industry That Feeds on It* (New York: Dutton, 1997), 284.

RESOURCES

Books

Abner, Allison, and Linda Villerosa. *Finding Our Way: The Teen Girls' Survival Guide.* New York: HarperCollins, 1995. A multiracial and multicultural guide. See chapter 1, "Good Bodies."

Browne, Susan, et al., eds. *With the Power of Each Breath: A Disabled Women's Anthology.* Pittsburgh, PA: Cleis Press, 1985. Excellent collection of stories, essays, and poetry by women with disabilities.

Brown, Laura S., and Esther Rothblum, eds. *Overcoming Fear of Fat.* Binghamton: Harrington Park Press, 1989.

Campling, Jo, ed. *Images of Ourselves: Women with Disabilities Talking.* London: Routledge and Kegan Paul, 1981. In this excellent book, women with various disabilities write informatively and movingly about their lives.

Chapkis, Wendy. *Beauty Secrets: Women and the Politics of Appearance.* Boston: South End Press, 1986. Insightful analysis of the roles of sexism, racism, and classism in shaping images of beauty for women.

Cooke, Kaz. *Real Gorgeous: The Truth About Body and Beauty.* New York: W. W. Norton, 1996. Cartoons and humor to help us laugh about the body prisons society tries to put women in.

Cupolo, A., K. Corbette, and V. Lewis. *No More Stares: A Role Model Book for Disabled Teenage Girls,* 1982. Disability Rights Education Defense Fund, 2032 San Pablo Avenue, Berkeley, CA 94702.

Duffy, Yvonne. *All Things Are Possible.* Ann Arbor, MI: A. J. Garvin and Associates, 1981.

Edison, Laurie T., and Debbie Notkin. *Women En Large: Images of Fat Nudes.* San Francisco: Books in Focus, 1994.

Erdman, Cheri K. *Nothing to Lose: A Guide to Sane Living in a Larger Body.* San Francisco: Harper San Francisco, 1995. Has an excellent section exploring the myths and realities of body image issues.

Fine, Michelle, and Adrienne Asch, eds. *Women with Disabilities: Essays in Psychology, Culture and Politics.* Philadelphia: Temple University Press, 1988.

Freedman, Rita. *Bodylove: Learning to Like Our Looks—and Ourselves.* New York: Harper & Row, 1990.

Friday, Nancy. *The Power of Beauty.* New York: HarperCollins, 1996.

Herron, Carolivia. *Nappy Hair.* New York: Alfred A. Knopf, 1997.

Hirschman, Jane, and Carol Munter. *When Women Stop Hating Their Bodies.* New York: Fawcett Columbine, 1995.

Howell, Jhana, ed. *Skin Trading: Women, Complexion and Caste* (forthcoming). Anthology focusing on themes of gender, race, ethnicity, class, and sexuality. For information on publication write 89 Walden Street, Cambridge, MA 02140; E-mail: jhana@msn.com

Hutchinson, Marcia G. *Transforming Body Image.* Trumansburg, NY: Crossing Press, 1985.

Hyman, Jane Wegscheider, and Esther R. Rome. *Sacrificing Ourselves for Love.* Freedom, CA: Crossing Press, 1996. Examines how women and girls risk health and well-being in order to please others. Contains good discussions about cosmetic surgery and breast implants.

Kano, Susan. *Making Peace with Food: Freeing Yourself from the Diet/Weight Obsession.* New York: Harper & Row, 1989.

Keith, Lois, ed. *What Happened to You? Writings by Disabled Women.* New York: The New Press, 1996.

Krotoski, D., et al., eds. *Women with Physical Disabilities: Achieving and Maintaining Health and Well-Being.* Baltimore, MD: Paul Brookes, 1996.

Lyons, Pat, and Debby Burgard. *Great Shape: The First Fitness Guide for Large Women.* Palo Alto, CA: Bull Publishing Co., 1990.

Neely, Barbara. *Blanche on the Lam.* New York: St. Martin's Press, 1992.

———. *Blanche Among the Talented Tenth.* New York: St. Martin's Press, 1994.

Newman, Leslea. *Some Body to Love: A Guide to Loving the Body You Have.* Chicago: Third Side Press, 1991. Writing exercises about body image and eating.

Panzarino, Connie. *The Me in the Mirror.* Seattle: Seal Press, 1994.

Polivy, Janet, and Peter Herman. *Breaking the Diet Habit.* New York: Basic Books, 1983. Sound advice on how to stop dieting and eat normally.

Resources for Rehabilitation: *A Woman's Guide to Coping with Disability,* 2nd ed., 1997. 33 Bedford Street, Suite 19A, Lexington, MA 02173; (617) 862-6455.

Rodin, Judith. *Body Traps: Breaking The Binds That Keep You from Feeling Good About Your Body.* New York: William Morrow & Co., 1992. Explores several "traps": vanity, shame, competition, food, dieting rituals, fitness, and success—and how to free ourselves from them.

Saxton, Marsha, and Florence Howe, eds. *With Wings: An Anthology of Literature by and About Women with Disabilities.* New York: Feminist Press, 1987.

Schoenfielder, Lisa, and Barb Wieser, eds. *Shadow on a Tightrope: Writings by Women About Fat Oppression.* San Francisco: Aunt Lute Books, 1983. Anthology of all the best articles about fat liberation.

Thompson, Becky. *A Hunger So Wide and So Deep: American Women Speak Out on Eating Problems.* Minneapolis: University of Minnesota Press, 1994. Excellent analysis.

Villarosa, Linda, ed. *Body & Soul: The Black Women's Guide to Physical Health and Emotional Well-Being.* New York: HarperPerennial, 1994.

Wolf, Naomi. *The Beauty Myth: How Images of Beauty Are Used Against Women.* New York: Doubleday, 1992.

Woman of Power. Women's Bodies. Issue 18, Fall 1990.

Articles

Arnold, Georgina. "Coming Home: One Black Woman's Journey to Health and Fitness," in Evelyn C. White, ed., *The Black Woman's Health Book,* 2nd ed. Seattle: Seal Press, 1994.

Hershey, Laura. "Choosing Disability." *Ms. Magazine,* July/August 1994.

Summer, Nancy. "The Making of Young Activists: Bringing Size Awareness to the Classroom." *Radiance,* Issue 45 (winter 1996): 10–14.

Walker, Alice. "Beauty: When the Other Dancer Is the Self," in Evelyn C. White, ed., *The Black Woman's Health Book,* 2nd ed. Seattle: Seal Press, 1994.

"The World at Large: Size Acceptance Efforts Outside the U.S." *Radiance,* Issue 45 (winter 1996): 34ff.

Periodicals

Fat Girl Magazine
2215-R Market Street, #193; San Francisco, CA 94114
E-mail: solo@sirius.com
Web site: http://www.fatso.com/fatgirl
"A 'zine for fat dykes and those who admire them."

Fat!So?
P.O. Box 423464; San Francisco, CA 94142
Web site: http://www.fatso.com

Healthy Weight Journal
402 145th Street; Hettinger, ND 58639; (701) 567-2646; Fax: (701) 567-2602

Hues
P.O. Box 7778; Ann Arbor, MI 48107; (800) 483-7482
E-mail: hues@branson.org
Web site: http://www.hues.net
Hues' mission is to expand the definition of womanhood to include women of all shapes, sizes, cultures, lifestyles, and sexualities; regular section on body issues.

Radiance: A Publication for Large Women
P.O. Box 30246; Oakland, CA 94604; (510) 482-0680
E-mail: radmag2@aol.com
Web site: http://www.radiancemagazine.com
A magazine that celebrates large women. Good articles on body acceptance, health, and well-being.

Audiovisual Materials

The Body Beautiful (video/film), 23 minutes. Available from Women Make Movies, Inc., 462 Broadway, Suite 500, NY, NY 10013; (212) 925-0606, for purchase or rental. Examines effects of body image and racial/sexual identity on a white woman and her black daughter.

The Famine Within (video), 2 hours. Documentary by Katherine Gilday. Available to groups and organizations through Direct Cinema, P.O. Box 10003, Santa Monica, CA 90410; (800) 525-0000.

Fat Chance (video). Bullfrog Films, P.O. Box 149, Oley PA, 19547; (800) 543-3764. In Canada call (800) 267-7710. E-mail: bullfrog@igc.org

Mirror Mirror (video/film), 17 minutes. Explores women's quest for the "ideal body." Distributed by Women Make Movies (see address at *The Body Beautiful*).

No Apologies (video), 30 minutes. Powerful video with skits about women with disabilities, body, and sexuality issues. Produced by Peni Hall. Sliding scale for purchase. Contact Wry Crips Disabled Women's Reader's Theatre, P.O. Box 21474, Oakland, CA 94620; (510) 601-5819.

Nothing to Lose. A Performance by the Fat Lip Reader's Theater (video). Poignant, funny and warm performance of poetry and of humorous and dramatic skits about self-acceptance from an activist perspective. Available from Fat Lip Reader's Theater, P.O. Box 299963, Oakland, CA 94604; (415) 583-1649.

Nothing to Lose: Women's Body Image through Time (video). Available from Wolfe Video c/o Customer Service, P.O. Box 685195, Austin, TX 78768; (800) 850-5951.

Size 10 (film), 20 minutes. By S. Lambert and S. Gibson. Australian-made 1978 film shows how women's body image has been formed and deformed by advertising and sexism. Available from Women Make Movies (see address at *The Body Beautiful*).

Skin Trade: Women, Complexion and Caste (videos). Three-videotape set of selected presentations from the March 1997 symposium of the same title, including the original schedule and information packet from the conference. Contact Skin Trading Video Series, 89 Walden Street, Cambridge, MA 02140; (617) 354-8657; E-mail: jhana@msn.com

Still Killing Us Softly (16-mm film), 30 minutes. Based on a lecture/slide show by Jean Kilbourne. Powerful and provocative presentation of the advertising industry's objectification of women's bodies. An excellent film for colleges, schools, church groups, women's centers. Available from Cambridge Documentary Films, P.O. Box 385, Cambridge, MA 02139; (617) 484-3993; E-mail: cdf@shore.net; Web site: http://www.shore.net/~cdf

Organization

Abundia
P.O. Box 252; Downers Grove, IL 60515; (738) 897-9796

Programs for the Promotion of Body-Size Acceptance and Self-Esteem

Association for the Health Enrichment of Large People (AHELP)
P.O. Drawer C; Radford, VA 24143; (703) 731-1778; (800) 368-3468; (800) 572-3120 (Virginia only)
Web site: http://www.nrv.net/~ahelp/

Body Image Task Force
P.O. Box 934; Santa Cruz, CA 95061; (408) 457-4838
E-mail: datkins@blue.weeg.uiowa.edu

Council on Size and Weight Discrimination
P.O. Box 305; Mt. Marion, NY 12456; (914) 679-1209

Guerrilla Girls
Box 105, Cooper Station; New York, NY 10276
E-mail: guerrillagirls@voyager.com
Web site: http://www.voyagerco.com/gg/gg.htm

Largesse, Resource Network for Self-Esteem
P.O. Box 9404; New Haven, CT 06534; (203) 787-1624
E-mail: 75773.717@compuserve.com
Web site: http://www.fatgirl.com/S/

National Association to Advance Fat Acceptance (NAAFA)
P.O. Box 188620; Sacramento, CA 95818; (916) 558-6880
E-mail: naafa@world.std.com/largesse
Web site: http://www.naafa.org
   Many local chapters, a newsletter, and Web site.

National Center for Overcoming Overeating
315 W. 86th Street, Suite 17B; New York, NY 10024-3180; (212) 875-0442
Fax: (212) 874-6596

No Diet Day Coalition
P.O. Box 305; Mount Marion, NY 12456; (914) 679-1209

Additional Online Resources *

About Fat Acceptance
http://www.bayarea.net/~stef/fat.html

African-American Woman's Web Guide
http://robynma.simplenet.com/nianet

Disability Cool: Women's Stuff
http://www.geocities.com/HotSprings/7319/woman.htm

FDA Cosmetics Safety Page
http://vm.cfsan.fda.gov/~dms/cos-toc.html

gURL Headquarters!
http://www.tsoa.nyu.edu/gURL/hq/index.html#menu

Soc.support.fat-acceptance   and   Alt.support.big-folks Home Page
http://www.comlab.ox.ac.uk/oucl/users/sharon.curtis/BF/SSFA/home.html

* For more information and listings of online resources, please see Introduction to Online Women's Health Resources, p. 25.

By Maria Bettencourt and Christina
Economos, based on earlier work by
Esther Rome

WITH SPECIAL THANKS TO Trisha Brown,
Patricia Cooper, Marilyn Figueroa, Bonnie
Gage, Deb Levine, Bonnie Liebman, Ruth
Palumbo, Caterina Rocha, Judith Stein,
Margo N. Woods *

Chapter 2

....

Food

F*ood touches practically* every aspect of our lives and affects how we feel physically and emotionally. By eating we take care of ourselves at the most basic level. Eating has tremendous emotional importance for women because even as we are faced with many stresses and responsibilities in life, we are still most often the ones who take care of budgeting, planning, and cooking for others. For women, food is closely tied in with nurturance.

I like baked chicken, mashed potatoes, jellied cranberry sauce, salad, and milk—they make me feel cared for. When I cook it for myself I become both my mother and me as a child.

Because we don't control the production and availability of food, it can be a source of problems as well as pleasure. It is not always easy to get practical and reliable information about what to eat and what to avoid. Even when we know how to make good choices we may not have enough money to eat well, or nutritious foods may be difficult to find. There is a great deal of information about what to eat, and it can be very confusing.

I try to buy fresh fruits and vegetables, but it is hard to afford them since I lost my job. We eat canned and frozen vegetables, since they are more affordable and always available at the store in our neighborhood.

About 80% of people living in poverty in this country are women and children. Budget cutbacks decrease the availability for women and children of food subsidy programs like food stamps, school breakfast and lunch programs, meals for the elderly, and so on. These programs, even when most heavily funded, have never been adequate. The Women, Infant and Children supplement program (WIC) at its height covered only 39% of the people eligible for it. One study estimated that for every dollar spent on this program, three dollars were later saved in reduced medical

* Over the years since 1969, the following women have contributed to the many versions of this chapter: Judy Norsigian, Marsha Butman, Tricia Copeland, Demetria Iazzetto, Bonnie Liebman, Vivian Mayer, Ruth Palumbo, and Christine Rugen.

costs. Food stamps cover about half the cost of an adequate meal for healthy people and make no provision if special diets are needed.

Many of us want to share the responsibility for choosing, buying, and preparing food in our household. This may mean changing our eating and cooking patterns, encouraging a partner or husband to participate in shopping and cooking, getting children to help out, and sharing meals with friends. For many women, a fast-paced lifestyle means eating out or on the run, eating prepared foods, and preparing quick and easy meals.

When my husband and I first decided to take turns cooking, it was very hard for me to let him take the responsibility. I would suggest recipes and look over his shoulder while he cooked, giving him helpful hints. Since he was unsure of himself, that only encouraged him to ask me how to do something every few minutes. When I realized that I might as well have been cooking myself, I decided to make sure I stayed in a different room and answered most questions with "why don't you experiment?" Now he's just as good a cook as I am. We have the added benefit of more variety, since he makes different kinds of things than I do.

EATING WELL

Our Changing Diet

With the abundance and variety of food in this country, you might be surprised that many nutritionists think we eat more poorly now than at the turn of the century. Even people in the U.S. who have enough money to buy whatever food they want make choices that are not the best nutritionally because of barriers to knowledge or access. We eat highly processed foods with too much fat, salt, and sugar.[1-3] We used to eat more whole foods, such as whole-wheat rather than white flour. In general, food was minimally processed or changed little from its original state, and the changes usually involved the kind of cooking or preserving that could be done in a home kitchen. Our current technology changes our food radically, split-

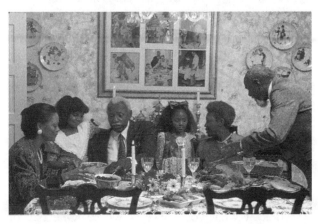

Tom McCarthy/Picture Cube

Disease	Possible Cause from Diet and Lifestyle
Heart disease	Too many saturated fats, cholesterol, and calories; lack of fiber and physical activity
Some cancers	Too many calories, alcohol, fats; lack of fiber, fruits, and vegetables, and physical activity
High blood pressure	Too much salt, alcohol, calories; lack of potassium and physical activity
Diabetes	Too many calories and simple sugars; lack of fiber and physical activity
Osteoporosis	Lack of calcium, vitamin D, and weight-bearing activity
Cavities	Too much sugar
Gallstones	Lack of fiber
Diverticulosis and constipation	Lack of fiber and physical activity
Anemia	Lack of iron, vitamin B_6, folic acid, or vitamin B_{12}

ting it into components and transforming, rearranging, and adding to it. We used to eat more complex carbohydrates, foods with a lot of starch and/or natural sugars, and fiber; now we eat more foods that have been highly processed with refined carbohydrates like cane sugar, or foods with fat and sugar substitutes[4,5] and with little fiber.

Diet and Illness

These dietary changes may be making us more susceptible to various diseases. Current research indicates links between diet and chronic diseases such as heart disease, diabetes, and some cancers.[6,7] Many of us have found this research compelling enough to change what we eat. Others of us who have had health problems have found that changing what we eat improves our health. Few doctors have any special expertise about the effects of diet and illness, and although some progress has been made, the nutrition education offered in medical schools is generally insufficient.

Government Guidelines for Good Health

General Eating Guidelines

Because our changing eating habits have been linked to various diseases, the government has developed suggestions on how and what to eat for good health. The U.S. Department of Agriculture (USDA) developed the Food Guide Pyramid,[8] a simple graphic used to represent modern thinking about healthful eating. The pyramid uses the USDA's *Nutrition and*

Your Heath: Dietary Guidelines for Americans (1995)[9] as its guiding principle and offers the best nutrition information currently available.

- *Eat a variety of foods.* Individuals should adopt eating styles that are consistent with their own lifestyles and that will supply all the nutrients needed for good health.
- *Choose a diet low in total fat, saturated fat, and cholesterol.* Decrease fats to less than or equal to 30% of calories. Reduce saturated fats to 7 or 8% of calories.
- *Choose a diet with plenty of vegetables, fruits, and whole-grain products.* Increase the level of complex carbohydrates to 55% of total calories, and increase fiber to 25–30 grams per day. Aim for five to nine servings of fruits and vegetables every day.
- *Choose a diet moderate in sugar.* Decrease refined sugar intake to no more than 10% of calories.
- *Use salt and sodium in moderation.* Try to consume less than 2,400 mg of sodium per day.
- *If you drink alcohol, do so in moderation.* Moderation means one 5-ounce glass of wine, a 12-ounce bottle of beer, or 1½ ounces of hard liquor.

Over the past few years, several different pyramids have been developed, in addition to the USDA's pyramid, that reflect different cultural eating practices. In the Asian Pyramid, red meat is regulated to one or two servings a month, poultry and fish are eaten a few times a week, vegetable oils including peanut oils are emphasized, and plant foods like rice, noodles, fruits, vegetables, and legumes constitute the foundation of the diet. In the Mediterranean Pyramid, red meat is limited to a few servings a month; poultry, fish, and eggs are eaten a few times a week; olive oil is emphasized; and plant foods like bread, pasta, whole grains, fruits, vegetables, and legumes constitute the foundation of the diet. In the Latin Pyramid, red meat is allowed weekly (or less often); poultry, fish, pork, and eggs are eaten several times a week; and plant foods

like maize, potato, rice, tortilla, whole grains, sweet potato, cassava, pumpkin, and plantain are emphasized. Fruits, vegetables, and legumes constitute the foundation of the diet.[10]

The authors of this chapter also recommend these measures:

- Cut protein to 10 to 15% of total calories, unless you have specific need (e.g., pregnancy, growth, or when fighting or recovering from illness).
- Limit caffeine to less than 200–250 milligrams a day. Caffeine is found in coffee, chocolate, black tea, some herb teas, many soft drinks (especially colas), and some over-the-counter drugs.
- Shop for organic foods when you can, since pesticides are widely used in the growing of most foods. Wash nonorganic fruits and vegetables thoroughly.

MAKING CHANGES

Would you like to see whether you can feel healthier and more energetic by eating differently? First of all, assess why you like the foods that you do and what factors influence your food choices. Do you use lots of sweet, salty, and fatty foods as rewards? Do you eat when you're not hungry? Do you always eat certain foods when you are depressed, angry, or upset? Are you nostalgic for certain foods you associate with childhood, special holidays, or childhood rewards? Do you eat more when you are alone? With others?

Sweets, especially ice cream, were always a treat and comfort food in my family. I had changed my diet in all kinds of other ways like eliminating white flour, but I did not seriously consider cutting out sweets, even though I knew they weren't good for me. I figured I would always have a sweet tooth. Then one day my doctor told me that my blood sugar was high, and I noticed my weight had really crept up over the years. A friend suggested I decrease the sugar in my diet. I felt so scared I was willing to give it a try. It was hard to do, so I took it one day at a time at first. Now I have stopped craving sweets most of the time. I only eat ice cream on rare occasions, which I never thought I could do.

Tips to Make the Guidelines Work for You

1. Introduce changes slowly, as they aren't always easy to make. Experiment with one thing at a time so you won't feel overwhelmed. This will help overcome resistance if you are cooking for others and will give your digestive tract a chance to adjust. Also, if you change too fast, you might find yourself craving what you are used to, which may lead to overeating.

2. Look at what you eat as a whole. One day of high-fat, high-sugar foods won't hurt you. (The

---

BALANCE FOOD INTAKE WITH PHYSICAL ACTIVITY

Putting food into your mouth is only one part of nourishing yourself. You need to be active, too. The U.S. Surgeon General's report on physical activity and health (1996)[11] recommends that every U.S. adult accumulates 30 minutes of moderate-intensity activity on most, preferably all, days of the week. See chapter 4, Women in Motion.

exception to this is if you have trouble regulating your blood sugar, as with diabetes or hypoglycemia.) Think about what you eat over a one- or two-week period. Don't judge yourself for indulging in less healthy foods. Given time, you will find a balance that's right for you.

3. Try new things when you aren't rushed.

4. Increase the whole foods in your diet. Generally, whole, minimally processed foods have a higher nutrient density than refined, highly processed foods. This means that for every calorie of food you eat you are getting more vitamins, minerals, and other important goodies than in a low-nutrient-density food. Vegetables tend to have very high nutrient densities, and foods high in fats and/or refined sugar are often low.

5. Change the snacks you keep around the house. Try fruits, vegetables, or whole-wheat or rice crackers. Popcorn can be made either plain or with seasonings like chili or garlic powder. Use nuts, seeds, and dried fruit in moderation. (They contain important nutrients but also a lot of fat or sugar.)

6. Gradually reduce the amount of processed foods you buy. They often are "convenience food" and tend to be high in salt, sugar, and fats, often saturated. They also are more likely to have artificial colors, flavors, and other questionable ingredients. You generally get less per dollar for the nutrients in heavily processed foods than in whole foods. Beware that the new fat-free foods often contain added sugar or sugar substitutes to boost the flavor lost by removing the fat.

7. Bring your own food as often as possible rather than relying on fast-food restaurants, vending machines, and food trucks (see no. 6 above). If you eat from them regularly, you won't get enough fresh vegetables, fruits, or whole grains.

8. Get together with your friends and help each other figure out how to eat healthy foods when away from home.

9. If you eat in restaurants, you can request and often get foods prepared just for you. You can also ask about the method of preparation and the ingredients.

10. Next time you watch TV, notice what kinds of foods are advertised, and consider how they help or hurt your body. This can be fun to do with children.

11. When you travel, pack your own snacks, and call airlines in advance to order low-fat or vegetarian meals and snacks. In bus and train stations, airports, and roadside restaurants, search for healthy alternatives to junk food such as fruit, bagels, grilled chicken sandwiches, salads, pretzels, and yogurt.

12. Cultivate your taste buds to identify new flavors from herbs and spices to add more interest to your food without fat.

Increasing Unrefined Carbohydrates

1. Make sure the bread label says "100% whole wheat" or "whole grain" and not just "wheat." Caramel and molasses may be added to make white bread look like whole wheat when it isn't. Use whole-wheat and colored pastas instead of white-flour ones.

2. Try eating more kinds of legumes (peas and beans). Also try using soy protein (tofu) or other vegetable sources of protein.

3. Strive for Five-a-Day. That means at least three servings of vegetables and two servings of fruit every day. A total of seven servings is even better. A serving is 1/2 cup of cooked or 1 cup of raw vegetables or one piece of fruit. Orange, yellow, and dark green vegetables and fruits are especially nutritious.

4. In baking, substitute pastry or all-purpose whole-wheat flour for white flour. Whole-wheat pastry flour, which has less gluten (the wheat protein) than bread flour or all-purpose whole-wheat flour, will make lighter-colored and lighter-textured baked goods. Note that unbleached flour is white flour.

5. Try using some whole grains like brown rice, buckwheat (kasha), or bulgur (a form of cracked wheat). They may take about twice as long to cook (40 minutes for brown rice, compared with 20 for converted white rice), but this is mainly a matter of remembering to start cooking them as soon as you begin to prepare the meal. You can use a pressure cooker to reduce preparation time.

6. For long-cooking foods, make twice as much and either freeze the leftovers or make them into something else the next day. You can buy many beans precooked in cans. Rinse to reduce added salt.

Decreasing Refined and Added Sugars

1. Check the sugar content of processed foods, which often have many types of sugar in them. The following are all names for different forms of sugar: HFCS (high-fructose corn syrup), invert sugar, molasses, honey (evaporated by bees), corn sweetener, caramel, corn syrup, sucrose, lactose, maltose, dextrose, levulose, fructose, maple syrup, brown sugar, turbinado, rawkleen sugar, jam, and jelly. As a rule of thumb, "ose" means sugar.

2. Drink more water or real fruit juice instead of soda or juice drinks. If you still want something fizzy, add seltzer to real fruit juices.

3. Drink 100% fruit juice and not "juice drinks," "juice blends," "juice-ades," "juice coolers," or "juice beverages," which may contain as little as 5 or 10% real juice. Check the label. Unless the drink is just "fruit flavored," which can mean zero juice, the percentage of juice must be listed on the label. "No sugar added" means just that.

4. Some people find honey, molasses, or malt syrup much sweeter than sugar and so use less of them than they would sugar. *Blackstrap* molasses has some good nutrients, like iron, but it is still a highly concentrated sugar. So far, honey has no measurable benefits over sugar.

5. Substitute sweet whole foods or real fruit juices for sugar in recipes. Try mashed cooked sweet potatoes; raisins soaked or boiled in water, then pureed in a blender; or very ripe mashed bananas instead of sugar where they can be substituted. That way you get other vitamins, minerals, and fiber with sweetness.

6. If you use cold cereals, choose less sugary ones and less processed ones. Check the labeling on the side of the box for the number of grams of sucrose and other sugars per ounce of cereal. Hot cereals, such as regular or quick (not instant) oatmeal, cracked wheat, cornmeal, and buckwheat (kasha), take no more than 15 to 20 minutes to prepare. They are minimally processed and contain no sugar unless added by you.

7. Use sweet spices and flavorings like cinnamon, ginger, cloves, allspice, and vanilla to replace some of the sugar in the food you prepare.

8. Try not to use sweets as a reward for kids (or adults!). They fill you up so you don't have room for nutritious foods. Ask relatives and friends to bring love, good stories, and fruit rather than sweets for the children. If they persist, suggest they pick up the tab on dental bills.

Decreasing Fats and Changing the Ratio of Fats in Our Diets

1. Check label for "saturated fat." Limit foods that contain 4 grams or more of saturated fat per serving, which is 20% of a day's worth (20% of the Daily Value [DV] for saturated fat). Avoid ingredients listed as animal fat, shortening, tallow, lard, hydrogenated oil, or coconut, palm, or palm kernel oil.

2. Increase your use of fish instead of meat, but keep in mind that eating contaminated fish flesh or fish by-products can be harmful. Ask where the fish you are buying came from and whether it was inspected by a government agency.

3. When eating poultry, remove the skin. That's where 25% of the fat is.

4. Try vegetarian meals a few times a week. Use those that rely on grains, vegetables, and legumes (see "Vegetarianism," p. 50).

5. Substitute 1% low-fat or nonfat milk or buttermilk, and nonfat or low-fat yogurt for some or all of the whole milk you drink. (Does not apply to very young children.)

6. Cut back on red meat, since it is high in saturated fats even if none is visible. About a third of the fat in U.S. diets comes from meat. If your meals don't feel as substantial, remember it's the fat, not the protein, that makes you feel so full after a meat meal.

7. Avoid processed meats like bacon, sausage, and regular cold cuts, which are high in fat and salt. Substitute low-fat hot dogs, cold cuts, and turkey bacon instead.

8. Cut back on the use of hard and processed cheeses, which are higher in fat. Try some of the tasty lower-fat and softer cheeses now on the market.

9. Instead of frying, try sautéing in vegetable broth or using smaller amounts of canola, olive, or other unsaturated oils. Keep the oil below smoking temperatures, and don't reuse it if it has darkened at all, because any oil may become carcinogenic through overheating. Try boiling, baking, stewing, or stir-frying instead.

10. Cut back on the butter, mayonnaise, cream, and salad dressing you add to foods. Try the lower-fat alternatives. Eliminate all use of margarine.

11. Eat fewer fried foods like French fries, potato chips, doughnuts, and fried fish and fried chicken. Substitute with low-fat alternatives, and bake with low-fat ingredients and substitutions.

Reducing Salt

1. Check the label for "sodium" and look for foods with less than 140 mg per serving. Limit foods that contain more than 20% of the day's worth (20% DV) of sodium.

2. Roughly 75% of the sodium we consume comes from processed foods. Reduce foods cured in salt, most condiments, processed cheeses, salty nuts, soy sauce, monosodium glutamate (MSG), bouillon, and many canned foods and soups.

Fat Facts

Saturated fats are solid at room temperature (70°F). Animal fats, hydrogenated (hardened) fats, and three vegetable fats—coconut, palm, and palm kernel—are saturated fats. Most of our saturated fats come from red meats, cheese, ice cream, whole milk, and cakes, cookies, pies, and other pastries. Polyunsaturated fats are those which are liquid (oils) and derived from plants like corn, safflower, or sesame. Omega-3 fatty acids are polyunsaturated fats that we obtain through fish and marine foods as well as from many nuts, canola oil, flax seed, and flax seed oil. Our bodies need omega-3 for numerous important functions, including the formation of cell membranes, the prevention of skin abnormalities, and the regulation of the production of prostaglandins. These polyunsaturated fats have also been found to have numerous beneficial effects on the cardiovascular risk profile. Fish is the one flesh food that has a protective effect against heart disease by virtue of these omega-3 fatty acids, and studies have documented low rates of coronary artery disease in people consuming large quantities of fish in their diets. Monounsaturated fats, like peanut, canola (rapeseed), and olive oil, are also liquid at room temperature but solidify easily in the refrigerator.

The term "trans fat" is used to describe a fatty acid chain and the type of bond that holds the chain together. A "trans fat" contains bonds in the "trans" configuration versus the "cis" configuration, which is how the bonds usually occur in foods. Trans bonds form when liquid polyunsaturated fats are partially hydrogenated (hydrogen is added), which makes them more solid at room temperature. A common example is the making of margarine from vegetable oil. Many processed foods contain trans fat, especially baked products. Trans fats appear to have an effect on blood cholesterol similar to that of saturated fat, elevating total cholesterol and LDL cholesterol. To avoid trans fats, avoid foods that list "hydrogenated" or "partially hydrogenated" fat on the ingredients section of their labels. Europeans have removed trans fatty acids from margarine; U.S. manufacturers have not.

3. Some people use less salt when adding it during cooking. Others use less if they cook without salt and add some if necessary at the table. You can see which works better for you.

4. Don't add softeners to drinking and cooking water because they add sodium to the water.

5. Check the sodium level of your tap water. If you are part of a municipal system, the water department will know what it is. If you have a well, you can get the water tested.

6. Substitute plain herbs, spices, onions, and garlic for salt. Use oil and vinegar or lemon or other fruit juice to flavor salads and other vegetables.

Understanding Nutrient Guidelines

While it is still not clear what an optimal diet is, the government makes an effort to determine what it is and offers information to consumers in a variety of ways. The Recommended Dietary Allowances (RDAs) are determined by a board of respected scientists, the Food and Nutrition Board of the National Academy of Sciences.[12] The RDAs are not fixed; the numbers of nutrients (vitamins, minerals, and protein) and amounts recommended are updated regularly as new information becomes available.

The Daily Values (DVs) are reference numbers set forth by the Food and Drug Administration (FDA), a government agency, specifically for use on food labels. The DVs represent two sets of standards: Daily Reference Values (DRVs) help determine the upper limits on the amounts of certain nutrients (total fat, saturated fat, cholesterol, and sodium) and optimal amounts of others (carbohydrates and fiber). The Reference Daily Intakes (RDIs) are used as a label reference for vitamins, minerals, and protein, reflecting the needs of the most sensitive population or those who need the greatest amount of that nutrient. These DVs differ from person to person because most are based on the number of calories one should eat to maintain a healthy weight. The food label DVs, seen on food packages under "Nutrition Facts" (see "Reading Labels," p. 50), are based on a 2,000-calorie reference

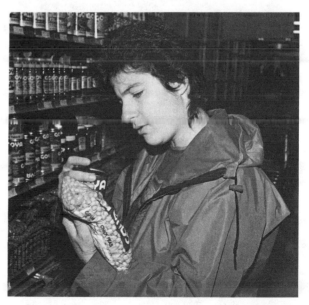

Elizabeth Shapiro

READING LABELS [13] *

1. Read the ingredients. The ingredients are listed in order of amount by weight used in preparation; there's most of the first ingredient and least of the last. Standardized foods must have full ingredient labeling, and the ingredient list now contains FDA certified color additives by name, sources of protein hydrolysates used as flavors and flavor enhancers, and declaration of caseinate as a milk derivative in foods that claim to be nondairy. These requirements allow people who may be allergic to such additives to avoid them. Nutrition labels are required for *most* processed food items sold in the grocery store.

2. Check serving size. Serving sizes are now uniform (similar foods have similar serving sizes, making comparisons easier) and more realistic than they used to be, reflecting the amounts that people actually eat. All of the nutrient information on the label is based on the serving size, so if you eat the equivalent of two servings, you will receive double the amount of nutrients listed on the label.

3. "Percent Daily Value" tells you the percent of a day's worth of fat, sodium, etc., provided by the food in the context of a 2,000-calorie diet. Some DVs are upper limits (try to eat no more than 100%), while others are optimal amounts (try to eat 100%). *Simple advice:* if a food has 20% or more of the DV, it's "high" in that nutrient. "Low" means no more than 5%.

4. "Calories from fat" helps you see how fatty a food is. Fat, saturated fat, and fiber are listed in grams and as a % DV; sugars are listed in grams only.

5. "Enriched" means that some of the nutrients removed during processing have been replaced to approximately the same levels found in the original food.[14] However, other vitamins and minerals and fiber in whole grains are not restored to such foods as enriched flour, breads, and pasta.

6. "Fortified" means that nutrients have been added to foods. These nutrients, such as iodine in salt or calcium in fruit drinks, may not normally be found in the food. They may be added in amounts greater than those that naturally occur, such as large amounts of vitamins and minerals added to breakfast cereals.

7. Although the labeling must be truthful, a product's advertising can be misleading. Nutrient content descriptions such as "free," "low," "lean," or "light" require a bit of research to interpret correctly. In addition, "cholesterol-free" on a label may disguise that it is still high in saturated fat. Products advertised as "light" or "100% natural" may still contain high amounts of saturated fat and sugar.

8. On cans, look at how weight is listed. "Net weight" includes any liquid used for packing. "Drained" or "filled" weight tells you what the actual food weighs.

9. Check the date to see how fresh the food is.

10. If you need more information, write to the manufacturer or distributor. The name and address must be on the label.

* In response to growing consumer concern, Congress enacted the Nutrition Labeling and Education Act (NLEA) in 1990 requiring food manufacturers to relabel food products. It was not until 1994 that the FDA enforced the NLEA with stricter and more truthful labeling requirements. Almost all processed foods are now required by law to have a "Nutrition Facts" section on their packaging. "Nutrition facts" provides mandatory and consistent nutrition information, enabling consumers to make informed choices. Nevertheless, some foods are exempt from standard requirements. If you want to know the ingredients, labeling, or grading requirements for any food, call or write to your local U.S. FDA office in the nearest major city.

diet. Your own DVs may be higher or lower depending on your calorie needs. The percent DVs indicate how far a serving of a particular food goes toward meeting the 2,000-calorie diet each day. The percent DVs can be valuable for comparing the nutritional value of different foods. Most people take the Daily Values too literally, thinking that if they follow them, they are protected. But DVs are not intended to assess individual needs, which may vary widely. Furthermore, we know that over 28 vitamins and minerals are essential in some way, but since deficiency diseases do not pose a risk to the majority of the population, labels are required to list only vitamin A, vitamin C, iron, and calcium. Researchers think that other nutrients are essential but haven't turned up final proof, and no doubt there are some yet to be discovered. Phytochemicals are an example of naturally occurring chemicals in foods like vegetables, fruits, and soy. Phytochemical-rich foods seem to protect against heart disease and some cancers.

VEGETARIANISM

Many of us today are interested in vegetarianism and are eating less meat or none at all. A recent study revealed that over 12 million people in the U.S. consider themselves vegetarians. We may do this for health reasons such as reducing our risk of heart disease, diabetes, and certain cancers; to eat more cheaply; to stop killing other living beings; or for religious reasons. The 1995 U.S. Dietary Guidelines support vegetarianism as a healthy way to eat. A plant-based diet is promoted as protective against many of the chronic illnesses faced by Americans.[15]

As a child, I never liked to eat meat and followed mostly a vegetarian diet with occasional eggs and some dairy. This was before the time when people understood this diet well. I knew that it was right for me and quickly became labeled stubborn, a fussy eater, etc. But when the household came down with seasonal colds and flus, I was running around quite happy and healthy with an excellent resistance.

A vegetarian diet is one that excludes meat, fish, and poultry. There are many variations of the vegetarian lifestyle. The most popular is the lacto-ovo vegetarian diet, which includes dairy products ("lacto") and eggs ("ovo"). Another growing type of vegetarian diet is the vegan, which avoids all types of animal products, including dairy products and eggs. Most vegetarians eat both eggs and dairy products. It is absolutely possible to live a healthy life and never eat any animals.

Getting enough protein on a vegetarian or vegan diet is not difficult if you eat enough of a *variety* of foods throughout the day to meet your caloric needs.[16] Proteins are made up of building blocks called amino acids. Of the 20 amino acids in foods, our bodies can make 11. The other nine are considered essential; that is, we can get them only through the food we eat. All foods, including plant foods, are plentiful in protein and contain all the essential amino acids. However, plant sources contain limited amounts of any one essential amino acid. For instance, beans are low in the essential amino acid methionine but are high in lysine, while white rice is high in methionine and low in lysine. So combining these foods increases their protein quality, although it is not necessary to combine them at each meal. Legumes team up perfectly with any grain, nut, or seed, and grains are a perfect complement with nuts and seeds. Most of the world's population eats a diet consisting of combinations of plant proteins.

Another nutritional concern often linked with the vegetarian diet, especially the vegan type diet, is vitamin B_{12}. Vitamin B_{12} is not found in plant products. Eating fortified plant products such as tempeh, miso, or some soy milk will help you meet your vitamin B_{12} needs, or you can take a vitamin B_{12} supplement if you don't eat fortified plant products.

Most children, adolescents, pregnant women, and nursing mothers need to be especially careful to get enough nutrients, particularly protein, calcium, zinc, folic acid, and iron, and sufficient calories to support their special developmental and growth needs. Older people need all of the same nutrients as do their younger counterparts. Since their caloric needs may be less, it is important to plan a diet that is very nutri-ent dense, with few foods that have limited nutritional value. A well-planned, varied, vegetarian diet can support the special nutritional needs of these groups. If you are concerned that your diet is not meeting your needs, consult a nutritionist knowledgeable about vegetarianism, or one familiar with a vegan diet. Your local dietetic association should be able to help you to find a nutritionist in your area, or you can contact the Vegetarian Resource Group for help with your questions (see Resources).

SHOPPING WISELY

Supermarkets plan their layouts to slow you down and encourage buying. If you understand how stores are laid out, it can help you be a wise shopper.

1. Outside aisles carry the freshest, healthiest food items; inside aisles carry the more processed, high-sugar, high-fat items.

2. End-of-aisle displays—great savings items—can entice you to buy less nutritious foods.

3. Products advertised most often are less nutritious.

4. Expensive, low-nutrient choices are put at eye level to catch your attention.

5. Candy and snacks are strategically placed at checkout counters.

6. Automated electronic scanners often make errors that add to your food bill. Check your receipt.

Follow these guidelines to avoid supermarket gimmicks and spending on unnecessary items:

- Plan your weekly meals in advance. Use store circulars to identify any healthy sale items.
- Prepare shopping lists from meal plans.
- Don't go shopping when you are hungry. It can lead to impulse buying.
- Shop in large grocery stores for the best bargains. Consider store brands for staple items.
- Read food labels and unit pricing to compare nutritional value and cost of foods.
- Use store and manufacturer coupons for additional savings. Avoid using coupons for items that you will not use.
- To avoid spoilage, purchase food in amounts that make sense for you and your family.
- Choose minimally processed foods. Shop the outside aisles.

PROTEIN COMBINATION CHART

To turn nonanimal foods into high-quality protein it is best to combine them with one of the foods pointed to. No arrows point out from the animal foods because they can stand alone but will enhance other groups.

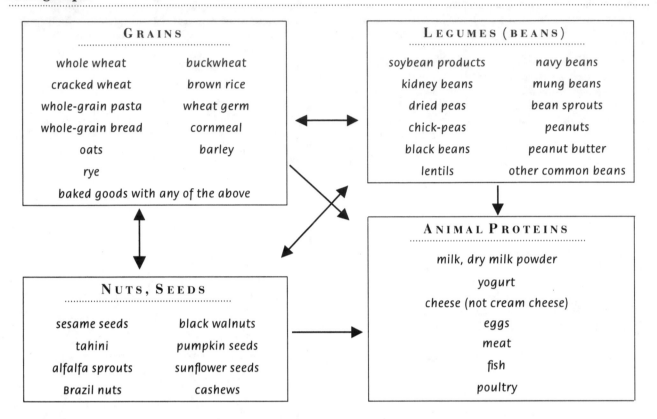

From Nikki Goldbeck, *As You Eat, So Your Baby Grows,* Woodstock, NY: Ceres Press, 1997.

SHOULD YOU TAKE SUPPLEMENTS?

No one really knows whether people without an obvious vitamin or mineral deficiency disease should take supplements. Individuals vary in their ability to absorb and use nutrients. At particular times you are likely to need specific extra vitamins and minerals—from birth through adolescence, if you take birth control pills, if you are pregnant and nursing, if you are sick, and after menopause, when you slowly become less efficient at absorbing nutrients. Some supplements may be particularly important for women. The average woman between the ages of 25 and 50 needs 1,000 milligrams of calcium a day. Younger women and postmenopausal women need up to 1,500 milligrams of calcium a day. This is equal to about five glasses of regular milk or calcium-fortified soy milk. Postmenopausal women who live in the northern parts of the country get too little sunlight for their bodies to make vitamin D during the winter and early spring months (October through May); they may need to take 400 international units (IU) of vitamin D a day during that time, along with enough calcium, to minimize bone loss. Women of child-bearing age need a minimum of 400 micrograms a day of folic acid to reduce the risk of having a child with neural tube defects, such as spina bifida. The greatest benefit of folic acid occurs in the first month of pregnancy, which makes it important not to wait until you are pregnant to get enough folic acid. It is best to get your nutrient needs from food, but if this is impossible, you may need a vitamin supplement. The amounts of vitamins you need (with the exception of calcium) are usually found in an ordinary multivitamin supplement. Read the label to determine whether the supplement provides 100% RDA for the vitamin or mineral.

Research suggests that some compounds found in plants, known as antioxidants, may reduce the risk of cancer, heart disease, cataracts, and another age-related eye disorder called macular degeneration. Antioxidants are beta-carotene and vitamins C and E. Beta-carotene is converted in the body into vitamin A, and unlike vitamin A, beta-carotene is not considered dangerous at high doses when taken by healthy individuals. Newly described compounds found in plant-based foods, known as phytochemicals, are also thought to be protective against cancer. Antioxidants are available in pill form. It is not possible to get phytochemicals in pill form yet, but they may be available in the future. Still, the best way to get these nutrients is to eat plenty of fresh fruits, vegetables, and soy products like tofu and miso, which are rich in these compounds. (See the table "A Partial List of Important Nutrients" for more information on food sources.)

In the U.S. today, 25% of what we eat is often made up of foods that provide calories and not much else, like soda, sugary snacks, and alcohol. Eating these nutrient-poor foods, combined with foods stripped of nutrients through processing or for other reasons, may mean we are not getting enough of all the nutrients we need. Your specific needs are based on a combination of your unique biochemical inheritance, which currently is difficult to assess; the environmental stresses in your life; your health status; how physically active you are; and how well you eat.

Particular stresses may be putting you at nutritional risk. Smokers have a higher metabolic turnover rate for vitamin C, so they will need at least 120 mg (twice the RDA) to meet their bodies' needs. Many drugs affect vitamin and mineral use. Aspirin affects folic acid absorption and depletes tissues of vitamin C; steroids increase the urinary output of calcium, and birth control pills and estrogen replacement therapy can result in folic acid and vitamin B_6 deficiency.

You may think you can find out whether you are deficient in one or more nutrients by experimenting with supplements, but take caution. There are numerous considerations in taking this route. For instance, nutritional status is not the only factor that influences your health, well-being, or disease resistance. Furthermore, taking supplements opens up the potential for toxicity. It is well known that fat-soluble vitamins, such as vitamins A and D, can be harmful if taken in excess because they are stored in the body. But water-soluble vitamins may also be harmful in large doses. High doses of vitamin B_6 have been shown to lead to partial paralysis, and high levels of niacin have been known to cause liver disease in some individuals.[17] A study done on male heavy smokers revealed that men taking beta-carotene had an 18% higher incidence of lung cancer, and vitamin E reduced the risk of prostate cancer but raised the risk for stroke.[18] Also, many supplements are useless or are less effective if taken by themselves. Furthermore, you can't get fiber easily from pills. Fiber is found in foods such as whole grains, fruits, vegetables, and legumes.

It is still not understood how vitamin supplements interact with the many compounds in foods. Some of these compounds may be more effective than the vitamins themselves. Supplements contain only one form of the vitamin rather than the many forms found in the food. Even though supplements are fast and easy to take, they cannot substitute for food.

Laboratories that will determine levels of certain nutrients in your body may be the wave of the future, but as yet there are still problems associated with them. First, they tend to be very expensive, and second, "the tests may measure what's there at the moment your blood is drawn . . . but nutrient levels can vary from day to day and from month to month."[19]

A diet of whole, minimally processed foods; regular exercise; and avoidance of smoking and negative stresses is your best bet for health. If you want to take a daily supplement, choose one at or below the recommended dietary allowances (RDAs). (See chart, "A Partial List of Important Nutrients.")

HELPING KIDS EAT WELL

Mothers and others often have a lot of challenges when feeding kids. Even strangers may condemn us if our kids are "too" fat or skinny, though how we feed them may have little to do with how they look. Knowledge of good nutrition and the provision of appropriate nutritious foods during the different stages of your child's growth and development will help ensure that she or he is eating well. Ellyn Satter, in her book *Child of Mine,* provides parents with the following advice: You as a parent are responsible for the quality of and amount of food you offer your child, and your child is responsible for how much she or he eats.

One way to interest kids in eating better is to set an example by eating well ourselves. Children do remember what they eat at home and can learn to make good choices, especially if you explain the reasons for the choices.

I tell my four-year-old that some foods help him grow better than others, and he wants to grow as fast as he can.

Kids of all ages eat a significant portion of their food in the form of snacks, just like adults. This is fine if the snacks are nutritious. Older kids, especially teenagers, just need a lot of food. Cookies can be made with wheat germ, whole grains, dried fruits, and nuts. Milk shakes can be made from yogurt, banana, crushed ice, and vanilla. Stock up on fruits, vegetables, peanut butter, and/or slices of soy cheese. When kids are hungry, they'll eat what's there, so make the snacks worth eating and enjoyable.

It's important to let kids decide when they are hungry and when they are full. They eat different amounts at different times depending on how fast they are growing, how active they are, and whether or not they are sick. Helping them to trust themselves in this way teaches them an important lesson they can use in regulating their eating all through life.

Involve children in growing, buying, and preparing foods. Have them read product labels for you in the supermarket. Try to find a small space, even if you are in the city, to grow something. Have older kids take turns at cooking meals. Younger kids usually will be eager helpers. Even a three-year-old can chop soft vegetables for a salad with a table knife, spread nut butters, help mix batters, or add ingredients to almost any recipe.

Since most mothers work outside the home today,

A Partial List of Important Nutrients

NUTRIENT/RDAs	CHIEF FUNCTIONS	IMPORTANT SOURCES	COMMENTS
PROTEINS 44–50 gm.	Provide nitrogen and amino acids for body proteins (in skin tissues, muscles, brain, hair, etc.), for hormones (substances that control body processes), for antibodies (which fight infections), and for enzymes (which control the rates of chemical reactions in our bodies)	Milk, cheese, yogurt, eggs, fish, poultry, meat, beans, tofu, certain vegetable combinations, seafood, soy products (tempeh, TVP® [textured vegetable proteins])	Recommended intake is 30% of total daily caloric intake
FATS	Provide concentrated sources of energy Carry fat-soluble vitamins (notably, A, D, and E) and essential fatty acids Provide insulation and protection for important organs and body structures Store calories to provide for pregnancy and nursing needs	Whole milk, most cheeses, butter, margarine, oils, nuts, meats	Recommended intake is 30% or less of total daily caloric intake
CARBOHYDRATES	Keep proteins from being used for energy needs, so they can be used primarily for body-building functions; also necessary for protein and fat utilization Provide our main source of energy Provide the glucose vital for certain brain functions	Grains and cereals, bread, vegetables, beans, fruits	Recommended intake is 40% of total daily caloric intake
VITAMIN A (fat soluble) 8,000 IU	Helps prevent infection Helps eyes adjust to changes from bright to dim light (prevents night blindness) Needed for healthy skin and mucosal tissues, such as the inside of the mouth and lungs, bones, and teeth	Fish liver oil, liver, whole milk, fortified margarine, butter, whole-milk cheeses, egg yolks, dark green, yellow and orange vegetables and fruits	Toxic in large doses; may cause birth defects in large doses
VITAMIN D (fat soluble) 200–400 IU	Regulates calcium and phosphorus absorption necessary for strong bones and teeth	Sunlight on bare skin, fortified milk, fish liver oil; small amounts in sardines, tuna, salmon, egg yolks	Toxic in large doses
VITAMIN E (fat soluble) 8 mg.	Helps preserve some vitamins and unsaturated fatty acids (acts as an antioxidant) Helps stabilize biological membranes	Vegetable oils (wheat germ, corn, and soybean), wheat and rice germ, egg yolks, legumes, corn, almonds	Destroyed by freezing

NUTRIENT/RDAS	CHIEF FUNCTIONS	IMPORTANT SOURCES	COMMENTS
B VITAMINS (water soluble) including thiamine (B_1), riboflavin (B_2), niacin, pyridoxine, folic acid, cobalamin (B_{12}), choline, etc.	Needed for steady nerves, alertness, good digestion, energy production, healthy skin and eyes, maintenance of blood, disease resistance Needed for protein, fat, and carbohydrate metabolism	Whole-grain breads and cereals, liver, wheat germ, nutritional yeast, green vegetables, lean meats, milk, cheese, molasses, peanuts, dried peas and beans, nuts and seeds, eggs, poultry, potatoes, fish	Heat, air, and sometimes light destroy B and C vitamins; most water-soluble vitamins are *not* stored in the body for long periods, so you need some every day
THIAMIN (B_1) 1–1.1 mg.	Aids in the release of energy from food; important for healthy brain and nerve cells	Whole grains, enriched grain products, legumes (beans and peas), dark green leafy vegetables, brewer's yeast, nuts, fish, meats	Enriched flour products and cereals are fortified with thiamin
RIBOFLAVIN (B_2) 1.2–1.4 mg.	Aids in the release of energy from food; used in production of red blood cells, important for health of skin and eyes	Fortified cereals, enriched white flour, animal products (meat, poultry, fish, eggs, dairy products), green vegetables	Found in all enriched flour products
NIACIN (B_3) 13–17 mg.	Helps release energy from food; helps maintain healthy skin, digestive system, and nerves	Nuts, brewer's yeast, enriched grain products, peanut butter, dark green leafy vegetables, legumes	Found in all enriched flour products
PYROXIDINE (B_6) 1.6 mg.	Aids in use of proteins and carbohydrates; helps form red blood cells in nerve and brain function	Whole grains, bananas, beans, nuts, brewer's yeast, chicken, fish, liver	
FOLACIN (B_{12}) 400 mcg.	Important in DNA synthesis, growth and protein metabolism; manufacture of red blood cells; proper function of nervous system	Meats, dairy products, eggs, and fortified soy products	Also referred to as folate, folic acid; important in prevention of birth defects (esp. spina bifida)
VITAMIN C (ascorbic acid) (water soluble) 60 mg.	Needed for healthy collagen (a protein that holds cells together), tendons, and bones Helps wounds to heal; needed for iron absorption Spares or protects vitamins A and E and several B vitamins	Citrus fruits, sweet peppers, leafy greens, broccoli, cauliflower, tomatoes, fresh potatoes, berries, melons, bean sprouts	If you are taking large doses and want to stop, taper off gradually to avoid scurvy
CALCIUM 1,000–1,500 mg.	Needed for building bones and teeth, for blood clotting, for regulating nerve and muscle activity	Milk and milk products, leafy greens (except as noted), broccoli, artichokes, blackstrap molasses, ground sesame seeds, canned fish containing bones, tofu made with calcium lactate, soups made from bones plus a little vinegar or lemon juice	Too much phosphorus and leafy vegetables that contain oxalic acid (chard, spinach, beet greens) reduce calcium absorption

continued on next page

A Partial List of Important Nutrients (cont.)

NUTRIENT/RDAs	CHIEF FUNCTIONS	IMPORTANT SOURCES	COMMENTS
PHOSPHORUS 800–1,200 mg.	Needed to metabolize fats and carbohydrates into energy in the body Makes up part of all the body's cells Needed with calcium for building bones and teeth	Milk, cheeses, lean meats, eggs, fish, nuts and seeds, poultry, legumes, whole grains, soft drinks	
MAGNESIUM 280–320 mg.	Required for carbohydrate metabolism Helps regulate body temperature, nerve impulses, and muscle contractions	Whole grains, leafy greens, beans, seafood, nuts	Large amounts lost in food processing
POTASSIUM AND SODIUM (no RDA)	Needed for healthy nerves and muscles Regulate fluid in cells Balance between these important	Potassium: fresh ripe fruits and vegetables (bananas, potatoes, dark leafy greens), legumes (limas, peanut butter), blackstrap molasses, fish, poultry, meat, milk Sodium: table salt, condiments (see tips on reducing salt, p. 48)	Sodium is recommended at no more than 2 gm. per day for adults
IRON 18 mg.	Makes up an important part of hemoglobin, the compound in blood that carries oxygen from the lungs to the body cells	Lean meat, liver, egg yolks, leafy greens (dandelions and kale), nutritional yeast, wheat germ, whole-grain and enriched breads and cereals, blackstrap molasses, legumes, oysters, turkey, dried fruit	Daily intake is important for menstruating women, pregnant women, and children
WATER	Not really a nutrient, but an essential part of all tissues Often supplies important minerals such as calcium and fluorine	Tapwater, tea, coffee, juice, soups, fruit, vegetables	Most people need six to seven glasses of fluid a day to keep good water balance in the body
FIBER (no RDA)	Also not a nutrient, but important for stimulating the intestinal muscles, encouraging the growth of certain intestinal bacteria, and regulating absorption of nutrients	Fruits, vegetables, whole-grains, bread and cereals, legumes, wheat germ	There are two kinds: insoluble, like cellulose; and soluble, like gums and pectins; both are important. Recommended intake is 20–30 gm. day

we may not be able to supervise our children's eating as much as we like. With young children we may have to make sure that the caregiver does not undermine our desire to feed our children healthy foods. Once children are in school, what they eat is influenced by what is available in the school cafeteria. In 1996, the U.S. Department of Agriculture (USDA), the government agency that sets standards for school meals, mandated that school meals meet the new dietary guidelines of no more than 30% overall fat and 10% saturated fat as well as a decreased amount of salt and sugar in prepared meals. There is also a grass-roots effort promoting plant-based school meals. The environmental group Earthsave (see Resources) works with communities to encourage schools to offer vegetarian and vegan options as part of the school menu. The group advocates for use of a variety of organic and unprocessed produce and provides schools with menus that meet the dietary guidelines for less than 30% fat.[20,21]

Even with the current emphasis on improving the nutritional quality of school meals, there is still the

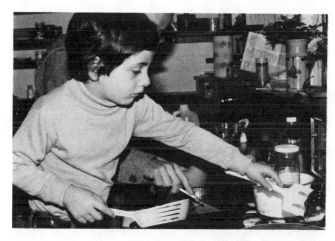

Esther Rome

overwhelming task of encouraging schools to include healthy snack food in school vending machines, offer healthy foods at school events, and change the types of foods sold at fund-raisers from sweets to more nutritious foods. When school football uniforms are purchased with the money collected from selling candies and cookies, and the coach doesn't believe that healthier foods will sell, we have our work cut out for us.

One way to influence what foods are offered in your child's school is to become involved and to get other interested parents involved in school activities. You can work with your child's school to develop a schoolwide nutrition policy that includes a commitment to offering healthy foods at school events, fund-raisers, and vending machines. The Centers for Disease Control and Prevention (CDC) has developed a guide for schools to help them develop schoolwide nutrition policies.[22]

Our children are often under a lot of peer pressure to eat the foods advertised on television or to get a candy bar on the way home from school even though they know we may disapprove. We can decide what foods our young children eat, but as they mature we have less control. The guidance we provide early on will influence them to make healthy food choices in their later years.

TRADITIONAL EATING PATTERNS
AND IMMIGRATION

Food is a basic need for human survival. Although all of us require the same nutrients, what we eat and how much we eat is influenced by our environments and our ability to access food.[23] Most of the world's population eats the kind of diet that we are being advised to eat in the U.S.: a diet high in complex carbohydrates and low in animal protein. For example, a traditional staple food for most Central and South American countries is rice and beans. Animal products are added as available or for special occasions. A traditional Asian diet is rich in rice and soy-based foods and vegetables supplemented with small amounts of animal products. In Africa, staples include peanuts

combined with a variety of grain-based foods. Research has shown that diets composed primarily of plant foods are the healthiest. This type of diet is protective against many of the chronic illnesses so common in most industrialized nations: heart disease, cancer, and diabetes.

In traditional cultures, certain foods have social prestige and values attached to them that are not necessarily related to their nutrient value. This relationship is often tied to economics and the availability and accessibility of the specific food. As a family's economic condition improves, so does the amount of manufactured foods eaten.

Coming to this country [from Bolivia], the first year or first couple of years, I gained so much weight because I could eat all the potato chips and corn chips [that I wanted]. I could have chocolate cakes. I was going nuts with how easy it was to eat this junk food because in my country, it is expensive.[24]

Milk and meat have high social value in Latin America[25] because they are not readily available for most of the population. When economic conditions improve, so does increased consumption of dairy and meat products.[26] This is true of most cultures where dairy and meat are often too expensive for everyday consumption.

Immigrants to the U.S. often make an initial effort to hold on to their traditional eating patterns, but when faced with the lack of traditional food products or when the cost becomes prohibitive, they may abandon their traditional food habits. The younger generation, in their desire to be like their U.S. counterparts and facing the same marketing and advertising messages, will quickly begin to fill up on soft drinks, eat fast foods, and avoid traditional foods.

Studies on food intake of first- and second-generation immigrants demonstrate a healthier eating pattern and overall better health status in the first generation. A study conducted on first- and second-generation Japanese-American women demonstrated that the second generation of women were at a higher risk for osteoporosis because of their reduced consumption of calcium, even though the first generation consumed no milk at all. The first generation of women consumed greater amounts of foods, typical of a Japanese diet, containing significant amounts of calcium, including tofu, bean products, whole dried fish, and fish bones.[27] Adults in many cultures are lactose intolerant; that is, they do not have the enzyme necessary to digest lactose, the sugar found in dairy products. Nonetheless, women in these cultures do not appear to be at high risk for osteoporosis.

When researchers at the University of California at Berkeley studied the diets of first- and second-generation Mexican Americans, they found that the diets of the first-generation women were higher in protein, calcium, vitamins A and C, and folic acid compared with those of the second generation. The second-generation women's diets resembled the typical

American diet.[28] Studies in other populations have reached similar conclusions.[29,30] When the traditional diet is replaced with one that is high in fat and highly processed foods, like the typical American diet, people begin to suffer debilitating chronic diseases prevalent in the U.S. and other affluent nations. Also, foods that are promoted as ethnic in the U.S. are often prepared quite differently from the way they may be prepared in the homeland. The traditional Mexican cuisine is not fat-packed like the kind that is offered in Mexican fast-food restaurants across the U.S. Traditional foods are rich in vegetables, beans, and rice and are prepared with less fat.[31] Chinese restaurants not long ago also received poor marks for the high fat and salt content of their food from the Center for Science in the Public Interest. The traditional Chinese meal is very low in fat compared to what is served in U.S. restaurants.

A recent national survey on eating habits[32] demonstrated some interesting results related to differences in eating patterns between African Americans and their white counterparts. Although the diets of everyone in the U.S. are shown to be improving in general, it is interesting that the diets of wealthier whites are resembling more and more the healthy diets of poorer African Americans 30 years ago. In 1965, African Americans had the most healthy diets, eating less fat and more fruits, vegetables, grains, and legumes than whites of the same socioeconomic status. Whites of the higher economic status had a high intake of fat from dairy and protein sources. We need to find ways to support the traditional eating patterns of families coming into this country, encourage them to maintain their healthy staple dietary patterns, and expand their diet with a variety of wholesome food products instead of less nutritious processed foods.

THE ECONOMICS OF ACCESS TO FOOD

The nutrition problems of industrialized countries are often related to excessive food intake rather than insufficient food. Nonetheless, hunger is a reality for many families. Approximately 30 million people in the U.S. cannot afford a nutritious and adequate diet. Hunger is not new to this country, but in recent years there has been a significant increase in the gap between those who have access to resources and those who do not.[33] Poverty and hunger are fundamentally linked. Census Bureau data show that over the past 20 years, real income has dropped for the bottom two-thirds of American households. A full-time hourly minimum wage worker in 1996 earned only 70% of what it would take to lift a family of three out of poverty.[34] Happily, the minimum wage was raised on September 1, 1997, reducing, but hardly closing, the gap.

Federal food assistance programs were initiated as early as the 1930s to help meet the nutritional needs of hungry families. The U.S. Department of Agriculture (USDA) administers several programs; each targets different populations, and all have a role in the alleviation of hunger. They include programs for children (School Lunch, School Breakfast, Summer Feeding, Special Supplemental Food Program for Women, Infants, and Children/WIC); for elders (Elderly Nutrition Programs, Congregate Meals, Meals on Wheels); for pregnant and breast-feeding women (WIC); and for any low-income person who meets the income criteria (the Emergency Food Assistance Program/TEFAP and the Food Stamp Program). Women and children are the primary beneficiaries of these programs. Nationally, about one in six people participates in one of the USDA programs, which help to feed about 45 million people on a monthly basis.[35]

The Food Stamp Program, which provides coupons that are cashed at the grocery store for food, has been considered a major safety net for most low-income families. Until the recent welfare law changes, any legal resident or family who met the income guideline of 130% of the poverty level as established by the U.S. government would be eligible to receive food stamps. Studies conducted to assess the benefits of participation in these programs have demonstrated that they have been effective in improving the health and nutritional status of participants. Families that participate in the Food Stamp Program spend more on food and have better nutrient intakes. Children in those families are less likely to be deficient in nutrient intakes than children who do not participate. Participation in the WIC program has been shown to reduce anemia in preschool children and low birth weight in infants. Children who participate in the School Breakfast Program have significantly higher standardized achievement test scores than eligible nonparticipants, as well as reduced absence and tardiness rates. Participation in the School Lunch Program has demonstrated improved nutritional intake.[36]

The Welfare Reform Law of 1996 threatens the very security of these programs and their ability to meet the needs of hungry individuals and families. The law (1) limits the length of time a family can participate in any one program—unemployed individuals between 18 and 50 years without dependent children are limited to three months of food stamps in a three-year period; (2) places restrictions on who can participate—many legal immigrants will be excluded; and (3) reduces overall program funding levels.

PROBLEMS ASSOCIATED WITH EATING PATTERNS

Low-Calorie Dieting

Do you find yourself worrying about your weight or thinking all the time about how everything you eat is fattening? Could it be because your lover says you are getting middle-age spread, because you don't look like the fashion models, because the supermarket magazines feature a new diet every month? Everywhere we look we see ads for foods, devices, and diet support groups to help us lose weight. We spend over $30 billion a year in the hope of becoming slimmer. Most of us in the U.S. have been on at least one diet to lose weight, and many of us go on several a year. ("Dieting" in this section means low-calorie dieting.) For many years, dieting has been medically endorsed as a cure for "obesity." But dieting doesn't "cure obesity." (For more on the social consequences of fatness, see chapter 1, Body Image.)

Dieting is debilitating, a form of self-starvation. The World Health Organization defines starvation as a calorie intake of less than 1,000 calories a day; weight-reducing diets in this country commonly restrict calories to 700–1,000 a day. When you don't eat enough, your body reacts in specific ways to help you survive. It doesn't matter whether you deliberately choose to eat less or whether you can't get enough food. Starvation is starvation. The fewer calories you eat, the longer you stay on a diet, and the more often you diet, the more likely you are to do permanent damage to your body.

Over a five-year period, 98 to 99% of the women who diet regain their weight.[37] In fact, 90% regain more than they lost.[38] Dieting can make you fatter.

Dieting, losing, and regaining weight—or "yo-yo" dieting—can lead to depression, rebound weight gain, and even early death. Repeat dieting also increases your risk of early death. Yo-yo dieting leads to increase of fat around the abdomen, which is also a risk for heart disease.[39] Dieting can make you fatter. Your body's response to the reduction in calories is seen as a form of starvation. Your body will increase the enzymes that make and store fat and slow down metabolism. Finally, dieting reduces your ability to recognize when you are full; it increases bingeing and cravings due to food deprivation, and generally slows down the rate of weight loss.

Studies show that diets don't work in the long run and that regaining weight is not a personal failure but a physiological adaptation to stress that our bodies make to help us survive. After repeated dieting, many of us begin to feel we can never control our eating.

Although actual requirements vary with size and physical activity, the average woman under 50 needs approximately 2,200 calories a day, whereas an older woman needs 1,900 calories. At calorie levels below this, you can easily be lacking necessary nutrients, especially if you consume a quarter or more of your calories from alcoholic beverages, sweets, and other low-nutrient foods.

What happens when you diet? Initially, you may feel great! You've made a decision to lose some weight, and you are determined to do it successfully. After a few days, you are likely to feel physically listless. If you are on a low-carbohydrate diet, you may become apathetic if not enough glucose is getting to the brain. Glucose is the end product of carbohydrate metabolism. It provides energy and fuel for the brain. When you eat an inadequate amount of carbohydrates, the protein from your diet will be converted to be used as energy. Your body will also break down protein from lean body tissue to provide the glucose needed for fuel or energy. Protein breakdown leaves extra nitrogen as a by-product, placing a strain on your kidneys. The fat that is broken down from body stores for energy doesn't provide any glucose. Without adequate carbohydrates, fat metabolism leaves waste products called ketones in the blood. If the amount of ketones is too great, the critical acid-base balance of the blood can be upset. Extra blood ketones can make you feel headachy, lethargic, dizzy, high, or possibly light-headed. After a couple of weeks, the brain can adjust to using some of the ketones for fuel as a stopgap measure. You may feel irritable, partly because it is harder for you to control your blood sugar levels without adequate food. You may also find yourself depressed and less interested in sex. You may become preoccupied with thoughts of food, especially sweets and "quick-energy foods" and devour them uncontrollably as a way of replacing missing calories and glucose, the fuel for the brain. This carbohydrate craving may be especially severe if more than 10% of the diet is from protein. High-protein diets may actually generate cravings for carbohydrates and doom the dieter to periodic calorie-laden binges. One woman describes how she stopped bingeing (and didn't try to be thin):

I worked at ignoring the rules and eating whatever I wanted. In the first month of "liberated eating" I craved only sweets. In effect, I was still bingeing. However, I chose not to berate myself for eating so much sugar. I reminded myself of all the sweets I'd been denied, and let feelings of nausea and hunger, rather than guilt, determine when I should eat again and what I should eat. At that point nausea and hunger were just about all I could be sure of. A month later, meat and dark green vegetables appealed to me very strongly. I chose a diet very high in protein and vitamins for a while. I think that during this period I was recovering from tissue damage due to previous years of dieting and bingeing. In the year that followed, my cravings became more subtle and diverse. I ate smaller portions and greater varieties of food in one day.[40]

If you try to follow the often-cited rule that you'll lose one pound of body fat for every 3,500 calories you don't eat, you'll probably be disappointed. First of all, this calculation gives only average weight loss. For each month you continue eating the same low number of calories, your rate of weight loss is usually cut in half. As a way of adjusting to a lower calorie intake, your body becomes more efficient at using and storing calories. Your basal metabolism (the calories you burn to keep your basic body functions going) can slow down by as much as 30%. When you stop starving yourself, you will probably replace and even exceed your original weight quickly, mostly in the form of fat. Your body is more efficient now, burning off fewer calories immediately and storing more fat for later use.

Fat often replaces the lean tissue lost from muscle and organs. You may have as much as 40% more body fat than before you started dieting. During a total fast, as much as two-thirds of the weight lost is a result of losing lean body tissue. But usually muscle tissue can

> Most fat women believe that they eat more than their thin friends. On average, fat people do not eat more than thin people.

be developed through vigorous exercise. If you continue dieting or adopt a pattern of repeat dieting, you risk amenorrhea (suppression of menstrual periods), anemia, liver impairment, gout, and elevated blood fats. If you have diverticulitis, tuberculosis, gout, Addison's disease, ulcerative colitis, or regional ileitis, weight loss will make you sicker.

Furthermore, a 1992 National Institutes of Health panel examining the safety and effectiveness of weight control techniques found a link between weight loss and increased death rates.

Your general body shape probably resembles those of your relatives, perhaps because of heredity or learned eating patterns. If one of your parents was fat, you have an 80% chance of being fat. We don't really know why people are different shapes and sizes. We do know that people's basal metabolism rates are different and that vigorous exercise may increase the rate. We don't know whether fat people's cells (even when the person looks thin after weight loss) act differently from thin people's. Researchers have come up with many theories to account for different body types, ranging from psychological to physical reasons, but so far none is satisfactory.

Food and Weight

According to a recent study, 34% of all adult Americans are "obese."[41] This represents an eight-pound weight increase over a ten-year period. About one-third of all obese people are thought to be genetically disposed to fatness.

The numerous studies on obesity and associated health outcomes have convinced many experts that obesity is responsible for, or is a contributing factor to, many chronic illnesses, including heart disease, stroke, high blood pressure, diabetes, and cancer. A very large study that followed up 11,500 nurses for nearly 20 years (the Nurses' Health Study) found that women who gained between 11 and 18 pounds had a 25% increase in heart disease. However, most studies in this country relating disease to fatness are done on people who are chronic dieters. Short-term weight-loss programs have found that slimming can improve high blood pressure and diabetes,[42] but repeated or yo-yo dieting may make them worse. Sudden and repeated weight loss may well be responsible for many of the diseases associated with fatness, but many researchers don't consider this when drawing conclusions from their studies.

Weight gain is caused by an imbalance in the energy (kilocalorie) equation: more energy in than out. One misconception is that an increase in energy from fat is solely responsible for weight gain or that fat makes you fat. In fact, it is the total amount of energy —irrespective of whether it is from fat, carbohydrate, or protein—that if consumed in excess will lead to weight gain over time. In other words, weight gain is more an issue of quantity than of quality.

Even worse than dieting are the various types of surgery medicine offers to women labeled obese. They include liposuction, jaw-wiring, and various ways to make the stomach and intestines smaller, decreasing a person's ability to eat and thereby absorb nutrients. These operations are performed almost entirely on women, may have a death rate as high as 10% and are only moderately effective in achieving the stated goal of weight loss. Doctors performing them really believe they are improving the woman's health, but they actually impair her ability to nourish herself properly. After intestinal tract operations, a woman often gets severe diarrhea for several months and is at higher risk for getting gallstones and arthritis, two problems supposedly "cured" by weight loss.

A growing number of experts are less sold on obesity as the main culprit in many chronic illnesses. Research done at the Cooper Institute for Aerobics Research in Dallas, Texas, which followed up 25,000 men and 7,000 women, found that when physical fitness was factored in, the thinner participants who were out of shape were more likely to die young than the fatter participants who exercised regularly.[43] The researchers pointed out that dieting has proved fruitless for many obese people, that it can actually lead to more problems, that the kinds of chronic illnesses seen in obese people are shared by people of normal weight who are sedentary, and that fewer heavy people exercise than do thin people. In addition, no studies focusing on obesity and corresponding health risks have controls for obese people who exercise regularly. Rather than promoting weight loss, these professionals would rather focus on increasing physical activity and on improving eating habits and self-esteem.

Regardless where the experts find themselves on this issue, all agree that to improve one's health and reduce risk of disease, one must maintain a regular exercise program and eat a diet that is high in vegetables, fruits, and grains and low in fat.

Managing Your Weight

A healthy weight is different for every woman. You may not match the ideal weight you see on a chart. Too much weight may become a health risk if it affects blood pressure, diabetes, arthritis, or cholesterol. Some studies have shown that even a modest weight loss of 10 to 20 pounds can help reduce risk of chronic diseases. However, repeated weight loss can prove to be very dangerous, even fatal.

The authors of this book do not recommend low-calorie dieting for weight loss. We are aware that many women will continue to diet to try to lose weight even after learning about dieting's long-term ineffectiveness and possible adverse consequences. Instead, we suggest the following to help you manage your weight.

1. *Get active.* Become much more physically active. This may be the single most important change you can make in your life. It will increase your strength and suppleness and probably your self-confidence as well as lifting depression. It can improve cardiovascular health, help maintain lean body mass, and may even lead to weight loss without dieting. Be aware, however, if exercise becomes another obsession for you. (See chapter 4, Women in Motion.)

2. *Eat healthy.* Eat a wide variety of foods, and make every bit count nutritionally. Limit your intake of high-fat and high-sugar foods, including soda. Follow the general eating guidelines listed on p. 45.

3. *Set realistic weight goals.* You are more likely to be successful if you lose weight slowly and if you set your goal within 20 pounds of your present weight. Do not restrict your calorie intake more than 500 calories a day under what you eat when not on a diet. Even with careful eating, it is virtually impossible to get the nutrients you need from food on less than 1,200 calories.

4. *Forget the magic answers.* There are no magic foods or pills to help you lose weight. Most over-the-counter weight-loss pills contain phenylpropanolamine (PPA), which is a relative of amphetamine (speed) and may increase blood pressure or produce agitation and dizziness; it may even set off a stroke or bring on psychosis. Prescription medications also have significant side effects (see "Diet Pills," p. 63).

5. *Listen to your body.* Trust yourself and pay attention to your body signals. Eat when you begin to get hungry. Don't wait until you feel starved. Learn to listen to your body's hunger signals and feelings of fullness.

6. *Don't sabotage your efforts.* Don't weigh yourself more than once every one or two weeks. Body water fluctuates daily.

7. *Find support.* Join with other women to discuss dieting, feelings about yourself and your body, and societal issues, such as the way ideal body images, both sexual and medical, divert your attention from control over your life and from more productive work.

Eating Disorders

People in this county are fixated on weight. This fixation has resulted in an explosion of disordered eating patterns. There is increasing pressure on women to be as thin as the models portrayed in the media. Women are made to feel like failures if they don't measure up to the ideals. Negative stereotypes are associated with being overweight. Prejudice and discrimination in education, work, medical care, and social relationships against fat women is not uncommon. Children as young as five years old are expressing feelings of being uncomfortable with their weight, and severe eating disorders affect children as young as nine years old. Ten percent of teenagers have clinical eating disorders.

Most of us at one time or another have used food to numb or deny our feelings, to comfort ourselves, or to put some order into our lives. Who among us hasn't at one time either binged or felt nauseated when scared, angry, depressed, lonely, or sad? However, when we let food become the major outlet for expressing our feelings, we risk damaging our physical and emotional health. Eating this way is a common strategy for many women to cope with a variety of abusive situations like racism or sexual abuse, and it is on the whole a healthier strategy than alternatives like drug or alcohol abuse. "Figure control is one of the few forms of control that women have been allowed to exercise."[44]

Anorexia nervosa is a form of severe and deliberate self-starvation, sometimes leading to death. It is associated with an intense fear of fat. All major body systems are affected. Amenorrhea is common in women with anorexia, as well as osteoporosis and associated fractures. *Bulimia nervosa* is another form of eating disorder. It involves recurring episodes of bingeing and then purging. Women will eat large amounts of food in a short period of time and then vomit or use laxatives, diuretics, or enemas and even participate in excessive forms of exercise to keep their weight down. The act of bingeing and purging can seriously injure the intestines or esophagus, lead to severe tooth decay from regurgitated stomach acid, and seriously upset the body's electrolyte balance, which in itself can be life-threatening. A third type of eating disorder is *compulsive eating* or *binge eating.*

Women with eating problems often seem to be acting out the ultimate stereotype of the female role: extreme self-denial, repression of anger and conflict, the desire to remain child-like, and conformity to the idea that a woman must be thin. These problems reflect graphically the little control women many feel we have over our lives.

My body was my ultimate and, to me, only weapon in my bid for autonomy. It was the only thing I owned, the only thing which could not be taken away from me. . . . I had discovered an area of my life over which others had no control. . . . What was going on in my body was as unreal, as devoid of meaning, as were the events in the outside world. The two were part of one whole, a whole of which "I" was no part. "I" had shrunk to a nugget of pure and isolated will whose sole purpose was to triumph over the wills of others and over the chaos ensuing from their conflicting demands.[45]

Some women who were sexually abused as children report that binge eating initially gave them a way to become bigger and gain a sense of control over their bodies. Over time, however, eating large amounts of food became less a solution and more of a problem.

DISORDERED EATING PATTERNS

SIGNS AND SYMPTOMS	WHAT TO DO

Environmental

Change in personality or behavior. More withdrawn, secretive, depressed or irritable; spends a great deal of time alone or in bathroom; prone to tantrums; shoplifts or takes money from friends and family members to meet food needs; denies there is a problem

Unusual eating habits: stops eating with family, friends; is eating amounts larger or smaller than normal; stops eating entirely; engages in vomiting, use of laxatives, diet pills, diuretics, or rigorous dieting or fasting to lose or maintain weight

Compulsive exercising to the point of exhaustion

Physical

- Fails to gain weight during expected periods of growth (i.e., adolescence)
- Extreme weight change
- Growth of fine body hair: complains of being cold
- Insomnia
- Constipation
- Skin rash and dry skin
- Loss of hair and poor nail quality
- Dental cavities
- Cessation of menstrual cycle or delay in menstrual cycle
- Extreme sensitivity to cold
- Inability to think clearly; irrational thinking
- Chronic fatigue

Educate yourself about eating disorders: who gets them, why, what are the signs, symptoms, consequences, and how to get treatment. The following agencies have information on eating disorders:

American Anorexia/Bulimia Association, Inc.
418 East 76th Street
New York, NY 10021
(212) 501-8351

Anorexia Nervosa and Related Eating Disorders, Inc.
P.O. Box 5102
Eugene, OR 97405
(503) 344-1144

National Association of Anorexia Nervosa and Associated Disorders, Inc.
P.O. Box 7
Highland Park, IL 60035
(708) 831-3438

Overeaters Anonymous Headquarters
World Services Office
P.O. Box 92870
Los Angeles, CA 90009
(310) 618-8835

Check your yellow pages. You may have a local resource that addresses eating disorders

Seek help from a family member, clergy, school nurse, or a qualified health professional. Early referral to a counselor or health care provider can help early recovery

Be supportive
Help person feel good about herself; accept herself regardless of body size

Provide emotional support and contact with people with similar problems; give all the support you can and reassure the person that you love her for who she is

Be alert to crisis situations in individual's life. A crisis can trigger an eating disorder

DIET PILLS

Diet pills are not cures for fatness. They often lose their effectiveness after a few months; once they are no longer taken, people tend to gain the weight back. Drug companies spend millions of dollars researching and marketing weight loss pills. Often the side effects and long-term complications are not fully known until many people have been affected.

For example, in 1996, two new prescription anti-obesity drugs—dexfenfluramine (marketed as Redux) and fenfluramine (which is part of the two-drug combination known as fen-phen)—were approved by the Food and Drug Administration (FDA). Although the drugs were approved only for people whose weights were threats to their health and were not recommended for people who had only a few pounds to lose, they were widely prescribed (doctors wrote over 18 million prescriptions between 1996 and 1997) and were huge moneymakers for the drug companies, physicians, and diet centers that are part of the weight loss industry. In the fall of 1997, upon request by the FDA, the companies withdrew the two drugs from the market after research indicated that they may have caused heart valve damage in as many as 30% of the people who took them. Women who have taken Redux or fen-phen in the past should inform their health care providers.[46]

Because eating problems and sexual abuse are both body issues, I see them as connected. Both are acted out on my body, and the numbing—emotional and psychological—I did when I was sexually abused is not all that different from the numbing out of unpleasant feelings I used food for.

Learning other ways to express feelings of anger, frustration, and powerlessness can eliminate our need to use food to express what we feel. Building self-esteem, discovering a sense of control over one's life, and receiving support from others can be key factors for recovery.

Eating disorders are preventable and curable. Learn to recognize the symptoms in yourself or in others, and take the necessary steps to get help. The chart on p. 62 outlines some of the typical signs and symptoms and where to get help.

Tooth and Gum Decay

Many of us forget that good teeth and gums are a significant part of good health. Without them we cannot eat many foods that provide important nutrients. Teeth are alive. Your saliva nourishes them through tiny passageways in the tooth. Poor nutrition can cause dental disease just as it causes other diseases of the body. Vitamins A and D, calcium, phosphorus, and fluoride are important for tooth development. Reducing sugar in your diet is another way to keep your teeth healthy. Teeth are especially prone to decay in the six-month period after they come through the gums, before they are fully hardened.

Foods containing sugar cause tooth and gum decay in the following way. Certain types of bacteria found in saliva use sugar to make themselves a protective coating. This helps them cling to our teeth as a sticky substance called dental plaque, which saliva cannot wash away. These bacteria, tiny organisms known as streptococci, multiply rapidly and produce large amounts of acids, which dissolve the enamel and irritate the gums, causing disease. To remove the plaque and prevent this decay, it's important to brush and floss our teeth daily.

The least cavity-causing way to eat sweets is to have them with meals and not between. The number of times you eat sweets, rather than the total amount, determines how much acid the bacteria produces. But the amount of sweets influences the quality of your saliva. Avoid sticky sweets that stay in your mouth a long time. Also, try to brush and floss your teeth after eating sugary foods. Even rinsing your mouth with water is effective. Whenever possible, eat foods with fiber that scrape off plaque, acting as a toothbrush (raw carrot sticks, apples, celery sticks, whole grains, etc.).

Intestinal Problems

Adding fiber-rich foods, such as whole grains; pinto, black, and other beans; peas; and fruits and vegetables to the diet seems to help the intestinal tract. Appendicitis and diverticulitis are practically nonexistent in cultures that eat no refined foods. Different kinds of fiber help with diarrhea and constipation. Soluble fiber like pectin, found in many fruits, absorbs water and thickens the stool. Insoluble fiber like bran from whole grains softens the stool. Some researchers think that by decreasing the time it takes for food to go through the digestive system from one end to the other, fiber indirectly acts to hurry toxins through the system and to dilute them so that there is less likelihood of developing bowel cancer.

Allergies and Other Reactions

Sometimes it's hard to figure out whether you have a food allergy, since it can show up in so many different ways. Your symptoms could be caused by many other problems. You may have rashes, hives, joint pains mimicking arthritis, headaches, irritability, or depression.

The most common food allergies are to milk, eggs, seafood, wheat, nuts, seeds, chocolate, oranges, and tomatoes. Many of these allergies will not develop if these foods are not fed to an infant until her or his intestines mature at about seven months. Breast milk also tends to be protective.

Migraines can be set off by foods containing tryamine, phenathylamine, monosodium glutamate, or sodium nitrate. Common foods that contain these are chocolate, aged cheeses, sour cream, red wine, pickled herring, chicken livers, avocados, ripe bananas, cured meats, and many Asian and prepared foods (see "Reading Labels," p. 50). Some people have been successful in treating their migraines with supplements of B vitamins, particularly vitamin B_6 and niacin. (High doses of vitamin B_6, 200 milligrams or more per day, can cause nerve damage.)

Children who are hyperactive may benefit from eliminating food additives, especially colorings, and foods high in salicylates from their diets. Foods high in salicylates include almonds, green peppers, peaches, tea, and grapes.

Cancer (see also chapters 7 and 24)

Healthier diets may help reduce the risk of cancer.[47-49] Here's how:[50] Decreasing dietary fat, a nutrient too common in this country, is linked to decreased cancers of the colon, breast, prostate, pancreas, and ovary. Decreasing saturated fats, especially from red meat, seems to decrease the risk of colon cancer. Choose most of the foods you eat from plant sources. At least five to nine servings of fruits and vegetables every day will provide more of the nutrients that seem to protect against cancer (carotenoids, vitamins C and E, and fiber). Keep your diet high in yellow, orange, and dark green vegetables, citrus fruits, whole grains, and cruciferous vegetables (vegetables in the cabbage family like broccoli, cauliflower, Brussels sprouts, and cabbage). Reducing cured or smoked foods protects against stomach cancer. Exercise may reduce the risk for colon and breast cancer.[51] Avoiding obesity may decrease the risk for postmenopausal breast and endometrium cancer. Limiting alcoholic beverages can reduce the risk of breast, liver, esophagus, mouth, and throat cancer. Not smoking or using smokeless tobacco will decrease the risk of lung, pancreas, stomach, bladder, esophagus, mouth, and throat cancer.

Certain food substances are likely to *increase* our chances of developing cancer. They may be natural constituents of our food, they may have been added to our foods purposefully by the food industry, or they may be contaminants in our diets. Sodium nitrite is used to cure and preserve meat and fish and to give the food a pinkish color. It doesn't have to be added at all, because now there are other less harmful ways to preserve food, such as freezing. The nitrites combine with amines, found in the food or even in our saliva, to form nitrosamines, which are carcinogenic substances. Smoked foods are an additional source of nitrosamines. Vitamin C decreases the production of nitrosamines in the stomach. Some manufacturers of products that use nitrites are adding vitamin C to those products.

Saccharin and many artificial colors derived from coal tar have been linked to cancer or organ damage in animal studies but are still certified for use by our government because of pressure from the food industry.

Naturally occurring carcinogenic contaminants also exist. Aflatoxin is produced by a mold that thrives in damp weather. It most commonly occurs on peanuts but can also be found on corn, figs, grain sorghum, cottonseed, and certain tree nuts. It sometimes gets into cows' milk from the grains the cows eat. Some aflatoxin reaches the marketplace and we eat it, although proper drying and storing of food can minimize it. Cutbacks in FDA funding have resulted in contaminants like these being less closely monitored.

Osteoporosis

Osteoporosis, a disease caused by the thinning of bones usually as we age, can be prevented and managed through diet and exercise. A calcium-rich diet, achieved by daily consumption of foods such as lowfat milk and dairy products, tofu, orange juice fortified with calcium, collard greens, kale, broccoli, and nuts can help prevent osteoporosis. Vitamin D is important for the absorption of calcium. You need at least 400 IU of vitamin D, which can be consumed through fortified milk, egg yolks, liver, multivitamins, and other fortified food products. Your body can make vitamin D because skin contains a precursor of vitamin D, and when it's exposed to sunlight (ultraviolet light), the precursor is changed to vitamin D, but the amount of precursor in the skin declines as people age. Small amounts of sunlight (ten minutes per day) can satisfy your vitamin D requirements. Women who stay indoors need roughly 400 to 800 IU a day of vitamin D year round.

SAFE, HEALTHY FOOD— WHAT ARE YOUR OPTIONS?

Agriculture in the United States is inextricably linked to world food policy and production. The production, marketing, and distribution of food (agribusiness) is big business. In this country, 18.6 million jobs are

Calcium Counts[52]

Age	Optimal Daily Intake (mg)
1–5	800
6–10	800–1,200
11–24	1,200–1,500
women 25–50	1,000
women 50–65 taking estrogen	1,000
women 50–65 not taking estrogen	1,500
women over 65	1,500
pregnant or lactating women	1,200–1,500

based in agriculture and 88% of consumer dollars goes to agribusiness.[53] In an age where much of the food available to us is highly processed and fabricated and where our agriculture and food business is based on making a profit, we have a problem. Many of the most immediately profitable methods of producing food deplete the nutrients in the soil, which results in less nutritious and more expensive food.

Planting practices may leave fields bare for periods of time, allowing precious topsoil to wash or blow away. Herbicides may be used to clear fields. The widespread use of herbicides, pesticides, and inorganic fertilizers destroys the organisms that control the structure of the soil and balance the availability of nutrients to the plants. This creates poisoning hazards for agricultural workers and contaminates groundwater. Irrigation practices may leave salts poisonous to plants in the soil or use up groundwater faster than it can be replaced.

An increasing number of farmers are interested in agricultural practices that conserve water, soil, and wildlife. Many are learning new farming methods that use less pesticides. The use of nonchemical methods or methods utilizing fewer chemicals, such as integrated pest management (IPM) and crop rotation, are two alternatives currently in use. An example of IPM is the control of damage from fruit flies to crops in Florida; the farmers released a harmless breed of insects to feed on the larvae of fruit flies, eliminating the need for pesticides. The use of organic farming methods is also on the increase. Although the number of organic farms has not changed substantially over the years, more land is being used for organic farming. The state of California alone has doubled the number of organic farms since 1988. Consumers can support this trend by buying organically grown produce when possible from stores or local farmers' markets, as well as encouraging Congress to increase the small amount of money for research on sustainable agriculture.

As consumers we contribute to poor agricultural practices by demanding blemish-free produce, which makes pesticides a necessary component of commercial agriculture. Business responds by making foods that are as uniform as possible and can withstand the abuse of mechanical harvesting and long-term shipping and storage. Land-grant colleges, supported by tax dollars and run by states, respond to the influence of agribusiness by researching ways to develop more processed foods and using labor-saving machines on large farms while paying little attention to the nutritive qualities of the foods they develop or the needs of the small farmer or consumer. Agricultural research has been partly responsible for the extraordinary decrease in the numbers of types of crops and varieties of seeds grown in the U.S. and elsewhere.

One product of agribusiness—the mechanically harvested tomato—took 20 years to develop. It is designed to be tough and is reputed to withstand an impact of 13 miles per hour without splitting. New gene-splicing techniques transform plants faster than was previously possible into "improved" products that often taste worse. Fuel-guzzling machines that harvest these tomatoes displace the farmworkers.

Our food supply has become more and more centralized. In the last 50 years, five million farms have gone out of business. Farmers grow most food in very few places in the country and ship it long distances. California produces 25% of the dollar value of the nation's food and 42% of the dollar value of domestic fruits and vegetables. New England imports 85% of its food.

The length of travel from one part of the country to another can be substantial: an average of five to seven days; up to two weeks for fruits and vegetables to get to New York from California. In that time, fruits and vegetables lose nutrients. In two days, for example, 34 percent of the vitamin C in refrigerated broccoli is lost.

The length of time food is stored after arrival and how it is stored during that time are also important. Canned juice loses as much as 70% of its total vitamin C when stored in a hot warehouse, while juice stored at 45°F keeps most of its vitamin C.

THE PROLIFERATION OF PROCESSED FOODS

The more the food is processed and made more "convenient" for the consumer, the more profit there is for the manufacturer. This results, for example, in the marketing of Hamburger Helper and the synthesis of entirely new foods such as nondairy imitation whipped cream. Slight differences from one product to the next also help increase profits. Wheaties are sprayed with two cents worth of vitamins and sold as Total for a substantial price increase.

The food industry adds many substances to processed foods to reduce manufacturing costs, replace costlier ingredients, improve appearance and texture, ease manufacture and transportation, and increase shelf life (how long the product is good after picking, processing, etc.). Yellow coloring gives bread the appearance of having eggs in it. Cheaper nonnutritive thickeners like modified food starch replace nutritive ones, perhaps eggs, because the parts don't separate as quickly, giving the illusion of a fresher product. Preservatives do the same thing by increasing shelf life, sometimes indefinitely. We no longer can observe the original color, smell, and texture of many foods to help us judge whether they are good for us.

Whenever a food is prepared, whether at the manufacturing level or in your home, some nutrient loss is inevitable. Even minimal processing of foods usually involves some nutrient losses. Frozen vegetables have to be blanched first and thereby lose B and C vitamins. Vitamin E is reduced by freezing. Sulfur dioxide on dried fruits destroys vitamin A, and sulfites destroy B vitamins. Minerals, unless physically removed from food as in flour refining, usually are not lost. Canning has generally been considered the least nutritious way to keep vegetables because they are heated long enough to destroy many nutrients. However, new methods of preserving nutrients—such as flash freezing, which involves freezing vegetables right after harvest, and new can-lining technologies—help retain most of the vitamins in processed fruits and vegetables. Processed fruits and vegetables can be more nutritious than fresh produce if the produce has been trucked across country and stored for long periods of time. If you buy from a local farmers' market in season, you can be assured of fresh produce, often picked the morning of market day.

You can also reduce nutrient loss when you prepare foods at home. Keep fresh vegetables whole until ready to use them; don't overcook vegetables and use small amounts of water to prepare them; cook vegetables with the skin on and peel afterward (if necessary). Use the liquid in canned vegetables, and keep the cooking water from fresh vegetables, because nutrients are often leached into the water.

More Is Less

Advertisements suggest that the large number of processed foods available represent a wide variety of food choices. In reality, our nutritional choices are severely limited. We see a small number of basic foods transformed into many different forms, none of which are nutritionally equivalent to the original foods. A raw or baked-in-its-skin potato (slightly less than a cup in volume) contains 50% of the RDA for vitamin C. Prepared potato flakes have 20% or less of the original amount. Synthetic potato chips like Pringles, which have been freeze-dried, reconstituted, molded, fried in oil, salted, flavored, and packed in fancy boxes contain 10% of the RDA for vitamin C in a serving. In addition, a pound of Pringles costs 20 to 25 times more than a pound of whole potatoes (1992 prices).

These types of highly processed foods are high in sugar and fat and provide little more than calories to our diets. Leave the highly processed foods for occasional use. You will benefit nutritionally and also save money.

Residues

During food preparation, processors sometimes add chemicals that they don't intend the food to contain when it is eaten. Vegetable oils are usually chemically dissolved out of the plants that they come from by solvents, such as gasoline or carbon tetrachloride. Although the solvent is then boiled off before the oil is bleached chemically and deodorized by heat, chemical traces may remain. Some of the pesticides and herbicides applied in the fields remain on the food at harvest time. Manufacturers ship chemicals banned for agricultural use in the U.S. to other countries, and

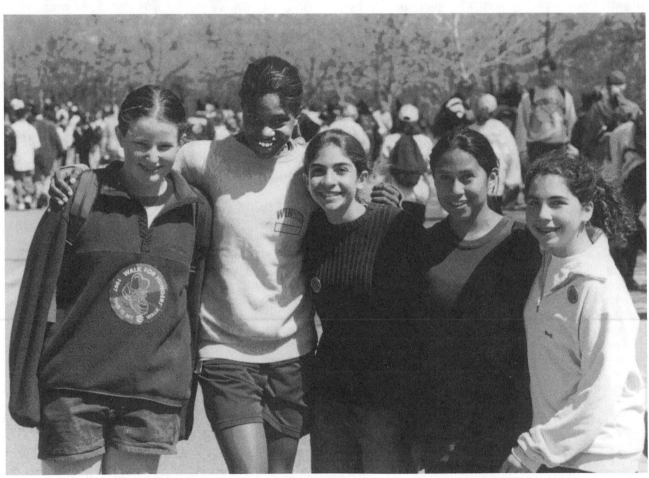

Project Bread's Walk for Hunger/John Hancock

farmers and farmworkers who may not know of their hazardous nature use them freely. Imported foods, including tropical fruits and vegetables available in winter, can contain these residues. One examination of coffee beans showed that almost half had pesticide levels higher than is allowed by U.S. law. It is always wise to wash all produce thoroughly before preparing it to eat. Antibiotics that farmers add to animal feed to promote growth are considered a factor in the increasing resistance of microbes to antibiotics in humans. These contaminants are in our foods because of the focus of large food corporations on increasing the efficiency and amount of food production.

The FDA and the USDA

It is the responsibility of our government to make decisions on behalf of the public interest. The FDA and the USDA are two government agencies that have that role as it relates to food policy, but they are sometimes not nearly as effective as we think they are or wish they were. The food industry influences how these agencies are run in several ways. Over 85 food industry groups maintain lobbyists in Washington to keep track of and influence pertinent legislation and regulations. These groups propose many of the regulations and supply test results when needed for the approval of new substances. Often people take jobs at the regulated industries after working at the FDA or USDA. Congress does not allot enough money in the federal budget for the FDA and USDA to allow them to do much independent testing and to enforce their own regulations very efficiently.

But several public interest groups keep an eye on food policy legislation and serve as strong lobbyists on behalf of the consumer. Examples of these lobbyists include consumer groups (e.g., Public Voice for Food and Health Policy) that work to form coalitions for specific issues to provide a united consumer lobby; nutrition, food safety, and quality groups (e.g., Center for Science in the Public Interest/CSPI) that support research on issues related to diet and health; antihunger lobbies (e.g., Food Research and Action Council/FRAC), concerned with issues related to food security and resources; and resource and environmental groups (e.g., Environmental Defense Fund), whose focus is on issues related to water quality, pesticide use, and endangered species.[34] All of these groups are strong lobbyists on behalf of consumers' interests. They will not go away and will continue to work to challenge the influences of agribusiness as they relate to our nation's food policies.

Advertising and Market Share

Through advertising, food companies influence us to buy certain foods—especially the most highly processed, least nutritious foods—because they are the most profitable. Advertising appeals not so much to our desire for a healthy or reasonably priced meal as to our desire for status, reward, popularity, satisfaction,

ARTIFICIAL FOODS

Fake Fats

Responding to the obsession with dieting in this country and the Surgeon General's advice to reduce the amount of fat that we eat, agribusiness multinationals are waiting to lap up the consumer's dollar with new fabricated fat substitutes, such as Z-trim and Olestra. The increased use of fat substitutes, however, may increase deficiencies of the fat-soluble vitamins A and E.

Fat substitutes are made by transforming foods lower in calories than fats into globules that slide over each other to give the feeling of fat in the mouth. Manufacturers are developing two categories of fat substitutes. One is made from starches—often from by-products of the processing of other foods—like cornstarch, cellulose gel from wood pulp, whey, or oat bran. A combination of heating, filtering, and high-speed mixing forms it into rounded particles. Companies claim that the body metabolizes these substances just as it does any other starch, but of course they are pretty much stripped of the vitamins and minerals that usually accompany minimally processed starches.

The other type of fat substitute combines proteins, sugars, and edible fatty acids from egg whites and whey to make molecules so big that they pass through the digestive system unchanged. Manufacturers claim that there are no adverse effects. The FDA approved the use of one of these substitutes, Olestra, in 1996 for use in potato chips, tortilla chips, and crackers. The products made with Olestra will carry the warning "Olestra may cause abdominal cramping and loose stools" on it. Many health and nutrition experts opposed the approval of Olestra because of the potential health risks linked to its use. In response to Procter and Gamble's plans to add vitamins A, D, E, and K to the product, a nutrition advocacy group responded, "the odds are that Olestra's adverse consequences would not be detectable for at least several decades, during which time enormous harm could have been done."[55] The safest course is to avoid fake fats, gradually reduce the amount of fat you eat and use in cooking, and start to incorporate dishes from cuisines generally using less fat, as many of the Asian diets do.

Aspartame

Although approved for use in 1974, aspartame, marketed as Nutrasweet or Equal, contin-

continued on next page

ues to be under a cloud of suspicion. Studies submitted to the FDA by the manufacturer, Searle, never clearly proved its short-term safety. Brain tumors in rats resulting from aspartame ingestion have never been satisfactorily explained. Recent data analyzed by the National Cancer Institute revealed a 10% increase in brain tumors since the mid-1980s. The research raised the possibility that "the rise in brain tumors in the mid-80s shortly after the introduction of Nutrasweet onto the market, could have been caused by the sweetener."[56] Virtually nothing is known about its long-term safety. The FDA has received over 7,000 complaints from consumers related to eating foods with both high levels and low levels of aspartame. These include allergic reactions, such as hives and rashes; behavioral disturbances, such as depression, hyperactivity, or sleep problems; seizures; loss of vision; headaches; diarrhea; severe abdominal pain; menstrual irregularities; intense thirst; loss of control of diabetes, and severe joint pain. As much as 10% of the population cannot digest the components that aspartame breaks into during metabolism: aspartic acid, phenylalanine, and methyl alcohol. High levels of phenylalanine in the blood of a pregnant woman can lead to retardation of the baby. Because it may break down from heat or long storage, aspartame is frequently combined with saccharin, a known animal carcinogen. Nothing is known about the safety of this combination.

increased fun, increased sexual potency, or an illusion of superior quality. The most pernicious ads are aimed at kids and emphasize the fun of eating nonnutritious snacks. Some large companies use children by linking sales of a certain brand to a cause. Campbell, for instance, offers a school sports or play equipment if students collect a certain number of labels. This offer usually ends up costing more than if the equipment were bought directly.

Corporations need to continually introduce new products to get a larger market share. This proliferation of new products, 80% of which fail, requires the company to advertise and to create needs for nonessential products. Food companies also encourage and capitalize on trends. For example, the companies that manufacture and market fat-free and low-fat foods are cashing in on our current preoccupation with counting fat grams.

Advertising tries to convince the consumer that a brand-name product is superior to unbranded ones. In advertising wars, conglomerates force out local companies, since they have more resources. Particular strategies include coupon saturation and price cutting.

Large corporations don't limit sales and advertising to this country. Pepsi and Coke are known worldwide and are considered high-status drinks, even among people living in poverty. Infant formula is another example. In Indonesia, processed foods account for 15 to 20% of the family food budget, even of very poor people.

Food Costs

Concentration in the Food Industry

Increasingly fewer corporations control food production, processing, and distribution. Once a small group of companies controls 40% or more of the market (called an oligopoly), companies set prices beyond their costs according to what they think they can get for a product.

Conglomerates buy up companies involved in every link of the food chain, from seed to supermarket shelf. For many commodities, the people who plow the fields no longer control farming. To gain more control over raw materials, large corporations own and manage their own farms or hire farmers and specify how and what they grow and for what price, while the farmers assume the risks of financing and growing the crop. Farmers are not getting a share of the increased prices paid in the supermarket. Only 6% of the rise in food prices in the past 20 years has gone to the farmer. While we're taught to believe that in farming "bigger is better," the most efficient farms in terms of food produced per acre are family farms big enough to be able to use technology but small enough to run without outside help. But deliberate government policies have encouraged farmers to "get big or get out."

Other Factors Affecting Cost

Some of the other factors in the supermarket price of food include such things as financing, labor, taxes, the world export market, government price supports for some commodities, maintaining the corporate bureaucracy, lobbyists in Washington, and the price of crude oil, which affects the costs of fertilizers, pesticides, fuel, and transportation.

For every dollar spent on food in 1994, 79 cents (76%) went toward marketing services, including labor, packaging, transportation, advertising, taxes, interest, repairs, and fuel. Consumer costs for farm products increased substantially from 1984 to 1994, primarily because of marketing. In 1984, the cost of marketing was $242 billion, whereas in 1994 it was almost twice as much: $401 billion.

Power to control and profits from food production in this country are more concentrated than ever. Sixty years ago, 40% of the population were farmers. Today, less than 1% of the population are farmers.

Packaging is the second largest component of the marketing bill, accounting for eight cents of every dollar. In 1994, the costs of packaging increased by 7%, primarily because of costs associated with shipping boxes, food containers, and plastic materials.

WOMEN WORKERS IN THE FOOD SYSTEM

On family farms in the past, women generally were equal partners in decision making as well as work. As farms become larger and are increasingly mechanized, men are trained to run the machinery and women are pushed out of farmwork. Women are often forced to supplement the farm income with low-paying non-farm jobs like waitressing or factory work. In food factories, it's often women who do the repetitive low-paying jobs, such as disemboweling and dressing turkeys in the assembly line, where it is cold, smelly, noisy, and wet. Mechanization will most likely eliminate even these jobs. While more women are attending agricultural school today to go into large-scale farming, it remains to be seen whether we'll get the jobs we want.

Of those who are agricultural workers, migrant women are the hardest hit. Low wages make it difficult for them to buy sufficient food and other necessities. Most fields do not have toilets or provisions for water, making the women, particularly, more susceptible to many infections. Pesticide and herbicide exposure, harmful to all adults and children, is even more so to pregnant women. When nitrogen from fertilizers leaches into well water or reservoirs, it can poison infants who drink formula or other foods prepared with that water. Maternal and infant mortality is more than 100% higher than the national average among migrant workers. At the end of a long, grueling day in the fields, the women are expected to cook and clean and raise their children under the usually squalid circumstances found in migrant labor camps, over which they rarely have control. In addition, U.S. agribusiness companies sometimes perpetuate unacceptable working conditions for women in developing countries.

CHANGES

On a personal level, each of us can work to make our diets more nutritious. Many cities have urban gardening programs through which you can get a plot of land to garden or get help with gardening in your yard or rooftop or porch (beware of problems with heavy metals, such as lead, in the soil).[57] If you have no gardening experience at all, get help or advice from someone who has gardened before. Often you can raise all your own vegetables and sometimes fruit in season this way. Not only is it cheaper, but it is also fresher.

Organized farmers' markets are now quite accessible. There may be farm stands if you live in a rural area. When you buy at these places, you support local

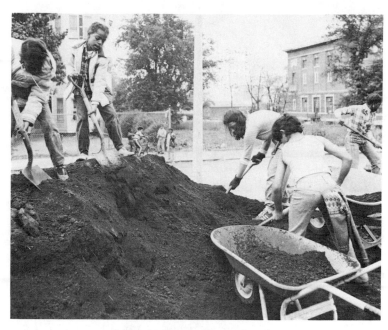

Boston Urban Gardeners/*Read D. Brugg*

agriculture, which benefits farmers, the land, and yourself. Consider preserving some of the foods through freezing, canning, or drying. These processes are surprisingly quick for some foods. (See Resources for cookbooks.)

The next level of activity involves forming or joining a group. On the local level, look for a food co-op or form your own. Find other concerned parents who want to improve the school breakfast and lunch program or to try to get rid of junk food from school vending machines. Introduce education about nutrition in the classroom or workplace. Work with others to improve the quality and choice of food in your college or workplace cafeteria or from vending machines and food trucks. Make a special request when you eat in restaurants to alert the management to the demand for healthy menu choices. Work with or support one of many groups advocating and helping small farmers. There are many organic farming and gardening associations.

Learn about and support local, regional, and national political advocacy and information groups. They inform the public about what is going on in big business and government, give expert testimony before Congress, and sometimes institute lawsuits in the public interest. Groups like these have done important work around such issues as land-use policy, water rights, working conditions of farmworkers or food-processing plant workers, the effects of tax law on land ownership, ways co-ops help or hinder cooperative behavior, energy use in agriculture, and getting food to the hungry.

The food industry is powerful. The only way to challenge it is to work together so that we become powerful.

NOTES

1. U.S. Department of Agriculture, U.S. Department of Health and Human Services, *Nutrition and Your Health: Dietary Guidelines for Americans,* 4th ed. (Washington, DC: U.S. Government Printing Office; 1995). *Home and Garden Bulletin No. 232.*
2. U.S. Department of Health and Human Services, *Healthy People 2000: National Health Promotion and Disease Prevention Objectives* (Washington, DC: U.S. Government Printing Office, 1990).
3. *The Surgeon General's Report on Nutrition and Health: Summary and Recommendations,* DHHS (PHS) publication no. 88-50211 (Washington, DC: U.S. Government Printing Office, 1988).
4. U.S. Department of Health and Human Services, *Healthy People 2000.*
5. *The Surgeon General's Report on Nutrition and Health.*
6. U.S. Department of Agriculture, U.S. Department of Health and Human Services, *Nutrition and Your Health.*
7. National Center for Health Statistics, *Monthly Vital Statistics Report* (October 1994).
8. U.S. Department of Agriculture, U.S. Department of Health and Human Services, *The Food Guide Pyramid.* (Washington, DC: U.S. Government Printing Office, 1995). Home and Garden Bulletin 252.
9. U.S. Department of Agriculture, U.S. Department of Health and Human Services, *Nutrition and Your Health.*
10. Oldways Preservation & Exchange Trust, Cambridge, MA.
11. U.S. Department of Health and Human Services, *Physical Activity and Health: A Report of the Surgeon General* (Washington, DC: U.S. Government Printing Office, July 1996).
12. National Research Council, *Recommended Dietary Allowances,* 10th ed. (Washington, DC: National Academy Press, 1989).
13. The information on the food label reflects the final regulations as published in the *Federal Register,* January 6, 1993, subsequent amendments, and a special report published in *FDA Consumer,* May 1993.
14. W. H. Sebrell, "A Fiftieth Anniversary—Cereal Enrichment," *Nutrition Today* (January/February 1992): 20–21.
15. U.S. Department of Agriculture, Department of Health and Human Services, *Nutrition and Your Health.*
16. V. Messina and M. Messina, *The Vegetarian Way: Healthy Eating for You and Your Family* (New York: Crown Trade Paperbacks, 1996), 76–85.
17. P. Thomas, "Food for Thought about Dietary Supplements," *Nutrition Today* 31 (April 1996): 46–54.
18. Ibid.
19. K. Terry, "Now There's a Test to Tell You Whether You're Getting What Your Body Really Needs," *Health* (January/February 1996): 81–84.
20. M. Friedman, "Stopping the Food Fight," *Vegetarian Times* (September 1996): 80–85.
21. "Plan-Based Menu Option Adopted in Some Schools," *CNI Nutrition Week* (August 23, 1996): 6.
22. Centers for Disease Control. "Guidelines for School Health Programs to Promote Lifelong Healthy Eating," *Morbidity and Mortality Weekly Report* 45, RR-9, (June 14, 1996).
23. U.S. Department of Agriculture, Department of Health and Human Services, *Nutrition and Your Health.*
24. D. C. Eliades and C. W. Suitor, *Celebrating Diversity—Approaching Families Through Their Food* (Arlington, VA: National Center for Education in Maternal and Child Health, 1994).
25. Diva Sanjur, *Social and Cultural Perspectives in Nutrition* (Englewood Cliffs, NJ: Prentice Hall, 1982).
26. Eliades Suitor, *Celebrating Diversity.*
27. D. Matsumoto et al., "Osteoporosis Risk Factors in First and Second Generation Japanese American Women," *Journal of Gender, Culture and Health* 1 (1996): 135–49.
28. "The Paradox of Plenty," *UC Berkeley Wellness Letter* (July 1995).
29. "The Champion Diet," *East West* (1990).
30. "Westernized Food Habits and Concentrations of Serum Lipids in the Japanese," *Atherosclerosis* 100 (1993): 249–55.
31. "America's Healthiest Fare?" *Health* (May/June 1995): 18.
32. U.S. Department of Health and Human Services and National Center for Health Statistics, *Third National Health and Nutrition Examination Survey, 1988–1994, NHANES III* (Hyattsville, MD: Center for Disease Control and Prevention, 1996).
33. M. J. Cohen and D. Reeves, "An Economic Explanation of U.S. Poverty," *CNI, Nutrition Newsletter* (October 18, 1996): 4–5.
34. Center on Hunger, Poverty and Nutrition Policy, "Kids Count Data Book," *State Works* (June 26, 1996). Focuses on child poverty and the working poor.
35. E. Kennedy, P. McGrath Morris, and R. Lucas, "Welfare Reform and Nutrition Programs: Contemporary Budget and Policy Realities," *Journal of Nutrition Education* 28 (April 1996): 67–70.
36. P. L. Splett, "Federal Food Assistance Programs: A Step to Food Security for Many," *Nutrition Today* 29, no. 2 (March/April 1994): 6–13.
37. Alvan Feinstein, "How Do We Measure Accomplishment in Weight Reduction?" in Louis Lasagna, ed., *Obesity: Causes, Consequences and Treatment* (New York: Medcom Press, 1974): 86.
38. Llewellyn Louderback, *Fat Power* (New York: Hawthorn Books, 1970): 143, quoting Norman G. Jolliffe, M.D., of the New York City Department of Health: "At least 90 percent of all the people who lose weight on a diet gain back more than they have lost." This phenomenon is corroborated by the testimony of many dieters and a 1992 National Institutes of Health panel.
39. A. R. Folsom et al., "Body Fat Distribution and 5 Year Risk of Death in Older Women," *JAMA* 269 (1993): 483–87.
40. Vivian Mayer, "Why Liberated Eating?" (ca. 1979): 14–15. Available through Fat Liberator Publications (see Resources).

41. U.S. Department of Health and Human Services and National Center for Health Statistics, *NHANES III*.

42. JoAnn E. Manson et al., "Body Weight and Mortality Among Women," *New England Journal of Medicine* 333, no. 11 (September 14, 1995): 677–85.

43. S. Blair et al., "Influences of Cardiorespiratory Fitness and Other Precursors on Cardiovascular Disease and All-Cause Mortality in Men and Women," *JAMA* 276, no. 3, (July 17, 1996): 205–10.

44. Vivian Mayer, "The Fat Illusion," *Hagborn* 1, no. 4 (Winter 1980): 3 ff. Also available through Fat Liberator Publications (see Resources).

45. Sheila MacLeod, *The Art of Starvation: A Story of Anorexia and Survival* (New York: Schocken Books, 1981), 56, 66, 98. A perceptive autobiography and analysis of anorexia.

46. Gina Kolata, "Two Popular Diet Drugs Recalled Amid Reports of Heart Defects, *The New York Times*, Sept. 16, 1997, p. 1.

47. J. H. Weisburger, "Nutritional Approach to Cancer Prevention With Emphasis on Vitamins, Antioxidants, and Caratenoids," *American Journal of Clinical Nutrition* (supplement), 53 (1991): 226–37.

48. A. T. Diplock, "Antioxidant Nutrients and Disease Prevention: An Overview," *American Journal of Clinical Nutrition* (supplement), 53 (1991): 189–93.

49. B. A. Miller et al., eds., *SEER Cancer Statistics Review, 1973–1990*. National Cancer Institute. NIH Publications No. 93-2789, 1993.

50. The American Cancer Society 1996 Dietary Guidelines Advisory Committee, *Guidelines on Diet, Nutrition, and Cancer Prevention: Reducing The Risk of Cancer With Healthy Food Choices and Physical Activity*

51. U.S. Department of Health and Human Services, *Physical Activity and Health*.

52. NIH Consensus Statement, *Optimal Calcium Intake* 12, no. 4 (June 6–8, 1994): 1–31.

53. R. Knutson et al., *Agriculture and Food Policy*, 3rd ed. (Englewood Cliffs, NJ: Prentice-Hall, 1995), 469.

54. Ibid., 99–109.

55. M. Karstadt and S. Schmidt, "Olestra, Procter's Big Gamble." *Nutrition Action Newsletter* (March 1996): 4–5.

56. "Study Raises Possibility of a Nutrasweet Link to Surge in Brain Tumors Since '80s." *CNI Nutrition Week* 26, no. 44 (November 22, 1996): 1, 6.

57. For more information on soil testing, send a self-addressed stamped envelope to: Soil Testing Lab, West Experiment Station, University of Massachusetts, Amherst, MA 01003.

RESOURCES

Nutritional/Wellness Information

Reading Material

Gebhardt, Susan, and Ruth Matthews. "Nutritive Value of Foods." *Home and Garden Bulletin No. 72*. U.S. Department of Agriculture, Washington, DC, 1981. Available from U.S. Government Printing Office, Washington, DC 20402.

National Research Council. *Diet and Health: Implications for Reducing Chronic Disease Risk*. Washington, DC: National Academy Press, 1989.

National Research Council. *Recommended Dietary Allowances*, 10th ed. Washington, DC: National Academy Press, 1989.

Rosenfeld, Isadore. *But Doctor, What Should I Eat?* New York: Random House, 1994. An excellent reference.

Stewart, Gordon W. *Active Living: The Miracle Medicine for a Long and Healthy Life*. Champaign, IL: Human Kinetics, 1994. (217) 351-5076. How to adopt a healthy lifestyle.

U.S. Department of Agriculture, U.S. Department of Health and Human Services. *Nutrition and Your Health: Dietary Guidelines for Americans*, 4th ed. Washington, DC: U.S. Government Printing Office, 1995. *Home and Garden Bulletin No. 232*.

U.S. Department of Health and Human Services. *The Surgeon General's Report on Nutrition and Health: Summary and Recommendations*. Publication No. 88-50211. Washington, DC, 1988. Available from U.S. Government Printing Office, Washington, DC 20402.

Vegetarianism

Reading Material

Akers, Keith. *A Vegetarian Sourcebook: The Nutrition, Ecology and Ethics of a Natural Foods Diet*. Denver, CO: Vegetarian Press, 1989. Lists regional vegetarian societies.

Klaper, Michael. *Vegan Nutrition Pure and Simple*. Paia, HI: Gentle World, 1990.

Lappe, Frances Moore. *Diet for a Small Planet*. New York: Ballantine Books, 1991. The popular vegetarian cookbook that explains protein complementarity.

Messina, Mark, et al. *The Simple Soybean and Your Health*. Garden City Park, NY: Avery Publishing Group, 1994. Readable and thorough.

Messina, V., and M. Messina. *The Vegetarian Way: Healthy Eating for You and Your Family*. New York: Crown Trade Paperbacks, 1996.

Moll, Lucy, and editors of *Vegetarian Times*. *Vegetarian Times Complete Cookbook*. New York: Macmillan, 1995.

Robbins, John. *A Diet for A New America*. Walpole, MA: Stillpoint Publishing, 1987.

Robertson, Laurel, et al. *The New Laurel's Kitchen*. Berkeley, CA: Ten Speed Press, 1986.

Yntema, Sharon. *Vegetarian Baby: A Sensible Guide for Parents*. Ithaca, NY: McBooks Press, 1980.

Vegetarian Resource Group, *Vegetarian Journal's Guide to Natural Foods Restaurants in the U.S. and Canada*, 2nd ed. Garden City Park, NY: Avery Publishing, 1994. Also includes juice bars, delicatessens, vacation spots, and camps.

Wasserman, Debra, and Reed Mangels. *Simply Vegan*, 2nd ed. Baltimore, MD: The Vegetarian Resource Group, 1995. The most sound and scientifically accurate resource for the strict vegetarian.

Organization

The Vegetarian Resource Group
P.O. Box 1463; Baltimore, MD 21203; (410) 366-8343
Web site: http://www.vrg.org

Women and Food, Dieting/Weight Loss, Eating Disorders

Reading Material

Ample Opportunity. *Newsletter of Ample Opportunity.* 5370 NW Roanoke, Portland, OR 97229; (503) 245-1524. Focuses on health and happiness rather than weight loss.

Berg, Frances. *Afraid to Eat: Children and Teens in Weight Crisis.* Hettinger, ND: Healthy Weight Journal, 1995.

———. *Health Risks of Obesity.* Hettinger, ND: Healthy Weight Journal, 1993.

———. *Health Risks of Weight Loss.* Hettinger, ND: Healthy Weight Journal, 1995.

Cohen, Mary Anne. *French Toast for Breakfast: Declaring Peace with Emotional Eating.* Carlsbad, CA: Gurze Books, 1995. Refreshing and useful.

Freedman, Rita. *BodyLove: Learning to Like Our Looks and Ourselves.* New York: Harper & Row, 1990. Ways to overcome negative feelings about weight, food, beauty, and sexuality.

Hall, Lindsey, ed. *Full Lives: Women Who Have Freed Themselves from Food and Weight Obsession.* Carlsbad, CA: Gurze Books, 1993. A collection of personal essays by 16 women who are highly respected professionals in the disordered eating field.

Heresies Collective. "Food Is a Feminist Issue." *Heresies,* no. 21, 1987. Special issue contains essays, articles, stories, poems, photos, drawings, and cartoons examining women's involvement with food and the complexity of the relationship between women and their bodies.

Hirschmann, Jane R., and Carol H. Munter. *When Women Stop Hating Their Bodies: Freeing Yourself from Food and Weight Obsession.* New York: Fawcett Columbine, 1995.

Ikeda, Joanne, and Priscilla Naworski. *Am I Fat? Helping Young Children Accept Differences in Body Size.* Santa Cruz, CA: ETR Associates, 1992.

Jenson, Joan M. *Promise to the Land: Essays on Rural Women.* Albuquerque: University of New Mexico Press, 1991.

Kano, Susan. *Making Peace with Food.* New York: HarperCollins, 1989. Excellent analysis and workbook to help women free ourselves from food obsession.

Kinoy, Barbara P., ed. *Eating Disorders: New Directions in Treatment and Recovery.* New York: Columbia University Press, 1994. A readable and up-to-date collection of essays on anorexia nervosa and bulimia nervosa from Wilkins Center professionals.

Lambert-Lagace, Louise. *The Nutrition Challenge for Women: Now You Don't Have to Diet to Stay Healthy and Fit.* Palo Alto, CA: Bull Publishing Co., 1990.

Latimer, Jane E. *Beyond the Food Game: A Spiritual and Psychological Approach to Healing Emotional Eating.* Denver, CO: Living Quest, 1993.

Lyons, Pat, and Debby Burgard. *Great Shape: The First Fitness Guide for Large Women.* Palo Alto, CA: Bull Publishing, 1990. (800) 676-2855.

Radiance: The Magazine for Large Women. P.O. Box 30246, Oakland, CA 96404; (510) 482-0680. Affirming and accepting yourself no matter what your size. A good place to find other resources.

Steiner-Adair, Catherine. "When the Body Speaks: Girls, Eating Disorders and Psychotherapy," in A. Rogers et al., eds. *Women, Girls and Psychotherapy: Reframing Resistance.* Binghamton, NY: Haworth Press, 1992.

———, and Amy Purcell. "Approaches to Mainstreaming Eating Disorders Prevention," *Eating Disorders* 4, no. 4 (1996): 295–309.

Thompson, Becky. *A Hunger So Wide and So Deep: American Women Speak Out on Eating Problems.* Minneapolis: University of Minnesota Press, 1994. Excellent.

———. "Multiracial Feminist Theorizing About Eating Problems: Refusing to Rank Oppressions." *Eating Disorders* 4, no. 2 (1996): 104–14.

Wolf, Naomi. *The Beauty Myth: How Images of Beauty are Used Against Women.* New York: Anchor Books, 1991.

Zerbe, Kathryn J. *The Body Betrayed: A Deeper Understanding of Woman, Eating Disorders, and Treatment.* Carlsbad, CA: Gurze Books, 1995.

Videos

Bulimia and the Road to Recovery. 27-minute color video. 1988. Available from Women Make Movies, 462 Broadway, Room 500, New York, NY 10013; (212) 925-0606; Fax (212) 925-2052; E-mail: rnso@wmm.com. Interviews with health professionals and women working through their problems with food, body image, and sociocultural pressures. Excellent for college audience.

Haynes, D. *BodyTrust.* A video on healthy lifestyle regardless of size. 2110 Overland Avenue, Suite 120, Billings, MT 59101; (800) 321-9499.

Organizations
(see also "Disordered Eating Patterns" chart, p. 62)

Diet/Weight Liberation Project
CRESP
Anabel Taylor Hall Cornell University; Ithaca, NY 14853; (607) 255-4214
Nonprofit support and education group. Membership fee includes subscription to newsletter *Grace-Full Eating.*

Fat Liberator Publications
Judith Stein
P.O. Box 30, Kendall Square; Cambridge, MA 02142
An extensive list of well-researched publications.

National Association to Advance Fat Acceptance
Department GS

P.O. Box 188620; Sacramento, CA 95818; (916) 558-6880
E-mail: naafa@world.std.com
Web site: http://www.naafa.org

Focuses on size acceptance through education, support, and civil rights. Publishes newsletter. Many local chapters in the U.S. and Canada.

Agribusiness and Related Issues

Berry, Wendell. *The Unsettling of America: Culture and Agriculture.* Magnolia, MA: Peter Smith Pub., 1995. An important exploration of the impact society and agriculture have on each other.

The financial pages of any major newspaper—for example, *The New York Times* and the *Wall Street Journal*—keep you current on the workings of agribusiness.

Fowler, Cary, and Pat Mooney. *Shattering: Food, Politics, and the Loss of Genetic Diversity.* Tucson: University of Arizona Press, 1990.

Gussow, Joan. *Chicken Little, Tomato Sauce, and Agriculture: Who Will Produce Tomorrow's Food.* New York: Intermediate Technology Development Group of North America, 1991. (800) 316-2739. How agribusiness is pushing food production off the land and into the laboratory.

———, and Paul Thomas. *The Nutrition Debate.* Palo Alto, CA: Bull Publishing Co., 1986.

Knutson, Ronald, et al. *Agricultural and Food Policy,* 3rd ed. Englewood Cliffs, NJ: Prentice-Hall, 1995.

Krebs, A. *The Corporate Reapers: The Book of Agribusiness.* Washington, DC: Essential Information, 1992.

Lappe, Frances Moore, and Joseph Collins. *Food First: Beyond the Myth of Scarcity.* Boston: Houghton Mifflin, 1977. How food for profit keeps the world hungry. Well documented.

Resources for Change

Readings

Greene, Janet, et al. *Putting Food By.* New York: NAL-Dutton, 1992. Comprehensive.

Harty, Sheila. *Hucksters in the Classroom: A Review of Industry Propaganda in Schools.* Washington, DC: Center for Study of Responsive Law, 1979. Available from Center for Study of Responsive Law, P.O. Box 19367, Washington, DC 20036. Excellent section on the food industry.

Organizations

Americans for Safe Food, a project of Center for Science in the Public Interest. See CSPI listing for address. Promotes sustainable agriculture through coalitions and education for changing policy and legislation on the state level. Encourages locally grown, organic food.

Appropriate Technology Transfer for Rural Areas
P.O. Box 3657; Fayetteville, AR 72702; (501) 442-9824; (800) 346-9140

Works with commercial growers to encourage sustainable techniques and promote local marketing of produce.

Center for Science in the Public Interest
1875 Connecticut Avenue NW, Suite 300; Washington, DC 20009-5728
E-mail: cspi@cspinet.org
Web site: http://www.cspinet.org

Publishes *Nutrition Action* magazine and a long list of valuable books and posters. Does research and prods government. Send for publications list.

Earthsave
Frederick Street; Santa Cruz, CA 95062-2206; (408) 423-4069
E-mail: earthsave@aol.com
Web site: http://www.earthsave.org

Institute for Food and Development Policy
398 60th Street; Oakland, CA 94618; (510) 654-4400
E-mail: foodfirst@igc.apc.org
Web site: http://www.netspace.org/hungerweb/food-first/index.htm

Publishes written and audiovisual material about the politics of food distribution and hunger.

National Center for Agricultural Law, Research and Information; School of Law; University of Arkansas; Fayetteville, AR 72701; (501) 575-7646

Free information on agricultural legal issues, from pesticide drift to commodities markets.

The National Gardening Association
180 Flynn Avenue; Burlington, VT 05401; (802) 863-1308
E-mail: nga@garden.org
Web site: http://www.garden.org

National gardening advocacy group. Contact it to find out about gardening groups in your area. Publishes magazine and other literature.

Pesticide Action Network
116 New Montgomery, #810; San Francisco, CA 94105; (415) 541-9140
E-mail: pana@pana.org
Web site: http://www.pana.org/pana/

Publishes the quarterly *The Global Pesticide Campaigner.* Helps groups in the U.S. and abroad to implement sustainable agriculture.

Public Documents Distribution Center
Pueblo, CO 81009; (719) 948-3334

Distributes government pamphlets, including several on food and related topics. Many free. Send for list.

Rodale Press
33 E. Minor Street; Emmaus, PA 18098; (617) 967-5171
Web site: http://www.rodale.org

Books on organic gardening, self-help, and nutrition. Also sponsors Cornucopia Project, an education project to help agriculture toward self-sufficiency. Ads and notices in *Organic Gardening* magazine will lead you to other groups.

Society for Nutrition Education
2850 Metro Drive, Suite 416; Minneapolis, MN 55425;
(612) 854-0035
E-mail: lansioo@gold.umn.edu
  For professionals. Publishes journal.

Helping Your Kids

  Satter, Ellyn. *Child of Mine, Feeding with Love and Good Sense*. Palo Alto, CA: Bull Publishing Company, 1991.
  ———. *How to Get Your Kids to Eat . . . But Not Too Much*. Palo Alto, CA: Bull Publishing Company, 1987.

Culture

  Sanjur, Diva. *Hispanic Foodways, Nutrition and Health*. Englewood Cliffs, NJ: Prentice-Hall, 1995.
  ———. *Social and Cultural Perspectives in Nutrition*. Englewood Cliffs, NJ: Prentice-Hall, 1982.

Additional Online Resources *

Ask NOAH About: Nutrition
http://www.noah.cuny.edu/nutrition/nutrition.html

Cath's Eating Disorders Resources on Internet
http://www.stud.unit.no/studorg/ikstrh/ed/ed.html

Diet & Nutrition Resource Center
http://www.mayo.ivi.com/mayo/common/htm/dietpage.htm

Dietary Guidelines for Americans
http://www.wellweb.com/nutri/usdaguid/contents.htm

Food Pyramid
http://www.ganesa.com/food/index.html

Health Information About Fatness
http://www.comlab.ox.ac.uk/oucl/users/sharon.curtis/BF/Inf/main.html

The Hunger Project
http://www.thp.org

Nutrition: Arbor Nutrition Guide
http://www.arborcom.com

Something Fishy's Eating Disorder Site
http://www.something-fishy.com/ed.htm

Tossed Salad Productions
http://www.tossed-salad.com

Veggies Unite!
http://www.vegweb.com

Yahoo! Health: Nutrition
http://www.yahoo.com/health/nutrition

* For more information and listings of online resources, please see Introduction to Online Women's Health Resources, p. 25.

CONTRIBUTORS INCLUDE Norma Finkelstein, Cheryl Kennedy, Janet Smeltz, and Caryn Kauffman, based on earlier work by Marian Sandmaier and Martha Wood

WITH SPECIAL THANKS TO Amy Rubin, Archie Brodsky, Denise Bergman, Suzy Bird Gulliver, Deborah McLellan, Wendy Sanford, and Jennifer Yanco*

Chapter 3

Alcohol, Tobacco, and Other Mood-Altering Drugs

Throughout history, people have used substances to alter their consciousness and change their moods. Women have used alcohol and drugs in a wide range of situations—as part of religious, social, and festive events; to feel included in a relationship or peer group; to avoid loneliness; to relieve financial or work stress, and to cope with physical or emotional pain, sadness, or depression.

Today, alcohol and other mood-altering drugs touch most women's lives. We may enjoy a drink once in a while, or we may drink every day. We may not drink at all but share our lives with people who do. We may have a partner, parent, child, or boss whose drinking or use of drugs hurts them and makes them untrustworthy or abusive. We may smoke and want to stop; we may smoke and not want to stop. We may suffer from chronic pain and might benefit from powerful drugs that we or our health care providers hesitate to use because they are potentially habit-forming. We may have an illness or disability requiring drugs that react badly with alcohol. We may have a daughter whose dates ply her with drinks to get her to have sex with them, or a gay or lesbian teenager who turns to alcohol or drugs to "escape" the pain of harassment. We may live in a community assaulted by poverty and racism, where neighbors and family turn to drugs and alcohol out of despair, and little is done by the dominant society to end the flow of drugs into the community or to make help available.

Alcohol and other mood-altering drugs can range from light, casual, or prescribed use to problematic or abusive use, to physical and/or emotional dependency, usually referred to as addiction. When is substance use simply an enjoyable part of life? When is it a problem? How can we know the difference? Are there special issues for us as women? This chapter attempts to be of use to women who have these concerns.

* Thanks also to the following for their help with the 1998 version of this chapter: Nancy Miriam Hawley, Judy Norsigian, and Yvonne Rushin.

SPECIAL ISSUES FOR WOMEN

Women are increasingly likely to use as well as abuse substances, and we are starting to smoke, drink, and use drugs at earlier ages than ever before.[1] Our modern-day culture promotes easy solutions and quick relief, and many of us, including young women, are lured into the promises of what these drugs can do. The influence can be peer pressure, the desperate need for short-term relief from a long-term problem, or the hope of an "extra edge" on ordinary activities.

Patterns of substance use, abuse, and dependence are different for women than for men. While men drink more frequently in groups and in public, a woman more often drinks privately and alone. On the other hand, women with alcohol and other drug use problems are more likely than men to be living with a partner who abuses alcohol or drugs, and to be influenced by a partner or friends to drink or use drugs. These situations also make relapse more likely for women trying to address their substance abuse.[2] In general, women depend more than men do on support networks for help. However, when a woman in a relationship with a man has an alcohol problem and goes for treatment, the man is much more likely to be unsupportive or to leave (when the man has the problem, more often the woman will stay and try to help).

Using alcohol and other mood-altering substances can make us especially vulnerable as women, leading us to place our bodies and our safety at risk. For example, using alcohol or drugs can make us more vulnerable to physical abuse from husbands or partners (especially, but not only, those who have drug and alcohol problems themselves), and it can affect what we do sexually. We may forget to use protection and put ourselves at risk for sexually transmitted diseases and HIV infection as well as unwanted pregnancy. Sexist assumptions linking the use of alcohol to women's sexual availability remain strong. Men often expect drinking women to be easier to seduce and more willing to engage in sex than nondrinking women. We become more vulnerable to rape and other physical violence. This is highlighted by the use of the tranquilizer Rohypnol (Roofies, date rape drug): slipped into a woman's drink as a "Mickey," Rohypnol can create a drunk-like state in only 10 minutes.

DEFINITIONS

The term *addiction* usually refers to both psychological and physical dependence on a drug. *Psychological dependence* is characterized by a preoccupation with and continual seeking (craving) for a substance, in spite of the havoc it has played with one's life. *Physical dependence* occurs when your body becomes used to the presence of a drug, including alcohol, and experiences uncomfortable symptoms (called "withdrawal") when it is not present in the body. *Withdrawal* symptoms can range from the headache often experienced by coffee drinkers who

If you wonder whether you have a problem with alcohol or other drugs, or whether you are developing a chronic dependence, the questions in "Drugs and Alcohol—Getting Help," p. 81, may be useful. At the first sign of a problem, it is crucial to talk to someone—a friend, a counselor, a health care practitioner—about your concerns.

abstain from coffee, to shakiness and anxiety from the absence of alcohol, to irritability and difficulty concentrating from the absence of nicotine, to severe gastrointestinal symptoms from heroin withdrawal. Withdrawal symptoms are temporary, and they subside once the body gets used to the absence of the substance, though the desire for the substance may last for a long time. *Tolerance* is a characteristic of dependence, in which more of the drug is needed to produce the same effect, or the usual amount of drug does not produce as strong an effect as it once did. *Dependence* and *abuse* are terms used to describe alcohol and drug problems, although you don't have to be physically dependent on a substance to have a problem with it.

VARYING PERSPECTIVES ON ADDICTION

Just about every drug that is prescribed for us in a health care context has some effects that we desire and those that we don't. This is true, as well, of alcohol, smoking, and certain mood-altering drugs. These, however, are potentially addictive—that is, some individuals will develop dependence on them over time.* If we become physically or emotionally dependent on nicotine, alcohol, tranquilizers, or cocaine, we are less and less likely to notice when the negative effects are taking their toll or to be able to stop using the substance on our own. Many people use alcohol once in a while or moderately, with considerable pleasure and no negative impact on our lives. There is even evidence that for some, a glass of wine a day can help prevent heart disease. Yet, for some of us, drinking takes the place of making necessary changes in our lives, and that same glass of wine can be one step in a downward spiral of alcoholism. Similarly, modest use of tranquilizers and other mood-altering prescription drugs can help in a highly stressful time; overuse of them (and/or overprescription of them) can lead to serious problems. Yet, industries are built around providing and profiting from our use of these substances—it is challenging to be an "informed consumer"!

There are many schools of thought about addiction, and several frameworks have been proposed in attempts to understand it and to find solutions. One such framework is a moralistic one, which sees addiction as

---

* Most antidepressants have not been proved to be addictive, and there is currently no scientific evidence that long-term use of them is damaging.

a sin or a personal failing. Other, more helpful frameworks include psychological, behavioral, cognitive, medical, and self-help approaches. The majority of alcohol and drug treatment programs in the U.S. at this time define substance abuse as an illness. The "illness" model of addiction makes certain things possible. There is less moral stigma for those who suffer from alcoholism and drug addiction; the emphasis is on treatment rather than blame or punishment; treatment is covered by health insurance and, at least minimally, by public assistance. For some people, this model has been helpful. Others are critical of labeling addiction as an illness, believing that this unnecessarily medicalizes the response to alcohol and drug problems and leads people to look for a solution outside themselves.

Thoughtful people also differ about whether our society's distinction between legal and illegal drugs is helpful. All mood-altering drugs affect one's thoughts and feelings, and addiction to them also has similar characteristics: preoccupation with the drug, and family, social, financial, and medical problems. The two drugs most damaging to individuals and society are nicotine and alcohol, both of which are legal. Marijuana, on the other hand, may well have some beneficial use for people who are going through chemotherapy, but it is currently illegal. A health care provider who uses her easy access to prescription drugs in order to supply herself with addictive amounts of tranquilizers or pain medications is using a legal drug; she is more likely to be able to maintain a habit without resorting to petty crimes that get her a police record. Due to racism and classism in the enforcement of drug laws, people of color and people with low incomes are put in jail more frequently than middle-class white people for breaking the laws concerning drugs: for selling drugs, selling sex to get drugs, stealing to buy drugs. At the same time, there is a shortage of publicly funded treatment resources that could help individuals address their substance use problems.

ALCOHOL

Alcohol is made available to us—even pushed on us—in a dizzying array of situations. It is not surprising that approximately 59% of women in the U.S. drink alcohol, and 6% of us consume two or more drinks daily—an amount considered to be heavy drinking for women. The age when girls first begin drinking has shifted downward. Moderate drinking among 18- to 20-year-olds has also increased, and the percent of female college students who drink is now nearly equal to their male peers (75 to 79%).[3]

The multibillion-dollar alcohol industry has been quick to take advantage of women's changing social and economic status, including more women working outside the home, with an aggressive advertising campaign geared to the "female market." In many magazines, such as *Glamour* and *Essence,* we can scarcely turn a page without seeing ads offering a new kind of drink and with it the subtle promise of increased status, sophistication, or sexiness. In acknowledgment of the power of this advertising, ads for hard liquor and cigarettes were voluntarily removed from television.

The social and cultural context in which we drink has a profound effect on how much, when, and where we drink and whether it is seen as acceptable or outside the norms of our culture. In some cultures, acceptable use of alcohol (and other drugs) exists within clearly defined religious and social circumstances. Violation of these norms indicates abuse of the drug. In the U.S., socially acceptable use of alcohol has evolved over time, and alcoholism is a relatively new word and concept.

In a society that judges women more harshly than men for dependence on alcohol, women tend to hide and deny our alcohol abuse rather than seek needed help. Internalizing our culture's condemnation, alcoholic women suffer more guilt and anxiety than alcoholic men, have lower self-esteem, and attempt suicide more often. Women with drinking problems may also use other drugs, including nicotine, cocaine, and prescription drugs commonly prescribed by physicians for "nerves" or "depression."

The effects of alcohol on women are different from the effects on men. Women become intoxicated more quickly and with lower consumption. We have less water in our bodies to dilute alcohol's effects, and initial research suggests that our hormonal cycles affect the way we metabolize alcohol; these may explain why a woman's blood alcohol level is higher than a man's of the same weight drinking the same amount of alcohol. We also have less of a specific enzyme (alcohol dehydrogenase) that affects the breakdown of alcohol in the stomach, so that more alcohol enters a woman's bloodstream. Because of women's different physiological responses to alcohol, the U.S. Department of Health and Human Services and the Department of Agriculture have recommended a woman have no more than one drink a day, while a man should have no more than two.[4]

We often forget that alcohol is a powerful drug: a central nervous system depressant that slows down all our body's major functions. Alcohol use diminishes motor coordination, judgment, emotional control, and reasoning powers. Consumed to excess, alcohol can be very harmful and can cause adverse health consequences, including death. Even a single episode of binge drinking can result in alcohol toxicity, overdose, coma, and death. Excessive and/or chronic drinking can lead to alcohol abuse or dependence, which can be devastating to a woman's physical, as well as social and spiritual, well-being. Women develop alcoholic liver disease after a comparatively shorter period of heavy drinking than do men, and the death rate of female alcoholics is 50 to 100% higher than that of male alcoholics. Other health risks for women include hypertension (particularly for African-American women) and an increased risk of osteoporosis, stroke, heart disease, gastrointestinal problems, and certain cancers such as liver and stomach cancer. Everyone who both smokes and drinks is at a particularly high risk for developing cancers of the upper respiratory and digestive tracts. Alcohol can mask many diseases because the woman doesn't feel, notice, or address the symptoms while drinking.

Women who drink heavily during pregnancy increase their risk of hypertension and premature labor. They may give birth to babies with adverse conditions ranging from possible abnormalities in fetal growth and development to fetal alcohol syndrome (FAS) and fetal alcohol effects (FAE). Fetal alcohol syndrome is a pattern of irreversible abnormalities that may include growth retardation, mental retardation, and structural abnormalities, such as facial, skeletal, and organ defects.

If we are postmenopausal, one or two drinks a day

IF YOU DRINK

- Eat something before or while drinking. Sipping drinks, rather than gulping them, also slows down the rate at which the alcohol enters the bloodstream. A woman weighing between 100 and 140 pounds should allow about two hours for her body to metabolize or "burn up" each drink; a woman weighing between 140 and 180 should allow at least one hour between drinks. (A "drink" consists of 3 to 5 ounces of wine, 12 ounces of beer, or 1 ounce of hard liquor. Each contains the same amount of alcohol.) Be aware that many cough medicines contain alcohol.

- If you've been drinking, don't drive. Even small amounts of alcohol can seriously interfere with judgment, coordination, vision, and reaction time, all of which are esstential for safe driving.

- Avoid using alcohol within a few hours of using any other drug, including over-the-counter medications, such as aspirin and aspirin substitutes. When taken together, alcohol and many other drugs dangerously multiply each other's effects, with results ranging from headache, nausea, and cramps to potential loss of consciousness and even death. It is particularly dangerous to mix alcohol with another central nervous system depressant, such as a barbiturate or tranquilizer (see p. 80).

- Sometimes the body is especially vulnerable to alcohol. When you're feeling sick or tired, for example, alcohol can affect your system more powerfully than usual. Hormonal variations related to the monthly menstrual cycle also have been found sometimes to affect how we metabolize alcohol.

---

may decrease the risk of death from coronary heart disease. However, researchers also report a modest association between moderate alcohol consumption and breast cancer, usually among women who consume the equivalent of two or more drinks per day. It is not yet clear whether this association is causal; it may be due to an alcohol-related increase in estrogens.[5] A small study in Boston recently showed that women who take estrogen and drink alcohol may raise the blood levels of estrogen to more than three times the intended dose. If you are taking estrogen and you drink alcohol on a regular basis, you may want to discuss this with your health care practitioner.[6]

The link between alcohol and breast cancer affects younger as well as older women, but the beneficial effects of alcohol consumption on coronary heart disease appear to affect older (postmenopausal) women only. Therefore, a woman should weigh family history and other risk factors for coronary heart disease and breast cancer when examining the pros and cons of light to moderate alcohol consumption keeping in mind that the effects of alcohol abuse and dependence on a woman's physical and mental health are much more devastating than any mildly positive benefits.

MOOD-ALTERING DRUGS

Mood-altering drugs range from prescription medicines, such as antianxiety agents, to illegal drugs, such as cocaine and heroin. It is crucial that we have information about the effects of any drugs we use, their interactions with alcohol and other drugs, and their potential for addiction. Misuse of drugs takes many forms. We might, for example, overmedicate ourselves with a drug prescribed for us, or we might take drugs ourselves that are prescribed for another person.

Prescribed mood-altering drugs, such as antianxiety agents, antidepressants, and sedatives, have long been marketed as medicines primarily aimed at, and used by, women. In certain situations, these drugs have justifiable and effective uses, such as for severe depression or anxiety, and for some physical ailments. The use of prescription drugs can become problematic when they are prescribed to women to "treat" the ordinary stresses of daily life, to control behavior, to avoid more costly medical and psychiatric interventions, and when they are used by women to self-medicate. For example, in the 19th century, patent medicines containing dangerously large amounts of opiates were sold to women for relief of "female troubles." Today, women receive twice as many prescriptions for psychotherapeutic drugs, more multiple and repeat prescriptions, and more prescriptions for excessive dosages than men.[7] (See chapter 23, Women Growing Older, p. 569, for a discussion of overprescription of drugs for older women.)

In 1992, an estimated 4.4 million women in the U.S. used illegal drugs. This included 3.1 million women who used marijuana; 419,000, cocaine; 98,000, crack; and 88,000, heroin.[8] In addition to the legal risks of possessing an illegal substance, women using illegal drugs risk developing physical and/or psychological addiction. Each class of drugs produces specific physiological and psychological effects in use and withdrawal, and increases both maternal and fetal risks in pregnant women. See the "Mood-Altering Drugs" box, p. 80.

INFORMED USE OF PRESCRIPTION AND OVER-THE-COUNTER DRUGS

- Before accepting a prescription for any drug, mood-altering or otherwise, ask your health care practitioner these questions: What is this drug for, and what are some nonchemical alternatives to it? Exactly how does this drug work on my body and mind? What are the risks, benefits, and possible negative effects? Can I become dependent on this drug? How does it interact with other drugs, with certain foods, and with alcohol? Should I avoid certain over-the-counter drugs while I am taking this medication? What are the specific risks of using this drug during pregnancy? How do I take the drug —when, how often, for how long, with food or not? How do I store the drug? Ask the pharmacist any other questions you might have.
- If a prescribed drug comes with a patient information brochure, read it and follow the instructions carefully. If there is no brochure, ask your doctor or pharmacist to show you the information on prescribing and adverse effects that the government requires drug companies to provide for each drug, or check the *Physicians' Desk Reference* in your library.
- Pay attention to your physical and emotional responses to any drug you take. Even over-the-counter drugs can have unpredictable and hazardous effects and should always be used with caution.
- If you are or might be pregnant, consult the section in chapter 19, Pregnancy, p. 445, for guidelines about drug use.
- Never take any mood-altering drug within a few hours of using alcohol (including the alcohol in many cold and cough medicines) or any other drug. A combination of alcohol and tranquilizers, barbiturates, or other sedative drugs can be especially dangerous —even fatal.
- Use caution in storing over-the-counter sleeping and diet aids, as they can be found and misused by children and adolescents.

SAFETY FACTORS REGARDING THE USE OF NEEDLES FOR INJECTABLE MOOD-ALTERING DRUGS

Many diseases, including HIV/AIDS, hepatitis, and bacterial infections, can be spread by sharing needles and other equipment. Needles should never be shared. For safety factors regarding needle use, please see chapter 15, HIV, AIDS, and Women, p. 368.

Race, Class, Women, and the Enforcement of Drug Laws

Drugs pose serious problems for women in many ways: the physiological effects of the drugs themselves, associated poor nutrition and lowered resistance to disease, and increased risk of contracting HIV and hepatitis for women who inject drugs or exchange sex for drugs. Drugs can have a devastating effect on our sense of self and our ability to take charge of our lives.

Drug use exposes women to other dangers as well, not the least of which is ending up in prison. Punitive approaches to solving the "drug problem" have resulted in the U.S. having the highest rate of imprisonment in the industrialized world. Seventy percent of women now serving federal prison sentences are in on drug-related charges. Many women imprisoned on drug charges lose custody of their children.

The "drug war" has had its highest casualty rate in communities of color. A disproportionate number of men and women of color are in prison as a result of discriminatory law enforcement practices and sentencing laws.* Those of us who are of African descent are suffering the burden of trying to maintain our communities as they are systematically emptied of men through the alarming rates of imprisonment. The emotional, financial, and physical burden of men's absence adversely affects women's health in major ways.

Concerned citizens need to work to change these discriminatory laws, monitor racist enforcement practices, and lobby for increased treatment programs and for an approach to the drug problem that focuses on eradicating the social conditions that make drug use attractive and available in the first place.

* Although white Americans consume more than half the crack in this country, because of enforcement practices that target particular communities, African Americans made up 89% of those sentenced for crack crimes in 1995 (Derrick Jackson, *Boston Globe,* Op-Ed. [May 14, 1997]: A15). Minimum drug sentencing laws are highly discriminatory against users of crack cocaine; a dealer convicted of selling 5 grams of crack, and a dealer convicted of selling 500 grams of powdered cocaine, are both to be sentenced to 5 years imprisonment (Sue Mahan, "Crack Cocaine, Crime and Women," *Sage* [1996]: 31–32).

MOOD-ALTERING DRUGS *

Central Nervous System Depressants

ALCOHOL

This is the most widespread mood-altering drug in use in the U.S. (See the full discussion on p. 77.)

TRANQUILIZERS

Antianxiety agents include minor tranquilizers such as Valium, Librium, Xanax, Halcion, Tranxene, and Ativan, and anticonvulsants such as Clonopin. These drugs are effective in relieving tension, anxiety, and muscle spasm when prescribed and used appropriately on a short-term basis. However, the side effects include drowsiness, decreased muscular coordination, menstrual irregularities, nausea, constipation, changes in sexual drive, and confusion. Of serious concern is that women can become physically dependent within a few months, depending on the daily dose. Withdrawal symptoms range from restlessness to acute anxiety attacks. Behavioral treatments, with or without medication, are more effective long-term solutions to anxiety problems.

This category of drugs also includes Vistaril, an antihistamine, and BuSpar, neither of which has the side effects common to minor tranquilizers.

BARBITURATES

Prescribed by physicians primarily to treat insomnia and pain, seizure disorders, and anxiety, these depressant drugs include Amytal, Butisol, Nembutal, and Seconal. Considered the most dangerous central nervous system depressants used in medicine today, barbiturates can produce coma, depressed blood pressure, and death. They are highly addictive and extremely dangerous when combined with alcohol. Physical tolerance begins to develop after about two weeks. Once a physical tolerance is developed, the margin between a sleep-inducing dose and a fatal dose is dangerously narrow. Finally, physical withdrawal is severe. Barbiturates are a major factor in many suicides, suicide attempts, and accidental drug poisonings. Withdrawal must be undertaken gradually and under competent medical supervision, as abrupt discontinuation can cause possibly fatal seizures.

SEDATIVE-HYPNOTICS (NONBARBITURATE)

Among the most commonly prescribed of these sleep-inducing and muscle relaxant drugs are Quaalude, Dalmane, Doriden, Halcion, and Noludar. Originally hailed as safer alternatives to the barbiturates, these drugs have been shown to pose many of the same risks of physical tolerance, addiction, dangerous withdrawal symptoms, and overdose. Common side effects are headache, hangover, and dizziness; effects reported less often include nausea, vomiting, blurred vision, and nervousness and excitement. All these drugs are extremely dangerous in combination with alcohol.

OPIATES (NARCOTICS)

Narcotics such as Percodan, Demerol, Stadol, Dilaudid, Darvon, and codeine are prescribed as pain relievers. These drugs are psychologically and physically addicting. The use of narcotics with tranquilizers, sedative-hypnotics, alcohol, or tricyclic antidepressants may cause respiratory depression, profound sedation, or coma. Withdrawal symptoms include anxiety, flu-like symptoms, and perspiring; medical supervision of withdrawal is recommended.

HEROIN

The most common opiate on the street is heroin. Heroin can be administered through injection or inhaling, and it is addictive no matter which route is used. The immediate effects of heroin include euphoria and then sleep. Repeated use produces a tolerance that requires consistently larger doses to produce the same effects. Withdrawal, which begins within 8 to 12 hours after the last dose, can be severe and can include symptoms of clammy skin, slow and shallow breathing, gastrointestinal symptoms, convulsions, coma, and possibly death. Injecting heroin creates a high-risk environment for contracting HIV, hepatitis, and other infectious diseases when individuals share needles. If you are pregnant and using heroin, it is important for the health of your baby that you stop using. Methadone maintenance to block the physical craving for heroin is the most widely used approach and will probably be recommended to you by your health care practitioner (HCP). You may want to explore with your HCP other options, such as a detoxification or tapering approach. For infants of pregnant women who use opiates, including methadone, there is a serious risk of neonatal abstinence syndrome (NAS), a constellation of withdrawal symptoms in the newborn that include hyperactivity, tremors, sleeplessness, incessant high-pitched crying, sweating, and poor feeding. NAS requires medical intervention.

OVER-THE-COUNTER SLEEP AIDS

See "Informed Use of Prescription and Over-the-Counter Drugs," p. 79.

Central Nervous System Stimulants

AMPHETAMINES

Amphetamines ("speed," "ice," "meth") such as Benzedrine, Dexedrine, Preludin, and Ritalin are highly addictive stimulant drugs usually prescribed for weight loss, chronic fatigue, sleep disorders, and attention deficit disorder. Low doses of amphetamines temporarily decrease appetite; relieve drowsiness; and increase heart rate, blood pressure, and breathing rate. These drugs have been shown to have so little value in long-term weight reduction that several states have banned their use for this purpose. These drugs also have such a high potential for abuse and dependence that it is now recommended that use be discontinued if tolerance develops. Physical tolerance can develop within a few weeks of regular use, requiring increasingly large doses. Common effects include sweating, insomnia, blurred vision, dizziness, and diarrhea. Some amphetamines, like Ritalin, have been used successfully under medical supervision to manage attention deficit disorder (ADD). For some other amphetamines, extended long-term use can lead to brain damage, convulsions, and coma. Medical supervision of withdrawal may be necessary if depression results.

COCAINE/CRACK

Cocaine is an addictive drug that provides feelings of excitement and euphoria by stimulating the central and peripheral nervous systems. Administered by injection, smoking, or inhaling, cocaine also causes increased alertness, rapid heartbeat, marked rise in blood pressure, insomnia, and loss of appetite. Long-term use can lead to depression and paranoia. An overdose of cocaine can lead to convulsions, agitation, hallucinations, heart attack, and possibly death. Withdrawal from cocaine may bring about profuse sweating, agitation, extreme drug-craving and drug-seeking behaviors, and sometimes suicidal depression.

Crack is a processed, smokeable form of cocaine that is potentially highly addictive. It tends to be five or six times stronger than powder cocaine. Crack produces an immediate, short, intense high that is followed by a severe crash characterized by depression, anxiety, and a powerful craving for more crack. Increasing the dose of crack risks cocaine overdose or poisoning characterized by nausea, vomiting, and irregular breathing, leading to possible convulsions, coma, and death.

HALLUCINOGENS (PSYCHEDELICS)

The most frequently used hallucinogens are LSD, mescaline, and PCP ("angel dust"). Designer drugs such as Ecstasy have recently become popular. These drugs create euphoria, hallucinations, and distorted perceptions of time and depth. Adverse reactions include paranoia, acute panic, and psychosis. Long-term use can lead to uncontrolled "flashbacks"—psychological phenomena in which a person reexperiences the drug-induced state.

INHALANTS

Glue, freon, benzene, amyl nitrate, and nitrous oxide are inhalants that cause immediate intoxication. These drugs are known for also causing heart failure, asphyxiation, and brain damage.

MARIJUANA

Marijuana is the most widely used illegal drug in the U.S. The effects of marijuana are immediate and include euphoria, stimulation of appetite, distortion of time, and sometimes anxiety. Long-term use of marijuana has been shown to impair short-term memory and sometimes motor coordination. Withdrawal is mild, with symptoms of irritability and sleeplessness.

ANTIDEPRESSANTS

See chapter 6, Our Emotional Well-Being, p. 125.

* Many thanks to Amy Rubin for help with this box on mood-altering drugs.

DRUGS AND ALCOHOL—GETTING HELP

It is often difficult to recognize or admit when alcohol and/or drug use has become a problem. Once we recognize some of the early warning signs, we can begin to seek help. Here are some questions you can ask yourself:

- Has someone close to you expressed concern about your drinking or drug use?
- When faced with a problem, do you often turn to alcohol or drugs for relief?
- Are you sometimes unable to meet home or work responsibilities because of drugs or alcohol?
- Do you regularly drive when under the influence of alcohol or drugs?
- Has your drinking or drug use caused any problems in relationships with family, friends, or co-workers?
- Do you often take a drug or have a drink in the morning?
- Do you find that you have to take increasing amounts of drugs or alcohol to achieve the same effects?
- Have you had distressing physical or psychological reactions when you've tried to stop drinking or using drugs?
- Have you—or has anyone else—ever required medical attention as a result of your drinking or drug use?
- Have you often failed to keep the promises you made to yourself or others about controlling or cutting out your drug use or drinking?
- Do you ever feel guilty about your drinking or drug use, or try to conceal it from others?
- Do you find yourself spending a lot of time thinking about when and where you will next get a drink or use drugs?

If you answered yes to any of the above questions, your drinking or drug use may be interfering with your life in ways serious enough for you to seek help. The following are some of the many ways you can address alcohol and other drug problems. The sooner you get help, the easier it will be to free yourself from dependence on these substances.

Self-Help Groups

Some women find it particularly helpful when trying to overcome alcohol or drug abuse to have the support and advice of others who have "been there." There are a number of different kinds of self-help groups, with varying approaches and philosophies. Keep looking until you find the group that works best for you.*

Alcoholics Anonymous (AA).   Probably the best-known self-help group for recovering alcoholics is Alcoholics Anonymous (AA). It is the oldest and largest network of self-help groups in the U.S., along with Al-Anon and Alateen, which help the families and friends of problem drinkers and drug abusers. Narcotics Anonymous (NA) and Cocaine Anonymous are similar self-help groups for drug users, with Narc-Anon for family and friends. AA and NA include

* For more information, see Resources.

THE PUBLIC DEBATE ABOUT MARIJUANA

The passage of ballot initiatives in California and Arizona in 1996 permitting the medical use of marijuana has sparked a public debate about whether the U.S. Government's antidrug policy is denying people a potentially beneficial remedy. People who have not been helped by conventional medications have turned to marijuana for relief of glaucoma; nausea and vomiting caused by cancer chemotherapy; epileptic seizures; and debilitating muscle spasms. Some people taking AIDS medication use the drug to restore their appetite, counteracting the life-threatening "wasting syndrome."

In order for marijuana to be allowed for medical use, it would need to be reclassified from a Schedule I controlled substance (one with a high potential for abuse and no accepted medical use) to a Schedule II drug (which physicians can prescribe for specialized uses). Meanwhile, the Drug Enforcement Administration has been investigating physicians who recommend marijuana to patients.

women and men who use multiple substances, and many groups address both issues. In larger urban areas, there are often special meetings for women, gays and lesbians, and people of color, as well as meetings in Spanish. These groups are based on 12 steps to recovery, along with daily readings and slogans. They have a spiritual emphasis; participants are encouraged to admit and accept powerlessness over their drinking and drug use, and to turn to a spiritual higher power for help.

SMART Recovery.   SMART Recovery focuses on self-empowerment and personal responsibility as paths to sobriety. SMART stands for self-management and recovery training. SMART Recovery advocates an abstinence-based self-help program using cognitive-behavioral techniques. SMART groups are more frequently found in larger cities on the East and West Coasts.

Women for Sobriety   is a network of local support groups that focus on the special issues and needs of women with drinking and drug problems. Although the network currently has few active groups, it supplies very helpful literature that is oriented toward women's needs, such as enhancing self-esteem.

S.O.S. (Secular Organizations for Sobriety)   is a group similar to AA without references to a higher power and other spiritual attributes. SOS groups exist mostly in the Midwest.

Moderation Management is a self-help support network that helps some problem drinkers reduce their drinking via a controlled drinking approach. It is based on behavioral treatment principles used in other countries but is outside the mainstream in the U.S. (see especially Audrey Kishline's book, *Moderate Drinking,* in Resources).

Treatment

In addition to these independent self-help groups, formal treatment is available in many settings, often on an outpatient basis. These formal treatment programs provide medical care, individual and group counseling, and a range of other support services both to "get you off alcohol and/or drugs" and to help you better understand yourself, learn better coping skills, and create support networks that will enable you to lead a healthy life. If there is a treatment program in your community designed specifically for and staffed by women, you may find it particularly helpful. The need for a brief inpatient stay for detoxification should be determined in consultation with a health care practitioner skilled in that area. Unfortunately, publicly funded programs are few, finding a way to pay for these services may be difficult, and for incarcerated women the services are usually minimal if they exist at all.

Once you find a program, there are several questions you can ask: How long is the program? What kind of treatment is offered? Is there child care? Are there provisions that make the program accessible to women with disabilities? Are there women-only groups? Female counselors? Are there staff and other participants who share your culture and speak your language? Are there alternatives (day or evening treatment) if treatment conflicts with work? Does the program offer family involvement? Are you comfortable with any requirements there may be to attend additional self-help programs? What kind of help will you receive if you relapse or "slip"?

We all need to understand that just as with our struggles with cigarettes, a severe alcohol or drug problem does not go away overnight, or even with one episode of treatment, but with determination, perseverance, and support. Learning to live without drugs or alcohol is possible. It has everything to do with learning new techniques for coping with life's problems, accepting help and support from others, making a decision to quit, and learning from a slip. It has little to do with willpower or morality. Finding alcohol-free, drug-free places to socialize can be especially helpful. Friends and family may be particularly supportive, but they may also need education about these issues, how they can help, how long it may take before you feel secure in your sobriety, and how to support you over the long haul.

SMOKING AND EXPOSURE TO TOBACCO SMOKE

About 23% of women in the U.S. currently smoke, with the smoking rates highest among women at the height of their child-bearing years (ages 25 to 44).[9] About 90% of them started smoking before they were 19.[10] Twenty percent of young people ages 12 to 17 are current smokers, with young women now smoking at a similar rate to young men.[11] Between 1991 and 1994, the number of eighth-grade girls, 13 to 14 years old, who had smoked within the previous 30 days increased 36%, and in 1993, the number of high school senior girls *smoking daily* was almost 22%.[12] Three thousand young people in the U.S. try their first cigarette each day, half of them girls, whose average age of initiation is 14.6 years.[13] Yet, it is widely known and well-documented that cigarette smoking is harmful to health and that nicotine, the psychoactive substance in cigarettes, is highly addictive.

Young girls start smoking as the result of many pressures. Cigarette advertising—a $6.3 billion industry in the U.S. in 1995[14]—takes aim at girls, pointing the way to cigarettes as a way to resolve self-esteem and body

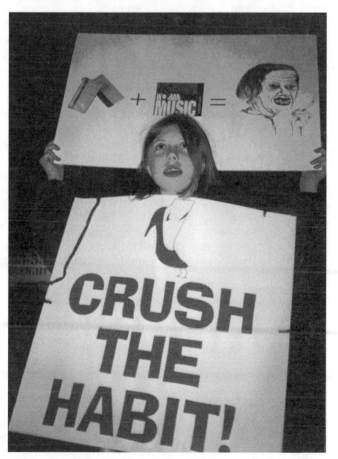

Young participant at a New York City "Virginia SLAM!" demonstrating against Philip Morris for trying to lure young women into the smoking habit through its new record label, "Woman Thing Music"/Rachel Shearer

image concerns. Since the 1920s, cigarette advertising targeted to girls and women has promoted smoking as a symbol of independence, emancipation, rebelliousness, and autonomy, and especially as a method of controlling appetite and weight. Indeed, challenging our society's current obsession with thinness needs to be a focus of any efforts made to reduce the rate of smoking among women and girls.

Both the short- and long-term health consequences of smoking are extremely serious, especially for women. Not only do women develop all the same smoking-related illnesses as men, but they also develop illnesses related to hormonal status, reproductive function, and pregnancy. Younger and newer smokers also experience shortness of breath, coughing, and decreased stamina. Recent studies have shown a drastic reduction in the development of lung function in adolescent smokers, with a more serious effect for girls.[15] In the U.S., smoking is the chief preventable cause of death. More than 152,000 women die each year of the health consequences of smoking, which include lung cancer, cardiovascular disease, heart attacks, and strokes.[16] In 1987, lung cancer surpassed breast cancer as the leading cause of cancer deaths in women in the U.S. Some studies suggest that women get lung cancer and other respiratory diseases after smoking fewer packs of cigarettes than men do, and develop lung cancer at younger ages.[17] Smoking doubles the risk of coronary heart disease. Women who use oral contraceptives and also smoke are at a tenfold greater risk of suffering a heart attack and at an increased risk of stroke compared with women who use oral contraceptives and do not smoke. There is a greater risk of cervical cancer in women smokers; studies show that the size of cervical lesions decreases when women stop smoking.[18] Women who smoke are also at greater risk for death from emphysema and suffer from higher rates of other chronic obstructive pulmonary diseases, such as asthma and chronic bronchitis. Women smokers are more likely than nonsmokers to develop chronic sinusitis, periodontal and gum diseases, peptic and duodenal ulcers, and severe hypertension. Smoking is also linked with decreased fertility in women and with early and more symptomatic menopause, ulcers, cataracts, and osteoporosis.

Exposure to the cigarette smoke of others is also a serious health hazard. In 1993, secondhand smoke, known as environmental tobacco smoke (ETS), was declared a carcinogen by the Environmental Protection Agency, which placed ETS in a category similar to asbestos and radon. Studies have shown that nonsmoking wives exposed to their husbands' cigarette smoke were twice as likely to develop lung cancer as nonsmoking wives of nonsmokers. ETS is a particular problem for certain groups, like Asian and Asian-American women, in which smoking prevalence is high among their male counterparts. Each year, an estimated 3,000 deaths due to lung cancer occur in nonsmokers exposed to ETS. Other studies have shown that children of parents who smoke are at higher risk

for middle ear infections and respiratory ailments such as bronchitis, pneumonia, and asthma, and tend to be hospitalized for these conditions more than children of nonsmoking parents.

During pregnancy, when chemicals in tobacco smoke are passed through the bloodstream to the fetus, smoking and exposure to secondhand smoke pose very serious health risks for the fetus as well as the mother. Smoking during pregnancy is associated with preterm delivery, low birthweight, premature rupture of membranes, placenta previa, miscarriage, and neonatal death. Newborns whose mothers smoked during pregnancy have the same nicotine levels in their bloodstreams as adults who smoke, and they go through withdrawal during their first days of life.

Low-tar and/or low-nicotine cigarettes do not lessen the risk of lung diseases, heart diseases, or risk to a pregnant woman and the health of her pregnancy. They may not even reduce the actual amount of tar and nicotine that enter the body because of how they are typically smoked. Other tobacco products such as cigars have been glamorized in print and electronic media, and marketed to women of all ages and classes. These products contain nicotine, are addictive, and can cause many or all of the serious health problems listed above, with increased risk of cancers of the mouth, tongue, throat, and lips. Non–nicotine-containing smoking products, such as clove cigarettes, lead to similar effects.

Quitting for Good

There are plenty of good reasons to stop smoking. The results are worth it. Quitters soon notice increased energy, endurance, self-esteem, and confidence. Stopping smoking during pregnancy shows immediate benefits for mother and fetus. The long-term benefits continue, and even if a woman was a heavy smoker, the risk of heart attack drops to nearly normal in three years. The risk of developing lung, kidney, and laryngeal cancer drops gradually, nearly equaling that of nonsmokers after 16 years.

More of us than ever are successfully freeing ourselves from addiction to nicotine, the organic compound that is the addictive component of tobacco. One of every three women who has ever smoked has now stopped, and since 1976 the percentage of women who smoke has declined from 33 to 25%. (Unfortunately, the rate of smoking is now rising among teenaged girls in many communities.) Nearly 80% of smokers say they would like to quit, and 65% have made at least one serious attempt. The addictive nature of nicotine requires that the motivated quitter have plans, strategies, and supports in place to deal with the initial period of physical and emotional discomfort that is present as the body detoxifies from nicotine.

Recovery from nicotine dependence is more complicated than a purely physical healing. Women who smoke associate most of their daily activities with smoking. A person who smokes a pack of cigarettes daily is delivering nicotine into her system 200 times a day and over 70,000 times a year. In stopping smoking, there is often the sense of losing a friend, a relationship, a constant companion. Developing a new self-image as a nonsmoker takes time. Some women do gain weight as the body's metabolism returns to a nicotine-free state. Exercise has been shown to minimize the weight gain and increase the likelihood that quitting will be sustained. Healthy food choices (more fruits, vegetables, and grains) and increased physical activity can offset the metabolic changes that come from quitting smoking. The time we quit smoking may also be the perfect time to set healthy eating habits in place (see chapter 2, Food).

It's a great feeling to be able to do so many of the things that were just out of the question while I was smoking—running around the park, dancing for hours at time, little things like enjoying the fragrance of my own clean hair. Just knowing that I'm healthier and my kids are probably healthier.

There's a great sense of accomplishment and power that comes from quitting—power to get hold of your own life. I still identify with being a smoker. I still smoke in my dreams. But I won't do that to myself any more.

The ability to quit smoking successfully depends largely on a strong commitment to stop, the belief that we can stop, and support from others. Many free or low-cost programs are available to those of us who are ready to think about quitting, including those offered through local chapters of the American Cancer Society and the American Lung Association. Some of these programs offer special support groups for women. Other low-cost programs can be found through hospitals, health maintenance organizations, schools, businesses, and community groups.

We will want to look at the timing of our quit attempt. We need to make space for not feeling so great for a few days. It helps if this is a time when we are not feeling overly stressed. Women also need to plan quitting around our menstrual cycles, as women who quit in the later phase of our cycle may have greater withdrawal symptoms than those who quit between day one of menses and day 15.

Ninety percent of those who have quit smoking in the U.S. have done it on their own. Whether we join a smoking cessation program or stop smoking on our own, it is important not to be discouraged or derailed. It is difficult to stop smoking. If you do "slip," think about the success you had up to this point as you ready yourself to continue. Now you know it is possible for you to be nicotine-free.

Withdrawal symptoms vary from person to person, and from one quit attempt to the next. Symptoms may include irritability, fatigue, insomnia, constipation and gas, coughing, dizziness, problems with concentrating, increased appetite, and depression. Withdrawal can be eased through natural methods, such as gentle exercise, drinking water, taking naps, talking with friends and support people, and deep breathing. Knowing that withdrawal eases after the first few days, and having the determination to become a nonsmoker, can make a big difference in how we feel. In addition, nicotine replacement therapy is now available over the counter in the form of nicotine gum and nicotine skin patches, and by prescription as a nasal spray. (A nicotine inhaler is currently going through the FDA approval process.) These can reduce withdrawal symptoms and ease the cravings for a cigarette when used according to directions. Used in conjunction with behavioral treatments or strategies such as those recommended in the package inserts, nicotine replacement therapy significantly increases success at quitting.

We can participate in one of the formal programs offered in our community or we can design our own support networks. Quitting can be done. It takes effort and planning, and it will challenge us. But it is one of the biggest favors we will ever do for ourselves and our health, and for the health of our families and friends.

NOTES

1. National Center on Addiction and Substance Abuse at Columbia University, *Substance Abuse and the American Woman* (New York: National Center on Addiction and Substance Abuse, 1996).
2. A. Rubin et al., "Gender Differences in Relapse Situations," *Addiction* 91 (Suppl.) (1996): S111–S120.
3. E. L. Gomberg, "Gender Issues," in Marc Galanter, ed., *Recent Developments in Alcoholism* 11 (New York: Plenum Press, 1993), 95–107.
4. *Substance Abuse and the American Woman.*
5. Marsha Reichman, "Alcohol and Breast Cancer," special handout in *Alcohol Health and Research World* 18, no. 3 (1994): 182–83.
6. E. S. Ginsburg et al., "Effects of Alcohol Ingestion on Estrogens in Postmenopausal Women," *JAMA* 276, no. 21 (1996): 1747–751.
7. S. Matteo, "The Risk of Multiple Addictions: Guidelines for Assessing a Woman's Alcohol and Drug Use," *The Western Journal of Medicine* 149 (1988): 742.
8. Center for Substance Abuse Treatment (CSAT), Women's and Children's Branch. *Practical Approaches in the Treatment of Women Who Abuse Alcohol and Other Drugs* (Rockville, MD: U.S. Department of Health and Human Services, 1994): 16–18.
9. Blumenthal, Susan. "Smoking v. Women's Health: The Challenge Ahead," *Journal of the American Medical Women's Association,* 51, nos. 1 & 2 (Jan. and April 1996).
10. U.S. Centers for Disease Control and Prevention, Of-

fice on Smoking and Health. *Data from the National Household Surveys on Drug Abuse* (1991).

11. U.S. Centers for Disease Control and Prevention. *1995 National Household Survey on Drug Abuse, Tobacco Related Statistics* (1996).

12. Lloyd Johnston, Patrick O'Malley, and Jerald G. Bachman, *National Survey Results on Drug Use from the Monitoring the Future Study, 1975–1995* (Rockville, MD: National Institute on Drug Abuse, 1996).

13. U.S. Centers for Disease Control and Prevention, Office on Smoking and Health, unpublished data as of September 1997.

14. U.S. Federal Trade Commission, *Federal Trade Commission Report to Congress for 1995 Pursuant to the Federal Cigarette Labeling and Advertising Act* (Washington, DC: The Commission, 1996).

15. D. Gold et al., "Effects of Cigarette Smoking on Lung Function in Adolescent Boys and Girls." *New England Journal of Medicine* 335, no. 13 (1996): 931–37.

16. U.S. Centers for Disease Control and Prevention, "Smoking—Attributable Mortality and Years of Potential Life Lost—United States, 1984," *Morbidity and Mortality Weekly Report* 46, no. 20 (1997): 444–51.

17. E. Zang and E. Wynder, "Differences in Lung Cancer Risk Between Men and Women: Examination of the Evidence," *Journal of the National Cancer Institute* 88, nos. 3–4 (1996): 183–91.

18. A. Szarewski et al., "Effectiveness of Smoking Cessation on Cervical Lesion Size," *Lancet* 347 (1996): 941–43.

....

RESOURCES
....

Readings

Bepko, Claudia, ed. *Feminism and Addiction*. New York: Haworth Press, 1991.

Black, Claudia. *It Will Never Happen to Me!* New York: Ballantine Books, 1987.

Covington, Stephanie. *A Woman's Way Through the Twelve Steps*. Center City, MN: Hazelden, 1994.

Gomberg, Edith L., and Ted D. Nirenberg. *Women and Substance Abuse*. Norwood, NJ: Ablex Publishing, 1993.

hooks, bell. *Sisters of the Yam, Black Women and Self-Recovery*. Boston: South End Press, 1993.

Jerome, Joan, and Lindi Bilgorri. *The Lost Years: Tranquilizers and After*. London: Virgin Publishing, 1991. An excellent self-help guide to avoiding, dealing with, and recovering from tranquilizer addiction.

Kasl, Charlotte Davis. *Many Roads, One Journey: Moving Beyond the 12 Steps*. New York: HarperPerennial, 1992.

Kishline, Audrey. *Moderate Drinking: The Moderation Management Guide for People Who Want to Reduce Their Drinking*. New York: Crown Trade, 1996. A self-help book by the woman who founded the Moderation Management support network.

Knapp, Caroline. *Drinking: A Love Story*. New York: Dial Press, 1996. Compelling personal account.

McGovern, George. *Terry: My Daughter's Life-and-Death Struggle with Alcoholism,* New York: Plume, 1997.

National Institute on Alcohol Abuse and Alcoholism. *How to Cut Down on Your Drinking*. Bethesda, MD: National Institutes of Health, 1996. NIH Publication No. 96–3770. Full text available at http://www.niaaa.nih.gov

Peele, Stanton, Archie Brodsky, and Mary Arnold. *The Truth About Addiction and Recovery: The Life Process Program for Outgrowing Destructive Habits*. New York: Simon & Schuster, 1991. Includes numerous non–12-step self-help techniques.

Roth, Paula, ed. *Alcohol and Drugs Are Women's Issues: Vol. 1—A Review of the Issues*. Metuchen, NJ: The Scarecrow Press, Women's Action Alliance, 1991. A comprehensive review of the issues with a strong multicultural orientation.

Sanchez-Craig, Martha. *Saying When: How to Quit Drinking or Cut Down*. Toronto: Addiction Research Foundation, 1993. A practical self-help guide.

Sandmaier, Marian. *The Invisible Alcoholics: Women and Alcohol Abuse,* 2nd ed. Blue Ridge Summit, PA: Tab Books, 1992. Explores why women drink, social attitudes, treatment needs, and how and where to get help. Includes in-depth interviews with diverse women.

Wilsnack, Richard W., and Sharon Wilsnack, eds. *Gender and Alcohol: Individual and Social Perspectives*. New Brunswick, NJ: Rutgers Center of Alcohol Studies, 1997.

Audiovisual Materials

The Last to Know, by Bonnie Friedman. A 45-minute 1984 film or videocassette. Available from New Day Films, 22D Hollywood Avenue, Hohokus, NJ 07432; (201) 652-6590. E-mail: tmcndy@aol.com. A powerful feminist film on women's experiences with alcohol and drug abuse.

Straight from the Heart: Stories of Mothers Recovering from Addiction, a 28-minute video. Six women of various ethnic and socioeconomic backgrounds support each other in a moving and powerful discussion about their addictions, ongoing recoveries, and how they got help. Produced by and available from Vida Health Communications, Inc., 6 Bigelow Street, Cambridge, MA 02139; (617) 864–4334.

Women of Substance. One ten-minute-long, one half-hour-long, and one hour-long advocacy video illustrating problems encountered by pregnant and parenting substance abusers seeking treatment, including issues relating to incarcerated women. Available from Video Action Fund, 1000 Potomac Street NW, Suite 202, Washington, DC 20007; (202) 338–3346.

Organizations

Al-Anon Family Groups
P.O. Box 862; Midtown Station; New York, NY 10010
Web site: http://www.Al-Anon-Alateen.org

Sponsors self-help meetings for spouses and children of alcoholics. For information, literature, and groups, contact your local Al-Anon office.

Alcoholics Anonymous
P.O. Box 459; Grand Central Station; New York, NY 10163
Web site: http://www.alcoholics-anonymous.org
   A worldwide self-help organization for recovering alcoholic women and men, with local chapters in most communities. To find meetings, contact AA headquarters or your local AA office.

California Advocates for Pregnant Women
P.O. Box 3029; Oakland, CA 94609; (310) 452-5968
   Conducts policy, legal, and educational outreach.

Legal Action Center
153 Waverly Place; New York, NY 10014; (212) 243-1313
   Provides legal and legislative advocacy, and legal and policy information regarding substance abuse, including issues surrounding HIV/AIDS.

Moderation Management
P.O. Box 27558; Golden Valley, MN 55427; (612) 512-1484
Web site: http://comnet.org/mm
   Self-help groups nationwide to help problem drinkers reduce their drinking.

Narcotics Anonymous/Cocaine Anonymous
Web site: http://www.wsoinc.com
   Call local information for phone numbers.

National Black Alcoholism Council
1629 K Street, NW, Suite 802; Washington, DC 20006; (202) 296-2696

National Clearinghouse for Alcohol and Drug Information
P.O. Box 2345; Rockville, MD 20847-2345; (800) 729-6686
Web site: http://www.health.org
   A federal information service offering free publications on alcohol and drug abuse.

National Council on Alcoholism and Drug Dependence
12 West 21st Street, 7th Floor; New York, NY 10010; (212) 206-6770
Web site: http://www.ncadd.org
   A national coordinating organization for local councils on alcoholism with publications on women and families. Local councils provide treatment referrals.

National Substance Abuse Help Lines
c/o Phoenix House; 164 West 74th Street; New York, NY 10023; (800) 262-2463

National Women's Resource Center
515 King Street, Suite 410; Alexandria, VA 22314; (800) 354-8824 (Information and referral line)
Web site: http://www.nwrc.org
   A federally funded national center offering information, including publications, regarding women and mental illness and substance abuse.

Secular Organizations for Sobriety, National Clearinghouse
5521 Grosvenor Boulevard; Los Angeles, CA 90066; (310) 821-8430 (24-hour help line)
   Self-help groups nationwide that emphasize personal responsibility and group support. No spiritual emphasis.

SMART Recovery (Self-Management And Recovery Training)
2400 Mercantile Road; Beachwood, OH 44122; (216) 292-0220
E-mail: srmail1@aol.com
   Self-help groups nationwide that focus on self-empowerment through changing beliefs about self and drinking. No spiritual emphasis.

Wisconsin Clearinghouse for Prevention Services
University of Wisconsin—Madison
1552 University Avenue; Madison, WI 53705; (800) 248-9244
Web site: http://www.uhs.wisc.edu/wch
   Offers low-cost, readable materials, including resources for lesbians and materials on fetal alcohol syndrome.

Women for Sobriety
P.O. Box 618; Quakertown, PA 18951; (215) 536-8026
Web site: http://www.mediapulse.com/wfs
   A national self-help organization for recovering alcoholic women. Write or call for referral to a local group.

Smoking

Readings

   Chollat-Traquet, Claire. *Women and Tobacco*. Geneva: World Health Organization, 1992. A review of the international issues concerning women and tobacco, including women-specific cessation tips.
   Delaney, Sue. *Women Smokers Can Quit: A Different Approach*. Evanston, IL: Women's Healthcare Press, 1989. Easy-to-follow book on cessation.
   Fielding, J. E., et al. "Smoking and Women: Tragedy of the Majority," *New England Journal of Medicine* 317 (Nov. 19, 1987): 1343–345.
   Greaves, Lorraine. *Smoke Screen: Women's Smoking and Social Control*. London: Scarlet Press, 1996 (available in the U.S. from Inbook, Division of Login Publishers Consortium, Chicago, IL).
   Janerich, Dwight T., et al. "Lung Cancer and Exposure to Tobacco Smoke in the Household," *New England Journal of Medicine* 323, no. 10 (June 6, 1990): 632–36.
   March of Dimes. "Give Your Baby a Healthy Start: Stop Smoking" 1990. Health hazards of smoking to the fetus, and tips on stopping smoking. Free from local March of Dimes chapters.
   National Institutes of Health. *Clearing the Air: How to Quit Smoking*. Washington, DC: National Cancer Institute, 1995. A readable guide with information on smoking-cessation programs. Available free from the National Cancer Institute, Bethesda, MD 20892; (800) 422-6237.

Orleans, Tracy, and John Slase, eds. *Nicotine Addiction: Principles and Management.* New York: Oxford University Press, 1993.

Slattery, Martha L., et al. "Cigarette Smoking and Exposure to Passive Smoke Are Risk Factors for Cervical Cancer." *JAMA,* 261, no. 11 (1989): 1593–598.

"Smoking and Women's Health" *Journal of the American Medical Women's Association* 51, nos. 1 & 2 (1996), special issue.

U.S. Department of Health and Human Services. *The Health Consequences of Smoking: Nicotine Addiction—A Report of the Surgeon General.* Washington, DC: U.S. DHHS, 1988.

Audiovisual Materials

Diary of a Teenage Smoker, a 26-minute 1991 videocassette. Young women speak about how they started smoking and how they want to, or have, quit. Comes with facilitator's guide. Canadian production. Available from East-West Media, 3716 Walker Creek Road, Central Point, OR 97502; (541) 899-7766.

The Feminine Mistake: The Next Generation, a 30-minute 1989 videocassette. Women and smoking. Available from Pyramid Media, P.O. Box 1048, Santa Monica, CA 90406-1048; (310) 828-7577.

First Time, Last Time, 30 minutes, 1988. Women from teenage to middle age discuss how they began smoking and their failures and successes at quitting. Available for free loan, or purchase from your local chapter of the American Cancer Society.

The Lady Killers, a 40-minute British documentary video explores why women smoke and barriers to quitting that are particular to women. Available from Biomedical Communications, Yale School of Medicine, 333 Cedar Street, New Haven, CT 06510; (203) 737-5282.

Organizations

Action on Smoking and Health
2013 H Street, NW; Washington, DC 20006; (202) 659-4310
Web site: http://ash.org
A citizen's group working for legislation to reduce the health toll of smoking and protect nonsmokers' rights.

American Cancer Society
(800) ACS-2345
Web site: http://www.cancer.org.
   Free and low-cost information available.

National Cancer Institute—Cancer Information Service
(800) 4-CANCER
Web site: http://cancernet.nci.hih.gov
   Low-cost materials and information are available.

STAT (Stop Teenage Addiction to Tobacco)
511 E. Columbus Avenue; Springfield, MA 01105; (413) 732-7828
E-mail: STAT@exit3.com

Tobacco Education Clearinghouse of California (TECC)
P.O. Box 1830; Santa Cruz, CA 95061-1830; (408) 438-4822
   Tobacco education materials, including materials for women and culturally diverse populations. Catalog available in English, Spanish, and several Asian languages.

Additional Online Resources *

Join Together Online
http://www.jointogether.org

Mental Health Net: Self-help Substance Abuse & Alcoholism Resources
http://www.cmhc.com/guide/substnce.htm

National Families in Action
http://www.emory.edu/NFIA

National Institute on Drug Abuse
http://www.nida.nih.gov

SAMHSA
http://www.samhsa.gov

Web of Addictions
http://www.well.com/user/woa

Welcome to The QuitNet
http://www.quitnet.org

* For more information and listings of online resources, please see Introduction to Online Women's Health Resources, p. 25.

By Suzanne Bremer, based on earlier
work by Janet Jones

WITH SPECIAL THANKS TO Maureen Ferrera
and Cindy Higgins of Boston Self-Help, Lynn
Jaffee of Melpomene Institute, Karen Kahn,
Jennifer Yanco, and Wendy Zinn *

A *lot more women* are out in the world moving around—and *it feels good.* We are swimming, walking, dancing, jogging, power lifting, Rollerblading, fencing, and hiking. We play basketball, softball, soccer, rugby, badminton, racquetball, volleyball, lacrosse. We are bowling, skiing, gardening, canoeing, wrestling, skating, rock climbing, wheelchair dancing, and sitskiing. We play tennis, football, ice hockey, golf. We are boxing, surfing, scuba diving, motorcycle racing. We practice archery, karate, yoga, tai chi, and gymnastics. We bike, skate, sail, ride horses, race cars, take aerobics, and skydive.

Women have not always exercised and done sports. Throughout history, women working on farms, in factories, and in the home doing domestic labor have led such physically demanding lives that "exercise" for its own sake has been meaningless and not really an option. During the 19th and early 20th centuries, exercise for middle-class women, for the most part, was deemed unladylike. Well-to-do women may have played golf or tennis, but they played corseted and gloved. Today, many women's lives may not be as physically demanding as the lives of our foremothers, but sedentary work is draining in its own way, and most women's lives are full of many stresses. Most of us have to work at getting the kinds of movement that a healthy body, mind, and spirit need.

Over the last 20 years, women have become more active, both because of our increased awareness of the health benefits of exercise and because the women's movement has raised our consciousness and created increased opportunities to participate in sports and exercise. Not all of us may be out there exercising all of the time—because there are still obstacles, both internal and external—but more of us are out there more often.

* Thanks also to the following for their help with the 1998 version of this chapter: Janet Jones, The National Black Women's Health Project, April Taylor, Kiki Zeldes, and all of you who responded to our survey. Over the years since 1969, the following women have contributed to the many versions of this chapter: Pat Lyga, Carol McEldowney, Mary Lee Slettehaugh, Judith Stein.

EXERCISE, SPORTS, PHYSICAL PLAY: WHAT THEY DO FOR US

Living is moving. Even when we lie still, all is in motion inside: the blood flows, the chest expands and contracts as we breathe, we digest food and eliminate wastes. The mind is full of thoughts, ideas, feelings, dreams. It is natural to want to move externally, too. We go outside and move around. Exercise is good for many systems in our bodies. Most women with chronic health problems and disabilities such as asthma or diabetes can benefit from some kinds of exercise.

The Cardiovascular System and Aerobic Exercise

When we move vigorously on a regular basis for 20 or more minutes at a time, the heart (a muscle) gets stronger and more efficient, pumping more blood with fewer strokes. Over time, this kind of *aerobic* exercise —that is, exercise that keeps us breathing hard (and thereby taking in more oxygen) while our blood is circulating rapidly—increases the actual number and size of blood vessels in our tissues and so increases their blood supply. When we exercise hard, blood circulates faster through these expanded vessels, bringing oxygen and nutrients to every part of us and taking wastes away more quickly. That's why we usually feel refreshed and invigorated afterward.

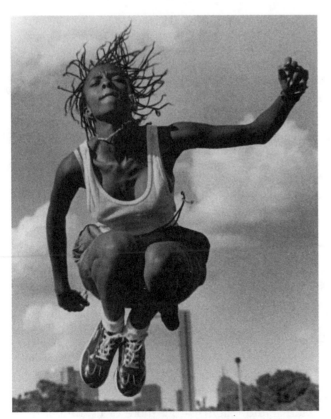

Yolanda McCollum/The Boston Photo Collaborative

WALKING FOR WELLNESS: THE NATIONAL BLACK WOMEN'S HEALTH PROJECT

Walking for Wellness, a health promotion and disease prevention program of the National Black Women's Health Project (NBWHP), was launched by NBWHP's founder, Byllye Avery, in 1992. The Walking for Wellness campaign encourages black women, their families, and their communities to take the initiative to improve and safeguard their health through their participation in an organized walking program.

Goals of the Program

- To increase the number of black women and their families in walking programs.
- To support and expand walking groups
- To increase awareness of the relationship between exercise and the reduction of risk factors associated with disease and disability.
- To support women in their efforts to make lifestyle changes.
- To provide ongoing education about health promotion and disease prevention.

Walking for Wellness encourages employers to allow employees to develop walking groups and walk during working hours. Walking for Wellness provides worksite walking groups, community walking groups, and individuals with

- Education, orientation programs, group support sessions and health information sessions.
- Preselected walking sites designed for 20- to 30-minute walks, three times per week; walking records so individual walkers can chart their own progress; and the opportunity to participate in the annual Walking for Wellness walkathon.
- Periodic health screening and confidential health risk appraisal, as well as ongoing program assessment.

Through a partnership with the American Heart Association and the National Conference of Black Mayors, the NBWHP held Walking for Wellness Days in Baltimore and Detroit in the summer of 1997 and will expand the program to ten cities in 1998. Walking for Wellness Days are day-long community-based, family events designed to encourage physical activity, preventive care, and health education in the community. To contact NBWHP, call (202) 835-0117 or E-mail NBWHPDC@aol.com.

Exercise has been shown to reduce hypertension (high blood pressure) and increase "good cholesterol" (see "Heart Disease, Heart Attack, Hypertension, Stroke, and Other Vascular Disorders," chapter 24, Selected Medical Practices, Problems, and Procedures, p. 644). African-American women in particular have high levels of hypertension. As a self-help strategy, the National Black Women's Health Project has created a "Walking for Wellness" program. With regular aerobic exercise, many women are able to keep their blood pressure at normal levels.

The Respiratory System

Exercising makes us breathe more deeply and regularly as more air moves rhythmically in and out of the lungs. The lungs develop a larger capacity, opening the air sacs up to the top and way down to the bottom of each lung for better gas exchange. We end up taking in more oxygen, which is essential for each cell in the body. If we practice rhythmic patterns of inhaling deeply, holding our breath, and exhaling all the air slowly, we strengthen the respiratory system while quieting the mind.

The Musculoskeletal System

Muscles increase in size when they are used regularly. Strong back and abdominal muscles are good insurance against the lower back pain that plagues so many of us these days. The abdominals also help hold the stomach and intestines in place and are critical to good digestion and elimination. Solid leg muscles get us where we are going and help the heart: when they contract, they squeeze the veins and so push the blood toward the heart, usually against the pull of gravity. Well-developed biceps and triceps muscles in the arms allow us to carry more and to perform everyday tasks with less effort and more independence. For self-defense purposes, more muscle power can sometimes help protect us. When our muscles are firm and flexible, they protect us in many ways from the stresses and strains of living. And besides, being physically strong feels good.

When we exercise, our bones get stronger, too. As muscles contract they pull on the bones, which increases bone strength over time. Also, the body lays down extra minerals in the bones along the lines of stress, decreasing our risk for osteoporosis (weakened bones due to gradual loss of calcium) later in life. If you walk or run, for example, the long bones in your legs will be gradually reinforced to meet the added pressure from your feet hitting the ground over and over again. This is true for women of all ages, even those who are postmenopausal (see also "Exercise and Growing Older," p. 93).

The Reproductive System

Far from "damaging our internal organs," as women were once taught, exercise helps them. Exercise will not hurt our breasts or cause a prolapsed uterus. In fact, the more active we are, the less premenstrual tension and painful menstruation are likely to interfere with our lives. Exercise can ease cramps, so unless we have excessive bleeding, nausea, or vomiting, we can go at it as hard as we like during this time of the month. Exercise during and after most pregnancies is highly recommended.

Those of us who run over 30 miles a week or exercise heavily in other ways may find that we menstruate less or not at all. One or more factors may be responsible: intensity of effort, length of workout, fat loss, and/or emotional stress. Amenorrhea is not healthy, particularly for young women. The hormones we produce during our menstrual cycles help to strengthen our bones and prevent osteoporosis. If you aren't menstruating, try cutting back on your workouts to see if you resume your cycles. And remember that you can become pregnant during long periods of amenorrhea.*

How Exercise Makes Us Feel

Whether we hate our jobs, are involved in a difficult relationship, or simply have too much to do while we try to juggle work, family, and friends, many women in late 20th-century North America feel anxious and stressed much of the time. Stress may seem natural—just a part of life—but it is dangerous to our health. Tense muscles in the neck can cause splitting headaches; in the leg, charley horses; in the gut, stomachaches. Overcontracted muscles restrict breathing, slow down or even cut off the blood supply in their vicinity by squeezing the vessels shut, and actually limit our strength and sap our energy.

Exercise is not the only answer to stress in our lives (you may want to tell off your boss or practice daily meditation), but it is a great way to release tension and take some time for ourselves. You may not be "flying" after working out, but you will almost invariably feel better than you did before: calmer, less tired, more refreshed.

Due to multiple sclerosis I haven't been able to run off stress in the conventional manner for years. But I have discovered a substitute that works for me. I have a motorized scooter and when the old urge to go for a run hits me, I get on my scooter and ride at high speed around the block a few times. The fresh air on me has the "feeling" of running and is a great stress buster.

I love the way exercise makes me feel—strong, confident, and relaxed. It is a fun activity for me, allowing me to let out tension and just go "nuts." It raises my

---

* See Melpomene Institute for Women's Health Research, *The Bodywise Woman: Reliable Information about Physical Activity and Health* (Champaign, IL: Human Kinetics, 1996). See chapter 12, Understanding Our Bodies: Sexual Anatomy, Reproduction, and the Menstrual Cycle.

spirit on a day when I'm feeling down and gives me a physical boost when I'm tired.

I have always had a poor body image. I have been on some weight loss scheme or another since age ten. Exercise has given me the power to actually enjoy listening to my muscles and inner rhythms and actually enjoy watching new muscles or contours. Although I will always have weight issues, I am not obsessed with them as before.

I feel energetic, in control and fit. . . . After exercising a huge sense of optimism overcomes me.

After a good workout, you feel that you have met your challenge for the day. And when you feel sore it is kind of good because you know it is working. The only problem is getting the energy and the motivation to get started.

OVERCOMING OBSTACLES

We all know that exercise is good for us. We feel better when we move around. But obstacles remain.

For every dollar men make, women make 75 cents. Our paychecks go for food, shelter, clothing, transportation, and medical care. By and large, women raise the children and run the household. Who has the time, money, or energy to run, to bike, to swim, or to dance?

These obstacles are real. Though we can find ways to exercise without spending a lot of money, time is a finite resource. But making time for ourselves is important, and exercise, by giving us extra energy, often adds hours to our day.

Old Myths and Prejudices

Even with a minimum of external obstacles, many of us still don't exercise regularly. This may be because of some old myths and prejudices that we need to throw out once and for all. Too many of us know well the long, cold stares and remarks like these:

- Big shoulder muscles are really ugly on a woman.
- Hey, fatty, you should get your exercise pushing away from the dinner table.
- You four girls are going to hog this court when we guys need a team practice? No way!
- Don't you know that sweating is unfeminine?
- You're 51 and you're taking up *what?!*
- Keep on pitching like a man, sweetheart—we know you're a dyke!
- What are these crippled women doing here? If I looked like that I wouldn't be caught dead in a bathing suit.
- Winning is everything—if you can't win don't bother playing!

We may have internalized many of these negative messages about women and physical activity. When

SOME GUIDELINES ON MOVEMENT FOR FAT WOMEN*

- Choose something that looks like fun. Don't worry about whether it's "good" for you or not, or if you do, think about improving your circulation and heart tone.
- Forget about losing weight or "firming flab."
- Find a place where you already see big women exercising, or do it at home.
- Go with a friend. Pick someone about your size or similarly new to the activity. Don't start out with a "jock."
- Give yourself leeway to be good or not so good at something.
- Get together with other fat women to find facilities. (Swimming is great, but locker rooms and bathing suits can be humiliating. A group of women in San Francisco rent a city pool a few hours a week for a fat women's swim, which makes all the difference.)
- Try walking, depending on your neighborhood; bowling, which requires no special clothes; social or ballroom dance classes, where you can have a friend as a partner.
- Wear comfortable clothes; don't worry about how you look.
- Good shoes appropriate to your sport can be especially important in preventing injuries.
- You have a right to remain physically inactive if you choose.

* From Judith Stein, cofounder of Boston Area Fat Liberation. See also Pat Lyons, *Great Shape: The First Fitness Guide for Large Women* (Palo Alto, CA: Bull Publishing Co., 1990).

we come to believe these myths, when they become stories that we tell ourselves, we run the risk of being diminished.

As women we tend to be particularly sensitive to issues of body image because we are so often judged by the way we look (see chapter 1, Body Image). The ridicule, hostility, and fear that greet us every time we walk down the street keep a lot of us immobilized. We may feel that we look too fat or too skinny, too black, too white, too ethnic, too poor, too old, or too butch. Learning to move around in public despite the harassment that we may face, learning to relax and take up the space that we are entitled to—these are victories over those who want us to feel ashamed of being who we are. All of us, regardless of size, age, ability, race, or class, deserve the health benefits of physical exertion.

Homophobia

Many of us once avoided sports, particularly team sports, for fear of being called lesbians. This was true whether we identified as heterosexual, lesbian, bisexual, or queer. Today, many lesbian coaches and athletes remain in the closet, often for good reason. As coaches and mentors of young athletes, lesbians fear losing jobs; for professional athletes, lucrative product endorsement contracts are at stake.

Thankfully, this situation has begun to change. Tennis champion Martina Navratilova, who is an open lesbian, has shown that athletes can come out. Once we all realize that not only is there nothing wrong with being a lesbian, but it doesn't matter if someone thinks you are one (even if you are not), then we are ready to make the playing fields safe for all women. Lesbian-baiting hurts all women athletes by making us all feel that we must always balance our athletic prowess with appropriate "femininity." We must work together to create an atmosphere where we can all be comfortable with who we are, so that we can play to the best of our abilities, whether as high school softball players, professional golfers, or Olympic triathletes.

EXERCISE AND DISABILITY

In this society, we tend to let professionals do our sports for us. When we think of basketball, we think of Michael Jordan and Rebecca Lobo. When we think of running, we think of Ben Johnson or Jackie Joyner-Kersee. Yet, sports (that is, exercise, play, movement) belong to all of us. While not everyone has a sneaker named after her, most of us can know the joy and sense of confidence and well-being that movement can bring. All women, whether we are physically fit or haven't moved a muscle in years, are able-bodied or living with a chronic illness or disability, are young or old, need to find enjoyable ways of being in our bodies and being active.

Women with disabilities are finding each other and the programs that we need. One very fine adapted yoga program takes place once a week at an urban self-help center. Women with a wide variety of disabilities, from multiple sclerosis to cerebral palsy and from angina to sickle-cell anemia, attend the program.

Linda spends her day in a wheelchair. Her leg muscles cannot hold her up, but her back muscles are okay. If she sits hour after hour with no chance to exercise, her back and abdominal muscles will wither away, and she will become even more disabled. Linda and several other women in wheelchairs are encouraged to walk several steps with help and then spend time on mats breathing, stretching, and doing visualization exercises. Loretta Levitz, the woman who developed and runs the program, explains:

I want people to stay as active as they can and then to start reclaiming the parts of their bodies that the doctor usually considers lost. The group is very important; so is healthy food.

Tosca, a woman with multiple sclerosis, has been a regular at the class for a long time. She explains that the class has taught her some important lessons:

About a year ago, one of my legs started "tremoring," as it often does. In anger I hit it. Then my other leg began shaking, too, but I decided to pat that one instead. The leg getting the loving treatment stopped its movement almost immediately, while the "abused" leg kept right on shaking. Relaxation and breathing have helped me expand my physical abilities, given me hope and renewed determination.

Swimming has always been a physical activity for those of us with differing abilities. Women of all ages and with a variety of disabilities (blindness, cerebral palsy, paralysis, and so on) can enjoy adapted swim classes. The instructors help their students get over fear of the water and then teach swimming and water safety skills. It is liberating to be free of the "hardware"—canes, crutches, wheelchairs—and to move into a medium that buoys you up. And these kinds of classes can be great places to meet people and make new friends.

EXERCISE AND GROWING OLDER

Our need for exercise continues, even increases, as we grow older. Research shows that physical activity can significantly improve our health even into our 80s and 90s.[1]

As our bodies age we can lose flexibility, muscle strength, and aerobic power. Joints can become stiffer because the fluid in them can begin to dry up; joint space can narrow and osteoporosis weakens bones (see p. 91). Muscles may sag more readily, and our minds, taking in all the ageist propaganda, may say, "Well, it's all downhill from here." We mustn't buy that line! Being active (perhaps with a longer warm-up period) may help keep joints supple, although the first movements at the beginning of a workout may be more painful than they were in our in younger years. We can walk, swim, jog, lift weights, take up a new sport. It is important to pay attention to your body and go slow, but *don't* let your muscles and bones, heart, and lungs deteriorate and your confidence with them. Woodie took scuba diving to celebrate her 54th birthday:

Why wait? I said to myself. It's something I've always wanted to do.

Maybe we can't be as undaunted as Ruth Rothfarb, who at 80 ran her first marathon (Ottawa, 1981)—but what a role model! At the end of the 26.2-mile course, her legs were tired, but, she says:

It was the greatest day of my life! I worked all my life in a store. I always liked the outdoors and enjoyed long walks, but there was never time for more. Eight or nine years ago I started jogging, and for the last five I have been competing.

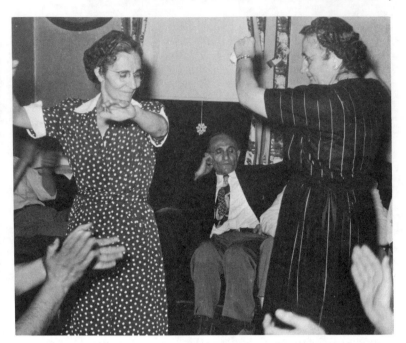

Varkey Sohigian

She runs about ten miles every day, walks a lot, and dances, too. The people in her apartment building used to think she was crazy, but now they encourage her with "Go, Ruthie!" She wishes they would get into exercise also, but so far very few have. She explains that women of her generation have many fears about their bodies, many don'ts and can'ts. Ruth guards her independence with a determined spirit, doing what feels right to *her:*

I need my sleep. I rest my arthritic leg when it bothers me, but I never miss that daily run.

Those of us in our 60s, 70s, 80s, and 90s who are not out running ten miles do not need to let Ruth's example make us feel defensive, but we can let it inspire us to do something at home, at our social center, or at our local Y.

EXERCISE AND ILLNESS

After surgery or a long illness, we need physical activity. Even hospital patients are encouraged to get out of bed as soon as possible. When we're ill, moving around gets the blood circulating, prevents painful bedsores, and stimulates the respiratory system as well. If you are bedridden, it's important to get help with exercising the movable parts of your body; even tensing and relaxing your muscles in a methodical way will help. Do some deep breathing at least once every hour.

I had a mastectomy four years ago and found the weights very important in gaining back my arm strength and sensation. I think that for women who have had mastectomies, working the arm and chest muscles is very important.

WHAT WE CAN DO

Exercise need not be time-consuming or expensive. There are lots of things we can do without much space or equipment. We can be active in the privacy and relative safety of our own homes. Clear a space so you don't feel hemmed in. Hang up a Nerf basketball hoop and shoot hoops in the hallway. Buy some two- or five-pound hand weights (expect to pay $2 to $10 each) and try strength training.

Stretch. Jump rope, run in place, work out with an aerobics or yoga class on TV or a videotape, do calisthenics, or ride an exercise bike. There is a lot of fancy exercise equipment on the market that you don't need to buy in order to get fit. See what you can do with the basics—walking, running, lifting hand weights—before investing in a treadmill or a $200 weight machine. You may want to look for a good used bike.

Try exercising to music. A steady upbeat makes you want to move; the slower rhythms are good for stretching, where the point is to hold to a count of 10 or 20 with no bouncing (repeat at least once). Stretch in quiet sometimes, though, so you can tune into your own rhythms and get a sense of what your body can and can't do. Visualizing how you want to feel and what you want your body to look like as you progress to more difficult feats is extremely helpful.

Women with older children can do physical activities with their kids. Vanessa used to manage a dance school started by her daughters:

I got a lot of pleasure out of joining those classes. Later I took karate with my boys at the community school night program. Even with a tight schedule, my motto is: you make time for what is important to you.

Carla jogs with her kids, especially on weekends, and this works well for them. If you jog with your children (from age six on), be sure it is *fun;* most children will run *playfully* for long distances without tiring (miles and miles) and will prefer this to sprinting.

At my son's suggestion, I got a baseball mitt when he was eight, and we've played a lot of catch since then, in addition to the jogging.

Sonya missed her every-other-day run so much when her baby came she decided she couldn't wait six, seven, or ten years.

After a few months, I put Charelle in a sturdy stroller and now I jog pushing her along. This way I can keep active and my daughter is getting a feel for movement right from the beginning!

Use what is close at hand. You may live near a bike path, park, lake, or municipal swimming pool or ice rink. If you love the outdoors, you might find places close by to hike or rent a canoe. If you're a nightlife person, look for local dance clubs (preferably smoke-free) where you can enjoy music and work up a good sweat at the same time. Look around for community centers and public recreational facilities. The Ys (YMCA, YWCA, YMHA, and YWHA) are low-cost alternatives to commercial health clubs. (Not all Ys have the same facilities or the same fees, so if you live in a city, you might call several in your area. Some may offer financial assistance.)

I have the tendency to have pain from an old back injury. When I exercise, I always feel more focused, that I have a better perspective. I breathe easier, have less back pain and more flexibility.

Exercise can also be good for our mental health. A growing body of evidence suggests that regular exercise can help those who suffer from mild to moderate depression or anxiety. We know that exercise increases the flow of blood to the brain; some researchers think that this increase in blood flow may have the same effect that some antidepressant drugs do.[2]

I have mental disability (depression, trauma). With exercise I feel that I have more power over my life; I'm less depressed and hopeless. Physically, I'm stronger, more toned.

Those of us who live in institutions also benefit from as much physical activity as possible, although we rarely get a fraction of what we need. Mental hospitals, nursing homes, and similar institutions (including prisons), with their understaffing and heavy reliance on drugs and/or lockups, often deny us the restorative power of exercise and play. As Crystal tells it:

I've been in the nuthouse twice and jail once. If you let out how you feel in a physical way—and believe me, you need to—they just drug your ass, that's it. Or put you in max. I lost my body in there, and my mind.

GETTING MOVING

Exercise Options

There are more ways of exercising than we can name. The key is to find something that you enjoy and then to stick with it for a while. Pick something that looks like fun and that suits your lifestyle, fits into your schedule, and doesn't necessarily involve buying a lot of fancy equipment or traveling long distances to start.

There are three basic types of exercise: *Cardiovascular exercise*, which burns calories and conditions the heart and lungs; *strengthening exercise*, which works to tone muscles, boost the metabolism, and strengthen bones; and *flexibility exercise*, which helps prevent injury and improves agility and range of motion. When considering your exercise options, you may want to balance your activities so that you include all three types of training.

Cardiovascular training
- walking, jogging, running
- aerobics, dancing, skipping rope
- rowing
- biking, cross-country skiing, in-line skating
- boxing, basketball, soccer
- swimming

Strength training
- free weights
- weight machines (Universal and Nautilus)
- resistance training
- calisthenics

Flexibility training
- stretching
- yoga
- tai chi
- ballet
- Pilates (stretching exercises popular with ballet dancers)

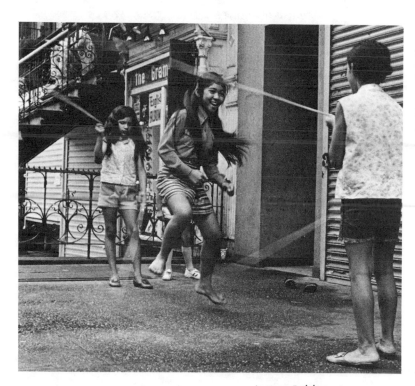

Jeanne Raisler

CLUBBING

Dancing is a terrific way to get your body moving. In the early '70s, dancing took on a whole new feel with the invention of Disco. In the '80s and '90s, that same spirit has redefined itself and has been transformed into what is known as clubbing. Clubbing hit the major dance spots of New York and spread like wildfire to cities like Newark, Chicago, and Los Angeles. Today, in most urban areas, you can easily find a crowd of young, artistic, expressionistic individuals dancing to the thunderous bass beats and the latest sounds of underground or house music.

In the club scene, you may see professional dancers, voguers (no, Madonna didn't start it!), and novice dancers, all out to have fun and to work up a good sweat—without inhibitions. Although you need to take care of yourself in the club scene (smoke, overuse of drugs and alcohol, and possible harassment by drunk men are a few of the hazards), the club scene is a good place to slip on some jeans or a leotard and just work out:

When I first started going to clubs in New York City and Newark, it was probably one of the most exciting experiences of my life. The music was pumping, the light show created a surreal effect, and the crowd was jamming. I always went with my girls and we watched each others' backs. If I danced, she watched my bag, my beverage, and the way I danced, and we would do the same for each other. The camaraderie and the fluidity of people dancing together, without any problems, created lasting bonds.

In any major city, one can find a good place to dance and relieve the stress of the day. If you're not quite sure whether a certain crowd is for you, ask around. You may find an all-women's club, a club for people under 21 or over 25, a club that strictly plays house music, or a club that does heavy metal or rock. You may even find a smoke-free and/or alcohol- and drug-free place to dance. The sky's the limit in the club scene.

For the greatest health benefits, drink seltzer or spring water so you don't get dehydrated when dancing. If you are a Saturday night dancer, add other forms of exercise such as a regular walk to your life, so that you get out and move around at least three times a week. Dance and enjoy!

Making It Happen

Be patient and diligent—the results won't come right away—but if you stick to it, you'll soon notice the difference. Don't, however, beat yourself up if you skip a workout. It is important to love and accept yourself no matter what stage you are at in any process. You are the only you that you've got, so be kind and gentle to yourself while you push your limits and stretch beyond what's comfortable.

To exercise regularly, you will need to make fitness a priority. Otherwise, "life" will always interfere. Exercising 20 to 30 minutes three times a week is what is generally recommended for fitness. *But exercising once or twice a week is better than not exercising at all.* Try scheduling time *(I put it in my datebook and treat it like any other meeting—no canceling)* or adding activity to your daily routine. You can take the stairs (or walk up a couple of flights and then take the elevator), park your car at the far end of the lot, take a walk on your lunch hour, run errands on a bicycle, or play catch with the kids.

Don't let any excuse you can fabricate stop you. The benefits outweigh any argument you can conjure up not to exercise. Last year I had a revelation and just changed my life through nutrition and exercise. I educated myself about food and committed myself to exercise. I had a lot of support, but I did it for myself. It's a lifestyle change; that is the only way to look at it.

I get up early in the morning before my family and do yoga for 15 to 20 minutes. I usually fit in an aerobic and Nautilus workout twice a week during my lunch hour (I work near the Y). My daughter is taking a kids' class at the Y, so I'm there on Saturdays, too.

Setting Goals

Start out with realistic, attainable goals. Meet them first, and then set a new set of goals.

The effect of any exercise program is determined by three things: frequency (the number of times each week that you work out), intensity (how hard you work), and duration (how long you work). Your exercise goals may be modest (to walk around the block three times a week) or more ambitious (to jog for 20 minutes at a moderate pace three times a week and to do a strength-training workout once a week). After you've grown comfortable with your new fitness program, you may "ramp up" to a 30- or 40-minute period of aerobic exercise and strength training two or three times each week. But the most important thing is to do what feels comfortable and possible for you.

You might want to chart your progress to remind you of how far you've come and give you a sense of success early on.

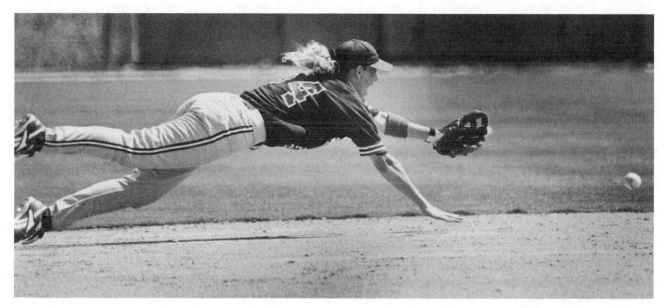

Laura Wulf/Stock, Boston

Team Sports

Team sports are wonderful. I've been seriously playing sports since high school. I've been rowing for eight years now. It gives me a close working bond with the other women on my team. It makes me feel that my body is a tool rather than an ornament.

I love to work out, especially on school teams— basketball, track, or volleyball. I feel accomplished after a workout. On a sports team, performing well is always a gratifying thing.

More and more of us are participating in group sports—practicing more often and developing our skills more seriously than ever before, whether in school or in city or town leagues. Basketball, volleyball, and softball have always been and continue to be very popular; soccer, rugby, and ice hockey are relatively new in popularity and growing. The challenge, excitement, and great satisfaction come when you're out there on the court or field or ice as a part of a group with everyone playing hard, and you make it all click. There is nothing else like it. And who would miss the socializing afterward—the jokes, the stories about last year, and plans for next season.

If you want to join a team, look for the one that is right for you. Some are very competitive—winning is all. Others are more fun-oriented: every woman gets to play in every game, people take turns playing different positions and help each other improve. You might want to talk to the coach or watch a practice; the coach often sets the tone for the whole team.

Some team sports give your body a well-rounded workout, and some don't. Basketball, soccer, rugby, and hockey are great for cardiovascular fitness and general body strength. They are strenuous, so you usually need to build up to them. Softball and volley-ball are less rigorous. If you play a sport where you stand around waiting for the ball to come to you, some aerobic activity would be a good adjunct. Pregame warmup for all group sports is essential.

TAKING CARE OF OURSELVES

It's important that we look out for our own safety and well-being when we exercise. Here are some suggestions to make exercise comfortable, fun, and safe.

- Wear clothes that are loose and allow you a full range of motion. Sweatpants, loose shorts, T-shirts, and leotards are all good options. For walking, you will need a good pair of comfortable shoes. For running, you will need well-fitted, well-padded running shoes (not sneakers); expect to pay anywhere from $40 to $90. For vigorous exercise, you may want to invest in a sports bra. If chafing is a problem, consider wearing exercise tights.
- If you have or suspect any physical limitations, check with your health care provider before embarking on an exercise program.
- For safety's sake, walk or run where and when there are people around. If this isn't possible, go with a friend or take a dog or a whistle. When walking or running alone, be aware of your surroundings (don't bliss out to the tunes on your Walkman). Watch out for cars, bikes, and "crazies." Act confident. Keep an eye on anyone who makes you uncomfortable. Be seen—wear something reflective after dark. Walk or run against the traffic; bike with the traffic.
- If bicycling, always wear a helmet. As with other sports, it's important to always wear well-fitted safety equipment. This may include helmets, padding, safety glasses, or mouth guards.

- In the cold weather, wear layers of clothing that you can shed as you warm up (remember that you lose a lot of heat through your hands and your head, so gloves and a hat may be key to a comfortable walk or run).
- Every sport, exercise, and activity has its own history and its own techniques. Consider taking a lesson and reading up on your sport.
- If it's helpful to you, find like-minded individuals to work out with. (*If I did not have my partner with me [at the gym] I would be at home now watching* ER *and eating Doritos.*) Or you may prefer to exercise alone, to use this time to think or relax.
- Always warm up and cool down to prevent injury. Start by stretching gently and then spend the first five to ten minutes warming up to your walk or your swim. This will loosen up your muscles and help prevent injury. Spend the last two to five minutes of your workout tapering off. After you stop, take the time to stretch again to prevent your muscles getting sore and tight (this is caused by the release of lactic acid during exercise). The ultimate luxury is to follow your workout with a long hot bath or shower.
- Vary the intensity of your physical activity. Some days it will be harder to exercise than others, so be sure to give yourself credit for being out there trying. Other days your workouts will be like magic; you will be amazed at your own strength, and you will work out a little bit harder.
- Drink plenty of water (or electrolyte-balanced sports drinks, if you prefer them). Try to avoid alcohol and caffeinated drinks, which increase dehydration.
- It is best not to eat heavily right before or right after exercising. In general, try to eat well and get enough rest.
- If you feel dizzy or faint, or if something really hurts, STOP.

Injuries

Occasionally you will stretch the ligaments of a joint too far, or maybe even tear them (a sprain) or pull a muscle or a tendon in much the same way (a strain). Unless the injury is severe, you can treat it yourself. As we get more in touch with our bodies, we are often able to sense what we can heal by ourselves and what needs professional help. For a sprain, think RICE: rest, ice, compress, and elevate the injured part. Apply cold immediately and for the next twenty-four to seventy-two hours. Ice for 20 to 30 minutes, then remove the ice for 20 to 30 minutes. Ice, along with wrapping the injured area (not too tight—you want to slow circulation, not stop it) and keeping it elevated, minimizes pain and swelling. At the end of this period you can switch to moist heat. Begin gentle movement as soon as possible; when you are ready to start full-scale exercising again, bind the area evenly (not too tight) for support and go easy. If in the meantime you are climbing the walls, be physical with the rest of your body; swimming might be a possibility, for example.

Here are some guidelines for avoiding injury:

- Warm up before your exercise.
- Start your activity slowly.
- Slow down and cool off after exercise.
- Drink plenty of water.
- Use the proper equipment for your activity.
- Don't overdo it.
- Increase gradually.
- Rest.
- Pay attention to the weather.
- Listen to your body.

Too Much Exercise?

You want physical activity to become a habit. In rare instances, however, it becomes an addiction: the activity controls the person, rather than the person controlling the activity. If you find yourself resentful at any interruption in your usual exercise program, such as illness, injury, bad weather, or other social arrangements, you may want to think about the place of exercise in your life. Are you trying to avoid problems such as a faltering relationship or a bad work situation by running 50 miles every week? Is exercise a way to make yourself so exhausted that you can't feel anything else? Are you keeping track of every ounce of weight, every contour, every inch of muscle and fat as you develop the "perfect" body? These are all signs that exercise has taken control of your life.

If exercise is becoming a problem, keep these points in mind:

- Rest is an essential part of a good exercise program; a day off gives you more, not less, control over your life.
- It is possible to be too thin; a certain amount of body fat is necessary to sustain life.
- Overexercise may lead to sports-induced anemia as well as changes in your menstrual cycle (see p. 91). It may also weaken your immune system, making you more susceptible to colds, flus, and other viruses.
- With exercise there is a point of diminishing returns; beyond a certain point, nothing can be gained by more exercise.[3]

THE POLITICS OF SPORTS

On the night of September 20, 1973, Billie Jean King played Bobby Riggs in an exhibition match in the Houston Astrodome; the nationally televised tennis match was seen by 40 million viewers. Riggs had earlier defeated Margaret Court in a similar exhibition. King arrived courtside carried on a sedan chair by four bare-chested men; Riggs entered riding in a rickshaw, pulled by several women known as "Bobby's Bosom Buddies."[4] Representative Bella Abzug quipped that

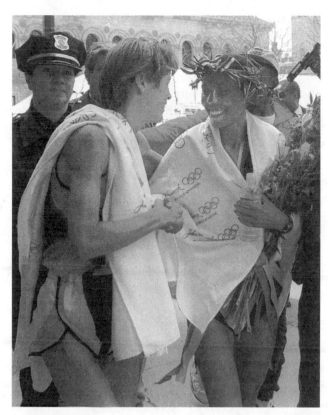

Three-time winner of the Boston Marathon Uta Pippig congratulates 1997 winner Fatuma Roba/*Jim Davis*/*Boston Globe*

the match afforded her the opportunity to "make book" with half a dozen of her fellow members of the U.S. Congress (yes, even our congressional representatives bet on sports!). It was great, good fun. And then they got down to playing. King bested Riggs (6–4, 6–3, 6–3). We finally had proof, in prime time, of what we had known all along: that a female pro tennis player could compete with a man and win. Much has changed since then. Or has it?

Title IX of the Educational Amendments of 1972, which mandated that educational institutions that receive federal funding provide equal opportunity for women athletes, is slowly changing women's scholastic sports. The commercial success of women's college basketball has lead to the formation of two professional women's leagues, complete with superstars,[5] and soccer is not far behind. We now have professional women's golf and tennis circuits. And we won't soon forget the starring role of women athletes in the 1996 summer Olympics. From gymnastics to track and field, softball, basketball, and soccer, U.S. women excelled in Atlanta. But while elite competition is exciting to watch, it is important that we become participants in sports, not just consumers. Each of us, no matter what age or color or ability, is entitled to experience the sheer joy that comes from movement.

But as women's sports increase in popularity and take their place on the national stage, we also need to ask ourselves some questions. What does it mean

when the big, burly coach asks the injured young woman gymnast to take her final vault to clinch the gold for the team? What does it mean when a male millionaire financially underwrites an all-women's America's Cup sailing team? Or when a brewing company underwrites a professional women's softball league? Why is it that the sports press titters about lesbians in the locker room and how a woman's breasts get in the way of a golf swing? Why is it, as Mariah Burton Nelson asks, that the stronger women get, the more men love football?[6]

These are questions that go deep into the heart of our society. Though women are taking to the courts and fields, sports is an industry controlled by men. We are breaking our way into a male cultural domain, and change comes slowly. We have much to contemplate as we lace up our shoes and go for a run, or nip off to the pool for a couple of quick laps.

NOTES

1. M. A. Fiatarone et al., "Exercise Training and Nutritional Supplementation for Physical Frailty in Very Elderly People," *New England Journal of Medicine* 330, no. 25 (1994): 1769–775. Also see Barbara Huebner, "Lift Weights, Lift Depression?" *Boston Globe,* Nov. 18, 1996, p. C1; and J. F. Nichols et al. "Efficacy of Heavy-Resistance Training for Active Women over 60: Muscular Strength, Body Composition and Program Adherence," *Journal of American Geriatrics Society* 41, no. 3, (March 1993): 205.
2. Huebner, "Lift Weights."
3. Jane E. Brody, "You Can't Exercise Too Much, Right? Wrong," *The New York Times,* Aug. 21, 1991. p. C10.
4. Allen Guttmann, *Women's Sports: A History* (New York: Columbia University Press, 1991), 210.
5. Tarik El-Bashir, "Women's N.B.A. Allocates the Superstars," *The New York Times,* Jan. 23, 1997, p. B14.
6. Mariah Burton Nelson, *The Stronger Women Get, the More Men Love Football: Sex and Sports in America* (Orlando, FL: Harcourt Brace, 1994).

RESOURCES

Books and Journals

Blais, Madeleine. *In These Girls, Hope Is a Muscle.* New York: Atlantic Monthly Press, 1995.

Cahn, Susan K. *Coming on Strong: Gender and Sexuality in Twentieth-Century Women's Sport.* Cambridge, MA: Harvard University Press, 1995.

Fahey, Thomas D., and Gayle Hutchinson. *Weight Training for Women.* Mountain View, CA: Mayfield Publishing, 1992.

Martins, Peter. *New York City Ballet Workout.* New York: Morrow, 1997.

The Melpomene Journal. Available from The Melpomene Institute (see "Organizations").

Nelson, Mariah Burton. *The Stronger Women Get, the More Men Love Football: Sex and Sports in America*. Orlando, FL: Harcourt Brace, 1994.

Nelson, Miriam E., and Sarah Wernick. *Strong Women Stay Young*. New York: Bantam Books, 1997.

Rodgers, Bill, and Scott Douglas. *Bill Rodgers' Lifetime Running Plan*. New York: HarperCollins, 1996.

Samuelson, Joan Benoit, and Gloria Averbuch. *Joan Benoit Samuelson's Running for Women*. Emmaus, PA: Rodale Press, 1995.

Simkin, Ariel, and Judith Ayalon. *Bone Loading: Exercises for Osteoporosis*. London: Prion, 1990.

Sports, Everyone! Recreation and Sports for the Physically Challenged of All Ages. Cleveland, OH: Conway Green Publishing, 1995.

Women's Sports and Fitness. Boulder, CO; (800) 877-5281 (subscriptions); Web site: www.women.com.

Organizations

Achilles Track Club
42 West 38th Street; New York, NY 10018; (212) 354-0300; Fax: (212) 354-3978
E-mail: achilles@aol.com
Affiliated with the New York Road Runners Club; encourages people with all types of disabilities to participate in running.

Melpomene Institute
1010 University Avenue; St. Paul, MN 55104; (612) 642-1951
E-mail: melpomene@skypoint.com
Web site: http://www.melpomene.org

National Black Women's Health Project—Walking for Wellness
1211 Connecticut Avenue NW, Suite 310; Washington, DC 20036; (202) 835-0117
E-mail: NBWHPDC@aol.com
A grass-roots effort that fosters community-based walking groups.

Special Olympics
1325 G Street NW, Suite 500; Washington, DC 20005; (202) 628-3630
E-mail: specialolympics@msn.com
Web site: http://www.specialolympics.org
Organizes sporting events for mentally and physically disabled athletes.

United States Organization for Disabled Athletes
143 California Avenue; Uniondale, NY 11553; (800) 25USODA

Women's Sports Foundation
Eisenhower Park; East Meadow, NY 11554; (800) 227-3988
E-mail: wosport@aol.com
A nonprofit, educational organization that promotes and enhances the sports experience for all girls and women. Send for their literature list.

YMCA/YWCA, YMHA/YWHA, and Community Centers
These organizations offer low-cost or no-cost fitness programs. Check your phone book for what's in your area.

Exercising for a cause: Many of us have found that we can exercise and raise money for the causes that we believe in at the same time. Not only are these events a lot of fun, but they can also help us to focus our training. In the Boston area, some of our favorite annual events are Project Bread's Walk for Hunger and the Boston–New York AIDS Ride. Events that take place nationally include the following:

Race for the Cure
Susan G. Komen Breast Cancer Foundation; (800) 462-9273
Sponsors three-mile road races and fun walks in more than 35 cities throughout the year.

Walktoberfest
American Diabetes Association; (800) 254-WALK
10-K (6.2-mile) walking events during the first weekend of October.

Many thanks to everyone who responded to our questionaires—you all are awesome!

Additional Online Resources *

Empowering Women in Sports
http://www.feminist.org/research/sports2.html

FitnessLink: The Health and Fitness Source!
http://www.fitnesslink.com

FitnessZone Searchable Fitness Library
http://www.fitnesszone.com/library

The Internet's Fitness Resource
http://rampages.onramp.net/~chaz

WWW Women's Sports Page
http://fiat.gslis.utexas.edu/~lewisa/womsprt.html

---

* For more information and listings of online resources, please see Introduction to Online Women's Health Resources, p. 25.

By April Taylor, with Claire M. Cassidy
(Acupuncture) and Ellen Fineberg
(Homeopathy), based on earlier work
by Pamela Berger and
Nancy Miriam Hawley

WITH SPECIAL THANKS TO Adriane
Fugh-Berman*

Chapter 5

Holistic Health and Healing: Navigating Your Way to Better Health

* Thanks also to the following for their help with the 1998 version of this chapter: Amy Crickelair, Donna Mills Currie, Pearlyn Goodman-Herrick, Margaret Henshaw, Karen Kirchoff, and Alexandra Todd; also Ted Chapman and Javier Olairu. Over the years since 1982, the following have contributed to the many versions of this chapter: Savitri Clarke, Rose Dubosz, Mary Fillmore, Jon Kabat-Zinn, Pamela Pacelli, Jane Pincus, Billie Pivnik, Lori Ponge, Susan Reverby, and Linnie Smith.

Many women today are excited by the increasing availability of a broad range of holistic health care methods that complement and challenge conventional Western medicine (also known as "biomedicine" or "allopathic") and expand our options for caring for ourselves. Some holistic methods, such as massage, herbal medicine, and spiritual healing, have been used by women for centuries to soothe and care for members of our families and communities, to assist during labor and birth, and to attend to people through long illnesses. Much of this information has been handed down from mother to daughter.[1] Other nonbiomedical healing methods such as acupuncture and tai chi, yoga and Ayurvedic medicine, which originated thousands

of years ago in China and India, respectively, involve more formal training of practitioners. These traditional Eastern methods of healing are practiced in many parts of the world.

In the U.S., these health care practices are often called "complementary" or "alternative." In much of the world, however, they are the most commonly used methods of healing. In this chapter, we name these methods of healing "holistic health care" because we believe that it is an important political act to acknowledge that the interconnection between body, mind, and spirit is fundamental to well-being and that these methods of healing were used by our ancestors long before the development of biomedicine.

The rapid spread of holistic health practices in the U.S. is evident everywhere and is attributable to the costs, inefficiencies, and limitations of biomedicine. Over the last ten years, we have seen a tremendous increase in the availability of books, articles, and research reports that address holistic health methods; in the number of health food stores and pharmacies that carry herbs, homeopathic remedies, and nutritional supplements; and in the number of practitioners offer-

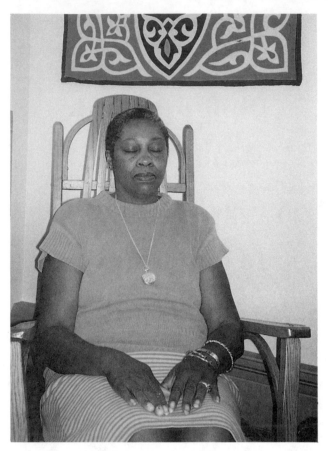

Elana Rosenbaum

ing holistic care. In 1992, the Office on Alternative Medicine was established at the National Institutes of Health, in Washington, DC, to study and research the efficacy and safety of a wide range of holistic health care methods. A year later, the *New England Journal of Medicine (NEJM)* reported that in 1990, Americans made 425 million visits to providers of "unconventional" therapy and spent roughly $10.3 billion out of pocket (i.e., not covered by health insurance) on these health care methods.[2]

It is important to learn and practice some holistic care methods ourselves, with the help of books and knowledgeable friends. We can also visit holistic care practitioners who have extensive training and expertise. Some of us may decide to go further, apprenticing with teachers and practitioners or, in some cases, taking courses that lead to diplomas and licensing. Holistic care can help us stay healthy when we are well, cure some illnesses, help us tolerate the side effects of biomedicine, and enable us to live more comfortably with disorders for which Western medicine has no known cures.

UNDERLYING ASSUMPTIONS
OF HOLISTIC HEALING

Fundamental to holistic healing is the idea that the body, mind, and spirit form an integrated whole and that the individual is deeply connected to herself, her

environment, and her community. Healing is based on the principle of rebalancing body and spirit.

Holistic healing begins with the following assumptions:

1. We are healthy when our body/mind/spirit exist in a balanced state of well-being.

2. In the broadest sense, our relations and interactions with ourselves, our families, and our communities affect and shape our health. Positive, loving, supportive relationships keep us healthy and give us opportunities to nurture and heal others. Equally important is the larger social, economic, political, and ecological context, which affects us through the nutritional content of our foods; the dangerous chemicals in the products we buy and are exposed to; the energy sources we use; the air we breathe; the hostility we face in the form of racism, sexism, homophobia and so on; and, most important, the financial and educational resources available to us. It is as crucial to try to achieve a balance between the individual and her surroundings as it is to balance body, mind, and spirit.

3. We have a great capacity for self-healing. Our cells are always engaged in the process of self-renewal, for our bodies continuously break down and build up structures, with tissues and organs replacing their cells in an ongoing process (with the exception of brain cells). We experience the physical body repairing itself in many ways—for instance, when scraped skin heals itself in a few days or when the eye tears and washes away a foreign particle. In addition, we may consciously use the mind to focus healing energies on those aspects of our being that are hurt or feel unbalanced. We can use physical touch, as with massage, to help us relax, release tension, and relieve pain.

We ourselves play a significant role in holistic healing. We must bring to the process a willingness to heal. While the desire to regain our health is not in itself necessarily sufficient for healing, it helps to fully focus our energies on restoring balance. At the same time, we must understand that sound health practices promote well-being (and may be a source of pleasure in their own right), but they do not guarantee longevity or freedom from illness.

A major piece of staying healthy is the condition of our immune system, which is our body's mechanism for fighting disease. Although we cannot always guarantee that our immune system won't be attacked by the toxins in the air we breathe or by the pesticides on the food we eat, we can strive to keep our immune system healthy by incorporating regular exercise and a healthy diet. Some of us may choose to use vitamin and mineral supplements, and medicinal herbs such as echinacea, ginger, or garlic. We can also try to limit our exposure to substances and situations that compromise our health and well-being. Though our ability to do so may be limited by our economic circumstances, the neighborhoods we live in, and the products available to us, we can always strive toward keeping healthy.

Though the words "heal" and "cure" are often used interchangeably, they are not synonymous. Sometimes no cures exist for particular diseases, yet people feel "healed"—that is, able to reconcile themselves to, accept, and live with the effects of chronic conditions or even terminal illnesses. Illness can provide opportunities for self-examination, growth, and change, as seen in the experiences of the following two women:

I was in my 44th year when I began experiencing what I called "fatigue." Weeks of "good night's rest" did not change my stiffness and pain on arising. I had a three-year-old daughter, two teenage sons, a husband, and a part-time job; I loved them all, I had no time to be sick or feel pain. When I found myself holding the wall as well as the banister to creep down the stairs one step at a time, I had to admit to myself that something was wrong. My wrists and fingers hurt; my elbows, knees, and ankles; my back, legs, and neck. An orthopedic surgeon told me that I had osteoarthritis.

Now I had to allow myself the luxury of time for exercise classes; a regimen of exercise and aspirin soon made life more possible. I still only resentfully recognized that I probably would never be completely pain-free again. . . . Some days the distance from car to store or bed to bathroom seems the longest and most painful ten miles I could ever walk. Nevertheless, some days are better than others. I have learned to rest on the bad days and to insist on some daily rest even on the good days.

Most important, in seeking to understand why I denied the pain so adamantly when I first felt it, I entered [psycho]therapy and learned how forcefully I had been denying emotional pain. My life is qualitatively different now—and better, even though lived with pain— as a result of my reevaluation of how I feel about myself, my goals, and my relations with others.

I had one of the more remarkable rites of passage experiences as an adult, when I had the experience of being touched by a healer from Maui, a woman who had two of the most powerful cultural and political backgrounds: Native American and African American. She was a Master Reiki and Shiatsu healer—she could help you manage any type of pain. At that time, my fibroids were interrupting my life in a big way, but before she laid her hands on me, she asked me about my life and certain circumstances. She connected to the inner part of my soul and touched upon childhood experiences which were in the way. She, as my Guardian, guided me through a maze of difficulty, and I now feel like I've connected with what caused me my fibroids and have worked myself away from unnecessary forms of negativity and pain.

Since the flow of energy is central to holistic healing, many methods encourage us to imagine our healing as taking place with the help of some form of *energy* that comes from a source within ourselves or from both an internal and external source such as a god or universal being:

As the acute stage of my asthma passes, I relax and further ease my breathing, reduce wheezing by feeling warmth and light flow through me, part of an energy I imagine to be universal energy of which we are all part. As I am able to breathe fully again, I picture myself giving that energy back into the larger cosmos. In a concrete way, this interchange enables me once again to be available to family, friends, and co-workers.

CHOOSING HOLISTIC METHODS AND PRACTITIONERS

Holistic health care is about self-healing and the process of aiming for wellness. We can use it to enhance our well-being in many endeavors of our lives. Thus, it is important for us as women to explore, research, and practice some holistic care methods on our own. We can read books, take courses, attend workshops at local community centers, or listen to the wisdom of our mothers or grandmothers. It is essential that we claim the wisdom and knowledge that is passed down to us—otherwise it may be lost forever.[3]

We must also recognize and reaffirm that women working together in self-help groups can do remarkable work together. These groups can offer support in staying healthy, in healing the wounds created by living in an oppressive and often violent world, and in researching different methods of healing. The National Black Women's Health Project and the Federation of Feminist Women's Health Centers offer support for self-help groups around the country (see chapter 27 Resources). Local institutions may also promote women's health through self-help. In Boston, the Women's Theological Center (WTC) sponsors a wide variety of programs, including a retreat for black women designed to help support our journey of self-healing. A poet who participated in a WTC retreat wrote the following poem affirming the strength and wisdom she felt in being among black women:

MEDICINE IS A WOMAN

I have walked among women, tall like mountains that many try to climb, but never master.
I am alive today because I have encountered such women every time I was near death and I
know such a woman will be there to walk with me to the other side when I die.
I have been hugged by the blazing sun, purified in the arms of such a woman. Her wisdom and affection have been a laying of the hands, midwifing the delivery of my soul into creation.

*When a woman walks towards you whose eyes
    burn like beacons, keep still.
The Egyptian bird of magic is anointing your
    heart, with the knowledge of life's possibilities,
and your power to realize your dreams.
Sink into her eyes, it is she who pollinates the
    petals of desire as she slips into your life singing
a magical incantation just for your ears.
Such women walk among us. Such women walk
    within me. I am such a woman.*

— LINDA KING

When seeking a holistic care provider, you will want to find someone whom you trust, whom you feel comfortable with, and with whom you can communicate. The best health care practitioners do not emphasize the conquest of disease but see themselves as facilitating the healing process and helping you maintain your health. It is important to find someone who works in partnership with you and whose ideas make sense to you. Ideally, you should come away from every encounter feeling more confident in your ability to promote healing in yourself and have the tools you need to make changes in your life.

As with any new endeavor in your life, when deciding on a healing method or a practitioner, you may find it helpful to speak to other people who have tried the method. Ask about the particular practitioner and about the negative as well as positive experiences people have had with this person. The suggestions listed below are good starting points to help advance your quest for better health.

- Form a women's self-help group that has a wide focus, or seek out other women in your community who are interested in getting information about how to approach and heal a certain illness. If there is a women's health center in your area, ask the women there for information, and support their work!
- Get your local library to order books pertinent to your interests and to subscribe to women's health and alternative health publications.
- Explore the politics of the method you want to use. Is it based on a sexist philosophy, or is the practice institutionalized in such a way that it is dominated by white men and members of other elite groups with patriarchal or racist attitudes? Is the particular setting inclusive of women or people of color? Is the practice/practitioner responsive to community needs (e.g., offers free classes, is located near public transportation, and/ or is in a building that is wheelchair accessible)? Ask yourself: Who profits from this mode of healing?
- Know that practitioners must be well trained in their own healing methods. Sometimes training is done through apprenticeship; sometimes schooling is required. If your practitioner is in training, make sure that she or he receives supervision from someone more experienced. A license or training certificate indicates a certain amount of knowledge and standardized training, but no piece of paper ever guarantees a person's ability to heal. Nor does the lack of one mean that a person isn't skillful or knowledgeable.
- You may want to look for practitioners who have sliding-scale fees or who are willing to barter services if you are unable to pay the full rate. A willingness to compromise on fees or a flat, low-income rate may indicate a commitment to accessibility. Often practitioners are able to charge less; though you may feel uncomfortable, it is perfectly acceptable to ask if someone is willing to adjust their fees.
- You may want to combine the least invasive of biomedical diagnostic techniques with the best that holistic methods have to offer. It's important to look for practitioners who are open to any information you may bring from Western medicine and who are able and willing to evaluate it with you.
- Find out how available your practitioner is. Is there a time when you can call to ask questions or discuss concerns?
- Beware of practitioners who offer miraculous cures. Even though you want definite answers, don't accept promises of magical cures any more than you would from practitioners of Western medicine. Occasionally, immediate and dramatic results do occur, but many holistic methods require time and patience.
- Seek out practitioners who listen carefully and are interested in the ways you present your health concerns. Practitioners should be willing to try different approaches and teach you the skills you need to maintain or improve your health. Good practitioners should be especially sensitive to the larger political and economic issues that affect women's health.

When I first sought holistic health care practitioners, I was a little nervous because many of the practitioners and clients didn't look like me, nor did they seem to have a broad cultural understanding. I remember walking into offices where people looked at me as though I were an intruder. But when other folks walked in the office, they were welcomed and greeted graciously. Nonetheless, after many attempts with practitioners who were afraid to touch me because of the color of my skin, I found people who looked like me, felt like me, and were eager to assist me in my struggle to keep healthy in a very unhealthy society.

I asked my friends for recommendations for a yoga teacher, and several suggested one man. When I went to meet him, a voice inside me told me this man was not the teacher for me. I said to myself, "I really want to do yoga; this teacher has been highly recommended;

*perhaps it's because I don't get along well with men."
But that voice kept saying, "I don't want to." I contemplated the matter by sitting down, closing my eyes, and just being quiet. The thought kept rolling through my mind, getting stronger and more persistent: This is not the right teacher for me. I dropped the idea of studying yoga with him.*

In general, when you are seeking any form of care or healing, be as informed and assertive as you can. There are many sincere, skillful, compassionate holistic practitioners and healers. As health care consumers we must look for them, ask them to share their skills with us, and tell our friends about them. While we don't want to become unnecessarily dependent on practitioners, when we work in partnership with them we can develop our ability to maintain a well-balanced body, mind, and spirit.

SOME PROBLEMS WITH HOLISTIC METHODS AND PRACTITIONERS

Holistic modes of healing seem to promise a richer way of practicing health care than the standard practices of Western medicine (drugs and surgery). However, holistic practices and practitioners have some of the same potential drawbacks: lack of accessibility, sexist and/or racist practitioners, practitioners who are unskilled or who practice unproven or unsafe therapies, and professionalization. In addition, just as people are beginning to learn, practice, and share their skills and knowledge, larger economic, social, and political forces are trying to control and regulate our healing methods. For example, many large drug companies (as well as some alternative businesses) are interested in cashing in on the recent popularity of herbs such as echinacea, St. John's wort, and ginseng.

Accessibility

The majority of the holistic practices discussed in this chapter are becoming more widely available to people via insurance, local cultural stores, and community workshops because of the demand from people who wish to stay away from the costly, invasive approaches of Western medicine. In many rural areas, however, the availability of holistic care is quite limited; the vast majority of services still seem to be concentrated on the East and West Coasts and can still be quite costly.

For those who have health insurance, there is a growing trend for some health maintenance organizations (HMOs) or community clinics to offer holistic health services. For example,

- In the state of Washington, health care insurers are required to cover any alternative health care treatment performed.

- In California, proposed legislation mandates that acupuncture be covered under workers' compensation benefits.
- Kaiser-Permanente, a California-based HMO, opened the Alternative Medicine Clinic in 1995, which provides acupuncture, nutritional advice, counseling, and relaxation therapy to Kaiser members.
- Blue Cross of Washington and Alaska, as a result of community pressure and perhaps because it sees an opportunity, has started coverage for alternative medicine including homeopathy, acupuncture, and naturopathy.[4]

The trend toward insurance coverage is certainly a sign that we are seeing the integration of holistic care methods into Western biomedical practices. However, insurance is not a panacea. Holistic care is based on the principle of maintaining balance and staying healthy (i.e., preventive care), while insurance is designed to pay for treatment when we are ill. The grafting of one model onto the other is fraught with difficulties. For example, insurance companies often restrict the duration of treatment, which may have an impact on the quality of care. In the Northeast, two new wellness-focused insurance plans, Oxford and Commonwell, provide alternatives that may prove to be more successful.

Insurance is not a perfect solution for other reasons as well. We live in a society where many people do not have health coverage and, as a result, have extremely limited access to health care or no health care at all. Seeing a holistic practitioner such as an acupuncturist, a homeopath, or a chiropractor can be expensive. The uninsured cannot reap the benefits of these forms of health care until we drastically change our health care system, including challenging the political and economic power of the insurance industry. We all need to work together for change by writing to our legislators, signing petitions, challenging the restrictive policies of our insurance companies, and organizing our own institutions.

Though many holistic care methods are marketed to those who can afford them—middle- and upper-middle-class people—we are also seeing the revival of indigenous healing knowledge. Many groups of black folk still maintain early forms of folk medicine, and Native American peoples have held firmly on to their traditions. As the population of the U.S. changes, emigrants from Africa, Asia, and Latin America bring with them their own family wisdom as well:

When I was a kid, I would always remember my mother boiling a big pot of herbs on the stove. I recall her telling me that many of the roots she knew in Puerto Rico didn't exist here, but there were a few she did know. We would search in local lots and she would find what we needed for an herbal bath, a cold, or just to keep us away from the "wrong" folk. These are the lessons and early foundations of self-care I will never forget and that I strive to keep alive.

Risks of Professionalization

Just as with Western medicine, you can learn a lot from professionals who have information you may need to stay well. However, we live in a time of excessive dependence on experts, which means we often turn to professionals for things we could do on our own. Try to avoid holistic practitioners who discourage the empowerment of their clients by setting themselves up as "experts" and refusing to share their knowledge. Be wary of those who try to get you to keep returning to them for additional services without improvement in your health or quality of life and without clear treatment objectives.

Lack of Social and Political Awareness

When holistic approaches identify the locus of healing only in the individual, as biomedical practice often does, they disregard political factors like poverty and racism as major sources of ill health. For instance, a practitioner might prescribe rest, exercise, and change in diet, and not attend to the fact that health problems might be caused by a dangerous on-the-job situation, the rigors of parenting, or daily encounters with sexism and racism.

Implicit in the practice of holistic healing is that you have a certain responsibility for keeping yourself healthy and for helping yourself get better. While trust in our capacity for self-healing is a welcome change from biomedicine's dependence on outside intervention, some writers and practitioners of holistic health place *too much* emphasis on the individual's responsibility for her own sickness and health. They seem to imply that if you get sick or if you don't get well, it's your fault. They may even ask why you "needed" to get sick. Your "wrong thinking," lack of will, personality defect (e.g., a "cancer personality") or insufficient faith in the practitioner is the real cause of your problems. Note the "blaming the victim" attitude of some early books on holistic healing:

We should not fool ourselves into thinking that disease is caused by an enemy from without. We are responsible for our disease.[5]

The only tyrant you face is your own inertia and absence of will—your belief that you are too busy to take your own well-being into your own hands and that the pursuit of self-health through a wellness promotive lifestyle is too hard, complicated, or inconvenient.[6]

This kind of thinking disregards political and social factors that affect health. Sometimes we become ill no matter how much we try to stay healthy. It is both cruel and inappropriate to blame ourselves or let others blame us for getting sick.

Sexism

Alternative health care does not automatically mean nonsexist or feminist. Like biomedicine, many of these methods are practiced by men and women who have not dealt with their sexism or with other oppressive attitudes and behaviors. Remember that both male and female practitioners can treat us badly, disrespectfully, and even harmfully. We should expect, and demand, that our practitioners treat us as equal partners in the healing process.

Racism and Elitism

When we look at the field of holistic health, we must be cognizant of the roles racism and elitism play in creating care for people of color—just as we must with any system where institutionalized practitioners are the more resourceful and "powerful" members of society. Study after study has shown that social class and race are major indicators to the kind of health care we receive in this country. In many health care settings, white people are in the majority, and many of these people have not dealt with their racism in a way that challenges them to change attitudes and beliefs, share resources, and deal with the painful historical legacy of racism and exclusion in this country. At the same time, it is important to recognize that many people of color have carried with them for many generations their own knowledge and wisdom, which has sustained them. Some institutions that are devoted to holistic health deal with the broader issues of the people they serve. For example, La Clinica de La Raza in California is one model where community-based education and service incorporates the practices of holistic health care services.[7]

Unfortunately, some holistic health centers, organized and operated primarily by people of color, have been targeted and dismantled because of the political affiliation of the founders, as in the case of the Black Holistic Health Center in Harlem.[8]

HOLISTIC APPROACHES

In this section, we describe some holistic healing approaches and give information and guidelines so that you can look further on your own. Because so many methods exist, we have provided information on those most widely available and useful for a wide variety of needs.

When you seek holistic health care, we strongly encourage you to seek support in your own community. Embarking on this journey may mean that you have to change some habits—the way you eat, the way you move, the way you think. Doing something new can feel strange.

I went for my first massage to someone recommended by a friend. Though apprehensive at first, I was quickly reassured by her strong, soothing hands.

Joining a self-help or research group and sharing knowledge with other women can help build your confidence. The more you understand about the methods of healing you choose, the more involved you can be in your own care. A support group can also help you withstand the cynicism and doubt you are likely to encounter from those who put all their faith in Western biomedicine.

I tripped on the sidewalk and hurt myself so badly that I couldn't walk or work. I was taken to the hospital and had X rays. The head orthopedist looked at the X rays and told me that there was nothing wrong with my foot. But I still couldn't walk. At that point I decided to see a chiropractor. I didn't know anything about chiropractors except that they were an alternative to medical doctors. My sister was the only one I knew who had used a chiropractor. When I went to the hospital to pick up my X rays, I told them I was going to visit a certain chiropractor.

"Don't go to him; he's a Communist," they said.

"I don't care what his political beliefs are if he can help me," I answered.

I made an appointment and after he adjusted my back and foot I could walk again in comfort.

Many women do not want to give up Western biomedical care completely, but find it doesn't meet their needs for preventive well-woman care. As a result, they seek out holistic approaches that they can combine with conventional ones:

How do I integrate different health care models in my life? I go to MDs mostly, but I understand their limits. I've done "talk" therapy and get (and give) massages. I take baths for aching muscles—water relaxes. Once in a while I experiment with herbs. I think about the food I eat, take some vitamins, and have done some work with the Alexander Technique, which has helped chronic back and shoulder aches.

One woman discussed her experience with a doctor:

I suffer from migraines, and my neurologist had me on all kinds of drugs for pain management and prophylactic care. It was my goal to get off of the meds I had to take every day, which were very strong blood thinners that supposedly opened the vessels in my brain. Needless to say, the side effects were unbearable. I discovered that feverfew [an herb] has many of the natural components of the synthetic drug I was on. I encouraged my doctor to read up on the herb. He did so, a bit reluctantly, but did confirm that feverfew would eventually give me relief similar to the very strong drug prescribed.

Just as there is no one right way to keep healthy, there is no one right way of healing. Bringing ourselves back into balance can mean something as simple as treating a cold by resting or as complex as totally altering our diet and other life habits to cope with chronic illnesses such as hypertension or arthritis. A method may work for one person or a particular health problem but not for another. Sometimes it is possible to figure out which approach helps the most; at other times it is not so clear, because holistic methods take time. We have to evaluate and make decisions about each situation as it arises; our own experience and intuition and the wisdom of trusted friends, family members, teachers, and professionals will be our best guides.

Holistic care methods include practices that we can learn about and use on our own, such as herbal medicine, meditation, visualization, yoga, tai chi, and some kinds of massage, and practices such as acupuncture and chiropractic, which require obtaining care from a trained practitioner. The latter may sometimes be expensive, but many of the former are accessible to anyone who wishes to learn about them.

Herbs

One very self-empowering way to supplement and maintain our health and well-being is with herbs. The use of medicinal herbs, sometimes known as phytomedicine (*phyto* is Greek for "plant"), has successfully maintained health in many cultures for thousands of years. Indian practitioners of Ayurvedic medicine use herbs; Chinese doctors prescribe herbs along with acupuncture and other forms of traditional Chinese medicine; and in parts of Africa, Europe, and the Americas, herbs continue to sustain and support our health as we go about our daily activities. Though we may think of herbs as a source of "alternative" healing, according to the World Health Organization, herbal medicine is the primary therapy for over three-quarters of the world's peoples.[9] About a quarter of our pharmaceutical drugs are derived from herbs.[10]

The key to using any herbal formula or remedy is knowledge and experience. Some herbs are very dangerous, and some may become toxic in the system if used for prolonged periods of time. Some are contraindicated for certain people but helpful to others. If you're using herbs for the first time, investigate and read as much as possible before beginning to use them. If at all possible, take a workshop or course to assist you in the process. When seeking out a professional, make sure you inform her or him of any medicines you are taking, of allergies, of foods you eat, of sleep and work habits. It is important for the herbalist to have a good sense of your overall health. In the U.S., many people are turning to Chinese medicine and its vast pharmacopoeia (over 2,000 herbs) of herbal medicine. If you decide to try Chinese medicine, it is important to find a practitioner who is knowlegeable about Chinese diagnosis. He or she will check your pulse and look at your tongue, skin, and eyes before deciding on an herbal formula, as the herbs prescribed will vary according to your constitution and pattern of symptoms.

Some herbs can be planted at home and dried for

future use, or they can be bought fresh or dried in many herb or grocery shops. Health food stores carry many herbs, along with vitamins and minerals, in capsule form. Some of the most popular herbs used today include garlic and goldenseal, which are natural antibiotics and immune enhancers; echinacea, which helps to cure colds and other upper respiratory ailments; ginger and peppermint, which help with digestion; and valerian, which reduces stress.

When I feel a cold coming on, I immediately take goldenseal and echinacea. Usually, within 24 hours, I'm fine. I used to often get bronchitis in the winter, but I haven't had it in years.

Women can use herbs for a wide range of health needs. In the area of reproductive health, herbs can be used to assist in toning and strengthening the uterus so that our reproductive organs function properly, to alleviate the symptoms of menstrual discomfort and pain, to help regulate our hormones, and to help with vaginal dryness and hot flashes during menopause.

Here are some of the herbs that can be used to keep our reproductive systems healthy:

- **For strengthening our uterus and ovaries:** raspberry, squaw vine, motherwort, false unicorn root, chaste tree, dong quai (except in the case of uterine fibroids).
- **For stimulating a normal menstrual flow:** yarrow, parsley, evening primrose, squaw vine, ginger, black and blue cohosh.
- **To soothe and calm us:** cramp bark, oats, skullcap, valerian, damiana, peppermint, chamomile.[11]

I suffered from excruciating menstrual cramps and had tried practically everything. A friend of mine who was studying to be an acupuncturist said I should try going to a Chinese herbalist for my problem. I didn't even hesitate. I walked into the office, and I was the only black woman in the room. Although my presence was quite noticeable, it didn't seem to faze the people sitting there. When I walked into the doctor's office, I could smell the strong mixture of herbs. He asked me what my problem was, then placed my hand on a black velvet cushion and took my pulse. He told me to stick out my tongue, which he said was heavily coated, and he looked at my skin. He told me not only of the problems with my period but asked me about diabetes, the pains in my neck and shoulders, and the lower left back pain I was experiencing. Girl, I almost fell out of my chair! He said he could write me a prescription for herbs to take every week for the next nine weeks—thereafter, he assured me I wouldn't have a problem. I did it—it tasted horribly bitter but I have noticed a tremendous difference. Now I'm considering going back to deal with those other problems.

Quieting the Mind

There are several holistic care practices that we can learn and practice on our own or with others. Many of them developed as spiritual practices in Eastern and South Asian cultures. Here we discuss meditation, yoga, and tai chi: practices in which we "quiet the mind" in order to be more present in our bodies and to renew the balance of body/mind/spirit. Recent studies have shown that these practices can slow the heartbeat, lower blood pressure, decrease muscle tension, and decrease the secretion of hormones related to stress.[12] Many people begin practicing meditation, yoga, or tai chi in order to deal with the health consequences of too much stress.

Meditation

Meditation gives us the opportunity to commune and connect with our inner selves. A simple definition of meditation is "the intentional paying of attention from moment to moment." In the words of a woman who has been meditating and teaching meditation for 15 years:

Meditation in its essence is different from every other human activity, but its essence is contained in every activity. Meditating, each one of us touches base with our deepest concerns, with the truth of our aliveness. . . . You could say it is acknowledging the radiant core of our being . . . our godliness, our Buddha nature, or whatever you like to call it.

Meditating, at its best, places us in touch with the moment and helps us respond directly to our innermost thoughts. If we are meditating, we are likely to be more alert and resourceful. People begin to meditate for different reasons: because it feels good, or because they want to feel calm, to diminish physical and mental stress or pain, or to get through a crisis. You might approach meditation only for practical reasons, then discover that something happens that makes you want to go deeper, to attain a different level of consciousness and a deeper, more gratifying state of relaxation.

There are many ways to meditate. Though you can meditate while you stand, walk, dance, or jog, many people sit or kneel in a quiet environment. Some meditate while carrying out daily activities such as washing the dishes. Some people repeat a word or sound over and over again to calm the mind; another method is to concentrate on your breath, focusing your attention on the rise and fall of your abdomen or on the feeling of the air entering and leaving your body. You can meditate at home indoors or outdoors, or in formal settings: churches, synagogues, mosques, temples, or ashrams. Some people enjoy meditating alone; others meditate in the company of family members, friends, self-help groups, or spiritual communities. Though meditation is a way of focusing one's attention inward, group meditation can create deep and lasting bonds between people.

You can learn meditation on your own using books or tapes, or you can work with a religious or secular teacher. As your practice develops, you are likely to find that meditation helps you pull your life together:

My early-morning meditation is part silence, part chanting. Sometimes I actively pray while I sit looking out the window at the rising sun. It's important for me to meditate every morning, if only for ten minutes to touch base with myself. I am continually surprised at how I get upset more easily on the days I don't meditate. Sometimes during the day when I'm silent or alone I find myself automatically feeling the tranquility I experience during meditation. This calmness helps me. Though usually my meditations are rather ordinary, on some days they are profound.

Yoga

The aim of yoga is to renew the body, focus the mind, and still the emotions. *Yoga* is a Sanskrit word that essentially means "union." Underlying yoga practice is the belief that "the body and mind are part of the continuum of existence, the mind merely being more subtle than the body."[13]

The basic aspects of yoga practice include *asanas, pranayama,* and concentrated thought. Asanas are physical postures that help stretch and limber the body. Pranayama are breathing exercises that increase the flow of oxygen, thereby relaxing the body. All the exercises emphasize awareness—awareness of the movements and the breathing, of areas of flexibility and tightness, and of applying your mind to the task.

When doing yoga postures, I was asked to move slowly into the posture, to hold it still for some time, and then to gradually release. This way of exercising has dramatic effects on my mind. I often begin in some turmoil, filled with the concerns of my day. As I focus my attention on my movements and my breathing, I experience my mind slowing down and relaxing. The practice gives me some distance from my problems. Doing the postures releases new energy, relaxes me, and allows for another perspective to emerge.

Studies demonstrate the benefits of regular yoga practice. These include physiological changes such as reduced blood pressure, lowered pulse rates, diminished stress, increased joint movement, and improved hormonal functioning. Several studies have confirmed that yoga has therapeutic value for respiratory ailments including chronic bronchitis and asthma.[14]

We can learn yoga on our own by using books, records, and tapes. However, there is no substitute for a good teacher who can provide individualized help with the various techniques. Yoga classes are taught in local Y's, adult education programs, college extension

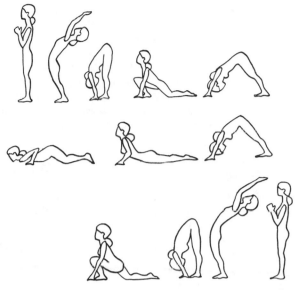

Jane Pincus

programs, dance and fitness centers. Whether you practice for 15 minutes a day or for more extended times, it is important to practice regularly.

The problems with yoga are the problems of any healing method applied improperly. If you feel pain, it is a good idea to stop, rather than pushing through to complete the exercise no matter what. You need to proceed at your own pace. In all these practices, it is important to pay attention to the fine line between simply exerting yourself and pushing beyond your limits—and this is different for everyone. Beware of perfectionism and athleticism. Benefits come from your efforts rather than from reaching a specific goal.

I get up in the morning and do the exercise "Salute to the Sun" [actually a series of 12 postures]. Whether I have a few minutes or a longer time to practice yoga, I benefit from the fullness of this exercise. I am cheered by the thought of saluting the sun. I am easily moved beyond the awkwardness of my body and the sleepy nature of my mind as I get into the movement of this exercise. After a while I am ready to welcome the day.

Tai Chi

Practiced for at least one thousand years, tai chi is a martial art form that originated in China.[15] Tai chi is a form of gentle movement, which anyone can do to condition and tone the body. The meditative grace of each movement is produced through concentration and the centering of the mind, which creates flows in energy. The person practicing tai chi is instructed on how to move the head and each leg, foot, hand, and arm in a deliberately graceful and coordinated movement. Tai chi can provide the health benefits of more strenuous exercise without straining the heart.[16]

I remember when a group of us were attending the Fourth World Conference on Women in Beijing in

1995. We were eager to see the Chinese practice the art form of tai chi in the early morning hours. The guide book told us to get to the parks at the crack of dawn to witness a number of techniques used. We all gathered around 5:30 in the morning, but the sun was already up so we had to hurry. When we arrived we saw the most breathtaking scene: many people, mainly elderly, were working in unison, gently swaying and chanting. . . . It was unforgettable!

As with yoga, tai chi instruction is often available through Y's or community health centers. You might also seek out feminist teachers of other martial arts who can teach you practical responses to verbal and physical assault while also training you in the mind/body concentration that is central to these practices.

Visualization

Visualization is somewhat similar to meditation practice in that it uses the mind to focus healing energy on the body. The practice of visualization has been formalized within biomedicine as *autogenic training*.[17] It is increasingly being used to modify blood flow, slow the heartbeat, and help us heal specific organs or conditions such as gastritis, gallbladder attacks, irritable colon, hemorrhoids, constipation, angina, headaches, asthma, diabetes, arthritis, low back pain, skin conditions, and thyroid disease.[18] Some cancer specialists use visualization in conjunction with drugs, surgery, and radiation to relieve stress caused by both the illness and its treatment and to help those living with the disease focus their energy on healing. Some studies indicate that meditation and visualization techniques can help us strengthen the immune system and, therefore, the body's response to cancer and other disease.[19]

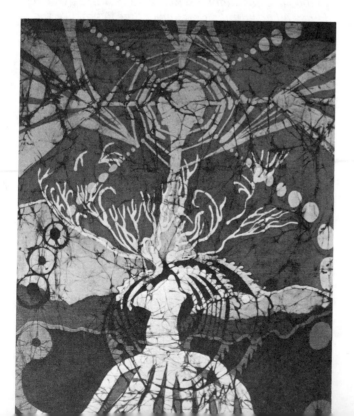

Many women find that visualizing a certain symbol, scene, or process has a positive healing effect on their bodies. Midwives have long used images and relaxation exercises to help women in labor relax, diminish fear or tension, and open up. The earliest records of visualization techniques used in healing date back to ancient Babylonia and Sumeria; many indigenous peoples continue to use these techniques today.

Visualization works in a general way by helping us relax. We are then more easily able to affect the involuntary systems of the body or to control pain. In the words of a scientist who underwent several operations for cancer:

The two years since I had the last operation have been the most productive of my life. I've had the opportunity to investigate healing in a way that I never did before. At first, when I felt the pain, I kept looking for an outside figure, a god figure, to help me, to care for me, to make it better. Then I said to myself, "Who's the most caring, best mother you know?" And I said, "I am." So I pictured myself cuddling myself. When the pain came, I went to it as a mother would to a child. I said, "How can I help it? How can I go to it?" Now when it comes, I say, "Poor baby." I tried to treat myself in a loving way. The more loving I was to myself, the more healed I felt. Now the pain is mostly gone.

Visualization involves relaxing; feeling at one with the object, scene, or process you imagine; and letting it expand to fill your consciousness until it becomes the only thing in your awareness. Hold your mind upon it. Sometimes it helps to have someone guide you. Some people must practice this meditative visualization; it is a skill to be learned. Others do it more quickly. Here is an example of a healing visualization:

Relax and let your attention go to the particular body part causing discomfort or pain, or which does not function as it should. Focus your attention on this place, and let yourself experience what it feels like right now. Don't feel pressured to achieve a specific goal. After a while, allow an image related to that area to come to your mind. It may be a detailed picture of what you think that part looks like, or it may be more abstract. Keep your mind focused until you are content with your image. Change it whenever you want. Now begin to visualize something happening within that part of your body to make it work better or start to heal. You might see energy, light, or color flowing into it; imagine it becoming warm or cool. A powerful image could help you feel better right away.

If visualization doesn't work for you, it may mean that you take in information in other ways than by using images. For example, you might do it through

One visual image: a strongly rooted tree
/Batik by Jane Pincus

your ears, so imagining sounds might be your way of "visualizing." Refer to the Resources at the end of this chapter to learn more and to discover other techniques that can help you use your mind to improve your health.

Bodywork

In this section, we discuss two forms of holistic care that focus on the muscles and skeletal structure of the body. Massage is a technique that we can sometimes do on our own (massaging those parts of our bodies we can reach) or with family or friends, or we can pay a trained practitioner; chiropractic care is done by licensed practitioners who adjust the alignment of our vertebrae to improve our overall health.

Massage

Touching is one of the most natural ways we have to communicate and to comfort one another. Whether it's with a simple hug or a complete body rub, we can help one another feel better:

Foot rubs are my favorite kind of massage. They bring back childhood memories of my father rubbing my feet; they feel so good to give and to get. My children often ask me to hold and rub their feet when I go into their rooms to say good night. Some of my friends and I exchange them as a way of being close and helping each other relax.

When done effectively, massage relaxes the body, releases muscle tension, improves joint flexibility, increases circulation and sensation, and generally enhances our well-being. Massage and manipulative techniques involve prolonged and intense touching, pulling, pressing, and rubbing. For this reason, you should not get a massage if you have phlebitis, skin infections, blood clots, redness, or skin that has become thin as a result of burn or injury. You should also check with your health care provider about having a massage if you have cancer that has spread throughout your body.

We can use many massage techniques on ourselves as well as on others. The massage methods most familiar to Westerners are Swedish (generally on the whole person, sometimes using deep pressure) and just general feel-good body rubbing. Asian forms of massage, which involve applying pressure to energy points, include acupressure and shiatsu, among others. Some forms of massage use oils to lubricate the skin, while other forms are done with the person fully clothed and do not use oils or other lubricants.

Practitioners often combine massage techniques and may also use visualization and aromatherapy (use of oils with particular odors for relaxation and stress reduction). Many people who do massage see themselves as channeling energy through their body and hands to heal and comfort the person they are massaging. A masseuse states:

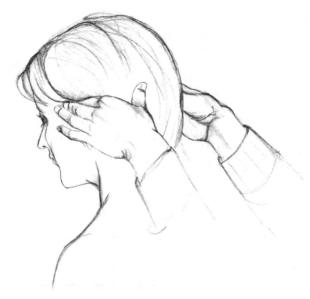

Christine Bondante

The way you touch someone is more important than the actual system you use. Whether you see yourself as channeling energy or are concerned with the muscle tone in your body and how you communicate it to someone else, you have to be rooted in your own body and pay attention to what is happening to you all the time you are giving the massage. While I give everyone the same massage in the order of things I attend to, my touch feels different to different people. It was wonderful when a woman told me she not only knew where her body was during the massage, but was aware of mine as well.

You don't need any special training to do general massage. Just get into a comfortable position and begin. Hold your friend's foot, head, hand, back, neck, or shoulders. Ask her where she wants pressure, whether you are applying too much pressure or not enough. With your thumb or whole hand, find and rub tender areas or sore spots.* Alternate gentle stroking with deep kneading and use visualization, too, if the person finds it relaxing. Avoid direct pressure on the spinal column; instead, press on either side. You don't necessarily need to massage the whole body—massaging one part, such as the foot or ear, can stimulate all the organs of the body. Breathe regularly and deeply while giving the massage.

While loosening our bodies, massage can also release painful emotions.

One of my first experiences with emotional healing and massage happened in a small and simple apartment in Cambridge. I had gone to see the masseuse (who worked at her home) because my body was filled with tension and I wanted some relief. When I arrived,

---

* Massage can be done with your hands, thumb, or feet, or with a massage ball. For an illustrated example of a massage for menstrual discomfort, see chapter 12, Understanding Our Bodies.

she suggested to me that I might be storing old emotional wounds in my body, as indicated by my posture. I asked her what she meant, a bit defensively. After all, I was doing yoga, walking, and eating well. I just had a lot of tension, that's all.

She didn't give a mental explanation. Instead, she asked me to lie down, and she began to massage the vertebrae in my neck. Massage, hold steady, massage, hold steady. At first I felt only the degree of tension in my neck; gradually I experienced a lump forming in my throat, my chest heaving and a bunch of old sensations returning to mind. I began to cry, small jerky sobs at first, like the opening of a faucet that has been shut off for a long time. Then a burst of tears, and finally several minutes of sobbing.

I was both terrified and relieved—terrified to think that there was so much deep emotion behind a stiff neck and relieved to know that it could be unlocked and soothed. At that moment I made a decision to see what else I could learn from this mysterious body that walked around with me all day.

If at some point you decide you want a professional massage or want to take a course or apprentice yourself to someone, you could get names from friends, your local woman's center, a health club, the Y, or a holistic health center if one exists in your area. A professional massage may cost anywhere from $30 to

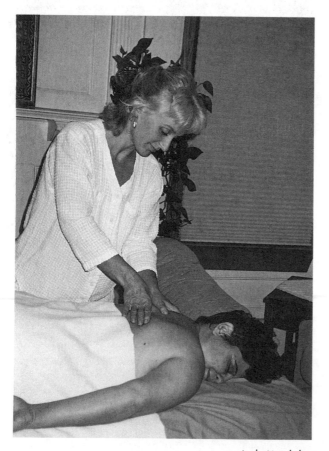

Judy Norsigian

$75 for one hour. Choose someone who uses techniques you like, and with whom you feel comfortable and can communicate well. Good two-way communication relaxes and energizes the masseuse as well. If you don't know much about a massage therapist you are considering, you can check to see if she or he was trained at a nationally accredited school, is certified, and is a member of the American Massage Therapy Association (see Resources).

Chiropractic

Many women visit a chiropractor for preventive health care. While the extraordinary flexibility of our bodies allows us to move with ease, it also makes it possible for our bodies to become unbalanced. The connective tissues that enclose our muscles and bones and give our body shape can become distorted by the ways in which we habitually sleep, walk, or sit, as well as by accidents. We accommodate to the distortions, but the longer we remain out of alignment, the more our movement becomes restricted. The resulting chronic muscle tension can affect us emotionally as well as physically; we sometimes lose our range of emotional responsiveness as we lose the flexibility of our physical movements.

Chiropractors believe that the human body works at its fullest potential only when the nervous system functions smoothly. The spinal column (the bony vertebral column that covers and protects our brain stem and spinal cord) is the "lifeline of the nervous system."[20] Chiropractors make adjustments (move the vertebrae) in the spine to restore proper nerve function and nerve conduction from the brain to muscles and organs of the body, making normal motion possible again. Spinal misalignments result from any of several causes: the way we habitually hold our bodies (for example, walking with our heads forward or standing with our knees locked); trauma from car, bike, motorcycle, or walking accidents; physical strain from overexertion or from sitting too long in one place; muscle tension from extreme mental and emotional stress; or poor diet or overuse of drugs.[21] Some chiropractors use X rays as a diagnostic aid, while others do not.

When I was pregnant, I visited my chiropractor once a month to be sure my back was aligned properly as my belly expanded and my weight shifted.

There are two distinct groups of practitioners within chiropractic. Believing that spinal misalignments cause diseases, the "straights" restrict their practice to spinal adjustments alone. The "mixers" have expanded their practice and offer other natural forms of treatment—suggestions about diet, exercise, meditation, visualization—in addition to spinal manipulation.

Chiropractors are also distinguished by style: "force" or "nonforce." "Force" technique involves more dramatic popping and cracking than "nonforce," which is more subtle and gentle. As with other alternative approaches to healing, women have a range of experiences with chiropractors.

I went to see a chiropractor recommended by several friends. He helped me with a specific back injury from running, but after a while I didn't like his attitude. Even though I was no longer having back problems, he suggested I keep coming more often than I wanted to. When I asked why, he said, "Well, there is always something to adjust."

"True," I said, "and I often feel better, but I can't afford the money."

So I looked and found another chiropractor who was willing to see me periodically for preventive care and in any crisis, too.

Dance and Movement Therapies

Movement and dance therapies are important components of the holistic approach to health care. Women have always danced and used movement for pleasure and relaxation. You find your own rhythm, experience control over your body, and discover the freedom to move in new ways. Many of us find that dancing—whether at clubs (see chapter 4, Women in Motion, p. 96), at home, or with friends—is a great way to throw off the stress of our lives. In indigenous cultures, dance is an important cultural and spiritual component of community. Some of us are learning the dances of our ancestors and of other peoples' traditions—Hawaiian, African, American Indian, and other indigenous forms of dance—to develop our sense of spiritual and physical well-being.

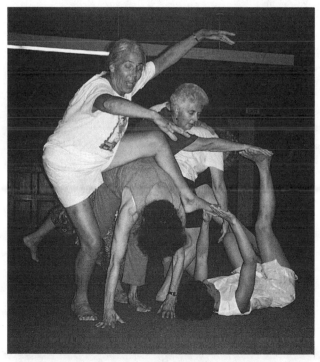

"Still dancing," Newton, Massachusetts, 1996/Doug Victor

Movement and dance also can also be used as more formal modes of healing. In the 1940s, dancer Marion Chace was the first American therapist to bring dance to a hospital setting. She observed that when traumatized soldiers could express their feelings through dance, they were able to leave the hospital more quickly. Chace set the path for other dance therapists to work with people who had a variety of severe psychiatric illnesses (e.g., children with autism, adults with schizophrenia) or who needed to counter the effects of powerful medications.*

Since that time, dance therapy, which is predominantly practiced by women, has become a popular mode of treating a variety of physiological and psychological conditions. Using movement rather than words, dance therapy addresses your physical body, emotions, mental attitude, and relatedness to the world. The therapist, by observing you and moving rhythmically with you, is able to mirror not only your physical movements but also the *feelings* behind those movements. As you learn to identify certain details of your physical and emotional states while you move, you can begin to alter your movements so that you feel more comfortable with yourself and with the people around you:

I was incredibly timid and anxious, so shy that I had trouble making friends or having any social life at all. I went to a dance therapist who worked with me in her office just moving, getting rhythms going. We began to breathe together, dance together, reach toward each other and move back. It was a way of communicating without needing to say anything. Once as we were moving I remembered my mother rocking me, and also the way I used to feel when she suddenly put me down to go take care of my brother. That memory released something in me and I started to cry. I never thought I could get such a feeling of release.

Dance and movement therapists also work with people who feel overweight and/or have eating disorders. They support you in your efforts to make fundamental changes in the way you relate to food and your body (see also chapter 2, Food, and chapter 4, Women in Motion):

As part of an exercise the group was physically lifting up a very large woman. This woman strongly believed that she always had to be supporting other people, but other people could not support her, especially because of her size. So the experience of being lifted up was a turning point for her. After this experience she could believe that she would be supported by people in other ways as well.

* Another school of movement therapy is based on the work of Rudolf Laban (see *The Mastery of Movement* [Boston: Plays, Inc., 1971]) and elaborated by Irmgard Bartenieff (see *Body Movement: Coping with the Environment* [New York: Gordon and Breach, 1980]).

Acupuncture

Acupuncture is the healing art central to the practice of Chinese traditional medicine. Developed and used over at least the last 2,000 years, acupuncture is now accepted in many places in the West as a method for maintaining health and healing illness. In acupuncture, the practitioner stimulates specific points on the body by inserting needles, applying heat using an herb (moxibusion), pressing, massaging (acupressure), or a combination of these.

Chinese medicine, which is intimately tied to the classical Chinese philosophy of Taoism (pronounced *Dawism*), aims to maintain or restore balance in the body to ensure health. Central to Taoism is the notion that the body has the power to repair and regenerate itself or to restore its own equilibrium. Acupuncture is thought to stimulate or awaken these natural healing powers within the body.[22]

Acupuncture is practiced according to many styles. The style common in Japan differs from the Korean, Chinese, French, and other styles. They differ in how much they treat the spirit and emotions as well as the body—that is, in how holistic their practice actually is. Although approaches may vary, the goals are the same: balance and improved energy.

In all styles of practice, the concept of yin and yang is central. These terms refer to the idea that all energy is in balance: dark (yin) is balanced by light (yang), heat (yang) by cold (yin), man by woman, moon by sun, and so forth. According to this philosophy, even though we may see one form as uppermost at a given time, the other form is always there in potential. Thus, in the dark of night, the potential for day is present; in the female person, there is masculine energy; and in the male person, there is feminine energy. Yin and yang are equally powerful forces; to label something "yin" or to label it "yang" does not imply any judgment about its goodness.

Unlike Western biomedicine, which emphasizes chemistry and anatomical structures, Chinese medicine has long focused on how people function: the dynamic aspects of the body, the "life force" that keeps the body alive and in healthful balance. They call this life force or vital energy *Qi* (or chi). According to Chinese medical theory, *Qi* circulates throughout the body along precise pathways or channels, the acupuncture meridians. The *Qi,* which controls the blood, the nerves, and all organs, must flow freely and be of an appropriate strength and quality in order for each organ and the person herself to function correctly. When the flow of *Qi* is impaired, a person experiences symptoms and becomes susceptible to disease.

Trauma, improper nutrition, stress, and many other factors can block or impair the flow of *Qi*. In acupuncture, stimulating certain points along the meridians controls the flow of *Qi* by attracting energy to a deficient area, dispersing an excess of energy, or dissolving a blockage, thereby lessening pain or strengthening the body's ability to maintain health.

A well-trained acupuncturist diagnoses the body's

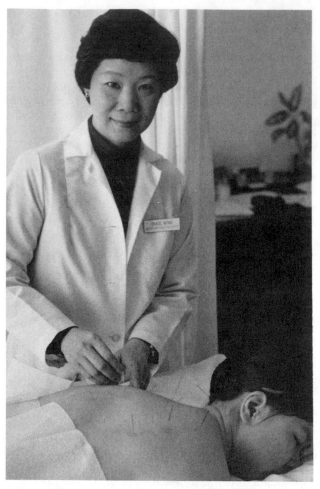

Grace Wong, Acupuncture Center of Washington (Bethesda, Maryland)

imbalance by a variety of techniques: questioning, observing, examining the tongue, listening (to breathing, voice, etc.), and reading the pulses. The latter is a primary diagnostic tool and is quite different from what a biomedical doctor does when listening to your pulse. Acupuncturists take your pulses at twelve different places on your wrist. They believe that each position corresponds to a functional organ system of the body. By reading the pulses, the acupuncturist can diagnose subtle fluctuations in the flow of energy and thus identify past, current, and potential problems.

Usually, an acupuncturist will take a complete health history and look for ways in which herbal remedies, changes in diet, exercise, and so on could complement the acupuncture treatments. Many acupuncturists in the U.S. work with biomedical physicians, and they may ask to see your medical records:

In my initial encounter with acupuncture, the acupuncturist was attentive and caring; even before I saw her, when I was just inquiring on the phone, she was taking notes. She sounded interested in my problem [heavy menstrual bleeding]. She thought that she could help me heal it. I had a good impression of her as a person and a healer.

When I walked into the acupuncturist's office for the first time there was an herb burning that smelled like pot to me, and the first thing that went through my mind was, What am I doing here? These are really "New Age" healers; this is more than I bargained for. I started to feel very nervous. I asked her what the smell was, and she told me that it was an herb called moxa [common mugwort], which they use to heat the needles and which adds to the treatment's effectiveness. I was ready to try something new, but I was also mistrustful.

After I sat down, the acupuncturist asked me a series of questions having to do with digestion, elimination, menstruation, sleep patterns, level of energy, emotional state, pain, other illnesses, diet, lifestyle. This was a lengthy initial question period. Now each time I come she asks me how I've been feeling that week, if there is anything out of the ordinary. She takes my pulse and looks at my tongue, skin, eyes. After gathering all this information, she adjusts the treatment to meet the specific needs I have that week.

During treatments the acupuncturist stimulates the appropriate acupuncture points with disposable hair-thin stainless steel needles. Needles vary in length from half an inch to several inches for use in different parts of the body. When the needle is inserted, you may feel a slight prick, tingling, numbness, pain, or nothing at all:

Part of the initial high of starting acupuncture was that I had expected it to be very painful because my image of it was that they used these big long needles and stuck them into people. When she actually did it, she used very small needles. The prick was quite mild and I got an almost euphoric feeling.

Acupuncture treatments have really minimized my problems with asthma. But I won't deny that the needles hurt as she was putting them in. Once in place, they didn't hurt anymore.

The needles rarely cause bleeding. Generally, from two to 15 needles are used. The hands, forearms, lower legs, feet, back, abdomen, and ears are the most common places to insert needles. Often the acupuncturist inserts the needle far from the symptomatic area or what you would think of as the site of the disease, because the meridians she or he wishes to affect run the length of the body. The Qi can be directed to bring back balance and harmony within the body from many places on the meridian. For acute ailments few treatments—sometimes just one—are needed. Chronic ailments usually require more treatments, but some people experience relief right away. Others initially feel worse and begin to experience improvement only after many sessions:

I am 60 years old and have severe arthritis, especially in my hands, feet, and hips. I had been pushing this pain out of my mind while I was taking care of my husband. He was very sick and if he knew I was in pain he would have wanted to go to the hospital. After he died I was very depressed, and when I went for psychological counseling the counselor suggested that I try acupuncture for the arthritis. He researched it and got me in touch with the acupuncturist. The acupuncturist told me that chronic pain like mine was deep-seated and harder to take care of. I had to go twice a week for a long time. It was expensive for me, and when after eight treatments I didn't feel any better, I didn't know what to do. Meanwhile, I had been put on a special arthritis diet by a nutritionist who worked with the acupuncturist. I decided I would go on with the acupuncture treatment, and when I got to 16 treatments I started to feel a little better. By 20 weeks I had found the acupuncture really helped me. Now the treatments have tapered off, one every two or three months, when I start getting sore. So it was definitely worth continuing with them. You either sink or swim, and I didn't feel like sinking.

Other people may not respond to treatments:

I saw a Chinese acupuncturist who came highly recommended. A friend of mine had been getting treated for a back injury and was getting some pain relief for the first time in months. The acupuncturist was warm and attentive and was sure she could help some of the symptoms of my chronic fatigue syndrome. We spent almost a year working together—she even called her teacher in China for a consult on me—but finally I had to acknowledge that I wasn't feeling any better. It was frustrating—I wanted so much for it to help and she seemed so sure that it could.

Acupuncture is a comprehensive health care system, which means it can address most illnesses—acute or chronic, physical, emotional, spiritual—as well as help keep a person well. It can also help with prenatal health and with childbirth. In a survey of 575 patients in five states, respondents said they most commonly used acupuncture care for

- pain relief in the muscles, joints, bones, head, and digestive system.
- mood care—to treat and prevent anxiety, depression, and anger.
- wellness care—to maintain good health.
- women's reproductive care—for menstrual and menopausal complaints, for infertility, and so forth.
- respiratory complaints, such as allergies, asthma, and hay fever as well as infections like colds, sinus infections, bronchitis, and pneumonia.
- care of other infections such as cystitis, hepatitis, HIV.
- substance abuse complaints—to get off heroin, cocaine, methadone, alcohol, nicotine, caffeine, and many prescription drugs.
- supportive care of autoimmune conditions such as diabetes, lupus, multiple sclerosis, and thyroiditis.[23]

Patients also report success using Chinese medicine to treat insomnia, simple and chronic fatigue, nausea (from pregnancy, or associated with chemotherapy), constipation and diarrhea, and disorders of the skin, sense organs, kidneys and urinary tract, heart and blood vessels, and male reproductive organs.

Scientific research that explains "how acupuncture works" is still in its infancy in the West. However, many useful reports exist, particularly supporting the use of Chinese medical care for pain relief, nausea, stroke care, respiratory disease, and substance abuse.[24] Look for these in your library, or if you have Internet access, try http://www.acupuncture.com.

Acupuncture, like any form of health care, cannot help everyone. You are more likely to get better results if you shop wisely for your acupuncturist. In some states, acupuncture may be done by only an MD. However, an MD's acupuncture training may be very limited (some states require 200 hours, but some have no laws requiring such training). Some states also allow chiropractors to perform acupuncture with as few as 50 hours of training. Check to see that the acupuncturist is certified by the National Commission for the Certification of Acupuncture (NCCA). Also, if you are unable to get a referral from someone you trust, you can contact the NCCA directly about certified acupuncturists in your area (see Resources).

Though reports of harm from acupuncture needles are rare, check to make sure that your practitioner uses disposable needles and sterile techniques. And remember that you should not experience lasting pain from needles.

Homeopathy

Homeopathy is a comprehensive system of medicine with a wide following in India and continental Europe and a smaller but dedicated clientele in the U.S. (1% of all adults in the U.S. use homeopathic remedies).[25] It is an exceptionally safe form of medicine that is based on the principle of stimulating the body to cure illness using natural substances found in minerals, plants, and animals. It can be used to treat a specific ailment or systemic problem or simply to maintain good health.

Samuel Hahnemann developed homeopathy (from the Greek *homoios* meaning "similar" and *pathos* meaning "suffering/disease") in the late 1700s in Germany. Hahnemann discovered that by using small doses of a substance that causes a disease, he could stimulate an infected organism to heal. This is known as the Law of Similars. Hahnemann tested and "proved" hundreds of substances, including cinchona bark, mercury, belladonna, arsenic, and silver nitrate, to name a few. Homeopathic reference books describe in detail the specific psychological and physical symptoms for each remedy. Contemporary research studies have also shown several of these remedies to be effective.[26]

One of the fascinating aspects of Hahnemann's discovery is that it takes only a small dose to stimulate

the body's healing response. In fact, if too much of the "cure" is taken, the patient may become even more ill. Homeopathic remedies are generally small pills with infinitesimal amounts of the healing substance suspended in a pleasant-tasting but inert glucose base. Doses with greater quantities of a healing substance have lower numbers—e.g., 6x or 15c—and are less potent than those with lower amounts of a healing substance. The lower the amount of the substance, the higher the numbers—e.g., 200c or x—and the more potent the remedy.

There are both lay and licensed practitioners of homeopathy. Medical and osteopathic doctors sometimes use homeopathic remedies, as do dentists, veterinarians, and midwives. Some states license naturopathic physicians who are trained in homeopathy.

I had been nursing my son, Michael, for a little over a year when I noticed soreness in my left breast while out doing errands with him. I didn't think much of it, but several hours later when we returned home, I began to have fever, chills, and sweating, and my breast was throbbing with pain. It came on quickly and was so severe that I called a relative to come over and take care of Michael. When help arrived, I managed to drive the two miles to the office of my homeopath. Within minutes she had diagnosed the problem as mastitis and prescribed the homeopathic remedy "phytolacca" [poke root], which I took immediately. It was difficult to drive home. It seemed as if every inch of my body ached. Within an hour the pain began to subside. Relief swept over me—the remedy was working! By that evening I had only slight tenderness in my breast and was able to nurse my son without pain. I was happy to have gotten better so fast and to have avoided antibiotics.

For those who can't afford to use a practitioner or simply prefer to learn on their own how to use homeopathic medicines for themselves and their families, there are a multitude of books to serve as guides (see Resources). Moreover, homeopathic remedies are inexpensive and readily available at many health food stores, at naturopathic pharmacies, and through practitioners. Originally, there were only single-substance remedies. Today, you can purchase combination remedies that use several single remedies together to address a condition (for example, menopause, migraine headaches, digestive problems, allergies, or vaginitis). Remedies are administered by placing pills under the tongue and allowing them to dissolve.

It is important to understand that homeopathy treats the whole person; two people with the same symptoms could very well require different remedies. Thus, an initial visit with a homeopath generally takes an hour to an hour and a half and is primarily used to discuss a person's overall condition, including eating and sleeping habits, psychological and emotional state, and family history as well as the specific ailments that are causing discomfort. A homeopath looks for those symptoms that are characteristic of the particular patient and define him or her as a whole person, such as certain fears, moods, and cravings. The homeopath prescribes a remedy and continues to monitor the patient to be sure that it is having the desired effect. Sometimes it takes months for a condition to be completely eliminated.

When my daughter was about five years old, she developed severe asthma. At first we used conventional medicine, but these powerful drugs altered her personality, making her more hyperactive. When the doctor suggested she be on these medications, including an inhaler, for years to come, we sought another option. The homeopathic doctor treated her without the unwanted side effects, and in a relatively short time, our daughter was symptom-free and has continued to be for ten years now. I was so impressed with homeopathy that I began to use it on my own. Today our family uses a combination of doctors and traditional medicines . . . homeopathy has given us a safe and reliable option for control of our health care.

Spiritual Healing

Scientific documentation is starting to become more available to establish evidence on spiritual healing, but in many communities, spiritual healing is a way of life that doesn't need any scientific explanation. There are on record incidents of physical healing that cannot be explained in purely medical, physical, or psychological terms.[27] Sometimes when a surprisingly rapid rate of healing or a total reversal of symptoms occurs, people attribute the healing to a nonphysical entity (spirit or deity), a group (prayer group, healing circle, church group), an individual (minister, shaman, psychic), or the person's attendance at a "miraculous" place (such as Lourdes). The techniques and rituals used in association with these incidents include meditation and prayer, touching with the intent to heal, communication with the spirit realm, and connecting with sacred deities or ancestors.

In many communities of color, spiritual healing has a strong religious base with roots in West Africa and indigenous communities of the Caribbean and the Americas. It can be called by many names, including Espiritismo, Curan-derimso, Santeria, and Voudon, and it is practiced with the assistance of individuals who have the gift of "sight" and touch. These cultural religious healing practices are used not only to assist in curing an illness but for general cleansing, safety, and spiritual guidance.

Espiritismo is one form, which is the syncretization of Yoruban (West African) and Afro-Cuban spiritual traditions.[28] Espiritismo is extremely popular in Puerto Rican, African-American, and Caribbean communities, where individuals will go to an Espiritista to find comfort, guidance, and help with health problems. An Espiritista may also assist in removing any negativity from the individual's person or home. Often people will go to a Centro Espiritista or to a Botanica for assistance, to seek out individuals who can offer a "read-

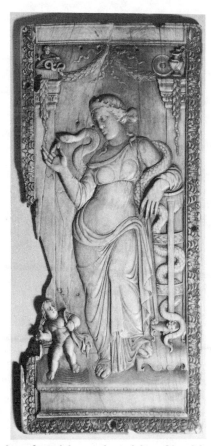

Ivory carving of Hygieia, ancient deity of health and healing/The Board of Trustees of the National Museums and Galleries on Merseyside (Liverpool Museum)

ing" and who can suggest ways of returning to a state of balance.

Therapeutic Touch is another method of spiritual healing. Studied and taught by Dolores Krieger and Dora Kunz, Therapeutic Touch is a way of channeling energy through yourself to help the healing process in another person. Therapeutic Touch has been effective in relieving stress-related conditions such as rashes, headaches, asthma, colitis, sleep disorders, high blood pressure, palpitations, and angina. A woman describes using Therapeutic Touch for the first time:

I have a long history of migraines. I went into the nurse's office as a migraine was just beginning. While I had heard about Therapeutic Touch, I had never tried it before. When the nurse offered me a choice of decongestants, pain relievers, Therapeutic Touch, or some combination, I decided to try Therapeutic Touch. (After all, I knew what the drugs could and couldn't do for me.) After the session my head felt lighter and less congested.

As the healer communicates her or his concern through physical touch, a strong "healing" intention, and ritual, you may be able to relax and let your body's healing energy take over.

One noted psychic healer emphasizes that a healer should focus on the whole person, not just on the particular part to be healed. He warns people to be wary of healers who charge money and/or promise a cure, and he cautions against the sleight-of-hand tricks some "healers" use to reinforce their clients' belief in them. He also requires that all his clients be in consultation with a physician.

To find a healer who is good for you, check with your friends, local Botanicas, herb shops, or Wicca (earth-based spiritual practice of old Europe) stores; they may be able to direct you to healing centers or even inform you where you can possibly become an apprentice and learn with an experienced healer.

NOTES

1. Murial J. Hughes, *Women Healers in Medieval Life and Literature* (North Stratford, NH: Ayer, 1977 [c. 1943]).
2. D. Eisenberg et al., "Unconventional Medicine in the United States," *New England Journal of Medicine* 328 (Jan. 1993): 246.
3. M. Singer and R. Garcia, "Becoming a Puerto Rican Espiritista: Life History of a Female Healer," In Carol Shepherd McClain, ed., *Women as Healers: Cross-Cultural Perspectives* (New Brunswick, NJ: Rutgers University Press, 1989). Gives an excellent story of a woman re-creating herself.
4. Maureen Minehan, "Alternative Health Care Eases into Insurance Coverage," *HR Magazine* 41, no. 4 (April 1996): 192.
5. N. Muramato, *Healing Ourselves* (New York: Avon Books, 1976), 4.
6. D. Ardell, *High-Level Wellness* (Berkeley, CA: Ten Speed Press, 1986), 2.
7. Kirk Johnson, "Elitism in Alternative Health," *East West Journal* (May 1986): 20–25.
8. J. J. Vander Wall, *Cages of Steel: The Politics of Imprisonment in America* (Washington, DC: Maisonneuve Press, 1992). Although this book is primarily about the U.S. penal system, one section outlines the political and economic consequences for black people who have tried to create healing institutions and what happens when "certain powers" do not like their efforts.
9. C. Clayton and V. McCullough, *A Consumer's Guide to Alternative Health Care* (Holbrook, MA: Adams Media Corp., 1995), 149.
10. Adriane Fugh-Berman, *Alternative Medicine: What Works?* (Tucson, AZ: Odian Press, 1996), 101.
11. David Hoffman, *The Complete Illustrated Holistic Herbal* (New York: Barnes and Noble, 1996).
12. Clayton & McCullough, *A Consumer's Guide,* 182.
13. J. L. Lasath, "Yoga: An Ancient Technique for Restoring Health," in Shepherd Bliss, ed., *The New Holistic Health Handbook* (Lexington, MA: Stephen Greene Press, 1986), 36.
14. Clayton & McCullough, *A Consumer's Guide,* 197.
15. Clayton & McCullough, *A Consumer's Guide,* 199.
16. Fugh-Berman, *Alternative Medicine,* 198.
17. W. Luthe, *Autogenic Therapy,* vol. 1 (New York: Grune & Stratton, 1969), 1.
18. E. Peper and E. A. Williams, "Autogenic Therapy," in Arthur C. Hastings et al., eds., *Health for the Whole Person* (Boulder, CO: Westview Press, 1980), 134.
19. O. Carl Simonton et al., *Getting Well Together* (New York: Bantam Books, 1978): 127–48, 183–85.
20. G. F. Rickeman, "Chiropractics." in Bliss, ed., *The New Holistic Health Handbook,* 348.
21. T. A. Vondarhaar, "Chiropractic in Theory and Practice," in Bliss, ed., *The New Holistic Health Handbook,* 349.
22. Stephan Chang, "Acupuncture: A Contemporary Look at an Ancient System," in Bliss, ed., *The New Holistic Health Handbook,* 48.
23. Claire M. Cassidy, "New Research: Patients Vote an Overwhelming 'Yes' for Acupuncture," *Meridians, Changing the Personal Experience of Health* 3, no. 2 (spring 1996): 28–34. Also Claire M. Cassidy, "Patients Point to What Makes Acupuncture Care Special," *Meridians, Changing the Personal Experience of Health* 4, no. 2 (summer 1997): 30–36. (*Meridians* is published by the Traditional Acupuncture Institute, Columbia, MD; 800-735-2968 for reprints.)
24. See D. Eskanazi, ed., "NIH Technology Assessment Workshop on Alternative Medicine: Acupuncture," *Journal of Alternative and Complementary Medicine* 2, no. 1, special issue (spring 1996); S. Birch and R. Hamerschlag, eds., *Acupuncture Efficacy, A Compendium of Controlled Clinical Studies* (Tarrytown, NY: National Academy of Acupuncture and Oriental Medicine, 1996); V. Brewington et al., "Acupuncture as a Detoxification Treatment: An Analysis of Controlled Research," *Journal of Substance Abuse Treatment* 11 (1994): 289–307.
25. Fugh-Berman, *Alternative Medicine,* 126.
26. J. Kleijnen et al., "Preparation for Childbirth by Homeopathy," *British Medical Journal* 302 (1992): 316–23.
27. See S. Krippner, "Psychic Healing," in Hastings et. al., eds., *Health for the Whole Person,* 169; D. Krieger, *Therapeutic Touch: How to Use Your Hands to Help or Heal* (Englewood Cliffs, NJ: Prentice Hall, 1979); and L. LeShan, *The Medium, the Mystic and the Physicist* (New York: Ballantine Books, 1982).
28. M. Singer and R. Garcia, "Becoming a Puerto Rican Espiritista," in McClain, ed., *Women as Healers,* 160.

RESOURCES

Books and Articles

Balch, J., and Phyllis Balch. *Prescription for Nutritional Healing.* Garden City Park, NY: Avery Publishers, 1997.

Bauer, Cathryn. *Acupressure for Women.* Freedom, CA: The Crossing Press, 1987.

Beinfield, H., and E. Korngold. *Between Heaven and Earth: A Guide to Chinese Medicine.* New York: Ballantine, 1992.

Benson, Herbert, M.D. *The Mind-Body Effect: How Behavioral Medicine Can Show You the Way to Better Health*. New York: Simon & Schuster, 1979.

Capra, Fritjof. *The Turning Point*. New York: Bantam, 1984.

Chopra, Deepak. *Ageless Body, Timeless Mind: The Quantum Alternative to Growing Old*. New York: Crown, 1994.

———. *Perfect Health: The Complete Mind Body Guide*. New York: Crown, 1991.

Consumer Reports. "Alternative Medicine: The Facts." *Consumer Reports Magazine*, Jan. 1994.

Cousins, Norman. *Anatomy of an Illness As Perceived by the Patient: Reflections on Healing and Regeneration*. New York: W. W. Norton, 1979.

Crawford, Robert. "Healthism and the Medicalization of Everyday Life." *International Journal of Health Services* 10, no. 3 (1980): 365–88.

Cunningham, D., and A. Ramer. *Spiritual Dimensions of Healing Addictions*. San Rafael, CA: Cassandra Press, 1988.

Domar, Alice, and Henry Dreher. *Healing Mind, Healthy Woman: Take Control of Your Well-Being Using the Mind-Body Connection*. New York: Henry Holt, 1996.

Eisenberg, David M., et al. "Unconventional Medicine in the United States: Prevalence, Costs, and Patterns of Use." *New England Journal of Medicine* 328 (1993): 246–52.

Fe Arriola, Maria, et al. *Isis and Other Guides to Health: Helpful Hints on the Road to Well-Being*. Manila: Isis International, circa 1996.

Fugh-Berman, Adrienne. *Alternative Medicine: What Works?* Tucson, AZ: Odonian Press, 1996.

———. "The Case for Natural Medicine." *The Nation* (Sept. 6–13, 1993).

Gauthier, I., and Lisa Vinebaum. *Hot Pants: Do It Yourself Gynecology*. Montreal: CAMCA, 1994.

Gawain, Shakti. *Creative Visualization: Use the Power of Your Imagination to Create What You Want in Your Life*. Novato, CA: New World Library, 1995.

Gladstar, Rosemary. *Herbal Healing for Women*. New York: Firestone, 1993.

Haas, Elson. *Staying Healthy with the Seasons*. Berkeley, CA: Celestial Arts, 1981.

Hoffman, David. *The Complete Illustrated Holistic Herbal*. New York: Barnes and Noble, 1996.

Hutchens, Alma. *Indian Herbalogy of North American*. Boston: Shambhala, 1991.

Kaptchuk, Ted. *The Web That Has No Weaver: Understanding Chinese Medicine*. New York: Congdon and Weed, 1993.

Kleijnen, J., et al. "Clinical Trials of Homeopathy." *British Medical Journal* 302, no. 6772 (1991): 316–23.

Krieger, Dolores. *Living the Therapeutic Touch: Healing as a Lifestyle*. New York: Dodd, Mead, 1987.

Lad, Vasant. *Ayurveda: The Science of Self Healing*. Santa Fe: Lotus Press, 1985.

LeShan, Lawrence. *The Medium, The Mystic and the Physicist: Toward a General Theory of the Paranormal*. New York: Ballantine, 1982.

Lockie, A., and Nicola Geddes. *The Women's Guide to Homeopathy*. New York: St. Martin's Press, 1993.

Lock, Margaret, and Deborah Gordon, eds. *Biomedicine Examined*. Norwell, MA: Kluwer, 1988.

Lu, Henry. *Chinese Systems of Food Cures, Prevention and Remedies*. New York: Sterling, 1986.

Martin, Emily. *Flexible Bodies: Tracking Immunity in American Culture from the Days of Polio to the Age of AIDS*. Boston: Beacon Press, 1994.

McIntyre, Anne. *The Complete Woman's Herbal*. New York: Henry Holt, 1994.

Mead, Kate Campbell. *A History of Women in Medicine from the Earliest Times to the Beginning of the 19th Century*. Haddam, CT: Haddam, 1938.

Micozzi, M., ed. *Fundamentals of Complementary and Alternative Medicine*. New York: Churchill Livingstone, 1996.

Mole, P. *Acupuncture: Energy Balancing for Body, Mind and Spirit*. Rockport, MA: Element, 1992.

Morrison, Judith. *The Book of Ayurveda: A Holistic Approach to Health and Longevity*. New York: Fireside, 1995.

Moskowitz, Richard. *Homeopathic Medicines for Pregnancy and Childbirth*. Berkeley, CA: North Atlantic, 1992.

Nissim, Rina. *Natural Healing in Gynecology: A Manual for Women*. San Francisco: Pandora Press, 1996.

Payer, Lynn. *Medicine and Culture*. New York: Viking Penguin, 1989.

Pelletier, Kenneth R. *Mind as Healer, Mind as Slayer: A Holistic Approach to Preventing Stress Disorders*. Magnolia, MA: Peter Smith, 1984.

Potts, Billie. *Witches Heal: Lesbian Herbal Self-Sufficiency*. Ann Arbor, MI: Du Reve Press, 1988.

Rick, Stephanie. *The Reflexology Workout*. New York: Crown, 1986.

Rose, J. *Herbs and Aromatherapy for the Reproductive System*. Berkeley, CA: Frog, 1994.

Scheffer, Mechthild. *Bach Flower Therapy: Theory and Practice*. Rochester, VT: Healing Arts Press, 1988.

Singer, M., and Garcia, R. "Becoming a Puerto Rican Espiritista: Life History of a Female Healer," in Carol Shephard McClain, ed. *Women as Healers: Cross Cultural Perspectives*. New Brunswick, NJ: Rutgers University Press, 1989.

Sobel, Dava. *Arthritis: What Works*. New York: St. Martin's Press, 1991.

Sobel, David S., ed. *Ways of Health: Holistic Approaches to Ancient and Contemporary Medicine*. New York: Harcourt Brace Jovanovich, 1979. Compilation of well-documented articles on health and healing.

Speight, Phyllis. *Homeopathic Remedies for Women's Ailments*. Woodstock, NY: Beekman, 1992.

Stein, Diane. *All Women Are Healers: A Comprehensive Guide to Natural Healing*. Freedom, CA: The Crossing Press, 1990.

Stein, Howard. *American Medicine as Culture*. Boulder, CO: Westview Press, 1993.

Teish, Luisah. *Jambalaya: The Natural Woman's Book of Personal Charms and Practical Rituals*. San Francisco: Harper San Francisco, 1988.

Trotter, Robert T., and Juan Antonio Chavira. *Curand-*

erismo: Mexican American Folk Healing. Athens, GA: University of Georgia Press, 1981.

Ullman, Dana. *Discovering Homeopathy: Your Introduction to the Science and Art of Homeopathic Medicine.* Berkeley, CA: North Atlantic Books, 1991.

Ullman, Dana, and Stephen Cummings. *Everybody's Guide to Homeopathic Medicines,* rev. ed. Los Angeles: Jeremy Tarcher, 1991.

Vanzant, Iyanla. *Value in the Valley: A Black Woman's Guide Through Life's Dilemmas.* New York: Simon & Schuster, 1995.

Weed, Susun. *Breast Cancer? Breast Health! The Wise Woman Way.* Woodstock, NY: Ash Tree, 1996.

Workshop on Alternative Medicine. *Alternative Medicine, Expanding Medical Horizons: A Report to the National Institutes of Health on Alternative Medical Systems and Practices in the United States.* Washington, DC: U.S. Government Printing Office, 1994.

Wright, Keith. *A Healthy Foods and Spiritual Nutrition Handbook.* Philadelphia: Health Masters, 1989.

Periodicals

Alternative Therapies in Health and Medicine
Innovision Communications; 101 Columbia Road; Aliso Viejo, CA 92656; (800) 899-1712
E-mail: altherapy@aol.com
Web site: http://www.healthline.com/alther.htm

HerbalGram
American Botanical Council; P.O. Box 201660; Austin, TX 78720-1660; (800) 373-7105
E-mail: custerv@herbalgram.org
Web site: http://www.herbalgram.com

Journal of Complementary and Alternative Medicine
2 Madison Avenue; Larchmont, NY 10538

Natural Health Magazine
Boston Common Press; 17 Station Street, Box 1200; Brookline Village, MA 02146; (617) 232-1000

New Age Journal
New Age Publishers; 42 Pleasant Street; Watertown, MA 02172; (617) 926-0200
Web site: http://www.newage.com/home/newage

Ta'i Chi Way Magazine
P.O. Box 3998; Los Angeles, CA 90039; (213) 665-7773

Vegetarian Times
1140 Lake Street, Suite 500; Oak Park, IL 60301; (800) 829-3340

Yoga Journal
2054 University Avenue; Berkeley, CA 94704; (510) 841-9200; (800) 334-8152

Associations and Organizations

Alternative Health Insurance Services
P.O. Box 6279; Thousand Oaks, CA 91359-6279; (805) 374-6003

E-mail: AltHlthIns@aol.com
Web site: http://www.alternativeInsurance.com

American Black Chiropractors Association
1918 E. Grand Boulevard; St. Louis, MO 63107; (314) 531-0615

American Dance Therapy Association
2000 Century Plaza, Suite 108; Columbia, MD 21044; (410) 997-4040

American Herbalists Guild
P.O. Box 746555; Arvada, CO 80006; (303) 423-8800
E-mail: ahg@herbalists.org
Web site: http://www.healthy.net/herbalists

American Holistic Nurses Association
P.O. Box 2130; Flagstaff, AZ 86003; (800) 278-AHNA
Web site: http://ahna.org/index.html

American Massage Therapy Association
820 Davis Street, Suite 100; Evanston, IL 60201; (847) 864-0123
Web site: http://www.amtmassage.org

Homeopathic Educational Services
2124 Kittredge Street; Berkeley, CA 94704; (800) 359-9051; (510) 649-0294
E-mail: mail@homeopathic.com
Web site: http://www.homeopathic.com

Kripalu Yoga Center
P.O. Box 793; Lenox, MA 01240; (800) 741-SELF; (413) 448-3152

The National Center for Homeopathy
801 N. Fairfax Street, Suite 306; Alexandria, VA 22314; (703) 548-7790
E-mail: nchinfo@igc.apc.org
Web site: http://www.healthy.net/nch

The National College of Chiropractic
200 E. Roosevelt Road; Lombard, IL 60148-4583; (800) 826-NATL; (630) 629-2000
E-mail: homepage@national.chiropractic.edu
Web site: http://www.national.chiropractic.edu

The National College of Naturopathic Medicine
11231 SE Market Street; Portland, OR 97216; (503) 225-7355
Web site: http://www.ncnm.edu

National Commission for the Certification of Acupuncture
1424 16th Street NW, Suite 501; Washington, DC 20036; (202) 232-1404
Web site: http://www.acupuncture.com

Office of Alternative Medicine, NIH
6120 Executive Boulevard, EPS Suite 4505; Rockville, MD 20852; (301) 402-2466

The Rosenthal Center for Complementary Medicine at Columbia University's College of Physicians and Surgeons
630 West 168 Street, Unit 75; New York, NY 10032
Web site: http://cpmcnet.columbia.edu/dept/rosenthal

ONLINE RESOURCES *

Alternative Medicine
http://www.altmedicine.com/altmenu.htm

The Alternative Medicine Homepage
http://www.pitt.edu/~cbw/altm.html

Complementary Practices
http://galen.med.virginia.edu/~pjb3s/
Complementary_Practices.html

Health & Healing News: Holistic & Alternative Healthcare Online
http://www.eskimo.com/~hhnews

MedWeb: Alternative Medicine
http://www.gen.emory.edu/MEDWEB/keyword/
alternative_medicine.html

Natural Medicine, Complementary Health Care, and Alternative Therapies
http://www.amrta.org/~amrta

Wellness Web: Alternative/Complementary Medicine
http://www.wellweb.com/altern/index.htm

Yahoo! Health: Alternative Medicine
http://www.yahoo.com/Health/Alternative_Medicine

* For more information and listings of online resources, please see Introducton to Online Women's Health Resources, p. 25.

By Nancy Miriam Hawley

WITH SPECIAL THANKS TO Cassandra Clay,
Nancy and Lang Keyes, Jeffrey McIntyre, and
Susan Yanow (box on "Depression: Choosing
Medication")*

Chapter 6

Our Emotional Well-Being: Psychotherapy in Context

Women have known for centuries that emotional well-being cannot be separated from physical health and spiritual aliveness. Since the inception of modern psychotherapy and marital and family therapy, women have been the primary consumers of these services. In this chapter, we explicitly place our emotional health in the broader context of our physical and spiritual well-being, envision psychotherapy in that larger context, acknowledge that many women use psychotherapy as one way to take care of ourselves, and offer guidance about how to be effective and proactive consumers.†

Many women are consciously or unconsciously affected by sexist discrimination. We may be carried by the force of cultural ideology into roles that squash our true selves. We may also face discrimination based on our social class; racial, religious, or ethnic background; sexual orientation; or physical and mental abilities. The world is not an easy place for women, and many of us carry around a great deal of pain from past traumas or present realities. Finding ways to move through that pain and take charge of our lives is important if we want to live in ways that make us feel alive, fully engaged, and satisfied with the choices we make.

Whatever our past and present realities, we *can* alter some aspects of ourselves and our lives and, in

* Thanks also to the following for their help with the 1998 version of this chapter: Amy Agigian, Jean Baker-Miller, Judi Chamberlain, Beth Damsky, Joan Ditzion, Cindy Irvine, Karen Kahn, Pamela Pacelli, Ester Shapiro, Peggy Wegman, and Evelyn C. White. Over the years since 1982, the following women have contributed to the many versions of this chapter: Judith Herman, Rachel Lanzerotti, Judy Norsigian, Catherine Riessman, Wendy Sanford, and Norma Swenson.
† This chapter does not address, in any comprehensive way, what in traditional medical settings is referred to as "chronic mental

illness." If you suffer severe emotional distress or a psychiatric disability, you can find help with a caring and well-trained therapist. However, you may need additional resources, beyond what you will find in this chapter. It is also important to know that a psychiatric disability falls under the Americans with Disabilities Act in cases of discrimination.

doing so, contribute positively to our overall health and sense of well-being. While each of us as an individual can consciously choose to behave differently, we may also need actively to engage and involve others close to us for advice, encouragement, and support. These healthy choices include

- **Wellness strategies** such as eating well, getting enough rest and exercise, learning about meditation, and finding ways to receive massages. A healthy body and a calm mind and spirit allow us to be more resilient day to day.
- **Creative activities** that we do alone or with others. Do you love to take walks, read, sing, dance, or drum? To paint, knit, write poems, or create in clay? Do you bird-watch, play softball, climb mountains, or canoe rivers? These are just a few of the activities that can stretch us, give us and others pleasure, and offer a space away from the daily challenges of our lives.
- **Friendships and community** with people who help and hold us in our lives. Do you make time to nurture your friendships? Do you have a community of others—family, friends, neighbors, religious, or spiritual—with whom you can both celebrate and grieve life transitions?
- **Support and self-help groups**. The women's movement sparked many kinds of support groups, from consciousness-raising to those focused on specific life events such as becoming a new mother, going through menopause, choosing parenthood as a lesbian, living with a particular illness or disability, or separating from a long-term relationship. Now we can find or create groups to address almost any concern we have. At their best, these groups help us see our individual concerns within the larger societal context. They also give us opportunities, while healing ourselves, to help heal others. In this tradition, anonymous self-help groups such as Alcoholics Anonymous and Al-Anon (and nonreligious-based alternatives sometimes termed "secular sobriety" or "rational recovery") offer invaluable assistance and support for individuals in recovery from addictions and for families affected by the addictions of someone they love.

In addition to exploring therapy, the authors of this chapter urge you to take a look at chapter 5, Holistic Health and Healing. Many women have found meditation, yoga, and other stress reduction approaches invaluable as parallel paths to emotional health and healing.

CHOOSING PSYCHOTHERAPY

When we focus more attention on our health, our friendships, and community activities, or join support or self-help groups, we often feel a greater sense of emotional well-being. Still, there are times in our lives when we feel depressed, anxious, or hopeless or when certain patterns keep repeating themselves. In these situations we may find help in talking with supportive family members, friends, spiritual advisors, or other members of our community. Sometimes, however, those closest to us are not able or willing to talk about what's wrong, offer too much advice, are too much part of the problem, are too upset to be helpful, or can't give enough time and attention. Then we may choose to seek out therapy.

Therapy sessions are facilitated by a mental health professional and occur one-to-one or in a couple, family, or group. Therapy involves an exchange between you and the therapist. Through these discussions we can experience and express our emotions, reexamine past experiences in order to understand our emotional lives more fully, tell our story and rewrite it, learn about our strengths to change behaviors and beliefs, place our concerns in the appropriate context (personal, interpersonal, societal), solve current life problems, communicate more clearly and effectively, learn about setting limits and establishing appropriate boundaries, and learn how to ask for help and what kinds of help we need to better understand ourselves.

While for some people therapy still carries the stigma and belief that you must be ready to be committed to a mental hospital, or at least out of touch with reality, *therapy is a sane, proactive choice for women facing any number of painful and difficult issues.* You may want to find a therapist because you feel desperate, are overwhelmed, or suffer from long-term emotional instability. You may also simply need someone to talk to about major life changes. It is important to understand that choosing therapy is not a sign of weakness, nor is it "putting your business out where everyone can see." All ethical therapy, whether individual or group, is confidential.

As women, we face many life transitions without adequate social support. You may find therapy helpful in the face of

- becoming a new mother (whether biologically or through adoption).
- getting into and out of relationships/partnerships.
- coming out as a lesbian/bisexual/transgendered woman.
- managing work roles inside and outside the home.
- grieving losses, including the loss of our own and others' capacities as a result of illness and aging.
- migrating to a new community.

For the past five years, my husband and I have been struggling with a life-threatening illness. I felt out of control, and I looked for a therapist who could help me with overwhelming feelings of helplessness, fear, and rage. While I have a large network of supportive friends, talking with them did not stop my spiral into depression. I found a friendly, direct woman with 40 years of experience. She helped me affirm and sort out my feelings and pointed me in a direction that enabled me to take action. My situation hasn't changed, and yet I feel more control over my life. Therapy is not a panacea, but it has been an instrument of enormous help in this very difficult life situation.

Therapy is also one tool that we can use when facing painful and debilitating issues, such as

- depression and isolation.
- anxiety and stress.
- past and/or present trauma caused by violence and abuse (emotional, physical, sexual).
- eating problems and body-image distortions.
- addictions—our own and those of people close to us.
- chronic illnesses/disabilities that cause pain, physical limitations, or emotional instability.
- relationships that are not working for us with family, colleagues, friends, and others.
- shame and anger about discrimination, abuse, and violence based on race, gender, sexual orientation, physical ability, or age (psychotherapy can help us in many ways, including supporting our work with others to take appropriate action to confront and to change discriminatory practices).

There was manic depression on both sides of my family. It's been eight years since I had my one episode of psychotic mania, which earned me two weeks in a mental hospital.

After my episode, I benefited a great deal from weekly individual meetings with a male psychiatrist. Sometimes it was frustrating because he wanted to avoid conflict or discussing my sexual abuse memories, but meeting with a male authority figure who treated me with caring and respect was also deeply healing.

Participation in a support group for manic depressives was wonderful for me. Our meetings were sometimes the only place I felt sane all week. "Oh you feel that way, too!" could be more soothing than any pill.

Currently, I see a therapist once a month, take very low doses of two mood stabilizers and two antidepressants, and practice daily meditation. This combination allows me to be an attorney with a full caseload.

I used to be dead set against all individual therapy and psychiatric medication. Now I figure if some therapy and some medication can keep me out of the hospital, and allow me to lead a relatively happy life, I'll do it.

DIFFERENT KINDS OF THERAPISTS

Some of us have a wide range of therapists to choose from; those of us who live in areas of the country with fewer services have to be more resourceful to find good mental health services, particularly a good fit with a therapist. A professional title is no guarantee of the quality of therapy or the kind of person a therapist is. Each group's members represent a spectrum of attitudes and beliefs about women and about healing and emotional health, and different degrees of awareness about the larger societal context. A therapist who

doesn't acknowledge power relations in the world may see the object of therapy as making you "fit in" better in a sexist, racist, and homophobic world—a goal you may not share. The specifics about different specialists may be useful to know, especially since they bear on insurance coverage. But ultimately you must trust your own perceptions and not under- or overestimate the title's meaning.

The categories of therapists that can be licensed by the state include marriage and family therapists, mental health counselors, nurses, psychiatrists, psychologists, and social workers. While psychiatrists (trained medical doctors) used to be the only practitioners who could hospitalize people as well as prescribe medications, now many social workers and psychologists also have hospital admitting privileges (though they cannot medicate). In addition, many nurses and nurse practitioners are now trained to counsel, and in many states can prescribe medications—a real boon to women who might have problems that require medications and who would value having more choices.

Other distinctions may be useful: Social workers are trained to consider the person in the context of the family and the community, psychologists are trained in psychological testing, and psychiatrists are knowledgeable about physical diseases and can factor that in when making an assessment. Marriage and family therapists and licensed mental health counselors have come much more into the forefront of psychotherapy in the last decade because of their skill in handling problems that are social as well as intrapsychic—e.g., divorce, single parenting, working with adolescents, school problems, and other problems that so many of us face throughout our lives.

While all these therapists may be licensed in your state, they may not all be reimbursed by insurance. You can check with the professional organizations or licensing boards for each specialty in your state to find out whether they can accept third-party reimbursement (see Resources). Be sure to ask about fees and insurance before you make a first appointment. Also, even if they are insurance-reimbursable, certain therapists may not be able to take the insurance you have.

Gender Bias

Among social workers, psychologists, and psychiatrists, you can find well-trained, open-minded, and creative therapists; you will also find incompetent, rigid, misogynist, and homophobic therapists. Gender bias in training and in practice is still common, and many therapists have inadequate knowledge about women's issues and women's perspectives. Even in what appears to be the best of circumstances, it is best to be cautious in selecting therapists who are trained primarily in a medical model that emphasizes pathology, not strength and resiliency. We want therapists to treat depression, for example, not just as a medical problem but as the response of a woman of a particular class and ethnic group to perhaps having survived years of abuse in an alcoholic family. We want therapists who are cognizant not only of our struggle and despair but of the resources we have already brought to our survival and can bring to our own healing. And we want therapists who understand the stresses in women's lives that are caused by the double burden of trying to earn a living and care for our families in a society in which women are often underpaid and criticized for whatever choices they make (we should be working if we're caring for children; we should be home with the children if we're working).

Types of Therapy

Therapists, regardless of discipline or professional title, use a variety of theoretical approaches and methods to work with people. Some of them have been influenced by feminist and holistic perspectives that take social context into account, and some have not. Here is a partial list of methodologies:

- Traditional approaches: e.g., psychoanalysis, psychodynamic, gestalt, Jungian, client-centered
- Cognitive and behavioral therapies: e.g., time-effective therapies
- Body-oriented and expressive therapies: e.g., creative arts, bioenergetics, psychodrama, massage and other forms of direct touch
- Hypnotherapy
- Approaches with a spiritual focus: e.g., psychosynthesis, transpersonal, the enneagram (a tool that uses the energy of the personality for spiritual purposes)
- Drug therapy: i.e., the use of psychotropic medications to alter brain chemistry

Group therapy, unlike the self-help groups discussed on p. 123, is facilitated by a trained practitioner. Guided by this skilled facilitator, you can find a safe and challenging environment in which to learn and practice new behaviors. General and specific groups (for example, groups may be offered for incest survivors, for recovery from addictions, for learning to live with chronic illness or stress) offer a community of support with multiple sources of feedback, a reduced sense of isolation, and a chance to make positive changes in your life. For many women, being in such a community of support is the most empowering form of therapy. Group therapy is an effective and economical form of therapy.

FINDING A COMPETENT AND CARING THERAPIST

The Quality of the Relationship

Not every female therapist is a feminist therapist. A feminist therapist is a person who wants women to fully empower themselves and who recognizes that we make choices in the context of our personal, social/political/economic, and spiritual realities. Some

DEPRESSION: CHOOSING MEDICATION

According to the National Institute of Mental Health, over 17 million people in the U.S., two-thirds of whom are women, suffer from depression. In recent years, large numbers of women have found relief with antidepressant medication.

Symptoms that *may* indicate you are suffering from depression include prolonged periods of fatigue; loss of pleasure in activities; feelings of worthlessness, sadness, or hopelessness; decreased or increased appetite; indecisiveness; tearfulness; and suicidal thoughts. These symptoms may be caused by biological factors such as hormonal or biochemical imbalances and/or by experiences such as abuse, oppression, or loss. If you believe that you are depressed, you may want to learn more about it by doing some research (see Resources). This will help you in making decisions about treatment options.

Medications for the treatment of depression are changing rapidly. In the 1990s, several medications that affect neurotransmitters in the brain (norepinephrine and serotonin) have come on the market. Most common are the SSRIs (serotonin selective reuptake inhibitors), including Prozac, Zoloft, and Paxil. (Be aware that names and types of drugs are constantly changing and evolving.) Newer drugs include Luvox (in 1997, not yet FDA-approved) and Effexor, which inhibits the reuptake of norepinephrine and dopamine in addition to serotonin. Because these drugs are apparently nonaddictive, have none of the health-threatening side effects of earlier antidepressants, and can be taken once a day, many women have been willing to try them. Especially when combined with psychotherapy, these medications often provide excellent relief of symptoms, though the side effects, including insomnia, nervousness, drowsiness, or reduced sexual desire do affect some women.

If you would prefer to try a nondrug alternative (if you have difficulty with these medications or are uncomfortable with taking drugs), you might consider the herbal remedy St. John's wort, prescribed and used widely in Germany and other European countries for mild depression. St. John's wort, usually taken one to three times daily in capsules that contain 0.3% hypericin, has been shown to be effective for people with mild depression.

If you decide to try medication, we recommend that you find a medical provider who can do a thorough evaluation and who is familiar with these medications. Usually it takes several weeks before you begin to feel the impact of the

continued on next page

drugs, and often you have to try several before you find the one that is right for you. For this reason, it is important to find a health care provider who will actively monitor your progress and, if you are seeing someone else for "talk therapy," who is willing to coordinate treatment with your therapist.

Controversy continues regarding the overuse of antidepressants, particularly by women. Some medical providers will prescribe these medications without doing a thorough evaluation to determine whether this is the right approach for you. Avoid providers who simply write a prescription and do not provide adequate followup. Research shows that drugs are best used in combination with talk therapy. Nothing is a substitute for compassionate helpers who can provide safety and guidance as we explore what we can change, what we cannot change, and how to know the difference.

men also take a feminist approach. In choosing a therapist, look for mental health professionals who make a good connection with you, your story and perspective, your concerns, and the changes you want to make.

The quality of the relationship is critical in healing. Be sure to use and trust your own responses to the initial interview about how the therapist's training and style might suit your needs. Comparison shopping for the right fit might feel overwhelming at a time when you are feeling emotionally vulnerable; yet, that is just when you have the greatest freedom to assess how different therapists handle the issues you present to them. This is a good time to think about what feels more or less constructive or supportive to you, and whom you feel the most comfortable with.

I've gone to a variety of therapists for shorter and longer periods of my adult life, by myself and with family members. The first time I went, I chose to see a woman, but men have helped me as well. The best of these therapists had these features in common:

They were gentle, friendly, and respectful.
They listened well and understood what I was saying.
They accepted the way I presented issues and didn't alter them to fit some theory.
Their own life problems didn't usually get mixed up with mine; when that happened, they were able to acknowledge it.
They helped me define my problems and see my way to making the changes I wanted to make.
They were open to my criticisms of them.
They cared that I succeeded without claiming responsibility for my success.

Working with the help of therapists who had these qualities, I felt stronger as a person and clearer about my life.

Finding a Therapist for You

Here are some places to begin looking for a therapist whose training, style, and personality are suited to your needs.

- Ask people whom you trust and feel comfortable knowing that you are seeking therapy: friends, family, colleagues, neighbors, religious or spiritual advisors, current health care practitioners.
- Look in women's newspapers or call a local women's center.
- For more anonymity, call the professional mental health organizations in your area, or national associations that may have listings of providers in your locale.
- Contact local mental health centers or places where therapists teach, such as colleges, therapy training centers, or hospitals.
- If you are in a managed care plan, try to find out as much as possible about the therapists available through the plan. You can ask the questions that follow to locate an appropriate person for you within the system. If you don't find a provider who fits your needs, there may be an appeal process that will enable you use an out-of-network provider. Culturally and linguistically appropriate mental health care is a protected civil right. Be assertive: your managed care plan has the responsibility to find someone for you to work with, even if it has to go outside the network.

After finding a possible therapist, here are some questions you may want to ask either on the phone or at an initial meeting:

- What is your training and theoretical orientation/approach?
- How do you prefer to work with people: individually, as part of a couple or family, or in a group?
- What is/are your specialties?
- Are you experienced in working with my specific concerns [name them]?
- How many years have you been in practice?
- Do you meet regularly with other colleagues to discuss your therapy work?
- Are you comfortable working with my particular [race, ethnic or religious background, sexual orientation, or disability]?
- How often would you suggest we meet, and would you have the time available?
- What are your policies about changing appointments? How much notice must I give?
- Do you charge for the initial meeting? If so, how much? Do you have sliding-scale fees?
- Can you be reimbursed by my insurance plan [identify specific plan]?
- What do you think about the use of psychotropic drugs?

As you speak to the potential therapist, how does this person sound to you? Does she or he answer your questions in a respectful manner? Is this person someone you would like to meet? Remember that you are looking for someone to help *you* make the changes *you* want to make. If you have the time and financial resources, interview several prospective therapists. You may work with this person for several months or even years, so it is worth taking the time to find a practitioner who fits your needs. Comparison shopping is more difficult when negotiating with a managed care company with a fixed list of providers. For example, you may be seeking a therapist who is a woman of color or a lesbian, but there is only one (or none) on the list. In these cases, we need to become advocates for change in the system and at the same time find a way to get the necessary services for ourselves or for a loved one.

Ethical Questions

State licensing boards and national professional organizations help maintain practice standards. You can use them to make sure the therapist you are considering is trained and follows ethical standards, and to determine whether a practitioner has ever been reported for an ethical violation. Many of the mental health professions have ethics review boards to ensure that a high standard of care is sustained (see Resources for names and numbers of professional associations). All licensed practitioners are accountable for maintaining the level of continuing education that will keep their work current, although these standards vary by profession and by state. Concern about the ability of a therapist to respond competently to your needs is an ethical concern.

You can also report ethical violations to these bodies. Some therapists—both men and women—do abuse their power. A practitioner may be lonely, need attention, or have unresolved problems of his or her own and try to create relationships with clients that meet those needs. Inappropriate behavior might include trying to create a social relationship outside of the professional context, discussing other clients by name or by other clearly identifying data, or revealing intimate information, either personal or about his or her relationships. Encouraging a client to become a friend or lover is wrong, as is other unprofessional behavior that interferes with your therapy. A therapist's job is to work for you and not in any way to use the relationship for her or his own personal needs or ends.

If you feel your therapist is acting inappropriately, there are places to get help. BASTA (Boston Associates to Stop Treatment Abuse), listed in this chapter's Resources, has an excellent checklist to help you determine whether your therapist may be crossing ethical boundaries. This organization also has information on filing complaints with licensing boards and professional organizations. Most important, if something about your therapy doesn't feel right to you, talk to

others about what is happening. Remember that you can end a therapy relationship at any time and find someone who can give you appropriate help.

CHALLENGES FOR CONSUMERS

While therapy can be a useful and life-giving tool, changes in the health care system are creating serious challenges for consumers of psychotherapy. Many of us no longer have health insurance coverage that includes good mental health care. Even those of us who are fully employed and insured through our workplaces may have limited mental health benefits that do not cover the kind of long-term care many of us seek when we begin work with a therapist. For women who have low incomes and/or do not have insurance, therapy is often completely out of reach. You may be able to find therapists who have sliding-scale fees, or as mentioned earlier in this chapter, you can seek out facilitated group therapy sessions or self-help groups. (For instance, there may be a local chapter of the National Black Women's Health Project in your area.)

FACING A CRISIS

There are moments when we don't have the time to go through a lengthy process to find an appropriate therapist. *If you, a family member, or a friend is in crisis*—i.e., in danger of committing suicide or harming another person—*go to the local hospital emergency room.* Be aware, however, that once at the hospital, you are subject to the possibility of involuntary commitment. Even if you sign into a hospital voluntarily, you may have difficulty leaving. If the hospital staff believe that you are a danger to yourself or others, they can keep you for 24 to 72 hours, depending on state law. After that time, if the hospital won't release you, you are entitled to a hearing before a judge. However, in all likelihood the judge will rule in favor of the hospital. Though managed care has made it less likely that a hospital will keep you indefinitely because of cost containment, as a patient on a psychiatric ward you do not have control over the situation, nor does your family. Psychiatric patients essentially lose their civil rights once they are committed to a hospital.* Involuntary commitment is on the rise again for Medicare and Medicaid patients, who are placed in psychiatric hospitals against their will to fill empty beds. Hospitals are then able to collect payment through these government-funded health plans.[1]

* See Judi Chamberlain, "Involuntary Interventions: The Call for a National Legal and Medical Response—Human Rights, Not Patients' Rights" (May 1994). Paper available from The National Empowerment Center (see Resources).

These can provide less expensive (and sometimes free) alternatives to individual therapy.

Managed care is having a particularly devastating impact on mental health services. Not only do we often have to choose our providers from an approved list, but insurers expect practitioners to quickly identify problems and find solutions (for a larger discussion of managed care, see chapter 25, The Politics of Women's Health and Medical Care, p. 696). Many of the values and guiding principles of good mental health care are in danger of being annihilated under the guise of "efficiency" and "cost-effectiveness." Managed care companies often devalue psychotherapy, which is most effective over a long period of time; instead, practitioners are encouraged to prescribe medication, which is cheaper and easier to manage but does not necessarily accomplish the same ends. While the use of psychotropic drugs, including antidepressants, has shown some success in the treatment of what were previously seen as purely psychological illnesses, these drugs cannot replace the human interactions and relationships that are at the core of good mental health care.

As medical and especially mental health consumers, we are facing changes that will often make it necessary to fight to get adequate care, to get the right kind of care, and to find a way to maintain the confidentiality of our relationships with the providers we are given and, if fortunate, able to choose. Although there continue to be instances in which some families and state authorities lock away assertive women of all classes and races by labeling us "crazy" (for more on involuntary commitment, see "Facing a Crisis," p. 127), the more common problem is not getting enough or the right kind of care, either because we don't have the money or our insurance carriers won't provide it. Prescribing psychotropic drugs to millions of women is not an adequate response to the pain that many women experience as a result of the complex social and economic realities of sexism, racism, homophobia, and other oppressions. Many of us have suffered physical or emotional abuse at some point during our lives, and recovery is a long process. We must continue to be proactive—individually and collectively—to get the care we need.

NOTES

1. Dolores Kong and Gerard O'Neill, "Locked Wards Open Door to Booming Business," *The Boston Globe* (May 11, 1997); and Mitchell Zuckoff, "Flawed Law Turns Patients into Prisoners," *The Boston Globe* (May 12, 1997).

RESOURCES

(Since space limited the number of our choices, we focused on self-help books. There are many excellent books oriented to practitioners and to theory that we were not able to include.)

Bass, Ellen, and Laura Davis. *The Courage to Heal: A Guide for Women Survivors of Child Sexual Abuse*. New York: HarperPerennial, 1994.

Bepko, Claudia, and Joann Krestan. *Too Good for Her Own Good: Searching for Self and Intimacy in Important Relationships*. New York: HarperCollins, 1991.

Bolen, Jean. *Goddesses in Everywoman: A New Psychology of Women*. New York: HarperCollins, 1985.

Boorstein, Sylvia. *Don't Just Do Something, Sit There*. San Francisco: Harper San Francisco, 1996.

Boston Lesbian Psychologies Collective, eds. *Lesbian Psychologies*. Urbana: University of Illinois, 1987.

Boyd, Julia A. *In the Company of My Sisters: Black Women and Self-Esteem*. New York: Dutton, 1993.

Breggin, Peter, and Ginger Ross Breggin. *Talking Back to Prozac: What Doctors Won't Tell You About Today's Most Controversial Drug*. New York: St. Martin's Press, 1994.

Cameron, Julia. *The Artists Way: A Spiritual Path to Higher Creativity*. Los Angeles: J.P. Tarcher, 1992.

Carter, Betty, and Joan Peters. *Love, Honor and Negotiate: Making Your Marriage Work*. New York: Pocket Books, 1996.

Castillo, Ana. *Massacre of the Dreamers: Essays on Xicanisma*. New York: New American Library/Dutton, 1995.

Caudill, Margaret A. *Managing Pain Before It Manages You*. New York: Guilford Press, 1994.

Dolan, Yvonne. *Resolving Sexual Abuse: Solution-Focused Therapy and Ericksonian Hypnosis for Survivors*. New York: Norton, 1991.

Duerk, Judith. *Circle of Stones: A Woman's Journey to Herself*. San Diego, CA: LuraMedia Press, 1989.

Edelson, Hope. *Motherless Daughters: The Legacy of Loss*. New York: Dell, 1995.

Gilligan, Carol. *In a Different Voice: Psychological Theory and Women's Development*. Cambridge, MA: Harvard University Press, 1993.

Greene, Beverly. "Lesbian Women of Color," in Comas-Dias, L., and B. Greene, eds. *Women of Color: Integrating Ethnic and Gender Identities in Psychotherapy*. New York: Guilford Press, 1994.

Hamilton, Jean A., et al., eds. *Psychopharmacology from a Feminist Perspective*. New York: Harrington Park Press, 1995.

Herman, Judith. *Trauma and Recovery*. New York: Basic Books, 1992.

Himber, Judith. "Blood Rituals: Self Cutting in Female Psychiatric Inpatients," *Psychotherapy* 31, no. 4 (winter 1994): 620–31.

hooks, bell. *Killing Rage: Ending Racism*. New York: Henry Holt, 1995.

———. *Sisters of the Yam: Black Women and Self-Recovery*. Boston: South End Press, 1993.

Jack, Dana Crowly. *Silencing the Self: Women and Depression*. Cambridge, MA: Harvard University Press, 1991.

Jamison, Kay Redfield. *An Unquiet Mind: A Memoir of Moods and Madness*. New York: Random House, 1995.

Jones, Anne, and Schechter, Susan. *When Love Goes

Wrong: What to Do When You Can't Do Anything Right. New York: HarperPerennial, 1992.

Jordan, Judith V., et al. *Women's Growth in Connection: Writings from the Stone Center.* New York: Guilford, 1991.

Kramer, Peter D. *Listening to Prozac.* New York: Viking, 1993.

Lee, Barbara. *Take Control of Your Money: A Life Guide to Financial Freedom.* New York: Villard Books, 1986.

Lerner, Harriet G. *The Dance of Anger.* New York: HarperCollins, 1989.

————. *The Dance of Intimacy: A Woman's Guide to Courageous Acts of Change in Key Relationships.* New York: HarperCollins, 1990.

————. *The Dance of Deception: Pretending and Truth Telling in Women's Lives.* New York: HarperCollins, 1993.

Lorde, Audre. *Sister Outsider: Essays and Speeches.* Freedom, CA: Crossing Press, 1984.

Louden, Jennifer. *The Woman's Comfort Book: A Self Nurturing Guide for Restoring Balance In Your Life.* San Francisco: Harper, 1992.

————. *The Woman's Retreat Book: A Guide to Restoring, Rediscovering and Reawakening Your True Self.* San Francisco: Harper San Francisco, 1997.

Maltz, Wendy. *Sexual Healing Journey: A Guide for Survivors of Sexual Abuse.* New York: HarperCollins, 1992.

Markowitz, Laura M. "Homosexuality: Are We Still in the Dark?" *Family Therapy Networker* 15, no. 1 (Jan.-Feb. 1991).

McGrath, Ellen. *When Feeling Bad Is Good.* New York: Bantam Books, 1994.

Middelton-Moz, Jane, and Lorie Dwinell. *After the Tears: Reclaiming the Personal Losses of Childhood.* Deerfield Beach, FL: Health Communications, 1986.

Miller, Alice. *The Drama of the Gifted Child: The Search for the Self.* New York: Basic Books, 1994.

Miller, Jean Baker. *Toward a New Psychology of Women,* 2nd ed. Boston: Beacon Press, 1986.

Palmer, Helen. *The Enneagram In Love and Work.* San Francisco: Harper, 1995.

Peurifoy, Reneau Z. *Anxiety, Phobias and Panic: A Step-by-Step Program for Regaining Control of Your Life.* New York: Warner Books, 1995.

Prochaska, James. *Changing for Good.* New York: Avon, 1995.

Roth, Geneen. *Breaking Free From Compulsive Eating.* New York: New American Library/Dutton, 1986.

Sanford, Linda T., and Mary Ellen Donovan. *Women and Self-Esteem: Understanding and Improving the Way We Think and Feel About Ourselves.* New York: Viking Penguin, 1985.

Schlessinger, Laura C. *Ten Stupid Things Women Do to Mess Up Their Lives.* New York: HarperCollins, 1995.

Siegel, Michele, Judith Brisman, and Margaret Weinshel. *Surviving an Eating Disorder: Strategies for Family and Friends.* New York: HarperCollins, 1989.

Simon, Clea. *Mad House: Growing Up in the Shadow of Mentally Ill Siblings.* New York: Doubleday, 1997.

Solden, Sari. *Women with Attention Deficit Disorder: Embracing Disorganization at Home and in the Workplace.* Grass Valley, CA: Underwood Books, 1995.

Weekes, Claire. *Peace from Nervous Suffering.* New York: New American Library/Dutton, 1990.

Weingarten, Kathy. *The Mother's Voice: Strengthening Intimacy in Families.* Orlando, FL: Harcourt Brace, 1994.

Wisechild, Louise M. *The Mother I Carry: A Memoir of Healing from Emotional Abuse.* Seattle: Seal Press, 1993.

OTHER RESOURCES

American Association of Marriage and Family Therapy
1133 15th Street NW, Suite 300; Washington, DC 20005; (202) 452-0109; (888) AAMFT-99
Web site: http://www.aamft.org

American Mental Health Counselors Association
801 N. Fairfax Street, Suite 304; Alexandria, VA 22314; (703) 548-6002; (800) 326-2642
E-mail: amhcahq@pie.org

American Nurses Association
600 Maryland Avenue SW, Suite 100; Washington, DC 20024; (202) 651-7060; (800) 637-0323 (to order publications)
Web site: http://www.nursingworld.org

American Psychiatric Association
1400 K Street NW; Washington, DC 20005; (202) 682-6114
E-mail: apa@psych.org
Web site: http://www.apa.com

American Psychological Association
750 First Street NE; Washington, DC 20002; (202) 336-5500; (800) 374-2721
Web site: http://www.apa.org

BASTA: Boston Associates to Stop Treatment Abuse
528 Franklin Street, Cambridge, MA 02139; (617) 661-4667
Responds to the needs of those abused in sexual ways by psychotherapists and other human service/health care providers.

Cochrane Collaboration, Depression, Anxiety and Neurosis Group
Ms. Carolyn Doughty, Coordinator
Department of Psychological Medicine; Christchurch School of Medicine; P.O. Box 4345; Christchurch, New Zealand
E-mail: cdoughty@chmeds.ac.nz

National Association of Social Workers
750 First Street NE; Washington, DC 20002-4241; (800) 227-3590; (202) 408-8600; (202) 408-8396 (TDD)
Web site: http://www.yahoo.com/Social_Science/Social_Work/Organizations/Professional/National_Association_of_Social_Workers

National Empowerment Center
(800) POWER2U
   Information and resources on self-help recovery for psychiatric survivors.

Stone Center
Wellesley College; 106 Central Street; Wellesley, MA 01281-8259
   This center produces working papers, audiotapes, and books based on a relational/cultural approach to understanding women's psychological development, problems, and treatment.

TELL (Therapy Exploitation Link Line)
(617) 964-TELL
   Victim support group, self-help model, meets monthly. Free.

   For additional resources, please see chapters 2, 3, 4, 5, 8, 9, 10, and 11.

Additional Online Resources *

The Anxiety-Panic Internet Resource
http://www.algy.com/anxiety/anxiety.html

Caregiver Survival Resources Home Page
http://www.caregiver911.com

Crisis, Grief, and Healing: Men and Women
http://www.webhealing.com

Dr. Grohol's Mental Health Page: Psychology Web Pointer
http://www.grohol.com

Emotional Support Resources
http://asa.ugl.lib.umich.edu/chdocs/support/emotion.html

Internet Mental Health
http://www.mentalhealth.com/p.html

Mental Health Net: Self-help Resources Index
http://www.cmhc.com/selfhelp.htm

National Women's Resource Center
http://www.nwrc.org

Office of Minority Health Resource Center
http://www.omhrc.gov/Welcome.HTM

Self-Help & Psychology Magazine
http://www.cybertowers.com/selfhelp

* For more information and listings of online resources, please see Introduction to Online Women's Health Resources, p. 25.

Chapter 7

Environmental and Occupational Health

ENVIRONMENTAL HEALTH BY Lin Nelson, based on earlier work by Patricia Logan

OCCUPATIONAL HEALTH BY Regina H. Kenen, based on earlier work by members of MassCOSH Women's Committee: Letitia Davis, Marian Marbury, Laura Punnett, Margaret Quinn, Cathy Schwartz, and Susan Woskie

WITH SPECIAL THANKS TO Dorothy Wigmore, Pat Hynes, Norma Grier, Carol Dansereau, Maureen Gorman, Elizabeth Gullette, Kristin Lacijan of NCAMP, Jacqueline Lapidus, Cheri Lucas-Jennings, Karen McDonell, Manju Mehta, Vernice Miller, Susan O'Brien, Ngazi Oleru, Cydney Pullman, and the thousands of women throughout the U.S. fighting for environmental justice *

We live in a small town. One morning a neighbor came over and said, "Don't drink the water," just after my husband and I drank two cups of coffee made from tap water. We had been drinking it for years, and we didn't know how long it had been contaminated. Then our neighbor said just how bad it was, how many milligrams of the chemicals were in it. No one knows where it came from or who caused it. I felt very angry. You pay your taxes —they get higher every year—and you've got people sitting down there in their offices letting things get that bad.

Everybody should have pure, clean water to drink. But what could I do about it? I don't know enough. And anyway, what about everything else? When you eat your chicken, how do you know if you get pure meat? Or what's in your vegetables? Or what's in your bottled water?

* Over the years since 1984, the following women and organizations have contributed to the many versions of this chapter: Judy Norsigian, The Shalan Foundation, Joan Bertin, Katsi Cook, and Maureen Paul.

Where and how we live and work affects our health in some obvious and not so obvious ways all the time. Sixty to 90% of all human cancers and high percentages of other lung, heart, nerve, and kidney disease as well as reproductive problems, birth defects, and even behavioral disorders are now thought to be environmentally caused. ("Environment" here includes our diet and living habits as well as our surroundings.)

Environmental hazards have increased tremendously in the last 50 years. To the accidents, stress, and disease that people have always encountered, 20th-century society has added toxic chemical and radioactive substances and fallout, and electromagnetic fields. Through their manufacture, processing, distribution, use, and disposal, these substances create a severe and unreasonable risk of injury to our environment and to our health.

NEW CONCERNS ABOUT WOMEN'S HEALTH

Scientific interest in women's health mushroomed in the 1990s, partly in response to women's grassroots campaigns for medical attention, legislation, and funding for research. The National Institutes of Health (NIH) have started a large-scale, long-term women's health study, the Women's Health Initiative. The Food and Drug Administration (FDA) now encourages the inclusion of women in study designs. The National Institute for Occupational Safety and Health (NIOSH) hired a coordinator of minority and women's health to help centralize and focus research on women's occupational health issues. The first International Women, Health and Work Congress, organized by the Centro de Analisis y Programas Sanitarias (CAPS, Health Programs and Analysis Center), was held in Barcelona, Spain, in 1993. There are now ongoing meetings of this International Women's Congress.*

Opinions differ about how much to emphasize biological gender differences and how extensive these differences really are. Women are in a bind. We want to be included in research studies, because we know our bodies are not necessarily susceptible in the same way as men's to all kinds of dangers and poisons. Yet, our history demonstrates that whenever differences between men and women are identified, women tend to be treated as second-class people. Some of the gender-oriented studies might be used against us—all in the name of "science."

There is an ongoing debate about which health hazards are more urgent: those caused by industrial practices and pollution, or those that result from the way we live our lives. We have chosen to focus in this chapter on some of each. It is easier for private corporations and government at all levels to blame individuals for making unhealthy "lifestyle choices" than to spend the money needed to clean up our communities and purify our food and water supply. Our "choices" are in fact limited by economic resources, family obligations, and the availability of alternatives. We can best begin by taking action about the risks we know, and press for more research on those we don't.

Connecting Occupational and Environmental Hazards

We need to remember that as we move among the places where we live different parts of our lives, our bodies respond to the total load of environmental influences, not just to each one separately. While occupational and environmental health are considered to be separate fields of study, and different government agencies deal with them,† many of the exposures to toxins and the problems they create are similar. We and our family members may be exposed to the same toxic substances or conditions in the workplace, at

home, and in our neighborhoods. One woman's "environment" may also be another woman's workplace. And we may be doubly exposed by working the "double shift"—as homemaker/caretaker and as an employee outside our homes.

In farm communities, for example, pesticides may affect both farm workers and everyone who lives and works in the area. Farm workers, community members, and even local physicians may not be aware of the particular chemicals being used or of their harmful effects.

I didn't really think about it at the time, but I lived where there was a lot of crop dusting. Every winter I got a sore throat as a reaction to this cotton defoliant they were spraying about the middle of December. That had nothing to do with the job. It had more to do with where I lived. When I remembered, I would always ask my doctor and he was reassuring, even when I was pregnant and due to deliver in January.

The connection to environmental conditions is strong in other occupations as well. As far back as 1941, 24 cases of beryllium poisoning were found among women making fluorescent lamps at a Sylvania plant in Salem, Massachusetts. Later, more cases were discovered in women living close to the plant, then additional cases in Ohio when emissions in the air were traced to a beryllium ore-extraction facility.[1]

There is currently more coordination between governmental agencies. For example, NIOSH and the National Institute for Environmental Health Sciences have a program through the National Toxicological Program whereby grants are given to medical schools to teach family physicians about occupational and environmental health so that they can answer basic questions and know where to refer their patients instead of claiming, as they too often do, that "it's all in your head."

Activists, researchers, and public health practitioners are now moving to make the connections in assessing the problems and developing responses. Organizations such as the Good Neighbor Project and the Labor Institute focus on "labor-neighbor" coalition building. Unions, such as the Oil, Chemical and Atomic Workers, and environmental organizations, such as the Center for Health, Environment and Justice, are increasingly effective in joining strategies. These collaborations can help us see the larger context of shared, continuous risk. Our communities need not make dead-end "choices" between safe jobs and a healthy environment.

Public Health and Responsibility

Environmental and occupational hazards affect entire populations, not just individuals. They are *public health issues*. The NIOSH sometimes emphasizes individual responsibility for prevention in its workplace safety and health programs, especially when eliminating the cause of the problem is claimed to be "economically infeasible." This approach raises serious

* For further information, contact CAPS, Paris 150, 08036 Barcelona, Spain. Phone: (343) 322-6554; Fax: (343) 410-9742. Follow the instructions in your phone book for international dialing.
† Both the Occupational Safety and Health Administration (OSHA) and the Environmental Protection Agency (EPA) were set up in 1970.

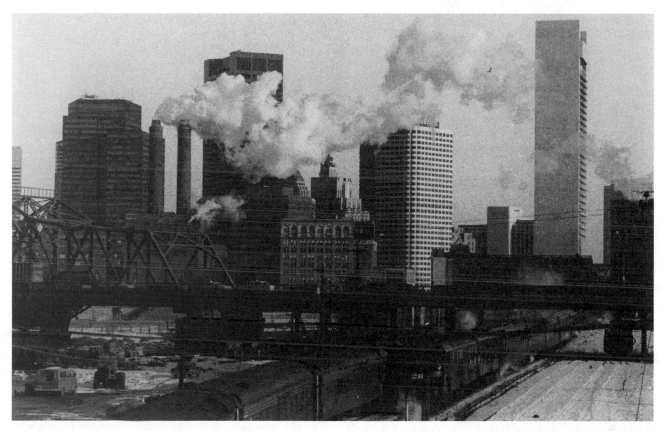

political questions about who profits from exposing us to danger at work or in our general environment. It also shifts responsibility for the dangers from public institutions and private corporations to us as individuals: we are told that our "lifestyle" or behavior is what makes us get sick or stay well. But we cannot avoid being exposed to toxic substances or dangerous conditions that we cannot control.

CHEMICALS

Between 50,000 and 75,000 chemical substances are in common commercial use in the United States. About a thousand new chemicals appear each year. The vast majority of them have not been tested, over time, for their potential ill effects, yet they are in our food, water, air, clothing, homes, and workplaces. Persistent and potentially harmful chemicals are globally distributed, contaminating both industrialized and developing countries as well as the earth's polar regions.[2]

Our sewers are loaded with acid and chemicals. You can see them cooking in there, coming right up in my cellar. I called the city officials and they said they have nothing to do with it anymore. It's up to the state. The state people came and took samples from the sewer. I have yet to hear the results. I have been going to the doctor for the past 30 years. I've got breathing problems, kidney and bladder trouble, my kid has a heart condition, my husband can't breathe. Every morning I get up

I know I am going to get that "sweet air" from the sewer disposal, and then I say, what's going to be next?[3]

Many common chemicals threaten our health:

- Car exhaust; particles, ash, and smoke from factories; emissions from chemical and nuclear plants; and drifting pesticides all contaminate our air. Chlorofluorocarbons and carbon dioxide pollute the atmosphere, leading to ozone depletion and global warming.
- Industrial chemicals, agricultural pesticides, herbicides used in forestry, and leaking dumpsites contaminate our waterways.
- Pesticides, fertilizers, preservatives, and additives undermine our food supply. The accumulation of contaminants in fatty tissue results in higher risks to those who eat animal products.
- Lead-based paint (now illegal) in pre-1978 housing can impair the development of young children who ingest it. Mothers with low incomes living in substandard housing may have a hard time getting their homes repainted as well as testing, protection, and treatment for their children.
- Household cleaning and personal care products, as well as chemicals used in dry cleaning, can produce toxic fumes and residues. Formaldehyde (in carpets, pressboard, insulation) and radon gas endanger homes, schools, and other public

buildings. Chemical vapors, carbon monoxide, and other air pollutants can disrupt moods and impair mental functioning.

RADIATION *

Available evidence suggests that low-level radiation from normally functioning nuclear power plants and from weapons facilities and testing contaminates our environment and our bodies in slow stages. The mining of uranium and disposing of the milling wastes (called tailings) and the spent fuel create even more hazards. Waste from a nuclear reactor or weapons plant remains radioactive for as long as 250 centuries.

Our immediate community has been threatened by the effluent from one of the largest uranium mines in this hemisphere. For many months this effluent contaminated our public water supply—our people drank, cooked with, and bathed in this water, which had radiation in excess of recommended exposures. It took litigation and thousands of dollars of taxpayers' money to remove this community from that contaminated water supply.

In the ultimate accident at a nuclear power plant, a meltdown, thousands die immediately of lethal radiation exposure; tens of thousands die within two or three weeks of acute radiation sickness; hundreds of thousands of cancers occur five to 30 years afterward. The meltdown at Chernobyl, now the most famous, is not the only accident in the past decade. And, of course, nuclear war itself is the ultimate environmental hazard. The U.S. still has 14,000 nuclear weapons, and over 28,000 exist throughout the world.[4]

The legacy of nuclear weapons production is particularly devastating for communities downwind of such installations as the Hanford Complex in eastern Washington State. Recent research findings suggest that women downwind of Hanford (in the area between the Cascade and Rocky Mountains in Oregon, Idaho, and Washington) are at greater risk for hypothyroidism and spontaneous abortion.[5]

Available evidence suggests that low-level radiation from normally functioning nuclear power plants and weapons facilities can pose serious threats to the environment and to our health. Mining of uranium, disposal of milling wastes, and spent fuel create even more hazards. While some people fear a full-scale accident at a nuclear plant, many others have already been subjected to dangerous radiation through nuclear testing. The U.S. government has downplayed the impact of nuclear testing on women's reproductive health in the Marshall Islands, while research findings from a study of 1,200 Marshallese women point to a pattern of difficult pregnancies, miscarriages, stillbirths, and birth defects.[6]

Many of us who work with computers in an increasing variety of jobs have been raising questions about radiation from video display terminals: Is it a danger to our health? How much exposure is tolerable? How long can it accumulate before health problems are detectable? Construction, delivery, health care, and social workers are as likely to be affected as those doing traditional office or data entry work (see Resources).

ELECTROMAGNETIC FIELDS

Electromagnetic fields (EMFs) are invisible lines of force created whenever electricity is generated or used. They are produced by power lines, electric wiring, and electrical equipment and appliances. Women's neighborhood groups have taken the lead in calling attention to the potential dangers of exposure to EMFs. Some studies have shown increased leukemia and cancer rates among workers exposed to high magnetic fields, but scientists disagree about the harmful effects of EMFs. They do agree that more investigation is needed.

Because of scientists' uncertainty, the federal government has not yet recommended any limits for worker exposure to EMFs. In the meantime, some simple and inexpensive measures can be taken to reduce EMF exposures. Magnetic fields often drop off dramatically beyond about three feet from the source, so work stations can be moved out of that range. The duration of exposure can be reduced. Layouts for office power lines can be designed so as to reduce EMF exposure for workers.

PERVASIVE RISKS, UNEQUAL BURDENS

Today, environmental hazards are so widespread that none of us can totally avoid them. Even snow in Antarctica carries residues of polychlorinated biphenyls (PCBs), dichlorodiphenyltrichloroethane (DDT), and lead.[7] Human breast milk contains high levels of some toxins, and human sperm samples contain PCBs.†

Although we encounter the most concentrated and dangerous hazards in the workplace, our general environment creates a toxic burden for everyone and an added burden for workers. While we are all involuntarily exposed to some environmental health hazards, and while toxic contaminants do cross regional, sex, class, and racial lines, there are very clear inequities. Economic and social power determines how much we can protect ourselves. Some people can afford to move away from a chemical dump or nuclear power plant; some can buy bottled water or food without additives or get better health care. Others at this point in our country's history cannot.

* For basic information on the health effects of radiation exposure and studies under way at nuclear sites, contact Physicians for Social Responsibility (see Resources).

† PCBs, once widely used in adhesives, paints, lubricants, electric insulators, and printing inks, can cause everything from skin discoloration to liver disorders to cancer; DDT causes cancer and endangers wildlife; lead damages the nervous system.

Racism and the Environment

The burdens of the toxic economy are shouldered more by some than by others. The Commission for Racial Justice (United Church of Christ) conducted an extensive landmark study and found that three of the five largest commercial hazardous waste landfills are located in mostly black or Latino communities, three of five black and Latino Americans live in communities with uncontrolled toxic-waste sites, and about half of all Asians/Pacific Islanders and Native Americans live near uncontrolled waste sites.[8] The clear identification of this environmental racism and the limited response of the mainstream environmental movement to this reality have inspired new thinking and action on environmental justice.[9]

In Pensacola, Florida, African-American neighborhoods were put at risk by the Escambia Treating Company, which left behind toxic deposits of pentachlorophenol. Nine years after the plant closed, the EPA excavated the area and stockpiled the dioxin-laced remains. Citizens Against Toxic Exposure (CATE), the community group that emerged to deal with this problem, believes that in a white community more effective protective action would have been taken more quickly. Their suspicions are supported by research on how communities of color face not only higher risks of hazardous exposure but also higher risk of negligence by agencies in responding to their needs. Through the dedication of CATE and the support of groups such as the Center for Health, Environment and Justice (formerly the Citizens' Clearinghouse for Hazardous Waste), the community waged an effective campaign to get residents out of harm's way. The EPA then agreed to relocate 358 families and set some limits on dioxin exposure in residential neighborhoods.[10]

Environmental health hazards are not only an urban problem. Rural people face heavy exposure to pesticides and herbicides, especially since agribusiness has taken over food production. Of the three million farm workers in the U.S., most are migrants, usually Latinos. Because only 25% are women, this occupational category often gets neglected as a women's health issue. However, it is an important one. Even if rural women are not agricultural workers themselves, they and their children live near the fields and are exposed to similar conditions.

Women throughout the world face common occupational and environmental hazards. How much prevention, protection, and enforcement of laws we can count on in each country varies by workplace and by the strength of labor unions in each country.

Many Native Americans live with persistent low-level radiation from the uranium mining that has taken over more and more of their land. Some companies have targeted their reservations for toxic-waste dump sites.[11]

In addition, pesticides, drugs and industrial chemicals and processes banned as too dangerous in the U.S. are exported for use in developing countries where regulations are nonexistent or not enforced.

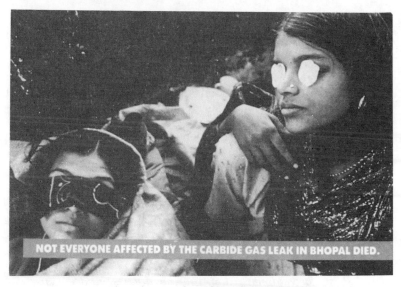

NOT EVERYONE AFFECTED BY THE CARBIDE GAS LEAK IN BHOPAL DIED.

Bhopal Group for Information and Action

Seven years after the 1984 toxic gas leak from the Union Carbide pesticide factory in Bhopal, India, 400,000 victims continued to suffer from untreatable or fatal illnesses (see Resources).

At the first Costa Rican Tribunal on Violations of Women's Rights in 1995, testimony was presented on behalf of a woman who handled fruit covered with toxins and sometimes scorpions and snakes. When no fruit was available, she was sent to work in a warehouse where dibromochloro-propane (DBCP), a chemical banned in the United States, and other such pesticides were stored. She reported headaches, severe menstrual cramps, vision loss, chronic allergies, and pains in her bones. She requested legal representation in the U.S. because some of the plantations belonged to a U.S. fruit company.[12]

As women we have had little to say about what we need or want. We have been targeted by industry and advertising as the consumers of the new technologies that create environmental hazards. Yet, women have been on the front lines in the struggle to curb hazards.

Official government and business statements about environmental hazards are almost universally reassuring: "Don't worry, no long-term dangers have been scientifically proved." They often put profit and prestige before people's health. Today we face the tragic consequences of trusting the reassurances of earlier decades —about DDT, for instance, or atomic testing. The authors of this book believe that we *must* be concerned about environmental hazards whether or not they are at present conclusively "proved" dangerous. We don't want ourselves, our loved ones, or anyone anywhere in the world used as guinea pigs in long-term safety experiments. We know our bodies, our workplaces, and our communities better than any scientist does.

When women get involved in environmental health advocacy, it is not necessarily because we are already dealing with a health problem of our own. Simply, many women are more likely than men to raise questions in our communities about the potential hazards of a sewage treatment plant, waste incinerator, or nuclear installation. Often we do this out of concern for the health of our own children or of those in the community. In spite of doubt and worry ("I'll only get myself and my family in trouble for raising this question or pushing to get that report"), we persist in community-based environmental advocacy, convinced that what we are doing needs to be done, and with growing confidence in our skills and strength.

HEALTH EFFECTS OF
ENVIRONMENTAL HAZARDS

At Love Canal,* they told us to go home and tend our gardens. But women are no longer at home tending their gardens because both have become unsafe. There are many effects of Love Canal chemicals, like central nervous system disease, including nervous breakdowns, migraine headaches, and epilepsy. We have not conducted a survey on cancer to see if the rate is abnormally high here, but we have found many women throughout the neighborhood with breast and uterine cancer. There are many cancers, and they are not just in middle-aged women. One 12-year-old child had a hysterectomy. We have many people with urinary problems, brain damage, and the list goes on. Cancers and other diseases may not surface for years.

To understand environmental health, we must understand that *everything* is connected—our body systems and organs, our life habits, our work, and our wider environment. Environmental hazards can attack a particular organ or body system, directly damaging it and/or leading to further complications. While scientists generally test substances in labs one at a time, in real life our bodies always deal with more than one hazard at once. The combined interaction of two or more hazards to produce an effect greater than that of either one alone is called *synergism*. The amount of exposure, the route of exposure, and the toxic substance(s) we are exposed to determine whether we will feel acute or chronic effects.

We can absorb toxic substances in three ways: through the skin, through the digestive system (eating or drinking), or through the lungs. Often toxins cause damage on first contact—burns, rashes, stomach pain, for example. Once in the bloodstream, they can damage many internal organs and systems.

In general, toxins affect women and men in the same ways: Anyone can have an allergic reaction or liver

* From the 1920s to the 1950s, the Hooker Chemical Company buried metal drums filled with tons of chemical wastes in the excavations in the Love Canal neighborhood of Niagara Falls, New York. In 1953, they covered the dump and sold the land to the Board of Education, which built a school on the site. Over the years, the drums rusted and chemicals seeped, mixed, and were spread by flooding and underground streams. Toxins killed plants, grass, and wildlife; sickened local residents; and caused birth defects and spontaneous abortions. In August 1978, the government declared Love Canal a national emergency area.

ENVIRONMENTAL HEALTH TERMS

- **Carcinogen (car-*sin*-o-jen):** A substance or agent that causes cancer, a condition characterized by usually rapidly spreading abnormal cell growth.
- **Mutagen (*mew*-ta-jen):** A substance or agent that causes (mutations) in the genetic material of living cells. When a mutation occurs in the egg or sperm (germ cells), it can be passed on to future generations. Recent research suggests that because genetic material controls the growth of cells, mutagens may either immediately or after a latency period cause abnormal cell growth, which becomes cancer.
- **Teratogen (teh-*ra*-to-jen):** A substance or agent that can cross the placenta of a pregnant woman and can cause a spontaneous abortion or birth disabilities and developmental abnormalities in the fetus.

All carcinogens are mutagens. Most mutagens are carcinogens. Many mutagens are also teratogens.

- An *acute effect* is a severe immediate reation, usually after a single, large exposure, like the nausea and dizziness of pesticide poisoning or the pulmonary edema (a blistering of the air sacs in the lungs) from the burns of toxic gases like ammonia or chlorine.
- A *chronic effect* is a recurrent or constant reaction, usually occurring after repeated smaller exposures.

Chronic effects can take years — the *latency period*—to develop. For instance, exposure to asbestos causes lung disease years later, and most cancers and progressive liver diseases develop only after 15 to 40 years. Many scientists believe that we will see more and more problems as the toxins introduced after World War II "come of age."

damage, chronic headaches or respiratory problems, mental retardation or lung cancer. Environmental hazards put extra stress on our bodies and compound any other health problems that we might have.

Skin Diseases

As skin is our body's largest porous organ, it is extremely vulnerable to chemicals and other contaminants and a frequent site of exposure. According to the U.S. Bureau of Labor and Statistics, skin diseases are the second most common type of occupational disease.

Prevention is very important, because a high percentage of both women and men who suffer from skin irritation eventually develop chronic skin disease. From 1983 to 1994, the rate increased from 64 to 81 cases per 100,000 workers. The actual number is probably higher, as skin diseases are severely underreported.[13]

Skin reactions to irritants may be immediate or may develop later. They may be one-time (acute), repeated (allergic), or ongoing (chronic).

Contact dermatitis—irritation from something that touches the skin—is caused by a wide variety of substances, including latex and some pesticides, which may also trigger allergic dermatitis. Latex is a major health hazard for women, who often use rubber gloves as a barrier against toxic chemicals, bacteria, or infected body fluids. The ruling by OSHA that requires the use of latex gloves as a precaution against HIV and other bloodborne infections has ended up causing another, different occupational hazard.

Respiratory Ailments

Nearly 30% of cases of chronic bronchitis, emphysema, and adult asthma may be attributable to exposure on the job.[14] Currently, more than 20 million workers are exposed to substances that can cause respiratory diseases. Asthma is now the most frequent respiratory disease diagnosis among patients in occupational health clinics; many people do not realize that preexisting asthma may be made worse by on-the-job exposure to polluted air. Also, new work sites are emerging as problem areas. Windows that do not open and air-conditioning systems that circulate air throughout office buildings, as well as chemicals used in synthetic building materials and furnishings, may contribute to breathing problems.

Coal, grain, and cotton dust are well-documented causes of respiratory ailments. Flour-permeated air in commercial bakeries is a hazard for women employed there. Dust in general may be an irritant, particularly for workers with other respiratory problems. Cigarette and cigar smoking interacts with other pollutants, making people sicker than when they are exposed to each separately.

The development of tests to identify substances and processes that may cause asthma or emphysema can help designers assure the safety of new materials before they are introduced, preventing disease. Research that identifies biomarkers or other early indications of risk can be used to justify transferring workers before they become disabled. However, such information can also be misused by employers to get rid of workers instead of cleaning up the workplace.

Multiple Chemical Sensitivities

People with multiple chemical sensitivities (MCS, also called environmental or ecological illness—see also chapter 24, Selected Medical Practices, Problems, and Procedures) have a chronic reaction to chemicals and irritants at levels generally regarded as "safe." The condition exhibits six features: (1) multiple symptoms affect many systems of the body; (2) symptoms usually follow identifiable exposure to chemicals; (3) symptoms come and go with exposures; (4) symptoms occur below exposure levels that are tolerated by most other people; (5) symptoms are triggered by substances commonly found in the workplace, household, and general environment; (6) other explanations such as asthma, hypochondria, or certain respiratory disorders can be ruled out.[15]

MCS can be triggered by ingredients in cosmetics and perfumes, newsprint, diesel fuel, solvent vapors, mattresses or other fabrics treated with flame retardant, pressboard, pesticides, molds, and permanent-press finishes. Symptoms can include the following: convulsions, lack of coordination, abnormal reflexes; personality changes, from depression to excitability; sensory effects, including vision and hearing disorders; memory loss; speech impairment; loss of appetite. A growing list of governmental authorities, court decisions, and professional organizations identifies MCS as a legitimate medical condition.

Support is available, however, for people with MCS (see Resources). The National Center for Environmental Health Strategies, which monitors medical, policy, and legal issues, also provides practical advice about improving indoor air quality, reducing exposure to chemicals, diagnosis and treatment, and defending patients' rights. If you have MCS, the Labor Institute can help you demand "reasonable accommodation" in the workplace under the Americans with Disabilities Act (see p. 149).

Infectious Diseases

Tuberculosis, hepatitis B and C viruses, and human immunodeficiency virus (HIV) pose a risk for health care and social service workers, corrections personnel, and people in other occupations who handle body fluids or hazardous waste. Laboratory technicians can also contract contagious diseases if they work with infected material. These hazards are particularly worrisome when they are transferred from patient to worker or from worker to worker through blood or through the air.

Women as consumers are alarmed by the increasing number of sicknesses and deaths because of bacterial contamination of food, notably by salmonella and E. coli. Cases involving unpasteurized apple juice and undercooked hamburgers have made headline news in recent years. Women in food-processing jobs may unknowingly be working with contaminated products, and may eat the unsafe food as well. A more reliable and efficient food inspection system would be a gain for women both as workers and as family members.

Reproductive Health Hazards

A reproductive hazard is any agent that has harmful effects on the male or female reproductive system and/or the development of a fetus. These hazards can be chemicals (like pesticides), physical agents (like X rays) or work practices (like heavy lifting).

Reproductive health hazards are probably the most controversial issues in environmental health. Because women bear children, reproductive hazards are too often considered "a woman's problem" involving pregnancy alone. This view ignores two important facts: that men are also affected by reproductive hazards, and that reproductive health means more than having healthy babies. All through life, men and women need healthy sexual and reproductive systems. As it is, reproductive hazards are often used as excuses to penalize women workers and permit management to avoid cleaning up the workplace.

Infertility in either sex, a spontaneous abortion early in pregnancy, and a baby with birth disabilities can all be early signs of a toxic environment. They can be important signals that something is wrong, since other signs like cancer can take a 15- to 40-year latency period to develop before they produce symptoms we can feel or see.

Fertility and Pregnancy Abnormalities

Reproductive disorders afflicting women include menstrual problems, reduced fertility, spontaneous abortions, and, in the babies we bear, low birth weight, premature births, developmental disorders, and birth defects. Men's reproductive disorders (impotence, decreased sperm count, defective sperm) affect the women with whom they are involved. Infertility (defined as the inability to conceive after one year of unprotected intercourse) is estimated to affect one couple in 12. Although numerous occupational hazards (such as lead, solvents, and some pesticides) are known to affect reproductive functions, their overall contribution is unknown. It is disturbing that more than 1,000 chemicals used in the workplace have been shown to affect reproduction in animals. Most of them have not been studied for their effects on humans. In general, most of the four million chemical mixtures in commercial use are still untested for such effects. Activities that upset the normal hormonal balance of the reproductive system, such as shift work, and substances that change estrogen levels or mimic the effects of estrogen, such as pesticides, need further study. Not enough attention has been paid to the effect on fertility and pregnancy of physical factors such as prolonged standing, reaching, or lifting, or to the interactive effects of workplace stressors and toxic exposures.

Other Reproductive Disorders in Women

When toxic substances disrupt the reproductive hormones, they can cause menstrual disorders, sterility, or loss of sexual drive.[16] Toxic substances may also directly damage the ovaries, eventually resulting in early menopause or ovarian disease. And, as with sperm cells, environmental mutagens can damage the genetic material in a woman's eggs, with the same effects: spontaneous abortion or birth disabilities. Recent animal studies show damage to the ovaries from polycyclic hydrocarbons (used in the petrochemical industry), alkylating agents (used in cancer treatment), and ionizing radiation. Exposure to lead, PCBs, and vinyl chloride can cause menstrual changes.

The Developing Fetus and Young Children

A fertilized egg and a fetus can sometimes react to toxins that do not appear to harm an adult. Some toxins affect the first three months of pregnancy, so early that you may be harmed before you know you are pregnant. During the first two weeks, the fertilized egg is so sensitive that an environmental hazard powerful enough to damage it will also destroy it. From the 15th to the 60th day of a pregnancy, the cells of the fetus multiply and differentiate into specific organs and systems. A toxin can disrupt this process, and there is no second chance for the system to establish itself. If the effect is very strong, the pregnancy often ends in a spontaneous abortion (miscarriage). If the fetus survives, the child may have a low birth weight or physical, developmental, or behavioral problems, some of which may not show up until years later.

A fetus is usually exposed to toxins in the environment or workplace through the mother's direct exposure. However, toxins can accumulate in semen as well. Some researchers think that having intercourse during pregnancy with a man who has had occupational exposure to toxins may also cause birth disabilities.[17] Pregnant women in this situation might consider ways of making love other than intercourse.

The developing fetus and young children are particularly susceptible to certain environmental hazards because their cells are dividing and growing rapidly. Yet the government still sets standards for "safety" levels of toxins based on effects on adults.

Breast Milk Contamination

The level of toxic contaminants in many American women's breast milk is often reported to exceed the FDA's "acceptable daily intake" levels for other foods. The World Health Organization acknowledges that few women around the world are without trace levels of industrial contaminants in their milk. Some women and their babies are at especially high risk. Among indigenous people in the high Arctic, where many still eat food from the land and sea, babies take in seven times more PCBs than the typical infant in Canada or the U.S.[18]

Infants are at risk of being exposed during their first year of life to fat-stored contaminants that are mobilized through lactation, at levels exceeding the EPA "safe dose." Some researchers track contaminant levels in breast milk because it is a significant "biomarker" for human exposure in general.

Public health practitioners, environmental advocates, and concerned parents all debate whether and how long to breast-feed. Because breast milk provides important immunological protection to babies, most environmentally concerned activists advise women to keep breast feeding if they want to. Also, bottle-feeding carries its own risks: contaminants in water used to make formula, chemical and hormonal additives in commercial formulas, and plant estrogens introduced through certain soy-based formulas. To limit the damage, nursing mothers can try to eat less fat of animal origin, avoid identified sources of contaminants (such as treated vegetables, or fish from certain areas), and avoid quick weight loss (which mobilizes fat-stored contaminants).

Endocrine Disruption

Are we being exposed to a wide array of industrial and pharmaceutical chemicals that mimic and distort the functioning of our endocrine system? The endocrine system is the body's complex array of hormonal messages that affect not only our reproductive health but also the thyroid gland and our neurological and immunological systems. Emerging research on endocrine-disrupting contaminants (EDCs), also called ecoestrogens or exogenous estrogens, is helping people to understand environmental threats to women's health.

Breast cancer and other cancers in women, breast milk contamination, and other reproductive problems (such as endometriosis, miscarriage, and tubal pregnancy) may be related to the presence of EDCs in our food supply, air, and water; in industrial discharges; and in certain products such as plastics. These EDCs mimic, block, or alter the body's normal estrogen functioning, thereby putting women at risk for disease. Despite debates about the contributing causes of breast cancer, most researchers concur that what determines the risk of breast cancer is the length and intensity of a woman's "life on estrogens." (See the following section, and chapter 24, Selected Medical Practices, Problems, and Procedures, for more on breast cancer.) The length of time between menarche and menopause, whether and when we bear children, and whether we breast-feed all affect our estrogen levels. If the body's own "natural" estrogen levels are augmented or altered in some way by chemicals that act like estrogens, then living in a "sea of estrogens" may be escalating our risk of breast cancer, endometriosis, and other diseases.

Groups like the National Coalition against the Misuse of Pesticides and the Washington Toxics Coalition (see Resources) can provide information about steps we can take to affect public policy and social change concerning the use of EDCs. Already, public relations firms connected to certain industries (the Chemical Manufacturing Association, the Chlorine Council) are trying to counteract these efforts by using spokeswomen, women-oriented "fact sheets," and outreach to women's publications.

Breast Cancer

Women in the United States have a one-in-eight chance of developing breast cancer at some point in our lives. A growing breast cancer movement is pressing for more research on the processes that result in breast cancer, and on the factors that may trigger them, so that preventive measures and better treatment can be developed. (For more information on breast cancer, see chapter 24, Selected Medical Practices, Problems, and Procedures.)

Recent research has found that certain chemicals, especially DDT, DDE, PCBs, methylene chloride (a common solvent), and atrazine (a widely used herbicide) are correlated with cancer in lab animals and/or humans. Dr. Mary Wolff at Mt. Sinai School of Medicine reported in 1993 that women exposed to DDT (a pesticide in the organochlorine family that also includes dioxin and some components of PVC plastics) are four times as likely to develop breast cancer. Diets high in animal fat may increase human organochlorine contamination. Over time, these compounds may trigger breast cancer by disrupting normal cell-regulation processes in sensitive breast tissue. A historical pattern of accumulation of organochlorine residue in the environment may account for the increasing numbers of women with breast cancer.[19] Other researchers have found that women workers with high exposure to dioxin have significantly elevated rates of breast cancer.[20]

As a result of lobbying by community activists, notably in New York and Massachusetts, studies are now being done on possible links between breast cancer and organochlorides. The Long Island breast cancer study, sponsored by the National Cancer Institute and the National Institute of Environmental Health Sciences, will test blood samples from 400 breast cancer patients and 400 healthy women for organochloride levels over time.

Still, of 722 NIH grants for breast cancer research in 1996–1997, only 33 (5%) involved a possible environmental connection.[21] The NCI and other research institutions have published articles stressing "prevention" that shift responsibility for cancer on to individuals by advising us to change our lifestyles, and the Harvard Report on Cancer Prevention[22] completely ignores the difficulties most women face in assuring our safety at work, or in avoiding hazardous chemicals that we may not even know are present in our environment. It is more important than ever for us to insist that government and industrial interests take responsibility for their contribution to environmental and workplace hazards that may cause cancer.

How Reproductive Hazards Affect Men

Environmental toxics can disrupt the production of male hormones in the testes, causing loss of sex drive and impotence. They can also cause problems with sperm production. A toxic agent can disturb sperm cells at any one of several stages of rapid growth, causing problems with fertility through a total lack of sperm, low sperm production, or malformed sperm. Toxins may be causing an overall decline in sperm counts in American men.

Men exposed to lead have decreased fertility and malformed sperm.[23] More than 50 currently used pesticides, including many products used in U.S. households, are linked to male infertility, as reported in laboratory and clinical studies.[24] In addition, men's sperm counts appear to be decreasing in many parts of the world. This is worrisome because it may be caused by exposure to chemicals, particularly the endocrine-disrupting contaminants described earlier.

Another problem for everyone's health is that some reproductive hazards are mutagens. When a mutation occurs in sperm cells, men can pass on damaged genes to future generations. Defective genes can produce spontaneous abortions or disabilities in children.

Environmental mutagens also pose dangers for the entire human species. Damaged genetic material, whether or not it causes visible damage, contributes its permanent changes to the total human gene pool. Genetically engineered plants and animals, produced by the new biotechnology industry, could affect human health in ways not yet known as they become part of our "natural" environment, food supply, and consumer products. Not only could a mutation rate increased by the effects of chemical and radioactive toxins produce a general decline in human genetic health, it could threaten human existence.

TAKING ACTION AGAINST ENVIRONMENTAL HAZARDS

As women, we are learning to be both more aware of environmentally caused problems and more confident about the power of such awareness. Often in the past we have just "accepted" a miscarriage or infertility or a chronically sick child. Now, instead of accepting, we're investigating. And when we do, we often find that the problems are environmentally connected. It's important not to just accept physicians' statements that "this is normal" or that we are "just being emotional." Environmental damage is often hard to prove. Persist. Don't just remain frustrated with your health care provider. Find a new one. Find someone you can talk to about it. And keep on learning to be more alert to things that can go wrong with your body because of environmental exposures. Don't discount your own knowledge of yourself, or your own power.

We can begin to minimize the effects of some environmental hazards by avoiding voluntary exposures and staying as healthy as we can. Taking action often seems complicated—bureaucracy to fight, chemistry and biology to learn, the power of polluters to deal with—but it is not impossible.

Environmental health is basically a community issue, one we cannot fight alone. Luckily, we don't have to. Recent polls have shown that the vast majority of Americans are increasingly concerned about environmental conditions—from polluted water to toxic landfills—and say they are willing to make sacrifices (e.g., pay higher taxes) to ensure a safer environment. The thousands of grassroots groups emerging across the country are evidence of this newfound determination. Because the manufacturers and agribusiness interests will not regulate themselves, we need a new era of environmental democracy with intense citizen involvement.

Strategies

Citizen action against environmental health hazards can take many routes. (See Resources for more information.) Experienced activists agree on some basic points:

1. *Be a careful consumer.* Avoid high-fat, high-on-the-food-chain diets and products containing EDCs and chlorine. Learn about and join boycotts and campaigns that affect occupational and environmental health.

2. *Investigate* environmental conditions where you live and work. Use the Toxic Release Inventory; demand information under worker and community right-to-know legislation; contact the Center for Environment, Health and Justice, the Good Neighbor Project, the Working Group on Community Right-to-Know, and other groups listed in the Resource section to learn about workplace and community monitoring and campaigning for preventive measures.

3. *Talk to your neighbors.* Develop "labor-neighbor" alliances concerned about toxic exposures from factories, landfills, waste shipment. Monitor health concerns, symptoms, and suspected exposures in the community. Conduct a community and workplace health survey. Watch for odd smells, bubbles or ooze, sick and dying wildlife and pets, abandoned oil drums, or trucks dumping at night. Find out whether local industries emit radiation. Pay attention to reproductive patterns in your area. Your community group may be able to get government or industry funding to support research and consultations with experts.

4. *Document your health* and that of your family. Keep a log of exposures, symptoms, and diagnoses. The health care providers you see should (and may not) be keeping an accurate medical and occupational/environmental history.

5. *Find out who paid* for the study when you or your group obtain information, statistics, or data. The answer should help you evaluate the data. Demand that information be presented in terms you can understand, not in the jargon of "experts." You can make effective use of industry or government

resources even if you doubt the motives of their sources.

6. *Use the consumer boycott.* Find out where pollutants come from and what products they're used in, and refuse to buy them. Women, especially, have enormous power as consumers.

7. *Work in coalition* with other organizations and movements. Don't limit your protest to "not in my backyard." Your community's efforts to protect itself will be more effective, just, and inspiring if they do not develop at the expense of others whose resources and power are more limited than yours. Organizations such as the Center for Health, Environment and Justice, the Environmental Health Network, the Labor Institute, and the COSH groups (see Resources) all help grass-roots groups. They can advise about the use of legal challenges, conducting surveys, building relationships with sympathetic scientists, getting a company to accept a "neighbors' inspection," and using national data systems and community right-to-know provisions. The CHEJ also provides workshops for women leaders. Increasingly, coalitions of environmental, labor, and other social justice groups are pushing beyond right-to-know (the basic right of access to certain information about on-site toxics) to right-to-act (the right to refuse work, change production activity, or enforce an emergency shutdown). Other groups provide support to parents investigating risks to children's health. See the Resource section for listings.

Women's Activism

Women have always been active in exposing and working to eliminate environmental health hazards.

- Ellen Swallow, the first woman student admitted to MIT, created the interdisciplinary study of nutrition, air and water pollution, architecture, waste disposal, and occupational health and safety. In 1892 she named this field "ecology."
- Rachel Carson's book *Silent Spring* (1962) exposed the widespread use and dangers of pesticides in our environment. Her work brought this problem to public attention, led to the ban on DDT in the U.S. and marked the beginning of the American environmental movement.
- Lois Gibbs organized the Love Canal Homeowners' Association and, with the women of Love Canal, forced the state of New York to recognize the problems. They signed petitions, did health surveys, embarrassed government and industry officials, picketed, blocked buses, and testified in Washington. Because of their work, the government evacuated 1,000 families, purchased their homes, and established a safety plan for the workers on site, a retroactive tax break, and a health fund to cover future problems.

- Bonnie Hill and seven other women correlated their miscarriages with the spraying of 2,4,5-T, a herbicide, near their homes in rural Alsea, Oregon. Their protests to the EPA led to the emergency ban in 1979 on the chemical for most uses in the U.S.
- Polly Heran, a member of the water board in Rocky Flats, Colorado, a community near a uranium mine and a nuclear weapons facility, discovered that the water supply had double the normal amount of uranium. Heran, along with a group of housewives, studied the issue. When they could not get the local authorities to act because there was no "conclusive" information on the radioactive effect of the uranium, they threatened to boycott and bankrupt the water department. They proved the toxicity of the uranium as a heavy metal rather than as a radioactive element, forcing the local government to take action.
- Sister Jacinta Fernandes and other community women conducted health surveys, marched, and held speakouts to complain about the Chemical Control Company dump in Elizabeth, New Jersey, which they suspected of contributing to their respiratory and other health problems. On Earth Day 1980, the dump exploded, forcing people from Elizabeth east to Staten Island to stay indoors while the chemicals burned. The group's pressure had forced cleanup of the worst chemicals from the dump *before* it exploded. Without their work, the fire would have been even more devastating.
- Lisa Crawford started asking questions about the "feed materials" plant, a uranium-processing site run by the Department of Energy, in Fernald, Ohio. With other women she founded Fernald Residents for Environmental Safety and Health (FRESH), now one of the most effective grassroots groups in the U.S. FRESH's efforts led to full disclosure of the plant's impact on the air and water, and Fernald was designated a Superfund site for cleanup funding. (The main purpose of both federal and state Superfund programs is the identification and remediation of hazardous waste sites.) As watchdog over the cleanup, FRESH inspires and advises other groups facing similar battles.[25]
- West Harlem Environmental Action (WHEACT), a coalition of young feminists and neighborhood elder women, challenged the placement of a sewage treatment plant in a section of New York City already treated as a "dumping ground." They fought to get testing for fumes in the air, identified the health implications of odors, and condemned the city's offer to build a much-needed park on top of the waste plant. WHEACT successfully sued the city, winning a sizeable settlement and the right to oversee the remedy. The legal victory also established a community's right to seek redress of a grievance—a fundamental element in environmental justice.[26]

As the women's health movement has shown, we must—and we can—take charge of our bodies, our health, our environment, and our lives.

WORK CAN BE HAZARDOUS
TO OUR HEALTH

The work we do affects our health not only while we are working but throughout the rest of the day, on weekends and vacations, and even in the years after we have left the job. The consequences of hazardous working conditions are severe. More than 100,000 workers die each year from known job-related diseases, and more suffer from other diseases not yet recognized as resulting from exposures on the job. Sixteen workers are killed and over 17,000 U.S. workers are injured on an average day in workplace accidents, and thousands more are disabled.[27] Our workplace is part of our environment. We cannot take poor working conditions for granted as "just part of the job." We have to think about why they exist, what they might be doing to us, and how they can be changed.

Workplace safety and health are usually associated with traditional "men's work," like mining, construction, and heavy manufacturing. But so-called women's work, such as cleaning, nursing, teaching, garment making, clerical work, and "service" work, is not so safe either.

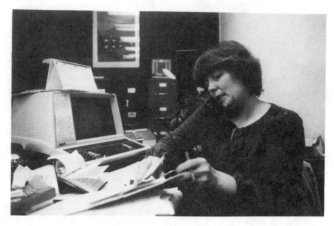
Ellen Shub

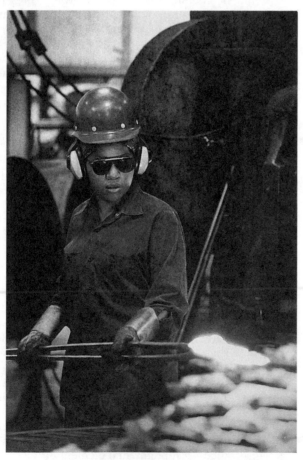
Robert Eckert/The Picture Cube

WHERE WOMEN WORK

According to the Department of Labor, 57% of all women in the U.S. work outside the home. Women make up 46% of the paid work force. The following list shows the distribution, by sector, of the female labor force.[28]

Agriculture 1%
Construction 1%
Finance, insurance, real estate 9%
Mining 0.4%
Manufacturing 12%
Public administration 4%
Service 48%
Transportation, communications, other public utilities 4%
Wholesale and retail trade 21%

While 48% of women workers are still employed in the service sector, the table shows that a majority of women in paid employment are now distributed across almost all sectors of the economy. However, women work in a narrower range of industries than do men. The tasks we perform and job titles we hold are often different from men's. Tasks and exposure to danger, as well as ways to prevent injury or illness, vary from job to job. Women's work often involves sustained, repetitive effort; or standing or sitting in a static position; without the rest breaks allowed to men who do heavy work. Female laundry workers, for example, lift as much as 4,000 pounds a day of wet laundry—more than men in many manufacturing or trucking jobs are required to lift.[29]

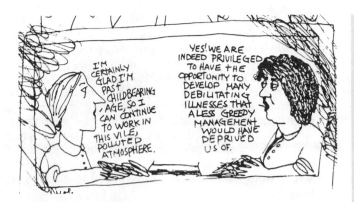

Nicole Hollander

I had worked at the hospital for four years as a housekeeper when I got sick with hepatitis. I found out that a patient on my floor had hepatitis and nobody had bothered to tell me what precautions to take. I filed a claim for worker's compensation and the hospital fought my claim! I never thought that a thing like that could happen. I was working in a place that was supposed to care about people's health and they never told me anything about protecting my health.

The growing number of women in heavy industry and construction jobs generally face the same, often dangerous conditions that men face. But women often feel pressure to prove that we are as good as the men we work with, and when we speak up about health and safety we're often seen as "too weak to take it." Yet, the problems we are concerned about also affect men, and women's vocal presence in these traditionally male workplaces is bringing a change in the way people think about health and safety issues.

Women have special concerns because of our social and economic situations. Sexist job discrimination puts a large majority of women into low-paying and stressful occupations. Many women carry the double duty of paid work *and* responsibilities at home, which makes it more difficult to get involved in after-work meetings about working conditions.

Women often have low seniority or jobs that place us in caretaking roles or require close working relationships with our bosses, making us hesitant to bring up complaints about hazards. In addition, only 16% of women workers belong to unions, which makes organizing more difficult. Women of color are more often stuck with dead-end, "no transfer" jobs in which we are exposed to more dangerous conditions for longer periods of time than our white counterparts. Women living in poverty, rural women, and women of color are prime candidates for the high-risk poultry industry. In North Carolina, the 70,000 rural women in the poultry industry endure unsafe machinery, speedup on the assembly lines, dull knives, slippery floors, and sexual harassment.[30] Despite a fire that killed many workers and that received national publicity, conditions have not changed.

A majority of migrant farm workers are young, and

SOME COMMON WORKPLACE HAZARDS

Potential Safety Hazards

No machine guards
Faulty switches, exposed wiring
Dangerous floors, doors, exits, aisles, stairs
Cranes, lifts, hoists
Poor lighting
Explosives
No fire extinguishers
No protective gear for emergencies
Poor maintenance of equipment
Lack of training in safe work practices and first aid
Speedup of work
No first aid equipment
Noise

Potential Health Hazards

Dusts, mists, gases, vapors, smoke
Heat, cold, dampness
Radiation
Uncomfortable or unsuitable workstations/ equipment
Noise, vibration
Repetitive movements
Shift work
Stress
Sexual and racial harassment and abuse
Multiple commitments to home, work, family

approximately 85% are people of color, mostly Latino. Migrant farm workers live and work under unhealthy, poverty-stricken conditions during their reproductive years. They rarely have access to worker's compensation, occupational rehabilitation, or disability compensation. While many are eligible for Medicaid and food stamps, few are able to secure these benefits because they are unaware of their eligibility and because most of the offices don't have Spanish-speaking employees or interpreters and do insufficient education and outreach. Some of the children are citizens and are eligible for benefits, but the parents are illegal immigrants who are afraid of being deported if they come to the attention of the authorities. Many have no health insurance.

Farm workers can suffer from accidents, pesticide-related illnesses, musculoskeletal and soft tissue disorders, and reproductive difficulties. They may also be vulnerable to cancer, birth defects, kidney and liver damage, and neurotoxicity as a result of exposure to chemicals. They also suffer from tuberculosis and other infectious diseases at a higher rate than other occupational groups. Women unable to get prenatal care are more likely to give birth to underweight babies. California is still the only state that requires doctors to report farm workers' occupational injuries, and lumping all agricultural workers into the categories of "immigrant" or "undocumented" labor for political reasons makes it more difficult to mobilize public support for their health needs.[31]

Recognizing Hazards in the Workplace

Management is supposed to provide a safe workplace, but this task is frequently low on its priority list. Improving conditions often costs money, and in addition, management may be afraid of giving up, or appearing to give up, control. Who controls the work-

WOMEN AT WORK: SOME HEALTH ISSUES

Women constitute nearly half (48%) of the U.S. workforce. Our median income is approximately 75% of men's income. Often we balance two jobs: wage earner and homemaker/caregiver.

Of women workers, 8% hold traditionally "masculine" jobs and 44% have gender-neutral jobs. Injuries, exposure to toxic substances, and improperly fitting protective clothing are key hazards.

Nearly half (48%) of U.S. women work in traditionally "feminine" jobs. Most hold clerical, service, health care, and teaching jobs. Stress, verbal and physical violence, repetitive motion disorders, and indoor air quality are key health issues.

Forty percent of physically demanding service occupations, such as nurses' aides, private household cleaners, machine operators, and agriculture workers, are filled by women of color. Hazards include lifting, exposure to dangerous chemicals, stress, and safety-related accidents.

Of employees in the U.S. health care industry, our fastest-growing service sector, 75% are women. Hazards include lifting, bloodborne infections, hazardous medications, violence, and adverse reactions to latex. Nurses' aide (90% women) ranks as the nation's third worst occupation (behind truck driver and construction laborer) for injuries involving lost work days.[32]

Homicide is the leading cause of death for women workers, although more men than women are murdered on the job. Health care workers, teachers, corrections officers, and social workers are the primary victims of assault at work. Strangers are overwhelmingly responsible for most physical and verbal attacks on workers.[33]

place is often an important, if unstated, issue in workplace health and safety struggles. If workers become knowledgeable about work processes and practices in order to make them safer, we are then more likely to question in general why and how things are done.

Recognition is the first step in eliminating hazards. You don't have to be an expert, but you do have to be persistent and thorough. A good way to begin is by talking with the people you work with. You and your co-workers are the best qualified to identify what the hazards and dangerous jobs are. Ask each other: Where does it hurt? What makes it hurt? How can it be fixed?

Some hazards are obvious. Just using your eyes, ears, and nose will help you pick out safety hazards such as obvious dust or fumes and excessive noise. Recognizing hidden hazards is often more difficult. See whether there is any pattern in who gets sick in your workplace. Talk to people or use a simple questionnaire to ask about mild symptoms, headaches, frequent illnesses, coughs, and so on. These activities will not only help identify problems but also help to build awareness and interest among fellow workers about job conditions.

Learn about the chemicals and other substances you work with. A trade name such as Wite-Out is not useful; you need to know the names of the actual chemicals in the product (in this case, trichlorethylene) because almost all information on chemicals is organized by the scientific chemical name. The Federal Hazard Communication Standard provides workers with certain rights of access to information—that is, management is supposed to provide training, appropriate labeling, and inventories of chemicals and material safety data sheets for each substance of exposure. However, the reality is otherwise. Employees too often do not know or act on their rights. Employers often intimidate workers into not asking the right questions. Manufacturers often do not tell the whole story about the substances they distribute.

Where to Start

- Find out how the Hazard Communication Standard affects your workplace—there are exemptions.
- Use whatever legal rights you have to the fullest. Management may try strong-arm maneuvers, and the manufacturer may cry "trade secret," but certain information is rightfully yours.
- Demand to see any exposure data your employer might have collected. You and/or your union have rights of access to your company medical records. You and fellow workers can conduct a survey to strengthen your understanding of your working conditions.
- Check with the Association of Occupational/ Environmental Health Clinics to find knowledgeable medical resources in your region. (Few physicians are sufficiently trained about toxic exposures.)

METHODS OF CONTROLLING WORKPLACE HAZARDS

1. Substitute

Can a safer substance or equipment (chemical or process) be used?
Use water-based correction fluid to correct typing errors instead of solvent-based fluid. Use natural, biodegradable cleaning products.

2. Change the Process

Can the job be done in a different and safer way?
Standing for most of the work day can lead to leg pain and varicose veins. If stools are provided and clerks can rotate sitting and standing, stress will be reduced.

3. Mechanize the Process

Is automating an operation the best answer to a dangerous job?
If mechanical lifting devices are provided and used, the back and shoulder strain caused by manual lifting will be avoided.

4. Isolate or Enclose the Process

Can the hazardous job be removed to a different area or time where fewer people will be exposed?
Can the worker be isolated from the operation, or can the process be completely enclosed?
If ventilating hoods are installed, fumes will be exhausted away from the worker's breathing zone.

5. Improve Housekeeping

In many operations, strict housekeeping is essential to keep toxic materials from being reintroduced into the air or to prevent safety hazards. Keep dust levels down to protect the lungs. Move obstacles out of the work areas and exits to prevent accidents.

6. Improve Maintenance

Is equipment regularly serviced and repaired?
Poorly maintained office machines, such as copiers, can give off irritating ozone gas.

PRIMARY HEALTH PROBLEMS AT WORK

Too often, concern's about women's occupational hazards focus on our traditional role as "babymakers." But many kinds of work-related injury and illness, unrelated to reproduction, affect women as well as men.

Hearing Loss

Hearing loss is the most common occupational disease in the United States. It is often accepted as normal in the workplace, but it is not. It can reduce alertness to safety warnings and severely impair the quality of a worker's life. While hearing loss can occur from an acute injury, it is more likely to develop gradually over time, as a result of exposure to noise, solvents, metals, asphyxiants, or heat. Loss of hearing usually occurs without pain or awareness on the worker's part. Once hearing loss has taken place, it is usually irreversible.

Most workers are unaware that exposure to certain kinds of chemicals can cause hearing loss. If you are worried about this possibility, find out what chemicals are in your work environment, call the NIOSH information line (800-35 NIOSH), and ask to speak to a hearing loss research expert or receive written information. The information is free of charge, and the people are usually very helpful.

No major studies have been done recently on the hearing status of people now working, so reliance on data gathered 30 years ago underestimates the amount of hearing loss due to occupational noise, especially if exposure is intermittent. Exposure to heat and chemicals have only recently been identified as a threat to hearing. Even if workers have ear protectors, removing them for as little as 15 minutes during an eight-hour work shift can cut protection by as much as 50%. Ear protectors must also fit properly to be effective. Women's ear canals are smaller than men's, so standard ear equipment may not fit us properly.

Back Disorders

Back pain is extremely common, and back disorders account for 27% of all recorded, nonfatal occupational injuries and illness involving days away from the job. About 30% of workers perform tasks that increase the likelihood that they will develop back problems. Many of these workers are women, especially women of color.

Any lifting over a barrier or in an awkward position can strain the muscles. Mechanical lifting devices, training, reorganizing tasks, and using a back belt may reduce risks. Redesigning materials, loads, and equipment can help those in occupations that involve lifting. New recommendations for lifting can be obtained from the NIOSH hot line (see Resources).

Foot and Leg Disorders

Many women suffer from lower back and leg pains from standing on their feet all day. These ailments are common among staff waiting on tables, salesclerks, nurses, nurses' aides, and household and office cleaners. Sometimes these jobs combine stooping and lifting as well. Blood tends to pool in your legs and varicose veins tend to develop. These jobs are particularly hard on pregnant workers. In addition, many of the jobs are particularly stressful.

For some jobs, like bank tellers, sitting on high chairs and stools can be substituted. For other jobs such as nurses' aides, frequent breaks to sit down are needed but rarely given. Upscale retail establishments often require their saleswomen to dress up and wear high heels, which exacerbate the problem. Request a chair to sit on, and if that is refused, ask to be rotated off the sales floor for part of the day so that you can alternate sitting and standing. If you are a household cleaner, request long-handled cleaning equipment that you can use standing up instead of kneeling on a hard floor.

Neck, Shoulder, and Hand Injuries

Women have always known about strain or injury caused by repetitive movements or awkward positions. Now, huge increases in the number of female workers suffering from repetitive strain injury (RSI) or cumulative trauma disorder (CTD) have led to growing interest in the science of ergonomics: designing equipment to meet the needs of the human body. Musculoskeletal disorders of the upper extremities—including such ailments as stiff neck and carpal tunnel syndrome—occur in food processing, automobile and electronics assembling, carpentry, computerized data entry, store checkouts, garment sewing, and many other occupations where repetitive, forceful work affects the soft tissues of the neck, shoulder, elbow, hand, wrist, and fingers. According to the Bureau of Labor Statistics, such injuries represent almost 65% of all reported illness at work.

Ergonomically designed equipment, sufficient rest, alternation of tasks, and reduced stress can greatly reduce these problems. Forceful movements, vibration, working in cold temperatures, and insufficient recovery time can make them worse. Unlike strains or sprains, which result from a single incident, repetitive motion disorders develop over time, and they can recur when we return to the task that produced the injury. The daily aches and pains that we ignore for all kinds of reasons, not least because we have to "get on with the job," paid or unpaid, may add up to long-term problems.

Indoor Environmental Quality

Many office and factory workers suffer from headaches, unusual fatigue, itching or burning eyes, skin irritation, nasal congestion, dry or irritated throats, and nausea caused by their workplace environment.

I take reservations for an airline. We have 800 people in the building, but only six or eight bathrooms. The windows don't open, so the air is never fresh. My section is supposed to be perfume-free, but people still use hair spray and aftershave. We take 90 to 120 calls a day, working eight and a half hours with only half

an hour for lunch. All the calls are timed. If you get up and walk around, the supervisor yells at you. You don't even have time to finish entering the last customer's data on the computer before the next call comes in. Also, we don't have designated work stations, so you're always sitting at a different keyboard, picking up everyone else's germs. I've had chicken pox and then bronchitis. I've had this cough for more than a year, and I think it's developing into asthma. I complained to my doctor about it, but she didn't refer me to a specialist. The health plan is cutting costs, but that means cutting care, too.

Many public facilities such as schools, office buildings, and subsidized housing projects have become dangerous indoor work environments because of flaking and peeling of old lead-based paint, or contain harmful chemicals in carpets, furnishings, or supplies. Even a new car may make the driver sick. But it isn't just in the air. Indoor environmental quality is now understood to include not only air contamination but also comfort, noise, lighting, work station and task design, and job-related psychosocial conditions such as monitoring, pace, and break time. A wide variety of workplaces, from factories to airplanes, provide an unhealthy environment for employees.

Work and Stress

In the garment shop where I work, a lot of us who've been sewing there for a while have been having pains in our hands or our legs. The union is collecting information to see if some jobs are worse than others (like hemming or making linings). We're hoping that we can find out whether there are any changes that would help, like changing the height of the tables or the angle of the machines. Anything that would make the job more comfortable would help my general level of tension! Between the noise from the steam presses, working fast enough to make a good rate, and bending over the machine all day without enough light, I'm lucky if I get out of there without my shoulders all bunched up and a splitting headache at the end of the day.

Management often tells us that stress is our fault, that we shouldn't bring our personal problems to work. But work conditions can *create* stress, which goes home with us and affects our personal lives, too.

Stress can result from physical factors, such as repetitive hand motions, poor seating conditions, excessive noise, heat or cold, eyestrain, or general work overload. Other causes of stress range from relations with the boss and our co-workers to sexual harassment and worry about safety and health hazards. Many women have jobs with low pay and no chance of promotion or retraining because of sexual and racial discrimination in employment and limited educational opportunities. Women who have children or want to have them must worry about maternity leave, child care, and loss of seniority.

HIGH-STRESS JOBS

Much publicity has been given to the Type A personality, typically a high-powered executive suffering from stress and a likely candidate for a heart attack. But these men have a lot of power and are usually happy and successful in their jobs. Research shows that jobs characterized by high demand annd low control, like those filled by millions of women, are the most stressful and most likely to be harmful to women's health.

Women in stressful jobs include cooks, salesclerks, typists, secretaries, library clerks, waitresses, bank tellers, cashiers, nurses' aides, receptionists, and sewing machine, telephone, office machine, and keypunch operators. Many of these women are poor and have full-time household and parental responsibilities as well. Many belong to groups that suffer from cultural prejudice and discrimination.

High-stress jobs exhibit the following characteristics:

- no control over speed of work
- no control over variety
- repetition of monotonous work
- not able to leave work station
- no control over decision making
- not enough time to complete assigned work
- not enough opportunity to obtain a promotion

Most women in jobs traditionally held by men have to deal with not being very welcome or accepted at the workplace, at least at the beginning. A black woman who works as a union carpenter's apprentice said:

It's difficult not to become paranoid that every insult or putdown comes from people's racist or sexist attitudes, even when you know that all apprentices get dumped on a lot.[34]

Stress can cause serious medical problems. We won't end stress on the job as long as job exploitation or racial oppression continue, but we can win some improvements, such as increasing the availability of information about the substances we work with, obtaining adequate staffing, and securing a say in decisions that affect our work conditions.

One of the most stressful things about our job at the phone company was the "clacker" that would start going CLACK CLACK CLACK whenever all the incoming lines were busy. The idea was to make us work faster. But it would make my stomach tie into knots and my hands get sweaty whenever I heard that thing.

So one day I got a big group of us to go in to the supervisor and say that we just couldn't work like that. There were so many of us that he had to give in.[35]

Though many companies today have "stress management" programs for employees, these programs define stress as an individual problem and allow the company to avoid changing the conditions that cause stress on the job.

Shift Work

Work on rotating shifts may cause physical and psychological hardship or make existing health problems worse. Digestion, the immune system, sleep, alertness, motor reflexes, motivation, and powers of concentration are all affected. Shift workers, on the average, smoke more heavily, are more likely to be obese, eat less nutritional food, have higher cholesterol and triglyceride levels in the blood (risk factors for heart disease), participate in fewer leisure activities, and are less involved in social networks than workers with a fixed eight-hour day.

Women who work shifts show high levels of job stress and emotional problems, more frequently use sleeping pills or tranquilizers, and are heavier drinkers than women with regular hours. Shift work is especially hard on family life and friendships, especially if there is nobody at home to help or if we can't afford paid child care. We may become more isolated and lose a valuable support network, increasing our level of stress.

Frequent rotation continually upsets the body's eating and sleeping cycles, like having permanent jet lag. If you are on a rotating shift, try to avoid daily or weekly rotation; if you can, stick to one shift for at least three weeks so your body can stay adjusted for a longer period of time. Try to get other workers to join you in demanding a less exhausting schedule. Unless you assert yourselves in a group, employers may resist making changes.

Harassment and Violence

Violence in the workplace is a serious health problem, though many employers and employees seem not to realize that. Industries that employ many women—such as bars, restaurants, hospitals, and grocery stores—report a large number of serious nonfatal injuries. According to the U.S. Bureau of Labor, 40% of the women fatally injured at work in 1993 were murdered. Homicide was the leading cause of occupational death for women (and the third leading cause of death for all workers) during the 1980s. While robbery is often the motive, homicides are also committed by disgruntled workers, former employees, clients, or male partners or ex-partners of women workers. A worker's risk for violence is increased if she exchanges money with the public, works alone or with few co-workers, works late-night or early-morning hours, or works in community settings.

A combination of relatively simple control mechanisms, such as changing workplace design to separate workers from the public, installing bulletproof barriers and alarm systems, adding staff, or forbidding employers to force women to work alone, can lower the risks. A Gainesville, Florida, ordinance requires two people on an 8 P.M. to 4 A.M. convenience store shift. Result: an 80% decrease in assaults, as well as increased sales because both customers and workers felt safer.[36]

Violence at work can be defined in various ways. Union actions now address such behavior as sexual and racial harassment and verbal abuse, which can also result in physical as well as psychological injury. Class action lawsuits against employers for sexual and racial bias are on the rise. Press coverage of sexual harassment charges against corporations (notably Texaco, Mitsubishi, and Astra), the armed forces, and the Citadel military school has finally brought this problem to widespread public attention.

A 21-year-old female Army recruit was subjected to attempted rape by her drill sergeant. She testified that as the sergeant tried to make her lie down she pushed him away, and he let her go.

I was so confused about the whole thing. He's my drill sergeant I'm supposed to obey him. . . . The whole thing made me sick to my stomach.

The drill sergeant was sentenced to five months in prison and discharged from the Army.[37] In another much-publicized case, a drill sergeant convicted of raping six female trainees was sentenced to 25 years in prison and given a dishonorable discharge. Unfortunately, sexual harassment in the military appears to be widespread, and this is increasingly alarming for women, who now make up 20% of Army recruits. Despite the recent flurry of concern, instances of harassment and violence in the workplace are frequently covered up, and cases are often settled out of court to silence plaintiffs and prevent publicity.

"Protecting" Women Can Cost Us Our Jobs

The distinction between protection and discrimination is often a fine one. For example, some states passed legislation after World War II limiting the number of pounds a woman could lift or the number of hours she could work on the job. While these laws were supposed to protect women from undue stress, the result was that women lost their jobs to returning servicemen.

In the 1980s, many companies instituted fetal protection policies that prohibited women of childbearing potential from working in areas where they might be exposed to chemicals so as to "protect the unborn child"; the result was that women lost access to jobs that had only recently been opened to them. It is no coincidence that companies or institutions that employ a largely female labor force, such as hospitals and the electronics industry, did not have such policies. When studies found that anesthetic gases might cause spontaneous abortions, hospitals didn't ban women workers from operating rooms. Instead, they installed devices that eliminated the problem.

Exclusionary policies ignore the fact that women are not pregnant most of their lives and that many exposures that may be harmful to a fetus are also harmful to an adult. Barring women from jobs instead of cleaning up the workplace diverts energy and attention from the real issue: the need to protect all workers from reproductive and other health hazards. Women's presence on the job may in fact raise awareness about hazards.

On my job as a field service technician, three women became pregnant and were immediately transferred to other jobs within the company. Three different doctors recommended this precaution because of the strong cleaning solvents that we use. Their situation has drawn everyone's attention to the possible dangers that we face on our jobs. Both men and women have been discussing symptoms they believe to be job-related.

Women won a major legal victory in 1991 when the Supreme Court ruled unanimously that the Johnson Controls fetal protection policy violated the Federal Civil Rights Act of 1964 prohibiting sex discrimination in employment. The successful lawsuit against Johnson Controls (the largest manufacturer of automobile batteries in the United States), brought by the United Auto Workers with the support of a coalition of labor, environmental, and women's groups, demonstrated that "fetal protection" policies, ostensibly designed to protect pregnant women from harm in the workplace, were designed more to protect the employer from being sued by injured workers.

If you are pregnant, it becomes more urgent to remove yourself from possible hazards. One possibility is to request a transfer to a safe job with the same pay, benefits, and seniority. If you have a union, this should be written into your contract. You may need to leave the workplace if no jobs without hazardous exposures are available. You may have certain rights to job transfer or paid leave under the pregnancy disability amendment to the Federal Civil Rights Act. Under this law, women "disabled by pregnancy" must be treated the same as other temporarily disabled workers, like those who have had heart attacks or accidents. ("Disabled" is a legal term meaning that one is unable to work.) Some states also have pregnancy disability acts.

When applying for a job, ask whether the company has a specific reproductive health policy, what it is, and whether it applies to both men and women. Some companies ask employees to sign waivers stating that they are aware of the job's possible reproductive hazards and will not hold the employer liable. Some lawyers think these waivers can be challenged in court. If your employer has a policy on fertility, pregnancy, childbirth, or any other issue related to reproductive health that seems unclear or unfair, contact a COSH or other occupational health advocacy group for support (see Resources for listings).

Male co-workers often think that reproductive hazards are just a woman's problem, and they must be educated to realize that this isn't true. Women are not expendable in the workplace, just as men are not expendable in the family. Job conditions should enable us to be both working people and parents. The U.S. is one of the few industrialized countries that fails to provide paid leave and monetary compensation for childbirth.

Useful Legislation

The Family Leave Act of 1993 requires employers to grant 12 weeks of *unpaid* leave for either parent to care for a new baby or seriously ill family member. This law applies only to companies with more than 50 employees. Many women work in smaller workplaces and cannot get maternity leave. Most other industrial nations do much better. Canadian workers receive 15 weeks of family leave at 60% pay, and French women get 12 weeks of maternity leave at full pay. Virtually every European nation provides support for new mothers.

The Americans with Disabilities Act (ADA) of 1990 prohibits discrimination against people with disabilities, in employment as well as many other areas. If you have a recognized disability, visible or not, and are otherwise qualified to do your job with or without "reasonable accommodation," you can obtain redress under this law.

Depending on the state you live in, your working conditions, and the availability of union support, the ADA may obtain support for "reasonable accommodation" for employees suffering from multiple chemical sensitivities. The ADA has also been used by workers with HIV/AIDS to sue employers for wrongful dismissal. For information and assistance, you can contact your union, the Job Accommodation Network, or the Equal Employment Opportunity Commission (see Resources for listings).

Legal Rights to a Safe Workplace

The major law dealing with workplace hazards is the federal Occupational Safety and Health Act, which requires employers to make their workplaces safe and free of health hazards "as far as possible." The law (first passed in 1970) established the Occupational Safety and Health Administration (OSHA), which sets standards for workplace conditions, inspects workplaces to see whether the standards are being met, and can impose fines on employers who violate standards and order them to clean up. Workers have a right to file complaints with OSHA calling for inspections and to ask NIOSH (see Resources) and state agencies to do health hazard evaluations.

Unfortunately, OSHA alone cannot solve all our problems. Few OSHA standards cover the hazards found in jobs traditionally held by women, and OSHA has seldom inspected offices, hospitals, or other predominantly female workplaces. OSHA's Hazard Communication Standard, passed in 1983 and expanded in 1987, gives workers the right to know about chemical hazards in their workplaces. The standard covers federal employees and workers in the manufacturing sector. Construction work is regulated by a separate version. As a result of a union lawsuit, the courts have now ordered OSHA to expand its standard to cover other workers. If you think your employer is violating this standard, write to your area OSHA office requesting a complaint form to fill out and sign. Your name will be kept confidential, and you are protected by law from harassment. If possible, get the advice and support of a union or COSH group about how to approach OSHA and how to make sure your rights are protected. A nationwide network of unions and COSH groups has been active in opposing anti-OSHA legislation in Congress as well as efforts within the agency itself to roll back protection for workers.

Other laws you should know about:

- *State workers' compensation laws.* All states have workers' compensation laws, which cover workers who are injured on the job or become ill as a result of work. These laws provide for the payment of medical expenses and part of lost wages.
- *State health and safety laws.* Some states have their own health and safety laws, which are particularly relevant to state and local government workers who are *not* covered under OSHA.
- *State and local Right-to-Act laws.* The purpose of these laws was to make sure that workers knew the hazards of the substances with which they worked. OSHA claims that the Federal Hazard Communications Standard (FHCS) overrides the state and municipal laws, which are sometimes stronger than the federal regulations.
- *National Labor Relations Act.* Provides some legal protection for concerted worker protests or job actions against unsafe working conditions. The act covers both unionized and nonunionized workers.

Women Taking Action

The Lowell mill girls struggled against hazardous conditions in the 1840s. In 1909, thousands of women in the garment industry in New York City went on strike to protest sweatshop working conditions and low wages. In 1943, 200 black women "sat down" at their machines in a tobacco plant in North Carolina in response to the death of a co-worker on the job, which the women saw as being the result of years of exposure to excessive heat, dust, and noise. In 1979, women led a strike to improve health and safety conditions and end sexual harassment at a poultry farm in

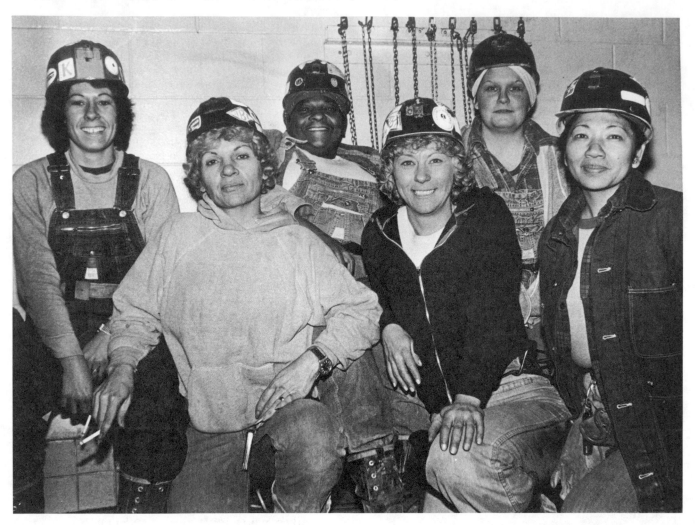

Coal-mining workers/Marat Moore

Mississippi. With a long history behind us, we continue to take action.

The process of workers coming together over a particular health and safety problem often starts informally. A woman who worked as a word processor at a major Boston bank contacted 9 TO 5 (an affiliate of Working Women) with concerns about her equipment, specifically the noise from the printers. She and her six co-workers met and discussed the problem with 9 TO 5 and came up with some reasonable solutions, which they presented to their supervisor. Eventually the company bought printer covers to reduce the noise. As one woman said, "While this may seem small, it is a big step for us. We've begun to talk together about our common concerns and now our supervisor is nervous that we may get together again on other issues."

When you organize at work, be sure to understand the difference between risk factors (dangers in the environment or workplace that may endanger health) and health outcomes (actual injury or sickness), and the consequences of focusing on one or the other. Try to show the connections. Show how a problem affects everyone. These are not individual issues, even if only a few individuals suffer at any given moment.

Whenever possible, it is most effective to form an ongoing workers' health and safety committee. Instead of just responding to emergencies, a committee can work preventively, uncovering potential problems before anyone gets hurt. A committee will have the task of approaching management, and there are lots of ways to get management's attention even when they don't want to listen.

I was working in a supermarket as a meat wrapper. We take the cut-up meat and wrap it in plastic. The plastic comes off a big roll that we cut to size by pulling it against a hot wire. A bunch of us were having asthma attacks and getting acne real bad. The health and safety committee met and decided that it was from the fumes of the plastic when it melted. We talked to our supervisor and he basically said, "Don't worry, ladies, it's all in your head." So we got mad and decided to try a new approach. We planned it so on one busy Saturday we all came to work with respirators on. After about an hour behind the meat counter with the customers staring at us in shock, the manager decided we were serious and agreed to meet with us and discuss what could be done.

Assess your group's strengths, weaknesses, barriers, and opportunities. You may find support in unexpected places. Ask what other workers in your shop or community can contribute to your campaign. For example, female clerical or health care workers battling unhealthy indoor environmental conditions might enlist male maintenance or security workers who could help with ventilation, furniture, machines, or safety issues.

Committees can gather information, educate themselves and their co-workers, help set priorities, and provide leadership and persistence to get things changed. Also, in groups we are less likely to be singled out as "troublemakers" and subjected to special harassment or even fired. A health and safety committee is most effective as part of a union. When you have a union, by law the company is obliged to talk to the union to negotiate about health and safety.

Class action suits have been used by groups of women to challenge sex discrimination and sexual harassment at work, as well as other health issues. Although more frequent nowadays, they are still difficult to win and are usually filed only against large companies that can afford to pay damages. In small companies, where many women of color and low-income white women work, this kind of legal action is less likely to be successful. Unions, COSH groups, the Labor Institute, and other advocacy groups listed in the Resource section can help you decide whether such a lawsuit is a good strategy for your group to pursue.

Sometimes *small acts of solidarity* on the part of many women from all racial and socioeconomic classes can lead to substantial gains in a campaign. For example, the AFL-CIO and the United Farm Workers are asking consumers to sign pledges supporting strawberry pickers' rights to a living wage, clean drinking water and toilets in the fields, job security, health insurance, and protection against sexual harassment and other abuses.[38]

Our work has more impact on our physical and mental health than we often acknowledge. Getting involved in improving working conditions is one more way that we as women can take control of our lives.

One of the best periods of my life was when we were on strike. We were all like one big family. Once I took a stand on what I knew to be right, I never felt freer in my life. Any average man or woman can do what we did. You can write press releases, push government, get things done. If you keep hammering the nail, eventually it's going to go in. I was "just a housewife." I'm proof that you don't need special talent or experience. I don't think people understand that. If I can get up and address 500 people, believe me, anyone can. If something has to be done, there are ways to do it. You don't need a college education—just determination.

NOTES

1. P. F. Infante and J. Pesak, "A Historical Perspective of Some Occupationally Related Diseases of Women," *Journal of Occupational Medicine* 36, no. 8 (1984): 826–31.

2. Staci Simonich and Ronald Hites, "Global Distributions of Persistent Organochlorine Compounds," *Science* 269 (September 29, 1995): 1851–854.

3. "Citizens Spoke Out on Chemical Control," *On CUE* 4, no. 6 (July 1987): 1. (Newsletter of the Coalition for a United Elizabeth, 135 Madison Avenue, Elizabeth, NJ 07201.)

4. "How About a Nuclear Weapons-Free 21st Century? It's Perfectly Possible." Fact Sheet, February 1997, Women's Action for New Directions (WAND), 110 Maryland Avenue NE, Suite 205, Washington, DC 20002.

5. Charles Grossman and Rudi Nussbaum, "Hypothyroidism and Spontaneous Abortion Among Hanford, Washington Downwinders," *Archives of Environmental Health*, 51, no. 3 (May/June 1996): 175–76.

6. "Marshall Island Stand at a New 'Crossroads'," *Health Research Bulletin* (PSR publication) 3, nos. 1–2 (Winter 1996).

7. Carol Sue Davidson, "Antarctic Lore," in *The Cousteau Almanac: An Inventory of Life on Our Water Planet* (New York: Doubleday, 1981); Tom Conry, "Chemical of the Month: Lead," *Exposure* no. 13 (December 1981): 6.

8. Commission for Racial Justice, United Church of Christ, *Toxic Waste and Race in the United States* (New York: Public Data Access, 1987).

9. *Race, Poverty and the Environment: A Newsletter for Social and Environmental Justice* 1, no. 1 (April 1990). San Francisco: Earth Island Institute.

10. Lois Marie Gibbs, "Turning Lemons into Lemonade," *Everyone's Backyard* 14, no. 4 (Winter 1996). 2.

11. Robert Bullard et al., *We Speak for Ourselves: Social Justice, Race and Environment* (Washington, DC: Panos Institute, 1990).

12. Y. C. Arguedas and C. B. Bustos. "Bitter Fruit: Health Woes of a Plantation Worker," *Women's Health Journal* (January–March 1996): 11–12. Santiago, Chile: Latin American and Caribbean Women's Health Network.

13. "NORA Priority Research Areas," 1996. National Institute of Occupational Safety and Health Web site.

14. Ibid.

15. *Multiple Chemical Sensitivities at Work: A Training Manual for Working People* (New York: Labor Institute, 1993).

16. See *Reproductive Health Hazards in the Workplace* (Office of Technology Assessment, U.S. Congress, 1985) for a helpful overview of reproductive effects.

17. Maureen Paul, "Reproductive Fitness and Risk," *Occupational Medicine: State of the Art Reviews* 3 (1988): 3.

18. Theo Colburn, Dianne Dumanoski, and John P. Meyers, *Our Stolen Future: Are We Threatening Our Fertility, Intelligence, and Survival?* (New York: Dutton, 1996), 106.

19. Virginia Soffa, *The Journey Beyond Breast Cancer* (Rochester, VT: Healing Arts Press, 1994), 78.

20. Joe Thornton, *Chlorine, Human Health and the Environment: The Breast Cancer Warning* (Washington, DC: Greenpeace, 1993).

21. Ellen Leopold, "Round Up the Usual Suspects," *Sojourner: The Women's Forum* 22, no. 7 (March 1997): 9.

22. Harvard Center for Cancer Prevention, Harvard School for Public Health, "Harvard Report on Cancer Prevention, Vol. 1: Causes of Human Cancer," *Cancer Causes and Control* no. 7 (1996).

23. Regina H. Kenen, *Reproductive Hazards in the Workplace: Mending Jobs, Managing Pregnancies* (Binghamton, NY: Harrington Park Press, 1993).

24. Caroline Cox, "Masculinity at Risk: Pesticides and Male Fertility," *Journal of Pesticide Reform* 16, no. 2 (summer 1996): 2–7.

25. Joni Seager, " 'Hysterical Housewives' and other Mad Women: Grassroots Environmental Organizing in the United States," in Dianne Rocheleau, Barbara Thomas-Slayter, and Esther Wangari, eds., *Feminist Political Ecology: Global Issues and Local Experiences* (New York: Routledge, 1996), 271–83.

26. Vernice Miller, Moya Hallstein, and Susan Quass, "Feminist Politics and Environmental Justice: Women's Community Activism in West Harlem, N.Y.," in Rocheleau et al., *Feminist Political Ecology,* 62–85.

27. National Institute for Occupational Safety and Health, *National Occupational Research Agenda Priority Research Areas.* 1997. Available on the National Institute for Occupational Safety and Health Web site: http://www.cdc.gov/niosh/nora.html#intro.

28. J. M. Stellman, "Where Women Work and the Hazards They May Face on the Job," *Journal of Occupational Medicine* 36, no. 8 (1994): 814–25.

29. K. Messing, B. Neis, and L. Dumias, eds., *Invisible: Issues in Women's Occupational Health* (Charlottetown, PEI: Gynergy Books, 1995).

30. Press Release from the Women's Center for Economic Alternatives (1987), 207 W. Main Street, Ahoskie, NC 27910.

31. A. R. Velasco, "Harvest of Shame Continues," *Pesticides and You* 16, nos. 1–2 (1996): 13–17.

32. National Institute for Occupational Safety and Health, *Workplace Health and Safety Issues for Women* (Cincinnati: U.S. Department of Health and Human Services, Public Health Service, Centers for Disease Control and Protection, 1997).

33. The Labor Institute, *Violence at Work: A Training Workbook for Working People* (New York: The Labor Institute, 1995). Available from the Labor Institute, 853 Broadway, Room 2014, New York, NY 10003.

34. *Connections: Network of Women in Trade and Technical Jobs,* Boston, MA, February 1982.

35. "Women at Work—Their Dual Role," Women's Occupational Health Resource Center, Columbia University.

36. The Labor Institute, *Violence at Work.*

37. Don Terry, "Testimony of Betrayal and Kisses at Army Drill Sergeant's Hearing," *The New York Times* (Nov. 14, 1996), p. A1.

38. National Coalition Against the Misuse of Pesticides, *Pesticides and You* 16, nos. 1–2 (1996). More information can be obtained from Jocelyn Shermank, UFW, (408) 763-4820; and Richard Greer, AFL-CIO, (202) 637-5279.

....

RESOURCES

....

Reading Material

General

AFL-CIO. Department of Occupational Safety and Health. *Safe Jobs: Promises Kept, Promises Broken: 25 Years of Worker Safety and Health in the United States.* Washington, DC: AFL-CIO, 1996.

Colborn, Theo, Dianne Dumanoski, and John P. Myers. *Our Stolen Future: Are We Threatening Our Fertility, Intelligence, and Survival?* New York: Dutton Books, 1996.

Firth, M., J. Brophy, and M. Keith. *Workplace Roulette: Gambling with Cancer.* Windsor, Ontario: Windsor Occupational Health Information Service, 1996.

Gottlieb, R., ed. *Reducing Toxics: A New Approach to Policy and Industrial Decisionmaking.* Washington, DC: Island Press, 1995.

Greenbaum, J. *Windows on the Workplace: Computers, Jobs, and the Organization of Office Work in the Late Twentieth Century.* New York: Monthly Review Press, 1995.

Linder, Marc, and Ingrid Nygaard. *Void Where Prohibited: Rest Breaks and the Right to Urinate on Company Time.* Ithaca, NY: ILR Press, 1997.

Moure-Eraso, R., et al. "Back to the Future: Sweatshop Conditions on the Mexico–U.S. Border: I. Community Health Impact of Maquiladora Industrial Activity." *American Journal of Industrial Medicine* 25 (1994): 311–24.

———, et al. "Back to the Future: Sweatshop Conditions on the Mexico-U.S. Border: II. Occupational Health Impact of Maquiladora Industrial Activity." *American Journal of Industrial Medicine* 31 (1997): 587–99.

New Solutions: A Journal of Environmental and Occupational Health Policy, P.O. Box 281200, Lakewood, CO 80228. Excellent resource on strategic linkage of workplace and environment.

Philadelphia Area Project on Occupational Safety and Health. *Getting Job Hazards Out of the Bedroom: The Handbook on Workplace Hazards to Reproduction.* 1988. PHILAPOSH, 3001 Walnut Street, Philadelphia, PA 19104. (215) 385-7000.

Service Employees International Union Eduation and Support Fund. *The HIV/AIDS Book: Information for Workers.* Washington, DC: SEIU, 1997. Available from SEIU. 1313 L Street NW, Washington, DC 20005. (202) 898-3443. One of the most widely used resources.

Sherman, Janette. *Chemical Exposure and Disease: Diagnostic and Investigative Techniques.* Princeton, NJ: Princeton Scientific Publishing, 1994.

Steingraber, Sandra. *Living Downstream: An Ecologist Looks at Cancer and the Environment.* Reading, MA: Addison-Wesley, 1997.

Steinman, David, and R. Wisner. *Living Healthy in a Toxic World: Simple Steps to Protect You and Your Family from Everyday Chemicals, Poisons and Pollution*. New York: Berkley Publishing Group, 1996.

United States Office of Technology Assessment. *Reproductive Health Hazards in the Workplace*. Philadelphia: J. B. Lippincott, 1988. Detailed documentation of research on reproductive hazards and the role of regulation, workers compensation and litigation.

Chemicals

Ashford, N., and C. Miller. *Chemical Exposures: Low Levels and High Stakes*. New York: Van Nostrand Reinhold, 1991. Key analysis of chemical sensitivity, diagnosis and treatment issues, and recommendations for improved prevention and care.

Dansereau, Carol. *Poisons in the Web of Life: The Case for Toxics Reform*. Seattle: Washington Toxics Coalition, 1996. Available from the Washington Toxics Coalition, 4516 University Way NE, Seattle, WA 98105. (206) 632-1545.

Citizen Action, Community-Based Advocacy and Worker's Training

Barnsley, Jan, and Ellis Diana. *Research for Change: Participatory Action Research for Community Groups*. Vancouver: Women's Research Centre, 1992. Available from Women's Research Centre, 2245 West Broadway, Suite 101, Vancouver BC V6K 2E4; (604) 734-0485.

Briskin L., and Patricia McDermott, eds. *Women Challenging Unions: Feminism, Democracy and Militancy*. Toronto: University of Toronto Press, 1993.

Brown, Phil, and Edwin Mikkelsen. *No Safe Place: Toxic Waste, Leukemia, and Community Action*. Berkeley: University of California Press, 1990.

Bullard, Robert, ed. *Confronting Environmental Racism: Voices from the Grassroots*. Boston: South End Press, 1993.

Cook, Katsi. "Use Science, But Trust Our Own Knowledge." *Native Americas* 12, no.14 (1995). Cornell's American Indian Program publication.

Dula, Annette, Sabrina Kurtz, and Maria Luz-Samper. "Occupational and Environmental Reproductive Hazards Education and Resources for Communities of Color." *Environmental Health Perspectives Supplements* 101 (Suppl. 2), 1993.

Gibbs, Lois. *Dying from Dioxin: A Citizen's Guide to Reclaiming Our Health and Rebuilding Democracy*. Boston: South End Press, 1995.

Hynes, H. Patricia. *Earthright: Every Citizen's Guide*. Rocklin, CA: Prima Publishing, 1990.

The Labor Institute. *Sexual Harassment at Work: A Training Workbook for Working People*. New York: The Labor Institute, 1994. Available from the Labor Institute (see "Organizations" below).

———. *Violence at Work: A Training Workbook for Working People*. New York: The Labor Institute, 1995. Available from the Labor Institute (see "Organizations" below).

Massachusetts Coalition for Occupational Safety and Health Women's Committee. *Confronting Reproductive Health Hazards on the Job: A Guide for Workers*. Boston: MassCOSH, 1992. Available from MassCOSH, 555 Amory Street, Boston, MA 02130; (617) 524-6686. Based on years of shop-floor experience, this booklet presents helpful information on the hazards, worker rights, and effective strategies.

Nelson L., R. Kenen, and S. Klitzman. *Turning Things Around: A Women's Occupational and Environmental Health Resource Guide*. Washington, DC: National Women's Health Network, 1990. A resource guide for women facing occupational and environmental problems at work, in the home, and in the community.

Wallerstein, Nina, and Harriet Rubenstein. *Teaching About Job Hazards: A Guide for Workers and Their Health Providers*. Washington, DC: American Public Health Association, 1993.

Pesticides

Briggs, Shirley. *Basic Guide to Pesticides: Their Characteristics and Hazards*. Bristol, PA: Taylor and Francis, 1992.

Carson, Rachel. *Silent Spring*. Boston: Houghton Mifflin, 1994, c. 1962. The book that started it all by explaining the effects of DDT.

Radiation

Bertell, Rosalie. *No Immediate Danger: Prognosis for a Radioactive Earth*. Summertown, TN: The Book Publishing Co., 1985. Careful, clear analysis of the radiation/health connection, examining military and industrial policies, key role of women in challenging nuclear establishment.

Technical References

Guillette, Lou, and Elizabeth Guillette. "Environmental Contaminants and Reproductive Abnormalities in Wildlife? Implications for Public Health?" *Toxicology and Industrial Health* 12, nos. 3/4 (1996).

Levy, B. S., and D. Wegman, eds. *Occupational Health: Recognizing and Preventing Work Related Diseases*, 3rd ed. Boston: Little, Brown, 1994. One of the key texts; directed to researchers, providers.

National Research Council. *Multiple Chemical Sensitivities: Addendum to Biologic Markers in Immunotoxicology*. Washington, DC: National Academy Press, 1992.

Needleman, H., and D. Bellinger, eds. *Prenatal Exposure to Toxicants: Developmental Consequences*. Baltimore, MD: Johns Hopkins University Press, 1994. In-depth evaluation of the effects of a variety of environmental toxicants on development. Also examines reproductive hazards in the workplace.

Paul, Maureen, ed. *Occupational and Environmental Reproductive Hazards: A Guide for Clinicians*. Baltimore, MD: Williams & Wilkins, 1992.

Shepard, T. H. *Catalog of Teratogenic Agents*, 8th ed. Baltimore, MD: Johns Hopkins University Press, 1995.

"Symposium on Women's Occupational Health." *Women and Health* 18, no. 3 (1992).

Women and Environmental/ Occupational Health

Diamond, Irene, and Gloria Orenstein, eds. *Reweaving the World: The Emergence of EcoFeminism*. San Francisco: Sierra Club, 1990.

Gibson, Pamela Reed. "Environmental Illness/Multiple Chemical Sensitivities: Invisible Disabilities." In Mary Willmuth and Lillian Holcomb, eds. *Women with Disabilities: Found Voices*. New York: Harrington Park Press, 1993.

Hynes, Patricia. *The Recurring Silent Spring*. New York: Pergamon Press, 1989. Feminist analysis of Rachel Carson and women/environment links, with focus on reproductive politics.

Kenen, Regina. *Reproductive Hazards in the Workplace: Mending Jobs, Managing Pregnancies*. Binghamton, NY: Harrington Park Press, 1993.

————. *A Woman's Guide to a Pregnancy Friendly Workplace* (tentative title). London: Pluto Press, forthcoming, 1998. Useful for women to understand protections that the European Community Directives provide for women workers as goal to be reached in the United States.

Klitzman, S., B. Silverstein, L. Punnett, and A. Mock. "A Women's Occupational Health Agenda for the 1990s." *New Solutions: A Journal of Environmental and Occupational Health Policy* 1, no. 1 (1990). Review of work conditions, proposals for protecting women's health, job rights.

Ratcliff, Kathryn Strother, ed. *Healing Technology: Feminist Perspectives*. Ann Arbor: University of Michigan Press, 1989. Reproductive technologies, health, occupational and environmental health, feminist strategies.

Rocheleau, Dianne, Barbara Thomas-Slayter, and Esther Wangari, eds. *Feminist Political Ecology: Global Issues and Local Experiences*. London: Routledge, 1996.

Shiva, Vandana, ed. *Close to Home: Women Reconnect Ecology, Health and Development Worldwide*. Philadelphia: New Society Publishers, 1994.

————. *Staying Alive: Women, Ecology and Development*. London: Zed Books, 1989. Path-breaking book on women, land, natural resources, development.

Soffa, Virginia. *The Journey Beyond Breast Cancer: From the Personal to the Political*. Rochester, VT: Healing Arts, 1994.

Women and Environments: The Journal for a Feminist Globe. Quarterly from Women & Environments Education and Development Foundation, 736 Bathurst Street, Toronto, Ontario, Canada M5S 2R4; (416) 516-2600. Web site: weed@web.net

"Women in the Movement." Special issue of *Race, Poverty and Environment* 1, no. 4 (winter 1991).

Audiovisual Materials

A Price for Every Progress: The Health Hazards of VDTs. Labor Institute, (212) 674-3322.

Assault on the Male, BBC, distributed by NOVA, 1995. 60 minutes. Focus is on endocrine-disrupting contaminants, including birth defects, reproductive health, breast cancer.

Chemical Birthright, University of Florida, 1996. 30 minutes. Endocrine-disrupting chemicals, human impacts.

Close to the Edge: Violence in the Workplace. 19 minutes, $15. Labor Institute (see "Organizations" below). Training video.

It Didn't Have to Happen: Preventing Cumulative Trauma Disorders. Labor Occupational Health Program, 2521 Channing Way, Berkeley, CA 94720.

More Than We Can Bear: Reproductive Hazards on the Job. 27 minutes, $15. Labor Institute (see "Organizations" below).

Multiple Chemical Sensitivities at Work. 28 minutes, $15. Labor Institute, 853 Broadway, Room 2014, New York, NY 10003; (212) 674-3322; Fax: (212) 353-1203. Training video.

Surrounded: The Occupational Hazards of EMFs (electromagnetic fields). 27 minutes, $15. Labor Institute, 853 Broadway, Room 2014, New York, NY 10003; (212) 674-3322; Fax: (212) 353-1203.

We All Live Downstream. 1995, Greenpeace. 30 minutes. On water quality, focused on Mississippi; citizen action, access to data.

Witness to the Future, 1996. Hour-long on employee/ citizen action on pesticides in California, toxics in Los Angeles, and nuclear hazards in Washington. From Video Project.

Two excellent sources:

The Media Network
39 W. 14th Street, Suite 403; New York, NY 10011; (212) 929-2663
E-mail: medianetwk@aol.com

The Video Project
200 Estates Drive; Ben Lomond, CA 95005; (800) 4-PLANET
E-mail: videoproject@igc.org
Web site: http://www.videoproject.org/videoproject

Organizations

Association of Birth Defect Children
827 Irma Avenue; Orlando, FL 32803; (800) 313-ABDC; (407) 245-7035
Web site: http://www.birthdefects.org/main.htm
Resources on environmental health.

Association of Occupational and Environmental Health Clinics
1010 Vermont Avenue, Suite 513; Washington, DC 20005; (202) 347-4976
E-mail: aoec@dgs.dgsys.com
Web site: http://152.3.65.120/oem/aoec.htm

Back Pain Hotline
Texas Back Institute
6300 West Parker Road; Plano, TX 75093; (800) 247-Back

Center for Health, Environment and Justice
See Citizen's Clearinghouse, below

Center for Science in the Public Interest
1875 Connecticut Avenue, Suite 300; Washington, DC 20009; (202) 332-9110
E-mail: cspi@cspinet.org
Web site: http://www.cspinet.org
   Special Project: Americans for Safe Food

Children's Health Environmental Coalition
P.O. Box 846; Malibu, CA 90265; (310) 573-9608
E-mail: chec@checnet.org
Web site: http://www.checnet.org
   Focus: linking citizens, practitioners, researchers, legislative strategists

Citizen's Clearinghouse for Hazardous Wastes (newly renamed the Center for Health, Environment and Justice)
P.O. Box 6806; Falls Church, VA 22040; (703) 237-2249
E-mail: cchw@essential.org
   Founded by Lois Gibbs; newsletter *Everyone's Backyard;* special reports such as "Empowering Ourselves: Women and Toxics Organizing," *Environmental Health Monthly,* "Community Health Surveys," Fact Packs (on cancer clusters, lead, PCBs, etc.)

Coalition of Labor Union Women
661 27th Street; Oakland, CA 94612; (510) 893-8766
   Resources, handbooks on job hazards and women's rights, especially regarding "fetal protection policy."

Commission for Racial Justice
United Church of Christ
Ms. Banice Powell Jackson (Executive Director)
700 Prospect Avenue; Cleveland, OH 44115; (216) 736-2164
   Special Project on People of Color and the Environment.

Committee for Nuclear Responsibility
P.O. Box 421993; San Francisco, CA 94142; (415) 776-8299
Web site: http://www.radical.com/radiation/CNR
   Resources on health effects.

COSH groups: Coalitions, Councils or Committees on Occupational Safety and Health. Union, worker, professional alliances providing technical and strategic support (example, South East Michigan COSH's fact sheet on "Reproductive Hazards in the Workplace"). For complete list of 30+ COSH groups, contact:
New York Committee on Occupational Safety and Health (NYCOSH)
275 Seventh Avenue, 8th floor; New York, NY 10001; (212) 627-3900

Earth Island Institute
300 Broadway Street, No. 28; San Francisco, CA 94133-3312; (415) 788-3666
E-mail: earthisland@earthisland.org
Web site: http://earthisland.org/e./index.htm
   Publishes *Race, Poverty and the Environment Newsletter.*

Environmental Consortium for Minority Outreach
1001 Connecticut Avenue NW, Suite 827; Washington, DC 20036; (202) 331-8387

Environmental Health Network
P.O. Box 1155; Larkspur, CA 94977; (415) 541-5075
E-mail: info@progway.org
   Published *Profiles on Environmental Health,* technical assistance, citizen/professional conferences. Special report: *Inconclusive by Design: Waste, Fraud and Abuse in Federal Environmental Health Research.*

Environmental Research Foundation
P.O. Box 5036; Annapolis, MD 21403-7036; (410) 263-1584
   Environment & Health Weekly, excellent report on relationship between health, environment, politics.

Food And Water
800-EAT-SAFE
   Focusing on food safety; *Food and Water Journal.*

Greenpeace
1436 U Street NW; Washington, DC 20009; (202) 462-1177
E-mail: info@wdc.greenpeace.org
Web site: http://www.greenpeace.org/~usa
   Resources, strategy, support on environmental health; *Chlorine, Human Health and the Environment: The Breast Cancer Warning,* by Joe Thornton, 1993

Highlander Research and Education Center
1959 Highlander Way; New Market, TN 37820; (615) 933-3443; Fax: (615) 933-3424
   Stop the Poisons School, cross-national labor/environment coalition projects, video (on capital flight and maquiladoras)

Labor/Community Strategy Center
The Wiltern Center
3780 Wilshire Boulevard, Suite 1200; Los Angeles, CA 90010; (213) 387-2800
E-mail: laborctr@igc.apc.org
   Labor/environment, including *L.A.'s Lethal Air; New Strategies for Policy, Organizing and Action*

Labor Institute
853 Broadway, Room 2014; New York, NY 10003; (212) 674-3322; Fax: (212) 353-1203
   Research and educational organization, which has been producing innovative training programs and print and video materials for workers for 20 years.

Latin American and Caribbean Women's Health Network
Casilla 50610; Santiago 1; Santiago, Chile; (562) 634-9827; Fax: (562) 634-7101
   Strong on environmental and occupational problems; *Women's Health Journal* (Spanish and English editions)

Mothers and Others for a Liveable Planet
Natural Resources Defense Council
40 W. 20th Street; New York, NY 10011; (212) 727-2700
Web site: http://www/nrdc.org
   Newsletter on children and the environment

National Association for Physicians for the Environment
6410 Rockledge Drive, Suite 412; Bethesda, MD 20817;
(301) 571-9791
E-mail: nape@ix.netcom.com
Web site: http://www.intr.net/nape.net

National Coalition against the Misuse of Pesticides
530 7th Street SE; Washington, DC 20003; (202) 543-
5450
   Health, environmental, legal, and community groups
lobbying and educating on pesticides

National Pesticide Telecommunications Network
Oregon State University
Weniger Hall; Corvallis, OR 97331-6502
E-mail: nptn@ace.orst.edu
Web site: http://www.ace.orst.edu/info/nptn

National Women's Health Network (see chapter 27 Resources)

Northwest Coalition for Alternatives to Pesticides
P.O. Box 1393; Eugene, OR 97440; (541) 344-5044
E-mail: info@pesticide.org
Web site: http://www.efn.org/~ncap
   Journal of Pesticide Reform; booklet "Getting Pesti-
cides Out of Our Schools"; many other resources

Physicians for Social Responsibility
1101 14th Street NW, Suite 700; Washington, DC 20005;
(202) 898-0150
E-mail: psrnatl@psr.org
Web site: http://www.psr.org
   Reports available on current research on nuclear im-
pacts on health, "Children's Environmental Health Report
Card," "Putting the Lid on Dioxins: Protecting Human
Health and the Environment."

Race, Poverty and the Environment Center
Project of the California Rural Legal Assistance Foundation
631 Howard Street, Suite 300; San Francisco CA 94105;
(415) 777-2752

Reproductive Toxicology Center
2440 M Street NW, Suite 217; Washington, DC 20037-1404;
(202) 293-5137

Safe Drinking Water Hotline
Environmental Protection Agency Waterdocket
4101 M Street SW, Room L-102; Washington, DC 20460;
(800) 426-4791

Sierra Club
85 2nd Street, 2nd floor; San Francisco, CA 94105; (415)
979-5500
   Projects/Web sites on hazardous waste, environmental
justice, endocrine-disrupting chemicals.

Southwest Organizing Project
211 10th Street SW; Albuquerque, NM 87102-2919; (505)
247-8832
E-mail: swop@igc.apc.org
   Newsletter *Voces Unidas,* also interfaith hearings on
toxic poisoning in communities of color; environmental
justice booklets.

Trade unions and local/regional labor councils: Check
with local unions and councils on key concerns, re-
sources, and activities in your area. Many national union
offices have health and safety staff, for example, AFL-CIO
Health and Safety Department (Washington, DC); the
Communication Workers of America (Washington, DC);
Service Employees International Union (Washington,
DC); Steelworkers (Pittsburgh); United Auto Workers
(Detroit); Oil, Chemical, Atomic Workers (Denver).

United Farm Workers
P.O. Box 62; Keene, CA 93531; (805) 822-5571
   Newsletter *Food and Justice* on impact of pesticides on
workers, communities, consumers.

Washington Toxics Coalition
4516 University Way NE; Seattle, WA 98105; (206) 632-
1545

Women's Environment and Development Organization
355 Lexington Avenue, 3rd floor; New York, NY 10017;
(212) 973-0325
E-mail: wedo@igc.apc.org
Web site: http://www.wedo.org
   Broad global focus and experience, including leader-
ship at population and women's summits; also, Action for
Cancer Prevention Campaign.

Working Group on Community Right-to-Know
U.S. Public Interest Research Group
218 D Street SE; Washington, DC 20003-1107; (202) 546-
9707
E-mail: uspirg@pirg.org
Web site: www.pirg.org/pirg

Government Agencies and Legal Resources

Centers for Disease Control (CDC)
Fax Information Service
NIOSH Directory
(800) 356-4674; (404) 332-4565
Web site: http://www.cdc.gov
   Ask for the Women's Office for occupational and envi-
ronmental information.

Consumer Product Safety Commission
Washington, DC 20207; (800) 638-2772; (301) 504-0990

Environmental Protection Agency (EPA)
Public Information Center
Community Right-to Know/Superfund Hotline
Indoor Air Quality Information Clearinghouse
401 M Street NW; Washington, DC 20460; (800) 555-1404
Web site: http://epa.gov
   Chemical and nuclear hazards in the general environment.

National Center for Environmental Health
Centers for Disease Control and Prevention
Mail Stop F-29; 4770 Buford Highway, NE; Atlanta, GA
30341-3724; (404) 488-7040
   Projects on breast cancer, reproductive health.

National Center for Environmental Publications and
Information
P.O. Box 42419; Cincinnati, OH 45242-2419; (800) 490-9198

National Institute for Environmental Health Sciences
P.O. Box 12233; 104 Alexander Drive; MD 3-04; Research
Triangle Park, NC 27709; (919) 541-4500
Web site: http://www.nih.gov
   Provides environmental justice community research grants.

National Institute for Occupational Safety and Health
(NIOSH)
4676 Columbia Parkway; Cincinnati, OH 45226-1198;
(800) 35-NIOSH
   For general occupational health information or to request help in evaluating potential hazards in your workplace.

Nuclear Regulatory Commission (NRC)
Office of Public Affairs
Washington, DC 20555; (202) 492-7715
E-mail: opa@nrc.gov
Web site: http://www.nrc.gov
   Regulating and licensing of nuclear facilities.

Occupational Safety and Health Administration (OSHA)
200 Constitution Avenue NW; Washington, DC 20210;
(202) 523-9700
   Rules on access to employee exposure and medical records. Guarantees access of employees and unions to certain company records regarding exposure and medical records. For a free copy of the OSHA Hazard Communication Standard, call your local OSHA office or write for a copy (29CFR 1920.20) to OSHA Office of Information, 200 Constitution Avenue NW, Washington, DC 20210; (202) 523-8151.

Toxicology and Environmental Health Information
Program
E-mail: tehip@teh.nim.nih.gov

Women's Bureau
U.S. Department of Labor
200 Constitution Avenue NW; Washington, DC 20210
Work and Family Clearinghouse: (800) 827-5335
Web site: http://www.dol.gov/dol/wb
   Information to employers, employees, and unions on developing work and family programs (child care, elder care). Ask for "Work and Family Resource Kit." Single copies are free with self-addressed label to the Women's Bureau.

Workers' compensation: Each state has an agency responsible for handling worker's compensation claims. Look in the state government section of the phone book under "Workers' Compensation" or "Industrial Accidents." If you don't find it there, try calling your state department of labor and asking for the name of the agency responsible.

Additional Online Resources *

At Work with Julie: Workers' Compensation Questions
and Answers
http://www.abag.ca.gov/govnet/julie/julie.html

The Center for Informed Decision Making
http://members.aol.com/cygnusgrp/index.html

EnviroLink Pre Home Page
http://envirolink.org

Environmental Health at the University of Edinburgh
http://www.ed.ac.uk/~rma/environ_health.html

Environmental Organization WebDirectory!
http://www.webdirectory.com

IGC: EcoNet
http://www.igc.org/igc/econet/index.html

Our Environmental Health
http://www.medaccess.com/environ/env_toc.htm

University of Washington: Department of Environmental
Health
http://dehmac.sphcm.washington.edu/DEHweb

Yahoo: Health: Workplace: Computer Related Health
Hazards
http://www.yahoo.com/Health/Workplace/Computer_
Related_Health_Hazards

* For more information and listings of online resources, please see
Introduction to Online Women's Health Resources, p. 25.

Chapter 8

Violence Against Women

By Marianne Winters, based on earlier work by Dina Carbonell, Lois Glass, Suzanne Gosselin, Carol Mamber, Jill Stanzler, Alice Friedman, Margaret Lazarus, Lynn Rubinett, Lena Sorensen, Denise Wells, Nancy Wilbur, Terrie Antico, Wendy Sanford

WITH SPECIAL THANKS TO Jackie Herskovitz, Judith Lennett, and Laura Tandara*

Violence against women is a worldwide yet still hidden problem. Freedom from the threat of harassment, battering, and sexual assault is a concept that most of us have a hard time imagining because violence is such a deep part of our cultures and our lives. Consider these facts:†

- Battering is the leading cause of injury to women aged 15–44 in the U.S.[1]

* Thanks also to the following for their help with the 1998 version of this chapter: Holly Curtis, Bonnie Gage, Marcia Gordon, Jackson Katz, Margaret Lazarus, Liza Rankow, Beth Richie, Vivianne Soto. Over the years since 1969, the following people have contributed to the many versions of this chapter: Gene Bishop, Andrea Fischgrund, Roxanne Hynek, Janet Jones, Freada Klein, Rachel Lanzerotti, Margaret Lazarus, Carol McEldowney, Judy Norsigian.
† This chapter focuses on male violence toward women, although we know that female-to-male and female-to-female violence happens as well. Men who are survivors have begun to speak out about violence that happened to them as children by men as well as women. Lesbians have begun to look at and address the extent of violence within lesbian relationships. (See chapter 10, Relationships with Women.)

- The FBI, which gathers data from law enforcement officials, indicated that 102,555 women were victims of rape in 1990.[2]
- In contrast to the FBI data, the *Rape in America* study estimates that 683,000 women are raped every year.[3]
- Approximately 50% of the homeless women and children in this country are on the streets because of violence in their homes.[4]
- One-fifth to one-half of U.S. women were sexually abused as children at least once, most of them by an older male relative.[5]
- Nearly two-thirds of women who receive public assistance ("welfare") have been abused by an intimate partner at some time in their adult lives.[6]

Given these facts, it is not surprising that the Vienna Declaration and Programme of Action calls violence against women a violation of the human rights of a majority of the world's population. Women are statistically safer out on the street than they are in their homes.[7] Violence against women is woven into the fabric of society to such an extent that many of us who are victimized feel that we are at fault. Many of those who perpetrate violence feel justified by strong societal messages that say that rape, battering, sexual harassment, child abuse, and other forms of violence are acceptable. Every day we see images of male violence against women in the news, on TV shows, in the movies, in advertising, and in our homes and workplaces. It is a fact of life for women of all ages, races, and classes.

I have never been free of the fear of rape. From a very early age I, like most women, have thought of rape as part of my natural environment—something to be feared and prayed against like fire or lightning. I never asked why men raped; I simply thought it one of the many mysteries of human nature.

In the broadest sense, violence against women is any violation of a woman's personhood, mental or physical integrity, or freedom of movement through individual acts and societal oppression. It includes all the ways our society objectifies and oppresses women. Violence against women ranges from sterilization abuse to prescription drug abuse, pornography, stalking, battering, and rape.* It includes the sexual and physical abuse of young girls and the abuse of elders.

Every form of violence threatens all women and limits our ability to make choices about our lives. Sexual violence is particularly insidious because sexual acts are ordinarily and rightly a source of pleasure and communication. It is often unclear to a woman who has been victimized and to society as a whole whether a sexual violation was done out of sexual desire or violent intent or whether these motivations are even distinguishable, because violence itself has come to be seen as sexual or erotic.

Thirty years ago, most forms of violence against women were hidden under a cloak of silence or acceptance. As more and more women talked with each other in the recent wave of the women's movement, it became apparent that violence against us occurs on a massive scale; that no woman is immune; and that

---

* We do not address the subject of pornography primarily because we disagree with one another and have not come to any clear positions on some crucial aspects of this issue. However, we all

- abhor all pornography that we find violent or degrading to women.
- believe it important to protest the existence of this type of pornography, though we would not seek government censorship.
- protest the fact that a huge pornography industry is making billions of dollars by objectifying, degrading, and dehumanizing women, children, and sometimes men. The work women are doing to expose this industry is central to our understanding of violence against women in cultures throughout the world.

We recognize that some of us will find offensive what others view as erotica, and vice versa, and that not all pornography represents "violence against women." But this need not keep us from speaking out against what we believe is degrading to women and, ultimately, to everyone.

family, friends, and public institutions have been cruelly insensitive about it. Over the past thirty years, women have mobilized to offer direct services to those who have encountered violence, to educate people about the range and nature of male violence against women, and to develop strategies for change. This chapter reflects the important work of some of these women.

TOWARD AN UNDERSTANDING OF MALE VIOLENCE AGAINST WOMEN

One man's violence against one woman may seem to result from his individual psychological problems, sexual frustration, unbearable life pressures, or some innate urge toward aggression. Though each of these "reasons" has been used to explain and even justify male violence, they oversimplify a complex reality: men have been taught to relate to the world in terms of dominance and control, and they have been taught that violence is an acceptable method of maintaining control, resolving conflicts, and expressing anger. When a boss sexually harasses an employee, he exerts his power to restrict her freedom to work and improve her position. When a battering husband uses beatings to confine his wife to the home and to prevent her from seeing friends and family or from pursuing outside work, he exerts dominance and control. When men rape women, they act out of a wish to dominate or punish.

Whether or not an individual man who commits an act of violence views it as an expression of power is not the point. The fact that so many individual men feel entitled to express their frustration or anger by being violent to so many individual women shows how deeply these lessons of dominance and violence have been learned.

Countless daily acts of violence create a climate of fear and powerlessness that limits women's freedom of action and controls many of the movements of our lives. The threat of male violence continues to keep us from stepping out from behind the traditional roles that we, as women, have been taught. Violence and the threat of violence keep us "in our place."

Now that I am on my own and living free of my abuser, I can see how my life was altered when I was being battered. Little by little, he isolated me from my friends, he convinced me to quit working, he complained about how I kept the house, he kept track of the mileage on the car to make sure that I wasn't going anywhere. Eventually, when the beatings were regular and severe, I had no one to turn to and I felt completely alone.

On the surface, it seems that men benefit from sexism—from this system of male dominance, control, and violence. On a deeper level, we know that sexism harms men as well as women. Sexism, and more specifically violence against women, harms men because it harms the women and girls in their lives and because

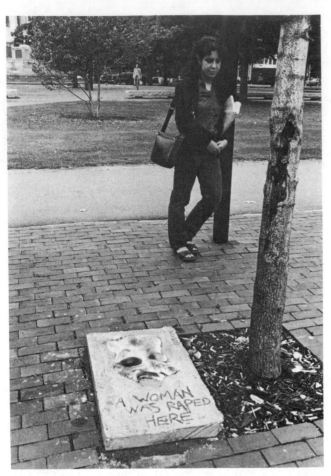

Ellen Shub

it keeps them from having positive and loving relationships with women. In recent years, some men have begun to recognize and acknowledge the ways in which relating violently toward women (and other men) harms them. Groups like "Real Men" and "Men to End Sexism" have been working to raise consciousness among other men and to teach men how to be allies of women in the effort to bring an end to violence against women.

RACE, CLASS AND VIOLENCE
AGAINST WOMEN

While violence is often targeted toward us simply because we are women, factors such as race, class, sexual orientation, and age put particular women at greater risk and with less access to resources. Women of color, older women, young women, lesbians, poor and working-class women, and women with disabilities, to name a few, are especially vulnerable to male violence. A married black woman who was fired for refusing to sleep with her supervisor said:

On many occasions Mr. ——— said to me, "For a colored girl, you are intelligent." I told him that if he has to refer to a color or race concerning me, I considered myself "black." He replied, "I don't believe in

black or all that stuff. To me you're colored, and that's it." One day he made a comment concerning my, as he called it, "voluptuous" shape. When I asked him politely to discontinue making such comments that include sexual overtures, he replied, "Why not? For a colored, you're very stacked, light-skinned, and pretty."

Too often, services that aim to serve victims of violence are not aware of or do not have sufficient resources to serve the widest range of women. For example, hotlines may be available only in English, police may hold racist attitudes toward women of color, courts may be inaccessible to women who have no telephones or transportation. Often, these institutions reflect society's racism and classism.

The man who raped me was white, and the cops here are all white. I didn't report it. I just told a few people I trusted. It helped, but I still feel scared, knowing he's out there and that nobody would do anything about it.

Most people take acts of violence less seriously if the woman is "poor," old, or institutionalized; or is a prostitute, a lesbian, or a woman with physical or mental disabilities. This is true for all women whose "male protectors" are nonexistent, invisible, or socially less powerful than other men. Older women have less freedom to fight sexual harassment at their jobs or to leave a battering husband, partly because age discrimination means they might not easily find other ways of supporting themselves.

Acts of violence against women are sometimes particularly motivated by racism, homophobia, or religious bias. These hate crimes can include beatings and verbal harassment (using ugly epithets) and vandalism of sacred spaces such as synagogues, churches, or cemeteries. Like other forms of violence against women, hate crimes can also include death threats, sexual assault, and murder. Perpetrators include white supremacist and neo-Nazi groups that attack people of color or Jewish people because of their intense hatred for these people. Open lesbians have been raped by men or groups of men angry at their social independence or because lesbians do not want them sexually.[8] Victims of hate crimes often experience intense fear and isolation, humiliation, and increased feelings of internalized self-hatred.

I guess the worst part of all this is feeling baffled by hate. Why—is the question that keeps running through my head. What have I done to deserve this?

Many states have specific laws about hate crimes.

BLAMING THE VICTIM

The most common emotional responses to sexual harassment, battering, and rape are guilt, fear, powerlessness, shame, betrayal, anger, and denial. Guilt is often the first and deepest response. Anger may arise only later; this is not surprising, because as women we often have no sense of a right to be free from these kinds of violence.

We may feel guilty about violence done to us because we are taught that our job is to make men happy, and if they aren't, we—not they—are to blame. Many of us heard from our parents, "Boys will be boys, so girls must take care"—the message being that we can avoid unwanted male attention if only we are careful enough. If anything goes wrong, it must be our fault. Blaming the victim releases the man who commits violence from the responsibility for what he has done. Friends or family may blame the victim in order to feel safe themselves: "She got raped because she walked alone after midnight. I'd never do that, so rape won't happen to me." WOMEN ARE NOT GUILTY FOR VIOLENCE COMMITTED BY MEN ON OUR BODY, MIND, AND SPIRIT. THIS VIOLENCE HAPPENS BECAUSE OF MEN'S GREATER POWER AND THEIR MISUSE OF THAT POWER.

SEXUAL HARASSMENT

Sexual harassment is any unwanted sexual attention a woman experiences. It includes leering, pinching, patting, repeated comments, subtle suggestions of a sexual nature, and pressure for dates. Sexual harassment can occur in any situation where men have power over women: welfare workers with clients, doctors with patients, police officers with women members of a police force, or teachers with students. In the workplace, the harasser may be an employer, a supervisor, a co-worker, a client, or a customer. Sexual harassment can escalate; women who are being sexually harassed are at risk of being physically abused or raped. Consider these facts:

- According to the U.S. Department of Labor, some 50 to 80% of women in the U.S. experience some form of sexual harassment during their academic or work lives.[9]
- In a survey of girls in middle schools and high schools that was distributed in *Seventeen,* 83% of the girls who responded reported instances of sexual harassment in school.[10]

Joan is a 43-year-old black woman who works as a waitress in a bar and restaurant. She often feels isolated, as many of her co-workers are white and have racist attitudes. A customer who comes in every day begins to flirt with Joan, making suggestive comments about her clothing and physical appearance. Unnerved by his comments, she tries not to show it because she doesn't want to lose any tip money. Often he grabs at her and touches her when she walks by. She feels so anxious at work that her stomach hurts, and she starts to call in sick more and more. She knows she needs to figure something out or she'll eventually lose her job.

One 16-year-old girl described her experience:

It came to the point where I was skipping almost all of my classes, therefore getting me kicked out of the honors program. I dreaded school each morning, I started to wear clothes that wouldn't flatter my figure, and I kept to myself. I'd cry every night when I got home, and I thought I was a loser. . . . Sometimes the teachers were right there when it was going on. They did nothing. . . . I felt very angry that these arrogant, narrow-minded people never took the time to see who I really was inside.[11]

Sexual harassment is a powerful way for men to undermine and control us. Attitudes of race and class superiority can result in a feeling by white men that they are entitled to sexually harass women of color or employees from a "lower" class or different background. There is an implicit (and sometimes explicit) message that our refusal to comply with the harasser's demands will lead to work-related reprisals. These can include escalation of harassment; poor work assignments; sabotaging of projects; denial of raises, benefits, or promotion; and sometimes the loss of the job with only a poor reference to show for it. Harassment can drive women out of a particular job or out of the workplace altogether.

Socializing at work too often includes flirting or joking about sex. Although it may be a pleasant relief from routine or a way to communicate with someone we are interested in, this banter can become insulting or demeaning. It becomes sexual harassment when it creates a hostile, intimidating, or pressured working environment.

There is such a taboo in many workplaces and schools against identifying sexual harassment for what it is that many of us who experience it are at first aware only of feeling stressed. We may experience headaches, anxieties, or resistance to going to work in the morning. It may take us a while to realize that these symptoms come from our being sexually harassed. We often respond by feeling isolated and powerless, afraid to say no or to speak out because we fear either that we somehow are responsible or that we won't receive help in facing possible retaliation. But when we take the risk and talk with other women, we often find that they are being harassed, too (or have been), and have similar responses to ours.

What You Can Do
If You Are Sexually Harassed *

Every instance of sexual harassment is different. The strategy you choose will depend on many factors, including how much you can afford to risk losing your

---

* The specific legal options for sexual harassment include filing charges of sex discrimination with your state's human rights commission or the Federal Equal Employment Opportunity Commission. In addition, women have used unemployment

job and whether you feel you can get support from your co-workers. Race and class differences may also affect how you respond, partly because these differences in a workplace can isolate workers from one another. As you think about whether and how you might respond to sexual harassment, here are some things to consider:

- Remember that you are not to blame. Sexual harassment is imposed sexual attention. No matter how complicated the situation is, the harasser is responsible for the abuse.
- Document what happens. Keep a detailed diary including dates, times, and places. Save any notes or pictures from the harasser—don't throw them away in anger. Keep a record of anyone who witnessed the harassment.
- Investigate your workplace or school policy and grievance procedure for sexual harassment cases. Know its overall records before you act.
- Generate support for yourself before you take action: Break the silence, talk with others, and ask for help in working out a response.
- Look for others who have been harassed who can act with you. Collective action and joint complaints strengthen your position. Try to use organizations that already exist, such as your union or employee organization, or an advocacy organization for your particular racial or ethnic group.
- Let the harasser know as directly and explicitly as possible that you are not interested in his attentions. If you do this in writing, keep a copy of your letter.

BATTERING

Battering, often referred to as domestic violence, is one of the most common and least reported crimes in the world. Battering happens to women of every age, race, class, and nationality. It is done by the men we marry or date who beat us; by our sons and nephews who bully us and slap us around; and by male relatives who verbally harass and degrade us.

Battering takes many forms and includes a range of threatening and harmful behavior. It may take the form of verbal and emotional abuse, with the direct or implied threat of violence. Battering may include control of finances and one's physical freedom. It includes the destruction of objects and harm to pets. Battering may involve severe and frequent beatings or may happen occasionally. It may include slapping, punching, choking, kicking, or hitting with objects. Stalking can be a part of battering, especially if the woman has left the relationship. Battering may escalate to sexual assault and can ultimately end in murder. Battering can happen in new relationships at the dating stage and may

continue into our elder years. As time passes, battering tends to increase in frequency and severity.

I have had glasses thrown at me. I have been kicked in the abdomen, kicked off the bed, and hit while lying on the floor—while I was pregnant. I have been whipped, kicked and thrown, picked up and thrown down again.

I have been slapped for saying something about politics, having a different view about religion, for swearing, for crying, for wanting to have intercourse.

I have been threatened when I wouldn't do something I was told to do.

I have been threatened when he's had a bad day—when he's had a good day.

Bringing an end to domestic violence is especially difficult because the men who batter us are also the men with whom we have been close or intimate, perhaps the fathers of our children. We may still be bound by strong feelings of love and loyalty. We may remain at home not only because the men physically stop us from leaving but also because we hope that the violent behavior will change.

Before I left I used to say, "Yeah, he punched and kicked me, but I'd said something to make him mad." Or "He only hits me when I argue." Now I see that everyone has a right to get angry—it's natural—but he had no right to express his anger so violently, to hurt me.

An all-too-common question asked about women who are battered is "Why do they stay?" This question itself takes the focus off of the real question, which is "Why does he beat her?" Battered women do not remain in the relationship because we enjoy the battering. We may feel trapped and unable to leave. Battering often escalates at the point of separation, and we may actually feel safer staying. If we have children, we may feel that we won't be able to support ourselves and our children if we leave. People whom we turn to for support—clergy, police, friends, family —may be uninformed about battering and may not take the situation seriously. We may know about the existence of shelters for battered women but may feel that moving to a shelter in a new neighborhood or city will cause too much upheaval for us or for our children (who may have to change schools while we take shelter). We may be afraid to leave if we believe our immigration status is dependent on the "good will" of the batterer. If we have been living with abuse for a long time we may be so worn down emotionally that we simply can't imagine a way out.

I went early in our marriage to a clergyman, who after a few visits told me that my husband meant no real harm, he was just confused and felt insecure.

---

compensation, civil or criminal assault, rape laws, union grievance procedures, and workers' compensation. Students have used the federal law, Title IX of the Education Amendments of 1972.

Things continued. I turned this time to a doctor. I was given little pills to relax me and told to take things easier. I was "just too nervous." I turned to a friend, and when her husband found out, he accused me of either making things up or exaggerating the situation. She was told to stay away from me.

Many battered women have had similar experiences of being challenged, patronized, or told that our problems are insignificant. In the face of such inexcusable treatment we must remember that NO WOMAN DESERVES TO BE BEATEN OR VERBALLY ABUSED. EVERY WOMAN DESERVES TO HAVE HER STORY TAKEN SERIOUSLY.

The Impact of Domestic Violence on Children

Children who do not see their mothers abused but who hear her screams and crying, the abuser's threats, sounds of the impact of fists hitting flesh, glass breaking, wood splintering, or cursing and degrading language do witness the abuse.[12]

The effects of growing up in the midst of domestic violence can be devastating for children. Children of battered women are very likely to be battered themselves. They live in constant fear and are often torn physically and emotionally between their adult caretakers: they may develop severe physical and emotional responses to the violence, including symptoms of post-traumatic stress disorder. Children of domestic violence learn that violence is an appropriate way to resolve conflicts, and they are likely to live out their childhood experiences of violence in their adult relationships and in their relationships with their own children.[13]

My very upper-middle-class, WASP father hit my mother drunkenly on an occasional Saturday night. Sunday morning she would explain away her bruises. I lived my whole childhood under this shadow—the possibility of violence, the sounds in the night, and the toll it took on me that she put up with it.

Many battered adult women heard verbal abuse or witnessed battering beginning in their early childhood. Some were physically or sexually abused by the same person who battered their mothers. Under these circumstances, it is easy to understand how we might come to believe the degrading and harmful messages we have received about ourselves. It is easy to understand how we might find ourselves in relationships with men who abuse us verbally and physically.

Most men began to learn violence at an early age. Many men who batter grew up witnessing their fathers abusing their mothers; they may well have been physically or sexually abused as children. They often came of age in families where male dominance was never questioned and where physical punishment "in the name of love" was accepted. When our families teach us to accept male dominance and violence as a way to relate to one another, this message is difficult to defy.

Efforts are beginning in many communities to break the intergenerational cycle of violence that exists in so many families. Often, these begin with community-based programs designed to intervene on behalf of children whose mothers are being beaten. Innovative programs that teach nonviolence and conflict resolution skills to preschoolers are being developed and duplicated in child care centers in diverse communities. Workshops on teen dating violence are being offered to middle- and high-school-age children. All of these efforts aim to teach girls and young women that we have a right to be free from violence and the fear of violence and to teach boys and young men a different way to relate to girls and women and to the world.

Elder Abuse: Battering of Older Women

Just as young children are especially vulnerable to violence from within our families, so too are older women at particular risk of being exploited and battered. In recent years, awareness has grown of the special problems facing older battered women, and this has resulted in special laws protecting elders from abuse in all fifty states.

Women who are battered in old age face many of the same problems as younger adult women struggling with abuse. In addition, we may be physically frail and dependent on the batterer for daily care. The nearest shelter for battered women may not be set up to accommodate our physical abilities.* We may well be fearful that if we seek help to end the abuse we will find ourselves forced into a nursing home. If the batterer is a spouse with whom we have lived for many years, it may be especially difficult to contemplate separation or ending the relationship. If the batterer is our adult child, calling for help from a social service agency or the police may simply be unimaginable.

Battered women's activists are becoming increasingly concerned about our ability to respond to older battered women. In addition to the challenge of making sure that our shelter services are physically accessible, there are conflicting mandates for those who serve older battered women. Most elder abuse laws are similar to child abuse laws in that they require service providers to report instances of abuse to public health authorities or social service agencies. This approach to domestic violence against older women may conflict

---

* The problem of accessibility of battered women's services for younger adult women with disabilities as well as elders is one that the battered women's community is beginning to address. Constructing barrier-free shelters and renovating existing shelters so that they are fully accessible to all battered women and their children is an important part of the effort to respond comprehensively to violence against women.

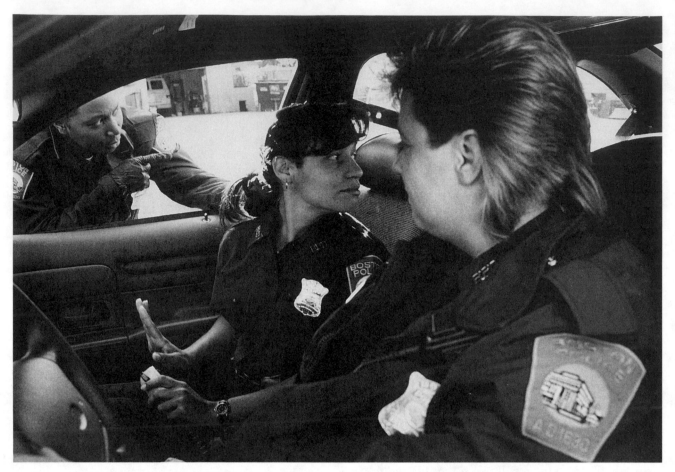

Carol Palmer

with the deep commitment of the battered women's movement to empowering victims of violence and protecting their right to privacy and confidentiality. Just as the battered women's movement has, from its earliest days, turned to battered women themselves in learning how to respond to domestic violence, so will activists and elder service providers want to listen to older battered women in working out how to meet the challenge of ending violence against elders.

What You Can Do
If You Are Being Battered

If you are in a violent relationship right now, there are things you can do that may help you to be safer, to assure the safety of your children, and to work toward ending the relationship if that is what you want to do. There are no right answers for every battered woman. The woman who is being battered knows best whether her actions may work to de-escalate the violence or incite further violence. Overall, your safety can increase the more you become aware, inform others, find support, and implement a safety plan.

During an attack, here are some things you can do to take care of yourself:

- Stay as calm as you possibly can.
- Try to shield yourself, especially your head and stomach.
- If you are able, and if it won't put you at greater risk, call 911 and get emergency assistance.
- Do the best you can to end the attack with the least amount of injury.

Safety Planning

Even if you are still in the situation and see no immediate way out, there are things you can do to plan for your safety:

- Become familiar with your state's laws and legal policies pertaining to domestic violence.
- Find out about restraining orders: how to get them and where to get an advocate if needed.
- Build a support network. Get connected with your local battered women's service, join a support group, and develop your network of friends.
- Learn and watch for warning signs of your partner's abusive behavior/attitude.
- Teach your children how to call for emergency assistance.

- Think through a safety plan and write it down. Let others know your plans when appropriate.
- If your abuser is drinking or drugging and you can get to Al-Anon meetings (see chapter 3, Alcohol, Tobacco, and Other Mood-Altering Drugs), you may find support and strength to make a change.

Making a safety plan while you are still struggling with a violent partner can help in two ways: First, it can give you a sense of hope in what so often feels like a hopeless situation. Second, it can actually bring you a bit closer to leaving a dangerous situation. There are battered women's service organizations in many communities. Most of these organizations help battered women develop safety plans. Safety plans include steps you can take to increase your own safety and the safety of your children.

There are alternatives to staying in a battering situation. More and more women are leaving men who batter, and they are finding help in making a new life despite economic hardships. Women everywhere have been organizing to help battered women leave abusive situations, to provide shelter and a more responsive legal system. Women have found the courage to tell their stories publicly. WE ARE NOT HELPLESS AND WE ARE NOT ALONE.

Legal Considerations

Men who batter can be prosecuted for crimes such as assault and battery. In addition, special laws protect battered women in all 50 states. These civil abuse prevention laws are very similar from one state to another. They give battered women the ability to go to a local court to obtain immediate protective orders against the batterer. Protective orders, often called restraining orders, can have several parts: They can order the batterer to stay away from us and our children; they can give us legal custody of the children; they can have a provision under which the batterer is ordered to pay support for us and our children. In addition to abuse prevention orders, more and more states are enacting anti-stalking laws. Recognizing that we are often at greater risk right after we leave the batterer, those laws impose criminal sanctions against a batterer who continues to harass us even after we have left.*

As a woman struggling to bring an end to battering, you are the only one who can decide whether or not to use your state's abuse prevention law. Some men are intimidated enough by the legal system to be stopped by a court order. If this is so, obtaining a court order may actually bring you a measure of safety. In some men, the tendency toward violence is so deep that no court order will stop them. In these instances, going to court may actually make you and your children less safe. Working on a safety plan with a coun-

---

* Since each state law is slightly different, contact a battered women's organization in your state to learn exactly how your state law works (see Resource section).

....
SAFETY PLANNING [14]
....

Increasing Safety While in the Relationship

- Carry important phone numbers for yourself and your children (police, hospital, friends, battered women's program) and a cellular phone or beeper if you can afford one.
- Find someone to tell about the abuse and develop a signal for distress. Ask neighbors to call the police if they hear noise of a violent episode.
- Think of four places where you can go if you leave in a hurry.
- Get specific items ready to take if you leave.
- Keep change for phone calls, open your own bank account, rehearse an escape route.
- Periodically review your safety plan and update it.

What to Take with You If You Decide to Leave

Money, checkbook, bank cards, credit cards; identification, driver's license, and car registration; birth certificates, Social Security cards, welfare identification; passport, immigration card, work permit; divorce or other court papers; school and medical records; house deed, mortgage; insurance papers and policies; medications and refill instructions; change of clothes.

Increasing Safety After You Leave

- If you have joint bank accounts, withdraw some money or transfer to a private account.
- Use different routes as you go home, to work, or to your daily tasks.
- Tell the people who care for your children who has permission to pick them up, and warn them if you think the batterer may attempt to kidnap them.
- At work, tell someone about the abuse and have that person screen your calls. If possible, show other people his picture and instruct them to call the police if he arrives at work.
- Avoid the stores, services, and banks that you know your batterer frequents.
- If it is right for you, get a protective or restraining order. Know what it orders and what would happen if he violates it. Keep it with you at all times.

selor at your area battered women's program will help you make this difficult decision. Whatever you do, it is important to remember that you are the best judge of your own needs.

SEXUAL ASSAULT

Sexual assault is any kind of sexual activity committed against a woman's will. Whether the rapist uses force or threats of force is irrelevant. Men use different kinds of force against women, from pressuring us for a goodnight kiss to withdrawing economic support from wives to using weapons. Rape is a legal term that is defined slightly differently in each state. Most state laws define rape in terms of penetration, with the use of force, and without the person's consent. Penetration can be with the penis or other instruments like bottles or sticks, and can be perpetrated in the vagina, anus, or mouth.

Sexual assault is always traumatic. When we are raped, survival is our primary instinct, and we protect ourselves as best we can. Some women choose to fight back; others do not feel we can. IF YOU WERE RAPED AND ARE NOW READING THIS CHAPTER, YOU DID THE RIGHT THING BECAUSE YOU ARE ALIVE.

Rape is more likely to be committed by someone we know than by a stranger.[15] Contrary to common stereotypes, the vast majority of rapes occur between members of the same racial group.[16] Most rapists lead everyday lives, go to school, work, and have families and friends.

Common Reactions
of Sexual Assault Survivors

Rape is frequently a private crisis owing to the isolation that many survivors feel because of a lack of support or the tendency of some to blame us. This creates a unique and difficult set of reactions that may also be experienced by women who have been battered, sexually harassed, abused as children, robbed violently, or hurt by other forms of violence. (In fact, sexual assault and battering often go hand in hand.)

While no two women respond in the same way, many feelings are common among survivors. You may experience a wide range of reactions immediately after the assault or years later. You are coping with a difficult situation that never should have happened in the first place. There is no one correct or preferred way to deal with the feelings and reactions you may find yourself having. As you move through a healing process, different reactions may intensify or lose intensity. You may experience feelings that you thought you had already addressed.

Self-blame and feelings of guilt. This is probably one of the most common reactions because of the false yet common myths about rape. We may feel humiliated, ashamed, or embarrassed about what we were forced or coerced to do. We often feel responsible for

decisions that we made before the assault that we (or others) may later think led to the assault. Even talking about the sexual assault can be difficult because we risk being disbelieved or rejected. THE TRUTH IS THAT RAPE IS NEVER THE FAULT OF THE VICTIM.

Like many victims of sexual attacks, I was silenced by my shame, guilt, and the mistaken belief, reinforced by the police and society in general . . . that I was "responsible" for what these men did to me. It is that silence that revictimizes rape and incest victims, over and over again, and I won't be silent anymore.

Fear, terror, and feeling unsafe. Intense fear may be experienced in many aspects of a woman's life. If you feared for your life or the lives of others during the assault, you may be afraid that the perpetrator will return. You may find that fear and terror become generalized to other areas or to situations that are similar to the assault.

There is nowhere that feels safe anymore. When I'm home I'm afraid that someone will break into my house; when I'm out, I'm afraid that I'll be attacked. My guard is always up.

Anger and rage. While it is normal to feel angry, this emotion can be difficult for women to express. We have been socialized to be nice, to hide our anger. For many women, directing anger toward the perpetrator may feel too threatening or may bring intense feelings of terror. You may sometimes direct your feelings of anger toward others in your life, where it feels safer. While this can be confusing for loved ones, it is normal.

I feel angry all of the time, even toward people who had nothing to do with the rape like my kids and my co-workers.

Anger turned inward. If you have a hard time recognizing or expressing anger, you may turn it inward. This can lead to forms of depression and suicidal thoughts, feelings, or even attempts. If you experience signs of depression that are long-lasting and don't seem to be alleviated by talking about it with friends, consider seeking help through counseling. Many communities have specialized mental health services for survivors of sexual assault.

I barely manage to function all day. When I wake up in the morning I just want to stay in bed. I feel like there is a dark cloud following me around. I feel sad and can't remember what it feels like to be happy.

Grief and loss. You may experience loss in many ways. For many women, rape or abuse may have conflicted with our ideas of whom we can trust or where we are safe. Throughout the healing process, you may experience grief over parts of your life that you felt you missed. Some survivors talk about a loss of innocence or a loss of their sense of power.

I feel like a part of me died, like my life will never be the same. Because I was raped by my boyfriend as a teen, I feel like I missed the chance to have a normal adolescence when everyone says those should have been the best years of my life.

Loss of control, powerlessness. Rape and sexual abuse rob women of the power and control that they have in that moment. You may feel powerless in general or in certain situations.

My life is not my own anymore; what's the use of making decisions when I have no power to change my life?

Isolation. You may feel as though no one can possibly understand. Or you may feel embarrassed that your healing process is taking as long as it is. Family members may be encouraging you to "just put it in the past" or "get on with your life" while your feelings are still very real and troubling. You may not want to talk to anyone about the rape for fear of being disbelieved or rejected.

I can't think of anyone that I can trust or talk to. I just want to be by myself even though I feel lonely.

Flashbacks and nightmares. Flashbacks and nightmares can feel overwhelming and frightening, although they are common and normal. A flashback is a memory that is experienced with one or more of the physical senses. A nightmare is a dream that sometimes involves aspects or pieces of the assault but can be combined with other events or aspects of the person's life.

I close my eyes to go to sleep and all I can see is the rape. I feel as though it is happening to me over and over.

Triggers: seasons, smells, circumstances. Survivors remember being raped with all of our senses. Triggers are circumstances that are the same or similar to those that occurred during the rape and that bring up feelings related to the rape. Certain smells, sights, places, or even times of the year may bring about feelings related to the assault.

Every year around this time I start to feel sad and have trouble sleeping. Because I was raped during the springtime, the signs that make everyone else happy make me feel isolated and nervous.

Changes in sexuality, intimacy. Changes in sexuality are common for women who have been sexually assaulted. While you may experience fear and aversion to sex and intimacy, on the other hand you may want to have more sexual experiences than before the rape. This may change throughout your healing process.

I want my partner's support, but I can't stand the idea of having sex. Even though it's been almost a year since the rape, I feel afraid of getting too close. I'm afraid that he'll touch me and that I'll react as if my partner is the rapist.

Spiritual crisis. Sexual assault often results in an intense spiritual crisis, especially for those who have operated within a spiritual framework before the rape. You may feel angry at a supreme being or may lose your faith completely. You may be told that the rape is a punishment for your "sins." The crisis of rape can create a crisis of self at a very personal and deep level.

The God that I believed in would never allow something like this to happen. I've lost my faith and sense of who I am.

Empowerment: Finding Ways to Regain Your Life

If you were sexually assaulted, you may have experienced any number of these reactions and others not listed here. The process that you are going through may feel overwhelming and never-ending. Yet, it is very much a process of healing and empowerment. You have had your sense of control taken away as a result of the rape, and healing can occur when you begin to regain a sense of power. Reflecting on the following points can help you move through the healing process:

Sexual assault was not your fault. Myths about sexual assault get expressed in any number of destructive ways: "It must have been who she was, what she was wearing, where she was. . . ." These have nothing to do with the fact that you were assaulted. You did not ask to be violated, and you did not do anything to deserve it.

You made the best choices and decisions you were able to make. You may have been forced to make life-or-death decisions before, during, and after the assault. Even if you feel you would make a different decision today, whatever you did at the time was okay.

There is no right way to feel or to heal. Your reactions and your healing process are connected to who you are as a person. Your culture and economic background can influence your healing process in both negative and positive ways.

You deserve support. Reach out to whomever you think can be a support person to you. There are rape crisis centers in most locations across the country. You may prefer to talk with a family member or friend, a clergy member, or a counselor. You may decide to find a support group, or try other kinds of healing support based on art, music, writing, physical activity, or meditation.[17]

Believe in your strength and your capacity to heal. While the process of healing may take time and may be difficult, you will find ways to reclaim the strong and capable parts of yourself.

Medical Considerations

If you have been raped, the first thing you may want to do is take a shower or bath and try to forget what happened. What you do is completely your decision, but consider two things:

- It is very important both physically and emotionally that you receive medical attention as soon as possible, even if you have no obvious injuries.
- Don't bathe or shower if you think you may later decide to prosecute, as you will wash away evidence that may be crucial to your case.

If you decide to go to a hospital, try to have a friend, relative, or local rape crisis counselor go with you to act as an advocate on your behalf. If you feel reluctant to go because you may not be able to afford it, be aware that most states have passed legislation that assures that rape exams are free of charge. If you go to the hospital, bring a list of any medications that you are taking, bring a change of clothing if you're still in the same clothes; if you have changed clothes, bring the clothing that you were wearing during the assault.

At the hospital, you have three basic concerns: your emotional well-being; medical care; and the gathering of evidence for a possible prosecution. You can refuse to be examined for evidence if you are absolutely sure that you will not want to prosecute. Some hospitals have specialized programs that attempt to assure that sexual assault survivors are given the best treatment possible. These programs are staffed by nurses or doctors who receive extensive training in the medical, legal, and emotional issues associated with sexual assault. They are set up to provide medical exams that are sensitive and provide the best evidence possible for prosecution.

Physical injuries to any part of the body can result from a rape; therefore, a thorough examination is necessary. That examination should include and/or result in the following:

A verbal history of the sexual assault and of related medical concerns. You will be asked to give a detailed description of the assault, which will be written down. While it may be difficult to talk about these details, they are important so that the medical provider will know where to check for injuries and where to document evidence such as bruises, scrapes, or other injuries. Pictures may be taken or evidence collected that wouldn't be noticed unless this information is known. Sometimes bruises may emerge later, in which case you should be encouraged to call the examiner back so that they can be added to your record. You will also be asked some questions that may seem unrelated, such as whether you have had sexual activity recently, whether you may be pregnant, and whether you use any birth control methods.

A pelvic exam. In collecting evidence, the practitioner will look for the presence of semen. (It is also possible to be raped vaginally with no semen or sperm present.) She or he will also comb your pubic hair for the possible presence of the man's pubic hair. All this medical evidence will be available to others, including the police, only with your written permission. You or the person with you at the hospital should check the record for accuracy and objectivity as soon as possible after the exam. If possible, do this while the doctor is still present. (If you were raped vaginally, see chapter 24, Selected Medical Practices, Problems, and Procedures, for more information about a pelvic exam. You will get a rectal exam if you were raped anally.)

Examination and treatment of any external injuries. The practitioner will examine you for any external injuries and may photograph bruises or other marks to document the assault.

Treatment for the prevention of sexually transmitted disease (STD). The practitioner will want to give you two shots of antibiotic in your buttocks. If you don't want this, be sure to say so. (Some women may not want to be given an antibiotic unless an STD is diagnosed; however, it is used as a preventive measure). Some STDs are not detectable until six weeks later, so it is a good idea to return for a six-week checkup (see chapter 14, Sexually Transmitted Diseases).

Treatment for the prevention of pregnancy. If you suspect that you will become pregnant as a result of the rape, the doctor or nurses may offer you emergency contraception (see chapter 13, Birth Control). A pregnancy resulting from rape cannot be detected until several weeks later. If you find that you are pregnant and are considering abortion, see chapters 16, Unplanned Pregnancies, and 17, Abortion.

Information about AIDS/HIV. There is a chance that you could contract HIV through a sexual assault. Should you want to, it may be possible to get immediate "morning-after" medication to treat potential HIV infection. If you are offered testing for HIV, be aware that it's too soon for HIV antibodies to show up from the assault. Also, testing results could become a part of your medical and legal record and could be used against you. For information see chapter 15, HIV, AIDS, and Women.

A follow-up exam. Although you may feel physically recovered shortly after the rape, a follow-up visit, to include tests and treatment for STDs and a pregnancy test if indicated, will assure you that you are taking care of yourself.

It is common for survivors of sexual assault to experience changes in overall physical health. Some find that their sleep and eating patterns change. Some experience headaches, body aches, stomach and intestinal problems, and fatigue. Some cope with the emotions with drugs or alcohol. While all of these are normal, it is important to take care of yourself and get help if any of them persist or get worse over time.

Ever since I was raped, my body doesn't feel like my own. I have pain in my back and I'm always on the alert for signs of sexually transmitted infections.

Legal Considerations

It is never easy to decide whether to prosecute a rapist. While improvements have been made in the legal system, prosecution can still be a painful and difficult process. Most communities have rape crisis centers that provide advocates as you move through the legal system. In many places there are victim/witness advocates in the offices of local district attorneys who can provide information and support. In some states you can report a rape anonymously or without prosecuting. Whether you report it or not, write down everything that you can remember, so that if you do decide to prosecute later on, your statement will be accurate. As you are deciding whether or not to prosecute, here are several things to keep in mind:

- Because the legal system can be confusing and difficult, it will help tremendously to have a friend or rape crisis counselor with you throughout the process.
- You will have to prove that you were sexually assaulted against your will and that the man used force or threatened force against you.
- Rape is a crime against the state. It is prosecuted by the district attorney's office. You will be the state's witness, and you will not have your own lawyer unless you can arrange for one to advise you.
- A trial can last from six months to several years. You will need to be prepared to continue thinking and talking about the rape for a long time, including giving an account of the event over and over while people judge whether you are telling the truth.
- You will need to prepare yourself for any outcome. Rape is one of the most difficult crimes to prove. Remember that even if your case does not end in a conviction, this does not mean that the rape didn't happen or that you didn't do your best to prosecute.

What to Do If Someone You Care About Has Been Sexually Assaulted

If you are a friend or family member of someone who has been sexually assaulted, you may feel that you don't know what to say, or you may have feelings of your own that get in the way of supporting her. You can be most helpful if you keep in mind that she is capable of healing and that you are capable of providing support. You are being supportive when you do these things:

Validate and believe her. If she feels ashamed or guilty, reassure her that the rape was not her fault and that her feelings are normal. Although you feel you might have reacted differently, remember that her reactions are uniquely hers.

Help create a safe place for the survivor. Help her to think about what changes, if any, she would like to make that will help her feel safer, whether related to her physical surroundings or to how she interacts with people at home or at work.

Allow her to express a full range of feelings. The feelings of a survivor of sexual assault can be very strong. Expressing these powerful feelings in a safe environment is an important part of the healing process. If you can feel comfortable supporting her in expressing her feelings, this can be very helpful.

Offer options, not advice. Survivors often struggle with important and complex decisions. You can be most helpful by helping her identify all of the options available and supporting her in her decision-making.

Dispel myths about rape. You can help empower a woman who has been sexually assaulted by being prepared to help her dispel destructive myths about rape and by assuring her that you do not believe these false ideas.

Advocate. She may need someone to help ensure that her feelings are validated and her rights are upheld in the medical or legal system.

Believe in the possibility of healing. Let her know that you believe that healing is possible and that she has the strength and capacity to heal.

Protecting Ourselves and Each Other from Rape *

Even though most sexual assaults are committed by someone we know rather than a stranger, we can take some steps to protect ourselves. Listing these sugges-

* Adapted from *How to Start a Rape Crisis Center* (1972) by the Rape Crisis Center of Washington, DC.

tions reminds us how wrong it is for women to be and to feel unsafe in our homes and our communities. Yet, until men stop raping women, we need to take precautions. The most effective protection comes from being with other women. Arrange to walk home together. Set up a green-light or safe-house program in your neighborhood. Get to know the women who live in your apartment building or on your street.

Safety at home. Make sure that entrances are well lit and that windows and doors are securely locked. Use only your last name on your mailbox. Find out who is at your door before opening it to anyone.

Safety on the street. Be aware of what is going on around you. Walk with a steady pace, looking as if you know where you are going. Dress so you can move and run easily. Walk in the middle of the street, avoiding dark places and groups of men. If you fear danger, yell "Fire," not "Help" or "Rape." Carry a whistle around your wrist. Always check the backseat of your car before getting in and keep the car doors locked while driving. Avoid groups of men on public transportation. If you can possibly avoid it, don't hitchhike; it is just too dangerous.

Safety in social situations. Pay attention to how you feel and trust your instincts. If you want to end a date or leave a party, say so, even if you are afraid or embarrassed. If you drink alcohol, keep an eye on your drink. Drugs are available that can be slipped into drinks to tranquilize a woman and create a blackout. For example, a drug called Rohypnol, or "Roofies," causes severe memory loss so that a woman can be raped but will not be able to remember anything.

These tactics can help you, but they are not foolproof. Practice tactics for the situations that make you feel most at risk and least powerful. Try to remain calm and to act as confident and strong as you can.

INCEST AND SEXUAL ABUSE OF CHILDREN

One common form of sexual abuse of children is incest, which has been defined as sexual contact that occurs between family members.* Most incest occurs between older male relatives and younger female children in families of every class and color. Other instances of sexual abuse of children are most often committed by friends who have access to children within the family setting and by people normally trusted by parents: doctors, dentists, teachers, and baby-sitters.[18] A sexually abusive relationship is one over which a child or young woman has no control. A trusted family member or friend uses his power, as well as a child's love and dependence, to initiate sex-

* Each state defines incest differently. In this chapter we discuss social attitudes and definitions regarding incest and the sexual abuse of children, not legal ones.

ual contact and often to ensure that the relationship continues and remains secret.

My barter with my brother was that he could do sex on me to practice for his girlfriends. I consented not because I enjoyed it but because I was afraid to be alone when my parents went out. . . . I never even thought of talking about it. That just couldn't be done.

Despite the fact that children are more likely to be sexually abused by an adult they know, parents teach children to expect danger from strangers and not from trusted authority figures. It is understandable, given this fact, that a violation of this trust is so terribly frightening and confusing.

The extent of incest and childhood sexual abuse is difficult to measure because of lack of reporting and lack of memory. One study in which adults were asked to report on past incidents found that one in four girls and one in ten boys experienced sexual abuse.[19]

Incest and sexual abuse of children take many forms and may include sexually suggestive language; prolonged kissing, looking, and petting; vaginal and/or anal intercourse; and oral sex. Because sexual contact is often achieved without overt physical force, there may be no obvious signs of physical harm.

Whether or not the signs of abuse are physical and obvious, sexual abuse in childhood can have lifelong consequences. As survivors, we often blame ourselves long after the abuse has ended—for not saying no, for not fighting back, for telling or not telling, for having been "seductive," for having trusted the abuser. Often there is no one to confirm that someone treated us cruelly and that this abuse was devastating to us.

For the next 20 years I will probably continue to walk around and ask other women, "What was your childhood like?" Hearing women say that no one touched them sexually at that young an age helps me realize that something in my childhood was really wrong.

Many of us have difficulty with sexually intimate relationships because of the memories they revive. Many of us desire sexual intimacy yet have difficulty trusting.

It's been really hard to figure out how this has affected me with men. I've had a hard time figuring out who is safe and who isn't. Now the only way I will sleep with someone is if I can have complete control. I need permission to feel uncomfortable with certain sexual acts.

Just as battered women and women who have been raped often blame themselves for the violence, those of us who have survived childhood sexual abuse struggle with self-blame. Teenagers with a history of incest might "sleep around" in order to feel accepted, or run away from our homes and communities. Depression is another common response to the abuse, and adult survivors often turn to drugs and alcohol to mask the pain. Some of us feel worthless.

I often feel hopeless and suicidal. My father treated me with such violence that this is the only way I know to treat myself. I'm learning better ways now, but it's difficult.

It is often very difficult to talk about incest or childhood sexual abuse. Some of us may never have told anyone, though the abuse may have continued for years. We may have dreaded family gatherings, where a particular uncle or family friend would come after us. For some of us, exploring our bodies with an older brother turned into a sexual encounter, after which we found ourselves feeling we had been taken advantage of. Sometimes a father, uncle, or teacher abused our sisters, and we didn't find out for years. Every survivor has her own story, and every story is valid.

Coping Mechanisms

Each of us responds differently to the pain and terror of incest and childhood sexual abuse. We struggle to find ways to cope that will permit us to keep on functioning and to survive. Too often, these coping mechanisms become problematic and don't serve the survivor well as an adult. Common coping mechanisms include self-injury, substance abuse, eating disorders, and dissociation.

Self-injury. Self-injury, much more common among women than men, occurs when we consciously hurt ourselves, by, for example, cutting, hitting, or burning ourselves. Because of the shame surrounding self-injury, women often keep this problem secret and do not reach out for support from others. Although self-injury is not usually done with the intent of suicide, it is a coping mechanism that, though understandable, can be seriously harmful to us.

There are many reasons why we injure ourselves. Some self-injury acts to block out emotional pain caused by childhood abuse. Many of us say that the physical pain evoked by self-injury diminishes intense emotional pain. Self-injury can also be a way of expressing anger and other strong emotions that were forbidden to us. Self-injury can begin as a way to replay an abusive experience in order to regain control of it emotionally.

Substance abuse. Many women who were sexually abused during childhood find that we have no outlet for the feelings associated with the trauma of sexual abuse. We may turn to alcohol or drugs to help us cope with strong feelings of terror, grief, and anger. After prolonged use or abuse of alcohol or drugs, we may find ourselves addicted and in need of help for a substance abuse problem. (See chapter 3, Alcohol, Tobacco, and Other Mood-Altering Drugs, for more information.) Those of us who enter treatment programs often find that our feelings related to the sexual

abuse come up when we stop relying on the substance. If this happens, it is essential to have support for the feelings connected to sexual abuse and for recovery from substance abuse. In recognition of the fact that so many women in substance abuse treatment programs are survivors of childhood sexual abuse, treatment programs are beginning to work with rape crisis centers and other experts on sexual assault to ensure that this special support is provided.

I thought that everything would be better once I stopped drinking, but now I have nightmares about the abuse I went through as a child. It makes it hard to keep to my promise to myself to stay sober.

Eating disorders. Problems with eating can develop in the wake of sexual abuse. These may take several forms, including bulimia, anorexia, and compulsive overeating. Each of these may serve as a different coping mechanism and may itself become a problem. (See chapter 2, Food, for more information on these eating disorders.)

Dissociation. Many survivors are familiar with dissociation. This is a process that produces an alteration in a person's thoughts, feelings, or actions so that for a period of time, certain information is not associated or integrated with other information.[20] A continuum of sorts, dissociation occurs when a child leaves her body and goes to the ceiling during the abuse. It can continue after the abuse: we may have trouble concentrating, experience detachment from ourselves, have dramatic mood shifts, and/or develop several distinct personalities.

If you find that a way you have coped with being abused is causing you problems as an adult, you can get help. Remember that you did what you did at the time in order to survive. Once your method of coping stops working, you can find other, healthier ways to respond to the violence you were forced to endure. Be as gentle with yourself as you can be, and know that you don't have to face these experiences alone. With gentleness toward yourself and with the caring help of others, you can build a support network and practice new ways of taking care of yourself.

Getting Help

To heal from the trauma of incest or early sexual abuse, we need to tell our stories to people who understand what we have experienced. Talking with others in counseling or in special support groups for women with a history of incest breaks the silence, helps us to gain perspective and know we are not alone, eases the pain and helps us feel healthier and stronger.

I now have a lot of compassion for myself because I know the implications of the abuse that occurred in my life. I owe myself all the understanding, patience, and acceptance I can find—a ton of it.

Some women find that they need to confront the family member who abused them. This is a frightening task, but if it is the right thing to do for your recovery, it can also be rewarding.

I feel empowered by letting him know I am aware that the incest occurred. I feel empowered by the fact that I didn't ask him if he remembered—I just told him. I knew he would deny it. I just wanted to say, "This happened." I did not expect results. Telling him was the total opposite of all that happened—what was invisible is now out in the open.

Those of us with a history of incest need to know that whatever we do or don't do is all right, because we have survived a childhood that wasn't like a childhood at all.*

Feminist Insights into Incest and Childhood Sexual Abuse

Years ago, "experts" who wrote about incest and child abuse blamed mothers for abandoning their children to sexually depraved husbands or accused young girls of being seductive or of fantasizing about sexual relationships with male relatives. For the past 30 years, feminists have been challenging these victim-blaming views. The factors that contribute to incest and sexual abuse of children are very complicated. When boys and men are supported in the belief that they have a right to dominate and control women and children, they may well decide that this includes the right to use us sexually. In a society that puts so much emphasis on sexuality as a measure of a man's worth, fathers, uncles, and brothers may try to bolster a low self-image by taking sexual advantage of the powerlessness of the children in their lives. In addition, in a culture in which male violence and sexuality are merged, men may become incapable of distinguishing between feelings of sexual desire and violent impulses —even when it involves their daughters, sisters, nieces, or neighbors. Whatever factors contribute to incest and sexual abuse of children, it is vital to remember that no child deserves to be sexually abused, and no child "invites" it.

As a result of recent challenges to long-held myths about incest and sexual abuse of children, reports of child sexual abuse have increased among adult women. One unfortunate result of this change has been an attempt to popularize the so-called false memory syndrome. This theory claims that many adults who remember sexual abuse as children are actually not remembering correctly. Research into the subject

of memories and how they work, however, confirms that children often repress their experience of trauma in order to survive and that this is a necessary and appropriate coping mechanism, not something that the child did wrong. This research is helpful in countering efforts to undermine those who are able to finally give voice to the violence they suffered as children.[21]

THE SEX INDUSTRY

Many women earn all or part of their living as sex workers or in other areas of the sex industry, including pornography, nude dancing, telephone sex, and computer pornography. Contrary to the ugly stereotypes of prostitutes as fallen women, dope addicts, or disease carriers,† sex workers are women at work—supporting children as single parents, trying to save money to go to school, surviving economically in a job market that underpays women at every economic level.

Once politically voiceless and isolated from other women, sex workers have organized over the past 25 years for support and political action.‡ As adult sex workers speak out, they expose the many forms of violence that they experience:§

- Poverty that forces women, especially women of color and runaway teenagers, into work as sex workers
- Sexism in the job market that means that even middle- and upper-class women can earn more in sex work than in most other jobs available
- Intimidation and beatings by pimps, to whom many sex workers must give their earnings in return for protection
- Police harassment and lack of police protection when we are victims of crime such as robbery, battery, and rape
- The arrest and prosecution of prostitutes while clients go free
- The racism and class bias that lead to the arrest and imprisonment of far more prostitutes of color and women with low incomes than white, middle-class women, even though the majority of sex workers are white and middle-class

As a middle-class white woman, trained as a registered nurse, I could work in a private call business instead of hitting the streets. I was arrested but never did time in prison; the system isn't aimed at putting me in jail. Women of color have less easy access to

---

* See especially Judith Herman's classic work, *Father-Daughter Incest* (Cambridge, MA/London: Harvard University Press, 1981).

† Only about 5% of STDs in the United States is spread by prostitutes.
‡ An example of such groups is COYOTE (Call Off Your Old Tired Ethics) in San Francisco. For more information, contact the National Task Force on Prostitution, P.O. Box 26354, San Francisco, CA 94126. Ask for the newsletter, *Coyote Howls*.
§ See, for instance, *Sex Work*, edited by Frederique Delacoste and Priscilla Alexander (Pittsburgh: Cleis Press, 1987).

places like upper-class hotels, where if you're a black woman and alone you're automatically tagged as a hooker. So they're in the streets and in the bars, where they are more visible and more vulnerable to exploitation and arrest—and they're the ones who end up in jail.

Some feminists have been critical of prostitutes for reinforcing sex-role stereotypes by allowing themselves to be sex objects or for participating in the sex industry, which many think contributes to violence against women. Many see sex work as violence in and of itself, especially when children and young girls are involved. (See chapter 26, The Global Politics of Women and Health, for more information.) Others insist that it is a legitimate way for women to earn money from men. As one prostitute said, "It's my body; why shouldn't I be the one to decide how I should use it?" Some sex workers find that the experience is generally positive, and the negative parts arise from the violence and harassment that they may be more at risk for because of their profession. Others enjoy parts of the work and hate other parts. Still others name their experience as violence. Prostitutes point out that they are no different from most women in having to sell their services to men. In the words of an ex-prostitute:

I've worked in straight jobs where I've felt more like I was prostituting my being than in prostitution. I had less control over my life, and the powerlessness wasn't even up front. People didn't see me as selling myself, but with the minimum wage so little and my boss so insulting, I felt like I was selling my soul.

Prostitutes have organized in the U.S. and Europe to demand decriminalization, the abolition of all laws against prostitution. With decriminalization, prostitutes would have more control over their work and the money they earn. Most of all, they would no longer go to jail for providing a service that society itself puts in such high demand and for choosing the highest-paying work available to them.

DEFENDING OURSELVES AGAINST VIOLENCE

Self-defense can increase the options and choices that we have in any given situation, including situations where we are at risk of violence. Self-defense itself is a choice that is made at a particular moment. Each woman will make the best choice that she can, based on her resources and knowledge at the time. Just as there is no one right way to respond to violence committed against us, there is no right way to defend ourselves. And, as much as self-defense may help in certain situations, the most important step in ending violence against women is to stop men from being violent and from allowing others to be violent.

In recent years the experiences of women who have been practicing self-defense have changed our ideas about what self-defense is and how we can use its techniques. If you decide to learn self-defense, be sure to think about the real possibility that the person you may defend yourself against may be your date, friend, husband, father, teacher, or co-worker.

Thinking about self-defense in this light, we can see that self-defense study actually includes any activity—assertiveness training, exercise, sports—that promotes self-confidence, self-knowledge, and self-reliance. In addition, the skills we tend to associate exclusively with self-defense can actually be of benefit in other areas of our lives. Self-defense classes teach us to shift our self-awareness so that we remember that we are the sources of our own energy and the initiators of our own actions. Instead of freezing in the face of assault, we learn to mobilize our thoughts, assess the situation, make a judgment about the level of danger, choose the response we wish to make, and then make it. (See Resources for information on self-defense classes, including "Model Mugging.") We can use this self-awareness in other life situations, such as medical examinations, job interviews, or communication with a difficult person.

I have experienced such profound changes in my self-image and in the way that I see the world and relate to people that I really can't separate my study of self-defense from the rest of my life.

Several myths can prevent us from defending ourselves effectively against a physical assault. They include the myth that the assailant is invulnerable, that greater physical strength will decide who will prevail, that we don't know how to defend ourselves. Yet, as women we have defended ourselves against attack in many instances. One woman frightened off three adolescent males who were following her along a city street by turning quickly and letting out a bloodcurdling yell. Another stopped a would-be assailant with a kick to the midsection. A young girl sitting on the train found a wayward hand on her knee. She took the man's wrist in her grasp, raised his hand high in the air, and said loudly enough for the entire car to hear, "Who does this belong to?" He got off at the next stop. There are countless stories like these, even though we don't see them on TV and we don't read them in the newspapers. When we do hear such stories we may attribute such escapes to luck or good fortune; too often we don't take credit for our own courage and resourcefulness. It is important to our self-confidence to reclaim those successes.

At this point, little is known about the value of self-defense for battered women. Street techniques, which depend upon surprise and causing damage, don't work as well against repeated assault by men we live with. Yet, other skills developed in the practice of self-defense may be useful, such as learning to work through the inner obstacles that come up when we are faced with a violent situation. As we begin to feel more self-confident, we will be able to consider how we

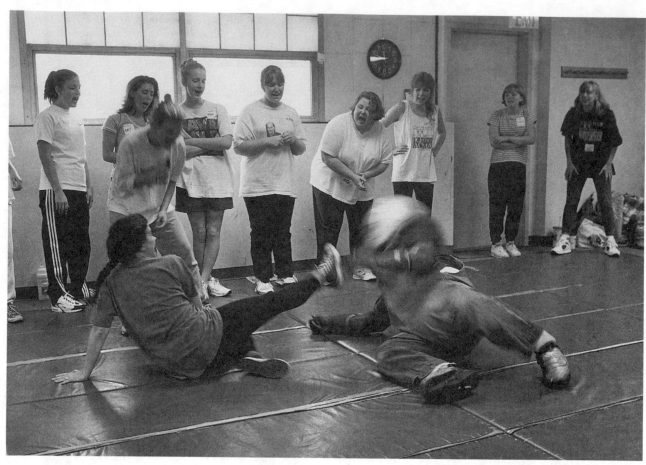

A **"Model Mugging"** class/*Carol Palmer*

might resist the battering or how we might eventually leave the batterer and the violence behind us.

Guidelines are needed for adapting physical techniques for use by women with various physical abilities. Furthermore, we need to support the work of all the organizations committed to our safety, because without them, self-defense is a piecemeal approach to women's safety.

ENDING VIOLENCE AGAINST WOMEN: NO WOMAN IS SAFE UNTIL ALL OF US ARE SAFE

Over the past 25 years, we have directed our collective outrage and concern into many kinds of action opposing violence against women.

- We organized consciousness-raising groups and discovered that our experiences of dominance by men were common and shared.
- We demanded that the public listen to us by demonstrating in large groups; holding public speakouts; and creating films, radio and TV shows, street theater, dramatic productions, books, pamphlets, newspapers, and articles.

- We set up educational programs for thousands of law enforcement and health professionals.
- In 1974, a group of feminists doing legal aid work in St. Paul, Minnesota, opened Women's House, the first U.S. refuge for battered women and their children. Current estimates suggest that there are more than 1,000 hot lines, shelters, and programs for battered women. Many states have formed coalitions to bring people together who work on these issues. The National Coalition Against Domestic Violence and the National Coalition Against Sexual Assault both have memberships of over 500 agencies and focus on public awareness and social change.
- Neighborhood groups have formed networks of refuges, called safe-house or green-light programs because participating homes are identified by green lights, where women harassed or attacked in the streets can find safety.
- We learned from feminists in other countries. The 1976 Tribunal of Crimes Against Women, held in Brussels and attended by women from all over the world, expanded the definition of violence against women to include dowry murders* and

* These occur when men marry women for their dowries and then kill them, as still happens in India.

genital mutilation. European feminists inspired both safe houses and "Take Back the Night" marches, which rally thousands of women yearly in cities across the United States to protest violence against women.

- Beginning in the 1970s, when the first state laws to protect women from abuse were enacted, we have worked diligently for improved legal responses to violence against women. The passage of the Violence Against Women Act in 1994 marked the first major attempt by the federal government to influence the enactment of strong state laws related to violence against women and to fund efforts to improve services, prosecution, law enforcement, prevention efforts, and community collaboration.
- At the United Nations Conference on Women in Beijing in 1995, violence against women was identified as one of the most pressing concerns of women worldwide.
- In the 1990s, women from Cape Cod, Massachusetts, began the Clothesline Project, a visual display of violence against women based on shirts made by survivors. The first national display bringing together all of the clothesline projects occurred in Washington, DC, in 1995.
- Men who have committed themselves to working to end violence against women have begun to form groups in which men help batterers deal with their violence. Recognizing that men who do not take action support the system that promotes violence against women, they talk about their socialization in relation to women, question the extent and consequences of male dominance, and listen to and respect the women around them.

We must continue to express a vision for a violence-free world loudly and clearly. We must work to maintain a strong network of services by and for women who have survived violence.

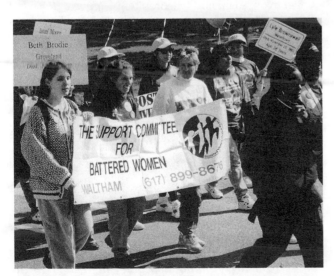

Jane Doe Walk for Women's Safety in Boston, 1996/Kate Schalk

We will continue to teach our daughters to expect equality for themselves and others. We will continue to teach our sons to question sexism and reject violence, to respect women as equals, and to work against all systems that are based on concepts of dominance. We will continue to support one another in protecting ourselves with ingenuity, strength, and pride. We applaud women who say no to male violence, who offer support to a friend, who protect one another, and who survive.

NOTES

1. Surgeon General, U.S., 1992.
2. U.S. Department of Justice, *Uniform Crime Reports for the U.S.* (Washington, DC: 1996).
3. National Victims Center and Crime Victims Research and Treatment Center, *Rape In America: A Report to the Nation* (Arlington, VA: National Victims Center, 1992). Available from National Victims Center, 2111 Wilson Boulevard, Suite 300, Arlington, VA 22201; (703) 276-2880.
4. U.S. Department of Housing and Urban Development, *A Report on the 1988 National Survey of Shelters for the Homeless* (Washington, DC: Office of Policy Development and Research, 1989).
5. Many studies have been published that present various estimates of the extent of child sexual abuse. These data can only be estimates because of the fact that many adult women do not remember being sexually abused or do not define childhood incidents as sexual abuse.
6. Mary Ann Allard, Randy Albelda, Mary Ellen Colten, and Carol Cosenza, *In Harm's Way? Domestic Violence, AFDC Receipt, and Welfare Reform in Massachusetts* (Boston: University of Massachusetts, 1997); Jody Raphael and Richard Tolman, *Trapped By Poverty Trapped By Abuse* (Chicago: The Taylor Institute, 1997).
7. Mary P. Koss et al. *No Safe Haven: Male Violence Against Women at Home, At Work, and in the Community* (Washington, DC: American Psychological Association, 1994).
8. Koss, *No Safe Haven*.
9. Hughes and Sandler, U.S. Merit Protection Board, as cited in "Facts About Sexual Harassment," U.S. Department of Labor, 1988.
10. Nan Stein, Nancy L. Marshall, and Linda R. Tropp, *Secrets in Public: Sexual Harassment in Our Schools—A Report on the Results of a* Seventeen *Magazine Survey* (Wellesley, MA: Center for Research on Women, 1993).
11. Nan Stein, "No Laughing Matter: Sexual Harassment in K-12 Schools," in Emilie Buchwald, ed., *Transforming a Rape Culture* (Minneapolis: Milkweed Editions, 1993).
12. National Center on Women and Family Law, *The Effects of Woman Abuse on Children: Psychological and Legal Authority* (New York, 1994). The National Center on Women and Family Law is defunct; however, their publications are available from the NOW Legal Defense and Education Fund in New York: (212) 925-6635.
13. For a detailed review and analysis of the literature on the impact of domestic violence on children, see Gover-

nor's Commission on Domestic Violence, *The Children of Domestic Violence: A Report of the Governor's Commission on Domestic Violence of the Commonwealth of Massachusetts* (Boston: Commonwealth of Massachusetts, 1996).

14. Adapted from *Domestic Violence: The Facts,* by Battered Women Fighting Back!, Inc. (Currently known as Peace At Home, Inc.) (Boston: BWFB, 1995).

15. Koss, *No Safe Haven.*

16. The Project on the Status and Education of Women, *The Problem of Rape on Campus.* (Washington, DC: 1978).

17. Adapted from Massachusetts Coalition Against Sexual Assault, *Supporting Survivors of Sexual Assault: A Journey to Justice, Health, and Healing* (Boston: Massachusetts Department of Public Health, 1997).

18. Andrea J. Sedlak and Diane D. Broadhurst, *Executive Summary of the Third National Incidence Study of Child Abuse and Neglect* (Washington, DC: U.S. Department of Health and Human Services, 1996).

19. *Congressional Quarterly Researcher,* Washington, DC, 1991.

20. Frank W. Putnam, *Diagnosis and Treatment of Multiple Personality Disorder* (New York: Guilford Press, 1989).

21. See Linda Meyer Williams, "Recall of Childhood Trauma: A Prospective Study of Women's Memories of Child Sexual Abuse," *Journal of Consulting and Clinical Psychology* 62, no. 6 (1994): 1167–176.

RESOURCES

For more information on violence in lesbian relationships, see chapter 10 Resources.

Books

Backhouse, Constance, and Leah Cohen. *Sexual Harassment on the Job.* Englewood Cliffs, NJ: Prentice-Hall, 1981.

Barry, Kathleen. *Female Sexual Slavery.* New York: Avon Books, 1979.

Bart, Pauline, and Patricia O'Brien. *Stopping Rape: Successful Survival Strategies.* New York: Pergamon Press, 1985.

Bass, Ellen, and Laura Davis. *The Courage to Heal: A Guide for Women Survivors of Child Sexual Abuse.* New York: Harper Perennial, 1994.

Brownmiller, Susan. *Against Our Will: Men, Women and Rape.* New York: Fawcett, 1993, c.1976.

Candib, Lucy M. "Violence as a Gender Issue," in M. K. Hendricks-Matthews, ed., *Family Violence: Toward a Solution.* Kansas City, MO: Society of Teachers of Family Medicine Publications, 1992.

Center for Women and Religion at the Graduate Theological Union. *Clergy Abuse Survivors Packet.* Available, for $5.00, from Center for Women and Religion, 2400 Ridge Road, Berkeley, CA 94709; (510) 649-2490.

Davis, Angela. *Violence Against Women and the Ongoing Challenge to Racism.* Latham, NY: Kitchen Table Women of Color Press, 1987.

Davis, Laura. *Allies in Healing: When the Person You Love Was Sexually Abused As a Child.* New York: HarperCollins, 1991.

———. *The Courage to Heal Workbook for Women and Men Survivors of Child Sexual Abuse.* New York: Harper & Row, 1990.

Dworkin, Andrea. *Pornography: Men Possessing Women.* New York: NAL-Dutton Press, 1991.

Fairstein, Linda. *Sexual Violence: Our War Against Rape.* New York: Berkley Publishing, 1995.

Finex House. *Escape: A Handbook for Battered Women Who Have Disabilities.* Finex House, P.O. Box 1154, Jamaica Plain, MA 02130; Attn: Chris Womendez.

Fortune, Marie M. *Sexual Violence: The Unmentionable Sin: An Ethical and Pastoral Perspective.* New York: Pilgrim Press, 1983.

Herman, Judith L. *Father-Daughter Incest.* Cambridge, MA: Harvard University Press, 1981. A classic.

Herman, Judith. *Trauma and Recovery.* New York: Basic Books, 1992.

Jones, Ann. *Women Who Kill.* Boston: Beacon Press, 1996.

Lerner, Gerda. "The Rape of Black Women as a Weapon of Terror," in Gerda Lerner, ed., *Black Women in White America: A Documentary History.* New York: Random House, 1992.

Levy, Barrie, ed. *Dating Violence: Young Women in Danger.* Seattle: Seal Press, 1991.

Lobel, Kerry, ed. *Naming the Violence: Speaking Out About Lesbian Battering.* Seattle: Seal Press, 1986.

Martin, Del. *Battered Wives.* New York: Simon & Schuster/Pocket Books, 1990.

Massachusetts Coalition of Battered Women's Service Groups. *For Shelter and Beyond: An Educational Manual for Working with Women Who Are Battered.* Boston: MCBWSG, 1992. Available from MCBWSG, 14 Beacon Street, Boston, MA 02108.

McEnvoy, Alan, and Jeff Brookings. *If She Is Raped: A Book for Husbands, Fathers, and Male Friends.* Holmes Beach, FL: Learning Publications, 1990.

Miller, Alice. *Banished Knowledge: Facing Childhood Injury.* New York: Doubleday, 1991.

Rush, Florence. *The Best Kept Secret: Sexual Abuse of Children.* New York: McGraw Hill, 1992, c.1980. Reviews the Bible, myths, fairy tales, and popular literature.

Russell, Diana E. H. *Making Violence Sexy: Feminist Views on Pornography.* New York: Teachers College Press, 1993.

Sanday, Peggy R. *Fraternity Gang Rape: Sex, Brotherhood, and Privilege on Campus.* New York: New York University Press, 1992.

Sanford, Linda Tschirhart. *Strong at the Broken Places: Overcoming the Trauma of Childhood Abuse.* New York: Random House, 1990.

Warshaw, Robin. *I Never Called It Rape: The Ms. Report on Recognizing, Fighting and Surviving Date and Acquaintance Rape.* New York: Harper & Row, 1988.

White, Evelyn. *Chain Chain Change: For Black Women in Abusive Relationships*. Seattle: Seal Press, 1994.

Wisechild, Louise M., ed. *She Who Was Lost Is Remembered: Healing from Incest Through Creativity*. Seattle: Seal Press, 1991.

Zambrano, Myrna, M. *Mejor Sola Que Mal Acompañada: For the Latina in an Abusive Relationship*. Seattle: Seal Press, 1985.

Article

Andrews, A.B., and L.J. Veronen. "Sexual Assault and People with Disabilities." In Deborah Valentine, ed. *Sexuality and Disabilities: A Guide for Human Service Practitioners*. Binghamtom, NY: Haworth Press, 1993.

Magazines and Newsletters

The Aurora: An Ongoing Forum for Women
P.O. Box 535; Plaistow, NH 03865
A quarterly newsletter for women.

The Cutting Edge
P.O. Box 20819; Cleveland, OH 44120
A newsletter by and for women who self-injure.

The Healing Woman Foundation, Inc.
P.O. Box 3038; Moss Beach, CA 94038; (415) 728-0339
E-mail: healingw@aol.com
Web site: http://members.aol.com/healingco/healing co.htm
Information, self-help, and support by and for women in recovery from childhood sexual abuse and related areas. Monthly newsletter.

Survivor Activist
Survivor Connections, Inc.
52 Lyndon Road; Cranston, RI 02905; (401) 941-2548
A quarterly newsletter.

Survivorship
318 Mission, No. 19; San Francisco, CA 94110
A newsletter for survivors of ritual abuse.

Audiovisual Materials

Breaking Silence, A Film on Incest and the Sexual Abuse of Children, 1985. New Day Films, 22-D Hollywood Avenue, Hohokus, NY 07432; (201) 652-6590; Web site: http://www.newday.com

The Confrontation: Latinas Fight Back Against Rape, 1983. Women Make Movies, 462 Broadway, Suite 500, New York, NY 10013; (212) 925-0606; E-mail: info@wmm.com

Dating Rights: Gang Rape on Campus. Available from Filmakers Library, 124 East 40th Street, Suite 900, New York, NY 10016; (212) 808-4988.

Delores, 1988. Domestic violence in Latino communities. Cinema Guild, 1697 Broadway, Suite 802, New York, NY 10019; (212) 246-5522; E-mail: cinemag@aol.com

Not a Love Story, 1981 film about pornography. The National Film Board of Canada, 350 5th Avenue, Suite 4820, New York, NY 10118; (212) 629-8890.

Rape/Crisis. An award-winning docudrama on the roots of sexual violence. The Cinema Guild. See *Delores*, above.

Rape Culture, 1975. Widely used. Cambridge Documentary Films, P.O. Box 390385, Cambridge, MA 02139; (617) 484-3993; E-mail: cdf@shore.net; Web site: http://www.shorenet/~cdf

Still Killing Us Softly, 1987. Explores violence and stereotyping in advertising. Cambridge Documentary Films. See *Rape Culture*, above.

We Will Not Be Beaten. The dynamics of battering, institutional response, and the role of shelters. Transition House Films, Box 530 Harvard Square Station, Cambridge MA 02238; (617) 354-2676.

Organizations

American Women's Self-Defense Association
713 North Wellwood Avenue; Lindenhurst, NY 11757; (800) 43-AWSDA
E-mail: awsda@nais.com

Covenant House Nine-Line
(800) 999-9999
24-hour national hot line for teens.

COYOTE (Call Off Your Old Tired Ethics)
2269 Chestnut Street, #452; San Francisco, CA 94123-2607; (415) 435-7950

Incest Survivors Resource Network International
P.O. Box 7375; Las Cruces, NM 88006; (505) 521-4260
E-mail: isrni@zianet.com
Web site: http://zianet.com/ISRNI

Mending the Sacred Hoop
206 West Fourth Street; Duluth, MN 55806; (218) 722-2781

Men Overcoming Violence (MOVE)
54 Mint Street, Suite 300; San Francisco, CA 94103; (415) 777-4496

Model Mugging
1168 Commonwealth Avenue; Boston, MA 02134; (617) 232-7900
An innovative course offered nationwide that teaches women self-defense in simulated rape situations against an instructor dressed as a mugger (with protective equipment).

National Alliance of Sexual Assault Coalitions
110 Connecticut Boulevard; E. Hartford, CT 06108; (860) 282-9881
E-mail: connsacs@linet.com
Web site: http://www.connsacs.org
Works on public policy issues.

National Center for Missing and Exploited Children
2101 Wilson Boulevard, Suite 550; Arlington, VA 22201;
(703) 235-3900
Web site: http://www.missingkids.com

National Child Abuse Hotline
P.O. Box 630; Los Angeles, CA 90028; (800) 422-4453
    A 24-hour hot line for adult survivors as well as children.

National Coalition Against Domestic Violence
119 Constitution Avenue NE; Washington, DC 20002;
(202) 544-7893

National Coalition Against Sexual Assault (NCASA)
125 N. Enola Drive; Enola, PA 17025; (717) 728-9740
E-mail: ncasa@redrose.net
    This membership organization sponsors conferences
and publishes a newsletter.

National Domestic Violence Hotline
(800) 799-SAFE
TDD: (800) 787-3224

National Network to End Domestic Violence
701 Pennsylvania Avenue NW, Suite 900; Washington, DC
20004; (800) 903-0111 ext. 3; (202) 434-7405

National Resource Center on Domestic Violence
6400 Flank Drive, Suite 1300; Harrisburg, PA 17112; (800)
537-2238

Network for Battered Lesbians/La Red Para Lesbianas
Abusadas
P.O. Box 6011; Boston, MA 02114; (617) 424-8611

S.N.A.P. (Survivors Network for Those Sexually Abused
by Priests)
P.O. Box 438679; Chicago, IL 60643-8679; (312) 409-2720

Stop Prisoner Rape, Inc.
333 North Avenue 61 #4; Los Angeles, CA 90042
E-mail: rwoods@worldnet.att.net
Web site: http://www.spr.org

Survivors of Incest Anonymous
World Service Office
P.O. Box 21817; Baltimore, MD 21222; (410) 282-3400

TELL (Therapy Exploitation Link Line)
P.O. Box 115; Waban, MA 02168; (617) 964-TELL
    Resources for those who have been abused by therapists.

VOICES (Victims of Incest Can Emerge Survivors)
P.O. Box 148309; Chicago, IL 60614; (800) 7VOICE8;
(773) 327-1500
E-mail: voices@voices-action.org
Web site: http://www.voices-action.org
    National network for incest survivors: literature, therapist referrals, conferences.

WHISPER (Women Hurt In Systems of Prostitution
Engaged in Revolt)
P.O. Box 5514, Rockefeller Center Station; New York, NY
10185

Women Against Pornography
P.O. Box 845, Times Square Station; New York, NY 10108;
(212) 307-5055

Additional Online Resources *

Anonymous Sexual Abuse Recovery
http://www.worldchat.com/public/asarc

Discord's Abuse Survivors' Resources
http://www.tezcat.com/~tina/psych.shtml

The Family Violence Prevention Fund
http://www.igc.apc.org/fund

Lambda Anti-Violence Project
http://www.duke.edu/~keri/avp.html

SafetyNet Domestic Violence Resources
http://www.cybergrrl.com/planet/dv

Sexual Assault Information Page
http://www.cs.utk.edu~bartley/saInfoPage.html

Victim Services: Something Happened
http://www.victimservices.org/visitor1.html

The Wounded Healer: Partners And Allies of Sexual Assault Survivors Resources List
http://idealist.com/wounded_healer/allies.shtml

* For more information and listings of online resources, please see
Introduction to Online Women's Health Resources, p. 25.

PART TWO:

Relationships and Sexuality

Introduction: Sexual Orientation and Gender Identity

By Wendy Sanford

With special thanks to Loraine Hutchins and Rebecca Rabinowitz*

Loving relationships are essential to our lives. When they involve sex, these relationships are intense, puzzling, and frustrating as well as energizing, comforting, and freeing. They raise issues of power and vulnerability, commitment and risk. Sexual relationships can be painful: a long-time union breaks up, a love affair promises much and then fizzles, a lover dies, a partnership turns abusive. Most of us want and need intimacy, and we usually recover from the hurt and try again.

This unit looks closely at our sexual relationships. What do they give us? How can we make them more what we want? What is unique to sexual relationships with men? With women? How can we understand our sexuality better and enjoy it more? How can we change the social structures and attitudes about age, disability, race, gender roles, sexual orientation, and class that keep us from freely loving others and ourselves?

The following prologues address sexual orientation and gender identity: two topics both separate and intertwined, that can affect our relationships with ourselves, each other, and the men and women we love.

* Thanks also to the following for their help: Emily Bender, Denise Bergman, Sara Burke, Anoosh Jorjorian, Lynn Rosenbaum, and Nina Solomita.

PROLOGUE I: OPENING UP SEXUAL ORIENTATION TO CHOICE

Many women today are moving beyond narrow definitions of sexual orientation and feeling freer to decide whom we want as sexual and romantic partners for brief relationships or for a lifetime. Some of us who choose relationships with men are finding that the choice feels freer when it's not the only socially acceptable choice. More women who have sexual relationships with women are being open about it, and some who have been lesbian for a decade or more are entering relationships with men. Bisexual women are insisting on recognition and acceptance. Some young women in high school have joined gay-straight alliances and proudly prefer to remain label-free. Some of us choose to call ourselves "queer" as an inclusive term that allows for many possibilities.

This fluidity in sexual orientation may be confusing at times, but it's promising, too. Despite a continuing backlash from people in conservative political and religious groups who believe heterosexuality should be the only norm, and resistance from some lesbians and heterosexual women who distrust bisexuals, this fluidity seems to be here to stay because it allows women (and men) to be more of who we really are and to love ourselves and others more fully.

More than 30 years ago, research by Alfred Kinsey showed that most people experience attractions to both women and men. Yet, in many of our families and schools, people either didn't mention lesbians, gay men, or bisexuals at all or joked cruelly about them. We were made to feel hesitant about some of our closest friendships.

When I was seven or eight, I had this best friend, Susan. We loved each other and walked around with our arms around each other. Her older sister told us not to do that anymore because we looked like lezzies. So we held hands instead.

In experiences like these, our culture teaches us to fear and hate homosexuality in ourselves and others. This homophobia hurts all of us, whether we are heterosexual, lesbian, or bisexual. It makes us reject aspects of our own personality and looks that are not "feminine" enough (assertiveness, muscular build, body hair, deep voice), because we are afraid that people will think we are lesbian. It turns us against friends and family members who have sex with women, depriving us of important relationships. It causes us to deny attractions that may be natural to us and it may prevent us from choosing the sexual partners who are right for us. It prevents us from publicly acknowledging our friendships with lesbian and bisexual women. It divides us from each other as women.

If we are lesbian or bisexual, homophobia puts us at risk of individual acts of antilesbian violence and discrimination. Heterosexism, the institutionalized assumption that heterosexuality is the only normal orientation, denies us legal, religious, and social privileges. We are prevented from getting married, filing joint tax returns, and being covered under a partner's health insurance (except in the rare companies and cities that allow coverage for domestic partners); we face job and housing discrimination and invisibility in the media. Homophobia and heterosexism are politically useful tools for those who want to preserve the "traditional" forms of family life and to suppress any alternatives.

When we see the price women pay for being lesbian, we can understand that for many of us heterosexuality is perhaps not so much a natural choice as compulsory.[1] If we were free to be with men, or women, or both, or to stay happily alone, many of us might choose to be with men, but we would be responding to what we genuinely want and not to what society tells us we ought to want.

With time, sincerity, willingness, and friendship, we can unlearn homophobia.

The main thing that finally helped me start letting go of my homophobia was getting to know a few lesbian women. As we became friends, the myths I'd heard about lesbians—that they are mannish, oversexed, undersexed, or out to seduce straight women—fell away. They were like everyone else.

Even after I became a lesbian at 35, I found that I had big doses of homophobia inside me. Sometimes I'd wake up after having sex with a woman I loved and have an attack of thinking that the wonderful thing we'd done was bad. Or I'd get upset when other dykes seemed too obvious in public. Slowly I've become prouder and more deeply affirming of lesbians and lesbianism—that is, of myself.

As those of us who are heterosexual struggle toward building more mutual and satisfying nonsexist relationships with men, we can use our privileged status as heterosexuals to challenge heterosexist laws and practices. For those of us who are queer, it's important to be ourselves and to be as public as we feel safe being, and to challenge heterosexism—with pride.

I think we must simultaneously build upon our sexual orientation identities to raise awareness and gain rights, as we continue to expand and blur the categories. This creates a necessary tension, which pushes us toward greater freedom.

PROLOGUE II: OPENING UP GENDER IDENTITY

Moving beyond the concept of two fixed gender identities is a new challenge for many of us and a very personal story for others. "Man" and "woman" are considered to be unassailable categories in the dominant culture of the U.S. In fact, men who "act" like women, and women who "act" like men, are primary targets of homophobia and gay-bashing, which in turn frighten many people into staying inside the two strict gender categories. Yet, is everyone either entirely a woman or a man? Is there nothing in between? Who gains, and who loses, when everyone is assumed to be—and is forced to be—all one or all the other? It starts with pink clothes and dolls for girl babies, blue clothes and trucks for boys. It starts earlier, when a newborn's genitals are checked and the pronouncement is made. It starts when intersexual babies (babies born with genitals that are not clearly male or female, formerly called "hermaphrodites") are taken away to be surgically changed—usually into anatomical females—sometimes even before their parents get to hold them.[2]

Gender Identity—A Few Definitions

Please keep in mind that these definitions are in a process of evolution; their specific usage and meanings may change over time.

Transgender: Most commonly used as an umbrella term, which includes all people who in some significant way defy or challenge stereotypical definitions of gender, or who have a conflict with or question about the gender they were assigned at birth. Some of the people this includes are transsexuals, drag queens and drag kings, cross-dressers, gender benders, and bearded women. "Trans" is an abbreviated term in current use.

Transsexuals: People who strongly believe that they are or ought to be the opposite sex, whose anatomy doesn't match their inner convictions and mental image of themselves. Many seek sex reassignment surgery.

Female to Male Transsexual (FTM): Someone who was born and raised as a female who identifies as a male.

Male to Female Transsexual (MTF): Someone who was born and raised as a male who identifies as a female.

Gender Bender: Someone who challenges and crosses traditional gender boundaries, often as a political statement of refusal to be governed by stereotypical gender-specific clothing, presentation, or gender roles.

Drag Kings: Lesbian women who cross-dress in male clothing for erotic and sexual pleasure or as a political statement, who identify as female or as in-between and don't want sex reassignment surgery.

Drag Queens: Gay men who cross-dress in female clothing, who identify as male or as in-between and don't want sex reassignment surgery.

Transsexuals

Transsexuals have a special relationship to gender: most feel that we were born in a body that doesn't fit our actual gender. According to medical science, we have a "gender identity disorder," with the word "disorder" implying that something is wrong with us. Solutions proposed have been medical and individual: hormones with sex reassignment (plastic reconstructive) surgery, hormones alone, and intensive retraining on how to walk and talk and present ourselves as the gender we feel we are inside. Medical science has developed ways of creating a vagina out of male genitals and (less successfully so far) creating a penis and scrotum out of female genitals. The surgery has been successful enough for thousands of transsexual women and men to achieve a better fit between our bodies and our identity, between our outside and our inside. Many transsexuals long for this surgery but cannot afford it; others are not interested in a medical solution.

The medicalization of transsexuality brings up several issues. We who are writing this book believe strongly that anyone who wants sex reassignment surgery should have access to full information, counsel-

ing, and treatment, and that expense should not be a barrier. Yet, as in the rest of this book, it is important to ask whether medical "solutions" actually reflect political and social biases. Transsexuals who want to be accepted for medical treatment must shape what we say in order to fit the guidelines set by physicians, so we speak about being in the wrong body—yet, is this always exactly how we feel? We may reassure the providers that we are heterosexual—yet, is this always how we feel? Would a medical solution always be necessary if the dominant society didn't punish people for stepping outside the two established genders? If a woman who looks like a man weren't harassed and beaten up when she tries to use the women's room, she might not choose to take male hormones in order to "pass" as male. If boys weren't harassed and beaten up for acting "feminine," they might not turn to a medical solution in order to live out that aspect of themselves. As an FTM asked,

If my position in society were accepted, or even revered, as an anatomical female with a male gender identity, would I still feel the need to change my body?[3]

Transgender

Throughout history, brave souls have crossed gender lines. (For a compelling account, see *Transgender Warriors* by Leslie Feinberg.) Today, many "gender benders" who are not transsexuals are stretching the strict categories. Some of us who have been raised as women may choose to dress in ways that men customarily dress. We may cut our hair very short. We may let our facial hair grow, and not tweeze it out or wax it off, although others may ridicule or attack us for not looking or acting "like women." We may bind our breasts or take male hormones. Some of us live our public lives as women and our private lives as men, or vice versa. We all pay a high price in a society that penalizes, often brutally, those who step outside the strict gender definitions. Transgender activist and drag king Leslie Feinberg portrays in a novel, *Stone Butch Blues,* the many times s/he was beaten by police as s/he grew up looking like a male in Buffalo, New York; more recently, Leslie was refused emergency medical treatment for a life-threatening illness when the physician on duty in the emergency room discovered that s/he was female.

The public often confuses gender identity and sexual orientation, thinking that all transgendered people are lesbian or gay. Transgendered people, including transsexuals, have varying sexual orientations: we may identify as heterosexual; as lesbian, gay, or bisexual; or as queer.

What if there are more than two genders? Most of us are so steeped in the two-gender mentality that the thought of moving beyond the man/woman split is disturbing.

At a workshop on transgender identities, I found myself staring at the panel trying to figure out who

they really were—a gay man in drag? a really butch dyke? It felt too uncomfortable not to know for sure if they were men or women. I realized then how much I determine my own ways of interacting with people based on whether I think I am speaking to a man or a woman. If I'm not sure who they are, then I'm not sure how to act.

We all might benefit from opening up our ideas of gender. The system of two rigid genders gives rise to the homophobic prejudices and practices that endanger the lives of lesbian, bisexual, gay, and transgendered people. It also sets the stage for sexism, for male privilege, and for violence against women. In the Resource section, you will find books by several leaders in a growing transgender movement: Leslie Feinberg, Kate Bornstein, Loren Cameron, Minnie Bruce Pratt, and others.

PROLOGUE III: FEAR OF LESBIANS, BISEXUALS, AND TRANSGENDERED PEOPLE, AND OUR UNITY AS WOMEN

Some women hesitate to join feminist projects because friends and family will assume that being a feminist means one is a lesbian. Some lesbians struggling for legitimacy and acceptance suggest that "straight" or bisexual women are less feminist than lesbians, or that "true" feminists wouldn't ally themselves with men in any way. Ultraconservative political and religious groups play on these divisions by portraying all feminists as overbearing man-haters as well as actual or would-be lesbians or bisexuals. Using homophobia as a tool to divide us and turn us against one another, they rob us of our energy and unity as a movement of women trying to build a more just society for everyone.

Transphobia (irrational hatred and fear of transgendered people) can divide us as well. For example, some women fear and distrust transsexual women who were born as males (MTFs). MTFs have been rejected from some women-only gatherings in the belief that they will inevitably try to claim the privileges they were used to as men, or because women who have experienced sexual abuse or other violence from men feel unsafe in their presence. Other women-born women wish to welcome MTFs, figuring that they have walked away from a lot of privilege in choosing to live as women. So the issues are complex, and they require care from all sides. MTF Kate Bornstein responds:

It took my becoming a woman to discover my "male behavior"... *[In the company of women] any act of mine that was learned male behavior stood out like a sore thumb. Things like leaping up and taking charge, even when it wasn't called for....I noticed I didn't have much remaining male privilege by the slow dawning of peacefulness in my life.*[4]

We who have written this book want our society to develop to the point where all women feel safe enough to affirm ourselves and each other as who we are.

I want to celebrate the beautiful incredible diversity of human sexuality and the richness and wonder of embracing all our variety, praising all life's expressions, not being afraid of or trying to control or suppress them, trusting and supporting each other.

When transgendered women and women of all sexual orientations can find friendship, growth, and power within the women's movement, we will without a doubt become a stronger and more vibrant force for social change.

NOTES

1. See Adrienne Rich's classic article "Compulsory Heterosexuality and Lesbian Existence," *Blood, Bread and Poetry,* (New York: W. W. Norton, 1986).
2. See Milton Diamond, Ph.D., and H. Keith Sigmundson, M.D., "Sex Reassignment at Birth, *Archives of Pediatric and Adolescent Medicine* 151 (March 1997): 298–304. See also the Intersex Society of North America's E-mail: info@isna.org; and Web site: http://www.isna.org.
3. Alex Coleman, "Adrift in the Nowhereland of Gender Ambiguity: Seeking Harbor in the Spectrum of Possibilities," *Sojourner: The Women's Forum* (Nov. 1995): 11.
4. Kate Bornstein, *Gender Outlaw: On Men, Women, and the Rest of Us* (New York: Random House, 1995): 110.

RESOURCES

For information on bisexuality see chapter 11, Sexuality; for information on lesbians see chapter 10, Relationships with Women. Thanks to the women of New Words Bookstore for their help.

Bornstein, Kate. *Gender Outlaw: On Men, Women, and the Rest of Us.* New York: Random House, 1995.

Brown, Mildred, and Chloe A. Rounsley. *True Selves: Understanding Transsexualism.* San Francisco: Jossey-Bass, 1996.

Cameron, Loren. *Body Alchemy: Transsexual Portraits.* San Francisco: Cleis Press, 1996.

Feinberg, Leslie. *Stone Butch Blues.* Ithaca, NY: Firebrand Books, 1993.

———. *Transgender Warriors: Making History from Joan of Arc to Dennis Rodman.* Boston: Beacon Press, 1997.

Kirk, Sheila, and Martine Rothblatt. *Medical, Legal and Workplace Issues for the Transsexual: A Guide for Successful Transformation—Male to Female, Female to Male.* Watertown, MA: Together Lifeworks, 1995.

Nettick, Geri. *Mirrors: Portrait of a Lesbian Transsexual.* New York: Masquerade Books, 1996.

Pratt, Minnie Bruce. *S/he.* Ithaca, NY: Firebrand, 1995.

Rothblatt, M. *The Apartheid of Sex: A Manifesto on the Freedom of Gender.* New York: Crown Publishers, Inc., 1995.

Wilchin, Riki Anne. *Read My Lips: Subversion and the End of Gender.* Ithaca, NY: Firebrand, 1997.

Organizations

American Educational Gender Information Service (for TG/TS)
P.O. Box 33725; Decatur, LA 30033-0924; (770) 939-2128 (business); (770) 939-0244 (hclp line)

Ingersoll Gender Center (for TG/TS)
1812 East Madison Street, Suite 106; Seattle, WA 98122; (206) 329-6651
E-mail: ingersollcenter@ingersoll.org

International Foundations for Gender Education
(for TG/TS)
P.O. Box 229; Waltham, MA 02154; (781) 899 2212; E-mail: ifge@world.std.com

For Web sites, see chapter 11, Sexuality.

By Sara Burke with Denise Bergman,
based on earlier work by Paula B.
Doress-Worters, and
Peggy Nelson Wegman

With special thanks to Maria Baez, Donna
Bright, Sharon Bright, Mayra Canetti, Leah
Diskin, Cheryl Majeed, Charlotte Mayerson,
Catherine Kohler Reissman, Rose Wright*

Chapter 9

Working Toward Mutuality: Our Relationships with Men

*O*ur relationships with men can be among the most rewarding in our lives. In a world where people are so sharply divided by gender, the connections we make across that line sometimes feel especially precious.

The best thing about my marriage is that I have a real friend. When you've done a lot of things together you have a commonality of ethics, a way of looking at the world that is terribly important, so I trust my husband a lot.

Eddie and I are really really really attracted to each other, and were from the beginning. Now that we've been together awhile, we also just adore each other. We're so much alike—it's intimate, it's comfortable, and it makes me feel that I have an outlet for all my perceptions of the world.

*Over the years since 1969, the following people have contributed to the many versions of this chapter: Nancy Miriam Hawley, Elizabeth Matz, Catherine Cobb Morocco, and Sandy Rosenthal.

When I met Pedro, he was really pursuing me, and I resisted because he didn't look the way I wanted him to look—he didn't have a ponytail, he wasn't six feet tall or a bodybuilder type. Now we live together and we're engaged. He's incredibly communicative, kind, and good. I feel so loved, in a warm, enveloping kind of way—all my ugly parts too. He wasn't the myth I was looking for, and when I put that aside, I got all of these rewards that I didn't even anticipate.

Those of us who look to men for love, friendship, intimacy, support, sex, or some combination of these often face big challenges to staying physically and emotionally healthy. How do we negotiate safer sex with our male partners? How do we protect ourselves from violence as we try to get to know potential lovers? How do we build long-term relationships that are equitable? How do we continue to develop our individuality and reinforce our strength as women, in spite of the messages that tell us we should count on men for everything? This chapter focuses on how, as heterosexual and bisexual women, we relate to the men

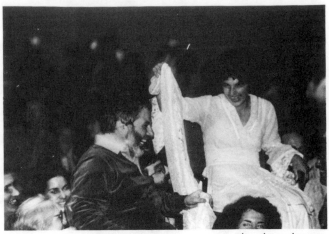

Cheryl Boudreaux

with whom we flirt, make love, or settle down—and on how we relate to *ourselves* in the process.

THE PERSONAL IS POLITICAL

In growing up, women and men are taught to behave and communicate very differently. Attitudes or actions encouraged in one sex are often not accepted in the other. Across cultures, we see that what men do is given more importance than what women do. We see men's needs taking precedence over women's needs, and women's worth being judged by how successfully we please men.

Fortunately, most women—and many men—have always known better. Real people are much more complex than stereotypes, and the rules we learn from our culture seldom give us everything we need to negotiate the relationships in our lives. In every place and at every time in history, some people have rebelled in small and large ways against their societies' gender-based codes, discovering new truths about how many different ways there are for a healthy person to be.

For many people, however, these ideas first came together in an organized way when the women's movement surfaced again in the 1960s. This feminist movement is still growing, and it continues to advocate for women's equality and empowerment in every area of our lives, from the most public to the most intimate. A wide variety of women today recognize, and act on, one of its basic principles: that our lives, work, ideas, and beliefs are as important as those of men and that society should be reorganized to reflect and support this principle.

The discovery of our power to make this stand can happen anywhere—on a girls' or women's sports team, in a labor union, while teaching or taking a class, at a meeting, around the kitchen table. When women and girls come together, we appreciate our abilities, increase our confidence, share warnings and strategies, and learn to trust and practice the solidarity of sisterhood. Wherever the impulse comes from,

whether we call it feminism or not, we remember our independence and ideas and become less willing to put them second to those of men. We hold our heads higher and break old patterns that made us feel ashamed or endangered. But these strengths are often met with resistance in our relationships with men who may feel profoundly threatened by our growth and change. Then we have to rethink what those relationships mean, which can be hard for both partners.

"The personal is political" expresses the belief that what seem like personal problems are often symptoms of larger social problems. For example, when women disagree with men and state our disagreement unapologetically, we often find that instead of responding to the substance of our opinions, men take issue with the way we express ourselves. We may be accused of coldness, arrogance, excessive anger. Words like "uppity," "bitch," and "castrating" are sometimes used to let us know we have crossed a social line. This is how, often unconsciously, individuals enforce our society's double standard: Only men are supposed to have strong opinions, and women are supposed to agree with them. Larger patterns like these, learned from childhood and perpetuated in many different ways, can make it challenging to talk about changes in our perceptions, even with men we like or love.

In high school I had a boyfriend I loved a lot, but sometimes he used to want me to look at pornographic magazines with him—he thought it was sophisticated for us to do this together, and he pretended that it was not all about getting turned on. But I didn't like it, and finally one time I said he could look through Playboy *if he wanted to, but I didn't want to do it with him, and I'd just go do something else until he was finished. Shortly after that, he broke up with me for being such a "radical feminist."*

No woman enters her relationships with men, or any other part of her life, with only her gender to think about. Our race and ethnicity, our age, how much money we have and how we get it, our politics, our sexual orientation—these are just a few of the infinite variables that form the unique weave of each woman's identity.

I believe that my relationships with men have been affected by my political ideas, by my status in society as a woman of color with a strong cultural and language background, by the difficulty that some men have in dealing with single mothers and independent women, and by the risk of dating and having sex in the times of HIV infection. In my opinion, Puerto Rican women should encourage and include our men in our struggles and organize toward societal changes and equality.

Our relationships with our lovers and life partners are often where we are most vulnerable. This makes them both the most important and sometimes the most difficult situations in which to speak our personal

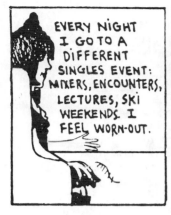
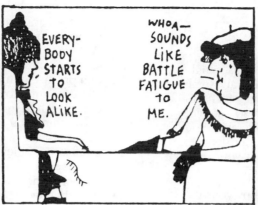
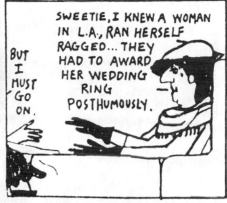

Nicole Hollander

truths. Change can be frightening, but with self-confidence and the support of our communities and with the trust that comes from sharing deeply, men and women can find new ways of being together that feel freer to all of us.

CHOOSING TO BE SINGLE

It would be nice to be in a relationship, but I don't really need that. My life is fine the way it is. And my life is full of love. In nine years of being single, I have never been lonely.

Staying single can be a normal, healthy, wonderful way to live, as many women discover in spite of all the negative messages to the contrary. Depending on how we choose to define it for ourselves, "being single" may mean having one or many lovers, an occasional casual sexual encounter, a committed relationship without marriage, or no sexual or romantic relationships at all. Whether being single is a temporary interlude or a life choice, these times can be among the most satisfying we ever experience.

I like the independence of being single, which for me means that I date men occasionally but don't sleep with them. Relationships are terrific, but for me, not being responsible for half the maintenance of a relationship means that I can spend time with more friends, and a lot more time thinking for myself about my own ideas and questions. In relationships I tend to let myself get wrapped up in my partner's issues, problems, and ideas, and don't think for myself as much.

I plan not to get involved in another exclusive long-term relationship. I am enjoying the lifestyle I am living now (I currently have about five men that I keep in contact with casually). I am always straight up with the men I date. In other words, I let them know right from the start that I have no intention of getting involved in a committed relationship. I do not want to mislead or hurt anyone. Most men are not used to that type of attitude from women, but most deal with it just fine. I do know that this will get old at some point, and

there are definitely lonely times involved. So what will my ultimate solution be? Time will have to answer that for me.

Although many communities admire independent single women, most of us are told from childhood that our lives will be incomplete until we find a man. Popular culture never tires of presenting single women characters who are desperate and lonely. Single women sometimes say that the hardest thing about being single is *not* loneliness but this constant societal onslaught.

I miss some things about being single, especially the spontaneity of not having to check in about another person's feelings before doing something, staying out late. What I don't miss is going to the movies, seeing some ideal love romance on the screen, and feeling as if my life is shit because I don't have that. Some movies should have a warning label for single people: "This movie will cause a large bucket of self-pity to rain down on you, even if you are perfectly happy."

I'm 30, and I'm not married. I get hints from people that they think I'm irresponsible, or that I must be a slut. When my parents and people at work ask me again and again if I've "met someone," I turn it into a joke, but inside I think, "I'm as happy as I can be right now, and you can't understand that."

When I broke up with my lover, I luckily had a circle of warm affectionate friends who would give me a hug or a pat on the back. Yet, I feel the lack of that very intimate whole-body contact. I didn't want to rush precipitously into a new relationship just because I felt so hungry to be touched. One answer was to get a massage every other week for several months.

When we are happy and strong on our own, we are better able to choose freely and carefully the men we do become close to. Creating a safe and equal relationship with a man can then become a challenge we accept out of mutual attraction, admiration, and love.

STAYING SAFE

Violence against women faces all of us. Single women confront particular risks. Here are some ideas you can use to be safer. You may feel self-conscious about such measures at first, but after a while they will become habit. Remember, you always deserve to be safe. If you take a risk once, or many times, you haven't forfeited your right or your ability to be safer the next time.

- If you live alone or are often out by yourself at night, take precautions against becoming a target for attack. (See "Protecting Ourselves and Each Other from Rape" in chapter 8, Violence Against Women.)
- If you are dating, take a man's number rather than giving him yours. Meet him in a public, well-populated place. Tell a friend where you will be and that you will call her the next morning to tell her you got in all right. Avoid excessive alcohol or drugs on the first few dates. If you pick up strangers, pay close attention to your surroundings and keep an eye on your drink; there are now illegal drugs available that cause short-term memory loss, and men sometimes administer them to women without their knowledge in order to rape them (see chapter 8, Violence Against Women, p. 170).
- If you are sexually active you may need to use birth control (see chapter 13, Birth Control). Learn about precautions against sexually transmitted diseases (STDs), including HIV (see chapters 14, Sexually Transmitted Diseases, and 15, HIV, AIDS, and Women). It can be difficult to discuss safer sex with a male partner, no matter how long or short a time you've known each other. Here are some things that might help:
- Learn beforehand about all the fun and satisfying sex you can have while protecting your health (see chapter 11, Sexuality). That way the conversation doesn't just have to be about the things you *can't* do.
- Know your own rules. Every woman who is sexually active makes choices about which risks she is willing to take and which isn't. Know *your* limits and requirements for protection before you get into a sexual situation, when your decision-making abilities may not be at their best.
- If possible, initiate a conversation with your partner about sex and protection *before* things get hot and heavy. If you have already started some sexual activity, take a break and start talking. Ask other women

how they approach this first-time conversation with a man.
- Become comfortable with the tools of safer sex. On your own, unroll a few condoms and practice putting them on a banana. Share useful information about sex and dating with friends you trust.
- If you think you will be unable to get your partner to use condoms for intercourse, think about other protection you can use that does not depend on the man's cooperation, such as the female condom (see chapter 13, Birth Control, p. 298). Remember, any protection is better than none.

With the help of our friends, thorough information, and our own good sense, we can take good care of ourselves. Only if we face such possibilities as date rape and sexually transmitted diseases can we rally our considerable defenses against these threats. And only if we face the danger honestly, and acknowledge that simply living our lives means taking some risks, can we get and give the support we need when we *are* hurt.

EXPLORING MAJOR AREAS OF TENSION IN RELATIONSHIPS WITH MALE LOVERS AND PARTNERS

Toward Shared Power in Relationships

Healthy relationships are part of healthy lives, and in healthy relationships, power is never misused or abused. However, women and men belong to groups that have different degrees of power—personal, physical, social, economic, intellectual, political—often determined by society. This imbalance influences the way we think, act, and relate to each other. How people perceive and treat us outside our relationships inevitably affects how we feel and act within them. Part of our struggle as we enter or continue to improve our intimate relationships is to dismantle these inequalities and separate ourselves from stereotypes and the expectations of others.

Social and Economic Power

Money, the most common source of power in our society, often symbolizes social power as well. Although women constitute nearly half the workforce in the U.S., our society continues to reward men's work a great deal more than women's work. Many of us whose partners are working cannot bring in an equal amount of money; women earn on the average only 75% of what men earn and the gap increases with age.[1] Downsizing, forced retirement, unemployment, and even salary increase can have major effects on our intimate relationships, especially when society maintains the traditional stereotype of the male as provider.

I am a Dominican woman with four children. I have resided in the U.S. for ten years. When I was growing up, my mother was the head of household. In my culture and country, men were supposed to be the head of household; women were to stay home and take care of the kids and spouse. Through the years, that has changed, and women are now more likely to go out and work also, depending on their social and family status and their career achievements. The way I am approaching the struggle of raising my girls is to follow my mother's example. What I expect from myself is no less than what I saw my mother do. In my relationship with my husband, I have my own money, and what I say, goes. This works for me. I would never let a man run my life or interfere with my plans. I have always worked full-time to give my girls and me all the material and abstract things that will make us happy. I expect and demand to be cared for because I am very caring to my partner and I am always willing to help him achieve his goals. I would never let a man be the head of household because it means losing control of what I want to achieve and where I want to go.

The history of enslavement, job discrimination, and racist patterns in imprisonment leave many African-American men with fewer options than the women who love them. A mother and her grown daughters reflect on the challenges of building mutual relationships with men in this context:

Because of the plight of the black male in the U.S., because he often is not there for families and women, we have over generations learned to be independent heads of households. This socialization, over time, has moved women into a powerful role: the traditional male role. When we are in relationships, it's difficult because we have to redefine those roles—that is, it's particularly difficult for black men because their position in society leaves their home the only place for them to be the "traditional men." The threat of strong black women, independent and on our own, creates tension.

Men frequently maintain that child care and housework are women's duties, even when those women are working outside the home as well. In many families the woman is a wage-earner, a caregiver, and a homemaker.[2]

Patterns of power are often revealed early in a relationship. Dating is a good example. The tradition that men pay for meals and tickets on dates feels comfortable to some women but not to others. Sometimes a man uses this tradition as a way to make a woman feel indebted to him, implying that she should "repay" him with sex.

A man took me out, and on the second or third date he wanted to sleep with me. So I told him I didn't want to be that intimate on so short an acquaintance. And he grumbled and said, "I just want to know if there's a pot of gold at the end of the rainbow."

Some men imply that paying for dates is burdensome, but they may be reluctant to give up the control that goes with paying when offered a chance to share expenses. Others may be more flexible. One woman says:

I believe in paying my share when I go out with a man. The man I'm involved with now earns a lot more money than I do, and he enjoys spending it on things that are fun. We often end up arguing about what kinds of things both of us can afford, which he feels limits us to what I can afford. Sometimes we compromise and he treats so we can do something special.

In each relationship we become involved in, however long or short, we will have social and economic power dynamics to contend with. It's going to be a long time before women get equal pay or equal work. Meanwhile, we must insist in our relationships that the contributions of both people be equally valued.

Developing Our Personal Power

I need to feel pride sometimes, the feeling that I have a talent and I'm using it. I feel that way when I'm singing or dancing, and when I'm talking about my job. I need that separate sense of my own giftedness.

I like to be able to be alone, and take care of myself. That's new, just in the past five years. It makes me feel stronger. It makes me feel great.

I'm a teacher, and I get a real sense of competency and pride from my job. The respect I get there fuels my sense of power, and I bring that into my relationship.

Some kinds of personal power are self-reliance, assertiveness, the ability to earn a living, independence, and self-confidence. Many of us were taught to find a man with these qualities and literally attach ourselves to him ("If you can't be one, marry one"). In this way, we could become complete. Creating an intimate relationship with a man was not to be simply a way to enrich our lives but the foundation of our identities as whole adult people. And so we faced a paradox: To feel stronger, many of us followed the best-traveled route and found a man; yet, we were stepping into a role that only served to undermine our inner strength.

Having an intense relationship with a man much older than me that I now know was abusive has affected every area of my life. Although it's been three years since the end of this relationship, I am still recovering and have been permanently changed by the ex-

perience of unknowingly giving up control of myself to another human being.

And what of physical strength?

One way men in my life used to have power over me was with body image—they would let me know that they didn't think I was thin enough, or fit enough to do the things they wanted to do.

Many women have been taught that to be physically strong is unfeminine, and a man's greater physical strength can pose an unspoken threat of intimidation that causes all sorts of problems, from feeling overpowered in a sexual encounter to being intimidated in an argument. Because we live in a society where violence or the threat of violence is ever present, it is not surprising that we have such feelings. When we refuse to accept the cultural image of women as lacking in physical strength and competence, we learn new skills and become physically stronger, and our self-esteem grows.

One of the things I plunged myself into at age 54 was to take tae kwon do [a Korean martial art]. I had always been fascinated by martial arts but never had enough nerve to try it. I was stirring up long years

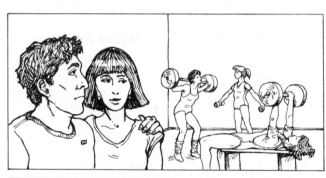

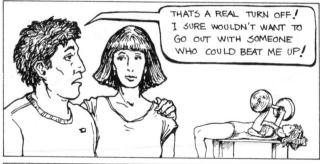

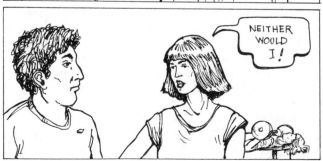

Greg Wenzel

of status quo; one more unorthodoxy didn't matter, I reasoned. All through our marriage I was never able to stand up to my husband, and I felt that taking a martial art might perhaps help me to become more assertive. My husband was totally put off by my taking up such a "masculine" activity. But I have persisted.

Women are taught to be uncomfortable with the idea of having power. (It is as unladylike as being physically strong!) Often when we do what is expected of us, we abdicate our power almost entirely.

When I started working on my graduate degree I was ambitious to become really well known in my field and fantasized being an adviser to members of Congress or even the President. Then I got involved with Dave and began to spend more and more time with him. He wanted total support for his work, and since we were in the same field I could help him a lot and be learning at the same time. But I definitely put my own ambitions on the back burner for about two years. I began to be more attached to the idea of staying in the city when I finished school so I wouldn't have to leave Dave, and I even began to fantasize about a less demanding job, maybe even just three days a week.

When we broke up, all my options opened up again, and I could reconsider my early ambitions. It was scary to consider the possibility of being as successful as my fantasies.

Getting Beyond Traditional Roles

One of the reasons I'm grateful for being bisexual is that it has opened up a lot of different models for me, and a lot of questions about what it can mean to be in a relationship. I still notice that when I'm with a man, I fall into patterns; part of me starts to have all these typical fantasies about marriage, a house, having children, staying together forever. But I don't forget all those questions opened up for me by same-gender relationships. My friends Bill and David love each other, and have been together for seven years, but don't live together. I know other couples who are not sexually monogamous but share a certain kind of intimacy only with each other. I don't necessarily want to do those things, but what I admire and learn from is that they made a relationship that works for them, instead of just following a script.

Roles are like parts in a play. We learn how to be a sexual partner, a wife, or a mother by following scripts that we learned as children. The scripts can lead us to drift into rigid roles without questioning them. Each partner begins a relationship with a set of experiences and beliefs that shape her or his notions about masculine and feminine roles. Some of us grew up with mixed messages.

I grew up in a household where we believed there were no distinctions between boys and girls. We were always told that girls were equal, and the five of us had exciting, far-reaching discussions and no-holds-barred, stimulating, intellectual arguments over dinner. But later I realized that while my father held court with us my mother was clearing the table. At some point he would call for his coffee to be brought to him. This affected my marriage. I feel intellectually equal or superior to Steven, but it's hard for me to feel okay about doing anything for my own work that demands or requires any adaptation by my family.

There are as many different ways to make peace with the lessons we learned in childhood as there are different women and men. Some women throw all the old ideas out and start from scratch. Others may be comfortable with some or all of what we learned. Many of us find that the relationships we like best are not the ones with the most familiar scripts, but the ones in which both partners are willing to improvise.

I grew up in a dysfunctional home, and I was the eldest kid, so I basically ended up running the house. It's still hard for me to let anyone else run things—in my house with my partner, I arranged all the furniture when we moved in, I do the bills, I say how clean the house has to be. Lately we've been talking about this, wondering together how much of it is because of my need for control, and how much is because we are falling into traditional man and woman roles.

We are taught gender roles not simply out of sentiment and tradition but because they fit us into existing social norms. As we struggle to change our relationships we must at the same time work to end sex discrimination at our workplaces, establish child care in our communities, and end the legal inequities women still face. In this transitional time we have the task of fitting the kinds of relationships we want into a society that may not only fail to support our vision but often actively oppose it.

Making Changes

We can begin to take small steps to change fixed roles. We can devise an action plan and take time for ourselves to build up our work skills, to work on something that interests us and brings in income. We can leave an unsatisfactory relationship or work hard toward changing our partner's attitudes and the structure of the relationship.

The change began for me as I prepared for a full-time job when all the kids were finally old enough to take some responsibility. I knew then I had to have Matthew as an active partner, though he preferred being passive and having everything done for him. My therapist told me to make a list of all the jobs that a family required in order to run. It was pages long; it just grew and grew. When I got it all written out after several weeks, it was clear that I did about 95% of it. And then I got very angry that I was the one who kept everything working around here. I basically decided I

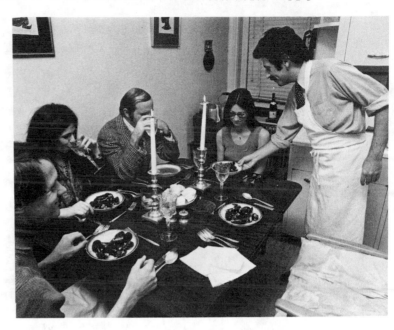

Cary Wolinsky/Stock, Boston

was going to go on strike. We began slowly and painfully to work out a more equitable system in the distribution of housework and cooking and parenting. Matt . . . felt that he "couldn't" do things that he didn't want to do, so it was painful. But I told myself it was worth it because it was the beginning. I was getting ready to start business school.

In the six months before I started school, I determined that I would teach the kids how to run the washer and dryer, to cook simple meals, to scrub the kitchen floor, to clean a bathroom. We set up job lists, and everybody had to do one thing a week: They would cook, and I would just be here if they needed help. And then I started business school full-time, and I was immediately overwhelmed. I was struggling. It was far more competitive than I had thought it was going to be. . . . I wasn't home after school; I had study groups late at night and on Saturday and Sunday. Things started to fall apart. Nobody liked it. The kids would grumble because other mothers didn't make their children do so much. We all need order in our lives, and it was chaotic for a while. By the time the first year had gone by, our job system was pretty well in place. This is really my break away from the house. I am no longer going to be here the way I have always been.

To create truly mutually supportive relationships we must realize that there is a difference between sharing *tasks* (taking turns calling for baby-sitters or paying the bills) and sharing *planning* (the overview—being aware of when sitters are needed, when a child needs to go to the doctor, and what the long-term financial plans are).

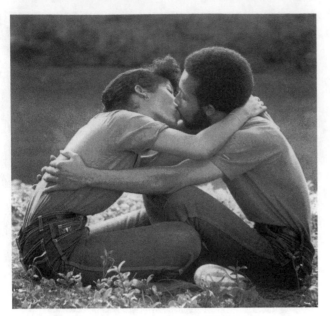

Willie Hill Jr./Stock, Boston

Understanding Some of the Barriers to Intimacy Between Women and Men

There are many different facets to knowing each other well and communicating on a deep level, letting our vulnerabilities show and our secrets be known, trusting enough to depend on someone and to allow that person to depend on us.

Intimacy is having someone in my life who I can get to know really deeply over time, who can get to know me and who I can be the best and worst of myself with.

Commitment means working on the relationship even when the early passion and urgency have evolved into a deeper if less dramatic kind of loving, and sticking through the hard, awful, painful, lousy, and deadening times (which can be dramatic in its own way!).

I'm still drawn to that rush of passion that I get early in a relationship, but now I'm old enough and I've been through enough with men to know that the rush doesn't last. We can rekindle it; there are times when I feel that passion with Don that always exists at the beginning, but I sure don't feel it 24 hours a day every day. It takes a lot of work and creativity to keep things sparking in a relationship. Sometimes I'm attracted to other men, but I think this has mostly to do with my fears about intimacy and with wanting the rush . . . and trying to disperse some of the intensity of being with one person. As I get older I'm more interested in whether this person is going to be with me. If the passion isn't there every night, it's okay.

Fearing Intimacy

We may fear too much closeness if in previous relationships we merged our own wishes, aspirations, and identities with those of our partner to such an extent that we lost sight of what we wanted for ourselves.

I wanted to be a satellite to him, revolving around him in his world . . . to let his life, his work, his friends, his energy pull me along. I was so relieved not to have to work anymore to build my own identity. This is what ultimately suffocated him and me and the marriage.

Often we experience conflicts between dependency and self-sufficiency, between the security of being in a good relationship and our need to remain separate.

One thing that's clear about my second marriage is that because I'm older and because of who Rob is, I am much closer to him than I was to my first husband. I am able to care for him much more deeply. And there are moments when he's away even overnight that are very painful to me. It's not "Oh, my God, I couldn't take care of myself," because I have and I can—but it's deeply, passionately missing somebody. And it's ironic because I had so strongly identified with the women's movement's "superwoman agenda" of being self-sufficient. Yet, it's come home to me just how painful it would be if something were to happen to Rob, how empty life would be. Not because my life isn't full in addition to him, but because I risked having a certain depth of commitment and feeling.

This society, which assigns active and dominant roles to men and passive or subordinate roles to women, exaggerates these conflicts. When we become conscious of men's greater power and prestige, we may fear the vulnerability that naturally comes with intimacy.

My work is lecturing and writing about pornography, child sexual abuse in battering situations, and other areas of female sexual slavery. I live two truths all the time: I live in a male-supremacist culture, yet I have a relationship with a man who is not a sexist. I used to feel that to be a totally strong woman and a feminist I should be alone, and I would feel guilty for having this real partner who loves me and helps me, whom I love and trust and depend on. But now I think, Why not just enjoy the special life I have and not worry about how I "should" be?

The stronger and more confident I feel about myself, the more able I am to be close to someone without fearing I'll lose myself.

We Learn Different Styles of Intimacy *

My idea about being intimate, more than making love, is having long, deep conversations. My fantasies of love affairs are about conversations like that. You just keep on talking and every once in a while something important or interesting will get said. John's idea is that you don't talk until you have something to say. I want to talk about everything from every possible angle. He considers that gossipy, repetitious, and intrusive. He's not secretive, but he wants to work things out for himself. His idea of intimacy is doing something together, like camping or canoeing. I sometimes think that John does not really know the part of me that I cherish most, and vice versa.

Frequently women value talking as a way of being close, whereas many men express intimacy mainly through physical activity or sexual closeness. Society holds up the "strong, silent type" as a masculine ideal. Many men find self-disclosure very threatening; showing one's softer side is not considered masculine. Because our sexist culture does not value a personal, "feminine" style of relating to others, most men are not motivated to learn it. This arrangement has cost men dearly: Many otherwise "successful" men are emotionally impoverished. It costs the women as well, who turn to these men for intimacy and find them seriously lacking. Very often women are responsible for the emotional climate in which a couple exists, and also, since many men have few or no intimate friends except for the women they are involved with, we end up having to give them a huge amount of emotional support. Again, a woman winds up doing "invisible" work. Her energy is sometimes so taken up with maintaining a relationship that she is diverted from her own personal achievement and development.

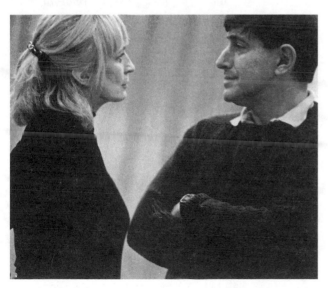

Jerry Berndt/The Picture Cube

* See chapter 11, Sexuality, for more information.

Many men have not yet caught up with women in terms of personal growth, knowing how to work on a relationship, or knowing how to be a good friend. Some men have begun to meet together in groups to talk about these issues, to develop the skills necessary for intimate personal relationships, and to learn how to pay more attention to their relationships with children, wives or lovers, and friends, even though nothing in our society encourages them to do so.

When it works, intimacy makes us feel so good that it enriches other parts of our lives and contributes to our energy and creativity.

MAKING IT WORK

In any long-term relationship, problems and painful issues come up regardless of how "right" we are for each other, of how hard we have worked to build the relationship, and even of how stable and solid we feel together. It can be frightening to look squarely at what is difficult and hurtful, for we want to believe that we chose a good partner and that we have made wise decisions. To become aware of aspects we were afraid to face, or to admit deep conflicts, may mean that we have made a major error. Sometimes, as we begin to get angry we become afraid that if we do not immediately squelch this anger, it will rage out of control and lead us inevitably to the end of the relationship.

Yet, avoiding confrontation is more likely to result in stagnation and resentment than in keeping the peace or making things better. *Conflict can be part of a creative process of working things out.* As a start we can identify the social aspects of our conflicts and avoid the common pitfall of blaming one another or blaming ourselves for everything that goes wrong.

Constantly Questioning Our Assumptions

We need to make a conscious and continuing effort to articulate what we really want in our intimate relationships with men, or the conventions of society will inevitably take over. One way to begin changing our relationships is to reconsider the kind of men we (think we) are looking for and our patterns of relating to men when we first meet them. Making changes at the beginning of a relationship may help us to shift the balance that gets set up in our future relationships.

I thought I was marrying this very exciting man, and I didn't see that his dynamism was an expression of the control he needed to have. I just saw the excitement, the energy. I didn't realize that it would make me feel smaller in the process. I learned that it's not just how "wonderful" the other person is, but how they make you feel. Now I pay a lot of attention to how I feel with someone at the beginning of a relationship. If I feel distinctly less wonderful in a man's presence, I don't care how sparkling or brilliant he is—I'm not interested.

But when a relationship has gone on for a long time, and patterns are already set, we may be scared to change or to have our partners change. If we were raised to believe that men should be strong and silent, we may feel uneasy when our partners express vulnerability, even though we have been asking them to talk about their feelings. We may want them to share caregiving chores but fear that they will encroach on our role, neglecting their paid work or being "unmasculine."

After 15 years of being a full-time homemaker, I decided to go to school. My husband and I divided up all the jobs and responsibilities so I could finish school and work at a fairly demanding job full time. Everything was working out fine, I thought, until one day Jim made some passing remark about one of our daughters and some problem she was having with her boyfriend. I was shocked to realize that something was going on I knew nothing about. I was no longer the "nerve center" of the family. That was a loss, because for many years knowing all those details had been my source of power within the family. Yet, on balance the change has been good for all of us. Being the nerve center was holding me back from developing other parts of myself, and as I moved out into the world Jim grew a great deal closer to the kids.

And we renegotiate these arrangements as time goes on.

We have been married 41 years, but because of the women's movement, there have been some recent changes in our relationship. My husband is a great theoretician. He may have read a hell of a lot more about the women's movement than I have, but to get him to cook dinner is a struggle!

By now we have struggled through the business about making dinner five or six times—different times at which decisions were made and they're acted on for a time, then something happens—like he goes away for three weeks, and when he comes back he's tired and he doesn't take the thing up again. So we have to negotiate the whole thing over again. At one point he said, "You know, the truth is I'm just lazy. It's just so much more comfortable not to have to do it." He can recognize that, but he doesn't prevent it from happening again. But the thing that makes it work is that he's open to being challenged about it.

Paying Attention to Each Other

So many things vie for our attention: work, friends, children, our various activities and chores. A new love eclipses almost everything else, but before too long the balance changes and it get squeezed in between the children's needs, the laundry, the car's transmission, and evening meetings.

An intimate relationship, while often background and sustenance for the rest of our lives, must at times have our full attention.

Several evenings a week since we married 11 years ago, we sit in the living room, each of us in our own favorite chair, and we have a glass of wine after the kids are in bed. And we talk . . . about the day, about ridiculous details of what happened at work, about some problem we've been having or whatever. Sometimes it's hard to take the time . . . the dishes need washing or there is a good show on TV or I just don't feel like it. But this, more than any other single thing, has kept us from getting too far apart without touching base.

We have long dry spells between us. . . . Sometimes I look at him, especially when he's upset about something and very silent and withdrawn, and it feels like I forgot what I was ever drawn to in this man. And then we take a morning off from work or we stay up until 2 A.M. trying to work out some big crisis, and then we might end up making passionate love, and then I remember, Oh! So this is what I love about you! But it's not the lovemaking so much as really talking about something other than whether today is garbage collection day or which check I forgot to enter in the checkbook. It's seeing "into his soul," into the person I am so close to.

There is no one "right" way to nurture a relationship; each of us must find what works best for us.

Enjoying Separateness

It seemed that I never had enough [time], and I couldn't figure out why. So I tried to examine my day and came up with the following percentages: friends, 5; family, 5; child, 15; work, 15; maintenance, 10; lover, 50.

I was appalled. As I looked at my list and tried to understand what it meant, I realized that there was no category for self. I had completely abandoned any organized attempts to spend time alone, enjoying and enveloping my own company, in favor or spending as much time as possible with the man who was closest to me. . . .

I wanted to know my own thoughts—away from all those absolutely-certain-about-everything male voices I knew. I wanted to hear myself singing. I began thinking about trying to structure some time alone with myself.

—Pearl Cleage*

It may feel natural for many of us to go on separate vacations or see separate friends. But other people often take it as a sign that something is wrong. Sometimes one member of a couple may be threatened when a partner's life excludes him or her in some way.

* From *Deals with the Devil and Other Reasons to Riot* (New York: Ballantine Books, 1993).

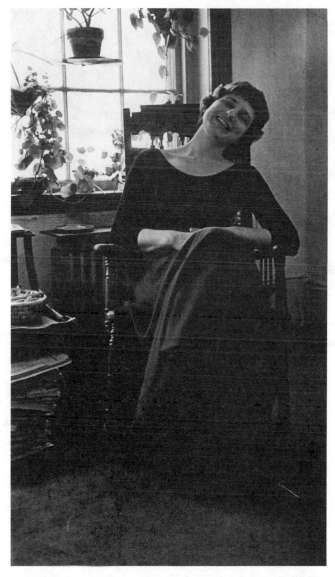

Vaughn Sills

very much, but that you'd love to come!" I have done this several times now; recently I even went out to dinner alone with a couple I particularly like. It's so much better than missing the parties and resenting Carl or dragging him along and having him sulk and then having to leave earlier than I want to. I resent it far less now when he watches sports on TV, which I dislike. I think that I wasted many years not doing what I enjoyed because sometimes it was different from what we enjoyed.

Martin and I have been together for 13 years. By together I don't mean married; it has always seemed sort of ridiculous to me to have the state involved in what is really a personal contract. And beyond that, I think that when you get married you begin to make a lot of assumptions and you don't even realize you're doing it. I use my relationship with Martin as a solid base to move out from. . . . I have a very active life independent of him . . . work and political meetings and seeing my friends. He and they are equally important to me—neither alone would be as good.

Keeping some distinct turf for ourselves, whether it's separate checkbooks or separate vacations, separate friends or not rushing into living together, does not have to threaten our relationship. In fact, it can be renewing to us and contribute to the vitality and growth of what goes on between us.

One of the reasons we have lasted together is that we have always lived in places where each of us could really build a whole life for ourselves—in terms of friends, work, interests—and not have to depend on each other for more than the other could give.

Having Other Friendships

Sometimes couples tend to close in on themselves. We may come to attach less importance to other friendships and let them drop. Yet, it is unrealistic to expect that one person can meet all our needs. Our friendships are crucial to our emotional well-being, our happiness, our growth.

Having deep friendships with other people creates a garden in which all of our potential can grow and flourish. We get a broader idea about who we are or can be and call upon different strengths. We are richer, more complex. What we learn through our intense friendships with others—about how to be close, how we seem to other people, how to fight constructively, what we enjoy—we can then weave back into our lives with our partners. Sometimes we have deep friendships with men, but more often our close friendships are with women. By expanding our intimate circles we relieve some of the pressure on our main relationships, and when times are hard other people can then give us support, nurturance and understanding. We don't have to depend only on our partners.

I have been seeing a man for almost a year now. I like him a great deal, but he is unable to understand my way of life. He is retired and enjoys just sitting with his feet up for the first time in his life. But I have a new volunteer job, and so I have a number of activities that to me are really stimulating. And these very things, which I've always wanted to do, make it seem to him as if I can't stay home and am always running around.

I remember years ago wanting so badly to go to a party we were invited to. But Carl really couldn't stand those people; he refused to go. What I really wanted was to go alone, and I would have had a grand old time, but in those days if you did such a thing people would surely have gossiped that you were on the brink of divorce! Several years ago our college-age daughter said to me, "Well, why don't you just tell them next time that Daddy really doesn't enjoy parties

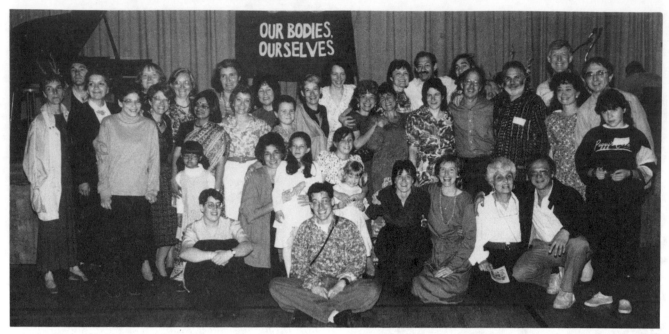

Some co-authors, family, and friends at the 20th-anniversary celebration of the publication of *Our Bodies, Ourselves* |
Ellen Shub

For black women, sisterhood is a major part of our lives. Friends, sisters, and mothers rely on each other. These are valuable and supportive relationships.

Sometimes Robert falls completely apart. He drags around the house in his bathrobe, doesn't shave, feels sick, and talks endlessly about it and generally comes unglued. This almost invariably happens when I am under the most pressure at work or when the kids are in shreds and demanding extra attention. I get so enraged at Rob for getting weak just when I need him that I yell and scream and berate him . . . just what he doesn't need—to be kicked when he's down. What I generally do is call up a friend I really love and trust. She has known me for six years and knows how to help me talk about things so that I get a better perspective on them. Having her to lean on when I feel overwhelmed or down also helps me to be less angry at Rob for falling apart at those times. I can go back to him able to say what I want to say much more clearly, having talked about it with Marie.

Women have always gotten together to talk with each other about the details of their personal lives. Though these gatherings have sometimes been considered trivial "chatting," what we are really talking about is the fabric of our lives. By spending time with other women, we see the potential power of articulating and clarifying what is going on in our lives. We learn that many of the issues we struggle with in loving and living with men are not unique to us.

Support groups can be helpful at all ages. Sheila has been married for 37 years.

I've been a member of a women's group for seven years now, and I think we came together out of a feeling that here we were, middle-aged. We didn't really fit into the women's movement totally. And yet there were things we wanted to talk about, and that was the only place they were getting talked about. We could recognize many of the things these women were talking about. And we looked at our lives and how not having a women's movement when we were younger had made an impact on our lives.

Some men, seeing the value of these groups, have set up their own. Other support groups include both men and women, such as single-parent, post-divorce and widow/widower groups, and groups that deal with a particular problem such as alcoholism or drug abuse.

Getting Help

Sometimes problems are very resistant to change, and it seems as if talking to our partner and to friends gets us nowhere. When we feel that we've gone around and around on the same issues with no improvement, we may become completely overwhelmed and believe that our problems are much worse than they ever were. But often it is simply that we get to a point where we are no longer willing or able to put up with the situation that has been going on for a long time. Profound changes can grow from these most desperate moments.

A few months ago things got to the point where, even though I loved Richard a lot, I just couldn't go on with this marriage the way it was set up. Richard refused to go to a therapist with me. In desperation I talked to two friends, each of whom has known us a real long time. And those conversations led to a mind-blowing realization that everything we did in our marriage had been set in the first six months of our relationship. I knew that I couldn't go on that way, so I told Richard how I felt. We stayed up all night talking and crying, then we slept and in the morning we cried again. He said he didn't want to lose everything he had ever loved and that he would try to change, and I said I would try but I couldn't promise and we would see. Right now things are much better between us and we are really trying to make it work.

But sometimes we get stuck in patterns that make it difficult for two people alone to make changes, or sometimes we just don't know how. Talking with friends may not always help enough. At this point, we may turn to therapy for help in understanding our own feelings and changing our behavior.

Therapy has helped me to focus on things I do over and over with men that result in my not getting what I need. For example, when I started therapy, I didn't realize how hard it was for me to ask for certain things. I didn't feel strong enough or confident enough to fight for myself. I found it hard to feel close, and I didn't understand how learning to get what I wanted would make me feel closer. It was a circle. . . . Now that I feel confident enough and aware enough of this pattern, it has changed.

We can use therapy to help improve communication about painful issues. But therapy for women can be a double-edged sword. Most often the women initiates the move to see a therapist, whereas the man may resist or refuse to go. But if we accept our cultural conditioning, which teaches us that our job is to maintain emotional relationships, take care of and give to other people, be sensitive, and work out problems, then turning to a therapist implies that we have "failed" at our role. Tragically, traditional therapy has often reinforced this perception (see chapter 6, Our Emotional Well-Being: Psychotherapy in Context). It is important to find a therapist whose definitions of health and normalcy are based on a worldview that sees women as having a full range of options, not on the premise that women's only or main role is to "service" men and take care of children.

After the first few months of couples' therapy, the therapist said to Matt, "So, you think the problem is that Anna is crazy just because she wants to go back to school, and if she would get 'better,' things would be okay again? Well, let me show you how you fit into Anna's problem." Then we began to look into Matt's part of it, how he wouldn't help take care of our four kids, how he needed to change for us to be able to work things out. For me that was enormously freeing, for the first time I saw that I wasn't the "crazy" one. And I began to feel that I could stay in my marriage and still grow and change in the ways I wanted to.

Not all relationships survive these profound changes. When a breakup seems likely, we have to ask ourselves which is more acceptable to us: the cost of leaving things as they are, or the risk that in trying to improve the relationship we may lose it.

Knowing When to Leave

Many of us struggle along for years in relationships that are not rewarding or affirming, wanting to make them better but not succeeding, and not yet convinced that we would be better off if we left. We may come again and again to the brink of leaving and then back off. This is not because things are not quite "bad enough"; even women whose men are violent toward them or are alcoholics or drug abusers or have incapacitating emotional problems often find themselves staying or struggling with whether or not to leave or how to leave. (See chapter 8, Violence Against Women, for a fuller discussion of domestic abuse.) What holds us back? Even with all the problems, we may still love our partner and be reluctant to lose him; we may feel loyal to him and perhaps not want to hurt him. Perhaps we think that breaking our commitment is a great personal failure, that we will be harshly judged by friends and family. We may try to stay together "for the good of the children" or may dread the prospect of being alone. And there is often the very real fear that we will not be able to support ourselves, and perhaps our children, financially. Yet, many women do ultimately decide that they want to end their relationships.

I once had a very bad relationship, but in other ways it was also very, very good. The two were evenly balanced, which made it hard to leave it. But eventually I decided that if I stayed, it would hurt like this forever, and if I left, the hurt I felt would get better eventually.

My relationship with Greg ended when I said that it was no longer working for us and that nothing we were doing was making it any better. He was not a person with whom I could fully engage. We never really learned to fight well together . . . not just having arguments but learning to compromise well. I felt turned off sexually, attracted to others, and the pleasure of being with him was gone. What was hardest about the divorce was that the family part of our relationship was good. . . . It was painful to let go of the father of my kids. It was scary to give my own needs so much weight.

The man I was living with began to undercut everything I did—to devalue my work, to be jealous of my friends and my small successes. When I got bogged down in a project, rather than encouraging me he would point out how the project was probably ill-conceived and not of much use anyway. The longer things went on, the more of my good creative energy went into trying to make the relationship work, and the less energy I had for my work and the rest of my life.

When I was first thinking about getting out of my marriage, I would think, Well, I get a lot of satisfaction out of being a parent and I'm very close to my kids. I get a lot of satisfaction from my friendships and I have a really good work situation. My relationship isn't so good, but maybe you just can't have everything. My husband had some serious problems, so I felt I couldn't blame him or just leave him. I never stopped to consider what it was doing to me to be spending years of my life with someone who was giving me so little. After a while I built up so much resentment that I just wasn't able to treat him in a loving way. And I began to be afraid that I would lose my capacity to love someone. I knew that I had a potential for loving that wasn't getting expressed. Yet it was a leap to assume that getting out of our marriage meant that I would have a good relationship again.

If you wind up accommodating your partner just to prevent fights rather than having some hope that it's worth while to sit down and try to work things out; if your relationship is based on evasiveness, deception, and withholding; if it is characterized by stagnation and a lack of room for change and growth; or if it just doesn't seem that your life is better in the relationship than it would be out of it, then it is time to consider ending it. You don't need to do this in isolation. Turning to friends, particularly ones who are wiling to talk openly about their divorces or hard times with their partners, can be an excellent source of support and insight. Individual or group therapy can help, as can support groups. There are also good books on the subject (see Resources). Much as we know it is important to work very hard to build a relationship,

it is also important to leave before we are damaged by it.

After a while in a bad relationship, I realize the nature of the relationship and bail out. Unfortunately, though, it takes me quite a bit of that hopeless waiting to be called, internalizing stress, and structuring my schedule totally around him to realize the disparity in the relationship. After being hurt for a while, though, I tend to get it—and the more times this happens, the earlier I recognize it. Now all I need to do is nip a bad relationship in the bud!

Conclusion

Though it may seem to be contradictory to advocate paying attention to our relationships and at the same time trying to be a separate person and seek other friendships, these multiple aspects of our lives can and do enrich rather than detract from one another. They also provide a balance that stimulates our growth and promotes our joy and well-being—our capacity for independence along with our capacity for intimacy.

We have been married for 13 years. . . . Daniel is not my best friend. We are quite different in many ways—have different friends, interests, and so on. There are ways in which I'm not even as intimate with him as I am with some of my women friends. But ever since I met him, I have not felt the excruciating loneliness that was the core of my life for 26 years. Being with him, knowing that we are partners in life, has permitted me to grow from an extremely unhappy, lonely person with little self-esteem and a lot of self-hatred into a happy, fulfilled, and self-loving woman. My identity is not derived from him, but being with him has enabled me to create a major transformation in myself.

NOTES

1. Institute for Women's Policy Research, *The Wage Gap: Women's and Men's Earnings.* "Table 1. Women's Earnings as a Percentage of Men's among Full-time Workers, 1955–1995," p. 1.
2. See Faye J. Crosby, *Juggling: the Unexpected Advantages of Balancing Career and Home for Women and Their Families* (New York: Free Press, 1991).

RESOURCES

Readings

Ahrons, Constance. *The Good Divorce: Keeping Your Family Together When Your Marriage Falls Apart.* New York: HarperCollins, 1995.

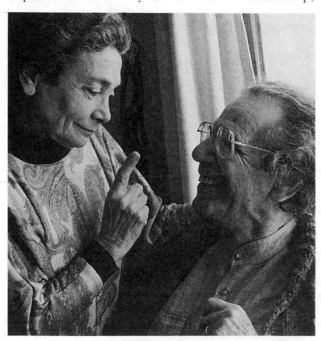
Anna Kaufman Moon/Stock, Boston

Arendell, Terry. *Mothers and Divorce: Legal, Economic and Social Dilemmas*. Berkeley: University of California Press, 1986.

Carter, Betty, and Joan Peters. *Love, Honor, & Negotiate: Making Your Marriage Work*. New York: Pocket Books, 1996.

Cleage, Pearl. *Deals with the Devil and Other Reasons to Riot*. New York: Ballantine Books, 1993.

Davis, Laura. *Allies in Healing: When the Person You Love Was Sexually Abused as a Child*. New York: Harper-Perennial, 1991.

Elkin, Larry. *Financial Self-Defense for Unmarried Couples: How to Gain Financial Protection Denied by Law*. New York: Doubleday, 1994.

Engel, Marjorie, and Diana Gould. *The Divorce Decisions Workbook: A Planning and Action Guide*. New York: McGraw-Hill, 1992.

Faludi, Susan. *Backlash: The Undeclared War Against American Women*. New York: Crown Publishers, 1991.

Findlen, Barbara, ed. *Listen Up: Voices from the Next Feminist Generation*. Seattle: Seal Press, 1995.

Golden, Marita, ed. *Wild Women Don't Wear No Blues: Black Women Writers on Love, Men, and Sex*. New York: Doubleday, 1993.

Grant, Gwendolyn Goldsby. *The Best Kind of Loving: A Black Woman's Guide to Finding Intimacy*. New York: HarperCollins, 1995.

Hauser, Barbara, ed. *Women's Legal Guide: A Comprehensive Guide to Legal Issues Affecting Every Woman*. Golden, CO: Fulcrum Publishing, 1996.

Hertz, Rosanna. *More Equal than Others: Women and Men in Dual-Career Marriages*. Berkeley: University of California Press, 1986.

Hochschild, Arlie. *The Second Shift*. New York: Viking Press, 1989.

hooks, bell. *Sisters of the Yam: Black Women and Self-Recovery*. Boston: South End Press, 1993.

Hutchins, Loraine, and Lani Ka'ahumanu, eds. *Bi Any Other Name: Bisexual People Speak Out*. Boston: Alyson, 1991.

Jones, Lisa. *Bulletproof Diva: Tales of Race, Sex & Hair*. New York: Doubleday, 1994.

Levy, Barrie. *In Love and In Danger: A Teen's Guide to Breaking Free of Abusive Relationships*. Seattle: Seal Press, 1993.

Malos, Ellen, ed. *The Politics of Housework*. Cheltenham, England: New Clarion Press, 1995.

Mayerson, Charlotte. *Goin' to the Chapel: Dreams of Love, Realities of Marriage*. New York: Basic Books, 1996.

Rich, Adrienne. *On Lies, Secrets and Silence: Selected Prose 1966–1978*. New York: W. W. Norton, 1995.

Riessman, Catherine Kohler. *Divorce Talk: Women and Men Make Sense of Personal Relationships*. New Brunswick, NJ: Rutgers University Press, 1990.

Rubin, Lillian. *Just Friends: The Role of Friendship in Our Lives*. San Bernardino, CA: Borgo Press, 1990.

Vaughan, Diane. *Uncoupling: How and Why Relationships Come Apart*. New York: Random House, 1990.

White, Evelyn C. *Chain Chain Change: For Black Women in Abusive Relationships* (expanded 2nd ed.). Seattle: Seal Press, 1994.

Periodicals

HUES (Hear Us Emerging Sisters) Magazine
P.O. Box 7778; Ann Arbor, MI 48107-9924; (800) 483-7482
E-mail: hues@branson.org
Web site: http://www.hues.net

Ms.
230 Park Avenue; New York, NY 10169; (800) 234-4486

Teen Voices
Women Express
P.O. Box 6009; Boston, MA 02114

*Additional Online Resources**

Ask Alice: Relationships
http://www.columbia.edu/cu/healthwise/cat8.html

B's Topics: Relationships
http://www.bguide.com/webguide/love

* For more information and listings of online resources, please see Introduction to Online Women's Health Resources, p. 25.

Chapter 10

Relationships with Women

By Emily Bender and Anoosh Jorjorian, with Peggy Lynch (Health) and Amelia Craig Cramer, Esq. (Legal)

BASED ON EARLIER WORK BY Barbara A. Burg, Loly Carillo, Sasha Curran, J. W. Duncan, Buffy Dunker, Deanna Forist, D. Hamer, B. J. Louison, Judy Norris, Gwendolyn Parker, Mariana Romo-Carmona, Wendy Sanford, Lynn Scott, Ann Shepardson, and others who, with regret and anger, felt they must remain anonymous to protect jobs, family relations, living situations, or parenthood

WITH SPECIAL THANKS TO Loly Carillo, Hannah Doress, Karen Kahn, Connie Panzarino, Gilda Bruckman, Liza Rankow, and Judy Brewer *

Being a lesbian for me is about the joy and wonder of loving women. It means being woman-identified, making women my priority. It is a way of life, so much more than a matter of who I want to sleep with.

Being a lesbian for me is about sex. I desire women, and I want to have sex with them.

Sometimes when I talk positively about being a lesbian, heterosexual friends say they hear me criticizing their choice to be with men. That's not true. For me, part of what's essential in being a lesbian is caring for other women, and this includes women who have made choices other than mine.

When I'm with a man there is a mystery in our gender difference. I know that he can never fully understand me. And sometimes I want that. But when I'm with a woman, we are similar in some very fundamental ways. It's the comfort of being truly known, with the vulnerability of having to be so honest.

I was disabled by an accident before I became a lesbian. As a woman in a wheelchair I felt something less than a person. But my nurse, who is a lesbian, told me I could have a strong self-image. She said that we are taught to hate ourselves because we are women and that we can love ourselves instead. I started spending time with lesbians. The closer I came to lesbianism the more I began to like myself.

The opportunities and possibilities for women who have intimate relationships with women have exploded in the past decade. Lesbian chic is in. Sports and entertainment figures are coming out in popular

* Thanks also to the following for their help with the 1998 version of this chapter: Beth Baron, Melody Brazo, Suzanne Bremer, Jenifer Firestone, Vicki Gabriner, Nancy Goldstein, Sasha Harris-Cronin, Beverly McGary, Jenna Milner, Carla Moniz, Corbett O'Toole, San Francisco COLAGE, Esther Sassaman, Tanya Seale, Melissa Shannon, Pam Sheridan, Dorothy Tan, and Sharon Wachsler. Over the years since 1969, the following women have contributed to the many versions of this chapter: Amy Alpern, Mary Bowe, Brenda Reeb, Holly Ellison, the Lesbian Mothers group at the Cambridge Women's Center, Jill Wolhandler, and a Boston Gay Collective (who wrote the original chapter, titled "In Amerika They Call Us Dykes").

magazines such as *Time* and *Newsweek;* an out lesbian, Roberta Achtenberg, ran for mayor of San Francisco and then became a top member of the Clinton administration; states are passing laws that protect the civil rights of gays and lesbians. At the end of the 20th century, women who love women are living our lives more freely and openly than ever before.

Women who have sexual relationships with women may identify as lesbian, bisexual, transgendered, or transsexual.* We call ourselves by many names: queer, gay, bi, dyke, lesbian, bulldaggers. This chapter uses the acronym "l/b/t" and, occasionally, the word "queer" to name inclusively lesbian and bisexual women as well as transgendered and transsexual women who partner with women. (For definitions of these terms, see the Introduction to Part Two.)

As the political and social climate changes, more l/b/t women are coming out and making ourselves known. Consequently, our diversity has never been more apparent. Although many still think of a lesbian as a masculine-looking white woman who drives a pickup truck and has a gravelly voice, they are discovering that they can no longer be sure if the black woman sitting next to them on the subway or the Latina working at the Girl Scouts office or the woman with the long hair and lipstick walking with her children is straight. We are the woman next door in the nursing home, the actress in the deaf theater production, your best friend from high school, the stripper dancing on the runway, your co-worker, the woman

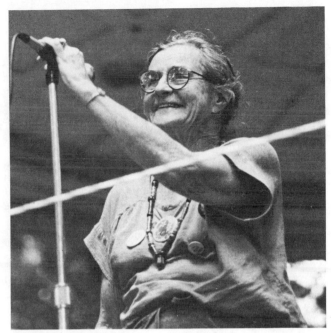

Ellen Shub

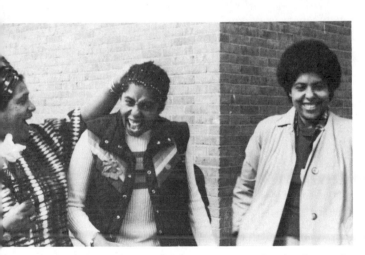

Longtime lesbian-feminist activists: the late Audre Lorde, Barbara Smith, and Beverly Smith/Tia Cross

* Although many, or even most, transsexuals identify as heterosexual, some identify as bisexual, lesbian, or gay in their sexual orientation. In the larger category of transgendered women, there are many women who identify as lesbian or bisexual. By including transgendered/transsexual women in a chapter that focuses mainly on lesbian and bisexual women, we don't mean to imply that all the progress that lesbian, bisexual, and gay people have made is shared by transgendered/transsexual people. We mean, instead, to express a vision that is inclusive of trans people in our continuing struggle to create a society in which we are all free to be ourselves and to love whomever we wish.

praying in the next pew. Some of us have disabilities. Some have or plan to have children; some have chosen not to have children. Some have relationships that last a lifetime; some are celibate. Some of us are married to men and cannot easily leave our marriages, yet we identify ourselves as lesbian. Lesbian and bisexual women in pop culture are no longer just the faces of singer k.d. lang, tennis champion Martina Navratilova, and actress Ellen DeGeneres but also the faces of musicians Me'Shell Ndegeocello and Ani Difranco and model Jenny Shimizu. As the breadth of who we are becomes more visible, we must change our definitions of what it means to be queer.

With diversity comes difference. As "our community" transforms into "our communities," we need to recognize that not all l/b/t women have the same experiences or concerns. Everything—from coming out to being with a lover to working in a political group— is influenced by an l/b/t woman's whole self, not just her sexuality.

In spite—or perhaps because of—our increased visibility and acceptance in the mainstream, homophobia continues to pervade our society. *Homophobia* is the irrational fear and hatred of homosexuality in ourselves and others. Like racism and sexism, this prejudice is institutionalized in our culture. We call the institutional privileging of heterosexuality over homosexuality *heterosexism*. So, for example, heterosexual marriage, the practice of providing "family discounts," and the denial of insurance benefits to gay couples all represent institutionalized heterosexist practices. These practices promote the belief that heterosexuality is the "moral," the correct, and/or the only way for people to have romantic relationships. As a result, l/b/t people who live openly risk losing our equality, our jobs, and even our friends and family. The freedom to live openly is a goal shared by queer folks across race, class, and other identity lines.

In this chapter, we want to reach out with information and support to women who are newly exploring their sexual identity and to l/b/t women who are isolated from a broad, understanding community. We also want to give heterosexual women a clearer picture of the lives of l/b/t women. But most of all, we would like to tell all women who desire intimate sexual relationships with women that they are not alone. We have written this chapter from our experiences and the experiences of women around us; we cannot even begin to encompass the lives and stories of all l/b/t women. If you do not see yourself reflected here, we want to encourage you to write your own words!

COMING OUT

Coming out is the process of coming to accept and affirm our sexual identity and deciding how open we will be about it. Coming out has changed dramatically over the past few years. In some places, especially in cities, women who love women can come out in relative ease compared with even five years ago. For an increasing number of us, our families embrace us, our co-workers accept us, and a community of women like ourselves welcomes us. This is hardly to suggest that this experience is the norm, but in writing this chapter, we want to emphasize the progress l/b/t women have made!

Still, for many l/b/t women, coming out is a long and difficult process. It can involve many stages: admitting to ourselves that we are queer, getting to know other l/b/t women, telling friends and family, marching in a gay-pride parade, being open at school or work. We face particular problems or dangers depending on our backgrounds, our age, our geographical location, or our health and abilities. Coming out may be especially difficult if we are transgendered or transsexual. Then we may be coming out about our gender identity as well as our sexual identity.

We spend a lot of energy deciding whether, when, how, and to whom we want to come out. When/if our society one day freely accepts women who partner with women, we will be able to use that energy in many other ways. In the meantime, we continue to work for a world in which l/b/t women can be open in all aspects of our lives.

Coming Out to Ourselves

Each of us has her own story of growing sexual awareness. Because we grow up in a culture that assumes everyone to be heterosexual, becoming aware of our identity and accepting it is often a gradual process. Coming out to ourselves can happen at any age or stage in our lives.

I didn't think about becoming a lesbian until at twenty-five I just fell in love with a woman and had to deal with it. As long as I was with her it was pretty simple, but when we broke up three years later, I finally had to ask myself, "Am I really a lesbian?"

I think I was always gay, but it took me seventy years to realize it.

I felt a strong political and personal commitment to women and a fascination for lesbians, but it scared me to think that maybe I wanted to love a woman—my parents would explode, my ex-husband would try to get custody of our kids, my friends might think I was out to seduce them. I was also afraid it would be a choice against men instead of for women. Finally, one day I said to myself, "For now, I am a lesbian," and some important piece of my identity clicked into place. I'm glad I chose to be a lesbian before I had a woman lover.

When I went to college there were only two other black students on the entire campus, and they came from comfortable middle-class families. I felt as out of place with them as I did with the middle-class white students. I began to become aware of an attraction to women, which I kept trying to suppress.

Since I was out of my element socially, I always came on as tough and aggressive to cover up, and people started accusing me of being a dyke. I was terrified that my fantasies were showing in some way, and I began dating to cover up. I knew that being a black woman gave everyone the right to walk on me (or try to, anyway), and I thought that being a black lesbian was some sort of capital crime.

The women's movement gave me support because I could see other women having the courage to change their lives. Their example gave me the courage to see that I was cheating myself by pretending to be straight. I reasoned that if a racist society wanted my head, they'd get it because I was black, and being gay wasn't going to make all that much difference. My life has been much fuller since then and a lot happier.

At first many of us try to deny our desire for women. It contradicts the expectations our families and society have for us—and, often, the expectations we have had for ourselves. Usually, all we've ever heard about "gays," "lesbians," "dykes," or "queers" is negative. We may not even know any openly l/b/t women.

In my little town in upstate New York I didn't know there were other dykes around at all. When I fell in love with a woman and became lovers with her at 16, she was the only person I knew who was gay. It was hard to say to myself, "I am a lesbian," when I didn't know any.

Stereotypes of l/b/t women may scare us away. But once we recognize and name ourselves, we can begin to define ourselves on our terms.

I remember the sting of words like maricón *[fag] and* tortillera *[lesbian]. I began to realize these words had something to do with me. But they didn't speak for me, for my feelings as a human being. . . . This was a time of incredible contradictions.*

We may want to reject our love for women because our sexist upbringing has taught us that women are inferior or because we know life will be hard or complicated (although possibly more satisfying) for us if we act on our desires.

Many of us have painful memories of trying to deny our feelings for women—dating men, getting married, consulting psychiatrists who tried to "cure" us, becoming dependent on alcohol or other drugs.

I was afraid that if I touched other girls I would like it and keep on touching them. So I became repulsed at the idea. I'm angry that I held the feelings down for so long that now I have a hard time just relaxing and touching someone I love.

Coming out to ourselves means learning to let go of the guilt, self-hatred, and fear that results from living in a homophobic society. Coming out means loving our whole selves as women who love women and being ready to celebrate our new-found sexuality.

When you first come out, it's like you're telling yourself something you don't want to believe. "You kissed that girl, didn't you? It felt good, didn't it? So what's wrong with it?" You finally begin to be honest with yourself. After that the rest of your life opens up.

When I came out, I didn't know any Asian lesbians in my city. I was raised in a very traditional Chinese family. Later I realized my sexual preference was for women, despite all the traditional Chinese expectations and the extreme homophobia of Chinese culture, along with all the other social expectations out there in American society.

I gradually began to integrate all three together: I tried to maintain my Chinese identity and to integrate that with feeling strong as a woman, tracing it basically through feelings of closeness with my grandmother, who was the matriarch of the family. I tried to pick out strong women in my personal past and to combine the traditions there that could help me to be strong as a woman and help me be able to feel strong about being a lesbian.

Coming Out to Friends and Family

Letting other people know we are attracted to women is usually more problematic than admitting it to ourselves. If we decide to be open about our sexuality, we become visible targets for physical and psychological harassment. We may be labeled sick, kept away from children, fired from our jobs. Yet, if we keep our sexuality hidden, we face insults and embarrassment when people assume we are heterosexual: Gynecologists want us to use birth control, friends want to fix us up with men, men make passes at us. We live with the fear that others will find out. We feel cut off from many of the people we love, and yet, full of new knowledge about ourselves, we want to share it with the people we are close to.

I want my family and friends to know I'm a lesbian because I want to be honest with them. I don't want to be hiding something from them, especially something so central to my life, something I'm glad about and proud of.

Many of us come out to friends first, choosing the ones who seem likely to be the most accepting.

One friend I came out to said, "I'm happy that you're in love. But I also feel that it's wrong, that you should have those feelings for a man." Once she said the negative part she seemed to let it go. From then on I asked my friends for their negative as well as positive responses, so they wouldn't try to be good "liberal" friends and hide the homophobic feelings that most everyone has somewhere.

My best friend for 13 years broke off our friendship several months after I told her, and I haven't heard from her in ten years. No matter how well you know someone, you can never know exactly what to expect from them when you come out.

Not being out to family is often particularly painful.

It's hard at family events when everyone is very heterosexual and brings their families and I'm not able to bring my lover. My aunts all ask when I'm going to marry.

Most parents have a hard time with the news.*

I look at my parents as being totally isolated. Who can they talk to about their daughter being lesbian? In this society people make very harsh judgments about gay people, and a judgment about a kid is taken as a judgment about the parents. My parents feel that they are responsible for the person I am, and they can get into guilt trips about what they "did wrong."

Thinking that lesbianism is something wrong and that it has a cause, parents may blame themselves.† Others don't take their daughter's choice seriously and keep hoping she'll meet a nice man and *really* fall in love.

---

* An excellent resource for parents is Parents and Friends of Lesbians and Gays (P-FLAG) (see Resources).
† The formation of sexual orientation (hetero, bi, or homo) is still not completely understood. Studies in the physical, social, and psychological sciences suggest that it is probably more fluid, less rigid, and determined by more factors than our society is currently willing to admit. Looking for a cause, however, usually implies that homophobic assumption that there is something wrong with being lesbian or gay. Who looks for causes of heterosexual orientation?

TEENAGERS COMING OUT

At fourteen I already knew I was different. All my girlfriends talked about was boys, and I wasn't interested. I dated a few guys, but mostly I skipped the social events. I picked out any strong women I could find and hung around with my coaches a lot. I was in trouble all the time—fighting with my parents, dealing drugs, drinking. I see now it was because I realized I was different and didn't know what to do about it.

The first thing I learned when I was a teenager coming out was to get a pair of dark sunglasses that no one could see through so I could look at all the cute girls without anybody knowing.

Some of us have always known that we are attracted to women, some of us discover that we are attracted to women as we get older. Maybe we recognize our attraction to a close friend, or we just know we're different, even, but we don't know how or why, or maybe we have romantic relationships with other young women.

During high school, you get all these messages about "your emerging sexuality." You could be exploring your sexuality in different ways: by yourself, with a boyfriend, or with a girlfriend. Wondering if your sexuality falls outside heterosexuality is called "questioning." Many of us went through a period of questioning before we came out. Usually, questioning is not easy. It can be hard to find friends who will listen to you without judging you or freaking out. Look for l/b/t groups in your area, or get online! It's totally normal to feel confused, depressed, or angry about being different, and it's important to find people who will understand and relate to you.

When I was 16, I told my boyfriend that I thought I might be attracted to girls. He said, "Great! Now we can have a threesome!" I was really pissed off because he didn't understand that it was about me, and not about him at all.

As you question and maybe even make the choice to come out, you will discover that there are many negative messages about gays. Remember that they come from narrow-minded people. These messages are not about you! You are a unique, wonderful person, and every aspect of your self contributes to that wonderful person. The world is homophobic (and sexist, and racist, etc.), but you can still lead a happy and fulfilling life.

Being different—whether it's because of your sexuality, or your background, or your personality—is a hard path to walk. It does get easier as you get older and gain more control over your life. But you have to be strong and stand up for who you are.

If you decide to come out to family or friends, think about what to expect before making your decision. Be strong, but don't set yourself up to get completely squashed. You might want to come out to people who are really close to you and who you think will accept you before you take on the rest of the world. Here are some things to think about.

1. Think about your family. Are your parents generally accepting? If your family is usually loving and accepting, they probably can handle this information. If not, you may not want to tell them. It's not easy to make your way as a teenager if your parents throw you out of the house, so err on the side of caution. If you do get thrown out (or you have to leave for your own protection), seek shelter with another family member or a friend. Try to call a gay hot line for information and support (see Resources).

2. Is there someone supportive that you could tell at school? A teacher, a guidance counselor? Is there a gay/straight alliance at school or a teen group in your area? Finding support is probably the best thing you can do for yourself. Many resources are listed at the end of this chapter.

3. If you feel depressed, do things that make you happy. Creative activities are sometimes helpful: keep a journal, draw, paint, take photographs. You might want to become involved in community work or political activism. You are likely to find people who accept your sexual orientation if you work with progressive groups like NOW or Amnesty International or if you do community service in places like battered women's shelters or homeless shelters.

4. Stay alive. Think about your future. If you don't make the choice to stay alive today, you won't have the choice tomorrow. If you feel like hurting yourself or committing suicide, call someone: a friend, a relative, a mentor, or a gay hot line. Talking to someone will help you through these times.

5. Look in the resource section of this chapter for teen talklines, teen centers, books, videos, and other resources that will help you get through this time. A book that you can probably find at your public library and is full of information is *Free Your Mind* by Ellen Bass and Kate Kaufman.

I can hear the tension in my parents' voices when they ask if the person I'm dating is a man or a woman. If I'm dating a man, they breathe a mental sigh of relief. . . . But if I'm dating a woman, they really don't know what to say.

Many parents react with anger, guilt, shame, hurt, and fear. Some react with violence: They may kick their l/b/t children out of the house, put them into mental institutions, kidnap and send them for deprogramming, disown them, or try to take their children away. L/b/t women with disabilities who come out to our families risk losing our family's care and their vital emotional and financial support. For l/b/t women of color, lack of family support can overflow into loss of community as questions of racial "loyalty" rise to the surface.

Some parents are accepting and supportive of their children who come out.

My mother's reaction was exceptional. She said, "I don't understand it at all, but I'm glad you're happy."

My father is afraid that I'll get hurt in a homophobic world, but he's trying hard to understand and support me. This year, he gave me two books on bisexuality for Christmas!

Coming out to family is often a process that takes several years. We change and grow as we come out, and our family changes with us, sometimes in congruence, sometimes in opposition. Some parents come to an understanding, even if they refuse any contact at first; some do not. Coming out makes family relationships more honest and sometimes more close than they would be if we kept living a lie. We may even be pleasantly surprised, as a lesbian grandmother reported: "One of my nineteen grandchildren said, 'I love telling my friends about my gay granny.'"

Beyond Friends and Family

How out is out? Some of us are comfortable with identifying ourselves to the world by our clothing, our appearance, or bumper stickers on our cars. Some of us believe that our sexuality is a private matter and should not be discussed in casual conversation. Each of us must decide for ourselves to what extent we want the world to know about our sexuality. Coming out—to our employers, doctors, supervisors, teachers, or clergy—can be risky.

Job discrimination, a problem for all women, hits l/b/t women hard. If we hide our sexuality in order to find a job, we fear being found out. Many l/b/t women keep totally "closeted" in the public eye, living a scrupulously careful double life. This is especially true for teachers and others who work with children, because gay people are stereotyped as child predators.

Yet, an increasing number of l/b/t women today are more open at work about our sexuality. In certain

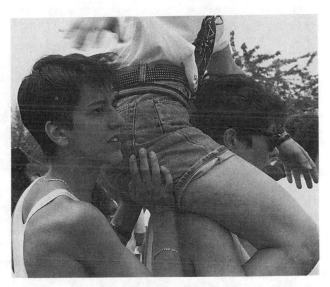

Women supporting women/Robin Melavalin

parts of the country, lesbian, bisexual, and transgendered/transsexual women and men have fought against job discrimination and won. Now, some employers even offer domestic partner benefits for same-gender couples. Employers in all fields need to learn that we'll work better at our jobs when we can be honest about who we are.*

Being a queer woman in a straight world is challenging enough. But many of us live outside "mainstream" U.S. society by virtue of our class, our race, our religious identity, or other factors in addition to our sexuality. When our identities overlap several communities, we often have specific cultural barriers to coming out and living openly and, as a result, conflicts within ourselves.

I identify as blue-collar, and I'm more comfortable with the working-class community. I relate to people who have struggled because I've struggled all my life. But a lot of blue-collar women don't accept me. The people I can be open with tend to be middle-class students. I'm very much an outsider.

People on the street deal with my disability sometimes, but no matter how butch I am or what buttons I have on, they won't deal with me as a lesbian.

L/b/t women of color often encounter prejudices within our home communities that are distinct from the prejudices we encounter in white society. We must grapple with two sets of stereotypes: that of our race and that of our sexuality.

Coming to womanhood as a Third World woman, regardless of your sexual preference, you have to deal with certain stereotypical images of Third World

* If you are interested in organizing in your workplace, contact Lambda Legal Defense and Education Fund (see Resources).

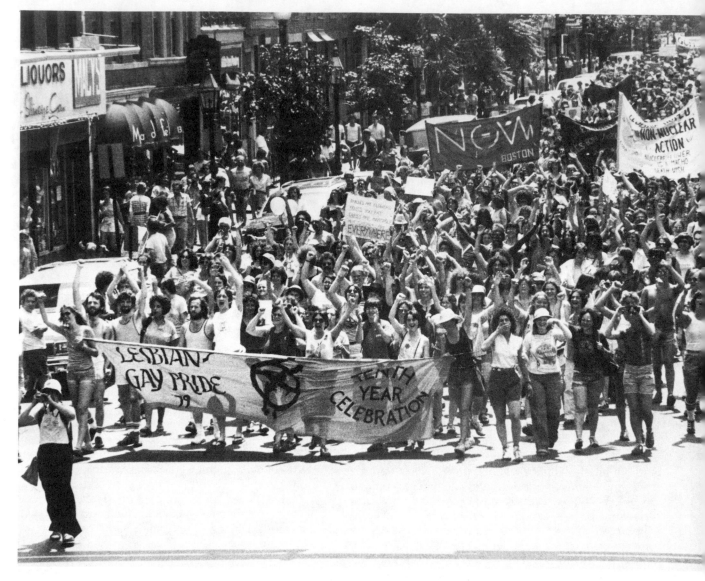

L/b/t women and our supporters have been marching for more than 20 years/Ellen Shub

women that are prevalent in this society. If you're a lesbian, it's even more difficult to struggle against these images. For a black woman, the images of the strong black woman who can carry everybody on her back or the earthy, sexy vamp are hard to fight against. Those images are unreal, confining, and racist, to say the least. Many people expect you to fit into some pre-conceived idea they have about what a black woman is supposed to be. They deny whole sides of you as a woman.

As women, and especially as Latina women, we have been programmed to be caretakers. Especially as lesbians, because we have never married, we often have to take care of everybody else, everybody else's family, everyone's needs. I'm taking care of myself now, too. I am affirming my life.

Some communities, particularly those that are marginalized in a bigoted society, draw strength and com-

fort from a strong, religious center. While some churches and synagogues have open doctrines, such as the Unitarian Universalist Church, the United Church of Christ, the Quakers, some Methodist churches, and some Jewish congregations, others teach that homosexuality is "immoral."

Despite this kind of institutionalized prejudice, many l/b/t women discover that tight family and friendship bonds prevail.

[In my experience,] in the black Christian church, they teach that lesbianism is wrong. But personal, individual homes is a different story. Black people don't disown [their children]. They're accepted. Families are not going to turn their child out of the house. . . . I was lucky. My parents were very accepting. If I wanted to bring someone home, it was no problem.

For me, there is no conflict between being Jewish and being queer. The culture of being Jewish applies to me

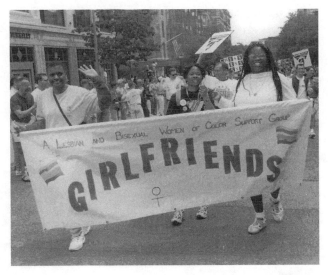

Ellen Shub

more than the laws do. Some people in my family would respond negatively [to my sexuality], not because they are Jewish, but because they are conservative.

The more l/b/t women are able to be visible, the more chance people have to see us realistically rather than stereotypically, to notice our support of each other, and to feel our strength. Our increasing visibility in numbers enables us to work more effectively against job discrimination and other kinds of oppression that have made many l/b/t women stay hidden.

I want us all to announce, "We're Lesbians!" all at the same time. People would be shocked to discover they know lots of lesbians, that they like us, respect us. If people were really aware of how many of us there are, they'd have a much harder time seeing us as abnormal.

I don't think I'm an alarmist when I say that I find it is more often not safe to be obviously out. In my experience, homophobia is as intense and pervasive as racial and sexual prejudice, plus it is still legally and socially reinforced. I don't think the answer is to act closeted. I think it is to be aware of the risks, evaluate them, prepare for them, and then take them.

FINDING OUR COMMUNITIES

Contact with other l/b/t women is crucial to feeling good about who we are.

I had already been in a relationship with a woman for two years when we discovered the lesbian community and its social, political, and cultural events. All of a sudden we felt like we belonged somewhere, and we started to identify as lesbians.

I didn't think there were any older lesbians in the whole city. Then two friends of mine gave a party and *invited all the lesbians they knew over 40 years old. It made me feel entirely different to look around that room and see how many we were. Now we meet every month.*

As late as the 1950s, most lesbians were extremely isolated from each other.

Unless you knew someone who knew someone else, the only place to meet lesbians was in the bars, and maybe you didn't like the bar scene. There were few books except lurid novels where lesbians were miserable and usually died unhappily, no newspapers that I knew of, no groups to go to. I was hungry for contact.

Thanks to the many gay, bisexual, and transgendered women and men who have struggled for our right to live and love openly and with pride, we now have many networks and organizing tools for reaching out to one another. Although the bars offer a place for some l/b/t women to meet openly and relax together, we now have gathering places that are not built around alcohol and night life and that reflect all the different interests we have. Daughters of Bilitis (DOB), founded in the 1950s, was the first to provide a place for lesbians to get together for sociability and discussion. Later, after Stonewall* and the emergence of the women's movement, organizations such as Lesbian Liberation and Radicalesbians focused on the politics of gay liberation and feminism. During the 1970s, we saw the emergence of a vibrant "women's" culture: lesbian music and books created by lesbian recording and publishing companies as well as woman-owned and operated restaurants, bookstores, banks, and community centers that catered to lesbians. Lesbians bought land in rural areas and created independent communities; they formed distribution networks to disseminate all the new books, magazines, and records; and they launched numerous women-only summer music festivals that continue to attract thousands of women every year.† In 1979, lesbians and gay men made their voices heard during the first national gay and lesbian march on Washington.

Since the 1980s, l/b/t groups have sprung up to match every interest. First, there are identity groups that provide queer women a safe space to meet and share experiences. There are groups for older women, women with disabilities, women of color, youth, and mothers, to name just a few. Second, there are groups

---

* The June 1969 Stonewall Riots are often cited as the birth of the contemporary lesbian and gay liberation movement. During a police raid on the Stonewall Bar in Greenwich Village, the patrons of the bar, mostly drag queens, fought back, setting off three days of rioting and ending an era in which gay people lived in constant fear of harassment. After the riots, numerous gay liberation organizations began to fight for full civil rights for gays and lesbians.

† In recent years, controversy over the presence of transsexuals and transgenders has divided the Michigan Women's Music Festival. Although more women express acceptance every year, the atmosphere is still unwelcoming to those who are trans.

that focus on politics and social change, ranging from the National Gay and Lesbian Task Force and the National Center for Lesbian Rights, which struggle to challenge the courts and change laws that oppress us, to the Lesbian Avengers and the Transsexual Menace, which are militant activist groups dedicated to humorous and/or confrontational tactics to promote l/b/t visibility as well as other progressive issues such as affirmative action. We have created our own religious communities, including the Metropolitan Community Church, Dignity (Catholic), Integrity (Episcopal), and Am Tikva (Jewish). Finally, there are groups that bring l/b/t people together to socialize and participate in a shared interest, such as country-western dancing, motorcycle riding, or choral singing. L/b/t women have organized around health issues, including AIDS, chronic fatigue immune deficiency syndrome (CFIDS), and breast cancer; have promoted and taught lesbian and gay studies courses; and have created l/b/t caucuses within other organizations. In the 1990s, we've seen the emergence of l/b/t culture on the Internet, a national Lesbian Conference held in Atlanta (1991), the establishment of an annual national female-to-male transsexual conference, and organizations promoting lesbian and gay marriage and the acceptance of gays and lesbians in the military. The 1993 March on Washington for Gay, Lesbian and Bisexual Rights, which according to organizers drew about one million people, may have been the largest civil rights march up to that point in history and was the scene of the first Dyke March, now a tradition during many June gay-pride celebrations.

The wide array of l/b/t groups and cultural and political events, particularly in large urban areas, offer chances to take that first step in getting to know other l/b/t women. (It's also a great way to find a girlfriend!) Of course, we may initially feel shy.

The first time I headed for the lesbian support group at the Women's Center I walked around the block four times and went home. I was scared to come out to a whole new group of people. The next month my need for friendship and support won out over my fears, and I went in.

Finding a "home" community is crucial for all l/b/t women, no matter how long we have been out. Meeting others gives us a mirror for our experiences and a sense of our own unique history.

When I came out in college, most of the queer women I knew were white, and some were African American. Then, when I moved to San Francisco, I saw a float in the San Francisco Pride Parade for Filipino gays and lesbians. I was amazed! The queen dancing on the float looked down, caught my expression, and smiled and beckoned to me. It meant so much to me to see others living proud, queer, and Filipino.

It's good to mix older and younger lesbians. When younger people get together more often with older lesbi-

ans and see that we're not doddering and so on, they'll be aware that there's not that much difference, and perhaps it will make it easier for them as they grow older.

If the first group you attend isn't for you, keep searching! There are so many options out there. You are bound to find the right place for yourself.

Differences and disagreements sometimes polarize different segments of the l/b/t community. Racism creates division and conflict, as it does everywhere in the United States. Lesbians of color often experience white lesbians as not respecting or sharing power with women of color in political groups and unwilling to confront their own racism. When white lesbians assume that their experience parallels that of people of color in this country, they ignore both their own privilege as white-skinned women in a racist society and the complex layers of discrimination that affect the daily lives of lesbians of color.

As a white, middle-class lesbian I can get very focused on the ways my family and the larger society discriminate against me and hurt me because of my sexual orientation. I do this because in most every other way I fit into the mainstream, dominant culture. It is easy for me to forget that other lesbians and bisexual women—women of color, women with disabilities, women who don't have my economic privilege—deal with many additional injustices, facing daily insults and dangers. Their sexual orientation is not their only or necessarily even their primary issue. To the extent that I forget this, it's not really possible for me to participate in building real coalitions.

Other issues divide us as well. Bisexual and transgendered or transsexual women have felt shunned or excluded from the lesbian community.

I rarely try to appear straight, [but] I feel pressure to be a lesbian. It's harder for me to hold onto my bi identity in a lesbian context than in a straight context. I'm afraid they'll say I'm "not queer enough."

L/b/t women with disabilities and chronic illness have had to struggle with able-bodied women to make them see the need to make community events wheelchair accessible, smoke- and scent-free, and sign-language interpreted.

Growing up I always felt there was something fundamentally wrong with me. Partly because I was a girl, partly because I am a dyke. When I developed a chronic injury, that was my frame of reference. I realized that it could no longer be my frame of reference if I wanted to heal. Growing up I also felt a sense of not belonging. Now I have multiple chemical sensitivities. The world is set up so I can't be there.

Most important, white middle-class lesbians and bisexuals have not always seen the need to join in the

RURAL L/B/T WOMEN

Meeting other women who desire romantic relationships with women in a small town or rural area can be very hard.

This is one section of the country where nothing different is accepted. It is a backwoods area. There aren't a lot of gay women here. If there are more, they are well hidden from the rest of us.

Some suggestions:

1. Read books and/or listen to records by and about lesbian, bisexual, and transgendered/ transsexual women who partner with women. They can make you feel good about your sexuality. (See Resources for mail-order women's bookstores.)

2. Contact the nearest lesbian, bisexual, gay, or trans organization (no matter how far away!). Check guides such as *Gaia's Guide* or *Places of Interest to Women,* or contact national lesbian, bisexual, and gay groups (see Resources). Ask to be on their mailing list. Organizations that are inaccessible because of distance may be able to tell you about nearby groups or give you the name of a woman who could put you in touch with other l/b/t women in your area.

3. Become involved in women's political activities. Is there a women's center near you, maybe in a university? Any feminist groups? Many l/b/t women are politically active, and most women's groups have l/b/t members.

4. Go to women's events such as concerts, conferences, and festivals. Many women's music festivals are held in the summertime in rural areas. Listings of upcoming festivals appear in feminist and lesbian and gay newspapers. Even if these events are not close to you, you might meet other l/b/t women from your area there, or someone who knows someone.

5. Start a fund for a gay getaway! Lesbian guides and women's newspapers will have listings of companies that offer cruises, outdoor adventures, and other getaways specifically for l/b/t women.

6. Get connected to the Internet. (If you can't afford your own computer, try the public library.) A World Wide Web search will turn up home pages for l/b/t groups and chat rooms for those who want to discuss everything from coming out to kinky safe sex techniques.

7. Look for cars with rainbow, lambda, or pink or black triangle bumper stickers. Many queer women and men use these symbols to identify themselves.

Have faith! We are everywhere!

wide range of struggles that affect women who face multiple oppressions.

There's been both sensitivity and a lack thereof in the lesbian community. We can confront other lesbians about things that wouldn't even come up in the heterosexual world—like not just getting wheelchair access to concerts but being able to sit with our friends. Yet where were other lesbians when we picketed inaccessible movie houses? Our power and strength are used for lesbian issues at lesbian rallies, but few women rally for us.

Often, what brings us back together is our solidarity in the face of attacks upon us. The right-wing has made anti-homosexuality the centerpiece of its agenda, actively working to appeal laws protecting the rights of gay, lesbian, bisexual, and transgendered people; campaigning against the right of gays and lesbians to marry or to teach in schools; and spreading lies about our lives. This aggressive attack on the queer community has led to increases in the number and the virulence of documented anti-lesbian and anti-gay hate crimes, but it has also promoted increasingly visible queer activism.* Because of the efforts of organizations like the National Gay and Lesbian Task Force, the 1996 Congress came within one vote of passing the Employment Non-Discrimination Act, which would have protected gays and lesbians against job discrimination. Still, in 1997, only ten states and the District of Columbia have passed civil rights laws prohibiting discrimination on the basis of sexual orientation in public or private institutions, leaving most l/b/t women vulnerable to the whims of landlords, employers, and people who simply can't accept our right to live freely, fully, and openly.

SEXUALITY†

Once a woman recognizes she's attracted to another woman, the missionary position goes right out the window.

* Some gay, bi, and trans women and men have joined the Pynk Patrol or Pink Panthers, groups similar to the Guardian Angels, which patrol the streets to defend queers against hate attacks.
† To enjoy sex with another woman while minimizing exposure to human immunodeficiency virus (HIV) transmission (the cause of AIDS) or other STDs, see chapter 14, Sexually Transmitted Diseases, and chapter 15, HIV, AIDS, and Women. For specifics about women's sexual response and more information on bisexuality, see chapter 11, Sexuality.

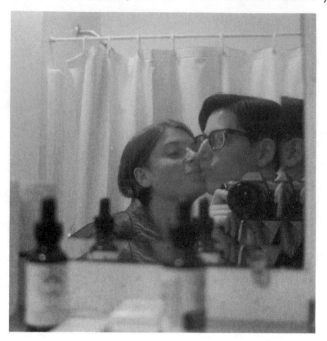

Hannah Doress

I am attracted to the same thing in both men and women: strength. If they can carry me to bed, I'm there.

People think disabled women are sexless. If I came out at work I don't know if they'd be upset or just laugh. They'd say, how can you be a lesbian if you don't have sex?

Sex with women invites us to redefine what having sex means. We may find that a whole new world of erotic possibilities opens up for us when we are intimate with another woman. Through sex we may express love, friendship, lust, nurturance, need, a sense of adventure, delight in our own bodies. We may kiss and hug a lot, caress our lover's body for hours, play with her nipples or clitoris, explore her vagina with our fingers or our tongues, touch our own bodies, reach orgasm or not. We may enjoy sex that is slow and gentle, or sex that is sometimes rough and aggressive. The possibilities are endless: massaging, hugging, licking, kissing, biting, rimming (oral to anal stimulation), spanking or whipping, caressing, direct clitoral stimulation, vaginal or anal penetration, nipple stimulation, fisting, oral sex, playing with power and roles, tribadism (rubbing a body part against your partner's genitals), erotic talk, or sleeping together without genital sex.

To enhance our sexual experience, some of us choose to use sex toys and other erotic materials. Sex toys can range from dildos to vibrators—in many shapes, sizes, and colors—to cucumbers, carrots, and candles, or anything else that strikes your fancy. Try experimenting with ice cubes, feathers, massage oil, or different foods (like whipped cream, chocolate, or honey). Watch erotic videos or read sexy passages of your favorite books. Let your fantasies lead the way.

Sex with my male lovers was always okay. But with Paula I'm amazed at the intensity. I want to touch and be touched, make love all the time, be rough, be gentle, penetrate her, feel her moving on me. I think I'm finally feeling the fullness and depth of my sexuality. I had always suspected there must be more to it, but hadn't figured out how to find it.

There is no one way to be sexual with another woman.

I want my lover on her back, my first two fingers curling up, as if to say "come here baby" inside her, my thumb on her clit, her voluptuous body shuddering. I like the same thing, but lying on my stomach. My lover says she loves hands because their possibilities are endless.

Making love with a woman for the first time usually involves a lot more than what happens sexually. We may feel suddenly freed as sexual beings. We may feel exhilarated and joyful and terrified out of our skins. It can take months and even years to learn about our shifting patterns in sex, what we like, and what our particular stumbling blocks are.

In finding out what turns my lover on, exploring her body, tasting her, learning her odors and textures, I am growing to love myself more, too.

I felt weird because [as a woman with a disability] I had to explain what my sexual needs were to anyone I wanted to sleep with until I realized that everyone has to explain what their needs are in order to get them met. I don't have sensation in my pubic area, but since there is no set standard to what lesbian lovemaking is, it leaves a whole world of sexuality and sensuality open to explore.

Although our woman lover has a body similar to ours, she may not like the same things we like. Our desires are as varied as we are. This means that sex with another woman is bound to be exciting, but also that it is not problem-free.

The more women I sleep with, the more I realize you can't assume what you like is what she likes. There are tremendous differences.

We had a wildly passionate sex life for a year and a half. When we moved in together, sexuality suddenly became an issue. It turned out our patterns were very different. My lover needs to talk, to feel intimate in conversation, to relax completely before she can feel sexual. I need to touch and to make a physical connection first before I feel relaxed enough to talk intimately. I'd reach out for her as we went into the bedroom and she'd freeze. We battled it out for months, both feeling terrible, before we figured out what was going on.

It doesn't help that most women, whether heterosexual or not, have internalized heterosexual models of sexuality that often make us insecure about our own desires. We may bring the following to lovemaking:

- The assumption that we owe it to our lovers to have sex when they want to.
- Distrust of our sexual responses—the conviction that we can't reach orgasm in sex with a partner.
- Little experience in being assertive or taking the lead in sex.
- The belief that we don't like sex much and are perhaps undersexed or "frigid."
- The feeling that sex is okay but not very profound.
- Shyness about touching ourselves in sex because we think (or we think our partner thinks) she should do it all.
- A focus on performance in lovemaking, including orgasm as a goal every time.
- Emotional scars from a history of sexual abuse.

In addition, our own sexual impulses and preferences may make us uncomfortable when they seem to follow a male model. We may feel uncomfortable with lust, for instance, or with acting aggressively, having fantasies of dominance or using erotic materials. Yet, these may be aspects of sexuality that we would enjoy. A dildo, for instance, is not a "penis substitute"; it may give us pleasure if we enjoy being penetrated in sex. As lesbians we have a chance to move away from male-defined sexuality and to reclaim all the dimensions of sexuality that deepen our intimacy, pleasure, and love.

For example, some l/b/t women practice bondage and domination (B & D) and sadomasochism (S/M)—that is, eroticizing the *consensual* exchange of power with the goal of safe, sane, and highly charged sex.* S/M and B & D allow us to experiment with sexualized power relationships within the realm of fantasy and role playing.

I'm a queer's queer. S/M is the erotic and philosophical center of my insistence upon a life of passion, presence, and hard truths. "Serious fun": that's what my lover and I call the world of forbidden eroticism in which we stage our most intimate and courageous moments.

Because women are so deeply socialized not to be sexually assertive or to seek pleasure openly, it can be a revelation to learn with a lesbian lover how to talk freely about what you both want in sex.

---

* These practices have been highly controversial within lesbian communities. For both sides of the debate, see *The Lesbian S/M Safety Manual,* by Pat Califia, ed. (Lace Publications, 1988), and *Sex Wars,* by Lisa Dugan (Routledge, 1996), as well as *Against SadoMasochism: A Radical Feminist Analysis,* by Robin Linden, Darlene Pagano, Diane Russell, and Susan Star, eds. (Frog in the Well, 1982), and *Lesbian Heresy,* by Sheila Jeffreys (Spinifex, 1994).

When I make love with a woman, the challenge is to be honest more often; to say what I am really feeling; to explore when I'm not feeling present instead of pretending that I am; if I am spacing out, to ask what's the fear.

Talking with our women lovers includes negotiating about safer sex—*before having sex.* Never having had to deal with birth control with a woman partner, we may feel awkward bringing up safer sex, but it's crucial. It is a dangerous myth that women who partner with women are not at risk of passing STDs or HIV infection to each other. We *are* at risk—and not because l/b/t women who partner with men "bring" HIV or other diseases into the community. This, too, is a dangerous myth. It makes us suspicious of each other and divides our communities. Many sexual practices transmit STDs and HIV. It is essential to protect ourselves by using appropriate barriers—latex gloves, finger cots, and dental dams—to prevent the sharing of bodily fluids. (See chapters 14 and 15 on STDs and HIV infection for more information on enjoying sex and staying healthy.)

For many of us, finding time and energy for sex seems to be the biggest problem of all.

It's all there: How are you feeling about your work? About the people you work with? Or about the fact that the house hasn't been vacuumed in two weeks, and the car needs something done to it? Gosh, it really would be nice to have a little time for sex now and then.

We need to feel free to be sexual, whatever form that takes for us. We are learning as women to balance what we give to others by taking time for ourselves: Maybe we also have to affirm the need for taking time for sexual pleasure.

People say lesbians don't have much sex. Well, I know a whole lot of lesbians who have a whole lot of sex, and good sex, at that!

If you or your lover(s) have problems with sex, you may want to join a discussion group or seek counseling. (See chapter 11 Resources.) But we might also feel comfortable discussing sexual problems, issues, and discoveries with our friends. "How's your sex life?" or "My girlfriend and I found this great edible body oil" can provoke helpful, therapeutic, and fun conversations.

RELATIONSHIPS

L/b/t women's relationships run the spectrum from celibacy to having many kinds of love in our lives to everything in between. We may be single; we may have one partner; we may have several partners. No matter what kind of relationships we have, however, most of us have grown up in a predominately heterosexual society, and our models of intimacy reflect that.

We are inundated with heterosexual images in the media, despite the fact that a few books and films and even TV shows are beginning to include openly lesbian characters.

Among these heterosexual models is the institution of marriage. Some of us choose to marry our same-sex partners because we see marriage as the way to demonstrate our commitment to each other. We want same-sex couples to enjoy the same rights and privileges as heterosexual couples; yet, at this time in the U.S., these rights and privileges are accorded *only* to *officially married* (i.e., heterosexual) couples. Others of us want to challenge the legitimacy of marriage (historically a religious institution) as the only "valid" relationship structure in the eyes of the state. We reject marriage because it unfairly privileges couples over those of us who choose to have deeply committed relationships with more than one person as well as those of us who prefer to remain single.

When I was married at 19, I knew exactly what I was supposed to do forever. I didn't have to think about it. When I entered into my first lesbian relationship, I didn't have any idea. Without role models, how we live has to come from our gut, and mostly I like it that way.

Being lesbian gives me a chance to do things differently from heterosexual couples I've seen. I've decided that I've got to be up front about my very human need for sexual dependability.

I am always surprised how many of my lesbian friends have ex-lovers as best friends. I wonder if it is because the community is so small, if women have a harder time letting go or if women simply are able to maintain better relationships with each other. It is not the same for my straight friends.

Of course, same-gender relationships raise many of the same issues that straight relationships do, but we are often more able to exercise the freedom to find our own solutions, thus creating examples for future generations of women, regardless of their sexuality. (For a more detailed discussion of intimacy and power in relationships, please refer to chapter 9, Working Toward Mutuality: Our Relationships with Men.)

Choosing Not to Be in One Major Relationship

Q: What does a lesbian bring to a second date?
A: A U-Haul.

—Lea DeLaria, comedian

As with heterosexual women, women who partner with women often place a tremendous emphasis on being part of a couple.

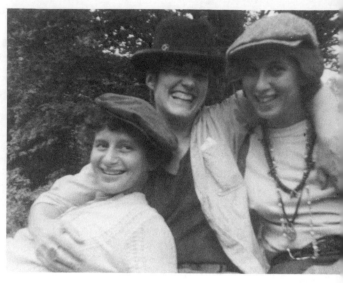

Shay Oglesby-Smith

The only thing that we have in our heads is: you meet a woman, you feel for her, you enter into a relationship, you relate only to her. It's been the downfall of many intimacies.

Yet some of us prefer to have relationships with women in ways that are not limited to the couple. We can choose to be single, to have many lovers, or to have more than one primary relationship.

We may choose singleness because we want some time alone, because we want to develop our independence, or because we feel more comfortable that way. Sometimes we look for satisfaction and approval from another person, and making alternative choices about one's life—being single or having many lovers—can help us find satisfaction within ourselves.

Usually after the end of a relationship, I take a period of time to be celibate. The last time I did it for six months, and I found it was a wonderful time to enjoy my sexuality without getting into any trouble, to learn about my habits and patterns in relationships, and to free up energy for personal growth and career development.

There are so many more women in my life now, so much room for so many more women.

I like the feeling of trying to create something new.

In choosing not to be in a couple, we do not necessarily distance ourselves from others. We still want, and have, intimate friendships. Some of us are sexually intimate with friends.

It's very hard for me to draw the line between friends and lovers, so I sleep with some of my very close friends. I find that really satisfying. A lot of the time I sleep with very close friends without having sex, which I find equally satisfying.

Choosing not to be in a primary relationship, for whatever reason, often gives us a chance to learn more about ourselves and to grow in ways that are sometimes stifled when we are absorbed in a couple. Intimacy can be found in many kinds of relationships, and we must all find what works best for ourselves.

Having One Primary Lover

Many of us choose to be in an intimate sexual relationship with one other woman, whether or not we live together. We build a relationship—planning our work and play so we can count on spending time together, helping each other through personal changes and difficulties, working through conflicts. We might stay together as lovers for a few months, a few years, or a lifetime.

I like being with someone who follows all the threads of my life, even the most mundane.

When I hear another lesbian talking about being involved as lovers and friends with lots of women, it excites me. I know that by choosing to be with one woman I am missing out on a certain kind of emotional adventure. But for my lover and me there is a kind of adventure I prefer at this point. Finally, after a few years, we are able to say to each other, "I need you," and know what that means. It doesn't mean, "I'm hopeless on my own—I can't let you go," but does mean risking a certain kind of interdependence that I haven't known before.

Alice and I grew up in different worlds—she in the '50s and I in the '20s. So much has changed, especially for women. What she wants for her life is not what I ever wanted or expected for mine. As long as both of us notice, respect, and understand these differences, we do well together. In a way, the age span is good— it makes us see that we can't be everything for each other, that we need friends our own age.

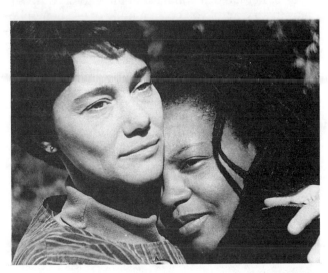

Alison Melavalin

Although there are endless differences between any two women, a certain closeness comes from being the same sex—similar body, similar socialization. When we are in a primary relationship with another woman, we can slip into being so close that there isn't enough breathing room. We have to work to find a healthy balance between closeness and distance, to define ourselves assertively, and to encourage each other to grow as individuals.

It's critical that my lover and I really understand our boundaries, where we want to say no and where we want to say yes. If I don't build my own privacy right away into a relationship, then the next thing I know I'm either spacing out or leaving.

If you get involved with a woman who lives far away or has to move for a job, you can't either of you assume the other is going to give up her home, friends, or job so you can be together. You both know how important all these are. My lover right now lives in another state. I hate the separation, but I value her independence as I value my own.

Keeping a long-term primary relationship alive and well takes work, and by refusing to acknowledge the significance of these relationships, straight society doesn't make it easier. Although much is changing (see "Oppression and Support," p. 214) lesbian relationships still lack the legal and social supports of heterosexual relationships. Fortunately, l/b/t women in long-term couples are sharing their stories through books, films, and other media (see Resources).

Butch-Femme Relationships

Many women who came out before the women's movement of the late 1960s and early 1970s were part of a gay culture where women were either butch (more "masculine") or femme (more "feminine"). Butch/femme was a dress code, a behavior code, but most of all an erotic partnership. Some people understand "butch" and "femme" as gender identities within the queer community, thus challenging the mainstream view that there are only two genders: man and woman.

I was a fem, a woman who loved and wanted to nurture the butch strength in other women. Although I have been a lesbian for over 20 years and embrace feminism as a world view, I can spot a butch 50 feet away and still feel the thrill of her power. Contrary to belief, this power is not bought at the expense of the fem's identity. Butch–fem relationships, as I experienced them, were complex erotic statements, not phony heterosexual replicas. They were filled with a deeply lesbian language of stance, dress, gesture, loving, courage, and autonomy. . . . Butch-fem was an erotic partnership, serving both as a conspicuous flag of rebellion and as an intimate exploration of women's sexuality.[1]

This complex gender system was rejected by lesbian feminists who came out in the post-Stonewall era. Lacking an understanding of the complexities of butch-femme relationships, these "new" lesbians saw butches as imitating men and femmes as playing "wife," thus reproducing the patriarchy in a lesbian world. Many of the women who were part of the "old gay" culture were excluded from the movement and considered antifeminist for wanting to maintain a gender system and a culture in which they felt comfortable. Although some women felt freed by the new politics of feminism and gay liberation, others felt that they no longer had a place as lesbians.

But lesbian feminists never eliminated the butch-femme culture; they simply sent it underground. As middle-class lesbian feminists became the predominant voices of the movement, working-class butch-femme couples were silenced.

Butches and femmes found their voices again in the 1980s as lesbians began to publicly debate issues of sexuality. In the 1990s, many younger lesbians have begun again to identify with this uniquely lesbian gender system. Today roles are less rigid, identities more fluid. Some women identify as femme, some as butch. Some identify as butchy-femme, some as medium butch, some as androgynous, and some as nothing in particular.

Neither drag nor political statement nor fashionable fad, my butch identity is my birthright, my heritage. It's the challenge of inhabiting a territory until recently uncharted and taboo. It's the gift of walking between and in both gender realms and loving the femmes who understand.

When I was in college, I felt I could never fit into the lesbian community there, because I didn't want to shave my head or wear men's clothing. Whenever I tried to adopt such a look, I felt uncomfortable. Identifying as a femme finally freed me to feel fully queer and fully myself. I love the variety of named and unnamed gender identities among queer women in the 1990s.

Oppression and Support

Most heterosexual couples can hold hands in public, go anywhere together, feel welcomed by their families and at religious services, and celebrate their relationships openly. Though some interracial couples may not share all of these freedoms, they, along with other heterosexuals, are able to make decisions for each other in times of sickness and provide for each other's material well-being in case of death. Women in intimate relationships with women can take none of these commonplace things for granted.

In the faculty room where I work, I hear the other teachers talking about their relationships . . . nothing real heavy, but they do give each other a lot of support. Since being out to them would mean losing my job, I can't let off steam all day; if Ann's sick and I'm worried about her I can't get any comfort at work. If we have a big decision to make, I can't ask for help in sorting it out. All this makes our lesbian friends terribly important, especially the ones who talk with us about our relationship.

It is important to support each other as l/b/t women. Today in simple, daily ways we can ask our friends how their relationships are going, give each other a chance to talk about fights, commitment, jealousy, work, housework, and all the other things people need to talk about. Some of us are finding religious or spiritual communities that honor our relationships and celebrate our commitments. We are creating our own rituals, where friends and family (sometimes blood relatives, sometimes alternative families, sometimes both) come together to affirm our identities, to honor our commitments, and to celebrate our families.

We are lucky to be living in a time when we are beginning to gain institutional support for our relationships. Soon, in the state of Hawaii, we may even gain the rights and privileges of marriage (see "Legal Issues," p. 221). We look forward to the time when we can all love more openly, more bravely, more outrageously, and more deeply, in as many ways as we can create.

Violence in Relationships

Despite the appealing image of love between women as somehow free of the painful misuse of power that plagues so many heterosexual couples, lesbian relationships can be marked by physical, verbal, or emotional abuse. Abuse can take many forms. Even if your lover does not actually physically harm you, you may be experiencing abuse in a relationship if you feel frequently insulted and demeaned by your lover or frightened by her physically or emotionally; if she uses intimidation of any kind to control what you do or how much time you spend with your family or friends; if she rages at you and blames you for problems in her life that you have nothing to do with. She may try to control you economically or use homophobia against you, threatening to tell others—for example your boss, ex-husband, family, or social service providers who control your economic status, immigration status, or the custody of your children—that you are an l/b/t woman.

You can look out for some warning signs that are common among batterers: excessive jealousy or romanticism, keeping you up all night by telling you how much she loves you and thereby depriving you of sleep so that you are more vulnerable. Even if you love each other, this kind of treatment is abusive, and you may want to seek help in getting free of the relationship.*

Battered women's shelters have struggled with the

---

* See Resources at the end of this chapter for a list of books on sexual abuse and battering, and the number for the National Domestic Violence Hotline. See also chapter 8, Violence Against Women.

long-hidden problem of lesbian battering. Initially, many lesbians who fled abusive relationships with women lovers found their problems misunderstood or overlooked by shelter workers. Though you may still encounter homophobia and heterosexism, more shelters are training their staffs and reaching out to battered lesbians. Still, it is often difficult to find a safe space. Your abuser may try to gain access to you at a shelter by claiming that she, the batterer, is really the victim. Confidentiality is important, especially in small communities. If your safety is at risk, seek help and tell as few people as possible where you are going.

We have only very recently begun to recognize rape as a possibility and a problem in our communities. Rape is any unwanted sexual act forced on one person by another. Unfortunately, many rape crisis centers do not recognize lesbian rape and do not offer help.

Sadly, many women who are battered or raped by women lose their community because they can never be assured of their safety. They may encounter their abuser at the local bar, at a concert, or at the meeting of a political group. Friends may feel confused, not wanting to "take sides." As l/b/t women, we must make an effort to create safe spaces for each other. Battering and rape in the l/b/t community has the same causes as battering in a heterosexual context: it is about one person's power over another (see chapter 8, Violence Against Women). You do not deserve to be controlled or hurt in any way. Seek out organizations that are specifically designed to help women in relationships with women (see Resources).

RAISING CHILDREN

Women who love women construct our families in a wide variety of ways. Some of us have long-term partnerships; others have multiple partners. Some of us have "chosen families" that include our lovers and our closest friends (male and female, queer and straight, single and coupled); some of us relate most closely to our biological families. Our families may look no different from a heterosexual nuclear family, or they may not resemble that institution at all. Often outsiders to our families of origin, we have used our energy and creativity to mold new concepts of family and community.

Choosing to raise children in the context of our l/b/t families is a relatively new trend. Until the 1980s, most children being raised by l/b/t women were from a previous relationship with a man (or, occasionally, a woman, in the case of male-to-female transsexuals). By the late 1980s, however, we began to experience what has come to be called the "lesbian baby boom." More and more l/b/t women, either alone or in couples, are choosing to become mothers. This shows how much we have come to accept and respect ourselves. Despite all the negative messages we hear about the "impact of homosexuality on our youth," as l/b/t women we know that we are just as capable as heterosexuals of loving and caring for children. What we have to remember is that it is also okay to choose to remain childless. Not all l/b/t women (or straight women for that matter) want to raise children—and that is an equally valid choice.

Some of us live with our children; some do not. Some of us are out to our children; others are not. Our support systems vary: Some of us are single parents; some of us co-parent with our female partners, some with our child's father, some with gay men; some of us live in communities where we all share in the care of one anothers' children. We receive very different amounts of support from friends, the child's father, and/or blood relatives. Some of us live in neighborhoods where we can be relatively open about our relationships with women; others among us have to keep our sexuality hidden from adult and child neighbors alike. In general, however, our daily family lives look pretty much like those of other families.

I leave today for a seven-day work trip. Meanwhile, back at the ranch, my lover is pretty miffed because along with the fact that I'm here and she and the baby are there, I spent my last day home at the computer, instead of being "normal" and spending the day after Thanksgiving buying a Christmas tree and shopping with my family. Ours is a typical overworked harried American post-modern lesbian family story.

Having Children

Choosing how to have a child and going through the process can be very challenging, time-consuming, and expensive. It is not uncommon for this process to take several years. Basically, for women who want to have children without having sex with a man, there are two choices: donor insemination or adoption.

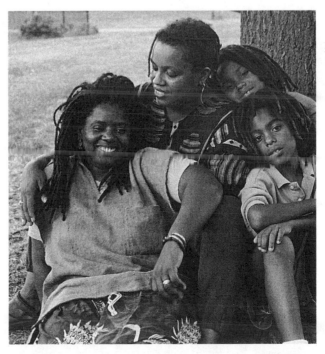

Gigi Kaeser

In both cases, it is extremely important for you and your partner to be aware of your custody rights. Birth mothers have strong legal claims to custody, but for female partners and foster mothers, the ties are much more tenuous. In some states, female partners can be granted second-parent adoption, which is a significant legal bond. An alternative option is co-guardianship, but guardianship rights can be withdrawn by the biological mother.

When considering your legal options, you may want to call an adoption agency or a lawyer outside your jurisdiction with whom you can openly discuss your situation and collect information. When you finally get in touch with the person you will work with, you will understand your options and can conceal your sexuality if necessary. For more complete information on insemination and adoption issues specific to l/b/t women, call or write to Gay and Lesbian Advocates and Defenders or the National Center for Lesbian Rights (see Resources). They can provide you with the laws and rulings specific to your state.

Donor Insemination *

You can choose to inseminate with a known or unknown donor. If you choose to inseminate using the semen of a family member (for example the brother of your partner) or friend or other known donor, you may face complex legal issues down the road. Many women like the idea of using a known donor either because they would like the donor to participate in the child's life (as a father, uncle, or family friend) or because they want to give their child the option of knowing their father in the future. However, there is always the risk with a known donor that the father could decide that he wants a greater role in the child's life (see "Legal Issues," p. 221).

If you choose anonymous insemination through a sperm bank, you will need to find a health care provider willing to work with single women and/or same-gender couples. Many health care providers will inseminate only women in heterosexual partnerships. There are, however, programs specifically designed for lesbian parents (see Resources). These programs can take you through the decision-making process and the actual pregnancy, and connect you with other women who are having children about the same time you are. If you choose to inseminate with an unknown donor, it is important to choose your sperm bank carefully.†

Insemination often takes many months and may take a year or more. This is often a stressful time for couples, because so much attention is focused on the insemination process and the goal of pregnancy. If you are the one not being inseminated you may find that you sometimes feel left out or as if you have no control over your life. You may find a support group or some form of couples' counseling useful during this stressful time. Books and other resources are listed at the end of this chapter.

Adoption ‡

Many l/b/t women are choosing to adopt children. Since it is often difficult for lesbians to adopt, many of us adopt simply as "single mothers." Some agencies will work with openly lesbian individuals or couples; you can call anonymously for information and ask about their policies regarding lesbian and gay parents, single parents, etc.

First, you need to decide which type of agency to use: public or private. The advantage to public agencies is that they are considerably cheaper than private agencies. The disadvantage is that public agencies handle only domestic adoptions, and the waiting list for babies can be very long. You may have to wait a few years before you have an adoption opportunity unless you are willing to take a child who is older or disabled. Also in some states, adoption and foster parenting by gays and lesbians is prohibited, making a public adoption impossible.

Private agencies handle domestic as well as international adoptions, and usually you have to wait only a year or so. Many gay and lesbian couples choose international adoption because it is far less likely that they will lose custody of the child to the birth parents than with a domestic adoption. However, the price of international adoption can run as high as $25,000, and there are many issues involved in raising a child from another culture. It is important to examine your economic and emotional resources before proceeding. Adoption, just like pregnancy, is a stressful process. Consider joining a support group.

Coming Out: A Family Issue

Coming out issues are different for families depending on whether we have children before or after we come to live our lives as a lesbian. We want our children to accept us for who we are and to feel comfortable in the world, but it isn't always easy. We may find it difficult to come out to children who have always known us as straight, and it is likely that our children will have to make an adjustment to this new situation. If we have children after we've come out, they don't know anything else and thus are usually accepting of our sexuality. The issues are also somewhat different depending on the child's family situation. Children in families with two female parents often must be "out" in kindergarten, at the doctor's,

* For the procedure, cost, and safety issues with donor insemination, please see chapter 18, Assisted Low-Tech and High-Tech Reproductive Technologies.
† Many women prefer to use the sperm banks in California because the state of California has the most explicit laws regarding the rights and responsibilities of the donor, the parents, and the children.

‡ Adoption is covered more fully in chapter 22, Child-bearing Loss, Infertility, and Adoption. For information on second-parent adoption, see "Custody," p. 217.

and with grandparents in a way that is not necessary for children in single-parent families. Children who live with their fathers or other relatives will likely have different issues from those who grow up in primarily lesbian households.

Being a lesbian mom, there's so much more to explain. [My son] gets called faggot and dyke, and he comes home from school with questions. You have to show your children you stand up for something. You have to talk about sex because that's what everyone thinks when they think about gay people.

Those of us who have children in same-gender couples can have age-appropriate conversations with our children at different points about the nature of our relationships and what they mean in the larger world. Being open with our children from the beginning may help them feel positive about their family even though it is unusual.

But living in a lesbian family may be problematic for our kids no matter how much we explain. Children may feel they have to hide our sexuality and resent it.

If they [other kids] knew about my mom I'm afraid they wouldn't like me. Sometimes I feel like I'm in the closet, too, and I'm not even gay.

If we come out after we have children, we are often concerned that our children will reject us. We wonder if coming out is worth the risk. But the closet carries risks as well. Being closeted means that we can never be fully honest with our children, that they may grow up believing there is something shameful about having same-gender relationships, that they may come to believe that we didn't trust them enough to tell them the truth about ourselves.

For all of us who are considering coming out to our children, finding support during this time can help us move toward a healthy, strong identity. Some of us think it is good for our kids to have a lesbian mother because they see the options. Our kids do not grow up believing the world to be heterosexual only; they have—right in the family—someone who is willing to be different. The better we feel about ourselves and our choices, the more we have to share with our kids and each other.

I have been out to my daughter as long as I have been out to myself. I heard her at four telling a communal sister that girls could fall in love with girls and it was okay for boys to fall in love with boys. Where is the revolution? Sometimes it's right in our own backyards.

Because we make ourselves open to our kids in this one area, we are open to them in a lot of ways. We dare to be different, and sometimes it hurts to be different. It also helps them understand prejudice. They begin to see that a kid who calls another kid some name about their religion or race is probably being as *bigoted and narrow-minded as someone who calls their mother a dyke. They can make connections that many people are never able to make.*

Custody

Leaving a Heterosexual Partnership

Custody issues vary among l/b/t moms depending on our situation. If you are leaving a heterosexual marriage and want to retain custody of your children, find out about the laws in your state, and bear in mind the political atmosphere. In recent years, numerous state courts have established legal precedents ensuring that lesbian mothers cannot be denied parental rights simply on the basis of their sexual orientation. However, blatant discrimination is not uncommon. The state of Virginia recently denied custody to a mother solely on the basis that she is a lesbian living with her life partner, who is a woman. Custody was granted to the maternal grandmother instead. And in the state of Florida, a child custody case was recently decided in favor of the father, a convicted murderer, over the child's lesbian mother. Consider all the factors that may affect your case. For example, your gender identity may be as problematic as your sexual orientation if you are transgendered or transsexual. If you are disabled, you may be in double jeopardy, as disabled mothers are often denied custody of their children. Once you have carefully considered your situation, try to find a lawyer who is supportive of lesbian mothers (see box, p. 218).

Having come out as a lesbian has been real difficult for me because my child was taken away by his father. I was granted visitation rights and because I didn't know to make it specific, I've gone for six months without seeing him. It takes that long sometimes for legal proceedings to work themselves out. It's amazing how the men—the fathers—get such special treatment. I mean, a battering husband is not treated the way a lesbian mother is. At the same time, though, it was being a lesbian and stepping out as a strong woman that made me able to withstand what followed.

Sometimes a father will win custody but sooner or later send the children back because he doesn't want the work of raising them. In addition, children who voluntarily leave may return to your home when they are older and clearer in identity. At the age of 14, regardless of previous custody arrangements, many courts will defer to the child's wishes regarding which parent they want to live with.

It is important to recognize that *not* living with our children may be what we need or want, though in this society it can be hard to admit. Some lesbian and bisexual women have left their children with their fathers, which is a courageous choice, since so many people believe that mothers should keep their kids. We need to be free to make the arrangements that are the most sensible and loving all the way around.

Sometimes I feel real guilty, like a lousy mother. You know: I should be able to handle it all. I should be able to raise two kids and not be overwhelmed all the time by being a mother. On the other side of that is that I feel real good that I could be clear about the decision that my younger son would live with his father. It has worked out for all of us.

SEEKING CHILD CUSTODY AFTER A HETEROSEXUAL PARTNERSHIP

Even if you think you may want your children to live with their father, it is often wise to establish custody at first so that you can retain control over that choice. If you do not want to live with your children but would like the option of spending time with them periodically, be sure the divorce/custody agreement includes specified visitation rights. If visits are left up to the children's choice, their father may pressure them into staying away from you.

It is invaluable to have a sympathetic lawyer, even if you don't expect that your sexual orientation will be an issue in the divorce and custody negotiations. Try if at all possible to find a lawyer who accepts lesbianism, has experience in custody cases (preferably with lesbian mothers), and is known and respected by the local court. Such an ideal person is often not available but worth looking hard for. Lesbians with limited financial resources and/or who live in nonurban areas may get some advice and assistance from the Lavender Families Resource Network or another lesbian organization (see Resources).

Prepare for a custody case with extreme care. You must demonstrate to the court as conclusively as possible that you are a competent, caring, dependable mother. A social worker may assess your mothering and present evidence at the hearing. You must seem reasonable, friendly, and cooperative to the social worker no matter what you are feeling. Keep records of events that will document your concern for your children: medical and dental care, school conferences and reports, clothing and food expenditures. Record your interactions. Gather as much support from your friends as you can during this stressful time, but if you have a lover, it is best not to move in together now, much as you want to. You may think of taking your children to another state, but this could be dangerous: The Uniform Child Custody Act makes it difficult to escape court involvement, and an attempt to take them away will reflect unfavorably on your case. Finally, expert witnesses like child psychologists are expensive but may be essential in case the opposition brings in its own "experts."

Leaving a Lesbian Partnership

As more of us raise children in lesbian partnerships, we need to clarify our roles as co-parents. Disputes over custody and visitation are becoming common when l/b/t parents split up. If your child is the biological or adopted child of your partner, you may find that you have no legal rights in relationship to the child you have parented for many years. This not only is hard on you as a parent but can be traumatizing to your child.

To protect ourselves, same-gender couples should put in writing detailed agreements establishing the rights and responsibilities of both parents, including what is to happen vis-à-vis custody and visitation in the event of separation. Although such an agreement won't necessarily hold up in court, it will demonstrate the basis for your partnership and establish your clear intent to parent together. If *second-parent adoption* is available in your state, this is your best protection. With second-parent adoption, both partners can become legal parents of their children, protecting both parent and child from financial and emotional loss (for example, without a second-parent adoption, a nonbiological/nonadoptive parent would not be guaranteed guardianship if the biological/adoptive mother died).

Support

So much of what we need as l/b/t mothers is the same as for all mothers.

I'm a single mother, and that's the most important factor in what makes it hard for me to be doing all that I'm trying to do.

My lover and I both work full-time. One of our daughters is in day care and the other's in kindergarten. It's a scramble. Some days, family life feels like an endless negotiation about who's going to be where, when.

For all mothers, help from friends is one thing that makes it easier to get through a day. Women who share a living space or live near each other can take some responsibility for each other's kids.

In other cases, other adults have built stable, regular relationships with our kids and cared for them on a regular basis, such as one afternoon a week or one weekend a month. In this way we have a break we can count on—a chance to relax a little, pull ourselves together, go out with our friends, or just be alone. Still another kind of support comes when groups or gatherings of women make plans for child care so mothers aren't the only ones with responsibility for arrangements. For mothers, the importance of adequate child care and reasonable locations and hours at l/b/t events cannot be overestimated.

Some of us have also been part of ongoing groups where we tell about our feelings and experiences as mothers. It has helped to know that other l/b/t mothers live with problems similar to ours, realize the problems aren't our fault, strategize new approaches, and

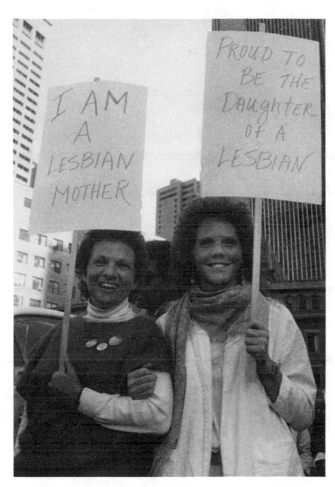

Ellen Shub

share the daily surprises and delights we get from our kids. It also helps our kids to get to know others like themselves, living in l/b/t families.

What I've always wanted for my children is a wider network of caring adults, and we're making one in this group. It's not enough just to come in and talk about being lesbian mothers; we include our kids, having parties for us all, going to the beach together. . . . The kids at some point look around the room and say to themselves, "All these kids have lesbian mothers" and feel less isolated.

HEALTH AND MEDICAL CARE *

Do women who partner with women have special health care needs? Are we at increased risk for certain health problems and decreased risk for others? It is difficult to answer these questions, as sexual orientation has not been included in demographic data collected in women's health research until recently, and

---

* This section was updated by Peggy Lynch. Particular health and medical problems as they affect l/b/t women appear throughout the book. Also, please see chapter 24, Selected Medical Practices, Problems, and Procedures, for more information on specific health problems such as breast cancer and chronic illness.

---

studies of lesbians are not representative of all women who partner with women.† Some health care providers (HCPs) and activists argue that lesbians are at increased risk for diseases such as alcoholism and breast cancer, while others feel that our biggest health problems are sexism, homophobia, and ignorance within the health care system—barriers that can be compounded by poverty, racism, and prejudice against immigrants.

Often, l/b/t women do not seek health care either because we don't realize the need or because we are uncomfortable with the sexist and homophobic attitudes of the health care system. Heterosexual women, because of their need for birth control, generally see HCPs more often than l/b/t women who partner with women. Some l/b/t women don't realize that it is just as important for us to have regular preventive care, such as Pap smears and mammograms, as it is for heterosexual women.

Getting good, sensitive health care is a challenge for all women. Most l/b/t women have the added disadvantage of having to depend on HCPs who know little about our lives and how our lifestyles may affect our health. We are often expected to educate our HCPs about what our particular needs might be. Even HCPs who are queer themselves may not understand or be sensitive to the needs of women who are less privileged, who work as sex workers, who have a different racial and/or cultural background, or who use drugs. Transgendered and transsexual women, whose gender presentation often doesn't match their biological sex, have an especially difficult time getting good health care. HCPs often don't know how to treat transsexuals or refuse to treat them. What happens if a female-to-male transsexual needs a pelvic exam? Often he is not taken seriously.

As l/b/t women, we must take extra care to find HCPs who are attentive to our needs. This can be a frustrating process, but one that will be worthwhile in the long run. Ask other l/b/t women you know if they have an HCP whom they like and to whom they can talk easily. Screen people on the phone ahead of time. Do not assume that the provider your friend likes is the right person for you. Explore all your options. If you live in a city, there may be a lesbian and/or gay health center (see Resources). You may also find that your choices are limited by your particular health plan—even so, you should look for a person who meets your needs. It is important that you feel that your HCP will listen to you and take you seriously, and that you are able to articulate your expectations to that person. If you have a disability or chronic illness, it is good to have a provider who will follow you attentively over the long term and who is willing to work with other providers if necessary.

It can be difficult to decide whether or not to come out to a health care provider and when it is necessary to do so. A good HCP should take a thorough health, family, and social history, and this conversation should

---

† The largest study of women's health, the National Nurses' Study, has recently begun collecting data specifically about lesbians.

give you the opportunity to disclose the intimate or family relationship you live in. In an emergency situation, HCPs should at least ask (in what is called the "review of systems") about sexual activity in the form of gender-inclusive, open-ended questions. This is becoming a standard of care, particularly among HCPs who have been educated in the last five to ten years. In addition, HCPs should ask what you prefer to include or omit from your medical record. (If you are not asked, be firm about what you want.) Most people agree that medical records are not fully confidential, if only because in medical settings, many people handle and file charts. Some request that HCPs not record the words "lesbian," "gay," or "bisexual" in the record, but be descriptive, as in "sexually active, female partners only" or "sexually active with male and female partners."

We have the right to expect professionalism from our HCPs, whether they are physicians, nurse practitioners, or physician's assistants, and from the other personnel in the health care settings. It is not our job to answer invasive questions about our lives. There is ample information in the medical and nursing literature from which an HCP can learn about health issues of lesbian and bisexual women. Several professional organizations, including the American Medical Association and the American Nurses Association, have taken relatively progressive positions on lesbian and gay health. Nonetheless, as patients we are more vulnerable if we do not fit someone's idea of "normal." Each of us must decide when and where to come out in our encounters with the health care system.

I would not come out in a medical situation unless there were compelling reasons to do so, because in the "patient" role I have so little power and am especially vulnerable to harassment. So I practice in advance how to maintain my privacy and still get the care I need—ways of refusing to answer offensive or unnecessary inquiries, and of asking direct, specific questions about what I need to know. For instance, if a practitioner says, "No sex for a month," I can ask whether I should avoid sexual arousal itself or just vaginal penetration. The book Lesbian Health Matters! *[see Resources] has helped me invaluably in dealing with medical visits.*

Some of us who are insured find our communities targeted as a "niche market" in the capitalist health care system, but those of us who are marginally employed, unemployed, or uninsured struggle to get health care of any kind. Seek out free care programs at public or nonprofit hospitals or community clinics, or find health centers or providers who have sliding-scale fees. Do not give up!

As l/b/t women and consumers of health care, we can take a few measures to improve our encounters with the health care system. (See chapter 25, The Politics of Women's Health and Medical Care, for more suggestions.) Know your own medical history and that of your family of origin. Take someone with you to act as your advocate when you have a health care appointment. Prepare yourself for emergencies or serious illness by preparing a legal document called a Health Care Proxy. Without this document, your closest blood relative will assume responsibility (see "Legal Issues," p. 221).

Some illnesses, like breast cancer, strike women exclusively, or, like chronic fatigue immune deficiency syndrome and multiple chemical sensitivities, seem to strike women more often than men. Those of us who partner with women, live primarily with women, and/or have women as our closest friendship circle are likely to encounter these illnesses in a partner or someone close to us sooner or later. We need to support each other and to make our events more accessible to those who are ill.

Breast Cancer

Although nearly 50% of lesbians surveyed in a 1987 National Lesbian Health Care Survey were or wanted to be mothers, fewer women who partner with women will be pregnant in their lifetimes than those who partner with men.[2] Few or no pregnancies translates into more years of the estrogen-progesterone cycle, which—in the context of increased estrogen in our environment—may be detrimental to the health of our breasts. This increased vulnerability to breast cancer is compounded by our lower incomes and the difficulty of finding free or low-cost mammograms in accessible locations. (Please see the long section on breast cancer in chapter 24, Selected Medical Practices, Problems, and Procedures.)

Alcoholism and Drug Abuse

Because oppression creates extra stress in our lives, some of us drink to excess or use illicit drugs. Drinking becomes a problem for anyone who can't control when and/or how much she drinks. Some drugs, especially heroin-based drugs, are extremely addictive. If you think you or a friend is addicted, please consult chapter 3, Alcohol, Tobacco, and Other Mood-Altering Drugs. A growing number of addiction support and recovery programs are willing to deal openly with women in lesbian relationships, and the more progressive ones respect lovers as family members. For example, many chapters of Alcoholics Anonymous, Narcotics Anonymous, and Al-Anon have l/b/t meetings. The PRIDE Institute, a residential treatment program in New York, provides services specifically for the lesbian and gay community (see Resources). Within our l/b/t communities we can all become more conscious about alcoholism and drug abuse. We can create drug-free spaces and serve inexpensive nonalcoholic drinks at bars to support recovering women and others who have problems with drinking.

Mental Health *

Almost everyone runs into times of emotional confusion; l/b/t women in this society face extra emotional stress. We may get help by turning to friends who listen well; by being in a women's or l/b/t support group; by asking an objective third person to mediate between us and a lover, co-worker, or housemate; and by trying to take better care of ourselves physically (see chapters 2, 4, and 5). When these sources of help aren't enough, we may choose to work for a time with a trained psychotherapist.

Historically, psychiatry has been anti-homosexual as well as sexist and male-dominated. In 1973, the American Psychiatric Association removed homosexuality from its list of illnesses to be "cured," but many conservative therapists still consider it abnormal. Transgenders and transsexuals must be particularly careful as new "gender disorders" are given official diagnoses. Be wary of a therapist who sees your sexual orientation as the source of your problems and therefore fails to take your real problems seriously.

Fortunately, today there are more openly lesbian and bisexual therapists (mostly in urban areas, so far) and more heterosexual therapists who are feminist and/or see lesbianism/bisexuality as a valid way of life. To find such a therapist, check with friends, a women's center, or in women's journals and newspapers. In your first interview, don't hesitate to ask about the therapist's views, training, and beliefs. (Chapter 6, Our Emotional Well-Being, suggests useful questions to ask.) Sometimes it's important to see a lesbian, but this isn't necessarily the most important criterion. One lesbian therapist said,

I don't care who my therapist sleeps with as long as she or he doesn't think sleeping with women is sick. Just because a therapist is a woman or even a lesbian doesn't mean she'd be the best one for you to work with.

Sometimes frightened or angry parents pressure or force a young woman exploring sexuality with women into therapy—or, worse, into a mental institution—in the hope of changing her sexual orientation. A young rural lesbian said, "My parents stopped giving me money for school when I came out to them. They said, 'We'll pay for a psychiatrist but nothing else.'" Obviously, therapy in such a situation is a mockery and a punishment. If you had this sort of bad experience, it doesn't necessarily mean you can't find a good, supportive therapist today.

LEGAL ISSUES †

As l/b/t women, we struggle for the legal rights and protections we deserve. This dilemma is compounded if we have low incomes, if we are women of color, or if we are imprisoned. Most legislators, judges, and lawyers in the U.S. judicial system are white, heterosexual men who exercise this society's bias against lesbians and other peoples different from themselves.

In the last 30 years, lesbians and gays have won recognition of our individual rights in some contexts and have seen new laws passed to expand our rights toward full equality in other contexts. The 1990s has been a time of increasing recognition of the individual and family rights of lesbian and gay people.

Individual Civil Rights

At the federal level, there is still no statute protecting l/b/t women from discrimination by private entities (private employers, landlords, and so on). However, in the landmark case *Romer v. Evans* (the case concerning Amendment 2 in Colorado), the U.S. Supreme Court ruled that the Constitution entitles lesbians, gays, and bisexuals to equal treatment under the law. This means that no federal, state, or local governmental entity (unlike a private entity) can legally discriminate against you because of your sexual orientation.

At the state level, as of spring 1997, ten states and the District of Columbia had passed civil rights laws prohibiting discrimination on the basis of sexual orientation by public or private institutions. These states are California, Connecticut, Hawaii, Massachusetts, Minnesota, New Hampshire, New Jersey, Rhode Island, Vermont, and Wisconsin. Similarly, dozens of cities have adopted ordinances that prohibit discrimination based on sexual orientation. Many of these cities, such as Denver and Boulder, Colorado, and Tucson and Phoenix, Arizona, are in states with no statewide protection.

These laws and ordinances generally help protect lesbian and bisexual women from discrimination in employment. A few protect lesbian and bisexual women from discrimination in housing and public accommodations. However, they do not guarantee us the same rights as heterosexuals with regard to marriage, family, and children. Full recognition of our rights as couples and families is essential to gaining full legal protection.

Our Rights as Couples

Marriage

Civil marriage is a state-recognized institution providing 1049 federal rights and responsibilities as well as hundreds more state rights and responsibilities, in-

---

* See chapter 6, Our Emotional Well-Being: Psychotherapy in Context, for more information on considering psychotherapy, and check the Resources in that chapter for l/b/t–related books.

† This section was updated by Amelia Craig Cramer, Esq., who at the time was the Executive Director of Gay and Lesbian Advocates and Defenders (GLAD). Founded in 1978, GLAD is New England's legal organization for lesbians, gay men, bisexuals, and people

cluding inheritance rights, hospital visitation rights, joint ownership and spousal support, joint tax returns, joint parenting and child support, joint insurance, joint pension and other benefits, joint decision making, exemption from property transfer taxes, and so on. Even with domestic partnership arrangements, health care proxies, and other legal documents, only about a dozen of these rights and responsibilities are available to same-gender couples.

For this reason, and the desire to have their partnerships receive social recognition and validation, three same-gender couples sued the state of Hawaii for the right to marry. It is likely that by 1998 same-gender couples in Hawaii (and those able and willing to travel there) will be able to obtain civil marriage licenses and certificates for the first time. There is a similar case pending in Vermont.

In response to the decision by the Hawaiian courts, the 1996 U.S. Congress passed the Defense of Marriage Act (DOMA), establishing marriage as a union between a man and woman and declaring that the federal government would not recognize same-gender marriages. In allowing states to refuse to recognize same-sex marriages licensed and certified by other states, the DOMA may violate the Full Faith and Credit Clause of the Federal Constitution. All this lays the groundwork for many years of legal battles as couples challenge their states and the federal government to recognize their marriages. Though not all l/b/t women want to marry, having the option to do so is important in establishing full legal and social equality for women who choose same-gender partnerships.

Domestic Partnership

Because same-gender couples are not able to marry, several cities have passed ordinances recognizing domestic partnerships. For the most part, these ordinances grant public employees family-related benefits such as insurance coverage, bereavement leave, and sick leave on behalf of loved ones. These ordinances don't guarantee these benefits if you are employed by a private company, but many companies, because of organizing efforts by lesbian and gay employees, are beginning to voluntarily offer domestic partner benefits. Companies such as Lotus, Levi-Strauss, and Ben & Jerry's have led the way.

Protecting Your Rights as a Couple

Without marriage or domestic partnership, our relationships have no legal standing. As a result, same-gender couples have explored other ways to protect our relationships.*

---

with HIV. GLAD's mission is to achieve full equality and justice for all individuals in these groups, primarily through impact litigation and education.

* A useful resource for couples is *A Legal Guide for Lesbian and Gay Couples* by Curry F. Hayden and Denis Clifford (Berkeley, CA: Nolo Press, 1991).

Relationship Contracts

If you are in or entering into a relationship that you think will last for some time, you and your partner can protect yourselves by working out a formal written agreement or contract about expenses, purchases, work, and so on. You may want your relationship agreement to specifically state how property will be divided if you decide to separate. Agreements regarding property, in the form of notarized contracts, may well stand up in court. However, going to court is painful and costly, and the outcome in lesbian cases is unpredictable. If you wish to separate and cannot solve property disputes, consider couples' therapy or mediation first.

Many of us who are lesbian lawyers encourage women to agree in their contract to community arbitration, thus avoiding the often sexist, homophobic legal system.

Health Care

In times of sickness or death, the law automatically entrusts your next of kin with the ability to make medical decisions. Your partner is legally powerless to visit you in the hospital, be informed of your status, make medical decisions for you if you are incapable, determine what will happen to your remains, or even be present at your funeral. You can, however, draw up legal documents to give your lover the right to make medical decisions for you while you are incapacitated and to determine the disposition of your remains if you die. These documents have different names in different states but are often called "Health Care Proxy" or "Health Care Power of Attorney" and "Power of Attorney for Disposition of Remains."

Joint Ownership of Property

Joint property ownership is not dependent on marriage, though it is not as financially beneficial if you are not married. You and your partner can jointly own real estate and personal property. However, tax record-keeping is difficult, and there are often tax disadvantages to doing so. Moreover, in the event of your partner's death, if you become sole owner of your jointly held real estate, you will be taxed on "transfer of ownership" even though surviving heterosexual spouses are exempt from such taxation. If your property is not owned jointly, you will want to make provisions for your partner in your will.

Our Rights as Parents †

Losing our children because of our sexual orientation is still a great fear for l/b/t mothers. Fortunately, though there still is blatant discrimination, some states have established legal precedents ensuring that lesbian mothers cannot be denied parental rights simply on the basis of their sexual orientation. Still, it is im-

---

† Many of the legal issues involved in parenting are discussed in the section "Raising Children," p. 215.

portant to be very careful if you are separating from a heterosexual partnership and want to retain custody (see "Seeking Child Custody After a Heterosexual Partnership," p. 218).

Custody can also become an issue if you have had your child by alternative insemination with a "known donor" (see "Having Children," p. 215). If you choose a known donor, prior to having the child you will want to determine who among the three should be considered legal parents and to make use of the state's legal procedures to arrange this. Lesbian couples and semen donors who fail to prepare for the legal parenting rights and responsibilities among themselves often run into conflicts later. Messy legal battles can ensue. And, even if you carefully construct a contract with a semen donor, in most states, as the "father" of the child, he can sue for custody.

Since many more of us are raising our children in same-sex couples, we also face issues of custody and visitation when our lesbian partnerships dissolve. In some states, such as Massachusetts, Vermont, and California, second-parent adoptions are permitted. Second-parent adoptions are the absolute best protection for you, your partner and your children (see "Raising Children," p. 215). If you cannot adopt the biological or adopted children of your partner, you may want to draw up a parenting agreement that states each parent's rights and responsibilities toward your children and custody and visitation arrangements in the case of separation or death. Also you will want to name each other in your wills and specifically state that your partner is to become the guardian of your children, if anything happens to you. Because our families are vulnerable to intervention by families of origin, a child's father, and/or the state, it is important to use the legal documents available to us to protect ourselves and our children as best we can, while we continue to fight for equal protection under the law.

NOTES

1. Joan Nestle. "Butch-Fem Relationships: Sexual Courage in the 1950s," *Heresies,* Sex Issue, 3, no. 4, Issue 12 (May 1981): 21.
2. J. Bradford and C. Ryan. *National Lesbian Health Care Survey.* Washington, DC: National Lesbian and Gay Health Association, 1987.

RESOURCES

Readings

Special thanks to Liza Rankow, Jenifer Firestone, and to Gilda Bruckman and the other women of New Words Bookstore in Somerville, MA (800-928-4788).

For resources on bisexuality and on sex boutiques, please see chapter 11, Sexuality. For resources on transgender and transsexual issues, see p. 182.

General Nonfiction

Anzaldúa, Gloria, ed. *Making Face, Making Soul/ Haciendo Caras: Creative and Critical Perspectives by Women of Color.* San Francisco: Aunt Lute Books, 1990.

Beck, Evelyn Torton, ed. *Nice Jewish Girls: A Lesbian Anthology.* Boston: Beacon Press, 1989.

Lim-Hing., ed. *The Very Inside: Writings by Asian and Pacific Islander Lesbian and Bisexual Women.* East Haven, CT: InBook, 1994.

Lorde, Audre. *Sister Outsider: Essays and Speeches.* Freedom, CA: Crossing Press, 1984.

Martin, Del, and Phyllis Lyon. *Lesbian—Woman 1991.* Volcano, CA: Volcano Press, 1991. Updated 1972 classic by the founders of Daughters of Bilitis (DOB).

Moraga, Cherríe, and Gloria Anzaldúa, eds. *This Bridge Called My Back: Writings by Radical Women of Color.* New York: Kitchen Table Press, 1984.

Osborne, Karen Lee, and William J. Spurlin, eds. *Reclaiming the Heartland: Lesbian and Gay Voices from the Midwest.* Minneapolis: University of Minnesota Press, 1996.

Penlope, Julia. *Coming Out of the Class Closet: Lesbians Speak.* Freedom, CA: The Crossing Press, 1994.

———, and Sarah Valentine, eds. *Finding the Lesbians: Personal Accounts from Around the World.* Freedom, CA: Crossing Press, 1990.

Pharr, Suzanne. *Homophobia: A Weapon of Sexism.* Inverness, CA: Chardon Press, 1988.

Pratt, Minnie Bruce. *Rebellion: Essays 1980–1991.* Ithaca, NY: Firebrand Books, 1991.

Raffo, Susan, ed. *Queerly Classed.* Boston: South End Press, 1997. Gay men and lesbians on class.

Ramos, Juanita. *Compañeras—Latina Lesbians: An Anthology.* New York: Routlege, 1994.

Ratti, R., ed. *A Lotus of Another Color: An Unfolding of the South Asian Gay and Lesbian Experience.* Boston: Alyson Publishers, 1993.

Rich, Adrienne. *Compulsory Heterosexuality and Lesbian Existence.* London: Onlywomen Press, 1981. A now classic and often-cited pamphlet.

Roscoe, Will, ed. *Living the Spirit: A Gay American Indian Anthology.* New York: St. Martin's Press, 1988.

Rose, Andy, ed. *Twice Blessed: On Being Lesbian or Gay and Jewish.* Boston: Beacon Press, 1991.

Segrest, Mab. *Memoir of a Race Traitor.* Boston: South End Press, 1993.

Silvera, Makeda, ed. *Piece of My Heart: A Lesbian of Colour Anthology.* Toronto: Sister Vision Press, 1991.

Trujillo, Carla. *Chicana Lesbians: The Girls Our Mothers Warned Us About.* Berkeley, CA: Third Woman, 1991.

Vaid, Urvashi. *Virtual Equality: The Mainstreaming of Gay and Lesbian Liberation.* New York: Anchor Books, 1995.

Vida, Ginny, ed. *The New Our Right to Love: A Lesbian Resource Book.* New York: Touchstone Books, 1996.

Lesbian/Bisexual/Transgender History

D'Emilio, John. *Sexual Politics, Sexual Communities: The Making of a Homosexual Minority in the United States, 1940–1970.* Chicago: University of Chicago Press, 1984.

Duberman, Martin, et al., eds. *Hidden from History: Reclaiming the Gay and Lesbian Past.* New York: NAL-Dutton, 1990.

Faderman, Lillian. *Odd Girls and Twilight Lovers: A History of Lesbian Life in Twentieth-Century America.* New York: Columbia University Press, 1991.

Kennedy, Elizabeth L., and Madeline D. Davis. *Boots of Leather, Slippers of Gold: The History of a Lesbian Community.* New York: Viking Penguin, 1993.

The National Museum and Archive of Lesbian and Gay History. *The Lesbian Almanac.* New York: Berkley Books, 1996.

Nestle, Joan. *A Restricted Country.* Ithaca, NY: Firebrand Books, 1987.

Older Lesbians

Adelman, Marcy, ed. *Long Time Passing: Lives of Older Lesbians.* Boston: Alyson Publications, 1986.

MacDonald, Barbara, and Cynthia Rich, eds. *Look Me in the Eye: Old Women, Aging and Ageism,* 2nd ed. Duluth, MN: Spinsters Ink, 1991.

Reyes, Karen, and Lorena F. Farrell, eds. *Lambda Gray: A Practical, Emotional, and Spiritual Guide for Gays and Lesbians Who Are Growing Older.* North Hollywood, CA: Newcastle Publishing, 1993.

Sang, Barbara, et al., eds. *Lesbians at Midlife: The Creative Transition.* Duluth, MN: Spinsters Ink, 1991.

Lesbian/Bi/Transgendered Women Who Are Deaf, Disabled, or Chronically Ill

(For more resources on disabilities and on chronic illness, see chapter 24, Selected Medical Practices, Problems, and Procedures.)

Luczak, Raymond, ed. *Eyes of Desire: A Deaf Gay and Lesbian Reader.* Boston: Alyson Publications, 1993.

O'Toole, Corbett J. "Disabled Lesbians: Challenging Monocultural Constructs." In D.M. Krotoski, M. Nosek, and M. Turk, eds. *Women with Physical Disabilities: Achieving and Maintaining Health and Well-being.* Baltimore, MD: Brookes Publishing, 1996.

Panzarino, C. *The Me in the Mirror.* Seattle: Seal Press, 1994.

Tremain, Shelley, ed. *Pushing the Limits: Disabled Dykes Produce Culture.* Toronto: The Women's Press, 1996.

Lesbian/Bisexual/Transgender/ Questioning Youth

Bass, Ellen. *Free Your Mind: The Book for Gay, Lesbian and Bisexual Youth and Their Allies.* New York: HarperPerennial, 1996.

Due, Linnea. *Joining the Tribe: Growing Up Gay and Lesbian in the '90s.* New York: Anchor Books, 1995.

Herdt, Gilbert, and Andrew Boxer. *Children of Horizons: How Gay and Lesbian Teens Are Leading a New Way Out of the Closet.* Boston: Beacon Press, 1996.

Heron, Ann, ed. *Two Teenagers in Twenty: Writings by Gay and Lesbian Youth.* Boston: Alyson Publications, 1996.

Romesburg, Don A., ed. *Young, Gay, and Proud.* Boston: Alyson Publications, 1995.

Singer, Bennett L., ed. *Growing Up Gay/Growing Up Lesbian: A Literary Anthology.* New York: The New Press, 1994.

Relationships

Berzon, Betty. *Permanent Partners: Building Gay and Lesbian Relationships That Last.* New York: NAL-Dutton, 1990.

Butler, Becky, ed. *Ceremonies of the Heart: Celebrating Lesbian Unions.* Seattle: Seal Press, 1990.

Clunis, Marilee D., and G. Dorsey Green. *Lesbian Couples: Creating Healthy Relationships for the '90s.* 2nd ed. Seattle: Seal Press, 1993.

Johnson, Susan E. *For Love and For Life: Intimate Portraits of Lesbian Couples.* Tallahassee, FL: Naiad Press, 1995.

McDaniel, Judith. *The Lesbian Couples' Guide.* New York: HarperCollins, 1995.

Slater, Suzanne, *The Lesbian Family Life Cycle.* New York: The Free Press, 1995.

Butch-Femme

Burana, Lily, et al. *Dagger: On Butch Women.* Pittsburgh, PA: Cleis Press, 1994.

Nestle, Joan, ed. *The Persistent Desire: A Femme-Butch Reader.* Boston: Alyson Publications, 1992.

Newman, Lesléa, ed. *The Femme Mystique.* Boston: Alyson Publications, 1995.

Sexuality

Bad Attitude, P.O. Box 390110, Cambridge MA 02139-0001. Lesbian bimonthly. S/M focus.

Bright, Susie. *Susie Sexpert's Lesbian Sex World.* San Francisco: Cleis Press, 1990.

Califia, Pat. *Public Sex: The Culture of Radical Sex.* Pittsburgh, PA: Cleis Press, 1994.

Caster, W. *The Lesbian Sex Book.* Boston: Alyson Publications, Inc. 1993.

Duggan, Lisa, and Nan D. Hunter. *Sex Wars: Sexual Dissent and Political Culture.* New York: Routledge, 1995.

Gomez, Jewelle, and Tristan Taormino. *Best Lesbian Erotica 1997.* Pittsburgh, PA: Cleis Press, 1997. Annual.

Kiss and Tell, Her Tongue on My Theory: Images, Essays and Fantasies. East Haven, CT: InBook, 1994.

Loulan, JoAnn. *The Lesbian Erotic Dance: Butch, Femme, Androgyny and Other Rhythms.* Duluth, MN: Spinsters Ink, 1990.

Morris, Kathleen E. *Speaking in Whispers: African-American Lesbian Erotica.* Chicago: Third Side Press, 1996.

O'Sullivan, S., and P. Parmar. *Lesbians Talk (Safer) Sex.* East Haven CT: InBooks, 1992.

West, Celeste. *Lesbian Polyfidelity: or How to Keep Nonmonogamy Safe, Sane, Honest, and Laughing, You Rogue!* San Francisco: Bootleg Publishing, 1995.

Sexual Abuse and Battering

See chapter 8, Violence Against Women, for more resources.

The Lesbian Caucus of the Massachusetts Coalition of Battered Women Service Groups. *Voices of Battered Lesbians.* Audiocassette. Available from the Network for Battered Lesbians and Bisexual Women, P.O. Box 6011, Boston, MA 02114; (617) 424-8611.

Renzetti, Claire M. *Violent Betrayal: Partner Abuse in Lesbian Relationships.* Newbury Park, CA: Sage Publications, 1992.

———, and Charles H. Miley, eds. *Violence in Gay and Lesbian Domestic Partnerships.* New York: Harrington Park Press, 1996.

Mothers

Clunis, D. Merilee, and G. Dorsey Green. *The Lesbian Parenting Book: A Guide to Creating Families and Raising Children.* Seattle: Seal Press, 1995.

Corley, Rip, and Jean Chang. *The Final Closet: The Gay Parents' Guide for Coming Out to Their Children.* North Miami, FL: Editech Press, 1990.

Martin, April. *Lesbian and Gay Parenting Book: Creating and Raising Our Families.* New York: HarperPerennial, 1993.

Wells, Jess, ed. *Lesbians Raising Sons: An Anthology.* Boston: Alyson Publications, 1997.

Weston, Kath. *Families We Choose: Lesbians, Gays, Kinship.* New York: Columbia University Press, 1991.

For Family and Friends

Elwin, Rosamund, and Michele Paulse. *Asha's Mums.* Toronto: The Women's Press, 1990. For children.

Fairchild, Betty, and Nancy Howard. *Now That You Know: What Every Parent Should Know About Homosexuality.* San Diego, CA: Harcourt, Brace, Jovanovich, 1989.

Griffin, Carolyn Welch. *Beyond Acceptance.* New York: St. Martin's Press, 1990.

Mohn, Richard D. *A More Perfect Union: Why Straight America Must Stand Up for Gay Rights.* Boston: Beacon Press, 1995.

Newman, Lesléa. *Gloria Goes to Gay Pride.* Boston: Alyson Publications, 1991. For children.

———. *Heather Has Two Mommies.* Boston: Alyson Publications, 1989. For children.

Rafkin, Louise, ed. *Different Daughters: A Book by Mothers of Lesbians.* Pittsburgh, PA: Cleis Press, 1987.

Valentine, Johnny. *The Daddy Machine.* Boston: Alyson Publications, 1992. For children.

Willhoite, Michael. *Families: A Coloring Book.* Boston: Alyson Publications, 1991.

Health-Related Material

(For more information, see other chapters in this book, including chapters 6, 15, 18, and 24.)

Butler, Sandra, and Barbara Rosenblum. *Cancer in Two Voices.* San Francisco: Spinsters Books, 1991.

Journal of the Gay and Lesbian Medical Association. Quarterly. Premier Issue Spring 1997. Gay and Lesbian Medical Association, 459 Fulton Street, Suite 107, San Francisco CA 94102; (415) 255-4547.

Lesbian Health Issues Newsletter. National Center for Lesbian Rights (see Organizations).

O'Donnell, Mary, et al. *Lesbian Health Matters!: A Resource Book about Lesbian Health.* Santa Cruz, CA: Santa Cruz Women's Health Collective, 1979. Available from Santa Cruz Women's Health Center, 250 Locust Street, Santa Cruz, CA 95060; (408) 427-3500.

Peterson, K. Jean, ed. *Health Care for Lesbians and Gay Men: Confronting Homophobia and Heterosexism.* New York: Haworth, 1996.

Plumb, Marj, and Laura Perry, eds. *Lesbian Health Fair Manual.* San Francisco: National Center for Lesbian Rights, 1996. Available from the National Center for Lesbian Rights (see "Organizations" below).

Rankow, Liza, ed. *Lesbian Health Bibliography.* San Francisco: National Center for Lesbian Rights, 1995. Available from the National Center for Lesbian Rights (see "Organizations" below).

Stern, Phyllis Noerager, ed. *Lesbian Health: What Are the Issues?* Washington, DC: Taylor and Francis, 1993. (To order, call 800-821-8312.)

White, Jocelyn, and Marissa C. Martinez, eds. *The Lesbian Health Book: Caring for Ourselves.* Seattle: Seal Press, 1997.

Legal Issues

Curry, F. Hayden, and Denis Clifford. *A Legal Guide for Lesbian and Gay Couples.* Berkeley, CA: Nolo Press, 1996.

Hunter, Nan, Sherryl Michaelson, and Thomas Stoddard. *The Rights of Lesbians and Gay Men: The Basic ACLU Guide to a Gay Person's Rights.* Carbondale: Southern Illinois University Press, 1992.

Partners: Newsletter for Gay and Lesbian Couples. Available from P.O. Box 9685, Seattle, WA 98109; (206) 784-1519. Adoption, child-custody, relationship issues.

Robson, Ruthann. *Lesbian (Out) Law: Survival Under the Rule of Law.* Ithaca NY: Firebrand Books, 1992.

———, et al., eds. *Gay Men, Lesbians and the Law.* New York: Chelsea House Publishers, 1997.

Guides to Meeting Places/Businesses/Resorts

Horne, Sandy, ed., *Gaia's Guide International,* 16th ed. New Montgomery Street, San Francisco, CA 94105.

Places of Interest to Women: The Women's Guide: USA & Canada. Ferrari Publications: P.O. Box 37887, Phoenix, AZ 85069.

Van Gelder, Lindsy, and Pamela Robin Brandt. *Are You Two . . . Together?: A Gay and Lesbian Travel Guide to Europe.* New York: Random House, 1991.

Women's Traveller. The Damron Company: P.O. Box 422458, San Francisco, CA 94142.

Fiction

Write to publishers, presses, and bookstores for current book lists. Our list is only a taste of what is available.

Levy, E.J., ed. *Tasting Life Twice: Lesbian Literary Fiction.* New York: Avon Books, 1995.

McKinley, Catherine E., and L. Joyce Delaney. *Afrekete: An Anthology of Contemporary Black Lesbian Writing.* New York: Anchor Books, 1995.

Nestle, Joan, and Naomi Holock, eds. *Women on Women 3: An Anthology of American Lesbian Short Fiction.* New York: Plume Books, 1996.

Ruff, Shawn Stewart. *Go the Way Your Blood Beats: An Anthology of Lesbian and Gay Fiction by African-American Writers.* New York: H. Holt, 1996.

Wolverton, Terry, with Robert Drake, eds. *Hers 2: Brilliant New Fiction by Lesbian Writers.* Boston: Faber & Faber, Inc. 1997.

African-American authors: Donna Allegra, Octavia Butler, Michelle Cliff, Jewelle Gomez, Audre Lorde, Kathleen E. Morris, Sapphire, Ann Allen Shockley, Alice Walker.

European/Euro-American authors: Dorothy Allison, Lisa Alther, June Arnold, Rita Mae Brown, Pat Califia, Sarah Dreher, Nisa Donnelly, Emma Donoghue, Katherine V. Forrest, Nicola Griffith, Jennifer Levin, Judith McDaniel, Isabel Miller, Kate Millett, Carol Queen, Jane Rule, May Sarton, Sandra Scoppettone, Sarah Schulman, Patricia Roth Schwartz, Barbara Wilson, Jeanette Winterson, Monique Wittig.

Asian-American authors: Mina Kumar, Larissa Lai, Sharon Lim-Hing, Anchee Min, Cecilia Tan, Kitty Tsui, Hsu Tzi Wong.

Jewish authors: Robin Berstein, Jyl Lynn Felman, Ellen Galford, Rebecca Goldstein, Judith Katz, Melanie Kaye/Kantrowitz, Joan Nestle, Lesléa Newman.

Latina authors: Denise Chaváez, Cherríe Moraga, Terri de la Peña, Achy Obejas, Emma Perez.

Native American authors: Paula Gunn Allen, Beth Brant.

Poetry

Because there are so many fine poets currently in print, we will list only names: Paula Gunn Allen, Gloria Anzaldua, Robin Becker, Becky Birtha, Olga Broumas, Stephanie Byrd, Chrystos, Cheryl Clarke, Jan Clausen, Michelle Cliff, Sandra Maria Esteves, Elsa Gidlow, Janice Gould, Judy Grahn, Marilyn Hacker, Joy Harjo, June Jordan, Willyce Kim, Irena Klepfisz, Joan Larkin, Audre Lorde, Renita Lynnet Martin, Nora Mitchell, Cherríe Moraga, Barbara Noda, Letta Neely, Pat Parker, Carol Potter, Minnie Bruce Pratt, Adrienne Rich, Kate Rushin, Sappho, Chocolate Waters, Fran Winant.

Periodicals

This is a representative sample.

Anything That Moves (Bay Area Bisexual Network) San Francisco, CA; (800) 818-8823
Web site: http://www.anythingthatmoves.com

Bridges: A Journal for Jewish Feminists and Our Friends Eugene, OR; (541) 935-5720
Web site: http://www.pond.net/~ckinberg/bridges

Dykes, Disability, & Stuff P.O. Box 8773; Madison, WI 53708-8773

Fat Girl: A Zine for Fat Dykes and the Women Who Want Them San Francisco, CA
Web site: http://www.fatso.com/fatgirl

Gay Community News: A Quarterly Journal for Gay Men and Lesbians Boston, MA; (617) 262-6969

Girlfriends San Francisco, CA; (800) grlfrnd
Web site: http://www.girlfriends.com

Lesbian Connection c/o Helen Diner Memorial Women's Center/Ambitious Amazons
P.O. Box 811; East Lansing, MI 48826; (517) 371-5257
Free to lesbians. Excellent resource for rural or traveling women.

Lesbian News Torrance, CA; (800) 458-9888 (outside L.A.); (310) 787-8658 (in L.A.)

off our backs: a woman's news journal Washington, DC; (202) 234-8072

Out New York, NY; (800) 876-1199

Sojourner: The Women's Forum Jamaica Plain, MA; (617) 524-0415
Web site: http//www.tiac.net/users/sojourn

Bookstores

Feminist and l/b/t bookstores need our business! To find the feminist bookstore closest to you, please contact Feminist Bookstore News at P.O. Box 882554, San Francisco, CA 94188; phone (415) 626-1556 or (415) 626-8970. Many stores accept mail, phone, and fax orders.

Presses and Publishers

This is a list of independent or small presses that focus on or include g/l/b/t books. For addresses, contact Feminist Bookstore News (listed under Bookstores). Alyson Publications, Aunt Lute Foundation, Circlet Press, Cleis

Press, Firebrand Books, Harrington Park, Kitchen Table: Women of Color Press, Naiad Press, New Victoria Publishers, Rising Tide, Sister Vision: Black and Third World Women of Colour Press, Seal Press, Spinsters Ink.

Archives/Special Collections/Information Clearinghouses

This list is a sampling.

Lesbian Herstory Archives (LHA)
P.O. Box 1258; New York, NY 10116; (718) 768-3953

West Coast Lesbian Collections
P.O. Box 23753; Oakland, CA 94623

Women's Collection—Special Collections Department
Northwestern University Library
Evanston, IL 60208-2300

Educational Film/Video

(Many distributors listed below have additional films.)
All God's Children, gay and lesbian people as full members of the black church. Available from Woman Vision, c/o Transit Media, 22D Hollywood Avenue, Hohokus, NJ 07423; (800) 343-5540.

Choosing Children: A Film about Lesbians Becoming Parents. Available from Cambridge Documentary Films, P.O. Box 390385, Cambridge, MA 02139; (617) 484-3993. Web site: http://www.shore.net/~cdf

Coming Out, Coming Home: Asian and Pacific Islander Family Stories. Available from A/PI-PFLAG Family Project, P.O. Box 640223, San Francisco, CA 94164; (415) 921-8850.

Gay Youth: An Educational Video for the Nineties. Available from Wolfe Video, Box 64, New Almaden, CA 95042; (408) 268-6782. E-mail: wolfe@wolfe.com. Excellent documentary comparing two teen stories.

It's Elementary. Teaching about lesbians and gays in schools. Produced by Women's Educational Media, 2180 Bryant Street, Suite 203, San Francisco CA, 94110.

Love Makes a Family: Gay Parents in the '90s. Fanlight Productions, 47 Halifax Street, Boston, MA 02130; (800) 937-4113. Web site: http://www.fanlight.com

Partnership Protection. Video about legal issues available from National Center for Lesbian Rights (see Organizations).

Pink Triangles. Excellent film about lesbian and gay oppression. Available from Cambridge Documentary Films (see *Choosing Children* above).

Organizations

Alcoholics Anonymous (Gay AA groups) (see chapter 3, Alcohol, Tobacco, and Other Mood-Altering Drugs)

Asian Pacific Lesbian and Bisexual Women's Network
P.O. Box 460778; San Francisco, CA 94146; (510) 814-2422

BI-Net USA/The Bisexual Network of the USA
P.O. Box 7327, Langley Park, MD 20787; (202) 986-7186

Bisexual Resources Center
P.O. Box 639; Cambridge, MA 02140; (617) 424-9595

Children of Lesbians and Gays Everywhere (COLAGE)
2300 Market Street, #165; San Francisco, CA 94114; (415) 861-5437; (702) 583-8029
Web site: http://www.COLAGE.org

Dignity USA (G/L/B/T Catholics)
150 Massachusetts Avenue NW, Suite 11; Washington, DC 20005; (202) 861-0017

Gay and Lesbian National Hotline
(888) THE-GLNH [843-4564]
Peer counseling, information, referrals. Toll-free and anonymous.

Gay and Lesbian Parents Coalition International (GLPCI)
P.O. Box 50360; Washington, DC 20091; (202) 583-8029
Web site: http://www.glpci.org

Gay, Lesbian, Straight Education Network (GLSEN)
121 W. 27th Street, Suite 804; New York, NY 10001; (212) 727-0135
Web site: http://www.glstn.org/

The Hetrick-Martin Institute
2 Astor Place; New York, NY 10003; (212) 674-2400
Publishes national directory for queer youth.

Lambda Legal Defense and Educational Fund (LLDEF)
121 Wall Street; New York, NY 10005; (212) 809-8585

Lavender Youth Recreation and Information Center (LYRIC)
127 Collingwood Street; San Francisco, CA 94114; Talkline: 800-246-PRIDE
Web site: http://thecity.sfsu.edu/~lyric

Lesbian AIDS Project (LAP) (see chapter 15, HIV, AIDS, and Women)

Mautner Project for Lesbians with Cancer
1707 L Street NW, Suite 1060; Washington, DC 20039; (202) 332-5536 (voice/TTY)

Momazons (for queer moms)
P.O. Box 82069; Columbus, OH 43202; (614) 267-0193
Web site: http://www.glbnet.com/business/oh/col/momazons/momazon2.html

National Black Gay and Lesbian Leadership Forum
1219 South La Brea; Los Angeles, CA 90019; (213) 964-7820
Web site: http://www.qrd.org/qrd/www/orgs/nbgllf

National Center for Lesbian Rights
870 Market Street, Suite 570; San Francisco, CA 94102; (415) 392-6257
The legal watchdog for g/l/b/t parents and others. Excellent publications.

National Domestic Violence Hotline
(800) 799-SAFE
 Referrals to lesbian or lesbian-friendly support and shelter services.

National Gay and Lesbian Task Force (NGLTF)
2320 17th Street NW; Washington, DC 20009; (202) 332-6483
Web site: http://www.ngltf.org

National Latina/o Lesbian and Gay Organization (LLEGO)
1612 K Street NW, Suite 500; Washington, DC 20006; (202) 466-8240

National Lesbian and Gay Health Association
(202) 939-7880

Old Lesbians Organizing for Change
P.O. Box 980422; Houston, TX 77098

Parents, Families, and Friends of Lesbians and Gays (P-FLAG)
1101 14th Street NW, Suite 1030; Washington, DC 20005; (202) 638-4200
Web site: http://www.plfag.org
 Local chapters throughout the country.

PRIDE Institute (for alcohol and chemical dependency)
101 5th Avenue, Suite 10D; New York, NY 10003; (800) 54-PRIDE

Project 10
7850 Melrose Avenue; Los Angeles, CA 90046; (818) 577-4553
 Support for l/b/t and questioning youth.

SAGE (Senior Action in a Gay Environment)
305 7th Avenue; New York, NY 10001; (212) 741-2247

Alternative Insemination

The organizations listed below are open to lesbian, bisexual, and single heterosexual women. The sperm banks listed ship sperm and give doctor referrals around the U.S.

California Cryobank
1019 Gayley Avenue; Los Angeles, CA 90024; (800) 231-3373

The Fenway Community Health Center
7 Haviland Street; Boston, MA 02115; (617) 267-0900
 Does office insemination, instructs on home insemination. Also serves as the required medical conduit for women from all over the U.S. who want to use a sperm bank but have no local doctor (one visit to FCHC required).

The Sperm Bank of California
2115 Milvia Street; Berkeley, CA 94704; (510) 841-1858

Additional Online Resources*

The Conception Connection
http://www.members.aol.com/altfamnet

A Dyke's World
http://www.qworld.org/DykesWorld

Lesbian.org: Resources for Lesbians
http://www.lesbian.org

LesBiGay & Queer Resources at igc
http://www.igc.org/lbg.resources.html

PlanetOut: Land On It.
http://www.planetout.com

Queer Resources Directory
http://www.qrd.org/qrd

Youth Action Online: Gay and Lesbian Youth
http://www.youth.org

For further information, see Jeff Dawson, *Gay and Lesbian Online* (Berkeley, CA: Peach Pit Press, 1996).

* For more information and listings of online resources, please see Introduction to Online Women's Health Resources, p. 25.

Chapter 11

Sexuality

By Lynn Rosenbaum and Wendy Sanford, with Janna Zwerner Jacobs, based on earlier work by Nancy Miriam Hawley and Elizabeth McGee

WITH SPECIAL THANKS TO Gina Ogden, Linda King, Judy Brewer, Denise Bergman, Eithne Johnson, and Curdina Hill*

O*ur powers* to express ourselves sexually last a lifetime—from birth to death. Whether or not we are in a sexual relationship with another person, we can explore our fantasies, feel good in our bodies, appreciate sensual pleasures, learn what turns us on, give ourselves sexual pleasure through masturbation. If we were taught to be embarrassed or ashamed of our sexual feelings, we may have spent a lot of energy denying them or feeling guilty. By the late 1990s, many women are learning to experience our sexuality without judging it and to accept it as part of ourselves.

We are all sexual—young, old, married, single, with or without disability, sexually active or not, transgendered, heterosexual, bisexual, or lesbian. As we change, our sexuality changes, too. Learning about sex is a lifelong process.

When we have relationships with other people, sexuality can be pleasure we want to give and get—communication that is fun and playful, serious and passionate. It can be a tender reaching out or an intense and compelling force that takes us over. It can get us into situations that delight us and ones we wish we could get out of. Sex can open us to new levels of loving and knowing with someone we love and trust. It can be a source of vital energy. Misused, it can hurt us tremendously. All of us as women face the troubling paradox of seeking to open ourselves to the deep vulnerabilities of sexual loving in a society in which we are often not safe or valued.

At times, sexual awareness and desires are quiet and other parts of our lives take center stage. Then, after a

* Thanks also to the following for their help with the 1998 version of this chapter: Emily Bender, Donna Bright, Sharon Bright, Gilda Bruckman, Mayra Canetti, Brenda Clark, Barbara Edelin, Vicki Gabriner, Irvienne Goldson, Marty Hackett, Sonja Herbert, Anoosh Jorjorian, Shelley Mains, Cheryl Majeed, Tom Medlar, Cindy Miller, Betsy Laitenen, Liza Rankow, Betsy Sandel, Marsha Saxton, Renae Scott, Marcia Sipski, Maria Tourreilles, Heidi Vanderheiden, Beverly Whipple, and Rose Wright. Over the years since 1969, the following women have contributed to the many versions of this chapter: Amy Alpern, Diana Chase, Francis Deloatch, Paula Doress-Worters, Bonnie Engelhardt, Mary Fitzgerald, Jean Gillespie, Ginger Goldner, Shere Hite, Janice Irvine, Nancy London, Jenny Mansbridge, Oce, Rosemarie Ouilette, Jane Pincus, Brenda Reeb, Marsha Saxton, and Jean Lastovica.

month or a year or ten years, the sexual desires may reawaken.

Although the majority of women explore sexuality in relationships with men, many do so with women or with both. Our sexual attractions may be fluid over time. When we affirm and support *all* women's choices of whom to love, we may understand and enjoy our own sexuality more fully.

The 1998 update of this chapter includes significant changes in the text and in the Resources. **Please consult chapter 15, HIV, AIDS, and Women, for important information on ways to enjoy sex with a partner without putting yourself, or your partner, at risk for transmitting HIV.**

SOCIAL INFLUENCES

Society shapes and limits our experiences of sexuality. We may learn, for instance, that if our looks don't conform to the ideal—if we are fat or old or have a disability—then we have no right to be sexual. Additional stereotypes confront many women. If we are black or Latina, for example, we are often portrayed as being more sexually available and active than we are or want to be.

The 1960s sexual revolution has had mixed results. Although it did encourage people to be less restricted about sex, it has also made many women feel we *ought* to be available to men at all times. And the double standard still prevails. Women are not really free, sexually or otherwise, as long as we remain socially and economically unequal to men. A dramatic example of this is the way men continue to use sexual violence as a weapon against women.

Nowhere in the world do women have full access to services crucial to our enjoyment of sex—sex education, protection from unwanted pregnancy and sexually transmitted disease, legal abortion when we need it. Current efforts by conservative religious and political groups threaten to limit our access even further, in an attempt to squeeze *all* our sexuality back into the boundaries of marriage and motherhood.

Breaking the Silence

When the women's movement surfaced again in the late 1960s, many women began speaking in small groups about sexual experiences and feelings. Talking more openly about sex is not always easy at first, but we have much to learn from each other. Such discussions can be funny, painful, and healing. We can affirm each other's feelings, help each other challenge society's distortions of our sexuality, encourage each other in our sexual adventures, and learn together to be more assertive about our own sexual needs and desires.[1]

Over the past 30 years, many of us have begun to redefine women's sexuality according to our own experiences and not what male "experts" have imagined. Wanting to do more than merely react to sexist patterns that we don't like, we ask: What do *we* want?

What images, fantasies, practices unlock the powerful erotic forces within us?

Sometimes our changing ideas and beliefs about sex do not match our sexual desires. Our desires have been partially shaped by the violent, sexist, and racist society in which we have grown up—even if we think that society is wrong. We may be faced with contradictions, such as thinking that pornographic magazines are harmful but still finding them enjoyable to look at. We might think that a man whistling at us on the street is degrading, but also like the attention it brings us. A particular sexual act may feel affirming in one situation but degrading in another. We may fantasize about sexual acts we would never wish to do. The *contexts* of our sexual lives affect our feelings of pleasure and well-being.

We are working for a society free of male/female inequalities, sexual violence, racism, homophobia, and media misuse of sex, so that our sexuality can be a source of refreshment, play, passion, connection, and energy.

Sexism and Power in Sexual Relationships with Men*

For those of us in sexual relationships with men, there are considerations that grow out of the power differences between men and women. Men as a group have more power in our society than women do. Even if you feel equal to your husband, male lover, friends, colleagues, or co-workers, our culture values men more. This supposed superiority (even though your sex partner may not feel superior at all) gets played out in sex in the following ways:

- You should make love when he wants to, whether you're in the mood or not.
- You should take care of birth control because condoms interfere with his pleasure, or you should not use birth control at all if he doesn't want you to.
- You should make yourself attractive to him when he gets home from work (this despite the fact that you have been working too, inside or outside the home or both).
- You should make sure the kids don't interrupt while you are making love.
- You should have orgasms to show him what a good lover he is.
- If you don't have intercourse, you should at least relieve him of his sexual tensions by oral sex or masturbating him. (It's no more painful for a man to go without orgasm than it is for a woman.)

I always used to see myself as there for a man's pleasure. I would do anything to please him. Just re-

---

* Most of these factors affect mainly male/female couples but may also arise in sexual relationships between women. See also chapter 10, Relationships with Women.

cently, at 23, I've realized that I have needs in sex and started to say something about it.

It's hard to say no to having sex with a guy when he's taken me out to dinner several times and given me so much.

I have a physical disability that makes me slow to feel sexual sensations in my genitals. With my husband I am finally going slow enough to get past my terror that I won't feel anything. But for five years I faked orgasms so men would think they were great lovers. I am angry now that I subjected myself to that kind of sexual pretense.

There are so many times I say yes when I don't really want to, just to avoid a long discussion about why not.

When I finally learned to have orgasms and wanted to make love more, my husband seemed to have less of a desire for sex. He wasn't used to my being so turned on and assertive. I think he missed the power he used to have in determining how our lovemaking would go.

Sex-Role Stereotypes

Traditionally, men are "supposed" to know more about sex, to initiate it, to have a stronger sex drive. Women are "supposed" to be passive recipients or willing students. Supposedly they want sex and we want love. Such rigid classifying of people by gender is false and damaging.

Perhaps what's at issue is not male sex drive at all but the fact that men are raised with different ways of expressing their emotions. Sexual intercourse is one of the few permissible ways for a man to be close to someone. For many men, it is the only acceptable place for their tender, loving feelings. It may be this limitation, rather than an innate, irrepressible sex drive that prompts men to initiate intercourse so often and leads to the false notion that women are less sexual than men. The sterotype may also arise from deep cultural fears of women's sexual passion and power. It may be that some women initiate other expressions of sex more often than men.

Conventional Definitions of Lovemaking

Most people learn to define sex with a man mainly in terms of intercourse, a form of lovemaking that is often well suited to men's orgasm and pleasure but is not necessarily well suited to ours.

In high school we had long making-out periods and I had orgasms all the time. When we "graduated" to intercourse I stopped having them so easily because we stopped doing all the other things.

I have orgasms easily during intercourse. Sometimes I love his thrusting deep inside me. Sometimes I don't want the penetration, I want something else. But he feels if we haven't had intercourse, we haven't actually made love.

I feel shy to ask for more foreplay when I know what he's really waiting for is the fucking.

Standard male definitions call all the touching, licking, sucking, and caressing that turns us on *foreplay* to the big act — *intercourse*. Some texts even call us *dysfunctional* or *frigid* if we don't reach orgasm *during* intercourse. This is not a female definition of sexual pleasure.

In a survey discussed in *The Hite Report* by Shere Hite (see Resources), 70% of women did not experience orgasm during intercourse, although most did during other kinds of sex play or masturbation. Many of us have learned ways of increasing our satisfaction in intercourse. But a more fundamental approach would be to change our definitions of lovemaking.

It took making love with women for me to see that all the other things — oral sex, having my breasts sucked, rolling around or just lying still and feeling the sensations, touching my lover and turning her on — all these are lovemaking for me. Now when I make love with men I do it more like making love with a woman — slower, more sensually and tenderly, sometimes without penetration at all.

Emphasis on Performance and Goals

Many sex books focus on techniques and say little about feelings. We worry about being sexy enough, about "doing it" well enough to please our partners. Orgasms, too, can become a goal: Some partners work at it for hours, wanting to please us or to show they are good lovers.

I feel vaguely guilty if sex isn't great all the time, as though if I'm a real woman I should have an incredible orgasm every time, instead of accepting that sometimes there will be little ones and sometimes big ones.

With sex coming at us from every direction in the popular culture, we may worry whether we are doing it enough. If we're single, we "should" be finding more sex partners. (Yet, women with many sex partners are often criticized.) If we're in a relationship, we "should" be making love a certain number of times per week.

Many couples these days report the "problem" of lack of interest in sex. This may reflect problems in their relationship or in ways of lovemaking. But what experts are calling insufficient interest in sex may actually be our own desires measured against today's escalated sexual standards. It may even be a reaction against the general hype about sex in the media. Or it may be simple skin hunger — the need to be touched by another human being without "going all the way."

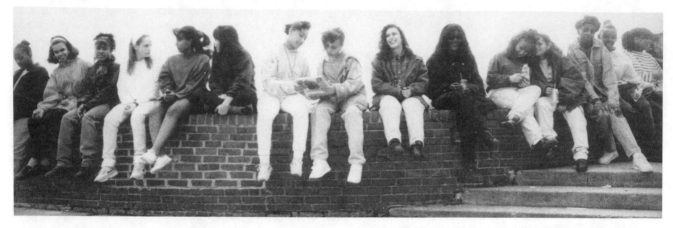

Shirley Zeiberg

Virginity and Abstinence

A virgin traditionally is someone who hasn't had sexual intercourse. Although men are virgins in this sense before they have had sex, the main pressure to be a virgin has been on women. Today we experience conflicting pressures about virginity.

My mother told me it's a gift I can give only once, so I'd better hold on to it.

Among my girlfriends during senior year of high school, I was the only virgin. This caused me embarrassment and teasing from my friends. I was branded as a nice girl, chicken, weird, etc., even though I did all the same things they did except have sex.

The idea of virginity is an old one. People in early Greece and Rome used the term to refer to a woman (or a goddess) who was autonomous, on her own, not "owned" by any man. Later it came to mean only sexual virginity and, ironically, to reflect the prevailing view of women as man's property. Remaining a virgin until she married guaranteed that a woman would uphold the family honor by passing from father to husband like unspoiled goods. Because there was no dependable birth control, it guaranteed also that babies would be born only to married couples.

Many parents today are less concerned about preserving their daughters' actual virginity than they are about ensuring safer sex and determining how soon or with whom their daughters have intercourse. Some parents respect and encourage a daughter's decisions about sex. But in many other families, the message is still "Stay a virgin!" We may "do everything but" have intercourse. This can be confusing to young women who technically remain virgins, yet may have become as emotionally and physically involved as we would with intercourse.*

Meanwhile, there is a lot of pressure today from the media, from popular music, and from peers for young women to be sexually active. Some teens have responded to this pressure by forming a movement for abstinence with the emphasis on sex as a *conscious choice*. We may choose to abstain from intercourse or other sexual activities because of fear of a sexually transmitted disease or getting pregnant, our religious beliefs, our traditional upbringing, or simply not being ready. Moreover, we may choose abstinence because we are focused on developing other parts of ourselves, such as our creative, intellectual, or athletic skills. We may be expressing intimacy in nonsexual ways through friendships and family relationships.

We must be free to have sex or not, as we think best. Having sex usually brings many changes in the relationship and in our life. Because it is often a big decision, it makes sense to think about it, talk it over with friends and the person we're involved with, choose a method of birth control if necessary. We have the right to say no to someone who is pushing us to have sex when we don't want to.

When we freely make choices about sex out of respect for our feelings and our bodies, we will be more likely to put ourselves into situations we can be glad about.†

Body Image‡

How we feel about our bodies is influenced by the messages we receive from families, lovers, co-workers, health care practitioners, coaches, and many others. We're affected by the images we see in magazines, music videos, TV, movies, and advertisements. We hear descriptions of women's bodies in popular music. We may dislike our own bodies because they don't live up to expectations or standards that we have internalized. All this can negatively affect our sexual lives.

For years I wouldn't make love in a position that exposed my backside to scrutiny, for I had been told it

---

* In order to remain "virgins," some young women may have anal intercourse instead of vaginal intercourse. Unprotected anal sex is a high-risk behavior for transmission of HIV/AIDS.

† For more on virginity and first intercourse, see *Changing Bodies, Changing Lives* by Ruth Bell et al.

‡ See chapter 1, Body Image, for a more thorough discussion.

was "too jiggly." Needless to say, this prevented me from being sexually assertive and creative and limited my responses.

We have a good sex life with lots of variety, fantasies, games. The fact that my disability prevents me from bending my leg limits us in some positions, but we just try different ones. Yet I don't have orgasms with my husband, only in masturbation. I am still struggling with my body. When I am unclothed I still feel like parts of me are really ugly. I think that when I can finish mourning and cry out my anguish over the disability, then sex will get better for me.

If we like the way we look and feel good about our bodies, we may feel better about making love.

One of the difficult things about being large is that more often than not other people are the problem, not me. Many times I have felt that people I know wonder at my friendship with my lover. They wonder how a thin person can make love to a large one. The idea, I suppose, is that large women aren't attractive. Nonsense, of course. I enjoy my body immensely when I make love, either to myself or my boyfriend. I never think about my largeness. I simply am it and positively luxuriate in it. I love my body when I make love. It is beautiful to me and to my boyfriend. For six years we have both exulted in good lovemaking.

Violence Against Women*

It is a cruel fact of our lives that many women are abused. Sex may be used as a weapon by both men and women. Incest, rape, sexual harassment by a boss or co-worker or teacher, battering in our homes—any of these can affect our sexual lives. If we don't experience violence directly, the possibility may leer at us from pornography, news stories, movies, crude jokes, and so on.

Sometimes when I hear about a rape that's happened, I can't make love with my husband, even though I love him and usually enjoy sex. I know he is a gentle person, but for a moment I don't see him; I see all the men who use their penises as weapons to dominate and hurt women.

I went through several one-night stands and I found that I did not have to love or really know the person to have sexual physical contact. In the past couple of years I have wondered why this detachment exists. The therapy I went through clarified many things for me. I wondered how my sexual assault experiences had affected my sexuality. I find now that I am much more deliberate about my sexuality, about balancing pleasure and intimacy. I think I am still capable of detaching feelings from sex, but I choose not to anymore.

* See chapter 8, Violence Against Women.

We must work for an equal, nonviolent society in which sex is used not for somebody else's profit or as an instrument of dominance, but in service of love—love of ourselves, love and friendship for others.

Racism

The combination of sexism and racism places heavy demands on those of us who are women of color as we strive to be and feel powerful. How this affects our sexuality is an immense and important topic, which is connected to our particular history of struggle in the U.S. and to the experiences of women of color worldwide. Within the limited space in this chapter, we can only scratch the surface.†

Many racial stereotypes focus on our sexuality through the use of racist myths. African-American women, for example, are stereotyped as sexually aggressive, oversexed, and "animalistic." Stereotypes of Asian-American women as existing to serve men's sexual needs are fostered by the rapid spread of sex tourism, sexual slavery, and forced prostitution in many Asian countries caused by militarism and changing global patterns of migration. (See chapter 26 for more on the international sexual exploitation of women.) Latinas and Native American women and other women of color confront equally demeaning stereotypes on a daily basis. The stereotypes that perpetuate racism and sexism often arise from contexts in which women and men of color were historically, or are in the present, subordinated, colonized, and enslaved by white people. During the enslavement of Africans in the U.S., for example, white slave owners and overseers raped African-American women freely, yet the stereotypes that developed at that time and continue to this day blamed the women rather than the men who raped them.

These and other destructive sexual stereotypes, along with the racial and sexual assaults that are a reality for many of us, influence the ways we do or don't assert our desires. They affect how others treat us, and when we internalize them and believe them, they affect how we treat ourselves.

When we consider the uses that this society has made of black women's bodies—as breeding machines, as receptacles for pornographic desires, as "hot pussies" to be bought and sold—surely our collective estrangement from a life-giving eroticism makes sense.[2]

Issues of power and sexuality are rarely separate from economic issues for us as women of color. One

† Most of the examples given here focus on African-American women who are heterosexual; we invite you to see where the issues are the same and different for women in other communities of color, and for those who have sex with women. The authors of this book welcome your ideas for the next revision of *Our Bodies, Ourselves.*

result of racial and economic discrimination is that many men of color are unemployed or underemployed, and this affects their self-esteem and the quality of their lives. Their relationships with women may be the only place where they can exert some power. Sometimes this makes us feel pressured to excuse behaviors that aren't in our best interest. We may not feel free to ask for what we want, or to insist on using condoms for protection from HIV. Or the man may want to be involved with more than one woman, and this may not be what we want. Many men of color are working two and three jobs, which interferes with the time to be a father and a husband, and there isn't the time to develop a fulfilling sexual relationship.

There just aren't as many black men around. On the whole, as I look at myself and my sisters and friends, I'd say that we don't have as much consistent sexual experience as we might like. We may have partners, but there's less stability over time. So there's less time to develop the trust and depth and safety to be more open sexually.

You add to this, that for me and my friends growing up as middle-class black girls, there was a big emphasis on educational goals. Black women could expect to be single for a big part of our lives, and our parents knew we had to be able to take care of ourselves. There was a big push to get our educations and to be successful—and this limited our sexual expression.

It takes love, support, and healing for us to embrace a full range of chosen sexual expressions, from exuberant to shy, from celibate to sexually active. Women have differing approaches to feeling good about ourselves despite the obstacles.

I think we should start with our feet, and remember how much they have carried us through. Bathing each other's feet is such a spiritual act. Also I learn a lot from women who are in recovery, how they learn to be loving to themselves again.

Talking about sexuality can be difficult because of the onslaught of stereotypes, but we can try talking with a couple of friends. We can learn to value the wholeness of our sexuality, informed as it is by spirituality and intelligence. We can focus on a particular relationship with a man or a woman, learning to bring our whole selves into that relationship.

Those of us with feminist awareness find that the experience of passion in a nonsexist context is amazingly healing. Without knowing that we hold within ourselves so much fear, we find in encounters with one another, with caring partners, that sexuality has often been a fearful site but that it can be a place where we can let fear go, where we can recover and come back to ourselves. . . . [We can] feel again the sense of wonder, of pleasure that there is a life-force within us charged with erotic power that can transform and heal our lives.[3]

We can be activists challenging the racism and sexism that attempt to define us. Chapters of the National Black Women's Health Project, the National Asian Women's Health Organization, the National Latina Health Organization, and the Native American Women's Education Resource Center, for example, educate women about our bodies and our sexuality. (See chapter 27 for more information on these organizations and how to reach them.) We can work for economic empowerment, knowing that improving the economic situation of women and men of color in the U.S. and worldwide can translate into healthier partnerships.

I think we're all angry about this, and often we talk in blaming ways about black men or black women. But really it's a community issue. And that's where the healing has to happen. African-American women need to find ways to get together to express our anger and sadness about all this, and then we need to come together with men to work it through.

Racism is one of many influences on our sexuality. As women of color we span a broad range of peoples, with many different traditions, cultural practices, ways of upbringing, and religions. Some of these cultural factors are a source of strength; others restrict or hurt us. For those who grew up in traditional families or traditional religions where men were expected to dominate women, coming into our own sexuality may require looking at ourselves—and at our mothers—in new ways. As a young Latina said in an open letter to her mother:

Mom, being a woman is more than what my grandfather taught you. It is true that part of being a woman is bearing and rearing children, making tortillas, smelling good, being quiet, being sweet, obeying, praying, going to church, and an endless list of tasks assigned to us by men to please men. Being a woman also includes many other things. . . . I refer to writing, singing, laughing, expressing your feelings in an open way, saying what you think without feeling awkward. I also talk about getting to know your body better, accepting your femaleness not as a tool to attract a nice-looking boy, but for yourself. . . . I hope I can remain as sweet as you have always been, without having to compromise my goals or my needs as a human, as a woman.

—Claudia Colindres[4]

GROWING UP

I watch my daughter. From morning to night her body is her home. She lives in it and with it. When she runs around the kitchen she uses all of herself. Every muscle in her body moves when she laughs, when she cries. When she rubs her vulva, there is no awkwardness, no feeling that what she is doing is wrong. She feels pleasure and expresses it without hesitation. She knows when she wants to be touched and when

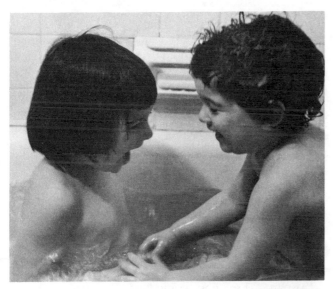

Annie Popkin

she wants to be left alone. It's so hard to get back that sense of body as home.

Childhood experiences and memories shape our sexuality. We may have learned to think of sex as forbidden, dirty, and shameful. Many of us have been sexually abused. It is most helpful for our families to talk comfortably and openly about sex and to respect our boundaries.

When we become teenagers, our developing bodies are usually a mystery to us.* We may discover that what the media, and most people, consider beautiful falls into a narrow range (see chapter 1, Body Image). We may lose respect for our uniqueness, our own smells and shapes. We may judge ourselves in relation to others. We may come to feel isolated.

It can take time—sometimes years and years—and positive experiences to get rid of these negative, often shameful, feelings. Many of us with young children want to help them grow up feeling good about their bodies and their sexuality, though sometimes it is hard to move beyond our own upbringing.

The other day I was taking a bath with my almost three-year-old daughter. I was lying down and she was sitting between my legs, which were spread apart. She said, "Mommy, you don't have a penis." I said, "That's right, men have penises and women have clitorises." All calm and fine—then, "Mommy, where is your clitoris?" Okay, now what was I going to do? I took a deep breath (for courage or something), tried not to blush, spread my vulva apart, and showed her my clitoris. It didn't feel so bad. "Do you want to see yours?" I asked. "Yes." That was quite a trick to get her to look over her fat stomach and see hers, especially when she started laughing as I put her finger on her clitoris.

* See *Changing Bodies, Changing Lives* by Ruth Bell et al.

Thanks in part to the women's movement, many of us with grown children and grandchildren talk with them more freely about sex now than we once would have. Many of us younger women have benefited from the openness of the women who raised us. "Growing up" sexually never ends.

BISEXUALITY†

Historically in the U.S., bisexuality has been stigmatized or simply not recognized. However, in the last 25 years, bisexual activists have helped to legitimize bisexuality as an acceptable sexual identity. In some instances, bisexual women have been able to build upon the work of the feminist and gay rights movements, though at other times, we have had to fight to be recognized within these communities.

Bisexuality can be defined in many different ways. One definition is to be sexually attracted to both men and women. This can take many forms, including being single, being married, being in a monogamous relationship, or having several lovers. Some of us choose to have sexual relationships with men at one point and with women at another point in our lives. We may become lovers with men only or with women only, without acting on our attractions to the other. For some, being bisexual means dating both men and women at the same time.

I've been in lesbian relationships for ages. Then suddenly last year I fell in love with a man. A total surprise!

When I first started getting involved with women as well as men, I wanted to be more intimate with them as an extension of being friends.

Sometimes, thinking of ourselves as bisexual is a safe stopping place in a transition from one identity to another.

For years I said to myself and my friends, "I think maybe I'm bisexual," meaning, "I'm probably a lesbian but I'm scared to death to admit it."

Yet, for many of us bisexuality is not transitional at all. We are comfortable with our desires and accept that we don't have to be *either* straight or gay.

There is a common stereotype that being bisexual means we are "promiscuous"—a negative expression for having many sexual partners. In fact, being bisexual may or may not include having multiple lovers (sometimes called nonmonogamy or polyamory).[5] Some women may have male and female lovers but still choose to identify as straight or as lesbian. And others prefer not to use any labels at all.

† For more on bisexuality, see chapter 9, Working Toward Mutuality: Our Relationships with Men, and chapter 10, Relationships with Women.

I've tried to define myself using labels of lesbian, straight, bisexual, and I didn't feel that any of them were mine. I think of it in terms of people I could love, not sexes I could love.

If we *do* choose to take on the bisexual identity, it can mean opening ourselves to discrimination and biphobia, but it can also lead us to connect with a growing bisexual community (see "Bisexuality" in Resources).

I'm aware of how being bisexual can make life difficult, but never once have I thought that it would be better not to be bisexual. I focus on how it's connected me to a community—particularly of women—that I really like. I love being bi! Just like being Jewish or being a woman—even though you can talk about the ways these groups are oppressed—it's just who you are. And it's not something I would want to change.

Being lovers with people of both sexes opens our eyes to social and political realities that may be new to us. If we were sexually intimate only with men before, a relationship with a woman may introduce us to the world of lesbian experience, with its particular satisfactions and oppressions. We may soon find that we have to be more careful in public than we ever dreamed of being; we may become aware of homophobia for the first time. Our friendships may take on new dimensions.

If we have been exclusively lesbian, being lovers with a man may allow us to experience some of the privileges of the dominant heterosexual culture, such as being able to show our love more freely in public. There also may be more struggles with sex-role stereotypes than we are used to. Before menopause, we may have the unfamiliar need for birth control.

Invisibility is a problem. Few people know that bisexuals exist, because we don't "fit" into either the heterosexual or the lesbian world. When we are open, both worlds may judge us. Heterosexual friends may be shocked and scared when we have a woman lover (see chapter 8, Relationships with Women). Lesbian friends may see our interest in men as being disloyal to the lesbian community. Lesbian lovers may distrust us, fearing that we will leave them for a man.

When I'm having trouble with a man and tell a lesbian friend, she usually gets a look in her eye that means, "What did you expect, being with a man?"

All these judgments isolate us. And we may feel pressure to choose: "I've had people press me to say I'm 'more' one than the other." As more women feel comfortable and safe in being open about bisexuality, we will create more of a community for ourselves, and we will further challenge both heterosexual and lesbian assumptions about whom and how women can love.

CELIBACY

Traditionally, celibacy has meant choosing not to marry. Today, many people use it to mean not having sex for a certain period of time. It can mean no sex with someone else or no masturbation as well. Sometimes we choose celibacy in response to our culture's overemphasis on sex, as a break from feeling we must relate to others sexually all the time: "I was tired of having to say yes or no." Or it can be a personal adventure.

I'm exploring myself as a sexual person but in a different way. My sensitivity to my body is heightened. I am more aware of what arouses my sensual interests. I am free to be myself. I have more energy for work and friends. My spirituality feels more intense and clear.

As part of a religious commitment (for nuns, priests, and others), celibacy offers a freedom to use one's energy for other people, not so much because lovemaking drains energy but because sexual relationships necessitate commitments, time, and attention. Yet, religious celibacy has often been misunderstood or ridiculed. A nun wrote as follows:

For many religious women sex means so much that we use it as a gift of our life in the service of a people. Not to engage in an active sex life or to marry is for the purpose of being free to be of service. It is painful and depressing when others speak of this gift as though to have made this decision is necessarily to have a warped personality.

When we choose celibacy, we can experiment with any form that offers what we want.

I spend part of each day in yoga and meditation. Sometimes I go for days without thinking about my sexual identity at all. I masturbate only when inspired, which is seldom these days. Yet in meditation last week I found myself having an orgasm. It was ecstasy!

In couple relationships, we may choose celibacy when we want some distance or solitude or when we just don't want to have sex for a while. This can be awkward and requires careful communication if a partner isn't feeling the same way.

I say to my woman lover, "I don't feel like making love this month, and I may not next month." Now, who does that? Is it okay? Am I allowed? The last thing we were ever taught was that it was okay to try what we want.

Some couples choose celibacy together, which allows both people to explore other dimensions of loving. It can help us get out of old sexual patterns, expand our sensual/sexual focus beyond genital sex if we want to, and make us feel more self-sufficient and independent, which can strengthen the relationship.

Sometimes being a parent to a new baby enforces a time of virtual celibacy. Sometimes we are faced with celibacy when we don't choose it—after a breakup or divorce, when a partner or lover dies, or simply during a dry spell. Though these circumstances may be painful, celibacy sometimes surprises us with its own satisfactions.

SEXUAL PLEASURE

Women experience sexual pleasure in many different ways: physically, emotionally, spiritually, and intellectually. We may enjoy a gentle caress, an erotic dance, or a sweaty orgasm. Traditionally, male researchers' descriptions of sexual pleasure have focused on genital sensations and stages of arousal. But pleasure and eroticism are much more than that. Sounds, sights, smells, and touch can arouse our sexual feelings, as do fantasies, a baby sucking at the breast, the smell of a familiar body, wearing a slinky dress, an engaging conversation, or a favorite song.

The erotic can be a positive source of power. The erotic not only is about what goes on in the bedroom but is about tapping into our deepest feelings and our creative energies, which run through all aspects of our lives. It can be about feeling connected—to our own strengths, to our lovers, to nature, to a higher power.*

For many reasons, however, we may not open ourselves fully to sexual pleasure. We may carry messages from our sexist, racist, and homophobic cultures that say our bodies and our feelings of pleasure are not valuable. We may feel physically or emotionally unsafe. We may fear getting pregnant or getting infected with HIV. We may have been sexually abused and find that certain situations bring on frightening memories. We may have to work so many hours in a day that we don't have much time or energy for sex.

For some of us, being able to communicate what we do want and don't want sexually—i.e., "setting boundaries"—allows us to feel a sense of safety and experience greater pleasure. By sharing our experiences of pleasure, while also acknowledging the limitations we face, we can move toward a greater understanding and fulfillment of women's eroticism.

MODELS OF SEXUAL RESPONSE

When I'm feeling turned on, either alone or with someone I'm attracted to, my heart beats faster, my face gets red, my eyes are bright. My whole vulva feels wet and full. My breasts hum. When I'm standing up I feel a rush of weakness in my thighs. When I'm lying down I may feel like doing a big stretch, arching my back, feeling the sensations go out to my fingers and toes.

* For more on the power of the erotic, see "Uses of the Erotic: The Erotic as Power" by Audre Lorde, in Resources.

As we become sexually aroused we go through a series of physical and emotional changes, sometimes called *sexual response*. In the 1960s, the researchers William Masters and Virginia Johnson developed a model of sexual response and orgasm, which became very popular. This model is physiological and focuses mostly on the genitals. Since that time, other researchers have developed different models to try to include a broader range of responses. Some of these basic patterns are described in this section.

It is important to remember, however, that there is no one "right" pattern of sexual response. What works, what feels good, what makes us feel more alive in ourselves and connected with our partners (if we have them) is what counts. Our sexual patterns, too, will change at different points in our lives. If the models proposed by sexologists and researchers (*or* feminists) don't fit our experiences of response, then we must trust ourselves and learn more from each other. These models are presented not to create a set of standards that we should try to follow, but rather to broaden our understanding of the various ways in which we may experience sexual pleasure.

Masters and Johnson observed and measured women and men engaging in sexual activities in a laboratory setting.[6] The activities were mostly masturbation and vagina-to-penis intercourse. This research, reported in *Human Sexual Response,* has contributed greatly to our understanding of sexual response, although it should be noted that the study had several limitations, including sample bias, an artificial setting, and experimenter bias. Their model describes four stages of physiological arousal: excitement, plateau, climax, and resolution. For drawings that may help you understand these stages, please see chapter 12, "Understanding Our Bodies: Sexual Anatomy, Reproduction and the Menstrual Cycle."

Early in sexual *excitement*, veins in the pelvis, vulva, and clitoris begin to dilate (open) and fill with blood, gradually making the whole area feel full. (This is called *vasocongestion.*) In the vagina, this swelling creates a "sweating" reaction, producing the fluid that makes the vaginal lips get wet—often an early sign that we are sexually excited. (In women who are past menopause, there may not be much lubrication.) The extra flow of blood also causes the uterus to enlarge and elevate within the pelvic cavity. Sexual tension rises throughout the body as muscles begin to tense up or contract *(myotonia)*. We may breathe more quickly, nipples may become erect and hard, and a flush or rash may appear on our skin.

If stimulation continues, we move into the *plateau* stage, according to Masters and Johnson. The responses continue to intensify. The inner two-thirds of the vagina continues to balloon while the outer third narrows and is quite sensitive to pressure. The uterus elevates fully. We breathe very rapidly and may pant. The clitoris retracts under its hood.

Enough stimulation of or around the clitoris and (for some women) pressure on the cervix or other sensitive areas cause pelvic fullness and body tension to build

Women's Sexual Response Cycle: Pleasure, Orgasm, Ecstasy in Ongoing Continuum

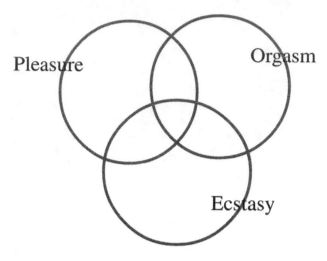

Pleasure

Orgasm

Ecstasy

Gina Ogden

up to a peak, or *climax*. Orgasm is the point at which all the tension is suddenly released in a series of involuntary and pleasurable muscular contractions that expel blood from the pelvic tissues. We may feel contractions in the vagina, uterus, and rectum.

If lovemaking doesn't continue, we enter the *resolution* stage. For one-half hour or more after orgasmic swelling decreases, the muscles relax and the clitoris, vagina, and uterus return to their usual positions.

In the 1970s and 1980s, several researchers and clinicians such as Helen Singer Kaplan[7] and Bernie Zilbergeld and Carol Rinkleib Ellison[8] expanded on the Masters and Johnson model.* They included emotional aspects of sexual response, such as desire, arousal, and satisfaction. Some models recognized that a peak emotional experience may or may not coincide with the physiological release during orgasm. David Reed developed a completely psychological model of sexual response called the Erotic Stimulus Pathway Model. He described moving through *seduction, erotic sensations, surrender, and reflection.*[9]

In her book *Women Who Love Sex*, Gina Ogden describes a very different sort of model.[10] Her work is based on descriptions by women themselves (though not a representative sample). Ogden visualizes sexual response as "three dancing spheres of energy": pleasure, orgasm, and ecstasy. These overlapping circles indicate that we may experience pleasure without orgasm or orgasm without ecstasy, and so on. In some cases, we may experience all three. Our sexual re-

---

* This section draws from the description of models of sexual response in *Exploring Our Sexuality* by Patricia Barthalow Koch (see Resources).

sponses are linked to intimacy, lust, fantasy, full-body stimulation, satisfaction, and more. In addition to physical and emotional responses, Ogden explores the spiritual aspects of sex. Ecstasy can be a transcendent experience or can be rooted deeply in the body and may be more easily described in poetic or mystical language than in physiological terms.

Professionals in modern society have enormous power to shape our understanding of ourselves. It is crucial that women remember that we do not have to rely exclusively on "experts" for accurate information about our sexuality. We can obtain powerful data by discussing our experiences in settings of our own making. In some cases, this information can be enhanced by research that attempts respectfully to scientifically record and measure our experiences.

Orgasm

Masters and Johnson asserted that all orgasms are physiologically the same (clitorally induced, with contractions occurring primarily in the outer third of the vagina). Yet, some women describe orgasms that don't fit this model. One such orgasm is brought on by penetration of the vagina and feels "deep" or "uterine." The buildup sometimes involves a prolonged involuntary holding in of one's breath, which is released explosively at orgasm. There do not seem to be any contractions of the outer third of the vagina. Many women with spinal cord injuries have no feeling in the pelvic area but report experiencing orgasm and its sensations elsewhere in the body (see "Sex and Disability," p. 248). Women without physical disabilities may also experience such sensations.

Searching for the one and only "right" model of women's orgasm does not reflect the diversity of experiences that women have.

The way I've heard about orgasms is there's supposed to be a big release, but that's not the way it works for me. I feel a really intense buildup that feels great, and then suddenly my clitoris becomes too sensitive to keep stimulating so I stop. I no longer have a desire to keep going and I just feel relaxed and tired, in a good way. I always wonder, did I miss the climax? Or was that not really an orgasm?

Orgasm can be mild like a hiccup, a sneeze, a ripple, or a peaceful sigh; it can be a sensuous experience, as the body glows with warmth; it can be intense or ecstatic, as we lose awareness of ourselves for a time.

Orgasm may feel different with a finger, penis, dildo, or vibrator in your vagina and different when you masturbate from when you make love with another person. It may feel totally different at different times even with the same person. Orgasm can be primarily physical but usually has emotional aspects as well. Feelings of intimacy can enhance our orgasms with a partner, and orgasms can enhance intimacy.

Often we become aroused at times when we can't get

enough stimulation to reach orgasm. Although sexual tension subsides eventually without orgasm, it takes longer, and our genitals and/or uterus may ache for a while. If we have been abused, sexual arousal may re-stimulate mental and/or physical memories of the abuse, and we may experience an aching sensation.

Quite a number of women have never had an orgasm. Some of us have "faked" an orgasm to please a partner or because media portrayals make us think we "should" be having more orgasms. Sexual, physical, or emotional abuse (past or present) may impair a woman's ability to have orgasms. Also, not being able to reach orgasm with a partner may be a clue that the relationship itself has problems and needs to change in some way.

Decreased orgasms, as well as lowered sexual desire, may be caused by the use of certain medications, substances, and antidepressant drugs such as Prozac and Zoloft.* For women who have not reached menopause, our sexual interest varies over the course of our menstrual cycle, usually peaking during ovulation. However, if we are taking oral contraceptives (the Pill), this cyclical nature of desire is suppressed. The specific effects of the Pill on women's sexual desire varies greatly among individual women.†[11]

With all the publicity about orgasms in the past years, many of us who don't experience orgasm believe that we're missing something pleasurable. We can try to reach orgasm by masturbating (see p. 240), reading books about it (see Resources), asking a partner to help, or joining a therapy group focused on sexual issues. A 53-year-old woman wrote to the Boston Women's Health Book Collective that after reading an earlier edition of this book she had masturbated and reached orgasm for the first time in her life. Yet, it's important that orgasm doesn't become one more performance pressure.

When I try too hard to have an orgasm it usually doesn't work and I end up frustrated and bored. For me it's best if I relax and let it happen if it's going to.

Some women can reach orgasm twice or more in quick succession. Knowing that multiple orgasms are possible has made some of us feel we ought to have them and that we are sexually inadequate if we don't. Men may expect it, too; one woman wrote that a man she knew was considering a divorce because the woman he was married to didn't have multiple orgasms. Yet, one orgasm can be plenty, and sex without orgasm can be pleasurable. Seek whatever feels best to you.

* See chapter 23, Women Growing Older, p. 564, for more on drugs and diseases that affect sexual desire in older persons. See chapter 6, Our Emotional Well-Being, for information on antidepressants. Also see *Sexual Pharmacology: Drugs That Affect Sexual Function* by Teresa Crenshaw et al. in Resources.
† See chapter 12, Understanding Our Bodies, p. 276, for more on the reproductive cycle. Also see *Women, Sex and Desire* by Elizabeth Davis in Resources.

The Role of the Clitoris

It may be arousing to stroke any part of our bodies, exciting to have our thighs caressed or our necks nibbled or our breasts sucked. We may find erogenous zones apart from our genitals, including fingers, toes, and ear lobes. For many women, the clitoris is the organ that is the most sensitive to stimulation and has a central role in elevating feelings of sexual tension.

Until the mid-1960s, most women didn't know how crucial the clitoris was. Even if we knew it for ourselves, nobody talked about it. Medical texts and marriage manuals (written by men) followed Freud's famous pronouncement that the "mature" woman has orgasms only when her vagina, not her clitoris, is stimulated. This theory made the penis central to a woman's sexual satisfaction. Following Freud, early psychoanalytic theories belittled women's enjoyment of masturbation as "immature" and labeled lesbian sex as a pale imitation of the "real thing."

Learning about the clitoris has increased sexual enjoyment for countless women and freed many of us from years of thinking we were "frigid."

The clitoris is sometimes called the joy button, which implies that it is one small spot. In fact, the clitoris has several parts. The glans (or tip, the part you can see) attaches to the shaft, which runs along internally from the glans toward the vaginal opening. The clitoris connects to a branching interior system of erectile tissue that runs through the genital area. (Erectile tissue responds to sexual arousal by filling with blood, becoming erect and hard. A penis also contains erectile tissue.) During sexual excitement, the clitoris swells and changes position.

You or your lover can stimulate your clitoris in many different ways—by rubbing, sucking, body pressure, using a vibrator. Any rubbing or pressure in the pubic hair–covered mons area or the vaginal lips (even on the lower abdomen and inner thighs) can move the clitoris and may also press it up against the pubic bone. Although some women touch the glans to become aroused, it is often so sensitive that direct touching hurts, even with lubrication. Also, focusing directly on the clitoris for a long time may cause the pleasurable sensations to disappear. As women grow older, the hood of skin covering the clitoris may pull back permanently, so that if you are past menopause you may need extra lubrication in order to tolerate having your clitoris rubbed.

Vagina-to-penis intercourse may give only indirect clitoral stimulation. As the penis moves in and out of the vagina it moves the inner lips, which are connected to the clitoral hood, and therefore may move the hood back and forth over the glans. When the inner lips become swollen and firm they can act as an extension of the vagina, hugging the penis as it moves back and forth and further increasing clitoral friction. To reach orgasm during vagina-to-penis intercourse, many of us need direct and sometimes prolonged clitoral stimulation both before and during intercourse.

Many women making love to other women focus directly on stimulating the clitoris. Many women who make love with men in their 60s and older find that if the men's erections happen less frequently, sexual pleasure increases, partly because penetration by the penis is no longer the focus of lovemaking. As more women begin to explore lovemaking beyond vagina-to-penis intercourse, it's likely that more of us will experience orgasm more often and more pleasurably with our partners.

The Role of the Vagina, Uterus, and Cervix

Women have the potential to respond to sexual arousal throughout the entire pelvic region. When we are aroused, the erectile tissue around the outer third of the vagina becomes full, and nerves in that area become more sensitive to stimulation and pressure. When the muscles around this part of the vagina (pubococcygeus muscles) are strong and well exercised, many women find that they reach orgasm more easily (see Kegel exercises, p. 274). Childbearing increases the system of veins in the pelvis, often making arousal quicker and stronger.

The G spot, or Grafenberg spot,[*12] is the area of spongy tissue surrounding the urethra, felt through the front wall of the vagina. It may feel like a small lump, halfway between the pubic bone and the cervix. It is filled with blood vessels and glands, and some of us find stimulation of this area pleasurable.

If you want to touch your G spot, one method is to sit on the toilet and insert your finger into your vagina. Explore along the upper front wall of your vagina, pushing up toward your navel. It can be difficult to reach this spot by yourself unless you have long fingers or a short vagina. When you first touch this area, it may feel as if you have to urinate, but this sensation may subside after a few seconds of massage. You can also have your G spot stimulated by a partner's finger or penis, a dildo, or a G-spot vibrator,. G-spot stimulation may contribute to our having orgasms. It is important to remember, however, that the G spot is not a "magic button" that automatically produces ecstasy when pushed. We can think of this as another area of our bodies to explore in enhancing our sexual pleasure.

Continuous stimulation of the G spot may also lead some women to ejaculate: to release fluid from the urethra. (Ejaculation can also occur without stimulation of the G spot.) Female ejaculation, which can occur with or without an orgasm, may feel wonderful or it may create anxiety that we have "peed" in bed. Chemical analysis has shown, however, that the fluid released in ejaculation is different from urine.

* The G spot was named by sex researchers Dr. John Perry and Dr. Beverly Whipple after Dr. Ernst Grafenberg, who wrote about it in 1950. For more on G-spot stimulation, see *The Good Vibrations Guide to Sex* by Winks and Semans and *The G spot* by Ladas et al., in Resources.

For drawings of a woman's sexual anatomy, please see chapter 12, Understanding Our Bodies, pp. 270–75.

Further up in the vagina are the cervix and uterus, which many women find crucial to orgasm. Although the inner two-thirds of the vagina and the cervix itself have little sensitivity, a penis, finger, or dildo pressing repeatedly on the cervix "jostles" the uterus and indeed the whole lining of the abdominal cavity (peritoneum). This can create a different kind of feeling internally before and during orgasm. Women who have had a total hysterectomy, in which the cervix and the uterus have been removed, may have to learn to focus on different kinds of sexual stimulation and feelings (see p. 242).

Masturbation

Masturbation is a special way of enjoying ourselves. When we were infants, touching and playing with our bodies, including our genitals, felt good. Then many of us learned from our parents, and later from our schools and religious institutions, that we were not to touch ourselves sexually.

Plenty of girls of color have had our hands smacked away from our genitals and been called naughty for playing with ourselves.

Some of us heeded their messages and some did not. But by the time we became teenagers, most of us thought masturbation was bad, whether we did it or not. We felt guilty if we did masturbate, or we suppressed it, or never discovered masturbation at all.

I never even knew about masturbation. When I was 21, a man-friend touched me "down there," bringing me to orgasm (I didn't know that word either). Then I had a brilliant thought—if he could do it to me, I could do it to me, too. So I did, though it was a long time before I could feel a lot of pleasure and orgasm.

Masturbation allows us the time and space to explore and experiment with our own bodies. We can learn what fantasies turn us on, the kinds of touch that arouse and please us, what tempo and where. We can learn our own patterns of sexual response without having to think about a partner's needs and opinions. Then, if and when we choose, we can tell our partners what we've learned or show them by guiding their hands to the places we want touched. As women who have for so long been taught to "wait for a man to turn us on," we achieve freedom by knowing how to give ourselves sexual pleasure.

For those of us who are women of color, masturbation may be one part of a larger effort to give ourselves the care we need. Some of us have spent so much time taking care of others that we have not been able

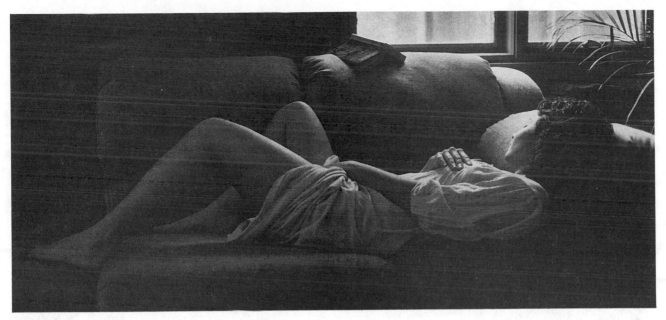

Michael Weisbrot/Stock, Boston

to attend to our own self-healing. We may have learned that our emotional needs were not as important as the need to collectively fight injustice. Valuing our personal needs is a step toward empowerment in our lives.*

I used to think masturbating was okay only if I didn't have a lover and only for a quick release. Now I see it's part of my relationship with myself, giving myself pleasure. My rhythms change. Sometimes I masturbate more when I have a lover. Sometimes I'll go for weeks without doing it.

Masturbation can help us enter a sexual relationship knowing more about what we want. We become less dependent on our partners to satisfy us, which can give them freedom, too. After menopause, masturbating also helps us keep our vaginal tissues moist and lubricating.

For me at 73, masturbation is better than a sexual relationship, as most of the time I'm more interested in nonsexual pursuits. Sustaining a relationship with all the time and thought involved would be a nuisance.

Learning to Masturbate †

If you have never masturbated and want to, you may feel awkward, self-conscious, even a bit scared at first. You may have to contend with voices within you that repeat, "Nice girls don't" or "A happily married woman wouldn't want to." You may fear losing control

* See *Sisters of the Yam,* by bell hooks, in Resources.
† Betty Dodson has been extremely influential in liberating masturbation for women. See Dodson, as well as Shere Hite and L. G. Barbach in Resources

of yourself, or you may feel shy or guilty about giving yourself sexual pleasure. Many of us have these feelings, but they can change in time.

Some suggestions: Find a quiet time when you can be by yourself without interruption. Make yourself as comfortable as possible: You are expecting a lover, and that lover is you! Take a relaxing bath or shower. Rub your body all over with cream, lotion, oil, or anything else that feels good. Slowly explore the shape of your body with your eyes and hands. Touch yourself in different ways. Put on music you like, keep the lights soft, light a candle if you want to. Think about people or situations you find sexually arousing. Let your mind flow freely into fantasy. Let your body relax. Of course, such a relaxed and special atmosphere isn't always possible—or necessary! Desire can overtake us at the most unexpected moments. We can find ourselves sexually aroused and masturbate while cooking a meal, traveling on a bus, working at a desk, riding a horse or bicycle, gardening.

Women have many ways of masturbating. We can moisten our fingers (with saliva, fluid from the vagina, or a lubricant) and rub them around and over the clitoris. We can gently rub or pull the clitoris itself; we can rub the hood or a larger area around the clitoris. We can use one finger or several. We can rub up and down and around and around, and try different kinds of pressure and timing. Some of us masturbate by crossing our legs and exerting steady and rhythmic pressure on the whole genital area. We may insert something into the vagina—a finger, room-temperature peeled cucumber, dildo. We may rub our breasts or other parts of our bodies. Some of us have learned to develop muscular tension throughout our bodies.

At 16 I gave up masturbation for Lent. Since I defined masturbation only as touching my genitals in a sexual way, in those six weeks I learned that I could have wonderful orgasms through a mixture of fantasy and quietly tensing up and relaxing the muscles around my vagina and vulva.

Still other ways of masturbating include using a pillow instead of your hands, a stream of water, an electric vibrator. (Vibrators are sold at many drug stores, often as body or neck massagers. For mail-order catalogs, see Resources.)

I can direct our shower nozzle so the water hits my clitoris in a steady stream. I have a real relationship with that shower! I wouldn't give it up for anything! It's nice when I get up for work and don't have time for sex with my lover but do have a little time for the shower. Those few minutes are real important for me.

Women experience a variety of sensations and feelings when masturbating. As you get sexually aroused your vagina may become moist. Experiment with what you can do to feel even more. Open your mouth, breathe faster, make noise if you want to, or move your pelvis rhythmically to your breathing and voice. As you become more aroused you may feel your muscles tighten. Your pelvic area may feel warm and full.

For me the most pleasurable part is just before orgasm. I feel I am no longer consciously controlling my body. I know there is no way I will not reach orgasm now. I stop trying. I like to savor this rare moment of true letting go!

It's this letting go of control that enables us to have orgasms. If you do not reach orgasm when you first try masturbating, don't worry. Simply enjoy the sensations you have. Try again some other time.

Masturbating opens me to what is happening in my body and makes me feel good about myself. I like following the impulse of the moment. Sometimes I have many orgasms; sometimes I don't have any. The greatest source of pleasure is to be able to do whatever feels good to me at that particular time. I rarely have such complete freedom in other aspects of my life.

Not everyone enjoys masturbating.

I have tried masturbating because I read about it, not out of natural desire. Sometimes it seems like a chore. I feel like I should take the time to explore my body but I quit after a few minutes because, quite frankly, I'm bored. It just doesn't seem to have the effect another person would.

If masturbating doesn't bring you pleasure, trust your own preferences and don't do it.

Masturbation with a Partner

When my fiance asked if he could help me masturbate, I thought it was kinky at first. Then I showed him how I do it, and he showed me how he does. We watch each other to see what feels good. He has trouble sometimes having orgasms inside me, and I know it's a relief to him that he can openly bring himself to orgasm after intercourse.

My lover rubbed her breasts and clitoris while I made love to her yesterday. After I got over feeling a little inadequate (I should be able to do it all), I found it was like having another pair of hands to make love to her with. It was a turn-on to both of us.

When one person in a relationship wants sex or orgasm more than the other, masturbation is a possibility. Here are some different views.

It's typical for my husband to want to make love at night, but I'm too tired. Then by morning I'm very horny and he wants to get up. I always tease him in the morning, ask whether he jerked off or not. Sometimes he did. Sometimes I'll be going off to sleep and feel the bed shaking.

I guess I'm old-fashioned enough to say that no husband of mine is going to have to masturbate because I wouldn't satisfy him.

Masturbation is such a private thing, and I want to keep it for when I'm alone with myself. Also, doing it with someone else would be the ultimate in showing that I'm a sexual person, and maybe I'm shy about that.

Exploring Lovemaking *

We have many ways of getting and giving pleasure with a partner: touching, caressing, looking, teasing, kissing, massaging, licking, sucking, penetrating.

My lover and I can spend hours—when we're on vacation or the kids are away on a weekend morning—looking at each other, stroking and cuddling each other, pulling and pushing and feeling our bodies stretch together. If we go past a certain point, we'll both know we want to "make love," but actually we have been making love the whole time.

What we do in sex is a matter of personal preference and ingenuity, whom we are with, how much love and understanding we feel, how comfortable we both are with our bodies, how each of us feels that day. At its best, lovemaking takes its shape as we and our partners move together by mutual (often unspoken) agreement. Sexual equality is as important in bed as it is everywhere else.

---

* For more on sexual techniques, see *The Good Vibrations Guide to Sex,* by Anne Semans and Cathy Winks, in Resources.

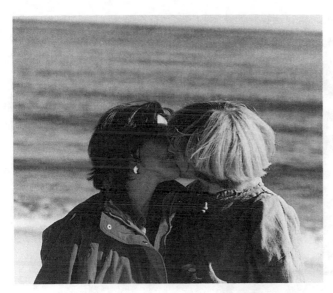

Jeffrey McIntyre

The hour or so after active lovemaking can be a special time.

After sex we talk tenderly, laugh deeply, whisper, cry, sleep like babies in each other's arms. Some of the most important conversations in our relationship have come in those satisfied and intimate moments.

Some sexual activities are riskier than others. See chapter 15, HIV, AIDS, and Women, for information on safer sex.

Touching and Sensuality

Massages, back rubs, foot rubs, head rubs—these are wonderful at any time. As part of lovemaking, they can make sex slower and more sensual.

Eric likes me to nibble his feet and suck his toes. I think that gives him as much pleasure or more than anything else we do in sex.

Tender touching can be a way of making love.

We always sleep right up next to each other naked. There's always a lot of touching and feeling, so even though we don't have intercourse that often, I consider us having sex all the time.

I yearn to feel the crook of her arm under my neck as I sleep. I long to stroke her face and enjoy how good it feels to wake up with her arms around me in the morning. The heat and passion of sex is great, but I think that a gentle caress is more personal. That's what I crave most right now.

When a couple has problems in sex, it may turn out that they have been focusing entirely on each other's genitals, and not taking time or learning how to touch and stroke each other lovingly all over. Many men are more focused on genitals than women are and need to learn the pleasures of touching.

One lover told me with great puzzlement at first that I made love slower than any woman he knew, and he didn't just mean it took me a long time to come. Later he got used to my "style" and said he liked it.

Vaginal Penetration

Some of us experience tremendous pleasure in having our male or female lover enter our vagina with fingers, fist, dildo, or other object (slang: fucking). If we are with a woman lover, we may enjoy entering her. Vaginal penetration can be gentle, playful, intimate, or passionate. (For penetration by a man's penis, see "Vaginal Intercourse," below.) Some women, however, do not like penetration at all and prefer to stick with external stimulation. As with all sex, it is important to communicate and respect both your partner's and your own desires.

Vaginal penetration can be thought of as reciprocal, with one of you enveloping the other's hand as it explores and penetrates. If you want your partner to enter you, make sure your vagina is wet with vaginal fluid or lubricants. If you want to go inside your partner, keep your fingers free of rings and your nails well filed. Wear an unpowdered latex glove or finger cot (resembling a cut-off finger of a glove) to protect against the transmission of HIV/AIDS through any cuts you may have on your fingers.

You can explore with your hands in many different ways: stroking, tapping, circling, thrusting. Experiment with different rhythms and speeds. Try stimulating her G spot (see p. 240). You can put one or more fingers inside her and, if you both like, gradually put your whole hand inside (called *fisting*). Inside her vagina, it can feel warm, wet, and wonderful.

Vaginal Intercourse

If you make love with a man, you may want to have intercourse—to feel his penis in your vagina (slang: fucking, screwing). Think of intercourse as reciprocal—you open up to enclose him warmly, you surround him powerfully, and he penetrates you. It can be infinitely slow and gentle, hard and thrusting, or both at its best, an exceptional part of lovemaking.

For information on intercourse as a means of getting pregnant, see Parts Three and Four of this book. If you do not want to get pregnant, you may need to use a form of birth control (see chapter 13, Birth Control).

I can so clearly remember moving in and around him and him in me, till it seemed in the whole world there was only us dancing together as we moved together, as we loved together, as we came together. Sometimes at these times I laugh or cry and they are the same strong emotions coming from a deep protected part of me that is freer now for loving him.

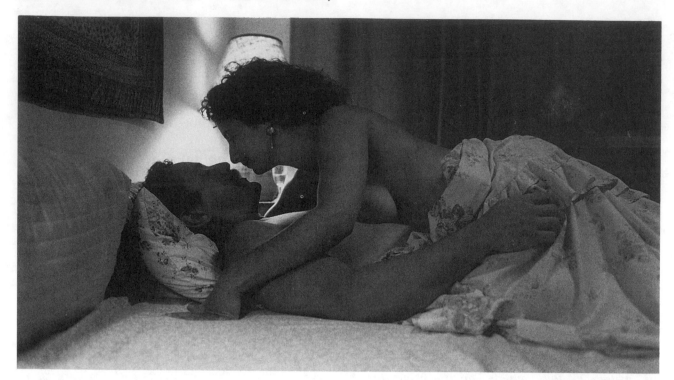

Michael Weisbrot/Stock, Boston

When I was trying to get pregnant, I found intercourse especially exciting because of the possibility that this might be the time his sperm met my egg. It was as if my vagina was beckoning his penis to come in for an intimate hug. I felt expansive and open in my whole body.

For intercourse to give you pleasure you must feel aroused, sexually excited, your vagina wet and open. Often it takes women longer—sometimes much longer—than men to become aroused. To add extra "juice," you or your partner can apply water-based lubricants or use a lubricated condom; some people use saliva. Do not use Vaseline or any oils. They destroy latex condoms and diaphragms.

If you are sexually inexperienced, frightened, not ready, not in the mood, or angry with your partner, or if you have a partner who practices only the "in and out" of intercourse and not the lovemaking that surrounds it, then penetration (especially when your vagina is dry) can be boring, unpleasant, even painful. Sometimes you will feel open and ready for intercourse immediately; more often you will want your partner first to touch, rub, kiss, or lick you vulva and clitoris, using his hands, mouth, or penis.

Certain positions at certain times will feel more exciting to you than others. The "man on top" is not a "naturally" better position at all. You can sit or lie upon him or lie side by side. Sit up with your legs over his and his penis in you. Or he can enter you from behind and reach around to caress your clitoris. If you want deep penetration and pressure on your cervix, choose positions that make these more possible. We are all different shapes and need to find positions that suit

us. If we have injuries or disabilities, being creative and using pillows for support may increase our comfort.

Intercourse is about pleasure and connection for both of you, and not necessarily orgasm. Many women don't experience orgasm during intercourse. Sometimes trying to have an orgasm makes you self-conscious and tightens you up. On the other hand, sometimes it's exciting to strive for orgasms.

If you are not ready for orgasm and the man is highly aroused when you begin intercourse, he might reach orgasm too soon for you if he moves back and forth inside you and you move your pelvis against his quickly. Both of you can slow your movements until you become more excited yourself. Experiment with holding your bodies still for a time when he enters you, then begin to move together slowly. Moving slowly can help men learn to delay ejaculation, which can make intercourse more pleasurable for both of you.

Pressure of the penis on the cervix can be the key to orgasm for some women, as are clitoral and vulval stimulation.

I love rubbing his penis against my clitoris and vulva. It gives both of us great pleasure and always brings me to the verge of orgasm.

It is best if you can communicate with words or movements what feels best to you. Yet, sometimes talking about it is neither easy nor possible.

He would come almost instantly when we began to make love after marvelous kissing. A little while later we'd make love again, when I'd be more aroused—aching for him, in fact. I never knew how to alter this pattern, never dared talk about it, and later on found out that he had resented "having" to make love twice.

Over time you and your partner can learn your mutual rhythms of desire and arousal and explore what gives each of you the most pleasure.

Oral Sex

Sometimes oral sex feels more intimate than any other kind of lovemaking. We can suck or lick our partner's genitals, which when done to a woman is called cunnilingus (slang: going down, eating, eating out) and when done to a man is called fellatio (slang: giving head, blow job, cock sucking). For some of us, oral sex brings orgasm more surely than other ways of making love.

We're really into oral sex and he's always ready and willing. He'll say, "Do you want to have an orgasm?" And he'll go down on me. It's terrific.

To enjoy oral sex it helps to like our partner's genitals and feel good about our own. Yet we are often ashamed of our "private parts."

At first I was repulsed by the idea of going down on a woman. I thought we smelled bad, that vaginas were nasty. It was a little pungent and intimidating in the beginning (though less so than a penis had been!). I soon learned to lose myself in the wonderful textures, tastes and formations of a woman's genitals. I realized that lesbian sex is about loving myself, overcoming my hatred of my own body.

For ages I thought my lover was doing me a favor when he did oral sex on me. I couldn't imagine that I tasted good. Finally he convinced me that he loves doing it. Also, I tasted my juices and they're not bad!

One of the pluses of oral sex with men is that we won't get pregnant. But with men or women, the risk of getting HIV/AIDS or another sexually transmitted disease still exists. We can have safer oral sex by using dental dams and/or condoms. And, like everything in sex, it's good only if we want to be doing it.

Often a guy I'm dating will say, "If you won't have intercourse, just give me a blow job." But if I didn't want him in my vagina, I probably don't want him in my mouth. Oral sex can feel like rape to me if I'm not in the mood to be doing it.

My husband likes me to do oral sex on him. Sometimes it's incredibly erotic for me to have his penis moving in my mouth. Since I don't enjoy swallowing his semen, I usually spit it out or let it flow out on the sheets, and that's fine. Sometimes, however, blowing him makes me gag—I don't want his penis filling up

my mouth at all. Then we do something else. Or we get in a position where I have more control, like being on top of him with the base of his penis in my hand.

What feels good in oral sex may differ from time to time and from person to person.

I like tongue, lips, moisture, not too much sucking and pulling, and time for exploring—my lover's got to be willing to stay with it for a while.

It can be done rather crummily! I hate it when I feel like he's eating me up with his teeth or when the pressure's too hard and it hurts or when he moves around from place to place and doesn't keep the stimulation steady.

For me there's no right or wrong place, just the places I want concentrated on on a particular day. I'm getting better at telling my lover where it feels best.

Anal Stimulation

The anus can be stimulated with fingers, tongue, penis, dildo, or any slender object. You can give or receive anal stimulation with a male or female partner. For many of us, it is a highly sexually sensitive area.

I like having something small in my anus during lovemaking—no pressure or movement, just there.

Having the area around my anus licked during oral sex is a real turn-on. And anal intercourse when I'm in the mood is incredibly sexy. I love the sensations deep inside me and the thrill of doing something so unusual.

The anus is not as elastic as the vagina, so be gentle. If you have anal intercourse, go slowly, wait until you're relaxed and use a lubricant—saliva or a water-soluble jelly such as K-Y Jelly, Astroglide, or Probe. Anal bacteria can cause serious vaginal infections and cystitis, so if you want your partner's finger(s) or penis or a dildo in your vagina after being in your anus, be sure they have been washed well first and have a male lover use a condom. If you or your partner want to use your tongue in the anus (sometimes called rimming), be sure to use a dental dam with lubrication to protect against getting a stomach infection or a sexually transmitted disease.

Anal sex is a very risky activity for HIV/AIDS transmission. The delicate tissue in the rectum is prone to small tears that make an entryway for the AIDS virus. Latex barriers (condom, gloves) must be used. See chapter 15, HIV, AIDS, and Women.

Anal intercourse isn't for everyone.

My husband wants to have anal sex a lot because he likes the tight fit and the exoticness of it. Once it happened and I almost didn't know it was happening. There was lubrication and everything was right and it felt fine. At other times I've really not wanted it, and a few times it's been almost painful and I've stopped it. I wish I liked it better because I'd love to give him that pleasure, but I have to be honest—I just don't enjoy it.

In our one great try at anal intercourse I ended up jumping three feet in the air and squealing like a stuck pig. This so terrified him that he completely lost his erection, and we laughed and laughed. I don't think it ever really got in or anything—somehow we hadn't quite worked out the logistics of it.

Fantasies

Today as I stretched out before my run, I closed my eyes and imagined my lover's naked body floating a few inches above me. I could feel her breasts on my face and in my mouth, our bodies reaching out, drawing close and then wrapped together. The images and feelings sailed me through an hour of strong running.

I had the fantasy of making love with two men at once. I pictured myself sandwiched between them. I acted on this one, with an old friend and a casual friend who both liked the idea. It was fun.

Nearly everyone has fantasies, in the form of fleeting images or detailed stories. They express depths within us to learn about and explore. The thoughts and images we carry in our minds can evoke strong physical responses. Some sex researchers assert that the *brain* is the most important organ of sexual pleasure, and some women report that they have orgasms from fantasy alone.[13] In fantasy we can be whatever we imagine. We may share our fantasies with a lover.

We've just started to talk about the fantasies we have during sex. At first it felt somehow "disloyal" that I've needed fantasies when the other person was such a good lover. Now we figure, the more pleasure the better.

Sometimes it can be difficult to accept sexual fantasies.

I imagined I was sitting in a room. The walls were all white. There was nothing in it, and I was naked. There was a large window at one end, and anyone who wanted to could look in and see me. There was no place to hide. There was something arousing about being so exposed. I masturbated while having this fantasy, and afterward I felt very sad. I thought I must be so sick, so distorted inside, if this image of myself could give me such intense sexual pleasure.

Many women have been brought up to think that sex should be "one way." We often decide we are bad or sick for imagining something different, or feel disloyal when we fantasize about someone other than the man or woman we are with. Yet, our fantasies treat us to *all kinds* of erotic experiences, including situations that seem "taboo." It takes a while to learn that this is okay and that we can enjoy these stories and images without having to act on them.

What about rape fantasies? Some people say that if we fantasize about having sex forced on us, that means we want to be raped. This is untrue: Totally unlike actual rape, fantasizing about rape is voluntary and does not bring us physical pain or violation. For those of us who grew up learning that "good girls" don't want sex, a fantasy of being forced to have sex may free us of responsibility and can be highly erotic. It can allow us the feeling of being desired uncontrollably.

In one of my juiciest fantasies, a woman and a man tie me up and make love to me and to each other. There is something extremely erotic in imagining being that powerless. In real life, my lover and I do at times feel totally vulnerable to what the other does or wants. This fantasy lets me play around with the power dynamics that are sometimes so intense between us.

We may distrust fantasies that seem to play into male pornographic images of women as submissive or masochistic, and imagine that in a less sexist future fantasies of dominance would come to us less often. Yet, this is difficult to predict. For now it seems important to accept that all kinds of fantasies may be erotic for us and free up our vital sexual energies.*

Role Playing

With our partners we can play act situations and fantasies that excite us, like being kids about to be caught or making love in a public place. We can dress up. We can be our child selves as well as our adult selves, our lusty and vigorous selves as well as our needy selves.

Sometimes when I'm feeling good I'll create a strip scene for my husband—and for me, since our mirror is strategically placed—and we both get very excited. Now he does it, too, standing in front of the bed, moving his body rhythmically, slowly taking off and throwing down his clothes. I love it. His strength and vulnerability come through at the same time.

In sadomasochistic (S/M) sex play, the playacting is based on fantasy situations of dominance and submission. Partners act out roles like master-servant, police-citizen, monarch-subject. One will enforce her or his will on the other, often experimenting with activities involving physical pain, until the other gives the signal to stop. The practice of S/M is highly controversial among feminists and has caused debate and division among lesbians. Women who support S/M point out that between partners who both fully want to be doing

---

* If you repeatedly have fantasies that disturb or scare you, they may be a sign that you need help. Talk about them with a trusted friend or a trained counselor.

it, S/M play can increase sexual pleasure and open up hidden issues of power, which are present in most human intimacy.*

S/M, like regular sex, allows people to share an intimate physical experience and an intimate emotional experience, but beyond that, S/M allows my partner and me to share a fantasy life, which is a deep kind of intimacy, very special and unique, which I would not trade for anything.

Others argue that dominance and pain infliction have no part in "healthy" sexuality. A major concern is that the many real inequalities in our society create a risk that S/M won't be just play, and that one partner will actually be dominant while the other feels forced to acquiesce. At times, S/M can camouflage truly oppressive behavior.

I was a battered wife. My husband, a professional with a good job, said he was into bondage. I bought into it at first. Toward the end he said that he could relate to me sexually only if he tied me up. At the end he was threatening to kill me. For him, bondage had to do with low self-esteem and wasn't a healthy expression of sexuality.

It's important to say no to anything we don't want to do. If we are confused or upset by pressure from a sex partner, we may want to discuss the situation with a friend or counselor who can help us decide how to respond.

Erotica

In recent years, women have begun to make inroads into the male-dominated industry of erotic entertainment. Much of traditional pornography has been based on men's fantasies and has depicted women's bodies as depersonalized objects. Today we can choose from a wider selection of sexually explicit videos, magazines, books, and sex toys created by and for women of all sexual orientations. Regarding these materials, there is a wide range of what different women consider to be erotic and what different women consider to be demeaning.

Sex toys and aids can spice up sexual encounters, make safer sex fun, and be an outlet for creativity. We can try edible body paints or chocolate-flavored condoms, an egg-shaped electric vibrator or a Venus-shaped dildo; an anthology of erotic short stories or a hot and sexy video. There are also instructional videos and books available on masturbation, orgasms, sexual intimacy, and much more. (See Resources for books, catalogues, and videos on erotica.)

Erotica can be bought in women's sexuality boutiques. These boutiques, the first of which opened in the 1970s, are often discreetly located and offer information and workshops for women and men. We may feel awkward or embarrassed entering a sex shop, and feel as if we are doing something bad. There continue to be attempts to censor and legislate sexually explicit material. However, there is nothing wrong with seeking information or buying products to make sex fun. The store clerks are used to answering questions from customers—you're probably not the first one to ask! For those of us who don't live near a store or don't feel comfortable going to one, many products are available by mail order. (See "Mail Order" in Resources for how to obtain catalogues.)

We all have different ideas of what is erotic. And of course we are not limited to what's available in a catalogue. A cucumber dildo, a shower nozzle spray, and looking at our own love letters and photographs can be intensely arousing. We can use our imaginations and resources to create our own erotic pleasures.

COMMUNICATING ABOUT SEX

Sexual Language

The true language of sex is both verbal and nonverbal. Sometimes our words and images are poor expressions of the deep feelings within and between us.

Few words in the English language seem appropriate to convey the attitudes and values we actually feel. Clinical, "proper" terms—vagina, penis, intercourse—seem cold, distant, tight. Slang terms—cunt, cock, fuck, ass—seem degrading or coarse. Euphemisms like "hooking up" and "making love" are vague. We use different words with lovers, children, friends, and doctors. Many of us are trying to put together a sexual language with which we are comfortable.

How to Say What We Really Want

We all face certain issues in a sexual situation, whether it's with a date, a longtime lover, or a spouse: How do I feel at the moment? Do I want to be sexually close with this person now? In what ways? What if I don't know—can I say I'm confused? Then can I communicate clearly what I want, what I don't want?

We may have been brought up to think that men, not women, should "make the first move," that "good girls don't initiate sex," and that "liberated women always want it." If we *do* initiate sex, we may face the possibility of being turned down. If we *don't* want sex, we often face (from men primarily) the assumption that "women don't really mean it when they say no." Or someone interprets our not wanting sex as a sign of rejection or "frigidity." The truth is that sometimes we love being coaxed into sex, and sometimes we hate feeling pressured. All we can do is try to be as fully aware as possible of our feelings at the moment, to be honest with ourselves about them, and to practice saying them, with clarity and no apologies, to the men or women we are with.

Communication about our sexual needs is a contin-

* For a guide to S/M, see *S/M 101: A Realistic Introduction*, in Resources.

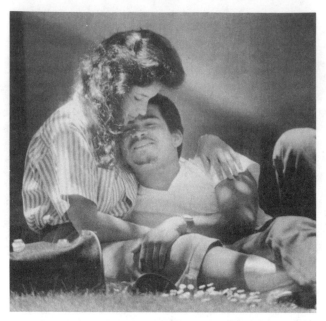

Spencer Grant/The Picture Cube

uous process. A woman who had found the courage to talk with her lover about their sexual relationship said in angry frustration, "I told him what I like once, so why doesn't he know now? Did he forget? Doesn't he care?"

Even in the most loving relationships, asking for what we want is hard.

- We are afraid that being honest about what we want will threaten the other person.
- Our partner seems defensive and might interpret our suggestion as a criticism or a demand.
- We are embarrassed by the words themselves.
- We feel that sex is supposed to come naturally and having to talk about it must mean there's a problem.
- We have been making love with the same person for years (sometimes several decades), and it feels risky to bring up new insights.
- We aren't communicating well with our partner in other areas of our relationship.
- We don't know what we want at a particular time, or we need to react to something our partner does.
- Even with willing partners, we may as women feel a deep inhibition about asserting our sexuality openly and proudly, which is what we'd be doing if we proclaimed our erotic needs and wishes. The barriers can be inside us, not just between us and our partners.

How do we work on better communication in sex? Making love is one of the special times when we can use more than words to reach each other. Taking a partner's hand and putting it in a new place, making the sounds that let him or her know we are feeling good, speeding up or slowing down our hip move-

ments, placing a firm hand on the shoulder meaning "let's go slow"—there are many ways of communicating if we will use them.

I've liked just saying, "Watch," and showing.

We were both really excited. My lover began rubbing my clitoris hard and it hurt. It took me a second to figure out what to do. I was afraid that if I said something about it, I would spoil the excitement for both of us. Then I realized I could just take my lover's hand and very gently move it up a little higher to my pubic hair.

We can practice saying what feels good while exchanging massages, for example, when the atmosphere is less intense. But communicating about sex doesn't happen overnight, and it doesn't always work no matter how hard we try.

For a discussion on communicating about safer sex, see chapter 15, HIV, AIDS, and Women.

SEX AND DISABILITY *

Some of the women speaking about sexuality throughout this chapter have a chronic disease or disability, which is either hidden, like diabetes or epilepsy, or evident, like muscular dystrophy or blindness. Those of us with illnesses and disabilities feel open and proud about being sexual people.†

Whether we were born deaf or with spina bifida or develop multiple sclerosis or lose a limb later in life, women with disabilities too often find other people assuming that we are not sexual beings.

I didn't go to the prom in high school and never dated. It wasn't until I got my first job that I felt like a member of my peers and gained the confidence to explore the social aspects of my life. I remember one week that I had a date with three different guys and my roommate was in shock.

In this culture people with disabilities are expected to be perpetual children, which means that sexual expression would not be appropriate and may be considered perverted.[14]

Those of us with disabilities discover early and more painfully something that all women face: that our identity as women and as sexual beings is measured according to our looks and our desirability to men.‡

* This section by Janna Zwerner Jacobs. See also the table on Sex and Disability later in this chapter, p. 251.
† See chapter 1, Body Image, for more on stereotypes of women with disabilities. Our special thanks to the women of Boston Self-Help and the Project on Women and Disability for their contributions to this section on sexuality and disability.
‡ It is ironic that with most disabilities we are considered asexual; yet, if we have a condition that makes us appear unintelligent— mental retardation or emotional or speech disability—we are often thought of as overly sexual. For instance, one argument against sex

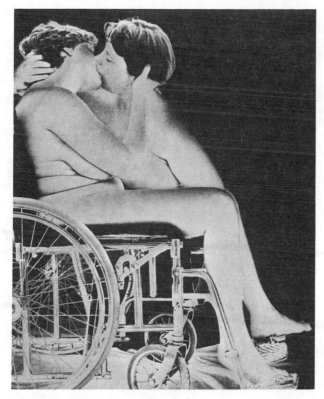

Tee A. Corinne

back, visualization, and meditation (see chapter 5, Holistic Health and Healing: Navigating Your Way to Better Health).

Reclaiming our bodies for our own experiences of sexuality takes time and patience.

My lover, who is a paraplegic, has been subjected to enormous amounts of insensitive medical attention all her life. Health care professionals have handled her body again and again without allowing her control over the process. So obviously it is difficult for her to let go of control of her own body and to entrust a lover with this control. I need to honor her experience, to know that it is not my fault or my inadequacy as a lover—or hers—that is the reason for sexuality being an issue in our relationship. We have discovered that honest and loving communication, with no blame or criticism, leads us to finding several ways to experience sexual pleasure with each other.

In my lesbian illness-support group we have to push past our own censored voices to discover what to do when the vulnerability of the body to pain and to medical manipulation numbs it to the touch of a lover.

I persist in feeling that my body is ugly when I'm naked. Yet, my husband clearly loves making love with me. I asked him one day if I made love with a limp. "Yes," he said, "you make love with a rhythm like your walking rhythm. It's nice."

A great deal of our sexuality relates to both verbal and nonverbal communication. Extra care may be needed in communicating when one partner is deaf or hard of hearing, or has a speech disability.

I worry about what weird noises my body is making that he can hear and I don't.[16]

Many of us seek fulfillment of our sexual desires and choose to be sexually active in spite of the barriers. We want to share in the experience of having a partner and share our experiences in the world with our partners. Intimacy and feeling connected keep us strong.

Being honest with a partner, especially if they are not disabled, is very important. I need to be comfortable to talk about what I like and can and can't do. You have to be really open and listen to their side of what they feel about you and your body. But I'm never ashamed of how I look undressed.

Vestibular problems [lack of balance] can enhance sex. You can get into a real floating kind of feeling. Learning disabled people are set up to feel the extremes. We under- and over-react. But whatever we do, it can be hard for our partners.[17]

We don't do much "hard-core sex" but find our greatest fulfillment in slow, deep touching and holding. We can't seem to get enough cuddling.

Recently I went to see a male doctor and told him I wanted to be tested for HIV/AIDS. Without even asking me any other questions, he just said, "No, no, people with your disability never get AIDS."

Growing up with certain disabilities can keep us from getting in touch with many of the dimensions of our sexuality.

Friends have said to me that getting their period for the first time was an important moment in their growing sense of themselves as womanly and sexual. Because my disability required my mother to catheterize me several times a day, she was the one who discovered my period. I understand now why it was so important to me a few years later to learn to change the pads myself.

Certain chronic diseases and disabilities such as chronic fatigue syndrome and some spinal cord injuries have associated pain, so there may be times when we want sex but just can't bear to be touched. Some of us have discovered that stimulating our genitals directly can help block the pain[15] and take our minds someplace else. For the many times when the pain threatens to take over our lives, some women are trying nonmedical alternatives like acupuncture, biofeed-

education for young people with certain disabilities has been that others didn't want to encourage their "natural promiscuity." This reveals an odd warp in our society's assumptions about sexuality.

I prefer to relate sexually to women because they are far less judgmental of my "odd" body and are really far more into sensual expression than men.

The logistics of lovemaking are often a challenge, especially with a severe disability. Between others' fears or unrealistic expectations, and physical spaces that aren't accessible or are poorly designed to meet our needs, simple issues sometimes become problems blown out of proportion. The cultural pressure for sex to be spontaneous is hurtful to those of us who need some accommodation to our disability.

You hear all these romantic stories about men "throwing their wives down" on the kitchen table and making love. My husband and I could never do that.

Even when sexually aroused, the spontaneity can soon disappear when your partner has to help empty your bladder and carefully clean and position you. . . . My sexual fantasies relate to spontaneous sexual behavior—sex in an elevator, in any room of the house, and in numerous positions—on the floor, up against the wall, and so on.[18]

Planning for sex in advance and frankly discussing needs and desires is usually helpful. Being honest and open to whatever makes us feel good can be a model for all lovers, whether or not they have a disability.

A personal care attendant or assistant may often be needed to help us prepare for sex, whether one or both partners has a disability. It might seem impersonal, but then our sex partner has a choice about how much of the preparation to be involved in, and we can feel more independent in the relationship. It is crucial to have an assistant who gives us space to be sexual and respects us; such a person may be hard to find. There is lots of negative pressure on everyone involved, since insurance companies and Medicaid won't pay for this kind of assistance, and some home health services have rules that don't allow aides to assist us in this way.

My husband and I are both disabled, so we need a lot of help. We decided that hiring a personal care attendant was too much of an invasion of our privacy, though. It is very frustrating, but we just don't have intercourse any more. We have our orgasms through oral sex now, and my husband says we are lucky and that other people would be jealous if they knew.

The prevailing medical beliefs and literature have served to undermine our sexuality in the past. If we experienced sexual response and orgasm despite a lack of sensation in our pelvic region, for instance, it was said to be a phantom orgasm, as though it were not quite real. Finally, the medical establishment has validated what we knew all along—that our orgasms are very real and can result from stimulating our genitals as well as other eroticized places on our bodies.[19]

I have erratic, vague sensation in my vagina and clitoris. When I have an orgasm, I feel most of the pleasure in my knees—it's a nerve transfer thing, I guess. I'm probably the only woman in the world whose knees come.

I have no sensation below my waist now, but for some reason my neck, ears, and armpits are much more sensitive than they used to be, and stimulation there is really quite exciting to me.

Until recently, most literature about sex and disability focused on men, their potency and performance concerns, and penis-in-vagina intercourse, and findings were generalized from men's to women's sexuality. It was assumed that sexual adjustment was easier for a woman, and the research focused on reproductive issues. More is now being published by women and people with disabilities.[20,21] Much of the latest research is more concerned with identifying the sexual needs and intimacy issues of women with certain disabilities, and with education and counseling to enable women with disabilities to pursue full and sexually satisfying lives.[22-25] Still, much more research needs to be done. (See "Sex and Disability" in Resources.)

A Lifetime of Sexual Relationships

Currents of sexual attraction and passion crisscross our lives and pull us into new relationships, deepen the ones we're in, and teach us about ourselves. We may act on them with a look, smile, touch, or kiss, or we may not want to act on them at all. When we make love with someone familiar or new, woman or man, we are often at our most open, most vulnerable, and also our most powerful. Sex can be dramatic, dull, comforting, scary, friendly, funny, passionate, frustrating, satisfying.

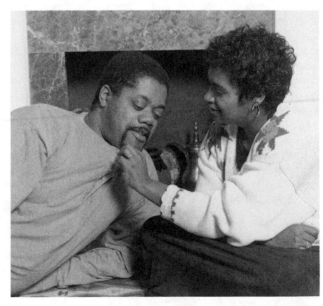

Jenny McKenzie

SEX AND DISABILITY

Many women with disabilities experience similar attitudinal barriers to sexual expression and difficulty accessing health care providers who are knowledgeable about the specifics of their disability as well as about sexuality. Certain disabilities and chronic diseases have a dramatic effect on sexuality, which may cause pain or medical complications when we engage in otherwise "routine" activities, such as making love, taking birth control pills, getting pregnant, or delivering a baby. Some of these disabilities have been chosen for inclusion on this chart.

CHRONIC DISEASE OR DISABILITY	EFFECTS ON OUR SEXUALITY	HELPFUL HINTS AND SPECIAL IMPLICATIONS
Cerebral palsy (CP)	Muscle spasticity, rigidity, and/or weakness may make certain sex acts and self-pleasuring difficult to impossible for us. Contractures of our knees and hips may cause us pain under the pressure of a partner, and spasms may increase with arousal. Some of us experience a lack of vaginal lubrication. Menstruation, fertility, and pregnancy are not affected. During delivery, those of us with severe CP might need a cesarean section.	Nongenital lovemaking, using different positions, and propping our legs up on pillows may help ease spasms. We can use a vibrator to make love alone or with another person if our arms and hands are involved. A water-soluble lubricant can often help if our vagina lacks lubrication. Inserting a spermicidal foam or a diaphragm may be complicated by spasms or poor hand control. Because of an increased risk of clotting, the birth control pill is not advisable for those of us taking seizure medication (anticonvulsants) or if our mobility is greatly restricted by severe CP.*†
Brain and cognitive disabilities (including epilepsy, traumatic brain injury [TBI], and stroke)	Our sexual abilities may vary depending upon the location of injury. We may experience a changed level of interest in sex as well as difficulty with vaginal lubrication and having an orgasm, sometimes caused by our medications or associated depression. Stroke and TBI may result in communication, cognitive, and visual-perceptive impairments, as well as loss of sensation, paralysis, and incontinence. Those of us with severe TBI may show sexual indiscretions and may be impulsive, while others of us may become confused about public versus private matters and act in ways some people find difficult to deal with in public. Many of us have irregular periods and may experience trouble getting pregnant. We may also go through menopause earlier than we expected.	If our balance, strength, or coordination is not good, it may help to engage in sexual activities that require little exertion. A water-soluble lubricant can help with a dry vagina. If we experience cognitive or behavior problems, social-skills retraining or help from a psychologist may assist us in better understanding our disability and gaining greater self-control and confidence. An understanding friend or partner will often be the best help during the slow recovery process. Birth control pills should be used with extreme caution if we have paralysis or circulatory disorders and are not advisable for those of us taking seizure medication.*†‡§
Diabetes	Most of the medical literature is about male sexual functioning, and the few reports show conflicting results. About a third of diabetic women in one study reported that their orgasms gradually became rarer and less intense. One possible explanation was that the threshold for orgasm increased because of damage to the nerve fibers in the pelvic region. A lack of vaginal lubrication and recurrent infections may make some lovemaking unpleasant.	Some women say that using a vibrator allows them to reach orgasm because the stimulation is more intense. Diabetes that is difficult to regulate may cause fertility problems and stop menstruation. Depending upon how stable our blood glucose levels are, pregnancy may be complicated and should be closely monitored. Birth control pills often aggravate other symptoms of our diabetes and should not be used because of possible cerebrovascular and cardiovascular complications.‖
Renal failure	In chronic renal insufficiency, menstruation may stop or become extremely irregular. Many women become infertile and rarely carry pregnancies to term. We may have difficulties becoming sexually excited, and as in diabetes, our orgasms may become rarer and less intense. Sometimes we have a decrease in vaginal lubrication and breast tissue mass.	Maintenance hemodialysis often brings on excessive and sometimes painful menstruation but may improve our desire for sex, though not necessarily sexual responsivity. Kidney transplants usually improve both our desire for sex and sexual response, and fertility improves dramatically. If our vagina is too dry, a water-soluble lubricant can help. Many of the drugs used to lower hypertension are likely to dampen our sex drive. The birth control pill is usually not advised.

continued on next page

SEX AND DISABILITY *(cont.)*

CHRONIC DISEASE OR DISABILITY	EFFECTS ON OUR SEXUALITY	HELPFUL HINTS AND SPECIAL IMPLICATIONS
Rheumatoid arthritis (RA)	Swollen, painful joints; muscular atrophy; and joint contractures may make it difficult for us to masturbate or make love in some positions. Pain, fatigue, and medications may decrease our sex drive, but genital sensations remain intact. Menstruation, fertility, and pregnancy are not affected, but birthing may be complicated if our hips and spine are involved. However, symptoms may improve during pregnancy because of changes in our immune system.	To avoid pain and pressure on affected joints, we can be creative in sexual positioning. If our symptoms respond to heat, we can plan sexual play after a hot compress or a hot bath with our partner. Choose the best time, when you have the least pain and stiffness, for lovemaking. Try sex instead of corticosteroids—it is said to stimulate the adrenal glands and so increases the output of natural cortisone, which alleviates painful symptoms. The birth control pill may not be good for us if we have circulatory problems or greatly restricted mobility.*†§
Systemic lupus erythematosus	Many difficulties are the same as in RA (above). However, because different people have quite different symptoms, often connected to other disorders, one cannot generalize. Research on the female sexual effects of lupus is scarce, despite the fact that nine out of ten people with lupus are women. Sometimes we also have sores in and around the mouth and vagina and a decrease in vaginal lubrication, so we may have pain during vaginal penetration.	For helpful hints, see RA (above). Also, we can use a water-soluble lubricant if our vagina seems dry. Choose birth control methods with extreme caution, especially if symptoms or complications other than RA exist. Birth control pills may not be advisable if we have circulatory or kidney problems or if our mobility is greatly restricted.*†§
Myocardial infarction (MI)	For those of us with very serious conditions, chest pain, palpitations, and shortness of breath may limit our sexual activities. However, many of us can resume regular lovemaking once we can climb two flights of stairs at a brisk pace without causing symptoms. (The cardiac responses during step climbing and lovemaking are similar, the average being 125 beats per minute.)	We should consult a physician to see when and if we can safely begin an exercise regimen. We can participate in lovemaking activities that require little or no exertion, especially with our arms (for example, on our side or back). Go slow in the beginning to minimize stress and fear of stress, because the majority of sexual problems arise from anxiety and misinformation about this ailment. Birth control pills should not be used.*§
Multiple sclerosis (MS)	Depending upon the stage and severity of MS, our symptoms will vary and may come and go. Some of us experience difficulty in having an orgasm, decreased genital sensitivity, dryness of the vagina, muscle weakness, pain, and bladder and bowel incontinence. There is no change in our menstrual and fertility patterns. The symptoms of MS often decrease during pregnancy but may increase slightly after pregnancy.	Because sexual difficulties may come and go with other MS symptoms, it helps to be creative. Some medication for spasms and topical anesthetics for pain may be helpful. If our balance is not good and we tire easily, we can use a vibrator or participate in lovemaking activities that require little exertion. A water-soluble lubricant can help with a dry vagina. Some women say that intercourse is painful but having their clitoris stimulated feels good. The birth control pill is not good to use if we have paralysis or restricted mobility, but a recent study showed that it may help symptoms in early stages of MS.*†‡§
Ostomy	More is still known about the sexual functioning of men with ostomies than about women, even today. Surgery should not impair our genital responsivity or fertility and often makes it safe to become pregnant, because a disease process, such as cancer or ulcerative colitis, has been wiped out. However, a few women report pain during intercourse or a lack of vaginal sensations after ileostomy and colostomy surgery.	An ostomy is a hidden disability until our clothes are off: therefore, it may help to find a comfortable way to tell potential partners before sexual relations begin. The opening or appliance may be covered or secured before lovemaking, both for aesthetic reasons and for support so it does not get in the way. We can use lovemaking positions in which we feel most secure that the bag will not get pulled out. If odors are a problem, we can bathe and empty the bag before making love. Consider alternatives to the birth control pill and consult a physician if taking it, because sometimes it is not absorbed properly.

CHRONIC DISEASE OR DISABILITY	EFFECTS ON OUR SEXUALITY	HELPFUL HINTS AND SPECIAL IMPLICATIONS
Spinal cord injury (SCI)	SCI may result in paralysis, spasticity, loss of sensation, incontinence, skin ulcers, pain, and a dry vagina, sometimes complicating making love with yourself or another. Changes in our ability to lubricate or feel genital sensations will depend on the level and severity of our injury. We may continue to have orgasms, regardless of the level or degree of paralysis. They may be similar to those before injury or may be diffuse, either in general or to specific body parts, such as our breasts or lips. Exploration is the key to discovering these changes. Our neck and ears and the area above the injury may become more sexually exciting. Arousal, self-pleasuring, and lovemaking may increase spasms and the risk of incontinence. Although we may stop menstruating for several months after the injury, fertility is not permanently disrupted.	It can help to make love in ways other than vaginal penetration, which may sometimes be difficult or painful because of increased bladder infections, spasms, and vaginal irritation and tearing. Be on guard for autonomic dysreflexia (AD), also known as hyperreflexia, which can lead to a life-threatening disruption of the autonomic nervous system marked by elevated blood pressure, headache, increased spasms, and chills. Taking our time and using a vibrator helps some women experience orgasm. Routine bowel and bladder programs can decrease the risk of "accidents" during sex, and a towel will help if there is any leakage. We can also tape our catheter down or move it out of the way so it does not get pulled out. Some spasm medications and a water-soluble vaginal lubricant may be of assistance. Pregnancy increases the risk of blood clot development and bladder infection, but many women have healthy and painless births. Be on guard for signs of AD during labor and delivery, and of uterine prolapse afterward. Take birth control pills only with extreme caution, if at all, and never if taking antihypertensive medication or if circulatory problems are present.*†‡§

* Many medications are directly responsible for the negative effects on our sexuality—often much more so than the disability itself! Examples of such drugs are antihypertensives (i.e., diuretics), antidepressants (i.e., serotonin reuptake inhibitors), tranquilizers (i.e., phenothiazines), spasticity medications (i.e., baclofen) and antiseizure medications (i.e., phenytoin), as well as medications such as lithium, digoxin, reserpine, and naproxen.
† The diaphragm may not be a good method of birth control if you have poor hand control, recurrent bladder or vaginal infections, or very weak pelvic muscles. If the use of your hands is limited, ask your partner or attendant to help insert the diaphragm. Also, devices are available that can make it easier to insert the coil-spring diaphragm, but some hand control is required.
‡ The IUD is not good to use for women with a loss of sensation in the pelvic area because of the risk that puncture or pelvic inflammatory disease may go unnoticed. Also, good hand coordination is needed to check the strings every month to make sure the IUD is still in place.
§ Birth control pills can increase the risk of clotting and cause serious medical problems such as embolism, deep vein thrombosis, and stroke. Birth control pills may also interact poorly or be rendered less effective when taken in combination with other medications. Be sure to inform your sexual health care provider about the medications and dosage you are taking when seeking contraceptive services.
Note: Table prepared by Janna Zwerner Jacobs.

Sex doesn't take place in a vacuum. We take struggles about other things—power, money, mutuality, competition—into bed with us. Sex in relationships can vary in meaning and intensity, and change over our lifetimes.

Sometimes I make love to get care and cuddling. Sometimes I am so absorbed in the sensations of touch and taste and smell and sight and sound that I feel I've returned to that childhood time when feeling good was all that mattered. Sometimes we tumble and tease. Sometimes sex is spiritual—High Mass could not be more sacred. Sometimes I make love to get away from the tightness and seriousness in myself. Sometimes I

want to come and feel the ripples of orgasm through my body. Sometimes tears mix with juices mix with sweat, and I am one with another. Sometimes through sex I unite with the stream of love that flows among us. Sex can be almost anything and everything for me. How good that feels!

Opening myself up to people sexually has always been hard. It was often easier to be sexual with people that I didn't know or with people who didn't treat me very well. I was too vulnerable if I actually cared about the person I was with and knew that they cared about me. Now, I'm in a committed relationship with someone I love very much. And I know that he loves me

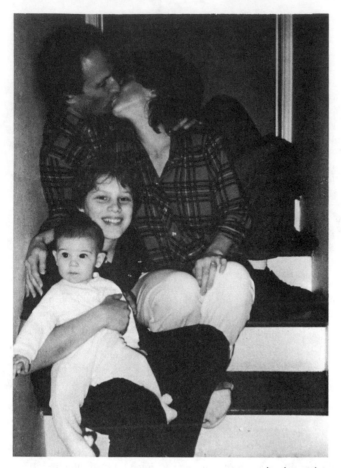

Louis Alexander

When I had my first daughter, my sexual energy entered a new path, a softer, more fluid flow. But because of our economic situation, I did the strong black woman thing and went back to work when all I wanted to do was be in that world of new sensual arousal and intuition.

Having a baby to take care of makes us both too tired to have sex much. Yet, nursing my daughter, touching her soft skin, feeling her sleeping body on mine—these are very sensual for me.

We've been married 32 years. I have no doubt that we'll be together until one of us dies. Yet, for the past ten years our libidos have been much lower than they used to be. It's possibly the effect of medications we are taking, my husband for a heart condition and I for high blood pressure. The ten years before that were my peak sexual years, and I don't think you suddenly go from a peak to a low. I don't mean we don't have sex; it just comes in spurts.

Sally and I have been together 17 years. Originally we had a sexual relationship. Then we broke up for five years, and when we got back together it never became sexual again. I'm really glad because I can't conceive of a happier relationship. We cuddle and kiss; we hold hands on the bus; we are affectionate all the time. But we don't have sex, and I don't miss it.

I've gotten so angry at him in fights we've had— little fights, big ones—that I could easier kill him than sleep with him. At first these feelings scared me. Now I know they pass and change and I feel loving again.

Deborah's and my lovemaking has been strong, deep, and varied since the first night we slept together. I've felt so sure of my sexuality with her, and increasingly trusting of the rhythms of our desire. Yet, last year when I went to live with her in her city away from my friends, work, women's group, my own turf, I suddenly became frighteningly dependent on

deeply and that makes sex with him difficult at times. There are times when a word he says or a way he touches me sets off a memory, and then I have to either call a halt to what we are doing or silently remind myself who I am with by saying his name over and over and over. I get frustrated and tired and angry that it has to be this way—that I can't just relax and let go of the fear even with a person I love and trust.

Just in the last two years—after 14 years of marriage—we've been able to talk to each other about sex. We experience a deep kind of uncrazy passion. When you are in love it's crazy passion—you want to swallow each other up and be swallowed. This, in contrast, is a relaxed openness. Anything goes, no hurry, free of guilt. We are more sexually connected than we've ever been in our lives and able just to be with each other.

After 20 years of being married I find myself thinking a lot about a sexual relationship with a woman.

My divorce (at 45) has me feeling like a teenager all over again. I go on dates; get crushes; wonder whether to sleep with someone for the first time, wait passionately for the phone to ring, hoping it's my current lover.

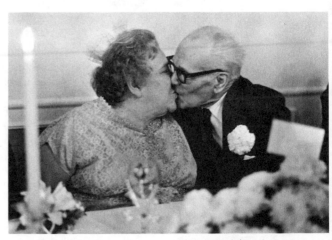

Jerry Berndt/Stock, Boston

whether she wanted to make love with me or not. When she did, it was wonderful because I was in touch with such deep places of need and sexual vulnerability in myself that our lovemaking was profoundly moving. But when she didn't—when she wanted to go to sleep or get up and do some work or go for a run or make some calls—I felt awful. I'd lie there feeling that I wanted sex "too much," afraid to tell her, angry, hurt, worried that she'd feel guilty. I finally dared to say something to her, only because our trust was deep enough for me to risk it. I cried as though a dam had broken. I began to see that when I'm away from my own world, the power in our relationship gets out of balance. Feeling out of touch with my own sources of strength and identity, I needed her to want me, as though her desire for me would actually make me exist. Sex and orgasm weren't the issue; identity was. We pulled out of this difficult time with a new respect for the power dynamics in our sexual loving.

APPENDIX

Sexual Health Care

Sexual health is a physical and emotional state of well-being that allows us to enjoy and act on our sexual feelings. We all need to follow certain procedures of routine care to stay sexually healthy.

- *A gynecological exam.* (See chapter 24, Selected Medical Practices, Problems, and Procedures, p. 591.)
- *Care of infections.* (See chapter 14, Sexually Transmitted Diseases, pp. 348–57.) If you get an infection of the vagina or urinary tract, you need to do something about it immediately.
- *Douching.* The vagina has a natural cleansing process. Unless you are instructed by a health care practitioner for a particular reason, you never need to douche (wash out the vagina). Frequent douching and the use of vaginal deodorants can change the acidic and alkaline balance in the vagina and lead to infections. Scents used in vaginal deodorants can also cause allergic reactions. Many of us have been taught that as women we need to douche. If that is something we want to continue to do, try douching once a month without harmful chemicals. Douching with vinegar and water, or plain yogurt and water, is suggested.
- *Genital cleansing.* Rather than douche or use vaginal deodorants, you simply can wash your genital area daily with warm water. Separate the outer lips and pull back the hood of the clitoris to clean away the secretions that collect around the glans. Our body secretions and smells are a natural part of us, and if you are in good health and wash regularly, you smell and taste good. However, some of us like to wash our genitals before lovemaking. Do what makes you comfortable.

- *Birth control.* (See chapter 13, Birth Control.) If you are fertile and do not want to become pregnant and you are having intercourse, you'll need to discuss with the man involved the use of birth control and who will use the selected method. If you cannot discuss it with him or he won't discuss it with you, you need to decide on a method of birth control to use yourself. Even if you are not having intercourse, if sperm is deposited anywhere near the vagina (even in the mons area), the sperm can swim into the vagina on vaginal secretions and up through the cervix to the uterus and fallopian tubes, and join with an egg.
- *Prevention against STDs and HIV/AIDS.* (See chapters 14, Sexually Transmitted Diseases, and 15, HIV, AIDS, and Women.)
- *Menstruation.* It's fine to have sex during your menstrual period if it feels comfortable to you. Some of us have found that orgasm relieves menstrual cramps.
- *Pregnancy.* (See chapter 19, Pregnancy.)

The Role of Testosterone in Sexuality*

Certain hormones play a role in sexual feelings, sexual activity, and intensity of orgasm. The most influential is testosterone, sometimes called the libido hormone and sometimes called the male hormone. Testosterone, like estrogen, is present in both men and women, though the proportions differ between the sexes. In women it is produced through the operation of both the adrenals (two small glands near the kidneys) and the ovaries.

The role of testosterone in sexuality is illustrated in several ways. When one adrenal is removed, women report a dramatic decrease in sexual interest, sensation, and frequency of orgasm. When ovaries are removed, many women report a similar loss.[26] Testosterone levels are lower in women after menopause or after ovary removal (oophorectomy) than in healthy young women with ovaries in place, suggesting less testosterone is produced as ovarian function slows or stops. There seems to be a significant correlation between blood testosterone levels and sexual responsiveness and satisfaction.†

Knowing the importance of testosterone, ovaries, and adrenals can alert us to protecting our sexuality from unnecessary removal of the ovaries or adrenals. For women who have tested below the designated normal range of testosterone levels (25ng/ml to 100ng/ml), testosterone replacement may be helpful in restoring sexual interest and arousal.[27] However, testosterone replacement is not the first solution to explore for those of us who experience decreased sexual desire. The most common causes of decreased sex-

---

* Prepared in part by Edith Bjornson Sunley.

† For more on hormones and desire, see chapter 23, Women Growing Older, and also *Women, Sex and Desire* by Elizabeth Davis, in Resources.

ual desire are relationship-based (see the following section), or are psychological or situational factors, not hormonal deficiencies. Antidepressant drugs may also cause reduced sexual desires and orgasms. In these cases, communication with a partner, ending a relationship that is not working, counseling, or switching medications may help us more than hormonal treatment.

Problems with Sex

At one time or another many of us have problems with sex. Read about the causes and treatment for the problem you are having, particularly if it is a severe one (see Resources).

Sexual problems in a relationship are often relationship problems. Some common causes are lack of information, poor communication patterns, male and female role expectations, a lack of trust or commitment, or unresolved conflicts. An abusive partner may use sex as a weapon to hurt or dominate us; in that case, the *abuse* is the problem. In addition, a history of sexual abuse for one or both partners may affect current relationships. (Male partners may also have been sexually abused.) See chapter 8, Violence Against Women.

How we think and feel about ourselves and sex powerfully affects how our bodies respond. Guilt, shyness, fear, conflict, and ignorance can all block or inhibit sexual responsiveness. If any of the following is a problem, we owe it to ourselves to explore further. We need not wait or be in total agony before we look for help. Sexual problems are common.

Problems with Orgasm *

Many of us experience difficulties reaching orgasm. Shame about exploring and touching ourselves keeps us from learning to bring ourselves to orgasm through masturbation. A variety of problems keeps us from having orgasms with another. Here are some of the reasons why:

- We don't notice or we misunderstand what's happening in our bodies as we get aroused. We're too busy thinking about abstractions—how to do it right, why it doesn't go well for us, what our lover thinks of us, whether our lover is impatient, whether our lover can last—when we might better be concentrating on sensations, not thoughts.
- We feel ourselves becoming aroused, but we are afraid we won't have an orgasm, and we don't want to get into the hassle of trying, so we just repress sexual response.
- We are afraid of asking too much and seeming too demanding.

* See especially Barbach's *For Yourself: The Fulfillment of Female Sexuality,* in Resources.

- We are afraid that if our lover concentrates on our pleasure we will feel such pressure to come that we won't be able to—and then we don't.
- We are trying to have simultaneous orgasms, which seldom occurs for most of us. It can be just as pleasurable if we come separately.
- We are in deep conflict about, or angry at, the person we are sleeping with. Unconsciously we withhold orgasm as a way of withholding ourselves.
- We feel guilty about having sex and so cannot let ourselves really enjoy it.

Lack of Interest in Sex: Sexual Aversion

For a few of us, the conflicts about ourselves and sex are so deep that we are never interested in sex. We may even feel an extreme, unpleasant sensitivity to touch or may feel so ticklish that we can't relax. Our bodies are reacting this way for a reason and protecting us from sexual experiences we can't handle at this point. This may well be a time to look for professional help.

Painful Intercourse or Vaginal Penetration

You may experience discomfort, even pain, with vaginal intercourse or penetration for the following physical reasons:

Local Infection
Some vaginal infections—like monilia (yeast) or trichomoniasis—can be present in a nonacute, visually unnoticeable form. The friction of a penis, dildo, or finger moving on your vulva might cause the infection to flare up, making you sting and itch (see chapter 24, Selected Medical Practices, Problems, and Procedures, p. 669). A herpes sore on your external genitals can make friction painful (see chapter 14, Sexually Transmitted Diseases, p. 351).

Local Irritation
The vagina might be irritated by a birth control foam, cream, or jelly you are using. If so, try a different brand. Some of us react to the rubber in a condom, diaphragm, or latex glove. Vaginal deodorant sprays and scented tampons can irritate the vagina or vulva.

Insufficient Lubrication
In most women, the wall of the vagina usually responds to arousal by "sweating," giving off a liquid that wets the vagina and the entrance to it, which makes penetration easier. Sometimes there isn't enough of this liquid. Some reasons: You may be trying to let the penis or object in (or your lover might be putting/forcing it in) too soon, before there has been enough stimulation to excite you and set the sweating action going. You may be nervous or tense about mak-

ing love (e.g., it's the first time, or you're worried about getting pregnant). If you are using a condom, you may need to add lubrication. Be sure to give the vagina time to get wet. If you still feel dry, you can use saliva, lubricating jelly (e.g., K-Y) or a birth control foam, cream, or jelly. **Never use Vaseline or other oil-based lubricant with a condom or diaphragm. It will deteriorate the rubber.** Hormone deficiency can also cause dryness. A lack of estrogen can affect the vaginal walls in such a way that less liquid is produced. This affects some women after childbirth (particularly if you are nursing your baby or if your stitches hurt) and some women after menopause. Try the lubricants suggested above, and see chapter 23, Women Growing Older, p. 564, for detailed suggestions.

Tightness in the Vaginal Entrance

The first few times you have intercourse, an unstretched hymen (if you have one) can cause pain. And whenever you are tense and preoccupied, the vaginal entrance is not likely to loosen up enough, and getting the penis, finger, or dildo in might hurt. Even if you feel relaxed and sexy, timing is important. If you try penetration before you are fully aroused, you might still be too tight, though you are wet enough. So don't rush, and don't let yourself be rushed.

Pain Deep in the Pelvis

Sometimes the thrust of penetration hurts way inside. This pain can be caused by tears in the ligaments that support the uterus (caused by obstetrical mismanagement during childbirth, a botched-up abortion, violent intercourse, gang rape); infections of the cervix, uterus, and tubes (such as pelvic inflammatory disease —the end result of untreated sexually transmitted disease in many women); endometriosis; cysts or tumors on the ovaries. All these may be treatable.

Clitoral Pain

The clitoris is exquisitely sensitive, and for many of us direct touching or rubbing of the clitoris (especially the glans, or tip) is painful (our partners may not know this until we tell them). Also, genital secretions can collect under the hood, so when washing pull back the hood of the clitoris and clean it gently.

Vulvodynia and Vaginismus

Vulvodynia is a chronic burning or stinging sensation in and around the vagina, which makes any kind of penetration, including entrance by finger, tampon, speculum, or penis, acutely painful. In some cases, this condition may be related to vaginismus, in which you experience a strong, involuntary tightening of your vaginal muscles, a spasm of the outer third of your vagina.* Please see chapter 24, Selected Medical Practices, Problems, and Procedures, p. 671, for more.

Whatever the cause, if penetration is at all painful,

don't put up with the pain! Find out what is causing it and do something about it. As an alternative to intercourse, we can also try "outercourse"—that is, pleasuring the rest of our bodies. The power that each of us has and the power that we have together to make our lives more satisfying is enormous.

Helping Ourselves

If you are feeling pain in your pelvic, genital, or vaginal area, get a thorough gynecological exam to find out whether there is a physical cause. Remember, however, that most doctors have not been trained to discuss sexual problems. Enlist the help of friends or a local women's group to find a sympathetic and competent health care practitioner.

Despite our knowledge about sex, and despite the support of friends and partners, sometimes we cannot work through our difficulties. If you need someone to talk with, call your local women's health center, free clinic, or the American Association of Sex Educators, Counselors and Therapists (AASECT) (see Resources) for the name of a recommended counselor or therapist in your area. Because there are men and women without adequate training who call themselves sex therapists, contacting AASECT may be better than consulting your yellow pages or, often, your health practitioner.

When there are sexual problems in a couple relationship, it is often the woman who seeks help first. This may be because culturally it is easier for us to admit to our sexual concerns. It may also be because we too often assume that if sex is a problem, it's we who are in need of help. But sexual problems usually reflect or express relationship problems.

You may have a difficult time finding a good health care practitioner or therapist. Those of us who are single or in lesbian relationships have even fewer resources than heterosexual couples. You may need to concentrate on working with friends or your partner or both, after reading the available books.

....

NOTES

....

1. For tips on how to start your own discussion or self-help group, see Barbara J. White and Edward Madara, eds., *The Self-Help Sourcebook: Finding and Forming Mutual Aid Self-Help Groups*, 5th ed. (Denville, NJ: Northwest Covenant Medical Center, 1995).
2. bell hooks, *Sisters of the Yam: Black Women and Self-Recovery* (Boston: South End Press, 1993), 119.
3. Ibid., 127.
4. Claudia Colindres, "A Letter to My Mother," in *The Sexuality of Latinas,* ed. by Norma Alarcón, Ana Castillo, and Cherríe Moraga (Berkeley, CA: Third Woman Press, 1993).
5. For information on the growing movement around responsible nonmonogamy, see *Polyamory: The New Love*

* See Linda Valins's book, *When a Woman's Body Says No to Sex,* in Resources.

Without Limits by Deborah M. Anapol and *Loving More* magazine in Resources.

6. William Masters and Virginia Johnson, *Human Sexual Response* (New York: Bantam, 1980), 21–22.

7. Helen Singer Kaplan, *Disorders of Sexual Desire* (New York: Brunner/Mazel, 1979).

8. B. Zilbergeld and C. R. Ellison, "Desire Discrepancies and Arousal Problems in Sex Therapy," in S. R. Leiblum and L. A. Pervin, eds., *Principles and Practice of Sex Therapy* (New York: Guilford, 1980), 65–104.

9. W. R. Stayton, "A Theology of Sexual Pleasure," *American Baptist Quarterly* 8, no. 2 (1989): 94–108.

10. Gina Ogden, *Women Who Love Sex* (New York: Pocket Books, 1994), 64–102.

11. Lorraine Dennerstein, "Female Sexuality, the Menstrual Cycle, and the Pill," in S. Zeidenstein and A. Moore, eds., *Learning About Sexuality: A Practical Beginning* (New York: Population Council, 1996).

12. Beverly Whipple, "How to Find the Grafenberg Spot" (Fact sheet available at the Boston Women's Health Book Collective), 1992.

13. Ogden, *Women Who Love Sex,* 128–48.

14. Nancy Mairs, *Waist-High in the World: A Life Among the Nondisabled* (Boston: Beacon Press, 1996), 140.

15. Barry R. Komisaruk and Beverly Whipple, "The Suppression of Pain by Genital Stimulation in Females" in *Annual Review of Sex Research* 6 (1995): 151–86.

16. Mairs, *Waist-High in the World.* 142.

17. Dale S. Brown, "Learning Disability: Unsure Social Behavior Means Insecure Sexual Relationships," *Disabled, USA* 3, no. 2 (1979): 1–5.

18. Jo Campling, ed., "Julie," in *Images of Ourselves: Women with Disabilities Talking* (London: Routledge and Kegan Paul, 1981), 17.

19. Marca L. Sipski, Craig J. Alexander, and Ray C. Rosen, "Orgasm in Women with Spinal Cord Injuries: A Laboratory-Based Assessment," *Archives of Physical Medicine and Rehabilitation* 76 (1995): 1097–102.

20. Mairs, *Waist-High in the World.* 40–63.

21. Beverly Whipple, Eleanor Richards, Mitchell S. Tepper, and Barry R. Komisaruk, "Sexual Response in Women with Complete Spinal Cord Injury: Achieving and Maintaining Health and Well-Being," in D. M. Krotoski, M. A. Nosek and M. A. Turk, eds., *Women with Physical Disabilities* (Baltimore, MD: Paul Brookes, 1996), 69–80.

22. Brown, "Learning Disability."

23. Sipski, "Orgasm in Women."

24. Margaret A. Nosek et al., "Sexual Functioning Among Women with Physical Disabilities," *Archives of Physical Medicine and Rehabilitation* 77, no. 2 (1996): 107–15.

25. M. Elizabeth Sandel, "Sexuality and Reproduction After Traumatic Brain Injury," in Lawrence J. Horn, and Nathan D. Zasler, eds., *Medical Rehabilitation of Traumatic Brain Injury* (Philadelphia: Hanley & Belfus, 1996), 557–72.

26. Helen Singer Kaplan and Trude Owett, "The Female Androgen Deficiency Syndrome," *Journal of Sex and Marital Therapy* 19, no. 1 (spring 1993): 3–24.

27. Ibid., 6–7.

RESOURCES *

For Resources on HIV, AIDS, and safer sex, see chapter 15, HIV, AIDS, and Women. For resources on lesbian sexuality, see chapter 10, Relationships with Women.

To add to the resources listed below, you can get extensive bibliographies on all aspects of sexuality from SIECUS, the Multi-Media Resource Center, and the Kinsey Institute for Sex Research (addresses in "Organizations," p. 261). Good sources of feminist books on women's sexuality are Down There Press (938 Howard Street, #101, San Francisco, CA 94103; 415-974-8985), Naiad Press (P.O. Box 10543, Tallahassee, FL 32302; 800-533-1973; E-mail: naiadpress@aol.com), Cleis Press (P.O. Box 14684, San Francisco, CA 94114; 415-575-4700; E-mail: cleis@aol.com), and for Spanish and English publications, Volcano Press (P.O. Box 270, Volcano, CA 95689; 800-879-9636; E-mail: sales@volcanopress.com; Web site: http://www.volcanopress.com). The Sexuality Library at the Good Vibrations mail-order store carries many other titles listed below (see "Mail Order," p. 261, for address).

Books, Journals, and Videotapes

Sexuality

Alarcón, Norma, Ana Castillo, and Cherríe Moraga. *The Sexuality of Latinas.* Berkeley, CA: Third Woman Press, 1993.

Anand, Margo. *The Art of Sexual Ecstasy: The Path of Sacred Sexuality for Western Lovers.* New York: Jeremy P. Tarcher, 1989. Exercises based on ancient Tantric sexual practices.

———. *The Art of Sexual Magic.* New York: Jeremy P. Tarcher, 1995.

Anapol, Deborah M. *Polyamory: The New Love Without Limits.* San Rafael, CA: IntiNet Resource Center, 1997. A guide to responsible nonmonogamy.

Anzaldúa, Gloria, ed. *Making Face, Making Soul—Haciendo Caras: Creative and Critical Perspectives by Feminists of Color.* San Francisco: Aunt Lute Books, 1990.

Barbach, Lonnie, G. *For Each Other: Sharing Sexual Intimacy.* New York: Signet, 1984.

———. *For Yourself: The Fulfillment of Female Sexuality.* New York: Doubleday/Anchor Books, 1976. For women who haven't had orgasms and would like to.

———, ed. *Pleasures: Women Write Erotica.* New York: HarperCollins, 1985.

Bell, Ruth, et al. *Changing Bodies, Changing Lives: A Book for Teens on Sex and Relationships.* New York: Random House, 1988. (Update due 1998.) Excellent sourcebook for teenagers and young adults.

Blank, Joani, ed. *Femalia.* San Francisco: Down There Press, 1993. Thirty-two photographs of women's genitals.

* Prepared by Lynn Rosenbaum, Janna Jacobs, and Amy Alpern with help from Diana Chace and Brenda Reeb. Thanks to Good Vibrations for use of their book descriptions, and to the staff at New Words Bookstore, 186 Hampshire Street, Cambridge, MA 02139; (800) 928-4788. E-mail: newwords@world.std.com.

————, ed. *First Person Sexual: Women and Men Write About Self-Pleasuring.* San Francisco: Down There Press, 1996.

————. *Good Vibrations: The Complete Guide to Vibrators.* San Francisco: Down There Press, 1989.

————. *The Playbook for Women About Sex.* San Francisco: Down There Press, 1989. A sexual self-awareness workbook.

Cline, Sally. *Women, Passion and Celibacy.* New York: Carol Southern Books, 1993.

Collins, Patricia Hill. *Black Feminist Thought: Knowledge, Consciousness, and the Politics of Empowerment.* New York: Routledge, 1990. Feminist academic analysis of African-American women's experiences, including sexuality.

Corinne, Tee. *The Cunt Coloring Book.* San Francisco: Last Gasp, 1988. Forty-two drawings of women's genitals.

Davis, Elizabeth. *Women, Sex and Desire: Exploring Your Sexuality at Every Stage of Life.* Alameda, CA: Hunter House, 1995.

Dodson, Betty. *Sex for One: The Joy of Selfloving.* New York: Crown Publishing Group, 1992. An inspirational guide to masturbation.

Eisler, Riane. *Sacred Pleasure: Sex, Myth and the Politics of the Body.* New York: HarperCollins, 1995.

Heyward, Carter. *Touching Our Strength: The Erotic as Power and the Love of God.* San Francisco: Harper & Row, 1989. A feminist theologian explores sexuality, power, and justice within a Christian context.

Heiman, Julia, and Joseph LoPiccolo. *Becoming Orgasmic.* New York: Fireside, 1992.

Hite, Shere. *The Hite Report.* New York: Dell, 1987. More than 3,000 women are surveyed about what they really do in sex.

hooks, bell, *Sisters of the Yam: Black Women and Self-Recovery.* Boston: South End Press, 1993.

Irvine, Janice. *Disorders of Desire: Sex and Gender in Modern American Sexology.* Philadelphia: Temple University Press, 1990.

Kahn, Ada P., and Linda Hughey Holt. *The A to Z of Women's Sexuality: A Concise Encyclopedia.* Alameda, CA: Hunter House, 1992.

Kaplan, Helen S. *The Illustrated Manual of Sex Therapy,* 2nd ed. New York: Brunner-Mazel, 1987. Contains valuable information but uses a heterosexual, medical model.

Kasl, Charlotte Davis. *Women, Sex and Addiction.* New York: Harper & Row, 1990.

Kitzinger, Sheila. *Woman's Experience of Sex.* New York: Penguin Books, 1985.

Koch, Patricia Barthalow. *Exploring Our Sexuality: An Interactive Text.* Dubuque, IA: Kendall/Hunt Publishing Company, 1995. A college textbook.

Ladas, Alice Kahn, Beverly Whipple, and John D. Perry. *The G Spot and Other Recent Discoveries About Human Sexuality.* New York: Dell, 1982.

Lorde, Audre. "Uses of the Erotic: The Erotic as Power," in *Sister Outsider.* Freedom, CA: Crossing Press, 1984. An important short essay.

————. *Zami: A New Spelling of My Name.* Freedom, CA: Crossing Press, 1983. Lorde's "biomythography."

Loving More. Quarterly magazine on responsible non-monogamy. IntiNet Resource Center, P.O. Box 4358, Boulder, CO 80306; (303) 543-7540. E-mail: pad@well.com; Web site: http://www.lovewithoutlimits.com

Martz, Sandra Haldeman, ed. *I Am Becoming the Woman I've Wanted.* Watsonville, CA: Papier Mache Press, 1994. An anthology on how women feel about their bodies across the life cycle.

Masters, William H., and Virginia E. Johnson. *Human Sexual Inadequacy.* New York: Bantam, 1981. Major research on the nature and treatment of sexual problems. The major drawback is the medicalized and performance-oriented approach.

————. *Human Sexual Response.* Boston: Little, Brown, 1970. See discussion in text of this chapter.

Morin, Jack. *Anal Pleasure and Health.* San Francisco: Yes Press, 1986.

Off Our Backs. 2337B 18th Street NW, Washington, DC 20009. A monthly women's news journal, which often runs articles on sexuality.

Ogden, Gina. *Women Who Love Sex.* New York: Pocket Books, 1994. Women's sexual pleasure in a context of cultural exploitation and abuse.

Reinisch, June with Ruth Beasly. *The Kinsey Institute New Report on Sex.* New York: St. Martin's Press, 1994. A comprehensive family book.

Snitow, Ann, Christine Stansell, and Sharon Thompson, eds. *Powers of Desire: The Politics of Sexuality.* New York: Monthly Review Press, 1983.

Tiefer, Leonore. *Sex is Not a Natural Act and Other Essays.* Boulder, CO: Westview Press, 1995.

Valins, Linda. *When a Woman's Body Says No to Sex: Understanding and Overcoming Vaginismus.* New York: Viking Penguin, 1992.

Villarosa, Linda, ed. *Body and Soul: The Black Women's Guide to Physical Health and Emotional Well-Being.* New York: HarperCollins, 1994.

Walker, Alice. *The Color Purple.* New York: Harcourt Brace Jovanovich, 1982. A powerful novel that touches on many aspects of black women's sexuality.

Walker, Rebecca. *To Be Real: Telling the Truth and Changing the Face of Feminism.* New York: Anchor Books, 1995. Essays by young feminists on many topics, including sexuality.

Winks, Cathy, and Anne Semans. *The Good Vibrations Guide to Sex.* Pittsburgh, PA: Cleis Press, 1994. An extensive guide to sexual techniques and toys.

Zeidenstein, Sondra, and Kirsten Moore, eds. *Learning About Sexuality: A Practical Beginning.* New York: The Population Council, 1996. International health care providers and researchers discuss the links between sexuality and reproductive health services, family planning, medical research, and more.

Bisexuality

Anything that Moves: The Magazine for the Inner Bisexual. Bay Area Bisexual Network; 2261 Market Street, #496, San Francisco, CA 94114; (415) 703-7977. A national, quarterly magazine with news, poetry, and fiction.

Binet News, P.O. Box 7327, Langley Park, MD 20787; (202) 986-7186. Quarterly newsletter published by a national activist organization, *Binet-USA,* which holds regional and annual meetings.

The Bisexual Anthology Collective, ed. *Plural Desires: Writing Bisexual Women's Realities.* Toronto: Sister Vision Press, 1995. Fiction, poetry, and essays, including many works by women of color.

Bi Women Newsletter. Bimonthly newsletter. The Boston Bisexual Women's Network, P.O. Box 639, Cambridge, MA 02140.

Hutchins, Loraine, and Lani Ka'ahumanu. *Bi Any Other Name: Bisexual People Speak Out.* Boston: Alyson Publications, 1991.

Ochs, Robyn, ed. *The Bisexual Resource Guide.* Cambridge, MA: Bisexual Resource Center, 1996. An international directory of organizations, publications, Internet resources, and more. To order, send $11.95 postage paid to Bisexual Resource Center, P.O. Box 639, Cambridge, MA 02140; (617) 424-9595.

Rust, Paula. *Bisexuality and the Challenge of Lesbian Politics: Sex, Loyalty, and Revolution.* New York: NYU Press, 1995. A sociological study on identity politics.

Tucker, Naomi, ed. *Bisexual Politics: Theories, Queries, and Visions.* New York: Harrington Park Press, 1995.

Weise, Elizabeth Reba, ed. *Closer to Home: Bisexuality and Feminism.* Seattle: Seal Press, 1992.

Sexuality and Sexual Abuse

Please see the Resources in chapter 8, Violence Against Women, for a more extensive listing.

Bass, Ellen, and Laura Davis. *The Courage to Heal: A Guide for Women Survivors of Child Sexual Abuse.* New York: HarperPerennial, 1994.

Davis, Laura. *Allies in Healing: When the Person You Love Was Sexually Abused As a Child.* New York: HarperCollins, 1991.

———. *The Courage to Heal Workbook: For Women and Men Survivors of Child Sexual Abuse.* New York: Harper & Row, 1990.

Maltz, Wendy. *Sexual Healing Journey: A Guide for Survivors of Sexual Abuse.* New York: HarperCollins, 1992.

Sex and Disability

Alexander, Craig J., and Marca L. Sipski. *Sexuality Reborn: Sexuality Following Spinal Cord Injury.* Videotape produced in 1993 by Kessler Institute for Rehabilitation, West Orange, NJ.

Crenshaw, Theresa L., and James P. Goldberg. *Sexual Pharmacology: Drugs That Affect Sexual Function.* Dunmore, PA: Norton, 1993.

Ducharme, Stanley H., and Kathleen M. Gill. *Sexuality After Spinal Cord Injury: Answers to Your Questions.* Baltimore, MD: Paul H. Brookes, 1996.

Duffy, Yvonne. *All Things Are Possible.* Ann Arbor: A.J. Garvin Associates, 1981. More than 75 differently abled women speak candidly about their lives.

Finger, Anne. *Past Due: A Story of Pregnancy, Disability and Birth.* Seattle: Seal Press, 1990.

Griffith, Ernest R., and Sally Lemberg. *Sexuality and the Person with Traumatic Brain Injury: A Guide for Families.* Philadelphia: F.A. Davis, 1992.

Haseltine, Florence P., et al., eds. *Reproductive Issues for Persons with Physical Disabilities.* Baltimore, MD: Paul H. Brookes, 1993.

Klein, Bonnie Sherr. *Slow Dance, a Story of Stroke, Love, and Disability.* Toronto: Knopf Canada, 1997. Only available in Canada through the Albert Britnell Book Shop: call (800) 387-1417.

Krotoski, Danuta M., Margaret Nosek, and Margaret Turk, eds. *Women with Physical Disabilities: Achieving and Maintaining Health and Well-Being.* Baltimore, MD: Paul H. Brookes, 1996.

Rogers, Judith G., and Molleen Matsumura. *Mother-to-Be: A Guide to Pregnancy and Birth for Women with Disabilities.* New York: Demos, 1991.

Saxton, Marsha, spec. ed. "Women, Disability and Reproduction." *Sexuality and Disability Journal,* Human Sciences Press, Summer 1994.

Erotica

Bright, Susie, ed. *Best American Erotica 1996.* New York: Simon & Schuster, 1996. Erotica by men and women.

———, ed. *Herotica: A Collection of Women's Erotic Fiction.* San Francisco: Down There Press, 1988.

———, and Joani Blank, eds. *Herotica 2.* New York: Plume Books, 1992.

———, ed. *Herotica 3.* New York: Plume Books, 1994.

Chester, Laura. *Deep Down: The New Sensual Writing by Women.* Boston: Faber and Faber, 1989.

———, ed. *Unmade Bed: Sensual Writing on Married Love.* New York: HarperCollins, 1993. Short story anthology.

Decosta-Willis, Miriam, Reginald Martin, and Roseann P. Bell, eds. *Erotique Noire: Black Erotica.* New York: Doubleday, 1992.

Friday, Nancy. *Forbidden Flowers.* New York: Pocket Books, 1991.

———. *My Secret Garden: Women's Sexual Fantasies.* New York: Pocket Books, 1991.

———. *Women on Top: Women's Sexual Fantasies of Power, Self-Exploration and Insatiable Lust.* New York: Simon & Schuster, 1993.

Kudaka, Geraldine, ed. *On a Bed of Rice: An Asian American Erotic Feast.* New York: Doubleday, 1994. An anthology of stories, essays, poems, and photos.

Libido: The Journal of Sex and Sensibility. P.O. Box 146721, Chicago, IL 60614; (800) 495-1988. Quarterly journal with erotic photos, stories, and poetry.

Olmos, Margarite Fernandez, and Lizabeth Paravisini-Gebert, eds. *Pleasure in the Word: Erotic Writing by Latin American Women.* New York: Plume Books, 1993.

Paramour: Literary and Artistic Erotica. P.O. Box 949, Cambridge, MA 02140-0008; (617) 499-0069. Published quarterly.

Pond, Lily, ed. *Seven Hundred Kisses: A Yellow Silk Book of Erotic Writing.* San Francisco: Harper San Francisco, 1997.

———, and Richard Russo, ed. *The Book of Eros: Arts and Letters from Yellow Silk*. New York: Crown Publishing Group, 1996.

Sheiner, Marcy, ed. *Herotica 4*. New York: Plume Books, 1996.

Sadomasochism (S/M)

Bannon, Race. *Learning the Ropes: A Basic Guide to Safe and Fun S/M Lovemaking*. San Francisco: Daedalus Publishing, 1993.

Califia, Pat. *Sensuous Magic: A Guide for Adventurous Couples*. New York: Masquerade Books, 1993.

Wiseman, Jay. *S/M 101: A Realistic Introduction,* 2nd ed. San Francisco: Greenery Press, 1996.

Videos

Educational and erotic videos can be obtained from women's sexuality boutiques (see "Mail Order," below), or you may obtain catalogues and videos directly from the following companies.

Fatale Video
1537 Fourth Street, Suite 193; San Rafael, CA 94901; (415) 454-3291
Lesbian erotic videos by and for women.

Femme Distribution
P.O. Box 268; New York, NY 10012; (800) 456-LOVE
Web site: www.royale.com
Includes the "Candida Royalle" series.

Focus International
(800) 843-0305
Clinical therapeutic techniques.

House O'Chicks
2215R Market Street, #813; San Francisco, CA 94114; (415) 626-6955
Videos on masturbation and female ejaculation, among other topics.

Multi-focus, Inc.
1525 Franklin Street; San Francisco, CA 94109; (800) 821-0514
Educational, includes videos about people with disabilities. Free catalogue.

The following is a short list of selected videos.

Becoming Orgasmic, Sinclair Institute, 1993. A woman is guided to orgasm.

Candida Royalle series, Femme. A line of heterosexual erotic videos with realistic characters and plots.

How to Female Ejaculate, Fatale Video, 1992. A group of women discuss their experiences and demonstrate ejaculation.

Selfloving: A Video Portrait of a Woman's Sexuality Seminar, Betty Dodson, 1991. A filmed version of Dodson's Bodysex masturbation workshop for women.

Sluts and Goddesses Video Workshop or How to Be a Sex Goddess in 101 Easy Steps, Maria Beatty and Annie Sprinkle, 1992. Humorous and daring challenge; includes sword dancing, a five-minute orgasm, passionate safer sex, and more.

Organizations

American Association of Sex Educators, Counselors, and Therapists (AASECT)
P.O. Box 238; Mt. Vernon, IA 52314; (319) 895-8407
This organization can help you find resources for sex therapy in your area.

Blacks Educating Blacks About Sex Health Issues
1233 Locust Street; Philadelphia, PA 19107; (215) 546-4140; Fax: (215) 546-6107

Information Service of the Kinsey Institute for Research in Sex, Gender, and Reproduction
313 Morrison Hall, Indiana University; Bloomington, IN 47405; (812) 855-7686
Send for their free list of bibliographies on many aspects of sexuality. Also available for a fee at http://www.indiana.edu/~kinsey.

National Black Women's Health Project (NBWHP)
1211 Connecticut Avenue NW, Suite 310; Washington, DC 20005; (800) 444-6472; Fax: (202) 833-8798

The Sexual Health Network
One Tamarac Ridge Circle; Huntington, CT 06484; (203) 924-4623
E-mail: mitch@aol.com
Web site: www.sexualhealth.com
Provides educational materials, information, and referral to sexual health professionals knowledgeable about a variety of disabilities and chronic diseases.

Sexuality Information and Education Council of the United States (SIECUS)
130 West 42nd Street, Suite 2500; New York, NY 10036-7802; (212) 819-9770; Fax: (212) 819-9776
E-mail: siecus@siecus.org
SIECUS publishes a bimonthly journal, annotated bibliographies, brochures, and other informational publications related to sexuality research, education, and legislation. Full list and order form are available upon request. Free bibliographies at http://www.siecus.org/pubs.

Through the Looking Glass
2198 Sixth Street, Suite 100; Berkeley, CA 94710-2204; (800) 644-2666
E-mail: tlg@lookingglass.org
Web site: http://www.lookingglass.org
Provides information, a newsletter, and support for women and parents with disabilities.

Mail Order

These women-owned sexuality boutiques offer a wide range of books, videos, vibrators, and sex toys, many of which are described in their catalogues.

Blowfish (mail order only)
2261 Market Street, #284; San Francisco, CA 94114-1600;
(800) 325-2569; (415) 285-6064
Web site: http://www.blowfish.com
   Also publishes the webzine Fishnet.

Eve's Garden International, Ltd.
119 West 57th Street; New York, NY 10019; (800) 848-3837
Web site: www.evesgarden.com

Good Vibrations
938 Howard Street, #101; San Francisco, CA 94103; (800)
289-8423
Web site: www.goodvibes.com

Grand Opening
318 Harvard Street, Suite 32, The Arcade Building; Brookline, MA 02146; (617) 731-2626
E-mail: grando@grandopening.com
Web site: http://www.grandopening.com

Additional Online Resources *

About Go Ask Alice!
http://www.columbia.edu/cu/healthwise/about.html

Bisexual Options
http://www.bisexual.org

The Coalition for Positive Sexuality
http://www.webcom.com/~cps/Home/index.html

Information About Isadora Alman's Site
http://www.askisadora.com/Info

Society for Human Sexuality
http://weber.u.Washington.edu/~sfpse

The Transgender Forum
http://www.transgender.org/tgfc.html

* For more information and listings of online resources, please see
Introduction to Online Women's Health Resources, p. 25.

PART THREE:

Sexual Health and Controlling Our Fertility

Introduction: Deciding Whether to Have Children

By Joan Ditzion

With special thanks to Merryl Pisha (Resources) and Denise Bergman

Our ability to protect our reproductive and sexual health, and to control whether and when we have children, is critical to our freedom—both to shape our lives and to express and enjoy our sexuality. This unit starts off with some basic tools for knowing our bodies better: It explains our sexual anatomy and the reproductive life span, the hormones of the menstrual cycle, and ways to deal with problems in menstruation. The unit discusses birth control and abortion: the two major tools available to women who have sex with men and do not want to have children right now. It describes how we can be sexually active and stay healthy—whether we are sexually active with men or with women—and offers ways to prevent sexually transmitted diseases (STDs), including AIDS. (For those who want to get pregnant someday, the information on STDs has extra meaning, as untreated STDs can cause infertility.) The unit offers guidance for making the difficult decisions surrounding an unexpected pregnancy. Finally, it addresses assisted reproductive technologies, looking at the latest scientific developments with a critical eye to both their positive and their negative impacts on women.

To know about the tools presented in this unit is not enough; we also need to develop the self-esteem and self-respect that allow us to feel we are worth caring for and worth protecting; the economic opportunities that empower us to plan our life choices; access to good health care; safety in our homes; and respect from our partners. There is work to be done in our society—on sexism, racism, and economic injustice, for example—before all women, including teenagers, women living in poverty, women of color, and women without health insurance, have equal access to the tools we need in order to protect our sexual health and decision making.

The following "Principles of Unity" from the former Reproductive Rights National Network (R2N2) express the many facets of complete reproductive freedom:

We believe that as women we have a right to control our own bodies and that we must organize to secure that right in the face of attacks by church, state, and the organized right wing. Therefore,

continued on next page

1. We support the right and access of all women, regardless of age or income, to abortion. We oppose . . . any attempt to cut off or restrict Medicaid funds for abortion, any legislation requiring parental or spousal notification, slanted "informed consent" ordinances and all other forms of restricting access to abortion.

2. We oppose all forms of sterilization abuse, including lack of informed consent, abuse of disabled persons, abuse in prisons and mental hospitals . . . and abuse resulting from the denial of abortion rights and the lack of safe, accessible forms of birth control.

3. We stand for reproductive freedom, including not only abortion rights and freedom from sterilization abuse but also good, safe birth control, sex education in the schools, the right to conduct one's sex life as one chooses, and an end to nuclear, chemical, and occupational hazards to our reproductive systems.

4. We support each person's right to determine his/her own personal and sexual relationships regardless of the sex of the people involved. We oppose the breaking up of families by the state in order to punish a parent for his/her sexual or political beliefs. We support the struggle for legislation guaranteeing civil rights to homosexuals.

5. Reproductive freedom depends on economics: equal wages for women, sufficient to support a family alone; a decent public health system; adequate welfare benefits; good housing; quality child care; and a public school system that meets children's needs.

6. We see our struggle for reproductive freedom as a worldwide one. We do not believe that overpopulation is a primary source of the world's problems. We oppose the racist population control policies of the U.S. government and agencies aimed at Third World peoples that limit their populations through forced sterilization and the distribution of dangerous drugs.

DECIDING WHETHER TO HAVE CHILDREN

Those of us who are original authors of *Our Bodies, Ourselves* came of age at a time of changing consciousness about having and raising children. Our grandmothers' generation had taken it for granted that they would have children no matter what their economic circumstances. Birth control was not readily accessible, it was ineffective, and the most socially acceptable life option was having children. Womanhood was equated with motherhood. While our mothers' genera-tion had more effective birth control, the vast majority of women assumed they would have children. Today, becoming a parent can be much more of a choice. Access to birth control and legal abortion make it possible for more of us to enjoy our sexuality and to control whether and when to have children. Increased longevity, improved prenatal care, donor insemination, and fertility treatments extend the child-bearing years into our late 40s and make it possible for more lesbians, single women, and infertile couples to have children when we choose.

Being able to control our fertility can give us the time to think deeply and fully about becoming parents. The decision to have or not have children can be one of the most crucial in a woman's life. Some of us know we want children. Some of us know we do not. For others of us, the decision goes back and forth, or it is clouded. We may have time to mull over all the options, or we may be under pressure to make a more immediate decision. There is a time limit, too. The decision not to become pregnant becomes final as we get older, although adoption continues longer as a possibility.

There is no way to predict how you might feel being a mother, what your child will be like, or how you will respond to a child. It can be useful to talk with many different kinds of women: mothers who are single and in couples, who have given birth and have adopted children, who had children at different times in their lives. You can talk with lesbian mothers, heterosexual mothers, and women who have decided not to have children at all. You can spend time with children of different ages, alone, with their siblings, with their families. Ask parents about the joys, sorrows, satisfactions, and strains. Find out how parents learn to care for children. Our age-segregated society makes it difficult for nonparents to have contact with children; yet, we as women are supposed to know instinctively how to take care of them. Ask women how their lives changed when they became mothers. Ask them what kinds of support help them in their role.

Consider asking yourself: Why do I want a child? When? What arrangements will I need to make so I can continue certain activities? What would my day-to-day life be like with a child? How will I juggle work and child care? What kind of health care will I have? What will the financial costs be? You might look into eligibility requirements for government subsidy programs, such as WIC, AFDC, or food stamps. These programs are undergoing a lot of change, and their ability to support parents in a reasonable manner is becoming more and more limited.

You can ask, too, What kinds of values would I want to encourage in my child, and who could help me do this? What kind of community would I want to raise children in? Am I ready to prepare a child to deal with the difficulties in life, like the racism that affects so many children, or the sexism and homophobia that distort the lives of boy and girl children alike?

If you have or adopt a child as part of a couple,

what if you find yourself single; are you prepared to parent alone? If you are single, how would having a child affect new relationships? Try to evaluate your emotional resources for parenting. One of the most critical things for parents to have is a good support system. Caring people can help you keep your perspective, your temper, and your sanity in the midst of the emotional chaos that sometimes occurs when one is a parent. Of course, there are no certain answers to all the questions you could ask yourself. But thinking about the details of parenting can help you get clearer about the impact a child or children will have on your life.

I hear two conflicting points of view. One that it is terrific to be a mother and the other—you'll regret it; your life will change! I am just beginning to find myself and grow. Having a child might stop that process, and I would feel so resentful. Everyone in my family is pressuring me to have a child. "Have one before I die," my grandmother says to me. I have to fight so hard not to give into pressures.

More and more women are acknowledging that we are not interested in becoming parents, and are challenging the cultural assumptions that motherhood is intrinsically gratifying. Although we are confident and happy with our decision, society can try to pressure us to feel guilty, unfeminine, or unsuccessful if we even *think* about not having children. At times, we may have to help people understand that our decision is legitimate.

It's too bad that young women think that they have to have children in order to be fulfilled women. I'm 56, never had kids, and feel as "fulfilled" as I could possibly be. Our lives can be rich with work, friends, and other people's children. I don't think that motherhood is the right choice for every woman.

For some of us, the decision not to have children is filled with regret. Perhaps we are infertile or have a genetic condition or disease that could be inherited, and we do not want to adopt a child. We may feel that we do not have enough money or economic stability. We may be single and want to raise a child with two parents.

It feels good to be clear about my priorities. Though I have a fine relationship with a man I love very much, I know I won't choose to live with him on a long-term basis if he doesn't want to share parenthood with me. I want very much to be a parent, though I don't want to take on this responsibility alone.

It is possible to not have children and still incorporate children into our lives. Children in many communities benefit from the friendship and guidance of women who are not their mothers. Lifelong relationships with children can be developed informally, with the children of family friends or relatives, or as part of formal structures or programs.

I do not have children, but I have a close relationship with my nieces and nephews and I baby-sit for children in my neighborhood.

Teaching high school means I have about 100 children. I see "my children" every day, and I can take a break on weekends.

My daughter and my friend Anna have developed a beautiful friendship. Audrey is now 16. She used to spread her toys on Anna's kitchen floor; now they go for long walks together. Kids value grown-ups who choose to be with them. They need their own relationships with adults they can trust.

Being a parent can have tremendous satisfactions. We can learn from our children as we watch them experience life. We can learn about ourselves as the dynamic relationship between ourselves and our children changes. Raising children is one way to be part of the continuity of life, to extend our spirit and our ways into the future. It can give us a new investment in making the world a better place.

I had a child at 46. Before that, although I loved being with other people's children, any time something went wrong and the child irritated me, I would think to myself, How could I ever stand the full-time responsibility of being a mother? Somehow, becoming a mother changed that. There is an intangible, indescribable bond intrinsic to the relationship, that in the long run transcends the petty everyday irritating occurrences.

She was so new—and I remember gazing at her and feeling such wonder. Part of that wonder came from my belief that she, and every new baby, would change the world. Twelve years later I still believe that, but I've learned that it's hard and challenging and rewarding work for me as a parent; it doesn't necessarily come naturally.

Many women wait to have children. We might want to understand ourselves better emotionally before becoming parents, to reach certain goals in our work or personal lives, or to have certain things in place, such as an education, a job, a relationship, or any number of experiences. Some women postpone having children until their 30s and 40s. At this age, our fertility is known to decrease, and becoming pregnant might take longer. But with a history of good nutrition, good health, and early prenatal care, women who become pregnant in midlife have an excellent chance of giving birth to healthy babies. See *The New Ourselves Growing Older* for a discussion on child-bearing in midlife.

Cultural definitions of mothering and our expectations of ourselves as mothers are often so impossibly idealized that we may never feel "ready" to have children. But not all the conditions for raising a child need to be ideal, and children can be very resilient.

The decision to become a parent seemed so right. Sometimes you must listen to your heart. It has been nearly six years since that decision has been made, and my life has changed considerably. Control and freedom are no longer part of my life, but a deep deep love that has never been felt before is now there every day. To care for a child and see the love and trust she has for you is the most rewarding feeling I have ever experienced. My daughter has given me new hope. Whoever thought that a child could teach an adult so much about living? You want to be there for your child. I am in awe of how intense our love is and how very, very tired and happy I am.

Parenting is hard work, both emotionally and physically, even for women who share child-raising with partners. Balancing parenting and a job can be difficult and stressful. Our technological fast-paced society does not serve the complex needs of parents and children, nor does it truly support and value the caregiving functions of families. In order for women to balance the demands of family and work, we need a public commitment to family policy that is consistent with feminist ideals, and that puts women's and children's needs as a priority. For example, the Family and Medical Leave Act of 1993 mandates that companies of 50 or more employees provide career continuity in the form of the right to return to employment at the same level following a caregiving leave. Yet, most women work in smaller companies, and the mandated leaves are unpaid. We need expanded policies. All workers need paid parental leaves with job protection for parents; gradual return to the work force with no penalties; affordable quality day care for infants, toddlers, and preschoolers; reentry programs to the same level of positions for parents who take time off to raise children; parental leave for sick children; part-time, flex-time, flex-place work, and job-sharing options.

Whether or not we individually choose to have children, child-rearing is important and valuable work that deserves social and economic support. Advocacy for better family policies is strengthened by interdependency between parents and nonparents and by our shared stake in the next generation.

RESOURCES

Books and Other Publications

Barnett, Rosalind, and Caryl Rivers. *She Works/He Works: How Two-Income Families Are Happier, Healthier, and Better Off.* San Francisco: Harper, 1996.

Bartlett, Jane. *Will You Be Mother? Women Who Choose to Say No.* New York: New York University Press, 1995.

Bombardieri, Merle. *The Baby Decision: How to Make the Most Important Choice of Your Life.* New York: Rawson, Wade, 1981.

Boston Women's Health Book Collective. *Ourselves and Our Children.* New York: Random House, 1978.

Cain, Madelyn. *First-Time Mothers, Last-Chance Babies: Parenting at 35.* Far Hills, NJ: New Horizon Press, 1993.

Comer, James P., and Alvin Poussaint. *Raising Black Children: Questions and Answers for Parents and Teachers.* New York: Plume, 1992.

Crosby, Faye J. *Juggling: The Unexpected Advantages of Balancing Career and Home for Women and Their Families.* New York: Free Press, 1993.

Delanzo, Elizabeth M. *Guide to Starting an Older Mom's Support Group.* Send $5 to Elizabeth M. Delanzo, 405 Waltham Street, Suite 114, Lexington, MA 02173.

Derman-Sparks, Louise. *The Anti-Bias Curriculum: Tools for Empowering Young Children.* Washington, DC: National Association for Education of Young Children, 1989. (Organization also has videos.)

Gay, Kathlyn. *I Am Who I Am: Speaking Out About Multiracial Identity.* New York: Franklin Watts, 1995.

Hochschild, Arlie. *The Second Shift.* New York: Avon Books, 1990.

Hopson, Darlene Powell, and Derek S. Hopson. *Different and Wonderful: Raising Black Children in a Race-Conscious Society.* New York: Simon & Schuster, 1992.

Jenness, Aylette V. *Families: A Celebration of Diversity, Commitment and Love.* Boston: Houghton Mifflin, 1993.

Keshet, Jamie. *Love and Power in the Stepfamily.* New York: McGraw-Hill, 1987.

Lang, Susan S. *Women Without Children: The Reasons, the Rewards, the Regrets.* Holbrook, MA: Adams Publishing, 1996.

"Lesbian, Gay, Bisexual and Transgender People and Education." *Harvard Educational Review* special issue 66, no. 2 (summer 1996). Useful for parents.

Lowe, Paula C. *Care Pooling: How to Get the Help You Need to Care for the Ones You Love.* San Francisco: Berrett-Koehler, 1993.

Pipher, Mary. *The Shelter of Each Other: Rebuilding Our Families.* New York: Putnam, 1996.

Reddy, Maureen T., ed. *Everyday Acts Against Racism: Raising Children in a Multicultural World.* Seattle: Seal Press, 1996.

Rizzo, Cindy, et al., eds. *All the Ways Home: Parenting and Children in the Lesbian and Gay Communities: A Collection of Short Fiction.* Norwich, VT: New Victoria Press, 1995.

Ryff, Carol D., and Marsha M. Seltzer, eds. *The Parental Experience in Midlife.* Chicago: University of Chicago Press, 1997.

Taylor-Jones, Christi. *Midlife Parenting: A Guide to Having and Raising Kids in Your 30s, 40s and Beyond.* Van Nuys, CA: Veracity Press, 1993.

Thompson, Becky, and Sangeeta Tyagi. *Names We Call*

Home: Autobiography on Racial Identity. New York: Routledge, 1996.

Umansky, Lauri. *Motherhood Reconceived, Feminism and the Legacies of the 60s*. New York: New York University Press, 1996.

Walter, Carolyn Ambler. *The Timing of Motherhood*. Lexington, MA: Lexington Books, 1986.

Weems, Renita. *I Asked for Intimacy: Stories of Blessings, Betrayals and Birthings*. San Diego: LuraMedia, 1993.

Video

Ten Keys to Culturally-Sensitive Child Care. "Essential Connections" series. Sacramento, CA: Far West Laboratories, 1993.

Organizations

See Resources in chapters 10, 21, and 22.

Chapter 12

By Esther Rome (1945–1995) and
Nancy Reame, with Wendy Sanford

WITH SPECIAL THANKS TO Abby Schwarz,
Katherine Saldutti, Cindy Irvine, and Nancy
Woods*

Understanding Our Bodies: Sexual Anatomy, Reproduction, and the Menstrual Cycle

FINDING OUT ABOUT OUR SEXUAL ORGANS

In talking with other women about our bodies and learning the biological facts, we arrive at a new respect for the beings we are. We equip ourselves with information of use to us in our daily lives and become active participants in our own health and medical care.

It's important to become as familiar with the appearance and function of our sexual organs as we are with other parts of our bodies. We can help reduce the risk of many women's health problems—like breast cancer, depression, and sexually transmitted diseases —if we understand the way our reproductive system works, how it interacts with other body functions, and how it in turn is influenced by our lifestyle, environment, and general well-being. We have found that with just a mirror we can see how we look on the outside. We can also look inside at our vaginal walls and cervix (lower part of the uterus) using a mirror, a

flashlight, and a clean plastic speculum† that we insert into the vagina and gently open up. We find that the vagina is very clean and that normal touching, as in a self-examination, is not painful or uncomfortable. We can do self-exams alone or with others, once or often. With practice we can see how the cervix and vaginal walls change with the menstrual cycle, with pregnancy or with menopause, and learn to recognize various vaginal infections.‡

It has taken a while for some of us to get over our inhibitions about seeing or touching our genitals.

When someone first said to me two years ago, "You can feel the end of your own cervix with your finger," I was interested but flustered. I had hardly ever put my

* Thanks also to the following for their help with the 1998 version of this chapter: Denise Karuth and April Taylor. Over the years since 1969, the following women have contributed to the many versions of this chapter: Leah Diskin, Nancy Miriam Hawley, Barbara Perkins, Toni Randall, and Abby Schwarz.

† A speculum is the instrument used by health care practitioners to separate the vaginal walls during a vaginal examination so they can get a clearer view of the cervix; plastic ones can be purchased from the Feminist Health Center of Portsmouth, NH (603-436-7588), for approximately $2.00 plus postage and handling.
‡ Please see the index to find more on topics mentioned in this chapter.

finger in my vagina at all and felt squeamish about touching myself there, in that place "reserved" for lovers and doctors. It took me two months to get up my nerve to try it, and then one afternoon, pretty nervously, I squatted down in the bathroom and put my finger in deep, back into my vagina. There it was, feeling slippery and rounded, with an indentation at the center through which, I realized, my menstrual flow came. It was both very exciting and beautifully ordinary at the same time. Last week I bought a plastic speculum so I could look at my cervix. Will it take as long this time?

DESCRIPTION OF SEXUAL AND REPRODUCTIVE ORGANS: ANATOMY (STRUCTURE) AND PHYSIOLOGY (FUNCTION)

Pelvic Organs

The following description will be much clearer if you look at yourself with a mirror while you read the text and look at the diagrams. It is written as if you were squatting and looking into a hand mirror. If you are uncomfortable in that position, sit as far forward on the edge of a chair as you comfortably can. Make sure you have plenty of light and enough time and privacy to feel relaxed. You may want to see more with a speculum.

First, you will see your *vulva,* or outer genitals. This includes all the sexual and reproductive organs you can see in your crotch. Too often we confuse the vagina—only one part—with the whole area. The most obvious feature on an adult woman is the *pubic hair,* the first wisps of which are one of the early signs of puberty. After menopause, the hair thins out. It grows from the soft fatty tissue called the *mons* (also *mons veneris,* mountain of Venus, or *mons pubis*).* The mons area lies over the *pubic symphysis.* This is the joint of the pubic bones, which are part of the pelvic bones, or hip girdle. You cannot feel the actual joint, though you can feel the bones under the soft outer skin.

As you spread your legs apart, you can see in the mirror that the hair continues between your legs and probably around your anus. The *anus* is the outside opening of the rectum (the end of the large intestine, or colon). You can feel that the hair-covered area between your legs is also fatty, like the mons. This fatty area forms flaps, called the *outer lips (labia majora),* which are more or less pronounced for different women. In some, the skin of the outer lips is darker.

---

* The formal medical term is included in parenthesis if it is different from the English term. We are not including slang terms in the text. They often represent a male view of a woman's body and have been used to put women down. We can make up words of our own, find old words with a gentler sound, like *yoni,* or use the common words, like *pussy* or *cunt,* in a more positive and loving way.

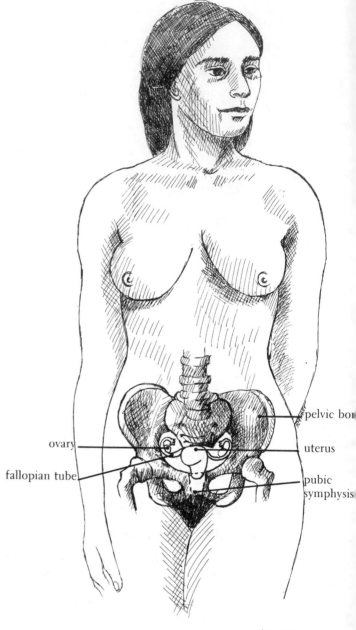

ovary —

fallopian tube —

— pelvic bon[e]

— uterus

— pubic symphysis

Nina Reimer

The outer lips surround two soft flaps of skin that are hairless. These are the *inner lips (labia minora).* They are sensitive to touch. With sexual stimulation they swell and may turn darker. The area between the inner lips and the anus is the *perineum.*

As you gently spread the inner lips apart, you can see that they protect a delicate area between them. This is the *vestibule.* Look more closely at it. Starting from the front, right below the mons area you will see the inner lips joining to form a soft fold of skin, or *hood,* over and connecting to the *glans,* or tip of the *clitoris* (*klit*-or-iss).† Gently pull the hood up to see the

---

† The glans of the clitoris is commonly referred to as "the clitoris." We will follow that convention, but please remember that the

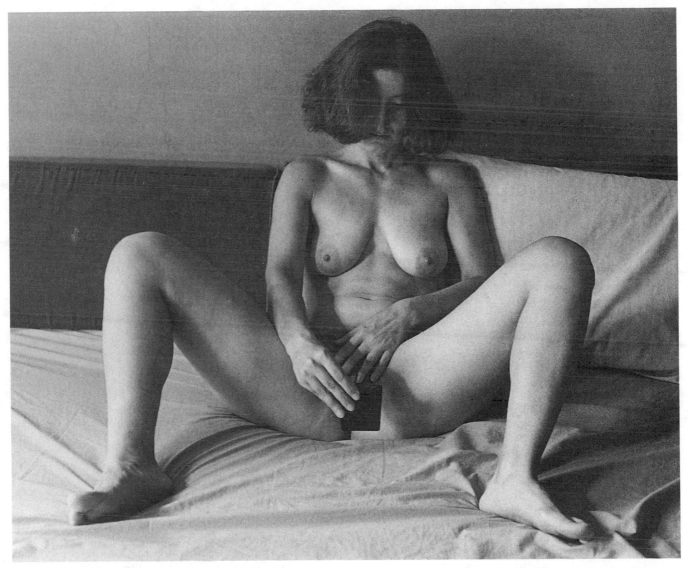

Hazel Hankin/Stock, Boston

glans. This is the most sensitive spot in the entire genital area. It is made up of erectile tissue that swells during sexual arousal. Let the hood slide back over the glans. Extending from the hood up to the pubic symphysis, you can now feel a hardish, rubbery, movable cord right under the skin. It is sometimes sexually arousing if touched. This is the *shaft* of the clitoris. It is connected to the bone by a *suspensory ligament*. You cannot feel this ligament or the next few organs described, but they are all important in sexual arousal and orgasm. At the point where you no longer feel the shaft of the clitoris, it divides into two parts, spreading out wishbone fashion but at a much wider angle, to form the *crura* (singular: *crus*), the two anchoring wingtips of erectile tissue that attach to the pelvic

bones. The crura of the clitoris are about three inches long. Starting from where the shaft and crura meet, and continuing down along the sides of the vestibule, are two bundles of erectile tissue called the *bulbs of the vestibule*. These, along with the whole clitoris and an extensive system of connecting veins and muscles throughout the pelvis, become firm and filled with blood (pelvic congestion) during sexual arousal. Some pelvic congestion, giving a feeling of fullness or heaviness in the pelvic region, can occur during the menstrual cycle right before your period comes. Both the crura of the clitoris and the bulbs of the vestibule are wrapped in muscle tissue. This muscle helps to create tension and fullness during arousal and contracts during orgasm, playing an important role in the involuntary spasms felt at that time. The whole clitoris and vestibular bulbs are the only organs in the body solely for sexual sensation and arousal.

Did you know that the clitoris is similar in origin and function to the penis? All female and male organs,

clitoris is really a much more extensive organ, consisting of the glans, shaft, and crura. The Federation of Feminist Women's Health Centers deserves much of the credit for this important redefinition of the clitoris. (See their book, *A New View . . .* in Resources.)

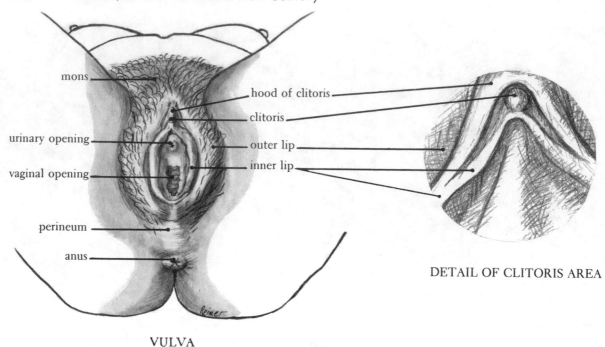

mons

hood of clitoris

clitoris

urinary opening

outer lip

inner lip

vaginal opening

perineum

anus

VULVA

DETAIL OF CLITORIS AREA

Nina Reimer

including sexual and reproductive organs, are developed from the same embryonic tissue (homologous) and similar in function (analogous). In fact, female and male fetuses appear identical during the first six weeks in the uterus. The glans of the clitoris corresponds to the glans of the penis, just as the outer lips of the vagina correspond to the scrotum.

In some parts of the world, there has been the cultural practice of excising a girl's clitoris and sometimes even sewing the labia together. This practice, often referred to as female genital mutilation, has been harmful to millions of girls and women (see chapter

24, Selected Medical Practices, Problems, and Procedures, p. 643).

The *vestibular* or *Bartholin's glands* are two small rounded bodies on either side of the vaginal opening and to the rear of the vestibular bulbs. They sometimes get infected and swell. You can feel them then. Once these glands were thought to provide vaginal lubrication during sexual arousal, but it is now known that they produce only a few drops of fluid.

Let's return to what you can see with the mirror. Keeping the inner lips spread and pulling the hood back again, you will notice that the inner lips attach to the underside of the clitoris. Right below this attachment you will see a small dot or slit. This is the *urinary opening,* the outer opening of the *urethra,* a short (about an inch and a half) thin tube leading to your *bladder.* Below that is a larger opening, the *vaginal opening (introitus).* Because the urinary opening is so close to the vaginal opening, it can become irritated from prolonged or vigorous sexual activity, which may lead to some discomfort while urinating. Around the vaginal opening you may be able to see the remnants of the *hymen.* When you were born, it was a thin membrane surrounding the vaginal opening, partially blocking the opening but almost never covering it completely. Hymens come in widely varying sizes and shapes. For most women the hymen stretches easily—by a finger as well as by a penis or a dildo. Even after it has been stretched, little folds of hymen tissue remain.

Now insert a finger or two into your *vagina.* Notice how the vaginal walls, which were touching each other, spread around your fingers and hug them. Feel the soft folds of skin. These folds allow the vagina to

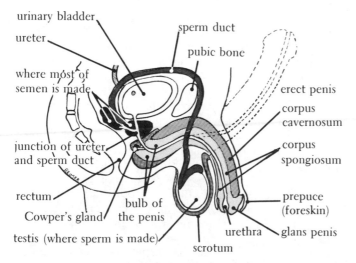

urinary bladder

ureter

where most of semen is made

sperm duct

pubic bone

erect penis

corpus cavernosum

corpus spongiosum

junction of ureter and sperm duct

rectum

Cowper's gland

bulb of the penis

prepuce (foreskin)

testis (where sperm is made)

urethra

glans penis

scrotum

MALE PELVIC ORGANS (side view)

Nina Reimer

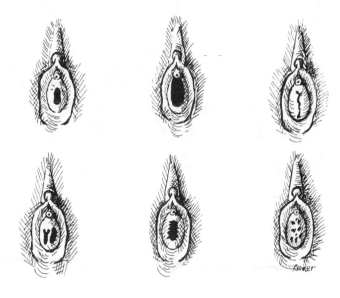

Nina Reimer

nancy, and during sexual arousal. These continuous secretions provide lubrication, help keep the vagina clean, and maintain the acidity of the vagina, which helps to prevent some infections. Push gently all around against the walls of the vagina, and notice where you feel particularly sensitive. For some women it is only the outer third; in others it is most or all of the vagina. Now put your finger halfway in and try to grip your finger with your vagina. You are contracting the *pelvic floor muscles*. These muscles hold the pelvic organs in place and provide support for your other organs all the way up to your diaphragm, which is stretched across the bottom of your rib cage. Strengthening these muscles can help you in many ways. See the box on p. 274.

Only a thin wall of skin separates the vagina from the rectum, so you may be able to feel a bump on one side of your vagina if you have some stool in the rectum or a small hemorrhoid.

Now slide your middle finger as far back into your vagina as you can. Notice that your finger goes in toward the small of your back at an angle, not straight up the middle of your body. If you were standing instead of squatting, your vagina would be at about a forty-five degree angle to the floor. With your finger you may be able to just feel the end of your vagina. This part of the vagina is called the *fornix*. (If you are having trouble reaching it, bring your knees and chest closer together so your finger can slide in farther. However, some women still may not be able to do this.) A little before the end of the vagina you can feel your *cervix*. The cervix feels like a nose with a small

mold itself around what might be inside it: fingers, a tampon, a penis, or a baby during childbirth. Notice that your finger slides around inside the vagina as you move it. The walls of the vagina may be almost dry to very wet. Dryer times usually occur before puberty, during lactation, and after menopause as well as during that part of the menstrual cycle right after the flow. Wetter times occur around ovulation, during preg-

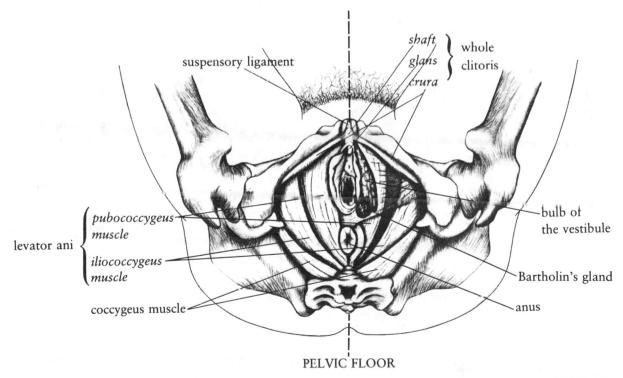

suspensory ligament

shaft
glans } whole clitoris
crura

levator ani {

pubococcygeus muscle

iliococcygeus muscle

coccygeus muscle

bulb of the vestibule

Bartholin's gland

anus

PELVIC FLOOR

Christine Bondante

STRENGTHENING THE PELVIC FLOOR MUSCLES (KEGEL EXERCISES)

Strengthening the pelvic floor muscles can increase a woman's ease in reaching orgasm and giving birth. It helps to prevent problems controlling urine flow (urinary incontinence) and prolapse of the uterus (see chapter 24, Selected Medical Problems, Practices, and Procedures, p. 661). You can do the exercises anywhere—in the car, on the phone, even as a wake-up exercise. A good way to locate your pelvic floor muscles is to spread your legs apart and start and stop the flow of urine, or tighten your vagina around one or two inserted fingers.

To start, tighten the muscles, holding for two to four seconds, and relax for ten seconds. Repeat five times. Do this three times a day. Work up gradually until you can hold the contraction for eight seconds and ten repetitions. Then you can add three or four short, fast but strong twitches at the end of each long contraction. Also, you can think of your bladder and uterus as an elevator, which you are raising little by little to the top floor. When you reach the top, go down floor by floor, gradually relaxing the muscles. (Be sure you do not contract your abdominal or buttock muscles, or hold your breath, while doing the exercises.)

FEMALE PELVIC ORGANS (side view)

Nina Reimer

dimple in its center. (If you've had a baby, the cervix may feel more like a chin.) The cervix is the base of the *uterus,* or womb. It is sensitive to pressure but has no nerve endings on its surface. The uterus changes position, color, and shape during the menstrual cycle and during sexual excitement as well as during puberty and menopause, so the place where you feel the cervix one day may be slightly different from where you feel it the next. Some days you can barely reach it. The dimple you felt is the *os,* or opening into the uterus. The entrance into the uterus through the cervix is very small, about the diameter of a very thin straw, and closed with mucus. No tampon, finger, or penis can go up through it, although it is capable of expanding enormously for a baby during labor and delivery. For information on how to see your cervix through self-examination, see chapter 24, Selected Medical Problems, Practices, and Procedures, p. 593.*

Reproductive Organs You Can't See

The nonpregnant uterus is about the size of a fist. Its thick walls are made of some of the most powerful muscles in the body. It is located behind the bladder, which is beneath the abdominal wall, and the rectum, which is near the backbone. The walls of the uterus touch each other unless pushed apart by a growing fetus or an abnormal growth. The top of the uterus is called the *fundus.*

Extending outward and back from the sides of the upper end of the uterus are the two *fallopian tubes* (or *oviducts;* literally, "egg tubes"). They are approximately four inches long and look like ram's horns facing backward. The connecting opening from the inside of the uterus to the fallopian tube is as small as a fine needle. The other end of the tube is fringed *(fimbriated)* and funnel-shaped. The wide end of the funnel wraps part way around the *ovary* but does not actually attach to it. It is held in place by connecting tissues.

The ovaries are organs about the size and shape of unshelled almonds, located on either side of and somewhat below the uterus. They are about four or five inches below your waist. They are held in place by connective tissue and are protected by a surrounding mass of fat. They have a twofold function: to produce germ cells (eggs) and to produce female sex hormones (estrogen, progesterone, and many other hormones, only some of whose functions we understand) as well as the male hormone, testosterone, which plays a role in sexual desire throughout a woman's life. The small gap between the ovary and the end of the corresponding tube allows the egg to float freely after it has been released from the ovary. The finger-like ends *(fimbria)* of the fallopian tube sweep across the surface of the ovary and wave the egg into the tube after ovulation. In rare cases when the egg does not enter the tube, it can be fertilized outside the tube,

---

* See Suzann Gage's drawings, and Silvia Morales's photos of cervical changes during the cycle, in *A New View of a Woman's Body,* listed in Resources.

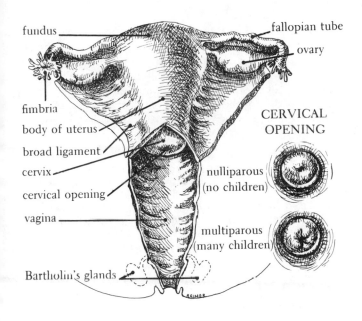

Nina Reimer

resulting in an abdominal pregnancy, which is very dangerous for the woman.

Our Breasts

When we look at our breasts in the mirror, we will most likely notice that they are not the same size and shape. Sometimes the right one is smaller than the left —a variation that is especially noticeable just after puberty. If we observe the shape of our breasts over time, we will also notice that they usually become droopier over the years as our skin becomes less elastic and our milk glands get smaller. This happens even faster after menopause, when the milk glands are no longer stimulated to grow. Because the breast is a receptor for the sex hormones produced by the ovaries, most of us notice pronounced changes during the menstrual cycle, with the most fullness right before our periods. This fullness can produce tenderness in some women and can be felt down into the armpit in the part of the breast called the "tail." Also, during pregnancy and nursing our breasts can enlarge considerably. Examining our breasts regularly can help us learn our usual patterns as well as detect anything out of the ordinary.

In the middle of the breast we notice a circle of darker skin. The color can be light pink to almost black. During pregnancy it may become larger and, in light-skinned women, darker. Sometimes the changes are permanent. This darker skin is made up of the *areola* and *nipple*. The areola may have small bumps on it. These are *sebaceous* or *oil glands*, which secrete lubricant that protects the nipple during nursing. Hairs often grow around our areolas and may increase over time or with the use of the birth control pill. Our nipples may stick out, lie flat, or be inverted (go inward).

All these configurations are normal. The nerves enter the nipple near the bottom of the areola. The only muscles in our breasts are directly under the nipple and areola. In response to cold or touch or sexual arousal, the areola may pucker and the nipples become more erect.

The inside of each breast consists of *fat, connective tissue,* and a *milk-producing* (mammary) *gland*. The gland is made up of *tiny milk-producing sacs and tubes,* or *ducts,* which during lactation carry the milk to the nipple. During the reproductive years, even when we are not nursing, these glands can periodically produce small amounts of clear fluid that flow from the nipples.

With the great increase of sex hormones during adolescence, the milk-producing gland in each breast

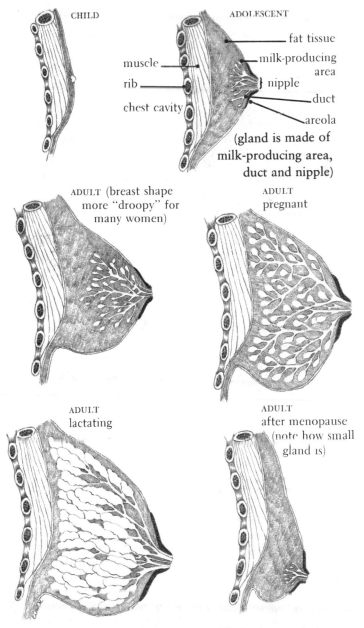

Breast changes over a lifetime/*Peggy Clark*

starts to develop and increase in size to about the amount of a spoonful. All women have approximately the same amount of milk-producing tissue at the same points in their reproductive life cycles. Most of the breast consists of fat that surrounds the gland, and connective tissue. The amount of fat in the breasts is partly determined by heredity. This fat makes breast size vary, and explains why breast size is not related to the sexual responsiveness of the breast or to the amount of milk produced after we have given birth. Because sex hormone levels change during the menstrual cycle, when we start and stop birth control pills, during pregnancy, during lactation, and after menopause, there can be variations in a particular woman's breast size and shape. The best time to have a mammogram is the first three to seven days after your period starts, when any fullness has gone away and the glands are easiest to see by X ray. (See chapter 24, Selected Medical Practices, Problems, and Procedures, pp. 608–9, on the decision about whether and when to have a mammogram.)

STAGES IN THE REPRODUCTIVE LIFE CYCLE

In childhood our bodies are immature. During puberty we make the transition from childhood to physical maturity. In women, puberty is characterized by growth of the breasts and the pubic and armpit (axillary) hair, and a growth spurt that results in increased height and weight, followed by the end of bone growth. Ovulation and menstruation (menarche) start near the end of puberty, generally when we are about 12½, though any age from nine to 18 is normal. To menstruate, a girl probably needs her body fat to be about one quarter of her total weight. Some experts believe that this is because the hormone leptin, produced by fat cells, must reach a certain level in the blood to help start menstrual cycles and to help maintain them after puberty. To sustain regular cycles, we also need to eat a balance of fat, carbohydrates (sugars and starches), and protein.

Menstruation and ovulation continue until age 50, on average, but any time between 40 and 55 is normal. When periods stop, *menopause* has occurred. The body changes that occur between the reproductive and postreproductive phases of our life, called the *climacteric,* often take place over as many as 15 years.

This entire reproductive process is regulated by hormones, chemicals in the bloodstream and in the brain that relay messages from one part of the body to another, setting off effects in receptor tissues. The levels of sex hormones are low during childhood, increase tremendously during the reproductive years, and then become lower and differently balanced after menopause. The signs and symptoms of menarche and menopause are thought to be caused by the changing levels of hormones.

I like the idea that we experience two *transitions, one into our reproductive years and one out of them. Menopause can be seen as another kind of puberty!*

During the reproductive years, monthly hormone rhythms determine the timing of ovulation and menstruation. This cycle, the menstrual cycle, regulates our fertility, allowing for the possibility of pregnancy a few days every month. By keeping track of our bodily changes during the cycle, we can know when we are most fertile or when a menstrual period is likely to come.

The Ovarian Cycle: Ovulation

I like to get away from the traditional medical model of the menstrual cycle, where everything is a hierarchy with hormones up in the brain controlling the hormones down in the ovaries. Things just aren't that simple. Instead, I like to think of the menstrual cycle as a symphony played by a hormonal orchestra with the brain as the conductor. All the right signals have to be brought together with the right timing and rhythm so as not to be off-key. Just as in music, fertility is dependent on the fine-tuning of the rhythm, melody, and tenor of the song, rather than on the absolute presence or absence of any one hormone.

Both ovaries at birth contain about 1,000,000 follicles, which are hollow balls of cells, each with an immature egg in the center. The ovaries absorb about half of these during childhood. About 300 to 500 of the 400,000 follicles present at menarche will develop into mature eggs across the reproductive life span.

Each month during our reproductive years, ten to 20 follicles begin maturing under the influence of hormones (see the Appendix for more details). Usually only one develops fully. Our bodies reabsorb the others before they complete development. Some of the cells in the follicle secrete the hormone called estrogen. The follicle, with the maturing egg inside, moves toward the surface of the ovary. At ovulation, the follicle and the ovarian surface open over the egg, allowing it to float out. About this time, some women feel a twinge or cramp in the lower abdomen or back, sometimes with a small amount of extra vaginal discharge, perhaps bloody. The symptoms can be severe enough to be confused with appendicitis or ectopic pregnancy. This is *Mittelschmerz* ("middle pain"). A few women have headaches, gastric pains, or sluggishness. Other women feel better at the time of ovulation. Cervical mucus changes at this time, too (see p. 277).

Just before ovulation, the same cells in the follicle start secreting progesterone as well as estrogen. After ovulation, the empty follicle is now called a *corpus luteum* ("yellow body," referring to the yellow fat in it). If the cycle is interrupted by pregnancy, the hormones produced by the corpus luteum help to maintain the pregnancy. If no pregnancy occurs, the follicle is reabsorbed. After ovulation, the released egg is swept into the funnel-shaped end of one of the fallopian tubes (oviducts) and begins its several-day journey to the uterus, moved along by wave-like contractions of the muscles in the tube (peristalsis). Each tube is lined with microscopic hairs *(cilia)* that

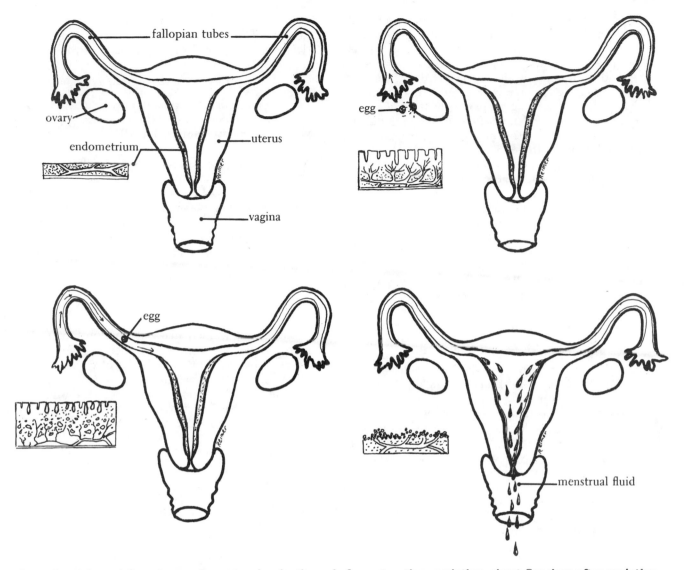

The endometrium at four stages of menstrual cycle: the end of menstruation, ovulation, about five days after ovulation, and menstruation/Nina Reimer

beat constantly. If the woman has had unprotected sexual intercourse with a man, or donor insemination, these cilia propel the seminal fluid in the direction of the ovary, carrying the sperm toward the egg.

If fertilization occurs (the union of an egg from a woman and sperm from a man), it usually takes place in the outer third of the fallopian tube (nearest the ovaries). Fertilization is also called conception and usually occurs within one day of ovulation. It takes a fertilized egg approximately five to six days to reach the uterus. If the tube has been scarred or unusually twisted by infection resulting from an IUD, endometriosis, or pelvic inflammatory disease, the fertilized egg might implant itself in the fallopian tube, resulting in a dangerous tubal (ectopic) pregnancy (see chapter 22, Child-bearing Loss, Infertility, and Adoption).

If the egg is not fertilized, it disintegrates or flows out with the vaginal secretions, usually before menstruation. You won't notice it.

The Uterine Cycle and Menstruation

Cervical Changes

The kind of mucus produced by your cervix changes through the cycle in response to hormones. Although there are general patterns, you can follow your own cycle to find out what yours is by feeling the entrance to the vagina with your finger, looking at the secretions, being aware of vaginal wetness or dryness, and recording these characteristics every day for several cycles. You may also wish to taste your secretions. They can be sour, salty, or sweet, changing during the cycle in a pattern typical for you. If you looked at it under a microscope, the mucus would usually look like a maze of tangled fibers. It is extremely difficult for sperm and many other organisms, like bacteria, to get through it. However, at ovulation, under the influence of estrogen, the mucus changes to form longer strands, more or less aligned, which can guide sperm into the uterus. Thus, the mucus is a kind of gatekeeper for the uterus. At ovulation, it is profuse enough to coat the vagina and protect sperm from the acid secretions produced there. After ovulation, as progesterone counteracts estrogen, cervical mucus thickens, and your vagina gradually becomes drier. Menopausal women may find that watching the changes in their cervical mucus is a simple way of monitoring their estrogen levels.

If you look at your cervix with a speculum, you may notice that about the time of ovulation the cervix is pulled up high into the vagina. It may also enlarge and soften, and the os may open a little.

Endometrial Changes and Menstruation

Estrogen, made by the maturing follicle, causes the glands of the uterine lining *(endometrium)* to grow and thicken, and increases the blood supply to these glands (proliferative phase). This part of the cycle can vary greatly in length, from six to 20 days. Progesterone, made by the ruptured follicle after the egg is released, stimulates the glands in the endometrium to begin secreting embryo-nourishing substances (secretory phase). A fertilized egg can implant only in a secretory lining, not in a proliferative one.

If conception has not occurred, the leftover follicle, or *corpus luteum,* will produce estrogen and progesterone for about 12 days, with the amount lessening in the last few days. As the estrogen and progesterone levels drop, the tiny arteries and veins in the uterus close off. The lining is no longer nourished and is shed. This is menstruation: the menstrual period, or flow. During menstruation, most of the lining is shed; the bottom third remains to form a new lining. Then a new follicle starts growing and secreting estrogen, a new uterine lining grows, and the cycle begins again. (It is possible to have a menstrual period—called an anovulatory period—without ovulating, even after cycles have been established. In young women, anovulatory cycles average once a year, increasing to eight to ten a year as menopause approaches.)

Any menstrual cycle that is more or less regular is normal. The length of the cycle usually ranges from 20 to 36 days, the average being 28 days. (The word *menstruation* is from the Latin *mensis,* for "month.") Some women have alternating long and short cycles. There are spontaneous small changes, and there can be major changes when a woman is under a great deal of stress. As you get older or if you have a baby, you may notice marked changes. An average period lasts two to eight days, with four to six days being the average. The flow stops and starts, though this may not always be evident. A usual discharge for a menstrual period is about four to six tablespoons, or two to three ounces.

Recent research suggests that eating soy products (tofu, soybeans, miso, tempeh) can lengthen the menstrual cycle. Soy contains *phytoestrogens,* natural chemicals that act like weak estrogens in the body and may reduce the risk of breast cancer, perhaps by lengthening the menstrual cycle and by an antitumor effect. Japanese women, who eat a lot of soy, have a lower incidence of breast cancer than women elsewhere.[1]

The Menstrual Fluid

The menstrual fluid contains cervical mucus, vaginal secretions, mucus, cells, and endometrial particles, as well as blood (sometimes clotted), but this mixed content is not obvious, since the blood stains everything red or brown. This regular loss of blood, even though small, can cause anemia. The fluid usually does not smell until it makes contact with the bacteria in the air and starts to decompose.

Products for Handling the Menstrual Flow

Women in different cultures handle their menstrual flow in many ways. Since earliest times, women have made pads and tampons from available materials, often washing and reusing special cloths or rags. Today, some women make them from cotton balls, gauze, or flannel. Most women use commercial menstrual napkins and tampons, most of which are made of rayon and cotton blends.

Commercial tampons raise some significant health concerns. *Toxic shock syndrome* (TSS—see chapter 24, Selected Medical Problems, Practices, and Procedures, p. 649) is a rare but life-threatening blood infection, which has been linked to the use of tampons, especially to high-absorbency tampons made with rayon and other synthetic ingredients. (All-cotton tampons have not been associated with TSS; TSS has been associated with diaphragms, the Keeper, and sponges, though rarely.)[2] To avoid TSS, do not use tampons between your periods or ones that are more absorbent than you need during your period, and do not use them overnight. Check the absorbency rating on the tampon boxes to help you select the lowest absorbency you need. A tampon is too absorbent if it is hard to pull out or shreds when you remove it or if your vagina becomes dry. When used under those circumstances, tampons can cause sores on the vaginal walls that you may not notice. Familiarize yourself with the signs of toxic shock syndrome, and if you experience them, remove the tampon immediately. One woman wrote,

I try to limit myself to using tampons only when I think I really need to—for working out, long meetings, travel, swimming. It works out to three to five tampons a month.

Menstrual product companies are always introducing "new, improved" products. Avoid *deodorized* or *scented* tampons, napkins, and feminine deodorant sprays. Many women have allergic reactions to the chemicals in them. If any of them cause problems, stop using them immediately.

ACTIVISM REGARDING DIOXIN AND MENSTRUAL PRODUCTS

You may want to become politically active about this health hazard. U.S. Representative Carolyn Maloney (D–NY) introduced a Women's Health and Dioxin Act in Congress in 1996 and 1997, to require the National Institutes of Health to assess the health risks to women—including ovarian and cervical cancer, and endometriosis—from dioxin residue in tampons and menstrual pads. Organizations involved in these issues include Women and Environments Education and Development Foundation (WEED) and Mothers and Others (see Resources).

In addition to the risk of TSS, some women experience vaginal irritation, itching, soreness, unusual odor or, in rare cases, bright red bleeding while using tampons. If you notice any of these conditions, stop using tampons, use a lower absorbency, or change brands to see if that helps. There is no premarket safety testing of tampons, and most research done by the manufacturers is kept secret.*

Dioxin residue in menstrual products. Most commercial napkins and tampons are bleached with chlorine to make them whiter and, in the case of rayon, more absorbent. Chlorine leaves residues of dioxin in the tampons and pads, as well as in the environment through waste water and landfill disposal. Dioxin is a harmful chemical that has been implicated in cancer and other health problems. In addition, most cotton production involves large amounts of pesticides, traces of which may remain in tampons and pads made from cotton that is not organically grown (without pesticides). Dioxin and pesticide residues are especially serious in menstrual products because the vaginal lining is much more absorbent than skin and because women wear tampons and pads for hours at a time (see Armstrong and Scott, *Whitewash,* in Resources).

Alternatives to commercial tampons and pads. Because of TSS, as well as chemical residues, many women use alternative products: all-cotton (preferably organic) chlorine-free tampons, chlorine-free disposable pads, washable cloth pads, and devices that collect rather than absorb the menstrual fluid (see below). Some of the large commercial tampon manufacturers market "all-cotton, chlorine-free" tampons, but there have been lawsuits claiming false advertising, and pesticides remain an issue. All-cotton and all-organic cotton, chlorine-free tampons are often sold in health food stores and by mail order.†

Some women use natural sponges (small sea sponges sold for cosmetic purposes), which are reusable and economical. Unfortunately, many pollutants are dumped into the oceans. We don't know how much pollutant a given sponge has absorbed, or whether residual pollutants may cause us problems. Almost no testing has been done.‡ Boiling a sea sponge for at least five minutes before use may help. Clean it after use in a mild vinegar-and-water solution, rinse well, and air dry.

Some women prefer products that collect rather than absorb the menstrual fluid. The Keeper is an elongated cup made of gum rubber held in place by suction in the lower vagina to collect menstrual fluid. It can be worn during swimming and other physical activities but not during intercourse or other penetrative sex. It is available only by mail order.[3] Some women use a diaphragm or a cervical cap in the same way as a Keeper.

"Instead" is a relatively new disposable device worn in the upper vagina to collect the menstrual flow.[4] The rim softens in response to body temperature and creates a seal to protect against leakage and slipping. "Instead" claims to be usable during strenuous physical activity and penetrative sex.

Laboratory tests have shown that rubber and latex can increase the production of small amounts of the TSS-causing toxin.[5] With rubber or latex collection devices (like the diaphragm and the Keeper; we do not know about "Instead"), there is a minimal risk of TSS, though it is much less than with the synthetic fibers in tampons.

A method developed and used by women in advanced self-help groups is menstrual extraction (see chapter 17, Abortion, p. 391).§

Those of us with disabilities that limit our mobility and our ability to do self-care—for instance, who have limited sensation in the lower part of our bodies, who don't have the use of our hands, or who use wheel chairs—often find all of these methods either irritating or difficult to use. We have to put together existing products in solutions that come the closest to what we need. There are, for example, very large pads, diapers, and pantliners designed for urinary incontinence that may be used; but these often use plastic, which can be a skin irritant, and most are bleached with chlorine bleach. We hope the burgeoning industry in different forms of protection will result in products we can use with more satisfaction.

* Report any tampon-related problems you have to the U.S. FDA (see chapter 25, The Politics of Women's Health and Medical Care, p. 717).
† One source is Seventh Generation, (800) 456-1177.
‡ Different researchers, using only a few sponge samples each, have gotten contradictory results. Caribbean and Florida sponges grow in *generally* less polluted waters than Mediterranean sponges.
§ See *A Woman's Book of Choices* in Resources.

Attitudes About Menstruation

Cultural, religious, and personal attitudes about menstruation are a part of our menstrual experience and often reflect our society's attitudes toward women. Consider for a moment the ways you have been influenced by attitudes and customs about menstruation. How did you first hear about it? How else have you found out about it: family, friends, advertising, lovers, books, films, teachers, nurses, doctors, taboos, slang, names, jokes? What particular experiences stand out in your mind? How did they make you feel? Are your current experiences different? How is menstruation a part of your life now?

Certain cultures have isolated women entirely or put them only in the company of other women during their periods, because people thought that menstrual blood was unclean, or because they thought menstruating women had supernatural powers. These powers were sometimes seen as good, but more often they were feared to be destructive. Women themselves may have started these practices to give themselves time for meditation or to give older women a chance to pass on their knowledge to younger women.

Taboos in the dominant culture today include refraining from exercise, showers, and sexual intercourse, or hiding the fact of menstruation entirely. Examine the wording in media ads for menstrual products to see how this is reinforced in our country.

In the belief that the menstrual cycle makes women unstable or less capable, some people deny jobs to women and treat us as inferior. Both women and men experience mood swings, but for women the changes are seen as a sign of inherent instability. This negative attitude leads us to deny admitting the changes for fear of being discounted. The idea that women lose a lot of time from work is largely unsupported. For example, one study of nurses shows that they lost very little

time because of menstrual problems.[6] Most women do not show important differences in their thinking capacity or in their ability to perform tasks throughout their cycles. We still work where we are "needed"—at home, in factories, in offices—with no concessions in schedules or routines to take account of individual differences in our cycles.

Feelings About Menstruation

Many of us were scared or even embarrassed when we first started to menstruate. We grew up with little or no knowledge about where the blood and tissue were coming from, why it came, and why it sometimes hurt. Some of us thought we were dying when we first saw our menstrual fluid. Some of us were desperately afraid that a teacher or boy would notice when we had our period. On the other hand, some of us felt inadequate if we didn't menstruate.

I used to worry about having my period. It seemed that all my friends had gotten it already or were just having it. I felt left out. I began to think of it as a symbol: When I got my period, I would become a woman.

Beginning and ending menstruation will always be different for each person—welcome to some, not to others. We do know that as we feel better about our bodies and learn more about ourselves, our experiences of our cycles can change. During times when we feel especially good about ourselves, we may experience our periods as self-affirming, creative, and pleasurable. Or we may have contradictory feelings at the same time.

I really love getting my period. It's like the changing seasons. I feel a bond with other women. I feel fertile and womanly and empowered because of my potential to make a life. I even like the little aches I get because it's a reminder of having my period.

As I entered menopause, my periods started coming much less often. After several period-free months, another period would surprise me, and back I would be, scrambling for tampons and a heating pad. I'd feel, "Oh my God, isn't this finished?" At the same time I'd feel nostalgic and a little sad, like this might be the last period I'd ever have.

Some of us will pay less attention to menstruation; others will explore it further through art, songs, writings, and new rituals.

Menstrual Problems

Menstruation is a normal, healthy occurrence for many years of a woman's life. Yet, many women, across a range of very different cultures, experience menstrual problems that range from mild discomfort to acute pain. For those of us who have these prob-

---

LEARNING MORE ABOUT YOUR CYCLE

A good way to start learning more about your own cycle and what is usual and normal for you is to keep a simple chart. Note the start of your flow on a calendar. Add whatever else you are interested in, or make a separate chart or journal. Some things you might consider looking at more carefully are color, texture, taste, clots, cervical changes, breast changes, or fluctuations in your general physical, emotional, or sexual state. You may find no pattern where you thought there was one, or you may find that some changes occur at particular times in your cycle. Remember to look beyond your menstrual cycle to your social cycles—rhythms associated with the days of the week or month—for possible links to any physical or emotional changes.

lems either occasionally or often, it is important to understand the problems and deal with them.

Menstrual problems may not be inevitable. More research is needed for us to understand enough about the interactions of our physical and emotional states with our external environment (physical and social) and our internal environment (including cyclically changing body chemicals and heredity) to know why some women have problems and others don't. We also need more studies into why certain remedies work for some and not for others. The Society for Menstrual Cycle Research is a group of women's health researchers who believe that menstrual health problems should be studied within the bigger picture of a woman's life, to fully understand their causes and treatments.*

Although most women have some physical or emotional changes or discomforts linked to our menstrual cycles, a smaller number (about 5%) find that the problems are more serious, and we may seek some kind of treatment. In the past, many doctors have attributed cramps and other menstrual problems to psychological causes. As a result, medical prescriptions sometimes include things that don't necessarily help us: general painkillers (when other medication may work better), hormones (sometimes in the form of birth control pills), tranquilizers, a "pat on the head," a hysterectomy, or an inappropriate recommendation to see a psychiatrist. Included in the following section are treatments and home remedies that have worked for many women. As home remedies are generally cheaper and less invasive, many women try them first. In addition, acupuncture has helped many women with menstrual problems.

Home Remedies for Menstrual Problems—An Overview

Women have been sharing menstrual remedies for centuries. Some of us have gained new respect for our own knowledge after trying traditional remedies and exploring new ones. Listed in this chapter are only those most frequently reported to work. *Because each woman is unique and has different reactions, pay attention to how the remedy you choose affects you.* Whatever specific remedies you may choose, the three that follow have wide application for all menstrual problems.

Food: It helps if you can eat food that is varied, sufficient, and balanced. Many women find that it helps reduce premenstrual bloating and fatigue to eat *more* whole grains and whole flours, beans, vegetables, fruits, and brewer's yeast and *less* or *no* salt, sugar, alcohol, and caffeine (in coffee, tea, chocolate, and soft drinks) (see chapter 2, Food). Also, you may

* The Society for Menstrual Cycle Research is a major advocate for reframing research subjects in women's health studies as co-researchers who participate actively in the design, collection of data, and interpretation of the research results. For more information, contact the Society (see Resources).

need to eat small, frequent meals or snacks rather than two or three bigger meals. Fiber is important, as some women report mild constipation just before menstruation.

Sleep: It helps if you can get the right amount for *you.* Your rhythms may change during your cycle. As much as you can, allow time for extra sleep if you need it.

Exercise: Moderate exercise helps many women feel more comfortable before and during menstruation. For some ideas about exercise, see chapter 4, Women in Motion. Yoga (especially the cobra position) and tai chi can be particularly helpful. Experiment with different positions to find out what helps you (see chapter 5, Holistic Health and Healing).

Approaches to Specific Premenstrual and Menstrual Problems

Premenstrual Changes

Women can have a variety of sensations or experiences for several days before and sometimes during the first day of menstruation. Among these are mood swings, depression (frequently mild and occasionally severe), bloating, breast tenderness, and headaches. Sometimes these premenstrual experiences disrupt our lives significantly. Sometimes, they are mild. For example, some women report feeling more energetic and creative premenstrually, and some find the milder mood swings tolerable and even interesting. All efforts so far to find a biological basis or uniform definition for the problems of premenstruation have failed, but these problems are very real nonetheless.

"Premenstrual syndrome" (PMS) is a medical term currently in use for a wide range of premenstrual experiences. The term "PMS" is often used with terms like "symptoms" and "treatments," as though premenstrual changes were an illness. The authors of this book are concerned that some medical professionals and drug companies have picked up on "PMS" and use it as an excuse to prescribe, and to sell, more medications to women. Many of the treatments prescribed for "PMS" are expensive (progesterone, fluoxetine) and can have serious side effects when taken in large doses over long periods of time (vitamin B_6, fluoxetine). None of the popular therapies, such as progesterone, high-dose vitamins or minerals, or evening primrose oil, have been shown to work better than a placebo (an inactive test substance like a sugar pill) in well-controlled trials. Hormone suppressants have not had careful clinical trials. Since the studies so far suggest that most of these treatments and the placebos *all* seem to work equally for many women, at least for a few months, it may make sense to try the least expensive and invasive approaches first.

For those of us with premenstrual problems, it is important that our health care providers, our families, and our co-workers take them seriously. Yet, the term "PMS" may encourage us to relate to more and more of our premenstrual experiences as medical problems. If we help each other increase our self-esteem, and feel more comfortable with our moods as well as our anger, we may experience many of our premenstrual signs differently. We may also feel more empowered to define what our specific premenstrual problems are, and to explore appropriate care for them without accepting a medicalization of the whole experience.

Mild Premenstrual Depression

Those of us who get depressed premenstrually often find, when we think about it, that we are concerned with problems that have been there all the time. We just can't ignore them as well during our premenstrual days. It is important to keep track of the problems that bother us, even if it means writing them down, so that when we're feeling better we remember to work toward solving them.

A week before my period comes I go through a few days of feeling more helpless, stuck, or down about things in my life that have been there all along. Sometimes I appreciate being more in touch with the underside of my feelings. Other times it really gets to me. The voices inside my head which are overly critical of what I do get much more insistent when I'm premenstrual. Recently I've identified them more quickly. I'll start to get down on myself for not being a good enough mother, friend, worker, daughter, and so forth, and I'll say, "Those are your critical voices—go easy on yourself!" It helps.

You might plan to get support for yourself for the times when you feel worst. Ask close friends to drop by, involve the rest of the family more in running the household, or ask someone to help with the kids. You might start a self-help group by advertising in the paper. See p. 281 for suggestions about food, sleep, and exercise; many women are too busy to do much for ourselves during this time, but whatever you can do might help.

Severe Premenstrual Depression

When premenstrual depression is more than the blues and interferes noticeably with your daily life (you can't get out of bed, miss work, or have suicidal thoughts), this is the time to seek advice from a mental health professional who has the skill and experience to distinguish serious premenstrual problems from other emotional problems. Recently the antidepressant drug fluoxetine (Prozac), which blocks the breakdown of the brain chemical serotonin, has been found to be effective for treating severe premenstrual depression.[7] This is the first time that any medication has been consistently superior to placebos in clinical trials, which suggests that this severe form of premenstrual problem may be related to a chemical imbalance in the brain. However, be aware that some health care providers prescribe Prozac for the milder emotional ups and downs of premenstruation; this is an inappropriate use of a medication that is expensive and can have significant side effects (including decreased sexual desire).

A natural compound found in St. John's wort, a flowering plant, has for some years been in wide use in Europe as a nondrug alternative for mild depression. It is much less expensive than Prozac and other antidepressant drugs, seems to have few side effects, and is effective in clinical studies, although it has not yet been tested scientifically in women with premenstrual depression. (See the box on depression in chapter 6, Our Emotional Well-Being.)

Dysmenorrhea (Menstrual Cramps)

You can do something about dysmenorrhea, the sometimes incapacitating cramping during your period. A particular constellation of symptoms, including cramping and often nausea and diarrhea, may be caused by an excess of a certain type of prostaglandin found in the uterus and perhaps "leaking" into the intestines. (One form of prostaglandins, which are substances found throughout the body, causes contractions of the uterine and intestinal muscles.) With too much prostaglandin, the usually painless rhythmic contractions of the uterus during menstruation become longer and tighter at the tightening phase, keeping oxygen from the muscles. It is this lack of oxygen that we perceive as pain. Anticipation often worsens the pain by making us tense up. It's not clear why some women have more prostaglandin in their uterus than others.

Severe cramping can also indicate endometriosis and pelvic inflammatory disease. The use of amphetamines and over-the-counter diet aids can also contribute to cramping.

Antiprostaglandins, a class of drugs developed for arthritis, constitute a medical solution that helps some women. In severe cases, you must take the drug before cramping begins; still, it may only lessen the pain. Some women find some of these drugs easier to tolerate than others. The most frequent complaint is upset stomach, which is often avoided by taking the drug with milk or other food. A few women have found that one drug ceases to be effective and that they must try another. Antiprostaglandins also reduce the amount of flow and shorten the period. We don't yet know how safe these drugs are for long-term, intermittent use, although they seem *relatively* safe so far.* It is probably best to start with home remedies. Acupuncture can also be helpful.

Home Remedies for Cramps and Backache. Herbs may help. Raspberry leaf tea is one most consistently recommended, but chamomile and peppermint are also good for general relaxation. Brew one tablespoon for each cup. Chinese herbs can help, too. Herbs, like

---

* The two most effective drugs seem to be ibuprofen (Motrin, Advil), and mefanamic acid (Ponstel). The side effects of ibuprofen are nausea and indigestion and, potentially, gastric ulcers; to avoid them, take it with meals and avoid alcohol. Naproxen (Naprosyn) and indomethacin (Indocin) are also presecribed; they tend to have more side effects. Please refer to the *PDR (Physicians' Desk Reference)* or a local pharmacy for side effects and contraindications. *Source:* C. Fogel and N. Woods, *Women's Health Care* (Newbury Park, CA: Sage, 1996), 541.

medications, should be used in moderation. (See Resources in this chapter and chapter 5, Holistic Health and Healing, for more on herbs.) Some women eat a lot of calcium-rich foods, or take calcium and magnesium supplements in a two-to-one ratio for several days before the flow or all through the cycle. Start with 250 milligrams of calcium and 125 milligrams of magnesium. (Do not take dolomite, which contains both calcium and magnesium, as it may be contaminated with lead or arsenic.) Heat on your stomach or lower back may help. Orgasm, with or without a partner, may work. Some women use nonprescription drugs such as aspirin, acetaminophen (e.g., Tylenol), or ibuprofen. Too much aspirin can thin your blood and make your flow heavier; see the footnote for the side effects of ibuprofen. Because the uterus is a muscle, relaxation exercises help, as do massage and sometimes biofeedback techniques (see "Menstrual Massage for Two People," p. 284, and look for other massages specifically for menstrual problems in yoga, shiatsu, acupressure, and polarity therapy books).

I have incapacitating cramps with every cycle, and so around my period I reduce stress on my body and mind as much as I can. Since wearing high heels exacerbates the pressure and tension in my legs, thereby aggravating the pain, I wear low heels. I eat less salt and red meat all month long, and less caffeine around my period. I take dong quai, a Chinese herb [not to be used if you have fibroids] and when I can afford it, I take cold-pressed evening primrose oil— 4–6 per day in the week before my period, and 4 a day during my period. I do tai chi regularly because it lowers my stress level. Around my period I listen to sitar music and other kinds of music, which puts me in a relaxed state of mind and lowers my anxiety levels. When I do all these things in combination, I can bring the pain down to where I don't have to take heavy pain-killing drugs. I believe acupuncture would help me, but it's too expensive right now and my health insurance doesn't cover it.

Heavy Periods and/or Irregular Bleeding
Very heavy periods can happen if you did not ovulate (e.g., if you are in menopause), if you are under severe stress, if you are using an IUD for birth control, if you are having a miscarriage, or if you have fibroids or a tumor in your uterus. Irregular bleeding—off-schedule menstrual flow—can be caused by entering menopause, by recent sterilization surgery, or by a health problem. Because heavy periods and irregular bleeding can signal serious health problems, it's a good idea to talk with a health care provider if you experience them.

Psychotropic drugs such as Valium and Librium, or "street" drugs, can also cause menstrual irregularities.

Home Remedies for Heavy Periods and/or Irregular Bleeding. Try eating foods or taking supplements with vitamin C *and* bioflavonoids (also called vitamin P). Most foods with vitamin C also contain bioflavonoids.

If this problem starts after you have stopped taking the Pill (see chapter 13, Birth Control) try 10,000 or fewer units of vitamin A—most safely taken in the form of beta-carotene. Excessive vitamin A is toxic; if you start to feel nausea, skin irritation, itching, or other changes, discontinue using it.

Amenorrhea
Another menstrual problem is amenorrhea, the absence of menstrual periods. Primary amenorrhea is the condition of never having had a period by the latest age at which menstruation usually starts (18); secondary amenorrhea is the cessation of menstruation after at least one period. Some causes are pregnancy; menopause; breast-feeding; excessive dieting or anorexia; starvation; heavy athletic training, especially during early adolescence; previous use of birth control pills; use of some drugs; a congenital defect of the genital tract; hormone imbalance; cysts or tumors; chronic illness; chromosomal abnormalities; stress; or emotional factors. Often amenorrhea is caused by a combination of several of these factors. Because amenorrhea is a frequent symptom of infertility, medical textbooks and practitioners pay considerably more attention to it than to premenstrual problems or painful periods, although the latter two are far more common.

Home Remedies for Amenorrhea. As a home remedy to bring on your period or for unusually light periods, you might want to try pennyroyal leaf tea (don't use the oil; it can be toxic). Brew one teaspoon per cup. (Do not use pennyroyal if you are or might be pregnant and want to keep the pregnancy.) Also, a weight loss of 10 to 15% below a healthy minimum can stop your periods; a return to *your* minimum weight or more will usually correct this. If you've taken the birth control pill and have trouble getting regular menstrual cycles back, be sure to get enough calories and vitamins, and try getting somewhat less exercise. You can also try supplements of vitamin B$_6$, folic acid, and vitamin E, and decrease the amount of protein you eat. Severe anemia can stop menstruation temporarily.

Breast Tenderness, Bloated Feeling
Home Remedies. Some women find vitamin B$_6$ or pyridoxine helpful. Start with 25 to 50 milligrams a day, and try up to 100 milligrams a day. Discontinue if you get tingling or other signs of temporary nerve damage. See chapter 2, Food, p. 55, for food sources of vitamin B$_6$. Use it with a general vitamin B-complex pill for better absorption. Try to decrease sodium by eating less salt, and increase potassium (see chapter 2, Food). Some women use diuretics: plain water, water-reducing teas, foods, herbs, or drugs. Use them with caution; most diuretics except water deplete the body of potassium. Avoid caffeine to reduce breast soreness.

Tiredness or Paleness
Check your iron level for anemia.

MENSTRUAL MASSAGE FOR TWO PEOPLE

by Esther Rome

Woman with Cramps:

A. Lie flat on your stomach, with or without clothes. Place a blanket or pad under you for extra comfort.

B. Have your arms straight out or slightly bent at the elbows. Point your toes inward if possible.

C. Tell the other person what feels good and what doesn't. It should feel good.

Person Giving the Massage:

A. Basic movement:

1. Remove your shoes (or kneel and use the heel of your hand).

2. Check to see if the woman is comfortable. You might gently shake her feet or legs to help her relax and to establish physical contact.

3. Stand, placing your outer leg next to the head and above the shoulder of the woman on the floor.

4. Put the heel of your inner foot against the edge of the top ridge of her pelvis, on the same side where you are standing (see diagram).

5. "Hook" your heel as much under the bone as you can. If you are not sure where the pelvic ridge is, feel for it first with your fingers. It may be higher up on her back than you think.

6. Keep both of your legs slightly bent.

7. Gently push away from you, toward her feet, at regular intervals of once or twice a second.
   a. When doing this, rock with your whole body by bending *only* at the *knee* and *ankle* of the leg you are standing on.
   b. Move forward and back. Avoid a circular motion.
   c. When you are pushing firmly enough, the whole body of the woman getting the massage will rock, too.
   d. Try not to push toward the floor with your inner foot. Keep your toes pointing upward to prevent this.
   e. Keep your heel in contact with her pelvic bone so the woman getting the massage won't feel bruised.

8. Increase the frequency and length of the push as long as the woman with the cramps says it is comfortable. You will probably need to work more vigorously than you first imagined.

B. When you feel comfortable with the basic movement:

1. Move your heel from side to side to different spots along the ridge of her pelvis on the side you are standing next to. Avoid her spine.

2. Stand on your other leg and repeat A and B-1.

3. Change sides as often as you like. Continue with the massage until the woman's cramps diminish or go away.

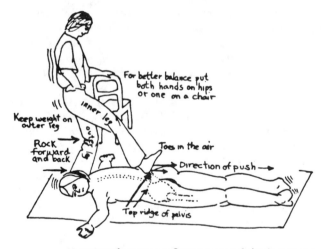

Menstrual massage for two people/Esther Rome

APPENDIX: HORMONES OF THE MENSTRUAL CYCLE SIMPLIFIED

During the reproductive part of a woman's life, baseline levels of all the sex hormones are continuously produced. In addition to those levels, there are fluctuations that establish the menstrual cycle. The main organs involved in the cycle are the *hypothalamus* (a part of the brain), the *pituitary* (also a part of the brain, located above the roof of the mouth), and the *ovaries*. (Both the pituitary and the ovaries are glands.) The hypothalamus signals the pituitary, which then signals the ovaries, which in turn signal the hypothalamus (feedback). The signaling is done by hormones secreted by the different organs and carried from one part of the body to another through the blood.

The hypothalamus and the pituitary are sensitive to the fluctuating levels of hormones produced by the ovaries. When the level of estrogens, primarily estradiol, drop to low levels, the hypothalamus increases its secretion of gonadotropin-releasing hormone (GnRH). This stimulates the pituitary to increase its secretion of follicle-stimulating hormone (FSH). FSH triggers the growth of ten to 20 of the ovarian follicles. Only one of these will mature fully; the others will be reabsorbed before ovulation. The ones that are reabsorbed are called *atretic*.

As the follicles grow they secrete estrogens in increasing amounts. The estrogens affect the lining of the uterus, signaling it to grow, or proliferate (proliferatory phase). When an egg approaches maturity inside a follicle, the follicle secretes a burst of progesterone in addition to the estrogens. The estrogens trigger the hypothalamus to increase GnRH. GnRH signals the pituitary to secrete large amounts of both FSH and luteinizing hormone (LH). The FSH-LH peak signals the follicle to release the egg (ovulation). Under the influence of LH, the follicle changes its function. Now called a *corpus luteum,* the follicle secretes estrogens and progesterone. The progesterone influences the uterine lining to secrete fluids nourishing to the egg if it is fertilized (secretory or luteal phase). Immediately after the peak that triggers ovulation, FSH returns to a baseline level. LH declines as the progesterone increases. If the egg is fertilized, the corpus luteum continues to secrete estrogens and progesterone to maintain the pregnancy. The corpus luteum is stimulated to do this by human chorionic gonadotropin (HCG), a hormone secreted by the developing placenta. HCG is almost chemically identical to LH, so it's not surprising that it has the same function.

If the egg is not fertilized, the corpus gradually stops producing hormones, paving the way for the release of the uterine lining. At this point, menstruation begins. When the level of estrogen reaches a low enough point, the hypothalamus releases GnRH and the cycle starts again.

Newly Identified Ovarian Hormones

Three recently discovered hormones—inhibin, activin, and follistatin—also help regulate the process of ovulation and may be especially important in the timing of the ovaries' normal loss of eggs, which brings on menopause. These hormones are proteins (not steroids like estrogen and progesterone). They either suppress (inhibin, follistatin) or encourage (activin) the secretion of FSH. An understanding of their function may lead to better ways to control fertility, treat infertility, and diagnose ovarian cancer.

....

NOTES
....

1. A. Cassidy, S. Bingham, and K. Setchell, "Biological effects of a diet of soy protein rich in isoflavones . . . on

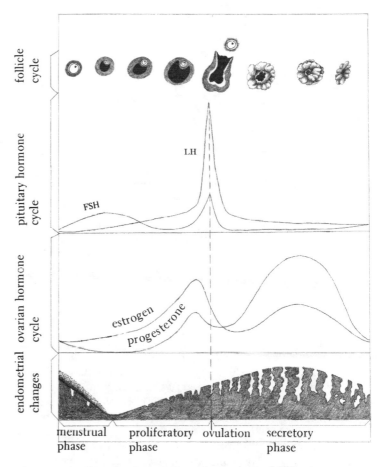

The menstrual cycle: the relationship between follicle development, hormone cycles, and endometrial (uterine lining) buildup and disintegration. The cervical mucus gets progressively wetter from the menstrual phase to ovulation, then becomes drier during the secretory phase /Peggy Clark

the menstrual cycle of premenopausal women," *American Journal of Clinical Nutrition* 60 (1994): 333–40.

2. See Philip Tierno and Bruce Hanna, "Propensity of tampons and barrier contraceptives to amplify *Staphylococcus aureus* toxic shock syndrome toxin-I," *Infectious Diseases in Obstetrics and Gynecology* 2 (1994): 140–45. Drs. Tierno and Hanna are rare examples of independent researchers, whose work is not paid for by the menstrual products companies.

3. For more information on The Keeper menstrual cap, write to The Keeper, Box 20023, Cincinnati, OH 45220.

4. "Instead" is produced by Ultrafem, Inc., 500 Fifth Avenue, Suite 3620, New York, NY; (800) 381-8138.

5. Personal discussion with Dr. Philip M. Tierno, Jr., Director, Clinical Microbiology, New York University Medical Center. See also Philip Tierno and Bruce Hanna, "Propensity of Tampons."

6. Jean Garling and Susan Jo Roberts, "An investigation of cyclic distress among staff nurses," in Alice Dan et al., eds., *The Menstrual Cycle,* vol. 1 (New York: Springer, 1980), 305–11.

7. Meir Steiner et al. "Fluoxetine in the treatment of pre-

menstrual dysphoria," *New England Journal of Medicine* 332 (1995): 1529–534.

RESOURCES

Readings

Armstrong, Liz, and Adrienne Scott. *Whitewash: Exposing the Health and Environmental Dangers of Women's Sanitary Products and Disposable Diapers.* Toronto: HarperCollins, 1992.

Ayalah, Daphna, and Isaac Weinstock. *Breasts: Women Speak About Their Breasts and Their Lives.* New York: Summit Books, 1979. Photos of breasts and women's feelings about their own.

Bell, Ruth, et al. *Changing Bodies, Changing Lives: A Book for Teens on Sex and Relationships.* New York: Vintage Books, 1987 (update due 1998). Excellent.

Blume, Judy. *Are You There, God? It's Me, Margaret.* New York: Dell, 1991 (1970). A wonderful adolescent novel with a positive attitude about menstruation.

Buckley, Thomas, and Alma Gottlieb, eds. *Blood Magic: The Anthropology of Menstruation.* Berkeley: University of California Press, 1988. Includes study of women in Borneo who use nothing to absorb blood during menstruation.

Chalker, Rebecca, and Carol Downer. *A Woman's Book of Choices: Abortion, Menstrual Extraction, RU-486.* New York: Four Walls Eight Windows, 1992.

Costello, Alison, Bernadette Vallely, and Josa Young. *The Sanitary Protection Scandal.* London: Women's Environmental Network, 1989. Environmental and health hazards of production, use, and disposal of women's sanitary products and disposable diapers.

Dalton, Katharina. *Once a Month: The Original Premenstrual Syndrome Handbook.* Alameda, CA: Hunter House, 1994. About PMS and progesterone treatment. Dalton has a dreadful attitude toward women and no interest in changing women's roles.

Dan, Alice J., and Linda L. Lewis, eds. *Menstrual Health in Women's Lives.* Urbana/Chicago: University of Illinois Press, 1992.

Delany, Janice, Mary Jane Lupton, and Emily Toth. *The Curse: A Cultural History of Menstruation.* Urbana/ Chicago: University of Illinois Press, 1988. A wide-ranging exploration of attitudes.

Federation of Feminist Women's Health Centers. *A New View of a Woman's Body.* Los Angeles: Feminist Health Press, 1991. Excellent drawings by Suzann Gage, as well as photos.

Ferrin, Michel, Raphael Jewelewicz, and Michelle Warren. *The Menstrual Cycle: Physiology, Reproductive Disorders, and Infertility.* New York: Oxford, 1993. Very accurate and well done.

Gardner-Loulan, J., B. Lopez, and M. Quackenbush. *Period.* Volcano, CA: Volcano Press, 1991. A good book for girls. Shows all kinds of body types.

Garrett, Laurie. *The Coming Plague: Newly Emerging Diseases in a World Out of Balance.* New York: Penguin, 1994. Excellent chapter on TSS.

Golub, Sharon, ed. "Lifting the curse of menstruation: A feminist appraisal of the influence of menstruation on women's lives," in *Women and Health* (special issue), 8, nos. 2 and 3 (summer/fall 1983).

———. *Periods: From Menarche to Menopause.* Newbury Park, CA: Sage, 1992. Comprehensive summary of research.

Harlow, Sioban D., and Sara A. Ephross. *What We Do and Do Not Know About the Menstrual Cycle: or, Questions Scientists Could Be Asking.* New York: Population Council, 1995. Argues for need for comprehensive program of menstrual cycle research.

Harrison, Michelle. *Self-Help for Premenstrual Syndrome.* New York: Random House, 1985.

Hubbard, Ruth. *The Politics of Women's Biology.* New Brunswick, NJ: Rutgers University Press, 1990.

Lander, Louise. *Images of Bleeding: Menstruation as Ideology.* New York: Orlando Press, 1988.

Lark, Susan. *Anemia and Heavy Menstrual Flow: A Self-Help Program.* Los Altos, CA: Westchester Publishing, 1993.

———. *Dr. Susan Lark's Chronic Fatigue Self-Help Book.* Berkeley, CA: Celestial Arts, 1995. Includes section on PMS.

———. *Dr. Susan Lark's Menstrual Cramps Self-Help Book: Effective Solutions for Pain and Discomfort Due to Menstrual Cramps and PMS.* Berkeley, CA: Celestial Arts, 1995.

Laws, Sophie. *Issues of Blood: The Politics of Menstruation.* New York: New York University Press, 1990.

Laws, Sophie, Valerie Hey, and Andrea Eagan. *Seeing Red: The Politics of Pre-Menstrual Tension.* London: Hutchison, 1985. Excellent political analysis of PMS.

Love, Susan M., and Karen Lindsay. *Dr. Susan Love's Breast Book.* Reading, MA: Addison-Wesley, 1995.

Love, Susan M., with Karen Lindsay. *Dr. Susan Love's Hormone Book: Making Informed Choices About Menopause.* New York: Random House, 1997. Hormones and menopause.

Martin, Emily. *The Woman in the Body: A Cultural Analysis of Reproduction.* Boston: Beacon Press, 1987. Excellent. How we conceptualize our body processes on the basis of our social organization.

National Women's Health Network. Packet on PMS. Order from NWHN, 514 10th Street NW, Suite 400, Washington, DC 20004; (202) 628-7814. NWHN packets are excellent and up to date.

Nissim, Rina. *Natural Healing in Gynecology: A Manual for Women.* San Francisco: HarperCollins, 1996.

Owen, Lara. *Her Blood Is Gold.* San Francisco: Harper San Francisco, 1993. Myth, tradition, and personal stories affirm the "positive power of the female cycle."

Parvati, Jeannine. *Hygieia: A Woman's Herbal.* Monroe, VT: Freestone Publishing, 1979. Dated, but it's a classic.

Rome, Esther R. "Premenstrual syndrome (PMS) examined through a feminist lens," in *Health Care for Women International,* 7, no. 1–2 (1986): 145–51.

Rome, Esther R., and Jill Wolhandler. "Can tampon

safety be regulated?" in Alice J. Dan and Linda L. Lewis, *Menstrual Health in Women's Lives*. Urbana: University of Illinois Press, 1992. 261–73.

Rome, Esther R., J. Wolhandler, J. Dieckmann, and R. P. Kahn. "Tampons: are they safe?" Boston: Boston Women's Health Book Collective, 1990. Brochure. For a copy, send a stamped, self-addressed business-sized envelope plus $1.00 to BWHBC, P.O. Box 192, W. Somerville, MA 02144. Also available in Spanish: "Tapones Vaginales."

Scambler, Annette, and Graham Scambler. *Menstrual Disorders*. New York: Routledge, 1993. Excellent on the overmedicalization of menstrual problems.

Sloane, Ethel. *Biology of Women*. Albany, NY: Delmar, 1993. Anatomy and physiology text with a feminist perspective.

Snowden, Robert, and Barbara Christian, eds. *Patterns and Perceptions of Menstruation*. New York: St. Martin's Press, 1983. Menstruation in different cultures.

Taylor, Dena. *Red Flower: Rethinking Menstruation*. Freedom, CA: Crossing Press, 1988.

Taylor, Diana, and Nancy Woods, eds. *Menstruation, Health, and Illness*. New York: Hemisphere Publishing Co., 1991.

Vines, Gail. *Raging Hormones: Do They Rule Our Lives?* Berkeley: University of California Press, 1994.

Weller, Stella. *Pain-Free Periods: Natural Ways to Overcome Menstrual Problems*. London: Thorsons, 1993.

See Resources in chapter 5, Holistic Health and Healing: Navigating Your Way to Better Health, for books on herbal remedies; in chapter 11, Sexuality, for other readings on sexuality; in chapter 23, Women Growing Older, for menopause.

Audiovisual Materials

Culpepper, Emily. *Period Piece*, a 10-minute 16-mm color film about attitudes, experiences, and images of menstruation. Available from E. E. Culpepper, Director of Women's Studies, University of Redlands, CA 92373; (714) 622-7624. E-mail: culpeppe@uor.edu

Mills, Sylvia V. *Is It PMS or Are You Really a Wreck?* and *Getting PMS Out of Your Relationships,* a set of two 1991 audiotapes on coping with PMS. Emphasizes ways to take care of yourself. Introduction mediocre, but most of the tape is empowering.

Starry Night Productions. *Under Wraps,* a 56-minute film made in 1996 that takes a candid look at menstruation from various personal, cultural, and artistic viewpoints. Covers evolution of tampons and TSS. Available

from Great North Enterprises, Suite #102, 11523-100 Avenue, Edmonton, Alberta T5K 0J8, Canada; (800) 290-5482. E-mail: gne@greatnorth.ab.ca

Organizations

Cochrane Collaboration Menstrual Disorders Group
Contact: Ms Ruth Jepson, Coordinator
Department of Obstetrics and Gynaecology, National Women's Hospital, University of Auckland; Claude Road, Epson; Auckland 3, New Zealand
E-mail: rjepson@auckland.ac.nz
(See chapter 25, The Politics of Women's Health and Medical Care, p. 710, for more information on Cochrane Collaboration.)

Mothers and Others
40 West 20th Street; New York, NY 10011; (888) ECO-INFO
E-mail: mothers@igc.apc.org
Produces an excellent newsletter that has covered the dioxin issue.

Society for Menstrual Cycle Research
c/o Alice Dan
Center for Research on Women and Gender; University of Illinois; 1640 West Roosevelt Road; Chicago, IL 60608; (312) 413-1924
Web site: http//www.wilpaterson.edu/wpcpages/icip/smcr

Women and Environments Education and Development (WEED)
736 Bathurst Street; Toronto, Ontario M5S 2R4, Canada; (416) 516-2600; Fax: (416) 531-6214
Campaigns to alert the public of the dangers of dioxin residue in menstrual products.

Additional Online Resources *

About Go Ask Alice!
http://www.columbia.edu/cu/healthwise/about.html

Information About Isadora Alman's Site
http://www.askisadora.com/Info

Teen Health Web Site
http://chebucto.ns.ca/Health/TeenHealth/index.html

Terra Femme: All-Cotton Tampon Company
http://www.biobiz.com/terrafemme/uspoltam.htm

* For more information and listings of online resources, please see Introduction to Online Women's Health Resources, p. 25.

By Susan Bell and Lauren Wise,
with Suzannah Cooper-Doyle
and Judy Norsigian

WITH SPECIAL THANKS TO
Felice Apter, Charon Asetoyer, Sara Dickey,
Anne Kelsey, Sophie Martin, Ava Moskin,
Cindy Pearson, Linda Potter, Judith Richter,
James Trussell, Kevin Whaley, and
Susan Wood*

Chapter 13

Birth Control

Birth control is fundamental to our ability to have autonomy in our lives, understand our bodies, control our health care, and enjoy our sexuality with a man. Today, most of us want contraceptives that are effective and dependable; have no harmful effects; involve no muss or fuss; protect us against sexually transmitted diseases, including HIV/AIDS; and can be used before the time of sexual intercourse. As we approach the end of a century filled with new technological wonders, it is ironic that many women view the current birth control options as far less than ideal. Many of us are dissatisfied with the choices facing us, and we still get pregnant when we don't plan to.†

Some new scientific advances have promising applications to the field of contraception. By itself, though, improved contraception is not enough. It cannot substitute for the crucial work of changing societal attitudes about birth control and sexuality, challenging the power imbalance between men and women, and ensuring that good information and a real choice of methods are available to all who want birth control. Real reproductive freedom depends on having the personal, social, and political power to choose freely whether, when, how, and with whom to have children (see introduction to Part Three, Sexual Health and Controlling Our Fertility, p. 263).

Current birth control technology has been shaped by many factors, notably the goal of population control. During much of the last part of this century, some government agencies and private organizations have attempted to develop birth control methods with the primary aim of reducing population growth.‡ Activists for social justice and women's health have long criti-

* Over the years since 1969, the following people have contributed to the many versions of this chapter: Ruth Bell, Susan Bell, Pamela Berger, Suzannah Cooper-Doyle, Jennifer S. Edwards, Charlotte Ellertson, Philip Hart, Nancy Miriam Hawley, Rachel Lanzerotti, Ken Legins, Pamela Morgan, Judy Norsigian, Barbara Perkins, Susan Reverby, Wendy Sanford, Abby Schwarz, Felicia Stewart, Alice Steinhardt, James Trussell, and Beverly Winikoff.
† The first section of the introduction is adapted from J. Norsigian, "Contraception Blues," *In These Times* 21, no. 7 (February 7, 1997): 17–19.

‡ See chapter 26, The Global Politics of Women and Health, for further discussion.

cized this "population control movement" and its precursor, eugenics (see "Sterilization," p. 331), for attempting to reduce the fertility of low-income women, women with disabilities, women of color, and women in less industrialized countries. Of particular concern has been the unsafe distribution of contraceptives, the availability of only one or two methods in many countries, and lack of adequate information about different contraceptives. Many have critiqued an undue emphasis on family planning over the provision of other primary health care services.

In the arena of contraceptive research, there have been promising developments. Partly in response to vocal women's health activists around the world, some major organizations that fund and carry out contraceptive research have taken greater care to investigate women's needs and priorities for birth control.[1] The World Health Organization, for example, has sponsored meetings that bring together diverse groups of women's health activists, advocates, and scientists. A group of women from different regions of the world, Women's Health Advocates on Microbicides (WHAM), has worked collaboratively with the Population Council on all phases of microbicide development and testing.[2] In general, there is now more emphasis on developing methods that not only prevent pregnancy but also prevent sexually transmitted diseases, infertility, and reproductive cancers.[3]

Examples of this new focus include:

- Lea's Shield, a one-size-fits-all barrier method in the final stages of clinical trials. It is shaped like a bowl, is made of silicone, and has a one-way valve that allows cervical fluid to flow out but blocks sperm from entering. Silicone is more resistant to heat, chemicals, and deterioration than is latex (used in most diaphragms, cervical caps, and most condoms for men).
- New vaginal microbicides that would not be too irritating to the vaginal lining and that women could use to prevent both pregnancy and sexually transmitted diseases (STDs), including HIV/AIDS. Noncontraceptive vaginal microbicides that would allow women to conceive and still prevent STDs are in the more distant future.
- Human monoclonal antibodies (MAbs) that would prevent both pregnancy and STDs. This type of microbicide relies on "passive immunization" (the delivery of antibodies directly to the mucus secretions in a woman's vagina). MAbs are *not* the same as the so-called antifertility "vaccines" (see p. 322), which cause a woman's immune system to produce antibodies.[4]

SOME OBSTACLES TO GETTING BIRTH CONTROL AND USING IT WELL

Birth Control and Sex Information

Negative attitudes toward pleasure and desire, and shame about sex, prevent many of us from seeking information. On a wider scale, these same attitudes serve to keep sex information from being distributed freely in schools and community organizations. Laws, medical practices, and public school policies still prevent us from getting the information and services we need, especially when we are young—in spite of many recent studies showing clearly that giving birth control information to teenagers does not make them more likely to have sex.

In the 1960s and 1970s, some legislatures and school boards reversed restrictive laws, and parents, teachers, and community people started good sex education programs in several U.S. school systems. More recently, groups such as the Moral Majority and Christian Coalition, supported by the policies of conservative federal and state governments, have attempted to reinstate the old restrictive laws or pass new ones and to stop existing sex education programs.

Birth Control— Who Protects Our Interests?

Women usually assume that when a birth control method is available through a doctor's office, medical clinic, or drugstore, its safety and efficacy have been proved. In the U.S., the Food and Drug Administration (FDA) regulates contraceptive devices and substances, deciding which ones are still experimental and which are legal to prescribe and sell. *All* birth control methods must be tested first on animals and then on women before the FDA approves them for marketing. Often, drug companies test new methods on women in Third World countries, or on low-income women and women of color in the U.S. When the effectiveness and safety of the method satisfy federal requirements, the FDA approves it for general distribution and marketing.

However, the recent history of women's contraceptives has shown that long-term complications and negative effects are rarely thoroughly understood when methods are approved. FDA requirements take up to ten years of work before a drug is marketed, but it takes 20 years or more for some complications to become apparent.

When we seek trustworthy advice about birth control in order to make careful choices, we find conflicting information and false reassurances. Some of us are prevented from gaining access to birth control; others are obliged to choose birth control without enough useful information. According to a WHO survey, different international agencies publish guidelines with inconsistent recommendations, and from one country to another, information given to physicians about a method's safety and effectiveness may be contradictory. As a result, "women seeking contraceptive services in many countries may be subjected to unnecessary tests, asked to return for follow-up more frequently than is appropriate, or told it is not safe for them to use a method when it would be safe."[5] Much of the available information about contraceptives comes from the drug companies that make them, and is biased accordingly. Health care providers may be influenced by drug company literature and sales personnel. Furthermore, physicians often recommend their own favorite method, which may not be the best one for us. And it is alarming that many physicians tend to recommend whatever methods they have available at the time of our visit.

A number of other factors can undermine our choices, including substandard health services and, in some countries, the need to obtain a husband's consent before we can get birth control. Thus, many of us find ourselves using inadequate or downright dangerous methods. Some of us, unwilling to go through the hassle, end up using nothing at all. A method that sits in a drawer or that isn't used properly won't be effective no matter how technically sophisticated it is.

Men and Birth Control

Most women and men assume that the responsibility for birth control should fall on women. One reason is that women have more at stake in preventing pregnancy than men do, for we bear the children and, in most cultures, are primarily responsible for raising them.

Placing *total* responsibility for birth control on women is inappropriate and unfair. It usually means that we must make arrangements to see a practitioner for an exam and a prescription, go to the drugstore, pay for supplies, and make sure they don't run out. With the Pill or IUD, we feel the effects and, more seriously, take whatever risks are involved. If we don't have some kind of birth control and a man presses us to have intercourse, we need to say no and make him accept our refusal. If we become pregnant, it is said to be our fault. Total responsibility often creates anger and resentment that can't help getting in the way of our sexual pleasure.

Many of us do not talk much about birth control with our partners. We may have sex with someone we've just met or don't know very well and find it difficult to bring up the subject, or we may be in a relationship in which communication is generally a problem. Yet, a man can share the responsibility of birth control in several ways. When no good method is available at the moment, a supportive partner will join us in exploring ways of lovemaking without intercourse.* He can use condoms and not just when we remind him to, help pay the doctor and drugstore bills,

* There are many ways to have sex with a man, but this chapter is about how to prevent pregnancy when sex includes vagina-to-penis contact and intercourse.

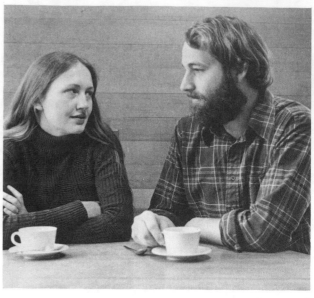

Page Bond

remind us to take the Pill each day, help to put in the diaphragm or insert the foam, check to see if supplies are running low. He can have a vasectomy, if we have a long-term relationship in which no children, or no more, are wanted. A man who truly shares responsibility for preventing pregnancy may gain our respect. We feel better about our relationship and use birth control better, as well.

Women and Birth Control

The increased availability and effectiveness of birth control methods can encourage friends, husbands, lovers to pressure us to have intercourse whenever they want to. We need to be assertive about *our* desires. Being protected from pregnancy does not always mean we want intercourse.

Many of us have found that we ourselves resist using birth control. Sometimes this is because of social and political factors such as poor sex education, a double standard concerning sex, or inequalities between women and men. For instance:

- We are embarrassed by, ashamed of, or confused about our own sexuality.
- We cannot admit we might have or are having intercourse, because we feel (or someone told us) it is wrong.
- We are unrealistically romantic about sex: Sex has to be passionate and spontaneous, and birth control seems too premeditated, clinical, and messy.
- We hesitate to "inconvenience" our partner. This fear of displeasing him is a measure of the inequality and our lack of control in our relationship.
- We feel, "It can't happen to me. I won't get pregnant."

- We hesitate to find a health care practitioner, who may turn out to be hurried, impersonal, or even hostile. If we are young or unmarried, we may fear moralizing and disapproval. We may be afraid the practitioner will tell our parents.
- We don't recognize our deep dissatisfaction with the method we are using, but we begin to use it haphazardly.
- We feel tempted to become pregnant just to prove to ourselves that we are fertile or to try to improve a shaky relationship, or we want a baby so that we will have someone to care for.

What Can We Do?

Each of us will have different opportunities for action, depending on where we live, how old we are, what resources are available to us, and how much political power we have. But all of us can learn for ourselves and teach one another about the available methods. By speaking openly and by carefully comparing experiences and knowledge, we can guide one another to workable methods and good practitioners. We can recognize when a practitioner is not thorough enough in examinations or explanations and encourage one another to ask for the attention we need. By talking together we can also get a better handle on our more subtle resistances to using birth control. We can begin the long but worthwhile process of talking with our male partners about birth control, encouraging them to share the responsibility with us. We can join together across state and national boundaries to insist that legislatures, courts, high schools, churches, parents, doctors, research projects, clinics, and drug companies change their practices and attitudes so that we can enjoy our sexuality without becoming pregnant. We can create self-help clinics and other alternative health care institutions where our needs for information, discussion, and personal support in the difficult choice of birth control will be better met. We can use the good clinics that do exist. We can campaign for decent housing, jobs, and child care for all, so that we can choose birth control freely instead of being forced to use it by our circumstances. We can insist that birth control methods meet the needs of all women, including women of color, women living in poverty, women with disabilities, and women in developing countries. Whatever we choose to do, we can act together.

HOW PREGNANCY HAPPENS *

Pregnancy depends on a healthy egg, healthy sperm, and favorable cervical fluid. For birth control to work, the process of conception must be stopped at some point along the way (see illustration on p. 292).

During sexual intercourse, sperm are ejaculated through the man's penis into the woman's vagina. In the presence of certain cervical fluid conditions, some of the sperm move, guided by the cervical fluid through the cervical opening (os), through the woman's uterus, and into the fallopian tubes. If the sperm encounter an egg in the outer third of the fallopian tube, one may join with the egg. The process of an egg and a sperm uniting is called *conception,* or *fertilization.* The fertilized egg takes several days to travel down the fallopian tube to the uterus, where, after one and a half to two days, it implants in the uterine lining and develops over the course of the next nine months.

It is also possible for sperm to be deposited in or near the lips around the vagina during ejaculation, even without intercourse. If fertile cervical fluid is present, sperm can move into the vagina and follow the same route to join with the egg. (This is even possible if the woman has an intact hymen or has never had intercourse!)

The egg leaves the ovary *(ovulation) approximately two weeks before the beginning of the next menstrual period.*† It can be fertilized for only about 12 to 24 hours. A woman can become pregnant from intercourse up to five days before ovulation if favorable cervical fluid is present. Although it is unusual, conception can happen after a woman has intercourse during her period if the cervical fluid begins during her menstrual flow, especially if she has an occasional short cycle.

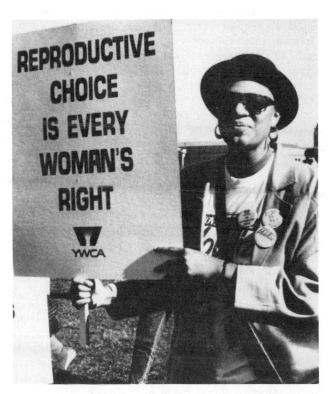

Ellen Shub

---

* See chapter 12, Understanding Our Bodies: Sexual Anatomy, Reproduction, and the Menstrual Cycle, for more details.

† A common misunderstanding is that the egg leaves the ovary at midcycle, halfway between menstrual periods. This is true only when the cycle is 28 days long—something that cannot be known for certain until that particular cycle is over and menstruation begins.

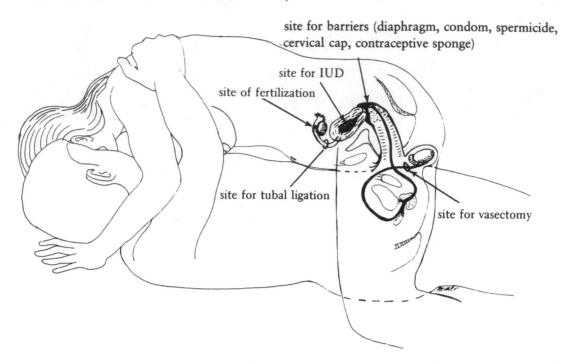

site for barriers (diaphragm, condom, spermicide, cervical cap, contraceptive sponge)

site for IUD

site of fertilization

site for tubal ligation

site for vasectomy

Nina Reimer

The Sperm

Sperm are made in the man's testicles ("balls"). Sexual stimulation makes blood flow into erectile tissue inside the penis, causing the penis to become stiff, hard, and erect. (The drops of liquid that come from the penis soon after erection probably do not contain sperm, although many people still think they do.) If stimulation is continued, the man usually has an orgasm. As orgasm begins, sperm travel up the sperm ducts, over the bladder, and through the prostate gland into the urethra and then are propelled out of the urethra by rhythmic contractions, which are very pleasurable to a man. This is called *ejaculation*.

About 300 million to 500 million sperm come out in one ejaculation. This large number is needed to ensure conception; even under favorable conditions, only about 200 sperm actually reach the egg.

Sperm move quickly and, depending on the cervical fluid, may reach an egg in as little as 30 minutes. Sperm cannot survive unaided in the acid environment of the vagina. Without cervical fluid to nourish and protect them, sperm die in half an hour to four hours. As soon as cervical fluid appears (during or after menstruation), sperm can survive in a woman's body for three to five days.

CHOOSING A BIRTH CONTROL METHOD

Because there is no one perfect method, our "choice" of a contraceptive will be something of a compromise. Safety and effectiveness are probably the most important factors. Convenience is also important to some. Those of us with medical problems, chronic illnesses, or disabilities may have additional needs to consider when seeking usable, effective contraceptives. Those of us who are healthy and fertile when we begin using birth control want to stay that way.

The table on p. 293 compares the risk of death associated with different birth control methods, pregnancy, and abortion. Be aware that this table does not take into account other factors such as social class, race, nationality, and pregnancy history. Birth control methods differ in how much protection they give against STDs (e.g., gonorrhea, herpes, chlamydia, and HIV) and pelvic inflammatory disease (PID). In general, barrier methods, especially condoms, provide good protection against most reproductive tract infections. *Note that inconsistent or incorrect use reduces the protection given by barrier methods.* The Pill provides some protection against PID; it may increase the risk of chlamydia. Its effect on STDs remains uncertain. The IUD offers no protection against STDs. For women at risk for STDs, use of the IUD increases the chance of developing PID. (See chapters 14, Sexually Transmitted Diseases, and 24, Selected Medical Practices, Problems, and Procedures, for more information on STDs and PID.)

When looking at *effectiveness* statistics in books and magazines, keep in mind that there is a difference between the *lowest expected failure rate*, which is based on consistent and correct use of the method, and the higher *typical failure rate*, based on records of actual use of the method over time. Typical user failure rates include accidents such as forgetting a pill, failing to put on the condom early enough, and removing the diaphragm within six hours after intercourse. The typical failure rate will give you a more realistic idea of how effective the method is and will invite you to

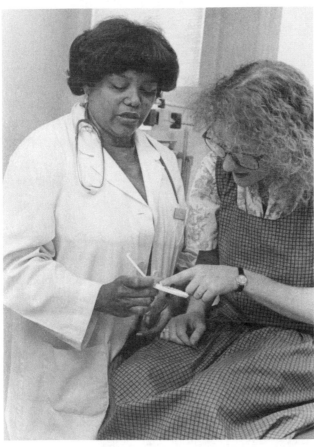

Gale Zucker/Stock, Boston

If you think your method of birth control is making you sick, go to a clinic or health practitioner. If the clinic or practitioner doesn't give you an adequate answer, get a second opinion. Stop using that method, and be sure to use another one to avoid pregnancy.

place them first. Most of us who use or have used birth control chose a diaphragm, cervical cap, or foam and condom, because they effectively prevent pregnancy, are safe, and offer some protection against STDs and PID (see chapter 14, Sexually Transmitted Diseases, p. 344). The safest way to control our fertility is to use barrier methods of contraception, with abortion as a backup in case of failure. If abortion is an unacceptable option for moral or religious reasons, then the overall safety of these methods—which are, in actual practice, less effective than hormonal contraceptives (Pill, Norplant, Depo-Provera) and the IUD—

consider the crucial question of how effectively *you and your partner* will use it. Recently, researchers have carefully reviewed studies of birth control effectiveness, and as a result of their reviews, they have revised their estimates of both lowest expected and typical rates of failure.[6]

The table on p. 294 gives the lowest and typical expected rates. A 5% pregnancy rate, or failure rate, means that studies in the past have shown that five women out of every hundred using that particular method have become pregnant during the first year of using it. By contrast, heterosexually active women using no method at all have an 85% pregnancy rate. Note that this table does not differentiate among groups of women on the basis of age, social class, and race. However, there are differences among these groups. Older women, for example, are more likely than younger women to use spermicides correctly and consistently and less likely than younger women to conceive if they do not use a method of birth control. Thus, the typical failure rate of spermicides is lower for older women than for younger women, and lower than the percentage reported in the table. Also, after the first year the failure rates for most methods are likely to be lower, since women who conceive in the first year are no longer included in the statistical calculations.

The primary authors of this book favor certain methods of contraception over others and have chosen to

RISK OF DEATH ASSOCIATED WITH BIRTH CONTROL METHODS, PREGNANCY, AND ABORTION

	Chance of Death in a Year
Birth control pills (nonsmoker)	1 in 66,700
Birth control pills (heavy smoker, 25 or more cigarettes per day)*	1 in 1,700
IUDs	1 in 10,000,000
Barrier methods	none
Natural methods	none
Sterilization:	
Laparoscopic tubal ligation	1 in 38,500
Hysterectomy	1 in 1,600
Vasectomy	1 in 1,000,000
Pregnancy:	
Terminating pregnancy:	
Illegal abortion	1 in 3,000
Legal abortion:	
Before 9 weeks	1 in 262,800
Between 9 and 12 weeks	1 in 100,100
Between 13 and 15 weeks	1 in 34,400
After 15 weeks	1 in 10,200
Risk per pregnancy from continuing pregnancy	1 in 10,000

* See chapter 3, Alcohol, Tobacco, and Other Mood-Altering Drugs, for other dangers of smoking.

Source: This table was adapted from R. Hatcher et al., *Contraceptive Technology,* 17th rev. ed. (New York: Irvington, 1998), Table 9-4. (The figure for the risk of illegal abortion is from R. Hatcher et al., *Contraceptive Technology,* 16th rev. ed. (New York: Irvington, 1990), 125.

LOWEST EXPECTED AND TYPICAL FAILURE RATES DURING THE FIRST YEAR OF USE OF STERILIZATION AND REVERSIBLE BIRTH CONTROL METHODS IN THE UNITED STATES

Method	Percentage of women experiencing an accidental pregnancy in the first year of use	
	Lowest expected *	Typical †
Chance ‡	85	85
Spermicides§	6	26
Periodic abstinence		25
Calendar	9	
Ovulation method	3	
Symptothermal″	2	
Postovulation	1	
Withdrawal	4	19
Cap		
Parous women +	26	40
Nulliparous women ++	9	20
Sponge		
Parous women +	20	40
Nulliparous women ++	9	20
Diaphragm	6	20
Condom—Female (Reality)	5	21
Male	3	14
IUD		
Progesterone T	1.5	2.0
Copper T 380A	0.6	0.8
Lng 20	0.1	0.1
Pill		
Combined	0.1	
Progestogen only	0.5	
Injectable progestogen		
DMPA (Depo-Provera)	0.3	0.3
Norplant and Norplant-2	0.05	0.05
Female sterilization	0.5	0.5
Male sterilization	0.1	0.15

* Among couples who initiate use of a method (not necessarily for the first time) and who use it perfectly (both consistently and correctly), this is the percentage expected to experience an accidental pregnancy during the first year if they do not stop use for any other reason.

† Among typical couples who initiate use of a method (not necessarily for the first time), this is the percentage who experience an accidental pregnancy during the first year if they do not stop use for any other reason.

‡ The lowest expected and typical percents are based on data from populations where contraception is not practiced and from women who cease practicing contraception in order to become pregnant. Among these populations, about 89% become pregnant within one year. This estimate is lowered slightly (to 85%)

in the table to represent the percent who would conceive among women now relying on reversible methods of contraception if they stopped using contraception altogether.

§ Foams, creams, gels, vaginal film, and vaginal suppositories.

″ Cervical mucus (ovulation) method supplemented by calendar in the preovulatory and basal body temperature in the postovulatory phases. With spermicidal cream or jelly. Without spermicides.

+ Parous: women who have given birth.

++ Nulliparous: women who have never given birth.

Source: This table is reprinted and adapted with the permission of James Trussell, from Table 31-1, Contraceptive Efficacy, in R. Hatcher et al., *Contraceptive Technology,* 17th rev. ed. (New York: Irvington, 1998).

is reduced by whatever risks pregnancy and childbirth might bring. Obviously, health problems associated with pregnancy and childbirth vary greatly among women and depend upon overall health status, access to appropriate care before and after birth, and social factors such as income and education. We believe that far greater use of barrier methods should be encouraged because they offer protection against STDs and, in the case of condoms, HIV. We must try to change the attitudes and prejudices that have kept us from using these methods in the past. Even when women choose the IUD or hormonal methods, barrier methods are important "companions" that help prevent STDs.

As you read, you will, of course, form your own opinions and make your choices. If you stop using one method, and you don't want to get pregnant, use another method.

THE DIAPHRAGM AND SPERMICIDAL CREAM OR JELLY

Before the diaphragm was invented in the 19th century, women had to depend on men (using condoms and withdrawal) to prevent pregnancy, and on crude abortion and infanticide for backup. The diaphragm was a major breakthrough, giving women responsibility over birth control and freeing us from unwanted pregnancies. It was popular until the 1960s—at one time, a third of all U.S. couples practicing birth control used it. By 1971, however, Planned Parenthood reported that only 4% of its clients were choosing diaphragms. What had happened?

In the late 1950s and 1960s, the drug industry, the medical profession, private foundations, and the U.S. government began to pour money into researching, developing, and distributing the Pill and the IUD, virtually excluding any research on the diaphragm and other barrier methods. Usually, these interests were more concerned with developing new technologies and/or making profits than with the health and well-being of women. Many of us believed the drug industry's and physicians' proclamations about Pill and IUD

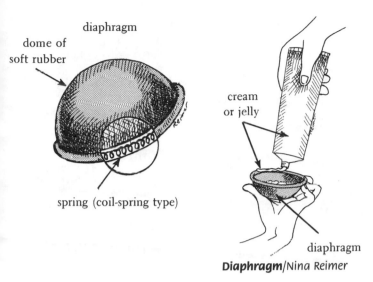

diaphragm

dome of soft rubber

spring (coil-spring type)

cream or jelly

diaphragm

Diaphragm/Nina Reimer

safety and hoped that the Pill and IUD would allow us more sexual spontaneity and protection against pregnancy than diaphragms.

Over the past 25 years, we have learned that diaphragms, correctly fitted and worn, prevent pregnancy, protect us against some STDs, and are safer than the Pill or IUD. Yet, there are still obstacles to diaphragm use. Only a practitioner can legally prescribe it. Some practitioners, especially physicians, do not include time for fittings in their schedules and often charge high fees for their services. A practitioner's attitudes about sexuality can affect her or his attitudes about certain methods of birth control and affect ours in turn. Many practitioners don't trust our ability to use a barrier method well; they frequently assume that IUDs or pills are better and that we wouldn't want to "mess" with the diaphragm. In 1995, less than 2% of U.S. women used diaphragms, and most of these were women over the age of 30.

Description

A diaphragm, which must always be used with spermicidal cream or jelly, is made of soft rubber in the shape of a shallow cup (see illustration). It has a flexible metal spring rim (arcing, coiled, or flat). When properly fitted and inserted, it fits snugly over your cervix, sitting in place behind the pubic bone and reaching back behind your cervix. It comes in a variety of sizes measured in millimeters, ranging from 50 to 95 millimeters, or 2 to 4 inches, depending on the size of your upper vagina.

How It Works

When the diaphragm is in place, holding spermicidal jelly or cream up to your cervix, the sperm cannot go into your cervical canal. Sperm may move around the rim of the diaphragm and be killed by the cream or jelly. Some women also smear jelly on the

outside of the diaphragm to help kill sperm remaining in the vagina. Always use a diaphragm with cream or jelly: *They* are the important contraceptives; the diaphragm exists mainly to hold them in the proper place.

Effectiveness

The diaphragm can have a failure rate as low as 6% if it is fitted properly, its use is carefully taught, and it is used correctly and consistently. Most likely, the 6% failure rate exists because the upper vagina can expand during intercourse, causing the diaphragm to move around a bit with frequent insertions of the penis. Also, there is a possibility that the diaphragm may move when the woman is on top during intercourse. The typical failure rate is higher: about 20%.

You can combine the use of the diaphragm with fertility observation (see p. 305). You can achieve almost 100% effectiveness with the diaphragm if your partner also uses a condom on your fertile days.

Reversibility

The diaphragm doesn't affect your fertility at all. Simply don't use it if you want to become pregnant.

Safety and Possible Problems

The diaphragm is almost completely safe. It cannot slide up inside us and disappear (as some of us may fear), because the vagina stops about an inch beyond the cervix. A particular cream or jelly may irritate your vagina or your partner's penis. Try a different brand if this happens. The diaphragm itself might push forward and cause cramps in your uterus, bladder, or urethra. For some women, this can lead to urethritis or recurrent cystitis. The diaphragm could also push backward on your rectum, which can be uncomfortable, too. If

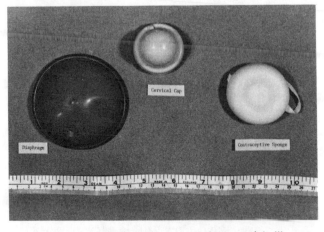

Diaphragm, cap, and sponge/Phyllis Ewen

this happens to you, it may mean that the diaphragm is the wrong size. Try out different types of diaphragms as well to see whether one is less uncomfortable than another. Inability to feel movement of the diaphragm during intercourse (because of paralysis, for example) might increase the failure rate for some women.

Some women get recurrent yeast infections when using the diaphragm, which you can avoid by making sure that you wash and dry your diaphragm thoroughly between uses. (For possible negative effects of jellies and creams, see p. 303.)

Who Shouldn't Use the Diaphragm

If you have a severely displaced uterus (severe prolapse, for instance), you cannot use a diaphragm. If you have curvature of the spine (scoliosis) or an incompletely formed spinal cord (spina bifida), you may not be able to use the diaphragm. Because diaphragms require manual dexterity, women with some kinds of physical disabilities might not be able to use them effectively without assistance from their partners. Women with chronic urinary tract infections or a history of toxic shock syndrome probably should not use the diaphragm.

If you don't feel comfortable touching your genitals and do not think you can get used to it, you will most likely have trouble using a diaphragm effectively. You may feel very squeamish and embarrassed the first time you put your finger into your vagina, but as you get used to it and realize that your body is yours to touch, you should get over any uneasiness about inserting the diaphragm. Starting or joining a self-help group may help you to discuss negative feelings about touching yourself.

How to Get the Diaphragm

The size of diaphragm you should use depends on the size and contour of your vagina and the muscle strength of the surrounding vaginal walls. In the U.S. it is usually a doctor, nurse practitioner, or other women's health care provider who measures (or fits) you for a diaphragm. The person fitting the diaphragm can choose one of the three kinds of metal spring rim (arcing, coiled, or flat) to fit your particular anatomy. If one kind doesn't fit, try another kind. Women who have a bladder that protrudes through the vaginal wall (cystocele) and/or a weakening in the wall of the rectum (rectocele), or less muscle strength in the vagina should try using a diaphragm with an arcing spring. These conditions are more likely to occur after childbirth or in midlife.

Very important: When you have been measured and fitted, practice putting the diaphragm in and taking it out before you leave the practitioner's office, so she or he can tell you whether you are doing it right. (Or go home, practice, and come back in a few days with the diaphragm in place.) Reach in and see what it feels like when it is in correctly, and get help immediately if you have problems, so that when you actually use it you won't be experimenting. Many practitioners neglect this important step.

The practitioner will have the diaphragm available right there or will give you a prescription for the proper size.

How to Use the Diaphragm

Like any tool, the diaphragm is simple to use once you've practiced with it. Putting it in and taking it out might feel awkward at first, but it will become easier and quicker every time. You must put the diaphragm in *within six hours** before intercourse or vagina-to-penis contact, because the creams and jellies may start to lose their spermicidal potency in the body after that time. The most conservative estimates say to put it in as close to intercourse as possible, but if you tend to get carried away with sexual intensity, it's probably best to insert the diaphragm in advance.

Preparation and Insertion

Put 1 teaspoonful to 1 tablespoonful of cream or jelly (3/4 inch from the tube) into the shallow cup (see illustration on p. 295). Spread the cream around. (Some books say to put the cream on the rim also; others say that cream on the rim makes the diaphragm slip. An effective compromise might be to put cream around the inside of the rim and not on top of the rim.) Then squeeze the cup together by pressing the rim firmly between your thumb and third finger. If you have trouble, you can buy a plastic inserter (good only with a flat-spring diaphragm). You can squat, sit on the toilet bowl, stand with one foot raised, or lie down with your legs bent. With your free hand, spread apart the lips of your vagina and push the diaphragm up to the upper third of your vagina with the cream or jelly facing up. If you have not used tampons or reached into your vagina before, remember that it angles toward your back (see illustration on p. 297). Now push the lower rim with your finger until you feel the diaphragm lock into place. You should then reach in to make sure you can feel the outline of your cervix through the soft rubber cup. Partners of women with certain physical disabilities can learn to insert the diaphragm and check it for accurate placement. (For more protection, some women insert a little extra cream or jelly with an applicator when the diaphragm is in place, but this is not necessary.) When it's in right and fits properly, you should not be able to feel the diaphragm at all. Your partner probably won't either, although some men notice that the tip of the penis is touching soft rubber instead of cervical and vaginal tissue. (This is not painful.) **Never use oil-based vaginal medication (such as common vaginal hor-**

---

* For more information on diaphragm use, see Hatcher et al., *Contraceptive Technology,* in Resources.

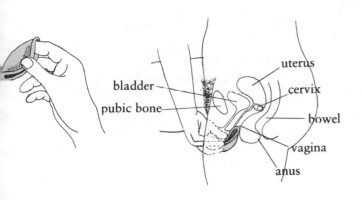

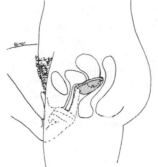

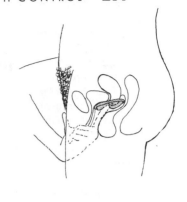

Insertion of diaphragm

Checking of diaphragm
/Nina Reimer

mones or vaginal yeast medications) or oil-based lubricant (like petroleum jelly or Vaseline) with a diaphragm, as they destroy the rubber.

Leave the diaphragm in for at least six hours after intercourse, because it takes the spermicide that long to kill all the sperm. You can leave it in for up to 24 hours, but not longer. Douching is unnecessary, but if you want to douche, you must wait six hours.

Subsequent Intercourse

If you have intercourse again, you must add more cream or jelly with an applicator. Put it into your vagina, leaving the diaphragm in place.

Removal

Remove the diaphragm by choosing a comfortable position, perhaps the same way you chose to insert it. If you have trouble reaching the diaphragm, try another position or bear down as if you were going to have a bowel movement. Slide a finger into your vagina and hook it under the lower rim of the diaphragm, either between the diaphragm and your vaginal wall or over the rubber dome. Pull the diaphragm forward and down. If you have long nails, take care not to rip the diaphragm.

Wash the diaphragm with mild soap and warm water, rinse and dry it carefully, dust it with cornstarch if you wish (but never talcum powder), and put it into a container (away from light). Don't boil it. Check it for holes every so often by holding it up to the light or filling it with water and looking for leaks, especially around the rim. If you poke the dome with your finger, it will be easier to detect possible cracks along the rim.

Life of Product

Get your diaphragm size rechecked every year or two. You may need a new size if you gain or lose more than ten pounds or have vaginal surgery and after pregnancy, abortion, or miscarriage. Diaphragms should be replaced every three years.

Cost

A diaphragm costs at least $20.* The medical examination for the diaphragm can cost from $50 to $150 depending on whether you go to a clinic or a private physician and the extent of the examination. Spermicidal jellies and creams vary in price from about $10, depending on the size of the tube. A 3.8-ounce tube contains approximately 12 applications.

Advantages

It is a good method if you have intercourse with a partner who is cooperative and helpful about using it and/or if you have intercourse relatively infrequently, because it only has to be used around the time of lovemaking. It is very effective if used well and every time. There are almost no side effects or dangers.

The diaphragm is helpful if you want to have intercourse during your period and don't want a heavy menstrual flow to interfere. Using a diaphragm can be a good kind of body education. If you are unfamiliar with what your vagina feels like, using a diaphragm will teach you. In the long run, the more familiar you are with your body, the more you will enjoy sex.

Repeated studies indicate that the diaphragm with cream or jelly reduces your chances of getting gonorrhea or trichomoniasis infections in the vaginal canal. It increases your protection against PID and cervical dysplasia and may help clear up adenosis.

Disadvantages

If either you or your partner wants sex to be uninterrupted and absolutely spontaneous, putting in the diaphragm can be a hassle if you don't put it in long before you start having sex.

You must remember to use it every time, be sure not to run out of cream or jelly, and have it with you when you need it.

* In some federally funded clinics, diaphragm kits (including diaphragm and jelly) can be had for $12 or even less.

The discharge of cream or jelly can be a nuisance, although it does not stain. Try different brands and, if necessary, use a pad or a tissue for leaking after intercourse.

Some people who enjoy oral sex find the taste of the jellies and creams unpleasant. One way around this is to wash carefully after putting in the diaphragm. Another is to put the diaphragm in after oral sex play and before intercourse. This is a definite interruption, however, and that increases the possibility that you won't put it in at all.

Some women find that they have more yeast and urinary tract infections while using a diaphragm. If urinary tract infections persist even after you have tried a different size or kind of diaphragm, you should stop using this method of birth control.

Responsibility

After you have been are fitted, you and your partner can share the responsibility of insertion, although a lot of women do the whole process themselves.

THE FEMALE CONDOM

Description

In 1993, the FDA approved the first condom for women—called Reality in the U.S. and Femidom in other countries (see illustration at right)—as an over-the-counter, nonprescription barrier contraceptive that also protects against STDs. The female condom consists of a soft, loose-fitting polyurethane sheath, which is closed at one end (this part covers the opening of the cervix). One flexible polyurethane ring is located at either end of the device, one at the closed end and one at the open end at the external edge (this remains just outside the vagina after insertion). When in place, the sheath lines the vaginal wall, creating a covered passageway for the penis. The ring at the closed end is inserted into the vagina, like a diaphragm. It then acts as an anchor inside the vagina, holding the sheath in place. The ring outside the vagina adds to the protective effects of the female condom by creating a barrier between the labia and the base of the penis and by keeping the female condom in place during intercourse. Like the male condom, it is intended for one-time use. The female condom does not contain spermicide and is prelubricated. It does not require precise placement over the cervix.

Effectiveness

The Reality female condom was designed to protect women against both pregnancy and STDs. As a contraceptive, it has a failure rate of about 5% when used consistently and correctly, similarly to the diaphragm and cervical cap. Typically, its failure rate is 21%. Consistent and correct use of the female condom gives more protection against STDs, including HIV infection, than either the diaphragm or the cap.

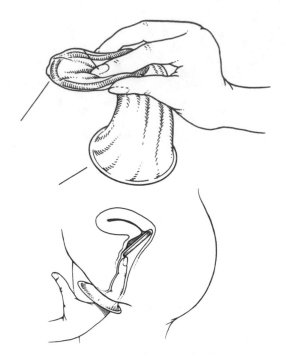

Insertion of Reality Female Condom

Reversibility

Perfectly reversible. To get pregnant, just don't use it.

How to Use the Female Condom

Insert the condom before any vagina-to-penis contact. Squeeze the inner ring and insert the female condom into your vagina just past the pubic bone, so that the inner ring covers your cervix. Check with your finger to make sure that the sheath is not twisted, so that it will be easy for the penis to enter into the vagina (see illustration above).

Advantages

Economic realities, violence, and power imbalances in sexual relationships make it difficult for women to ask men to use male condoms. However, when a woman can offer her partner a choice between using his or hers, the gender dynamics can change. The Reality female condom offers women protection against both pregnancy and STDs. In an era during which HIV infection among women is on the rise, this protection—although not 100% effective—is especially valuable.

Because it can be inserted up to eight hours before intercourse, it does not interrupt the flow of lovemaking in the way that the male condom can. A man doesn't need to have a fully erect penis when a woman uses the female condom. In addition, for men who are willing to use a male condom but find it difficult to keep an erection while putting one on, the female condom helps avoid what can be an awkward moment during lovemaking that includes intercourse. Also, maintaining an erection is not necessary for removal of the female condom.

The polyurethane lining in the female condom is stronger than the latex membrane used in most male condoms. It is soft and thin and more resistant to oils. Last, as an over-the-counter product, the female condom does not require a visit to a clinic or practitioner's office. It is, however, not available in many communities.

Disadvantages

The female condom is significantly more expensive than male condoms. Some women may find the female condom messy or inconvenient. It can make a "farting" noise. Men are usually aware of the outside ring, and you may have a problem if your partner objects to it. Using it requires his cooperation, which implies being able to talk and negotiate with your partner. This may not always be possible.

As with other female barrier methods, to use the female condom we do have to be comfortable touching our genital area, although a little practice is usually all we need to overcome any awkward feelings.

How to Get Female Condoms

You can find female condoms in drugstores and at family planning agencies. They are made in a standard size and can be purchased in packages of three for under $10 a package.

THE MALE CONDOM
(RUBBER, PROPHYLACTIC, OR SAFE)

With the exception of withdrawal, the condom is the only temporary means of birth control a man can use. It is also the only barrier method whose protection from HIV transmission during vaginal and anal intercourse has been documented. Because it can be purchased over the counter or found on a drugstore shelf, or even purchased by mail, men don't need to visit a medical facility to obtain a prescription. Furthermore, women can also easily buy and carry condoms. It should not be surprising, therefore, to find that the condom is the most frequently used barrier method in the U.S.

The condom, like all other methods, fell into disfavor when the Pill and the IUD appeared. Men could share in the spontaneity and relative sexual freedom brought about by the Pill and IUD without having to experience their negative effects. Today, the condom is viewed much more favorably, and the development and use of condoms have increased because people have learned more about heterosexual transmission of AIDS and other STDs.[7]

Egyptian men wore condoms in 1350 B.C. as decorative covers for their penises. The condom was popularized for protection against conception in the 18th

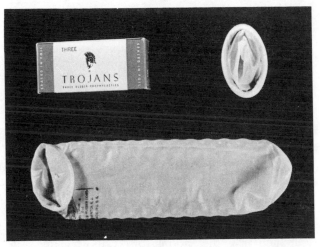

Condoms/Elizabeth Shapiro

century. It is a sheath, usually made of thin, strong latex rubber, designed to fit over an erect penis to keep semen from getting into the woman's vagina. A condom is usually about 7 or 8 inches long and 2 inches wide; it is usually rolled up before packaging. The open end has a rubber ring around it to help keep it on the penis, and the closed end is either plain or tipped with a little nipple to catch the semen and help to keep the condom from bursting. Plastic (polyurethane) condoms (sold under the brand name Avanti), which also protect against STDs, can be used by people allergic to rubber. Because "skin" condoms (made of lamb membrane) contain pores (microscopic holes) that let viruses pass through in laboratory studies, they are not recommended for protection against STDs. Now that more research attention is being given to condoms, there have been a few innovations in condom design. There are more than a hundred brands of condom in different sizes, shapes, thicknesses, colors, and scents, with or without spermicide or lubrication.

Effectiveness

A good-quality condom has a failure rate of about 3% when used as directed, but typically its failure rate is about 14%. Some condoms ("spermicidal condoms" or "spermicidally lubricated condoms") already contain spermicide. The concentration of spermicide in them is so low that they appear to be no more effective than condoms that don't contain spermicide. We suggest combining condoms with a spermicidal foam, cream, or jelly in your vagina for close to 100% protection if the condom is used correctly at every act of intercourse. Used with a diaphragm or cervical cap, condoms provide extra protection at ovulation.

Reversibility

Perfectly reversible. To get pregnant, just don't use condoms.

How to Use the Condom

The man or woman unrolls the condom onto the erect penis *before* any vagina-to-penis contact or intercourse. Long before ejaculation the male may discharge a few drops of fluid. This preejaculatory fluid is unlikely to contain sperm, but it probably can transmit HIV.

Cautions

Leave space at the end of the plain-ended condom for the semen: ½ inch of air-free space between the end of the penis and the condom will keep the ejaculate, which comes out fast, from bursting the condom. Catching air in the end may also cause bursting. After putting on the condom, check thoroughly for holes or tears, especially in the tip.

Lubricated rubber condoms minimize the risk of tearing but tend to slip off the penis more easily and have to be used extra carefully. Condoms that are preshaped or contoured may increase sensitivity for some men; they may also be less likely to slip. Some men and women have reported that the dyes in colored condoms stain and cause burning and irritation. Scented condoms may be irritating as well.

If you do not use a lubricated condom, use a water-based lubricant to prevent tearing—spermicidal foam, cream, or jelly or K-Y Jelly, but *never Vaseline* or other oil-based lubricants such as massage oils, suntan lotion, hand cream, or baby oil, which can corrode the rubber. Saliva is always available but may increase your chances of developing a monilial (yeast) infection. Apply the lubricant after the condom is on the penis.

One of you must hold the rim when you move away from him or he withdraws his no-longer-erect penis after ejaculation; otherwise the condom might slip off and sperm could get into the vagina.

In case of accident, insert cream or jelly or foam into your vagina as quickly as possible. Do not douche. You may want to consider using emergency contraception (see "Emergency Contraception After Unprotected Intercourse," p. 324).

Responsibility

The man uses the condom. It is much more enjoyable to use it if both partners join in putting it on. For a couple having intercourse more than a few times, condoms are a good way for the man to share in birth control. In a shorter-term relationship, when you may not know whether you'll be having intercourse or not, condoms can be very convenient. But don't expect the man to have a condom in his pocket—you may be disappointed. If you don't know him well enough to be sure he'll have a condom, it makes sense for you to have some with you. But it is hard for many of us to pull out a rubber and suggest that the man use it.

Advantages

It is fairly cheap, readily available, and easy to use. It is a method of birth control that gives good protection against some STDs (chlamydia, herpes, gonorrhea, hepatitis B virus, genital ulcers, PID, and HIV) when used in every instance of vagina-to-penis contact. It also prevents partners from reinfecting each other with an STD, such as trichomoniasis, during the treatment period.

If the man tends to ejaculate too quickly, a condom may decrease the stimulation of his penis enough to help him delay ejaculation and prolong intercourse. A condom catches the semen, so if the woman wants to go somewhere right after intercourse, she won't feel drippy.

It reassures some women to have this immediate, visible proof of protection against pregnancy and STDs.

You don't need a doctor's prescription to buy a condom.

Disadvantages

You have to use the condom right at the time of intercourse, which ruins the spontaneity of sex for some couples unless the woman puts it on the man and makes it a part of sex play.

It may lessen the man's sensation, as his penis doesn't touch the vaginal walls directly. Many men resist using condoms for this reason, forgetting the effects that women's birth control methods can have on a woman's enjoyment of sex. Some men say they do not feel such a great reduction in sensation.

The condom eliminates one source of lubrication for intercourse (the drops of fluid that come out when the man gets an erection), and the resultant friction can irritate a woman, especially during the entrance of the penis into her vagina. If this happens, use a water-based lubricant or a lubricated condom, preferably lubricated with a spermicide.

How to Get Condoms

You can find condoms in drugstores, at family planning agencies, in vending machines, and on many college campuses. There are different sizes of condoms (typically, condoms are 7 inches long, and the longest condoms are 8 inches) and they are sold in packages of 6, 12 or 36. "Large" condoms are usually about 8 inches long and a bit wider than other condoms. The cost varies, depending on the brand and the store, so shop around. Prices range from $4 to $11 for a package of six and from $13 to $22 dollars for a package of 36. Some high-quality latex condoms are sold under the brand names Ramses and Trojans.

Life of Product

Condoms have a shelf life of five years if they are kept dry, sealed, and away from heat, sunlight, and fluorescent light. Look for an expiration date on the package. Sometimes there is a date that isn't identified as an expiration date; in that case you can assume it is the date of manufacture. The tip (closed end) of a packaged condom generally deteriorates fastest because it's not rolled up protectively inside the rest of the condom. Because heat is one of the causes of deterioration in condoms, do not store them for longer than a month in a wallet or pocket.

THE CERVICAL CAP

The cervical cap was approved for marketing in the U.S. in 1988. It is a thimble-shaped rubber cap that fits snugly over the cervix. Like the diaphragm, it blocks sperm from entering the cervical opening. Usually, a small amount of spermicide is used on the inside of the cap to kill any sperm that might break through the suction seal. Used in some European countries, the cap was also used during the early 20th century in the U.S.* With the rise in use of the Pill and IUD, the cervical cap, like the diaphragm, declined in popularity.

The National Women's Health Network, feminist health groups, and a small number of physicians and nurses spent nearly a decade campaigning for the cap and shepherding it through the long process of review by the FDA. In addition, much of the research on the cap has been conducted at feminist health centers across the U.S. The availability of the cervical cap today represents a victory for women's health activists.

Description

The only cervical cap approved for use in the U.S. is the Prentif cavity rim, made of flexible rubber. It looks somewhat like a thimble with a rim and fits over the cervix the same way a thimble fits over your finger. It is about 1½ inches long and covers almost the entire cervix. Because cervices are different sizes, this rubber cap comes in four different sizes, from 22 millimeters to 31 millimeters in diameter (less than 1 inch to about 1¼ inches). Other kinds of caps not approved by the FDA are the vault (or Dumas) cap and the Vimule cap. The following information is about the Prentif cervical cap only.

How It Works

Like other barrier methods, the cervical cap keeps sperm out of the uterus. The cap is designed to create an almost airtight seal around the cervical opening. Suction, or surface tension, hugs it close to the cervix, and sperm can't move past the edge of the cap the way they can with the diaphragm. The spermicide both

---

* The idea of the cervical cap is thousands of years old. In ancient Sumatra, women molded opium into cuplike devices to cover their cervices. See Barbara Seaman and Gideon Seaman, *Women and the Crisis in Sex Hormones*, p. 190.

inactivates sperm and strengthens the suction seal between the cap and the cervix.

Effectiveness

For women who have never given birth, the cap is about as effective as a diaphragm. Its lowest expected failure rate is 9%; its typical failure rate is 20%. For women who have given birth, the cap is less effective. For women who have given birth and who use the cap correctly and consistently, its expected failure rate is 26%; its typical failure rate is 40%. A certain percentage of failures may be due to the cap being dislodged during intercourse by the penis thrusting against the cervix.

How to Get the Cap

Now that cervical caps have been marketed for almost a decade in the U.S., practitioners at many family planning clinics know how to fit them. You can get a list of practitioners and clinics that fit cervical caps from the Concord Feminist Health Center, 38 South Main Street, Concord, NH 03301, (603) 225-2739; Cervical Cap Ltd., 430 Monterey Avenue, Suite 1B, Los Gatos, CA 95030, (408) 395-2100; Boston Women's Health Book Collective, 240A Elm Street, Somerville, MA 02144, (617) 625-0271.

The cervical cap must be fitted to your cervix by a trained practitioner. When it fits properly, a cap should completely cover your cervix and grip it firmly. To insert it, you have to be able to reach your cervix with your fingers. Whenever you are fitted for a cap, be sure that the practitioner gives you time to try inserting and removing it.

How to Use the Cap

Most health workers advise using a small amount of spermicidal jelly or cream inside the cap. The cap should be filled about one-third full. If you use too much, it may break the suction. The spermicide should be spread around the inside of the cap but not on the rim. Some health workers recommend inserting the cap at least 30 minutes before intercourse or vagina-to-penis contact to allow suction to build up. You may insert it up to 40 hours ahead of time. For backup, some women insert cream or jelly into the vagina if they have intercourse after the cap has been in place for a few hours.

You *must* keep the cap in place for at least six hours after intercourse. Douching is unnecessary, but in any case, never douche while the cap is in place, since this could dilute the spermicidal jelly or cream.

Practitioners debate how often to remove the cap. Although some believe the cap can be worn continuously for 72 hours (three days) or longer, the FDA regulations state that it should not be left in place for longer than 48 hours (two days), partly because of the lack of good data on failure rates with longer use and concern about toxic shock syndrome.* Some women remove the cap once a day or every other day to allow cervical secretions to flow freely. This may help prevent infections and toxic shock syndrome. During your period, remove the cap often or don't use it at all, in order to reduce the risk of toxic shock syndrome and because the menstrual flow may break the suction seal.

Some women help prevent odors by soaking the cap for 20 minutes in 1 cup of water mixed with 1 tablespoon of cider vinegar or lemon juice. After soaking, rinse and dry the cap before using. For a month or two after you start using the cap, and whenever you have intercourse with a new partner, check it right before and after intercourse, and use extra spermicide in your vagina or have your partner use a condom for extra protection. Especially if the cap doesn't fit exactly right, and depending on the angle of penetration and your particular anatomy, the cap can become dislodged when a man's penis thrusts against your cervix. You may have to see if a different-size cap fits better, or switch to a diaphragm.

Who Shouldn't Use the Cervical Cap

Many women, even those who can't wear the diaphragm, can use the cervical cap, but the existing sizes may not fit all women. If you have a cervical erosion or laceration, you shouldn't use the cap because it doesn't allow the free flow of cervical secretions, which may be a cause of irritation. If you have a history of toxic shock syndrome, you should not use the cap.

It is possible for a woman's vagina to be so long that she can't reach deep enough inside to place or remove the cap easily. Some women have found that a diaphragm inserter/remover (similar to a giant plastic crotchet hook) can help with removal. Ask your practitioner to write a prescription for an inserter/remover if you need one and the local pharmacy will not sell it over the counter.

Other reasons for not using the cervical cap are the same as those for not using the diaphragm (see "Who Shouldn't Use the Diaphragm," p. 296).

Advantages

When used properly, the cap is very effective and you can insert it long before intercourse, which means it need not interfere with lovemaking.

The cap itself is relatively inexpensive, costing about $30, and the fee for the initial fitting can be $30 to $150. Because it requires so little spermicide, one tube will go a long way.

Because of its size, the cap may be more comfortable than the diaphragm. Also, because it requires less

cream or jelly, the cap is less messy, and women using it are less likely to feel the spermicide leaking after intercourse than women using the diaphragm.

It is a good choice for women who experience repeated urinary tract infections when they use a diaphragm if this problem is caused by pressure from the diaphragm rim. Cap users, however, also may have problems with urinary tract infections because of altered bacterial growth in the vagina.

It provides some protection against gonorrhea and chlamydia.

Like the diaphragm, the cap helps us to learn how our bodies change during our menstrual cycles and encourages us to get to know our bodies better.

Disadvantages

The cap may not available everywhere. It comes in only four sizes, so it does not fit all women.

The cap may cause an unpleasant odor if you don't remove it fairly often.

Some women dislike the idea of trapping cervical secretions for as long as the cap is worn because this may lead to infections.

Occasionally a partner feels discomfort if his penis hits the rim of the cap during intercourse.

You have to keep checking the cap carefully after intercourse to feel whether it has become dislodged. If the seal is broken, the cap's effectiveness is reduced.

Some women have trouble inserting and removing the cap.

It does not protect against most STDs.

THE CONTRACEPTIVE SPONGE

Investigation to develop a contraceptive sponge was prompted by several factors: women moving away from using pills and IUDs, a growing recognition by the medical establishment that women are seeking alternatives, a slight rise in publicly and privately funded research for improving barrier methods and producing new ones. In 1983, the FDA approved the sponge for general over-the-counter marketing. For 12 years (1983–1995), U.S. women could use a contraceptive sponge (Today Sponge). This barrier method is no longer available in the U.S., even though it is a safe and effective form of contraception. The only manufacturer of it, Whitehall-Robins Health Care, decided to stop making it after an inspection by the FDA in 1994 disclosed bacterial contamination in the water system used to make the sponge. The FDA did not object to continued production of the Today Sponge under appropriate manufacturing and hygenic conditions; unfortunately, Whitehall-Robins decided that the financial costs of bringing its factory into compliance with FDA regulations would be too high. We would like to see women's health needs taking precedence over company costs, especially in the light of increased attention to woman-centered research in pub-

---

* Some researchers have found high concentrations of *Staphylococcus aureus*, the bacteria involved in toxic shock syndrome, in women who have left the cap in for three days or more.

lic and private nonprofit contraceptive research organizations.

Another contraceptive sponge, Protectaid, is now manufactured and sold by AXCAN Ltd. in Canada. Unfortunately, it is not currently available in the U.S. The active ingredient in this sponge is a combination of three spermicidal agents (nonoxynol-9, sodium cholate, and benzalkonium chloride), each in quite low concentrations, thus reducing the risk of cervical or vaginal irritation.

VAGINAL SPERMICIDES: JELLIES AND CREAMS

Spermicidal cream or jelly is really designed for use with a diaphragm or cervical cap (and can be used for extra protection with a condom). The lowest expected failure rate for spermicides used alone (jellies, creams, foams, and vaginal suppositories) is 6%; the typical failure rate is 26%. Recent studies, on which this estimate is based, are mostly about suppositories and foam. Using spermicides with condoms gives much better protection, both against pregnancy and against some STDs.

Cream or jelly comes in a tube with a plastic applicator. Jellies are clear, creams are white. They are available without prescription at all drugstores.

Cream or jelly is deposited just outside the entrance to your cervix at the top of the vagina. In the U.S., the active ingredient in most spermicidal creams, jellies, foams, vaginal suppositories, and films is nonoxynol-9, a detergent that kills sperm.

How to Use Jellies and Creams

For use with a *diaphragm* or *cap,* see the earlier sections on these devices. For use with a condom: As short a time as possible (under 15 minutes) *before* vagina-to-penis contact or intercourse, you or your partner should fill the applicator, insert it into your vagina, and push the plunger. Use an additional full plunger for each additional act of intercourse. Leave the jelly or cream in for six to eight hours. If you want to douche, you must wait.

Possible Negative Effects

Vaginal spermicides probably increase your risk of getting yeast and urinary tract infections.

Controversy persists about the impact of spermicides on the risk for HIV. Spermicides used alone do not protect against HIV. Spermicides decrease a woman's risk slightly for gonorrhea and chlamydia, and this in turn may reduce her susceptibility to HIV. However, the active ingredient in spermicides (nonoxynol-9) can also irritate vaginal tissue, particularly with frequent or prolonged use of spermicides. Studies of commercial sex workers show that frequent or prolonged use of nonoxynol-9 makes the damage worse. This damage to the vagina may increase a woman's risk of HIV

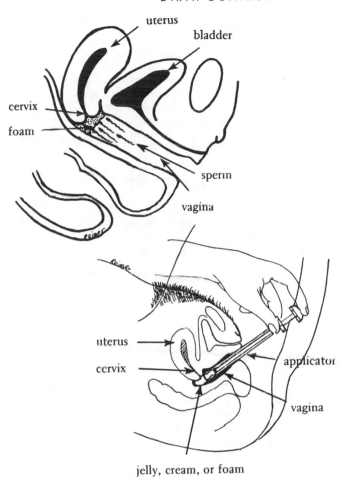

How to insert sperm-killing foam, cream, or jelly/Nina Reimer

infection. (See chapters 14, Sexually Transmitted Diseases, and 15, HIV, AIDS, and Women.)[8]

Repeated studies show that contrary to previous reports, there is no link between spermicide use and disabilities present at birth.

Advantages

Like condoms, cream and jelly are easy to get on short notice.

Spermicides with nonoxynol-9 increase your protection against gonorrhea, chlamydia, and trichomoniasis. They also appear to protect against PID and bacterial vaginosis. (See chapters 14, Sexually Transmitted Diseases, and 24, Selected Medical Practices, Problems, and Procedures, for more on these conditions.)[9]

Disadvantages

Cream and jelly can leak. Some women have allergic reactions to these products; try different brands if you have problems. Jelly may be less irritating but tends to be more gooey than cream. You or your partner may find the smell or taste unpleasant.

VAGINAL SPERMICIDES: FOAM

Description

Foam is a white, aerated cream that has the consistency of shaving cream and contains nonoxynol-9, which kills sperm. It comes in a 1.4-ounce can with a plunger-type plastic applicator and costs about $10. Three brands currently on the market in the United States are Delfen, Emko, and Koromex.

How It Works

Deposited just outside the entrance to your cervix at the top of your vagina, foam disperses into your vagina and covers the opening of your cervix, where it keeps the sperm from entering the cervix. Foam also immobilizes sperm.

Effectiveness

The lowest expected failure rate of foam used alone consistently and correctly is 6%, but the failure rate among typical users is 26%.

We strongly recommend using foam in combination with a condom. When used together at every act of intercourse, their effectiveness approaches 100%. Foam is also very effective when used as a supplement during the first week of the first time a woman takes the Pill.

Problems with effectiveness arise from using too little foam, not realizing that the container is almost empty, failing to shake the container enough, not inserting the foam correctly, or inserting it after vagina-to-penis contact has begun.

How to Use Foam

Insert no longer than 30 minutes before vagina-to-penis contact. If the foam is in a can, shake the can very well, about 20 times. The more bubbles the foam has, the better it blocks sperm. Also, the spermicide tends to settle in the bottom of the container, so it must be mixed. Put the applicator on top. When the applicator is tilted (Delfen) or pushed down (Emko and Koromex), the pressure triggers the release valve and the foam is forced into the applicator, pushing the plunger up. Some brands of foam come in preloaded applicators.

Lie down, use your free hand to spread the lips of your vagina, insert the applicator about 3 to 4 inches, and push the plunger. (See illustration on p. 303.) Then remove the applicator (without pulling on the plunger, or you may suck some of the foam back into the applicator). Insert one full applicator of Emko, Emko Pre-fil, or Because, or two applicators full of Delfen or Koromex. If you have never used tampons, you may want to practice inserting the applicator. You'll find that your vagina angles up toward your back, not straight up in your body. Your aim is to deposit the foam at the entrance of your cervix.

Wash the applicator with mild soap and warm (but not boiling) water before putting it away. You don't have to wash it immediately.

Cautions

Put in more foam every time you have intercourse or vagina-to-penis contact, no matter how recent the last time was. Leave the foam in for six to eight hours. If you want to douche, you must wait. If the foam is dripping and bothers you, use a minipad or tissue in your underpants.

Keep an extra can on hand. Some brands indicate when they're running out; others just come out of the can more slowly. Use foam with a condom for maximum effectiveness of both.

Negative Effects

Foam can irritate some people's genitals, leading to pain, itching, or the sensation of heat. Other negative effects are the same as for creams and jellies (see p. 303).

Responsibility

Basically the responsibility is the woman's, but either you or the man can put it in.

Advantages

When used with a condom, foam is a highly effective means of birth control. It works immediately and remains effective for at least an hour.

It is quick, taking about 30 seconds to use.

It is less drippy than cream or jelly.

It helps to prevent some STDs, as creams and jellies do.

Disadvantages

Alone, foam is rather ineffective.

Using it can be an interruption if you do not treat it as part of sex play.

It increases the risk of yeast and urinary tract infections.

Many people think it tastes terrible; it should not be inserted before oral sex.

Controversy persists about the impact of spermicides, including foam, on HIV.

How to Get Foam

You can buy it in a drugstore without a prescription.

Although you don't have to see a health practitioner to get foam, have a checkup if you think you've been exposed to an STD.

Try different brands. If one causes irritation, another may be satisfactory.

Other Vaginal Spermicides: Foaming Suppositories, Film, Tablets

There are three other types of foaming spermicides: suppositories, contraceptive film, and tablets. Spermicidal suppositories and tablets (Encare Oval, Intercept, Koromex Inserts, Prevent, Semicid) and vaginal contraceptive film (VCF) can be used alone *but we strongly recommend that you use them only in combination with a condom.* To use a suppository or tablet, unwrap one and insert it into your vagina up against the back, so it rests on or near your cervix, 10 to 30 minutes before vagina-to-penis contact. To use VCF, make sure your hands are dry, place one paper-thin sheet on your finger, and insert the film on or near your cervix 15 minutes before vagina-to-penis contact. The spermicidal suppository, tablet, or film will remain effective for no more than an hour. With repeated intercourse, you need to insert another suppository or film. These products melt inside the vagina and are left in, not removed, after intercourse. Suppositories, tablets, and film are considered to be as effective as the other spermicides. Suppositories and tablets don't seem to disperse into the vagina as well as the foams and creams do. Otherwise, the advantages and disadvantages of these products are the same as for creams and jellies.

FERTILITY OBSERVATION (NATURAL BIRTH CONTROL)

We can learn to understand our bodies' hormonal changes that are linked to fertility by observing three body signs: cervical fluid, basal body temperature, and cephalad shift (cervix changes). In this way, we can accurately determine whether we are fertile (able to conceive) or infertile (not able to conceive) on a day-to-day basis. It takes only a few minutes each day to make and record our observations.

Using Fertility Observation is a simple, accurate way to understand when you can and cannot become pregnant as your cycle unfolds. Unlike the Rhythm Method, which predicts, on the basis of past cycles, when the fertile time may occur in the future, Fertility Observation is based on actual physiological evidence (changes in your own fertility signs), rather than on prediction and guesswork. The Rhythm Method, which is notorious for its high failure rate, erroneously assumes that ovulation can be accurately predicted in the current cycle from information on the length of previous cycles. However, the length of time before ovulation can vary greatly from woman to woman and, for each woman, from cycle to cycle. The Rhythm Method is generally considered outdated and unreliable—particularly since the more effective, proven Fertility Observation method is available.

Observing our bodies' natural indicators, we learn that we are fertile during only about one-third of each menstrual cycle. Even if we aren't interested in birth control, this information can be used to understand our bodies better, to achieve pregnancy through intercourse or insemination, to identify and reverse infertility problems, or to predict menstruation.

The Three Fertility Signs

1. *Cervical fluid (mucus).* This is a daily method of identifying fertile and infertile times by simple observation, as the cycle unfolds. Cervical fluid tells when fertility begins and ends in each cycle, the times of highest fertility, and when ovulation and menstruation are approaching. Fertility begins when cervical fluid appears, and lasts through the evening of the fourth day past the cervical fluid peak (the last day of wet, fertile cervical fluid). Ovulation occurs anywhere from two days before to two days after this peak day.

Cervical fluid is a direct reflection of estrogen and progesterone levels in the body (the fluid is wet and fertile when estrogen, which comes from developing eggs in the ovary, rises and is dominant, and is sticky or dry when progesterone is dominant after ovulation). In this way, cervical fluid is an accurate, external way to identify internal hormone changes.

A simple way to understand this is to summarize a hormone cycle: Estrogen rises and drops, and you ovulate. Progesterone rises and drops, and you menstruate. In external signs, cervical fluid appears and becomes wetter, then ovulation occurs. The cervical fluid becomes drier or sticky for about two weeks, then you menstruate.

Cervical fluid identifies fertile and infertile days throughout the entire cycle, regardless of whether or not cycles are regular. This is especially valuable to women during times of breast-feeding, premenopause, and stress.

2. *Basal body temperature (BBT).* BBT indicates ovulation after it has occurred, identifies postovulatory infertile days, and confirms pregnancy. Temperatures are lower before ovulation and higher afterward. Before ovulation a woman's waking temperature is typically 97° to 97.5°F. After ovulation the range is typically 97.6° to 98.6°F. A sustained rise (up to three days) of at least $4/10$ of a degree Fahrenheit confirms that ovulation has occurred. If BBTs remain elevated for more than 17 days (and you have no fever or illness), pregnancy is confirmed.

BBT does not indicate when fertility begins or which preovulatory days are safe for vagina-to-penis contact or intercourse.

3. *Cephalad shift (cervix changes).* The cephalad shift represents a change in the position and feel of the cervix. When you are fertile, the cervix becomes softer and higher, and the os (opening) widens. When cervical fluid changes from wet to dry, the cervix becomes firm, lower, and less open. Cervix changes alone do not show when fertility begins and ends, nor do they indicate safe or unsafe days for vagina-to-penis contact and intercourse. However, they offer a valuable way to confirm the accuracy of cervical fluid and BBT observations.

The three fertility signs are simple to observe and record, requiring no more than a few minutes each day.

Avoiding Pregnancy Through Fertility Observation

To prevent pregnancy, you can use these three fertility signs in two ways:

1. *Natural family planning (NFP)*. This involves postponing all vagina-to-penis contact when you are fertile (about one-third of the cycle). Intimacy can be expressed in ways that prevent sperm from coming in contact with fertile cervical fluid on the labia or at the cervix. NFP is acceptable to people who do not wish to use artificial means of contraception for religious, medical, or philosophical reasons. It is most often taught by instructors and organizations affiliated with the Catholic Church.

2. *Fertility awareness method (FAM)*. During the fertile part of a cycle, FAM offers the choice of postponing vagina-to-penis contact, using barrier methods of contraception, or expressing intimacy in nonsexual ways. This nonreligious approach enables contraceptive users to know when a barrier method failure is more likely to result in pregnancy, so that contraceptives can be used even more carefully during these times. Women can also reduce barrier use with FAM knowledge because we can identify the two-thirds of the cycle when we are naturally infertile. Although jelly or foam in the vagina can temporarily mask indications of fertility (for a few hours), some women report no problems in combining a barrier method with fertility awareness, especially if the man is using a condom.

It is crucial to learn fertility observation methods directly from qualified instructors and to chart your observations daily. It is *not* advisable to learn a method just by reading a book. Although several books in the Resources can be very helpful and are recommended, books (including this one) cannot give you the personal feedback, support, and experience sharing that you need to ensure successful use of fertility observation. Because fertility observation places responsibility for reproductive decisions firmly in the hands of the user, successful use depends on learning the method correctly, understanding how to use it, and being clear with your partner about how you will use it. *Any intercourse during the fertile parts of your cycle is highly likely to result in pregnancy.* But if used correctly, fertility observation is as effective as the male condom and more effective than the diaphragm in preventing pregnancy.*

Check your local women's health center or write to the following nonreligious fertility awareness groups for more information: Ovulation Method Teachers Association (OMTA), P.O. Box 101780, Anchorage, AK 99510-1780; Fertility Awareness Network (FAN) P.O. Box 1190, New York, NY 10009. Both are feminist, prochoice groups that offer all fertility awareness options. For a free list of all fertility awareness books and groups (including which signs they teach, their philosophy, and options for preventing pregnancy), send a stamped, self-addressed envelope to Fertility Awareness Services (FAS), P.O. Box 986, Corvallis, OR 97339 (FAS specializes in compiling all available fertility awareness information). If you are willing or want to hear Catholic morality mixed in with the information, most Catholic hospitals or churches can help you find a teacher.

Here are some issues to consider in choosing a group:†

1. Is the teacher a woman with experience herself? A male-female couple? A medical person? A nun or priest?

2. Does the format include participatory classes or groups and more than one meeting?

3. Is there an option to learn in an all-woman group? If all classes are open to men, is the orientation toward monogamous heterosexual couples? What efforts are made to ensure support for other sexual lifestyles?

4. Can you get help from the teacher in the months or years after the training process is over?

5. Where does the registration fee go? (Are you unwittingly supporting a cause you would find offensive?)

6. What is the sponsoring organization's or teacher's position on birth control and abortion? Are you being pressured to follow one way of thinking, or do you feel you are being given all the options and allowed to decide which methods and reproductive choices you will apply to using Fertility Observation and birth control? It is important to connect with a teacher and organization that support your philosophy and needs. If you hear the term "pro-life" used, remember that this indicates an anti-abortion philosophy.

The Ovulation Method (Awareness of Mucus)

Thirty years ago, an Australian couple, Evelyn and John Billings, sought a method of child spacing that would be effective in preventing pregnancy and also

---

* Depending on which method you use, write down the day of your cycle; whether you feel wet or dry; and describe the color and consistency of any external fluid, your temperature, and changes in your cervix.

† Adapted from S. Bell et al., "Reclaiming Reproductive Control: A Feminist Approach to Fertility Consciousness," *Science for the People* 12, no. 1 (1980): 6–9, 30–35.

acceptable to the Catholic Church—one that would reinforce the Catholic philosophy about sexuality, marriage, and women. They developed the ovulation method, a way of interpreting the vaginal sensations of wetness or dryness and the consistency of the cervical fluid so as to determine whether you are fertile or infertile. The Ovulation Method is very effective. It has only a 3% failure rate if used consistently and correctly.

You may already be aware that you normally have a vaginal discharge that varies throughout your menstrual cycle. You may notice nothing for several days and then suddenly experience a discharge—a bubbling sensation, a stickiness or a feeling of your vaginal lips being wet. This is caused by cervical fluid, made in the cells of the cervical canal in response to your hormonal changes. Here is a brief outline of the relationship of cervical fluid to fertility (see also chapter 12, Understanding Our Bodies, p. 277).

1. *Menstruation.* A cycle begins on the first day of your period. Because cervical fluid can begin during menstruation (especially in women who tend to have short cycles), and because menstrual flow may mask the presence of cervical fluid, the menstrual period is not necessarily safe for unprotected intercourse or vagina-to-penis contact.

2. *Dry days after menstruation (if any).* Most women have several days of dryness (no cervical fluid) after their period ends. You may have no sensation of discharge, no cervical fluid present at the vaginal opening, and no noticeable discharge on your underwear, and your labia feel dry. These are called preovulatory (before ovulation) dry days. Intercourse is safe *every other evening after menstruation as long as you have been dry all day.* Allow a day after intercourse to ensure that seminal fluid is not masking the beginning of cervical fluid. If still dry on the day after that, you can again have intercourse, or vagina-to-penis contact, on the evening of that dry day.

You can check for cervical fluid either outside the vagina (labia) or inside the vagina (at the cervix itself). However, it is important to check the same way throughout a single cycle, so that your readings are consistent. If checking outside, wipe your fingers over the labia and pat them together a few times to determine the sensation of the mucus. If checking inside, insert two clean fingers inside your vagina (being careful not to touch the always wet vaginal walls), gently touch the cervix, and withdraw your fingers (again without touching the vaginal walls). Then pat your fingers together to determine the sensation of cervical fluid.

Note: When checking for cervical fluid, the most important thing to note is sensation (what it feels like). This is what identifies whether it is a fertile time in your cycle. Wet, slippery, creamy, slick are all "fertile" sensations; dry, sticky, tacky, gummy are all "infertile" sensations.

3. *Mucus days.* Fertility begins as soon as cervical fluid (mucus) appears. This usually occurs after the several dry days that follow menstruation, although cervical fluid can also begin during the last days of your period. Your fertile time begins when you feel a

sensation of wetness or creaminess outside your vagina, when wiping with toilet paper, or when you notice the presence of cervical fluid on your underwear. The important thing to notice is change from the feeling of dryness. The cervical fluid usually starts off with a day or two of sticky mucus, which becomes increasingly creamy and smooth, then wetter and more slippery. It can even become extremely slippery and stretchy, like egg white. *As soon* as cervical fluid appears, it nourishes and protects sperm until ovulation. Therefore, to prevent pregnancy, postpone intercourse or use barriers from the time cervical fluid appears to the evening of the fourth day after it changes to dryness or an infertile type of cervical fluid.

The last day of cervical fluid with any fertile characteristics is called the mucus peak day. Ovulation occurs anywhere from two days before to two days after the peak day. You are fertile from the time the cervical fluid appears until the evening of the fourth day after peak. The number of fertile days varies from cycle to cycle, although they usually last six to 12 days (about one-third of the cycle).

4. *Postpeak (luteal) phase.* After the peak day, your cervical fluid will change drastically, from wetness to a more sticky, tacky, or drier discharge. These dry or sticky days signal the beginning of the luteal phase, the ten to 16 days of dryness before your next period arrives. From the evening of the fourth day past the peak day until your period begins, you cannot conceive.

These descriptions cover a general pattern. Although every woman is unique and may differ slightly from this pattern, every woman can easily learn to recognize her own pattern.

If you have a vaginal infection, you may not be able to tell the difference between cervical fluid and the discharge from your infection or any medication you are using to treat it. *If you are ever unsure about whether you are fertile or not, always consider yourself possibly fertile and use other methods of contraception until you are sure of your observations.*

The Symptothermal Method

The symptothermal method (STM) combines basal body temperature and cervical fluid (mucus) observation. Some consider it to also include Rhythm Method use. However, because cervical fluid gives more accurate information about preovulatory infertile and fertile times, rhythm is no longer used by most fertility awareness groups.

When you use the STM, the cervical fluid (see previous section) indicates when fertility begins and ends. Basal body temperatures are low before ovulation and higher afterward. By taking your temperature on a basal body thermometer (which measures in tenths of a degree) each morning at the same time and recording it on a chart, you will see that your BBT rises slightly following ovulation and stays high until menstruation begins. (It falls as your period starts and stays low until the next ovulation.) Your fertile time ends either on the fourth day after the mucus peak or on the evening of the third day in a row of elevated temperatures, whichever is later. (Elevated temperature means 4/10 a degree Fahrenheit above the highest of at least six preovulation readings after the first four days of menstruation.)

Effectiveness of Fertility Observation

Some health professionals rate all natural methods of birth control as poor. In most cases, they have confused the word *natural* with the word *rhythm*. Recent studies (based on women avoiding all vagina-to-penis contact on fertile days) indicate that the ovulation method and STM can be extremely effective when taught carefully, understood thoroughly, and used correctly. When used consistently and correctly, the ovulation method's failure rate is 3% and the STM's failure rate is 2% during their first year of use. When the ovulation method is not used consistently and correctly, that is, when women and their partners have intercourse or vagina-to-penis contact during the fertile time or when there is misunderstanding of the rules or disagreement between partners about how to use the method, it has a much higher failure rate. Failure is also more likely during periods of stress.

You can use fertility observation to increase the effectiveness of barrier methods by avoiding any vagina-to-penis contact on fertile days.

Reversibility

Reversibility is excellent. Just have intercourse on fertile days.

Responsibility

Basically the responsibility is the woman's. It requires cooperation from the man.

Advantages

It has no negative effects.

Many of us enjoy being more aware of our body's cycles and have found this knowledge useful in making many other health care decisions. It is user-controlled and costs nothing to use.

It can lead, during fertile days, to exploration of other ways to give and receive pleasure, such as mutual masturbation and oral sex. (Be sure to avoid all vagina-to-penis contact.)

The cooperation necessary for this method can bring understanding and closeness between partners.

Disadvantages

The major disadvantage is the risk of pregnancy if you are not committed to using it correctly.

It *does not* protect you against STDs, including HIV infection.

It takes at least two to three cycles to learn and use confidently.

It may be impractical if you are not in a committed, cooperative relationship with your sex partner.

If you choose not to use a barrier method and instead abstain from intercourse and vagina-to-penis contact when you are fertile, it can be sexually frustrating unless you enjoy other forms of sex.

Mechanization of Fertility Observation

Numerous machines and devices are being developed to measure hormonal changes and to pinpoint fertility. They are based on the same principles as Fertility Awareness, but they're more expensive without necessarily being more accurate.

BREAST-FEEDING: LACTATIONAL AMENORRHEA METHOD (LAM)

In previous editions of this book, we warned that breast-feeding is not a reliable method of birth control. However, for some women, breast-feeding (LAM) can be a reliable method of birth control for up to six months after giving birth. After you give birth to a baby, it takes time for your body to begin ovulating and menstruating again. The length of time it takes depends on whether or not you breast-feed your newborn baby; it will take longer for women who breast-feed than for women who do not.

LAM is a newly accepted method of natural birth control that helps a breast-feeding woman prevent pregnancy. To use LAM correctly, a woman must be fully or nearly fully breast-feeding,* her body must not have begun menstruating again, and her baby must be under six months old. When used correctly, LAM has a failure rate of less than 2% in the first six months after a woman gives birth. Failure rates are lowest for women who are fully breast-feeding more than ten times each day.

LAM is very effective if used correctly. However, it does not protect against sexually transmitted diseases, and it is only effective for a short period of time after a woman gives birth. To prevent pregnancy, a woman must start using another method of birth control after her first menstruation OR after she begins to supplement breast-feeding with other liquids or solids OR after her baby is six months old.

BIRTH CONTROL PILLS

In 1960, the FDA approved the Pill for marketing in the U.S. without adequate testing or study. Although medical literature confirmed dangers of the original

---

* "Fully breast-feeding" means that a woman is nursing her baby on demand, in the daytime and at night, and that she is breast-feeding exclusively. "Nearly fully breast-feeding" means that she is nursing on demand day and night, supplementing with vitamins, and infrequently giving her baby water or juice. (See M. H. Labbock et al., "The Lactational Amenorrhea Method," in the Resource section for details on the method and its implications.)

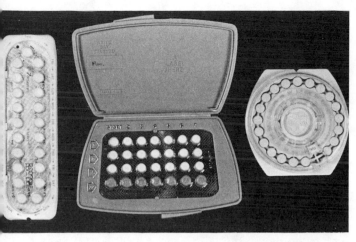

Pill packets/Elizabeth Shapiro

Pill as early as 1962, very few professionals cautioned against using it too widely or too quickly; to do so meant fighting against the prevailing ideology, which supported rapid development and distribution of new drugs generally, and risking the charge of holding back progress. To women, taking a Pill every day that was almost 100% effective in preventing pregnancy seemed like a wonderful alternative to the methods then available. Many women first heard about the dangers of the high-dose estrogen pill (blood clots, heart attacks, strokes, depression, suicide, weight gain, decreased sex drive) when they read Barbara Seaman's book *The Doctors' Case Against the Pill,* published in 1969. Many chose to stop taking the Pill or to find another alternative.

Efforts by women and consumer activists in the late 1960s, along with well-publicized congressional hearings, led to modifications of the Pill as well as special patient package inserts; since 1978 the FDA has required physicians and pharmacists to hand out comprehensive information sheets on its possible negative effects and complications. Because many of the most serious negative effects are associated with high dosages of estrogen, drug companies reduced the estrogen content of the Pill and also began to develop progestin-only pills. Today's low-dose combination Pill is safer than the high-dose Pill and even has some health benefits beyond contraception. Over 70 million women worldwide use the Pill. In the U.S., it is the most frequently used reversible method of contraception.

Recently, so-called third-generation pills have been approved for use in the U.S. Like other combination pills, they contain a lower dose of estrogen but a *different* type of progestin (see "How They Work," at right). In the U.S., third-generation pills now represent 15% of the market. In 1995, after three studies demonstrated a link between third-generation pill use and an increased risk of nonfatal blood clots, the Committee on Safety of Medicine in Britain recommended that women stop using these pills, but the FDA concluded that the risk does not justify switching to other

methods. In light of the controversy, we recommend that women avoid using third-generation pills until more research has been completed on their short-term and long-term effects.

In some countries, contraceptive pills are available without prescription; women in Mexico, for example, can purchase them at a pharmacy without first seeing a health practitioner. In the U.S., the Pill is only available by prescription. Some view the prescription-only policy as a "medical barrier," especially in settings where there is limited or no access to quality health care, or where the costs and inconveniences of visiting a doctor and undergoing tests discourage Pill use. Although it is probably true that over-the-counter availability of oral contraceptives would make it easier for some women—especially younger women—to obtain the Pill, the authors of this book believe that the Pill should not at this time become a nonprescription item. We simply do not know whether the health benefits of making oral contraceptives available over the counter (OTC) clearly outweigh the possible health costs.

First, OTC availability of the Pill would eliminate the clinical screening that could detect health factors making oral contraceptive use risky. Second, disease detection and prevention would be decreased as a consequence of fewer visits to health care providers. It is during the visit, when women come for oral contraceptives, that health care providers often detect sexually transmitted diseases or other problems requiring medical attention. Third, face-to-face exchanges between health care providers and women about choosing oral contraceptives would rarely take place with OTC availability of the Pill. Fourth, it is likely that OTC availability would decrease many women's financial ability to obtain the Pill. Women who now have insurance coverage for the Pill would have to purchase it out of pocket.

How They Work

To understand how birth control pills work, you need to know how menstruation works. Chapter 12, Understanding Our Bodies: Sexual Anatomy, Reproduction, and the Menstrual Cycle, and its appendix describe what hormones are and how the hormones estrogen and progesterone guide a woman's menstrual cycle.

The way the most widely used pills (combination pills) work to prevent pregnancy is outlined in the table on p. 311, which puts an average menstrual cycle and the Pill cycle side by side. It shows how the Pill alters your menstrual cycle by introducing synthetic versions of the female hormones. The seven-day "no-hormone" period built into monophasic combination pill cycles (see "How to Use the Pill," p. 317) produces bleeding, but this is not a true menstrual period; with these, the user is more likely to become pregnant if she misses a pill just before or after the hormone-free interval than if she skips one in the middle of the cycle.

Combination birth control pills prevent pregnancy

primarily by inhibiting the development of the egg in the ovary. During your period, normally the low estrogen level indirectly triggers your pituitary gland to send out follicle-stimulating hormone (FSH), a hormone that starts an egg developing to maturity in one of your ovaries. The Pill gives you just enough *synthetic estrogen* (ethinyl estradiol or mestranol) to raise your estrogen level high enough to keep FSH from being released. So, during a month of taking the Pill, your ovaries remain relatively inactive, and there is no egg to join with sperm. This is the same principle by which a woman's body stops ovulating when she is pregnant: The corpus luteum and placenta put estrogen into her blood, thereby inhibiting FSH. So, in a way, using much lower levels of hormones, the Pill simulates pregnancy, and some of the Pill's negative effects are like those of early pregnancy. If ovulation occurs, it is because your body needed a higher dose of estrogen than your Pill gave you to inhibit FSH, or because you have missed one or more Pills.

Synthetic progesterone, called *progestin,* is used differently in different varieties of the Pill. Progestin provides important contraceptive effects, including increased thickness of cervical fluid, slowed movement (motility) of sperm, slowed movement of the egg, and incomplete development of the uterine lining.

Monophasic oral contraceptives have constant doses of estrogen and progestin. Loestrin 1/20 (20 micrograms of *ethinyl estradiol* and 1 milligram of *norethindrone*) is the lowest-dose combination pill. The amount and type of progestin differs between Lo-Ovral (*norgestrel,* 0.3 milligrams) and Levlen (*levonorgestrel,* 0.15 milligrams), and Nordette (*levonorgestrel,* 0.15 milligrams); they each contain 30 micrograms of *ethinyl estradiol.* In 1993, the FDA approved Desogen and Ortho-Cept, which contain 30 micrograms of ethinyl estradiol and 0.15 milligrams of a new type of progestin, *desogestrel.* Desogen and Ortho-Cept are third-generation pills.

Triphasic oral contraceptives have three phases; in each third of the menstrual cycle the amount of progestin varies (Ortho-Novum 7/7/7, Ortho Tri-Cyclen, Tri-Norynl) or the amount of both estrogen and progestin varies (Tri-Levlen, Triphasil). The pills for each phase are a different color. In all triphasic pills, the progestin slowly increases throughout the cycle. In Tri-Levlen and Triphasil, estrogen also increases at midcycle. A full cycle of triphasic oral contraceptives has a low dose of estrogen and a lower dose of progestin than other types of combination oral contraceptives.

Biphasic oral contraceptives (Ortho-Novum 10/11, Nelova 10/11) are rarely used. They have two phases. They provide less progestin *(norethindrone)* during the first ten days of the cycle (1/2 a milligram) and more in the next ten days (1 milligram); the low dose of estrogen remains constant throughout the cycle (35 micrograms of *ethinyl estradiol*).

The *progestin-only pills* (Ovrette, Nor-QD, Micronor) are not quite as effective as combination pills in preventing pregnancy.

Combination Pills

Effectiveness

The combination pills have a very low expected pregnancy rate of 0.1%, but in typical use, they show a failure rate of 5%. Pregnancy is more likely if you forget to take your pill for one or more days, especially at the beginning or the end of the 21 active pills; if you don't use a backup method of birth control for the first seven days when you start your first packet of pills; when you miss two or more pills; or while taking the antibiotic rifampicin,* anticonvulsants, or some other medications; when experiencing severe vomiting or diarrhea; and occasionally if you change from one brand of pill to another. (Under these conditions, use a backup method of birth control for the rest of your cycle to prevent pregnancy.)

Reversibility

If you want to become pregnant, stop taking pills at the end of a packet. Most women soon become fertile again. It may be several months before your ovaries are functioning regularly, and your first non-Pill periods may be a week or two late or missed completely. If your periods were irregular before you began taking the Pill, especially if you are a teenager, you may have irregular periods for up to one year or longer when you stop.

Most women do have successful pregnancies after they go off the Pill. However, on average it takes one or two months longer for them to conceive than women who have not taken the Pill. If you have not conceived within one year of trying after going off the Pill, you might want to seek medical assistance (see chapter 22).

Safety

Many of us are uneasy about taking a medication that affects almost every organ in our bodies each day for months and years, because its effects have not been conclusively tested and may vary from woman to woman. Yet, some of us choose to take whatever risks are involved because we want a highly effective contraceptive method and absolutely don't want to become pregnant.

A great deal of information exists on both the benefits and adverse effects of the Pill, as the following pages demonstrate. In most cases of Pill-related injury or death, women had not been examined carefully enough by the doctor who prescribed the Pill for them, had taken the higher-dose Pill, had not had checkups while taking the Pill, or had not been told that they had some particular risks. Some women ignored pains

---

* Rifampicin is the only antibiotic that definitely interferes with the Pill's effectiveness. It is a good idea to use a backup birth control method whenever you are taking any antibiotic. The effect of antibiotics on Pill effectiveness seems to vary from woman to woman.

WOMAN'S MENSTRUAL CYCLE AND THE WAY THE COMBINATION BIRTH CONTROL PILL AFFECTS THAT CYCLE TO PREVENT PREGNANCY

Normal Menstrual Cycle*	**With the Pill**
Day 1. Menstrual period begins.	*Day 1.* Menstrual period begins.
Day 5. An egg in a follicle (pocket, sac) in one of your ovaries has begun to ripen to maturity. The egg starts developing in response to a hormonal message (FSH) from your pituitary gland, which in turn has been triggered indirectly by the low level of *estrogen* (an ovarian hormone) at the time of your period.	*Day 5.* Take your first pill. In the pill, you take two synthetic hormones every day: estrogen and progestin (synthetic progesterone).
Days 5 to 14. The follicle in which the egg is developing makes first a little, then more and more estrogen.	*Estrogen:* The pill contains more estrogen than there usually is in your body on day 5—enough to stop the usual message from your pituitary gland (FSH) for an egg to develop. By taking this amount of estrogen every day for 21 days, you prevent an egg from developing at all that month. Therefore, there is no egg to join with the sperm.
1. Estrogen stimulates the lining of your uterus to get thicker and the cells of your cervix to produce fluid that is receptive to sperm.	*Progestin:* A little progestin every day provides three vital backup effects:
2. As estrogen increases, it slows down and then cuts off FSH.	**1.** It keeps the plug of mucus in your cervix thick and dry, so sperm have a hard time getting through.
Day 14. Ovulation. Estrogen peak and a spurt of progesterone occurring during days 12 to 13 indirectly trigger ovulation. Ripe egg is released from ovary, starts four-day trip down fallopian tube to uterus. Conception with sperm from the man must occur in the first 24 hours.	**2.** It keeps the lining of your uterus from developing properly so that if an egg does ripen (if estrogen level of pill is too low for you or if you forget a pill) and sperm do join with the egg, the fertilized egg will not be able to implant.
	3. It inhibits activation of enzymes that permit sperm to unite with the egg.
Approximately days 14 to 25. The ruptured follicle, now called *corpus luteum* ("yellow body"), makes two hormones for about 12 days: *Estrogen* continues. *Progesterone* increases and peaks about day 22: 1. It makes your cervical fluid (plug of mucus in cervix) thick and dry, a barrier to sperm. 2. It stimulates the glands in lining of your uterus to secrete a sugary substance and further thickens the lining.	*Days 6 to 25.* Continue taking one pill a day.
Approximately days 26 to 27 to 28. If pregnancy is prevented successfully, *corpus luteum*'s manufacture of *estrogen* and *progesterone* slows down to a very low level. This drop creates an appropriate environment for reducing the excess layers of the tissue lining your uterus.	*Day 26.* Take your last pill.† *Days 27 to 28.* The sudden drop in estrogen and progestin creates an appropriate environment for reducing the excess layers of the tissue lining your uterus.‡
Approximately day 29 to day 1. Menstrual period begins. Low level of *estrogen* (see days 26 to 28) will begin indirectly to stimulate pituitary's egg-development hormone (FSH) to start a new cycle.	*Day 29 to Day 11.* Menstrual period begins. Your period is lighter than normal, because of effect 2 of progestin in the pill.

* This is a simplified version of the menstrual cycle. See the appendix to Chapter 12, Understanding Our Bodies, for a more thorough description.

† With the 28-day combination pill, you take pills without hormones in them from day 27 to day 5.

‡ Emily Martin, *The Woman in the Body* (Boston: Beacon Press, 1987), 52.

that were, in fact, warning signals, and sought help too late.

How Long to Take the Pill

If you are not now experiencing problems, you may want to enjoy the freedom of the Pill indefinitely. Yet, if you take the Pill for many years at a time, you are in a sense part of a huge experiment on the long-term effects of daily hormone ingestion in healthy women. Researchers disagree on how long a woman should continue to take the Pill. They agree that once you pass age 40, you are at higher risk of Pill-related death if you have an additional risk factor (see "Who Should Absolutely Not Use the Pill," p. 312). They also agree that taking periodic breaks from the Pill does *not* improve your future ability to have a baby. A few studies suggest that some young women who have used the Pill are more likely to develop breast cancer before age 35 (see p. 314 on the Pill and cancer).

Going Off the Pill

For women who stop taking the Pill because they want to become pregnant, it typically takes one to two months longer than it does for women who have not taken the Pill. Women who stop taking the Pill but do not want to become pregnant may feel awkward using another method of birth control, especially one of the safer barrier methods. It is a sad fact that many of these women get pregnant in the first few months after going off the Pill. We need discussion, information, and support in making the switch to another method. It helps to have a partner or partners who understand and appreciate our desire to change to a safer form of contraception.

Warning Signals

Any problem lasting more than two or three cycles should be reported to a physician or medical facility. The following can be symptoms of serious problems: severe pain or swelling in the legs (thigh or calf), bad headache, dizziness, weakness, numbness, blurred vision (or loss of sight), speech problems, chest pain, cough, shortness of breath, or abdominal pain. *Report these immediately,* for they may be signs of heart attack, stroke, or liver tumors and indicate that you should stop taking the Pill. (Some leg cramps may be caused by fluid retention induced by the estrogen in the Pill. Don't confuse this with severe leg pain, but also don't hesitate to call a medical practitioner if your leg cramps become painful).

Who Should Absolutely Not Use the Pill

The Pill is dangerous for women with the following conditions or situations:*

- *Any disease or condition associated with excess blood clotting.* Bad varicose veins, thrombophlebitis (clots in veins, frequently in the leg), pulmonary embolism (blood clot that has traveled to the lung, usually from the leg).
- *Stroke, heart disease or impairment, coronary artery disease.*
- *Hepatitis or other liver diseases.* As it is the liver that metabolizes sex steroids (progesterone and estrogen), no one with liver disease should take the Pill until the disease has been cleared up. Use a good alternative method of contraception, because pregnancy can be a great strain on the liver.

- *Heavy smokers.* Women who smoke 20 or more cigarettes a day and are over 35 years of age run a statistically higher risk of stroke, heart attack, and other blood clotting problems when they take the Pill.
- *Breast-feeding and less than six weeks after giving birth.* The estrogen in combination pills may dry up the mother's supply of milk, especially if administered soon after she gives birth, or decrease the amounts of protein, fat, and calcium in the milk. Some estrogen will also come through in the milk. At present this is a controversial subject, because no one knows the long-term effects of this substance on children.
- *Pregnancy ended within the past three weeks.* There may be an increased risk of thromboembolism during this period.
- *Liver tumors or liver cancer, cancer of the breast (or history of cancer of the breast) or of the reproductive organs, pregnancy, previous cholestasis during pregnancy, migraine headaches with focal neurologic symptoms ("classic migraines"), moderate/severe hypertension (blood pressure 160/100 or more), diabetes with certain vascular complications and/ or have used the Pill for more than 20 years, prolonged immobilization after major surgery.*

Who Should Use the Pill Only As a Last Choice

For women in the following situations or conditions, the risks of the Pill generally outweigh its advantages. Before choosing the Pill, carefully consider using another method and discuss the potential risks with a medical practitioner; if you take the Pill you should be carefully monitored for problems. Consider how severe your condition is, how available and acceptable other methods of birth control are, and whether you have access to emergency followup service.†

- *Women over 40 with a second risk factor, such as diabetes or high blood pressure,* run a statistically higher risk of thromboembolism and other complications when taking the Pill. Because such risks also increase during pregnancy, women over 40 should consider a barrier method, IUD, or sterilization—tubal ligation for you or vasectomy for your partner—instead of the Pill if you want to avoid pregnancy.
- *Women over 50* have an increased risk for heart disease and cerebrovascular disease, and the estrogen in the Pill increases their risk.
- *Smokers,* especially women who smoke 15 or more cigarettes a day and are over 35 years old, run a statistically higher risk of stroke and heart

---

* These conditions are contraindications for combination pills. See p. 318 for information about contraindications for progestin-only pills.

† These conditions are contraindications for combination pills. See p. 318 for information about contraindications for progestin-only pills.

attack when they take the Pill (see table on p. 293).

- *Diabetes or gestational diabetes during a previous pregnancy.* Sugar metabolism is extensively altered in women who are taking the Pill. Progestin tends to bind the body's insulin and keep it out of circulation, which increases a diabetic woman's insulin requirement. If you have diabetes, practitioners recommend that you take a progestin-only pill with norethindrone-type progestin and have regular blood tests. Many doctors do advise diabetic women to take the Pill because pregnancy is especially hazardous to them.
- *Breast-feeding,* partially (at least three weeks), fully (at least three months), and especially when breast-feeding fully for six weeks to six months after giving birth, because of the effects of estrogens and progestins on breast milk (see p. 312).
- *Migraine headaches that start after the Pill is initiated; mild hypertension (but blood pressure under 160/100); Gilbert's disease; active gallbladder disease.*

Who Should Consider Another Method Before Choosing the Pill

There is some disagreement about how risky the following situations or conditions are for women who wish to take the Pill. According to the World Health Organization, the advantages of using the Pill generally outweigh the disadvantages for women with these conditions. Others believe that the Pill should be used infrequently. Since individual women's risks vary, the authors of this book recommend that you consider another method and be carefully screened by a practitioner before choosing the Pill. You need to have access to a provider whom you can contact if you suspect any adverse effects.*

- *Sickle-cell anemia or trait.* Black women planning to take the Pill should have a sickle cell test. If it is positive, you should discuss the hazards of taking the Pill, which include an increased risk of intravascular blood clotting.
- *Conditions likely to make it difficult for a woman to follow Pill instructions reliably.* Major psychiatric problems, alcoholism, or other substance abuse, homelessness, or cognitive impairment.
- *Cardiac or renal disease or a history of these diseases, family history of high lipid levels, death of a parent or sibling (especially a mother or sister) due to heart attack before age 50, history of pregnancy-related jaundice, elective major*

surgery planned in the next four weeks, long leg casts or major injury to the lower leg; DES daughter (see chapter 24, Selected Medical Practices, Problems, and Procedures).

It may be unwise for women with the following conditions to take the Pill: depression, chloasma, hair loss related to pregnancy, asthma, epilepsy, uterine fibromyomata, acne, varicose veins, hepatitis B or C.

Complications and Negative Effects

The Pill enters our bloodstream, travels through the body, and affects many tissues and organs, just as natural estrogens and progesterone do. However, the hormones in the Pill are synthetic and have exaggerated effects on some women.

Although there is an FDA-required package insert, health workers and doctors must carefully discuss with us the risks we take in choosing the Pill. Unfortunately, they themselves don't always know or take the time. Also, they sometimes believe that effects are psychosomatic and that telling us what might happen will influence our perceptions. This attitude is insulting and dangerous. Find out what the risks are before you get a prescription for the Pill.

Many of us experience no effects or only a few effects from using the Pill. Some women have pregnancy-like symptoms during the first three months, but after that they don't notice anything. Also, many women choose to put up with mild effects in exchange for the Pill's convenience and effectiveness. If you want to use it, try it for a few months to see how your body responds.

The Pill and Cardiovascular Disease— Heart Attack and Stroke

Cardiovascular disease (heart attacks, strokes, pulmonary embolisms, other clotting disorders) is responsible for most Pill-related deaths and serious complications. More and more studies show that the risk of circulatory disease is low for healthy women taking low-dose pills, who don't smoke, and who are younger than 40.[10] The risk of cardiovascular disease is not related to the length of time that you use the Pill and disappears when you stop taking it. There is controversy about third-generation pills; several studies show an increased risk of nonfatal blood clots in women using them.[11] See p. 312 for warning signals.

The Pill and High Blood Pressure

Fewer than 5% of women on the Pill will develop hypertension (abnormally high blood pressure) and thus be at greater risk for heart attack and stroke. The incidence of high blood pressure is higher for older women, and increases the longer women take the Pill. Women who develop hypertension should stop taking

---

* These conditions are contraindications for combination pills. See p. 318 for information about contraindications for progestin-only pills.

the Pill; within a few weeks of stopping, blood pressure usually returns to normal. Women with moderate or severe hypertension should not use the Pill; those with mild hypertension are strongly advised by practitioners to choose some other form of birth control.[12]

The Pill and Cancer

The relationship between Pill use and cervical cancer is not entirely clear. Several studies, however, suggest that there may be some connection between the Pill and certain forms of cervical cancer. Because of this, practitioners strongly recommend that women taking the Pill have a Pap smear every year.[13]

Researchers disagree about the relationship between the Pill and breast cancer. Most studies show that women who take the Pill are not more likely to develop breast cancer than women who do not. However, several recent studies indicate that women who start using the Pill before the age of 25 and use it for more than four years are at an increased risk of developing breast cancer before the age of 35.[14]

The Pill decreases women's risk of developing endometrial and ovarian cancer for at least ten years after they stop taking it. Most of the studies demonstrating this protection are about high-dosage pills, but low-dose pills also seem to protect women.[15]

Although early studies found an association between the Pill and skin cancer (melanoma), more recent ones show no evidence of such a relationship.

The Pill and Your Present or Future Children

There does *not* appear to be an increased risk of heart impairments, limb reductions, or other problems present at birth for babies whose mothers were taking the Pill while pregnant or became pregnant within three months of stopping the Pill.

Don't use combination pills while breast-feeding (see pp. 312 and 313 and also "Breast-feeding and Contraception" in chapter 21, Postpartum, p. 509).

Children who find pills and eat them may become nauseated. We do not know what harm this may cause. You should go to or call a medical facility if your child swallows more than a few pills.

Other Effects

Nausea or Vomiting

Nausea is the most common early negative effect of the Pill; vomiting is rare. The estrogen in the Pill may irritate your stomach lining or make you feel sick to your stomach, just like a pregnant woman whose body is getting used to the high levels of estrogen that the placenta puts into her blood. Nausea usually goes away after three months. Taking antacid tablets or taking the Pill with dinner usually gives relief, and so

does switching to a pill with 20 micrograms of estrogen (e.g., LoEstrin-1/20).

Breast Changes

Increased breast tenderness or fullness may occur, but it usually lasts for only the first three cycles. Switching to a pill with only 20 micrograms of estrogen can offer relief.

Changes in Menstrual Flow

Your periods will be lighter with most pills (estrogenic pills cause more normal flow). Occasionally your flow will be very slight or you will miss a period. If this happens and you have missed any pills or were late starting your pill pack, have a pregnancy test. Missing a period does not necessarily mean you are pregnant; sometimes it is due to taking pills for a long time or taking progestin-only pills. If you miss two periods in a row or are especially worried, consult a practitioner and have a pregnancy test.

Breakthrough Bleeding

This is vaginal bleeding, spotting, or staining between periods. If there isn't enough estrogen or progestin in the pills you are taking to support the lining of your uterus at a given point in your cycle, a little of the lining will slough off. (This may also occur if you miss a pill.) With combination pills, it usually happens in the first three cycles and often clears up after that, as your uterus gets used to the new levels of hormones. If breakthrough bleeding doesn't stop after the first three cycles, be sure you are taking a pill every day. If it continues, see a practitioner to find out whether you need to try a different brand or whether you may have another problem. With progestin-only pills, this is more common. Breakthrough bleeding is more common among women who use low-dose combination pills. Breakthrough bleeding does not mean that the Pill isn't working as a contraceptive.

Headaches

Occasionally women taking the Pill develop severe, recurrent, or persistent headaches or more severe migraines.

Migraines are painful, throbbing headaches that result from a problem in the circulation of blood to the brain. Because *migraines can be a warning signal for impending stroke,* women who have them should consider discontinuing the Pill, especially if they are getting worse.

Depression

Possibly one woman in four is more irritable, anxious, or depressed when taking the Pill. These symptoms often continue instead of improving with succeeding cycles. Switching to a lower-dose pill may help. Vitamin B$_6$ supplementation can also help (see "Nutrition and the Pill," p. 316). If you have serious depression, stop taking the Pill, but switch to another method right away if you still need contraception.

Change in Intensity of Sexual Desire and Response

Many women feel and act sexier as soon as their fear of pregnancy is removed. But some women taking progestin-dominant, low-dosage estrogen pills don't feel like making love, reach orgasm less easily, and complain about dryness and less sensation in the vulva.

Urinary Tract Infection (UTI)

While some reports indicate that women taking the Pill tend to have more infections of the bladder and urethra (the tube that leads urine out of your body), more recent studies do not support this finding. Frequent sex is more likely to be the cause of urinary tract infection.[16]

Vaginitis and Vaginal Discharge

Vaginitis is a vaginal inflammation that may be caused by trichomoniasis or by infection with a fungus, bacteria, or a virus. The Pill changes the normal vaginal environment. Its effect on vaginitis is unclear. Vaginitis is treatable, but if it persists you may have to stop taking the Pill. The Pill does not seem to make the vagina more susceptible to the yeast monilia *(Candida albicans).* Increased vaginal discharge is fairly common, can be due to estrogen, and does not necessarily indicate infection—though if it is bothering you, you should have it checked.

The Pill can cause cervical ectropion, a condition in which cells that usually grow inside the cervical canal grow on the part of the cervix that sticks out into the vagina. This condition may make a woman more vulnerable to chlamydia infection.

Cervical Dysplasia

This problem, growth of abnormal cells on the cervix, is more common in women using oral contraceptives than in women not using the Pill.

Skin Problems

The Pill may be associated with eczema, urticaria (hives or rashes), or, more rarely, chloasma, changes in skin pigmentation, sometimes described as "giant freckles" or pregnancy mask.

The progestin-dominant pill can cause or increase skin oiliness in some women. An estrogenic pill can decrease acne.

Gum Inflammation

The Pill, like pregnancy, can cause gum inflammation. Women taking the Pill should brush their teeth extra carefully, use dental floss regularly, and see a dentist every six months to a year.

Asthma and Epilepsy

The Pill can aggravate existing asthma and may change the response to medications taken to treat this condition. It does not appear to aggravate existing epilepsy, but medications taken to control seizures can make the Pill less effective by interacting with it. Women with these conditions should stay under close medical supervision.

Interactions with Other Medications

The Pill interacts with some other medications so that neither works as it should. This can make the Pill less effective (the antibiotic rifampin; anticonvulsants such as griseofulvin, carbamazepine, phenobarbital, and other barbiturates); or change the strength of the other medication (oral anticoagulants, antidepressants, benzodiazepine tranquilizers, beta-blockers, corticosteroids, gypoglycemics, methyldopa); or increase the serum concentration of estrogen in the Pill, changing a low-dose pill into a high-dose pill (1 gram or more of vitamin C). Consult with a practitioner before mixing the Pill with these other medications.[17]

Liver and Gallbladder Disease

The Pill is associated with an increased incidence of gallbladder disease and of liver tumors (both benign and malignant). Jaundice may be an early symptom of liver complications, so at the first sign of jaundice you should stop taking the Pill. Benign liver tumors are rare, but they can increase rapidly in size and may rupture spontaneously.

Virus Infections

A slightly higher incidence of bronchitis and viral illnesses among Pill users suggests that the Pill may affect your body's immunity. Some researchers believe that the Pill impairs the immunity of cells in the vagina, making women more susceptible to the human papillomavirus (HPV), which causes genital warts (see chapter 14, Sexually Transmitted Diseases).

Other Problems

The Pill also has been linked to certain other health problems, but there is no conclusive proof that it causes visual disturbances, including discomfort or corneal damage among contact lens wearers; pleurisy; arthritic symptoms (swelling of joints); ulcers in the mouth; bruising; lupus erythematosus, an autoimmune disease of unknown origin (see chapter 24, Selected

Medical Practices, Problems, and Procedures); abdominal cramping during the first three months; changes in thyroid function; photodermatitis (sunlight sensitivity with hypopigmentation); one form of hair loss, called alopecia; excessive hair growth (hirsutism); benign growths consisting of muscular tissue; autophonia, an ear or nasal disorder that causes increased resonance of the voice, breath sounds, and so on. Nevertheless, if you encounter any of these problems, it might be connected with taking the Pill.

Beneficial Effects

Besides greater freedom from pregnancy, the Pill has several beneficial effects. Women taking it have shorter menstrual periods with less bleeding and cramping. Premenstrual tension tends to decrease. Iron-deficiency anemia is less likely, probably because of decreased menstrual flow. Benign breast growths are less frequent. Acne clears up for some women. The Pill also appears to protect against ovarian and endometrial cancer, some kinds of PID, and ectopic pregnancy. The Pill may help prevent rheumatoid arthritis and functional ovarian cysts (high-dose estrogen combination pills protected against them, but it's not clear whether low-dose pills have the same effect). Its effect on bone density remains controversial, but three recent reports suggest that long-term pill-users may have higher bone-mineral density.

Nutrition and the Pill

The Pill alters the nutritional requirements of women who take it, which may contribute to some of the complications and negative effects. Pill use has been linked to increased requirements for vitamins C, B_2 (riboflavin), B_{12}, and especially B_6 (pyridoxine) and folic acid (folate or folacin). Women who face the greatest nutritional risks are teenagers, low-income women who may lack access to nutritious foods, women recovering from a recent illness or surgery or who have just given birth, and women who have taken brands with moderate to high estrogen levels for two years or more. Because metabolic changes occur within the first few months after you begin the Pill, it is a good idea to have a physical exam and blood tests after you have used it for six months and if you suspect you have any particular deficiencies.

Studies show that women taking the Pill may have impaired glucose tolerance. This means that their carbohydrate metabolism is adversely affected, resulting in weight gain and/or elevated glucose and insulin levels (ranging from mild to diabetic). These alterations are less likely to occur with low-dose pills.

While taking the Pill, try to maintain a healthy nutritional balance:

1. Eat wholesome foods, especially those containing complex carbohydrates.

2. Reduce sugar intake.

3. Take vitamins, especially vitamin B-complex (but less than 25 to 50 milligrams of vitamin B_6 per day), vitamin C supplements (but less than 1,000 milligrams per day), and folic acid.

Doing the same thing for a few months after you stop taking the Pill is also a good idea, especially if you plan to become pregnant. A higher than average number of women who conceived within four months after discontinuing the Pill developed folic acid and vitamin B_6 deficiencies during pregnancy.

Water Metabolism and Weight

The Pill alters water metabolism. Estrogen can cause weight gain due to increased breast, hip, or thigh tissue. Both the estrogen and progestin in pills can cause fluid retention, a temporary (and usually cyclic) effect that usually begins in the first month as a result of increased sodium. You may experience swollen ankles, breast tenderness, discomfort with contact lenses, or a weight gain of up to five pounds. You can control water retention by changing to a pill with lower amounts of progestin or estrogen or reducing your salt intake moderately. (Diuretics are risky, so discontinue Pill use if the above methods do not work.)

Progestin-dominant pills (Ortho-Novum, Norlestrin, Ovral) can cause appetite increase and permanent weight gain because of the buildup of protein in muscular tissue. If you want to gain weight, this is helpful. Pill-related depression may also lead to increased appetite and weight gain.

How to Get the Pill

In the U.S., you need a prescription from a health care practitioner in order to get the Pill. Don't borrow pills from a friend. You do not necessarily need a complete physical exam to start taking the pill. However, as we have seen, certain physical conditions make taking birth control pills very dangerous, *so it is in your vital interest to have a careful exam before taking pills*. Be sure a practitioner checks your blood pressure and gives you an internal pelvic exam, breast exam, and Pap smear. She or he should ask you questions about your medical history of breast cancer, blood clots, diabetes, and migraines, as well as any medications you take. If you smoke, it's very important to discuss this too. If you were born between 1945 and 1970, find out whether your mother took DES while she was pregnant with you. If so, you should have a colposcopy test because you might have adenosis, a condition that the Pill can aggravate (see the section on DES in chapter 24, Selected Medical Practices, Problems, and Procedures). *Too many people prescribe and use birth control pills hurriedly; make sure you are carefully checked for each one of the contraindications.* When you are taking the Pill, you should have a checkup once a year.

How to Use the Pill

Combination pills usually come in packets of 28 pills, but sometimes in packets of 21. With 28-day pills, which give you 21 hormone pills followed by seven different-colored placebos (without drugs), you take one pill a day with no pause between packets. You will have your period during the time that you are taking the seven different-colored pills. The 28-day pill is good if you feel you would have trouble remembering the on-and-off schedule of the 21-day pill. With the 21-day pills, you take one pill a day for 21 days and then stop for seven days, during which time you will menstruate. There is no difference in the effects on your body between 28-day and 21-day pills.

You have a choice about when to start taking your first package of pills. If you take the first pill on the first Sunday after your menstrual period begins, you need to use a backup method of birth control for the first week you are using the Pill. If you take the first pill on the first day of your menstrual period, you do not need to use a backup method of birth control. Take one pill at approximately the same time each day. If you feel nausea, take the pill with a meal or after a snack at bedtime.

Here is an almost foolproof schedule: Take a pill at bedtime, check the packet each morning to make sure you've taken a pill the night before, and carry a spare packet of pills with you in case you get caught away from home or lose pills. Read the directions carefully.

If you are taking antibiotics for an acute infection, or if you get sick and have vomiting or diarrhea, it's a good idea to use another birth control method for the rest of the cycle to be safe.

If You Forget a Pill

The more hormone pills you miss, the greater your risk of becoming pregnant. If you miss only one, you do not need to use a backup birth control method. Take the forgotten pill as soon as you remember it, and take the next pill at its appointed time, even if this means taking two pills in one day. If you miss two or more pills, use an additional method (male or female condom, foam) and follow the instructions given in the patient package insert that is included with your pill package, and/or check with a health care practitioner.

You may miss a period after missing one or more hormone pills; this is normal. If you miss two menstrual periods in a row, you should have a pregnancy test because you might be pregnant.

Responsibility

Birth control pills are primarily the woman's responsibility. You see the doctor, get examined, remember to take them, feel the effects, and run the risks. It's important to understand fully both the risks and benefits as well as how to take the pills correctly. It helps to involve your partner as much as possible in helping you remember, using condoms to prevent sexually transmitted diseases, and using condoms or another backup method if you miss two or more pills.

Advantages

You have almost complete protection against unwanted pregnancy.

Regularity of menstrual cycles—a period every 28 days.

About 50% reduction in risk of PID.

Lighter flow during periods. This effect pleases most women and bothers some.

Relief of premenstrual tension.

Fewer menstrual cramps or none at all.

An estrogenic pill will clear up acne for some women. (The FDA recently approved Tri-cyclen, a triphasic oral contraceptive, to treat acne.)

You may enjoy sex more because the fear of pregnancy is gone.

Taking the Pill has no immediate physical relationship to lovemaking, which is especially relaxing if you are just starting to have intercourse and have a lot to learn about your body and a man's. Later on, when you are more comfortable with sex and more able to communicate openly with your partner(s), the interruptions involved in using a diaphragm or foam and condoms may not seem so prohibitive.

Disadvantages

Most of the disadvantages have been described under the section on effects. The only one to add is that you do have to remember to take a pill every day. Some women are forgetful or live lives that are too chaotic for them to remember to do so (pills are more likely to be missed on Friday and Saturday). Younger women who live at home and feel a need to hide their pills from their parents sometimes leave them behind or are unable to take them on time.

Differences Among the Several Brands

How do you and your practitioner determine which pill you should take? Be aware that different pills contain different kinds, strengths, and quantities of synthetic estrogen and progesterone. Low-dosage pills with less than 50 micrograms of estrogen are associated with a significantly lower incidence of serious negative effects than the older, high-dose pills, so practitioners have been prescribing pills with lower and lower doses of estrogen. Today, they typically begin by prescribing pills with 35 micrograms of estrogen or less.

Some monophasic combination pills containing 35 micrograms or less of estrogen are Loestrin 1/20, Loestrin 1.5/30, Lo/Ovral, Nordette, Levlon, Brevicon, Modicon, Ovcon-35, Norinyl 1 + 35, Ortho-Novum 1/35, Demulen 35, Genora, Nelova, and Ortho-Cyclen.

Third-generation monophasic pills (Desogen, Ortho-Cept 21) contain 30 micrograms of estrogen. The lowest-dose monophasic pills are Loestrin 1/20; these tend to produce more spotting between periods. Biphasic or triphasic combination pills with 35 micrograms of estrogen are Ortho-Novum 10/11, Ortho-Novum 7/7/7, Tri-Norinyl, Tri-Levlen, Triphasil, Ortho Tri-Cyclen, and Nelova 10/11.

The effects of a particular pill are related to the amount and potency of the progestin relative to the estrogen in that pill. The low-dose pills producing the most androgenic (masculinizing) effects—for example, hairiness, acne, and permanent weight gain—contain norgestrel (Nordette, Lo/Ovral, Levlen). Low-dose pills producing the least androgenic effects contain norethindrone (Ovcon-35, Modicon, Brevicon, Genora, Nelova). Third-generation pills were developed to reduce androgenic effects even further, as well as to reduce headache, nausea, breakthrough bleeding, and breast tenderness. These pills (Desogen, Ortho-Cept 21) have recently been associated with an increased risk of nonfatal blood clots.

Although the compounds vary in strength, the effectiveness of the actual dose is similar for all. Variations among women, and in a particular woman from cycle to cycle, are more important than the dosage. Also, each woman's body has its own normal estrogen and progesterone levels. You and your medical practitioner may want to experiment with different brands to minimize undesirable effects.

Progestin-Only Pills

Progestin-only pills are sometimes called minipills, but this term will not be used here in order to avoid confusion with the low-dose estrogen combination pill and with a pill that was taken off the market several years ago. Fewer than 1% of all U.S. women taking birth control pills take progestin-only pills.

Description

These pills contain small doses of the same progestins available in combination pills. Micronor and Nor-Q-D each provide 0.35 milligram of norethindrone, and Ovrette provides 0.075 milligram of norgestrel. They contain no estrogen. You take one a day continuously, starting on day 1 of your period, at the same time each day (particularly important), without stopping during your period, which may come irregularly.

Progesterone changes cervical fluid so that it blocks sperm, inhibits the egg's movement through the tubes, partially inhibits the sperm's ability to join with the egg, and partially inhibits implantation. You may feel safer taking these pills, knowing that they have no estrogen and a very small dose of progestin and that they may have about the same rate of effectiveness as an IUD. On the other hand, the irregular cycles may get you down, or you may not wish to be one of the testers of a very new pill.

Effectiveness

The lowest expected pregnancy rate is 1 to 1.25%, higher than that of the combination pill. The typical failure rate is 5.0%. The pregnancy rate may be lower for women who switch from the combination pill to the progestin-only pill than it is for women who have never taken the combination pill.

Contraindications

Women with the following conditions should *absolutely not take* progestin-only pills: pregnancy, unexplained vaginal bleeding, breast cancer. Women with the following conditions should use progestin-only pills only as a *last choice:* hepatitis, jaundice, cirrhosis, benign or malignant liver tumors, functional ovarian cysts, cardiovascular complications, history of breast cancer, women who are breast-feeding, women who are unable to take pills consistently and correctly. The progestin-only pill interacts with some medications (rifampin and most antiseizure medications) and becomes less effective. If you are taking another medication, consult with a health care practitioner before starting progestin-only pills.

Possible Effects

The most common complaint of women using progestin-only pills is irregular bleeding: spotting between periods and very irregular menstrual periods (amount and duration of flow and length of cycle); another is breast discomfort. There is an increased risk of ectopic pregnancy and functional ovarian cysts.

NORPLANT

Description

Norplant is a long-lasting hormonal contraceptive implant that has been marketed in the U.S. since 1990. In 1994, more than three million women from 26 countries around the world were using Norplant, including 900,000 U.S. women. Although Norplant was quickly adopted by many women in many countries (including the U.S.), use of this birth control method has declined dramatically. Requests for removal have increased, even from women who had been satisfied with the method.

Norplant consists of six match-size flexible nonbiodegradable Silastic rubber capsules, each containing the synthetic progestin levonorgestrel, which is present in some birth control pills. They are inserted in the fleshy part of a woman's upper arm, just under the skin, by a qualified, specially trained practitioner. The hormone is released slowly through the walls of the capsules until they are removed. The capsules can be felt, and sometimes noticed, as ridges or bumps. Norplant is designed to last for up to five years.

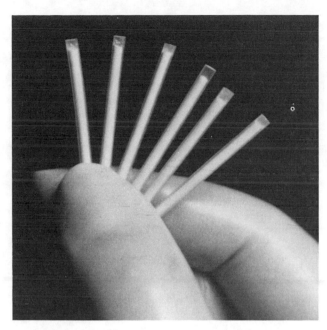

A set of six Norplant capsules/The Population Council

How Norplant Works

This progestin-only contraceptive method works in three ways: by inhibiting ovulation (so eggs are not released by the ovaries), by thickening and decreasing the amount of cervical fluid (which impedes sperm activity and prevents it from entering the cervix), and by endometrial thinning (making the lining of the uterus thinner so that implantation is prevented).

Norplant begins working within 24 hours of insertion and provides highly effective protection from pregnancy for up to five years. After that, effectiveness is significantly reduced, and there is an increased risk of ectopic pregnancy, so the capsules must be removed after five years. A new set can be implanted or another birth control method chosen if a woman still wants to avoid pregnancy.

Effectiveness

Norplant is extremely effective. The failure rate is 0.05% in the first year of use, 0.5% for the second year, 1.2% for the third year, and 1.6% for the fourth year, and 0.4% for the fifth year. The overall failure rate for five years of continuous use is 3.7%. Today, the company that manufactures Norplant (Leiras) produces only capsules made with soft tubing, and these appear to have a lower failure rate for all women than the earlier hard-tube ones. Women weighing more than 154 lbs. had a higher failure rate with the old capsules, but with the new ones there's less of a difference.[18]

Reduced Norplant effectiveness has been reported for women who metabolize steroids rapidly: those using antiseizure drugs such as phenytoin (Dilantin), carbamazepine, or phenobarbital or those taking rifampicin. If you take any prescription drugs, ask your health care provider for any new information about the possibility of drug interactions.

Reversibility

Norplant can be removed at any time, but cost factors and the availability of a trained practitioner may determine how freely a woman can make this choice. The pregnancy rates for women who have Norplant removed (and do not use any other method of contraception) are comparable to the pregnancy rates of women using no contraception. Most women begin ovulating and menstruating again during the first month after Norplant is removed.

Safety and Possible Problems

The hormone found in Norplant has been used in combined oral contraceptives for more than 20 years. Although the accumulated data are still insufficient to enable detection of rare or long-term adverse effects, the FDA has received a small number of reports of stroke, thrombocytopenia and thrombotic thrombocytopenia purpura (blood disorders in which the cells responsible for clotting are reduced, causing excessive bleeding and bruising), and pseudotumor cerebri (swelling inside the skull) in women using Norplant. The literature distributed with Norplant now includes a discussion of these reported adverse reactions. In spite of such reports, the FDA still affirms the safety and effectiveness of the hormone levonorgestrel for long-term contraception and the safety of the capsules used in Norplant. A patient acknowledgment form introduced in 1995 enables a woman to certify that she has been given information and the opportunity for thorough discussion about Norplant before it is inserted. (See p. 322 for information about the possible coercive use of Norplant, under "Disadvantages.")

In general, progestin-based birth control methods are not the first choice for breast-feeding women compared with nonhormonal methods. Some nursing mothers do use Norplant, but not earlier than six weeks after childbirth. So far, studies have shown no major effects on the growth or health of infants whose mothers used Norplant beginning six weeks after childbirth. (In contrast, estrogen-based contraceptives should never be used by nursing mothers.)

Studies show no increased risk of disabilities at birth in infants born to women who have used birth control pills during pregnancy, and the risk seems to be no different with Norplant use. However, if you become pregnant while using Norplant, you should have your implants removed if you want to continue the pregnancy. If you become pregnant and choose to have an abortion, discuss Norplant removal with your practitioner.

Norplant does affect thyroid and adrenal functioning, lipid and lipoprotein metabolism, and blood sugar level, as do oral contraceptives (the Pill). Because most birth control pills contain four to five times the level of progestin than is present in Norplant, it is assumed that progestin-related problems would be fewer with Norplant, which presents the lowest possible exposure to a hormone of any hormonal-based method.

Because the long-term safety of Norplant had not been established, the National Women's Health Network opposed Norplant's approval by the FDA in 1990. In 1994, nearly 200 lawsuits were filed against Norplant's U.S. distributor, Wyeth-Ayerst, 46 of them class action suits. The lawsuits are legitimate attempts by injured women to gain compensation for a variety of problems caused by the implant, ranging from scarring and emotional distress attributed to difficulties with removal to claims of autoimmune disorders resulting from exposure to the silicone in the implant's shell.

Who Shouldn't Use Norplant

Women should not use Norplant if they have or have had blood-clotting problems; a history of blood clots, heart attack, or stroke; liver disease; or breast cancer (confirmed or suspected). With the exception of breast cancer, all of these health conditions affect more women of color than white women. In addition, women who suspect they may be pregnant, who are breast-feeding infants younger than six weeks, or who have undiagnosed abnormal vaginal bleeding should not use Norplant, nor should women who are taking antiseizure medications or the antibiotic rifampin/rifampicin. Because it is not known whether progestin-only contraceptives, such as Norplant, increase the risk of serious cardiovascular problems for cigarette smokers, it is advisable for women smokers to avoid Norplant or quit smoking before using it.

Conditions That May Make Norplant a Riskier Choice

Women should check in regularly with their healthcare provider if they choose to use Norplant and have any of the following conditions: history of irregular menstrual periods; diabetes; high levels of cholesterol; migraines or other headaches; gallbladder, heart, or kidney disease; heart lesions; chest pain due to diagnosed heart disease; history of acne becoming worse; or an allergic reaction while using combination birth control pills.

How to Get Norplant

Many doctors, nurse-practitioners and family-planning clinics now offer Norplant. Make sure you get Norplant from someone who has had special training in how to insert the capsules, because improper insertion can make removal difficult. Ask your provider if he or she has attended a training course for insertion and removal of the implants; if not, obtain referral to someone who has. Get as much information as possible beforehand, and make sure that removal

will be available on demand and for a fee you can afford.

Norplant should be inserted within seven days after a woman's period begins (to ensure she is not pregnant) and under sterile conditions (to avoid the possibility of infection). A local anesthetic is injected into the arm and may cause some initial pain. After a small incision is made, the six small capsules are placed one at a time through this incision, just under the skin and in a fan shape. The procedure, done in a clinic or office, should take only 10 to 15 minutes but may take longer in cases when there are problems. The incision is covered with a protective bandage that can be removed after a few days. Discoloration, bruising, and swelling may occur in the implant area for several days.

When in place, Norplant should not cause pain or discomfort for more than a day or two. If it hurts, see your Norplant provider to make sure you don't have an infection.

Cost

Norplant is manufactured by Leiras Oy Pharmaceuticals in Finland and distributed in the U.S. by Wyeth-Ayerst, a private pharmaceutical company. In the U.S., implant and insertion materials are sold to most health care providers for $365 to $375. The total cost of Norplant, including counseling, insertion, removal, and followup, is between $615 and $715. More than 50 major HMOs and 1,000 other insurance plans in the U.S. cover part or all of the cost. Women with very low income and no private insurance might get it through Medicaid, the federal and state government program that reimburses health care practitioners for services rendered to eligible women. All 50 states now cover Norplant costs for women receiving Medicaid.*

Prices for removal can be much higher. Some providers charge $150 for each capsule (that's $900 to remove all six). In addition, some states have a "reversal of intent" law, which means that when the cost of implantation is covered by Medicaid, the cost of removal will be covered by Medicaid only if there is a medical reason for removing it. We know of several women who were uncomfortable after having Norplant inserted, but because their doctors did not think their discomfort was serious enough to be a "medical reason," these women could not get Medicaid coverage for removing the Norplant.

Despite many pleas to adopt a public-sector price for family planning clinics that serve low-income women, Wyeth-Ayerst never did so. However, the company established the Norplant Foundation, which

---

* Medicaid coverage for Norplant in all 50 states is a mixed blessing. It gives more low-income women access to Norplant, but it also raises the possibility of further abuse. According to a recent Planned Parenthood national survey, 12% of all clients at its clinics are Medicaid recipients, but 95% or more of the women getting Norplant at some of these clinics are Medicaid recipients.

reimburses doctors and clinics for Norplant given to a limited number of low-income women. Free Norplant kits are more difficult to obtain for rural women (where physicians are more scarce) and for women living in areas where physicians are limited to only ten free kits per year. Some women lose insurance coverage or Medicaid eligibility after Norplant is inserted, and must then pay a removal fee (from $150 to $200), which they often cannot afford.

The U.S. Agency for International Development (USAID) and the United Nations Population Fund (UNFPA) were able to purchase Norplant for only $23 per set from the manufacturer for use in so-called developing countries. Leiras was able to obtain the marketing rights for Norplant outside the U.S. in part because of its agreement with the Population Council, the developers of the method, to offer a public-sector price.

Averaged over five years, the annual cost of Norplant ranges from $125 to $150. Buying 13 cycles of the Pill, including one gynecological visit, amounts to a total annual cost of almost $300, or close to $1,500 over a five-year period. However, the cost of Norplant remains the same whether it is used for a few months or for a full five years, since most of the implant's final cost (implant and insertion) is billed at the time the method is purchased, not spread over a long period of use. Therefore, women who want birth control for only one year probably should not use Norplant, although there are times when unexpected circumstances cause a woman to stop using it.

An additional cost for women who experience unpredictable bleeding with Norplant (see "Complications and Negative Effects," at right) is the expense of panty liners or sanitary pads.

Removal

Norplant capsules should be removed at the end of five years, although they can be removed earlier at your request.

The key to successful removal is proper insertion. When the capsules become embedded in deeper tissue, they are harder and more painful to remove. Some women develop more scar tissue around the capsules than others, particularly African-American women, who tend to form keloids.

Removal is more difficult than insertion. Although removal can be a simple process taking no more than 20 to 30 minutes, complications do occur in rare cases. These complications can include a painful, difficult operation lasting two hours or more; serious bruising; scarring; and nerve damage. Sometimes, one or more of the capsules cannot be removed at the first attempt, requiring a return visit. Make sure your provider is trained in performing removals; if not, ask to be referred to a trained provider.

After removal, a woman should keep the area clean, dry, and bandaged for at least several days to avoid the possibility of infection. Bruises may appear, but usually they go away completely.

Care

No special care is necessary for Norplant, but you should not wet, bump, or strain the area for a few days after Norplant has been inserted.

Complications and Negative Effects

Irregular bleeding. The most common problem associated with Norplant is erratic, unpredictable bleeding, which sometimes requires frequent use of menstrual pads. In the first year of use, more than 80% of Norplant users report some irregularity in menstruation, usually amenorrhea (no bleeding), very light bleeding, or excessive bleeding (but rarely enough blood loss to produce anemia). Bleeding irregularities usually decrease during the first year of use. For many women, their periods return on a regular basis. If regular periods do return and then you miss a period, you should get a pregnancy test. Irregular bleeding is the most common reason given for discontinuing Norplant use.

Some people who are uncomfortable having intercourse when the woman has menstrual bleeding find that Norplant interferes with their sex life. You should consider this likely inconvenience when deciding whether to try Norplant.

Some clinics recommend trying a month or two of the progestin-only pill (see "Progestin-Only Pills," p. 318) before using Norplant. If you have irregular bleeding and find it too disruptive, then Norplant might be a poor choice for you.

Headaches, weight changes, and depression are common effects of Norplant. (In the U.S., weight gain is far more common than weight loss.) Usually these effects are not severe, but sometimes they are disruptive, and they are the second most frequently cited reasons why some women seek Norplant removal. Nervousness, acne, and hair loss associated with Norplant use can also be bothersome enough for women to want Norplant removed. Nausea and dizziness have also been reported by women using the implant.

Functional ovarian cysts. Norplant use increases the risk of functional ovarian cysts, which are usually symptom-free but may cause lower abdominal pain. These cysts usually go away spontaneously, but they do require surgery on rare occasions and can be a reason to have Norplant removed.

When to Seek Help

Women using Norplant should get medical attention if they experience any of the following problems: severe lower abdominal pain (a possible sign of ectopic pregnancy), heavy vaginal bleeding, arm pain, pus or bleeding at the insertion site, expulsion of an implant (when the implant comes out—very rare), delayed menstrual period after a long interval of regular periods, migraine headaches, repeated very painful headaches, or blurred vision.

Although pregnancy is rare among Norplant users, when it does occur, it is an ectopic pregnancy (outside the uterus) about 17% of the time. However, the rate of ectopic pregnancy has been much lower than the rate estimated for women in the U.S. who use no contraception. Ectopic pregnancy rates for Norplant users may be higher for heavier women, and may increase the longer a woman has Norplant in place. Also, the rate of ectopic pregnancies may differ substantially for women in different countries.

Advantages

Norplant is highly effective, long-lasting, and easily reversible (assuming that removal is problem-free), doesn't interrupt lovemaking, and enables women to avoid the negative effects of estrogen, which is found in all combination birth control pills. It also doesn't require a woman to do anything on a regular basis (like remember to take a pill). For some women, decreased menstrual bleeding is an advantage as well.

For women who do not want to have any more children, Norplant offers an important alternative to sterilization.

Disadvantages

The complications and negative effects described earlier are, of course, possible disadvantages.

Although Norplant is highly effective at preventing pregnancy, *it does not protect against any STDs, including HIV.*

Some have expressed concern that Norplant may trigger even further keloid formation (excessive growth of scar tissue on the skin) in African-American women and women of Mediterranean descent. This needs to be studied more.

Norplant's most serious disadvantage may be that (like the IUD and long-term injectable contraceptives) it is not fully in the control of the woman who uses it. Like the IUD, Norplant must be inserted and removed by a trained practitioner. This makes Norplant prone to abuse. It has been studied and used inappropriately, coercively, and even punitively.

Many cases have been documented of women who sought and were unable to obtain removal of Norplant. For example, in Bangladesh, women suffering from the side effects of Norplant were told that the implant was not removable. In the U.S., South Dakota law states that if Medicaid pays for insertion of Norplant it will not pay for removal unless there is a medical reason to do so. Even when removal is not refused, personnel trained in the removal technique are sometimes simply not available.

Dependence on a provider facilitates misuse in other ways. It can be subtle: Researchers or health care providers may withhold information about other methods of birth control and/or minimize the health risks of Norplant use. It can be more obvious: In the U.S., specific groups of women have been targeted for Norplant use in a coercive environment. Low-income women receiving public assistance have sometimes "chosen" Norplant over other methods of birth control to remain eligible for other welfare benefits or services. Norplant has been used as a condition of parole; all of the first four women receiving parole under these conditions were welfare recipients, and three of them were women of color. In 1994, six women who were convicted of child abuse or child abandonment were given the "choice" between using Norplant or serving several years in prison. This type of punishment and reproductive coercion resembles previous attempts in U.S. history to impose birth control or sterilization on women of color and low-income women.

The Brazilian Feminist Network for Reproductive Rights and Health began an international campaign against Norplant in 1994. The campaign grew in response to Norplant's introduction in Latin American countries, and in recognition of its disproportionate use in the southern hemisphere, where poverty is more widespread. In low-income communities, people tend to be less healthy generally and to have less access to medical services than in communities with more resources, so Norplant can cause greater damage to women's health. This underscores the importance of having an adequate system of family planning or health care services in order that Norplant can be provided appropriately.

Responsibility

A woman bears the total responsibility for Norplant use. However, men can take responsibility for preventing sexually transmitted diseases (including HIV) by using condoms.

A woman must remember to have Norplant removed after five years, if not sooner. Experience in many countries already demonstrates that some women forget to have it removed. In our mobile society, it may be difficult for clinics and other providers to follow up women after five years to remind them when it's time to have Norplant removed.

Every Norplant user should be given a card with the date of insertion and the recommended removal date. She should keep this card with her medical records. Her practitioner should also note these dates on her medical records kept in the office or clinic.

DEPO-PROVERA AND OTHER INJECTABLE CONTRACEPTIVES

Depot-medroxyprogesterone acetate (DMPA), better known as Depo-Provera, Depo, or "the shot," was approved by the FDA in 1992 for use in the U.S. as a progestin-only hormonal contraceptive.* It is administered as a deep intramuscular injection of 150 mg

---

* Other injectables, which are not marketed in the U.S. include NE10 (norethindrone enanthate or Noristerat) effective for two months, and Cyclofem and Mesigyna, both effective for one month. NET En, like DMPA, is a progestin-only injectable, while once-a-month injectables contain both progestin and estrogen.

every three months, but it actually provides up to 14 weeks of protection. Before 1992, DMPA was on the market for several other approved uses (for example, the treatment of uterine cancer).* Today, manufactured and distributed by the Upjohn Company, it is available in more than 90 countries and is used by an estimated 30 million women worldwide.

DMPA works by preventing ovulation. It also thickens cervical fluid, making a barrier to sperm. In the first year of use, it has a failure rate of 0.3%.

To use DMPA for birth control, have your first injection within a week after your menstrual period begins; it starts protecting you against pregnancy immediately. If you want to continue using DMPA for birth control, you must have a shot every three months.

Complications and Negative Effects

Like Norplant, the most common side effect of DMPA is an altered menstrual pattern: very heavy periods, irregular periods, or no periods at all (amenorrhea). About half of women using DMPA for a year report amenorrhea, and the longer a woman uses it, the greater the likelihood of amenorrhea. Menstrual disturbance is the most common reason for discontinuing its use.

Other side effects include weight gain, dizziness, headaches, depression, acne, moodiness, abdominal discomfort, decreased libido, hair loss, anxiety, breast tenderness, and backache. These effects may continue up to six to eight months after a woman's last injection.

According to several U.S. studies, DMPA does not increase the overall relative risk of breast cancer. However, a New Zealand study indicated that the risk of breast cancer is highest among women who use DMPA for more than six years. That study also suggests that DMPA may stimulate the growth of preexisting breast tumors in young women. On the basis of available data, the link between DMPA and breast cancer remains uncertain.

Using DMPA does not appear to increase the risk of liver, ovarian, or invasive cervical cancer, and may lower the risk of endometrial cancer. Although studies have not shown adverse effects on nursing infants, nonhormonal contraception is considered a safer alternative for women who breast-feed.

Reversibility

Unlike Norplant or progestin-only pills, DMPA can lead to delays in the return of fertility. A woman may have to wait an average of six months to a year to become pregnant after stopping DMPA because it has an extended effect on ovulation. Most women conceive within a year after their last injection.

* The practice of prescribing drugs for nonapproved uses is legal, but physicians who do this are supposed to obtain signed consent forms demonstrating that the drug's unapproved status, as well as potential risks, are known to the woman.

Cost

Upjohn provides single-dose disposable syringes to clinicians for $29.50. Including the cost of a gynecological visit, you are likely to be charged about $50 per injection (or $200 per year). The annual cost of using DMPA is similar to the cost of using birth control pills.

Advantages

DMPA is reversible, highly effective, can be used without a partner's knowledge or consent, does not interfere with lovemaking, and requires minimal responsibility on the part of the user (only a visit to a practitioner every three months for another injection). It reduces a woman's risk of ectopic pregnancy and, unlike birth control pills and Norplant, has demonstrated no interaction with antibiotics or enzyme-inducing drugs. DMPA decreases the frequency of seizures in women with seizure disorders, and the frequency of sickle-cell crises in women with sickle-cell disease.[19]

Disadvantages

DMPA has many hormone-related negative effects (see "Complications and Negative Effects," at left).

This is a provider-dependent method that is not in the control of the user. It leaves room for potential manipulation or coercion of women. Indeed, this has been documented—particularly among women of color, women with low incomes, young women said to exhibit "out-of-control behavior," and women who have physical disabilities or cognitive impairments. Doctors who assume that these women are not capable of complying with other birth control methods have identified them as "ideal acceptors," encouraging them to use DMPA and other long-acting methods instead of taking the time to explore different options. For example, in the U.S., DMPA was often given to African-American, Native American, and cognitively impaired women as a contraceptive before the FDA approved it for that purpose. One large Depo-Provera study at Grady Memorial Hospital in Atlanta (1967–1978) violated the rights of thousands of low-income women who were given this drug without informed consent or followup.

Depo-Provera provides no protection against STDs, including HIV. Some researchers suggest that the prolonged or irregular bleeding that may occur with DMPA may facilitate STD transmission, including HIV transmission.

Several small studies have shown that women who use DMPA are more likely to lose bone, or fail to build bone, depending on their age. Although bone mass can usually be regained if hormone use is stopped before menopause, it is possible that significant loss could occur, increasing the risk of fractures in old age. Women under the age of 16 probably should not use DMPA because loss of bone mass at this age may increase the risk of osteoporosis after menopause.

DMPA makes high-density lipoprotein (HDL, or "good" cholesterol) levels fall significantly. Allergic reactions (anaphylactic and anaphylactoid) may occur immediately following DMPA injections, but these severe reactions are rare.

Women Who Should Not Use Depo-Provera

Women with the following conditions should not use DMPA: known or suspected pregnancy, unexplained vaginal bleeding in the past three years, severe or acute liver disease or liver tumors, severe gallbladder disease, past or current breast cancer, severe high blood pressure, heart disease, diabetes, hepatitis. Aminoglutethimide (Cytadren), a drug used by people with Cushing's syndrome, decreases Depo's effectiveness. Women who are concerned about weight gain are not advised to take DMPA.

The Controversy

Many women's health activists have opposed the widespread use of DMPA because of concerns about its long-term health effects and its potential for being used coercively. The National Women's Health Network gave testimony in 1983 at a special FDA Board of Inquiry hearing, opposing the approval of DMPA for contraceptive use in the United States.* After the FDA approved it in 1992, several women's health organizations, including the National Latina Health Organization, the Native American Women's Health Education Resource Center, and the National Women's Health Network, documented the disproportionate use of DMPA in low-income women and women of color. They called for a moratorium on its use, and began to distribute an informed consent protocol that would provide consistent and up-to-date information about this contraceptive (contact the National Women's Health Network for a copy—see chapter 27 Resources).

Quickly and easily administered, injections may be attractive to both providers and users. However, for those of us who are not informed about DMPA and who are considered by providers as "ideal acceptors" for DMPA, it may not be in our best interests to have it widely available. Although we can stop using other methods immediately when we have problems, DMPA must remain in our system for at least several months until our body fully metabolizes it. Until we can be sure that true informed consent for all women will be the rule rather than the exception, misuse of DMPA and similar methods that a woman cannot discontinue by herself represent a serious threat to those women already most vulnerable to abuse.

* In mid-1984, this board recommended denying approval for contraceptive use of DMPA. Upjohn then withdrew its application, but reapplied in 1992 and obtained FDA approval to market DMPA for birth control.

EMERGENCY CONTRACEPTION AFTER UNPROTECTED INTERCOURSE

Emergency contraception (called the morning-after pill in previous editions) may be needed after unprotected intercourse by women who do not use any birth control because they forget to, choose not to, or do not have access to birth control; whose barrier method of contraception hasn't worked properly; or who are raped or sexually assaulted.

In previous editions of this book, we raised serious questions about the safety and effectiveness of various morning-after pills. Poorly designed studies with poor followup of women enrolled in them led us to question the claims made about the effects of these methods. We now believe that emergency contraceptive combination pills should be widely available and that information about them should be widely circulated. Our position has changed because new careful studies support the safety and effectiveness of this method of emergency contraception. For free information about preventing pregnancy after unprotected sex and to obtain names and telephone numbers of health care professionals in your area who can provide emergency contraception, call the Emergency Contraception Hotline: (800) 584-9911.

One of the biggest barriers to emergency contraception is ignorance. Most women and many providers do not know that it is available and works effectively. Combination pills, progestin-only pills, and copper IUDs are all marketed for birth control, but in many countries (including the U.S.) they have not been advertised or marketed for emergency contraception. In 1997, the FDA finally concluded that ordinary birth-control pills were safe and effective for emergency contraception and published the proper doses for six brands, paving the way for manufacturers to market them as "morning-after" pills.

The likelihood of becoming pregnant after a single act of unprotected intercourse is low. Depending on where you are in your menstrual cycle and your body's ability to conceive, the likelihood is between 0 and 20%. If a woman has a single act of unprotected intercourse, the risk of either partner transmitting a bacterial STD, such as gonorrhea, chlamydia, or trichomoniasis, is much higher than the risk of the woman becoming pregnant.[20]

The most frequently used method of emergency contraception is a special dose of combination birth control pills, taken within three days (72 hours) after unprotected intercourse. In North America and Europe, practitioners typically recommend 200 micrograms of the estrogen ethinyl estradiol and 1 milligram of the progestin levonorgestrel (or 2 milligrams of norgestrel) in two equal doses. The first dose is taken as soon as possible (up to 72 hours after unprotected intercourse), and the second dose 12 hours later. This form of emergency contraception is known as the "Yuzpe regimen" after the Canadian doctor who developed it 25 years ago.

The hormones used in the Yuzpe regimen are available in several brands of oral contraceptives. In Finland, Germany, Sweden, Switzerland, and the United Kingdom, pills are packaged and marketed specifically for emergency use; in the U.S., they are not. *If you use birth-control pills for emergency contraception, it is important to take only one brand of pill and only the number of pills recommended for each dose.*

This method works by changing a woman's hormone levels, which prevents pregnancy by disrupting the processes of ovulation, egg transport, fertilization, and implantation. It is very effective; it prevents pregnancy in about 75% of the women who would otherwise conceive after a single act of unprotected intercourse.

Even though the hormones used in this way for emergency contraception are the same as those in some birth control pills, they are used for such a short time that most women can take them safely, and no long-term complications have been reported. *Do not use this method of emergency contraception if you have a history or current case of migraine headaches* at the time you are seeking emergency contraception. If you could be pregnant already, it's a good idea to have a pregnancy test before using emergency contraception. If after taking both doses of the pills you become pregnant anyway, there is no evidence of potential danger to your offspring.

Nausea and vomiting are the most common negative effects of this method of emergency contraception; about half feel nauseated and about 20% vomit. For this reason, some practitioners advise taking the pills with food or with an antinausea medication. Other negative effects are breast tenderness, dizziness, abdominal pain, and headaches. Using combination pills for emergency contraception may also change the timing of your next menstrual period; it may begin a few days earlier or a few days later than usual.

Pills containing progestin alone (levonorgestrel) are also used for emergency contraception. Progestin may prevent fertilization by immobilizing sperm or prevent implantation by making the uterus unable to support the fertilized egg. The usual dose for emergency contraception is two separate doses of progestin (0.75 milligrams of levonorgestrel in each dose) 12 hours apart. The first dose should be taken within 48 hours of unprotected intercourse and the second dose 12 hours later. This dosage is about as effective as the Yuzpe regimen. Women using progestin alone for emergency contraception commonly experience vomiting, nausea, and breast tenderness, but less frequently than women using combination pills.

In many Eastern European countries (including Hungary, Bulgaria, the former Soviet Union, and the Czech Republic), some developing countries (including China, Kenya, Ecuador, and Malaysia), and a few Western countries (the Netherlands and the United Kingdom), progestin (sold under the brand name of Postinor) has been used by women who have intercourse infrequently.

A copper IUD can also be used for emergency contraception. It has proven extremely successful at preventing pregnancy if inserted within five days after unprotected intercourse. The IUD probably works by causing an inflammation of the uterine lining that prevents the implantation of a fertilized egg. Once inserted into the uterus, a copper IUD can be left in place and used as your regular method of birth control for up to ten years. Of course, women who should not use the IUD for birth control (see p. 327) should not use it after unprotected intercourse either.

If you have had unprotected intercourse, you may prefer not to use emergency contraception. You may prefer to wait to see whether you are pregnant and, if so, have an abortion.

THE INTRAUTERINE DEVICE (IUD)

Centuries ago, when camel drivers in the Middle East started out on a long journey across the desert, they would insert pebbles into the uterus of a female camel to keep her from becoming pregnant on the trip. A foreign body in the uterus seems to prevent pregnancy most of the time. The IUD became a popular contraceptive for women in the 1960s because it seemed to be the perfect alternative to the Pill. It was about as effective and didn't introduce synthetic hormones into women's bodies. Once the IUD had been inserted, women didn't have to worry about forgetting to use it. It was an inconspicuous method, so it couldn't be discovered by the wrong person. However, like other provider-dependent methods of birth control, the IUD left room for potential manipulation or coercion of women; it seemed especially "appropriate" for young women, women with low incomes, or Third World women, whom providers often viewed as uncooperative and/or irresponsible.

Worldwide, the use of IUDs has increased. Today more than 106 million women use them, 72 million of them in China and most of the rest in Third World countries. Unfortunately, poorer health and limited access to medical care exacerbate the risks and complications of IUDs. In the U.S. use of the IUD has declined dramatically from as many as 10% of all U.S. women using contraception in the 1970s to fewer than 1% today; most users are women over the age of 35.

When IUDs were first manufactured in the 1960s, the FDA was not required to review any medical devices (including IUDs) for safety and effectiveness before they were marketed in the U.S. In some cases, such serious problems emerged that IUDs were removed from the market. An extreme example is the Dalkon Shield, an IUD manufactured by the A. H. Robins Company and marketed from 1971 to 1975. The Dalkon Shield was soon implicated in many cases of pelvic inflammatory disease (PID) and spontaneous septic abortions (miscarriages). In the U.S., 20 women died as a result of Dalkon Shield–related septic abortions.

In 1981, and again in 1983, the National Women's Health Network filed a class-action lawsuit against A. H. Robins, seeking a worldwide recall of the Shield, then inside an estimated 550,000 women. The lawsuit

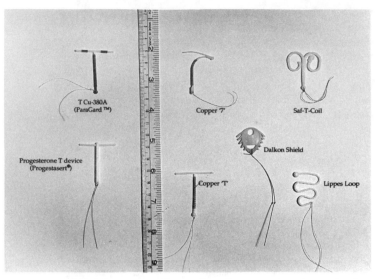

Different types of IUDs/Jennifer S. Edwards and Alice Steinhardt

provided an important means of educating the public about the Shield and about the need to hold corporations accountable for their defective products, not just in the U.S. but internationally. Thousands of women filed lawsuits against A. H. Robins. By 1985, the company had paid $250 million to settle approximately 4,400 suits and had been ordered by juries in 11 cases to pay $24.8 million in punitive damages. That same year, A. H. Robins declared bankruptcy and was ordered to set up a trust fund to compensate injured women. Ten years later, the Dalkon Shield trust had paid $1.42 billion to 185,000 women in the U.S. and 110 other countries.

Today, FDA approval is required before any IUDs can be marketed in the U.S. The two IUDs for sale in the U.S., the TCu-380A (ParaGard) and the Progesterone T device (Progestasert System), are more effective and safer than the Dalkon Shield. These IUDs may be more satisfactory than other methods of birth control for women who are in mutually monogamous, stable relationships and who are at low risk of STDs. For midlife women who want long-term contraception, IUDs may be preferable to sterilization, because over time, they appear to be just as effective. The information below is about the TCu-380A and the Progesterone T device, unless another type is specifically mentioned.

Description

IUDs are small devices that fit inside the uterus. Most contain copper or synthetic progesterone. One or more strings are usually attached to IUDs. When the IUD is in place, these strings extend downward into the upper vagina.* IUDs come in different sizes and shapes (see photo above).

---

* You can see the IUD string(s) if you use a speculum and a mirror to look at your cervix (see chapter 12, Understanding Our Bodies: Sexual Anatomy, Reproduction, and the Menstrual Cycle).

How It Works

No one is absolutely sure how the IUD works. The most widely accepted theory is that it prevents fertilization. *Copper* IUDs cause an inflammation or chronic low-grade infection in the uterus; the body's response is to produce higher numbers of white blood cells, prostaglandins, and enzymes in the uterus and fallopian tubes. These changes may damage or destroy sperm or interfere with its movement in a woman's genital tract, making fertilization impossible. They may also speed up the movement of the egg in a fallopian tube, causing the egg to arrive at the uterus too soon to be able to join with sperm. *Hormone-releasing* IUDs thicken the consistency of cervical fluid so that sperm cannot pass through it.[21]

Different Types of IUD

The TCu-380A (ParaGard) is a plastic IUD that has a thin copper wire wrapped around the vertical stem and a sleeve of copper on each "arm," with a clear or whitish string attached to it. Other IUDs containing copper that are available outside the U.S. are the Multiload-250 and Multiload-375 and various forms of Copper-Ts. Copper IUDs tend to increase bleeding during menstrual periods. The TCu-380A lasts for 10 years; other copper IUDs must be replaced more frequently.

The Progesterone T device (Progestasert System) is a plastic IUD containing synthetic progesterone and has a blue-black double string attached. (See "Possible Effects," p. 318, for contraceptive effects of progesterone.) Another hormone-releasing IUD is LNG-20, which can be left in place for up to five years and is used primarily in Scandinavia, western Europe, and Singapore. Hormone-releasing IUDs decrease bleeding during menstrual periods but are associated with a higher rate of ectopic pregnancies than are other IUDs. The Progesterone T must be replaced every year because the supply of progesterone in the device is used up after 12 months.

All plastic IUDs are coated with barium so that they will be visible under X ray (see "Perforation or Embedding," p. 328).

Effectiveness

The IUD is a very effective form of birth control. The lowest expected failure rate of the TCu-380A is 0.6% and of the Progesterone T 1.5% in the first year of use. The typical failure rate for the TCu-380A is 0.8%; for the Progesterone T it is 2%. Pregnancy rates for IUDs are lower among women over 30.

It is a good idea to use a supplemental birth control method for the first three months after IUD insertion, as that is the time when the IUD is most likely to be expelled and conception most likely to take place.

Expulsion

A major drawback of the IUD is its high expulsion rate. Within one year of use, between 1 and 10% of women using IUDs will have expelled them, sometimes without knowing it has happened. These women could be vulnerable to pregnancy without being aware of it. Younger women, women who have never been pregnant, and women who have heavier bleeding and/or cramping during their menstrual periods are more likely to expel IUDs.

If your body is not going to tolerate the IUD, it will usually expel the device during the first three months after insertion. This happens most frequently during menstruation. Because you might not feel it coming out, check for it in the toilet and on your tampon or sanitary napkin. Be sure to feel the length of the string a few times each month, especially right after your period.

Signs of IUD expulsion include an unusual vaginal discharge, cramping or pain, spotting, a longer string, or an ability to feel the IUD in your vagina or cervical os. When an IUD is being expelled, your male partner may feel pain or irritation during intercourse.

The longer your body retains the IUD, the better your chance of not expelling it.

Reversibility

Most women who stop using the IUD in order to become pregnant conceive as easily as women who have never used it. However, the IUD can harm our fertility. It can cause damage through perforation or embedding. Also, the few women who conceive with an IUD in place are more likely to have an ectopic pregnancy than women not using one. And, there's an increased risk of PID in the first few weeks after an IUD is inserted. These serious complications can cause impaired fertility or sterility and may lead to hysterectomy. Health practitioners should tell this to every woman who chooses an IUD as her form of birth control, especially to those of us who hope someday to have children.

Safety

Studies have documented serious negative effects suffered by IUD users (see p. 320). Women using IUDs have a greater risk of developing PID during the first few weeks after insertion. When the practitioner places the device correctly in the uterus and uses basic infection-prevention measures,* the risk of infection is low for healthy women. Because of the risks of infection and perforation each time an IUD is inserted, many practitioners recommend that women use the TCu-380A (which needs replacement every ten years) instead of the Progesterone T (which must be replaced every year).

Researchers agree that IUDs are a poor choice of

---

* Precautions should include washing hands, using gloves, cleaning the cervix and vagina with a water-based antiseptic, and using a "no-touch" technique for inserting the IUD.

birth control for any woman at risk of getting an STD, including HIV. IUDs may increase a woman's risk for HIV by changing the lining of the uterus. If a woman is HIV-positive, an IUD may increase her risk of transmitting HIV to her sexual partner(s). Researchers disagree about whether women using IUDs are more likely than those who aren't using them to develop PID after catching a sexually transmitted disease.

Warning Signals

The following are signs of serious problems: late period or missed period; abdominal pain; pain with intercourse; increased temperature, fever, or chills; noticeable or foul discharge; spotting; bleeding; heavy periods; clots. *Report these immediately,* for they are signs of infection, perforation, or pregnancy. Report any exposure to an STD and any problem lasting more than a few cycles to a health practitioner or clinic.

Who Should Absolutely Not Use the IUD

IUDs should *absolutely not* be used by women who are pregnant or who have genital tract cancer; undiagnosed abnormal vaginal bleeding; active gonorrhea or chlamydia; active, recent, or recurrent pelvic infection; or postpartum endometritis or who have had an abortion within the past three months followed by infection. (Remember that gonorrhea and chlamydia infections in women are often *asymptomatic*.)

Who Should Use the IUD
Only as a Last Choice [22]

For women with the following situations or conditions *the risks of the IUD generally outweigh the advantages:* women at risk of exposure to STDs/HIV (IV drug users, multiple sexual partners, or a partner who is an IV drug user or who has multiple sexual partners); difficult access to emergency treatment. Before choosing an IUD, carefully consider using another method and discuss the potential risks with a medical practitioner; if you choose the IUD you should be carefully monitored to watch for problems. Consider how severe your condition is, how available and acceptable other methods of birth control are, and what access you have to emergency followup services.

Who Should Consider Another Method
Before Choosing an IUD

There is considerable disagreement about how risky the following situations or conditions are for women who wish to use IUDs. The World Health Organization believes that for women with the following situations or conditions, the advantages of the IUD generally outweigh the risks of using it. Others believe that IUDs should be used infrequently by women with these conditions or situations, and then only after considering other methods of birth control and after being carefully screened by a practitioner. Such women then need to be able to contact a provider if they suspect any adverse effects. The authors of this book agree with the more cautious approach, and recommend that women with the following conditions should consider using another method: pregnancy in the future as a high-priority goal; blood disorders or impaired coagulation; impaired response to infection (in women with diabetes or taking steroids); inability to check IUD string or identify warning signals (for women with physical disabilities, such as spinal cord injury, rheumatoid arthritis, multiple sclerosis, or cognitive impairments); unresolved abnormal Pap smear; history of severe fainting or severe vasovagal reaction; anemia; sickle-cell anemia; severe menstrual cramps or bleeding; valvular heart disease; history of ectopic pregnancy (for women using hormone-releasing IUDs). Exposure to DES *in utero* (DES daughter), if it results in an alteration of the shape of the uterus, or certain other uterine abnormalities (bicornate uterus, cervical stenosis, endometrial polyps, leiomyomata, small uterus) may distort the shape of the uterus so much that inserting an IUD is impossible.

Complications and Negative Effects

Infections

Recent analyses show that pelvic inflammatory disease (see chapter 24, Selected Medical Practices, Problems, and Procedures) is twice as likely to occur in women using IUDs as in women using *no* contraception. PID most commonly occurs in the first few weeks after an IUD is inserted, probably because infection-causing organisms can be carried by the IUD or the instruments used to insert it into the uterus. The risk of PID can be reduced substantially if the practitioner inserting the IUD uses careful infection-prevention procedures. To prevent infection, some practitioners recommend the short-term use of antibiotics at the time of insertion.[23] PID is also caused by sexually transmitted diseases.[24] Women who have an STD while using an IUD are at high risk for pelvic inflammation. PID will not go away by itself. It can lead to tremendous pain, future ectopic pregnancy, sterility, and even death.

Women who become pregnant with an IUD in place may be more susceptible to an infected miscarriage, called a *septic abortion,* a rare condition that in most cases leads to hospitalization and can even cause death to the woman as well as the fetus. That is why most doctors recommend having the IUD removed if you become pregnant.

Excessive Bleeding and Cramping

The most common problem for women with IUDs is increased menstrual bleeding, sometimes excessive, and painful cramping and/or backache. Some women experience longer periods and bleeding or spotting and/or cramping between periods, too. Usually these symptoms are more intense during the first three to six months after the IUD is inserted. Approximately 10 to 15% of IUD users have the IUD removed within one year because of bleeding and cramping.

Copper-containing IUDs increase blood loss by 20 to 50%. Although heavier menstrual flow caused by an IUD can worsen anemia, it does not seem to cause anemia. Because many menstruating women are marginally anemic anyway, it is a good idea to have a blood test before you get an IUD and at each followup appointment. Eat plenty of iron-rich foods. *Hormone-releasing IUDs* decrease menstrual flow, but women using them may experience spotting or light bleeding between periods.

Perforation or Embedding

Although rare, these are potentially serious complications. *Perforation* can be partial, with some of the IUD pushing through the uterine wall and the rest staying in the uterus, or it can be complete, with the entire IUD pushing out of the uterus into the abdominal cavity. Perforation occurs or begins to occur most frequently during insertion, primarily because of a practitioner's poor technique. It happens less often when a uterine sound has been taken, so always insist on this procedure (see "Ultrasound" in chapter 19). *Unfortunately, there are usually no symptoms accompanying perforation.*

Embedding can happen when the lining of the uterus grows around the IUD. It occurs over time. If an IUD becomes partially embedded in the uterine wall, the device will usually still be effective, but embedded IUDs can cause more pain during removal. In some cases, you may need a dilation and curettage to get it out (see "Dilation and Curettage" in chapter 24, Selected Medical Practices, Problems, and Procedures, p. 594). In several cases we know of, women had hysterectomies because of embedded IUDs—a devastating blow for anyone who wants to have a child.

The first sign of perforation or embedding may be a shorter string or no string at all during your monthly check (a good reason to check the string more than once a month). If this happens, be sure to see a health worker immediately. You should also use another form of birth control, because if the IUD has left the uterus, you are no longer being protected against pregnancy. In fact, some women become aware of perforation only after finding out that they are pregnant. You can have the IUD replaced, or you may want to choose another method of contraception.

Missing String

Because a missing string can mean expulsion, perforation, or embedding, there is no way of knowing what has happened unless you see the IUD come out. Otherwise, there are several procedures available for trying to locate it. A medical practitioner can probe your uterus with a uterine sound or a biopsy instrument. If sounding fails to locate the IUD, an X ray or ultrasound (see "Ultrasound," chapter 19, Pregnancy, p. 462) may work. If the IUD is still in the uterus, she or he can then try to pull the string down to remove the IUD. This may involve dilating the cervix, which can be painful.

If no IUD can be located, it has probably been expelled. If you are pregnant and decide not to have an abortion, you should not have an X ray. Ultrasound may be used instead (see chapter 19, Pregnancy), although this procedure can be expensive.

There is disagreement about what to do if the IUD is located outside the uterus. Some researchers think it should be removed if the perforation is discovered in the first few weeks after insertion, but if perforation is discovered after that time, removal of the IUD may lead to further complications. Some researchers think removal is necessary only if a woman has abdominal symptoms. Removal of an IUD that is not in the uterus and not expelled requires surgery. This can often be done in the outpatient services of your hospital or clinic. A laparoscopy operation is performed in this case (see "Laparoscopy," chapter 24, Selected Medical Practices, Problems, and Procedures, p. 596). If the IUD is not accessible by laparoscopy, more extensive surgery may be required.

Pregnancy

If your period is late and you have an IUD, have a pregnancy test. If you know you are pregnant and you have an IUD in place, you should have the IUD removed *whether or not* you wish to continue the pregnancy. If you are pregnant and you do not have your IUD removed, you are more likely to have a pelvic infection or septic abortion. These are life-threatening conditions that must be treated. If you have the IUD removed, your risk of miscarriage is about 25%. If you don't, you have about a 50% chance of miscarrying, and during the second trimester your chances are ten times greater than normal. If you do not have a miscarriage, you are also more likely to have a baby born prematurely.[25]

Ectopic Pregnancy

If you become pregnant with a copper IUD in place, there is a 3% chance of ectopic pregnancy. Women who conceive with the Progestasert are about five times more likely to have an ectopic pregnancy than women using a copper IUD. *An ectopic pregnancy is a serious problem* that can cause hemorrhage and lead to infection, sterility, and sometimes death. Frequently it is misdiagnosed, so IUD users should be aware of possible symptoms of ectopic pregnancy (see chapter 22, Child-bearing Loss, Infertility, and Adoption, for more information).

Other Possible Effects

Women using IUDs may be more likely to develop nonspecific vaginitis. Copper IUDs do not appear to produce an allergic reaction or to have a negative effect on a developing fetus. There is no evidence that the IUD can cause cancer, but it has not been studied long enough to know the long-term effects of either the material it's made of (polyethylene) or the materials some IUDs contain (progestin and barium).

How to Get an IUD

Because of the risk of perforation and infection, a well-trained person must insert the IUD. Choose a practitioner who has experience with IUDs and find out in advance which device is used. If she or he doesn't insert IUDs or the kind of IUD you want, go to someone else.

If possible, have a full medical, pelvic, and breast examination, including a Pap smear, pregnancy test, and tests for STDs before being given the IUD. This is very important, because if you have a sexually transmitted disease or are pregnant, you should not use the IUD. That means at least two visits, because it takes a few days to receive results from the Pap smear and the STD cultures. In the U.S. your practitioner should give you an informed consent form to sign at this time (see "Our Rights as Patients" in chapter 25, The Politics of Women's Health and Medical Care).

The practitioner should do a sounding of the uterus to measure its depth and position. An IUD can be put into a tipped uterus.

Insertion takes place through the os (the opening in the cervix), which is about the size of a thin straw. Just before insertion, the IUD is straightened out in a plastic tube like a straw. The practitioner gently puts the tube into the vagina and up into the uterus through the cervix (see illustration below), then withdraws the

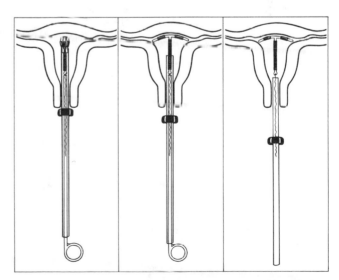

The insertion of Copper TCu-380A/The Population Council

tube while holding the inner plunger steady. This leaves the IUD in position. The practitioner then removes the plunger and the IUD stays in the uterus, with its string dangling into the vagina. Make sure that you understand how to check the string.

The process can hurt, sometimes a lot, because the inserter stretches the os open and the device irritates the uterus. You may have cramps during the insertion and for the rest of the day, especially if you have never given birth. Bring a friend with you if you can— someone who can accompany you home after the appointment. You might want to have a local anesthetic or take a mild painkiller, or you can pant quickly or relax and take deep breaths.

When to Get an IUD

This is controversial. Many providers say an IUD can be inserted any time during the menstrual cycle, if it is certain that the woman is not pregnant. This gives you more options to have the IUD inserted when it is most convenient for you. Insertion may be less painful during or just after your period because the os is slightly opened at that time. Also, the fact that you are having your period probably means you aren't pregnant (although sometimes women have one or even two scant periods during pregnancy). Some practitioners suspect there may be a greater chance of infection or expulsion during menstruation, and avoid inserting IUDs at that time. In the past few years, practitioners have changed their views about insertion of IUDs after childbirth or abortion. They now believe that IUDs can be safely inserted immediately after childbirth if a woman has had a normal labor and delivery, her uterus is firm, and the bleeding has subsided. However, there is a higher rate of expulsion at this time. They also believe IUDs can be safely inserted immediately after an abortion if the uterus is not infected.

The best time for insertion may be between periods and at least six weeks after childbirth or abortion.

Because expulsion and infection are most likely to occur in the first few months after an IUD is inserted, you should have a followup visit three to six weeks afterward, to make sure that your IUD is still in place and there are no signs of infection.

Checking Your IUD

At first you'll want to check your IUD string before intercourse (you may want to ask your partner to do it) and after each period. After three months or so, once or twice a month is enough.

You can try to feel the string with your finger or look for it during a cervical self-exam using a speculum (see "Self-Examination," chapter 24, Selected Medical Practices, Problems, and Procedures, p. 593). To check with your finger, squat, bringing your bottom down near your heels to shorten the length of your vagina, and reach into your vagina with your longest (clean) finger. The bathtub or shower is a good place, or bear down while you are sitting on the toilet. You may be confused by the folds in your vagina, but when you reach your cervix you will know it, as it is harder and firmer than anything else you'll touch. Find the dimple in your cervix; this is the entrance to your uterus, and the strings of the IUD should be sticking out a little way. Some days your uterus may be tipped in such a way that you can't reach the cervix or find the hole; try again the next day. If you cannot find the strings for a few days or if they are much longer or shorter, or if you feel a bit of plastic protruding, call your health practitioner or clinic.

Advantages

You don't have to worry about forgetting to take a pill, checking your signs of fertility, or using a barrier method at the time of intercourse.

Checking the string a few times each month encourages you to get to know your vagina and cervix and to feel comfortable about touching your genitals.

If you have an IUD containing progesterone, you will probably have less bleeding during your menstrual periods.

Disadvantages

Most of the disadvantages in terms of pain and risk have been described already. Note particularly the likelihood of infertility due to PID. The IUD offers no protection against sexually transmitted diseases, including HIV.

Responsibility

The woman sees a practitioner for insertion and three to six weeks later for a checkup. She experiences the insertion and any negative effects. The woman or her partner must check the string periodically and remember when it's time to have the IUD replaced.

Cost

An initial examination with screening and blood tests costs about $100. A second visit, including purchase and insertion of the IUD, costs from $215 at a clinic (for the two visits, the total cost is about $315) to $300 at a private doctor's office (total $400). The cost for removal of the IUD is about $100.

New IUD Design

Researchers are always designing new products to improve the effectiveness and reduce the problems of IUDs. View *all* new IUDs cautiously, because experience has shown that many of their long-term negative effects will show up only after they have been put on the market. Some new designs we've heard about include variations of the copper-bearing and progesterone-releasing IUDs (the Lng is already available in some countries), IUDs made without a rigid frame (the FlexiGard Device) and a frameless flexible copper device (GyneFix IUD) that attaches to the uterine wall.

WITHDRAWAL (COITUS INTERRUPTUS, "TAKING CARE" OR "PULLING OUT")

Withdrawal is used throughout the world as a folk method passed on from one generation to the next. Withdrawal involves removing the penis from the vagina just before ejaculation so that the sperm is deposited outside the vagina and away from the lips of the vagina as well.

Withdrawal is not very effective because the man cannot always withdraw his penis in time to avoid contact with the vagina and vaginal lips (when fertile cervical fluid is present, sperm can move all the way from the vaginal lips up into the fallopian tubes). Multiple acts of intercourse in a short period of time increase the likelihood of failure, because more sperm are mixed in with the lubricating fluid. It is not possible to give reliable failure rates for withdrawal because so few studies have been done.[26] However, researchers estimate that withdrawal has a lowest expected failure rate of 4% but a typical failure rate of 19%.

Withdrawal has several drawbacks in addition to its high failure rate. The man must stay in control and therefore cannot relax. When used over a long period, pulling out may lead to premature ejaculation. Withdrawal can also be uncomfortable for the woman: The man may have to withdraw before she reaches orgasm, interrupting the flow of her sexual response; also, she may be worrying whether he's going to withdraw in time, so that she, too, cannot relax completely. Some couples who have used withdrawal for a long time have been able to work out these problems. Finally, withdrawal does not protect you against STDs, including HIV infection; even the few drops of pre-ejaculatory fluid that come out of the penis long before orgasm can contain HIV.

STERILIZATION

Sterilization is a *permanent** method of birth control, available for both women and men. In women, the fallopian tubes are cut and/or blocked so the egg and sperm cannot meet. This is called *tubal ligation*. In men, the vas deferens is cut and/or blocked so sperm cannot mix with seminal fluid. This is called *vasectomy*. Today, sterilization is the most frequently used method of birth control in the world. For some women, the choice to be sterilized is a positive wish to avoid pregnancy forever. Some have already had children; others decide they never want children.

Choosing to be sterilized is a major step. As many as 25% of the women who are sterilized regret this decision later on, particularly if they are sterilized be-

fore the age of 30. Women are more likely to regret being sterilized when they are young, have less information about the procedure, or know about fewer other contraceptive methods before sterilization. Under whatever circumstances sterilization is chosen, the decision usually brings up deep feelings.

In some countries, especially those in which other methods of contraception are not easily available, population control advocates promote sterilization as the best form of birth control. In more highly industrialized regions of the world, about 11% of women who use birth control are being sterilized, whereas in less industrialized areas, 38% of women trying to prevent pregnancy are undergoing sterilization. Many women are having it done without adequate information about the possible risks and consequences involved, or under coercive circumstances.†

Some women turn to sterilization in desperation because there is no suitable form of reversible contraception for them. (Nothing else points out so clearly our need for better temporary methods of birth control.) Many feel they have no other choice: "The lack of employment opportunities, education, day care, decent housing, adequate medical care; safe, effective contraception and access to abortion all create an atmosphere of subtle coercion."[27] Refugees or victims of natural disasters are also living in situations that can create a coercive atmosphere.

Sterilization abuse—when women are sterilized without full informed consent—continues to be a problem in many parts of the world. In the U.S., women living in poverty or who are African American, Puerto Rican, Chicana, or Native American, or who have little or no understanding of English, have been more likely to be sterilized than white women from the same or higher socioeconomic classes.‡ Women with physical disabilities who are deemed "unfit to reproduce" by medical practitioners have also been abusively sterilized. Sometimes physicians consider women mentally unfit to use other methods of birth control and push sterilization on them.§ Physicians

---

† Most (but not all) documented cases of coerced sterilization in the U.S. involve women. Here we focus on the experiences of women.
‡ Sterilization abuse is not a new development. Beginning in the 19th century, people known as eugenicists tried to popularize the idea that social problems such as crime and poverty could be eliminated by preventing certain "unfit" people from having children. The eugenics movement, which has proponents even today, argued that criminals, "imbeciles," blacks, and immigrants would produce more "inferior" people like themselves if allowed to reproduce. Eugenicists urged the passage of laws empowering the state to sterilize such individuals against their will. These eugenics laws were passed in 37 states and still remain on the books in some.
§ A major investigation and report, produced only after great pressure from people such as Connie Uri, a Native American physician, found that large numbers of women living on Indian reservations had been sterilized without consent by government-sponsored programs. (See the U.S. General Accounting Office Report to Hon. James G. Abourezk, B 164031 [5], November 1976.) At a major teaching hospital in Los Angeles, a resident went to the local newspapers to expose cases of

---

* Although there have been some successful attempts at reversing both vasectomies and tubal ligations, the operation should be considered permanent and not reversible.

pressure women into giving consent during labor or childbirth, welfare officials threaten the loss of benefits if women refuse, or no one informs women that the operation is permanent. African-American women in the South are all too familiar with the "Mississippi appendectomy," in which the fallopian tubes are tied or the uterus is removed without their knowledge. Sometimes sterilizations are done primarily for the purpose of training residents or interns. Of the million hysterectomies done each year, perhaps one out of five is done for sterilization only, with no legitimate medical reason. Hysterectomy, a major surgical procedure, is unnecessary for sterilization purposes. The risk of death or complication from a hysterectomy is ten to 100 times greater than from a tubal ligation (see "Hysterectomy and Oophorectomy" in chapter 24). Especially if women are poor, public and private programs make it easier to get sterilization services than abortions, prenatal care, and financial assistance so that women can have healthy children; or practitioners refuse to perform abortions until women agree to be sterilized. Occasionally, physicians refuse to sterilize fully informed white middle-class women with no children who request this procedure.

For 25 years, feminists, health activists, and others have joined together to expose sterilization abuse and to organize against it in hospitals, communities, courts, and legislatures. In 1975, responding to this pressure, New York City became the first city in the United States to produce guidelines. On March 9, 1979, federal sterilization regulations went into effect.

The most important requirements of the federal regulations include the following:

Obtaining voluntary informed consent using a mandatory, standardized consent form in a person's preferred language.
Prohibiting overt or implicit threat of loss of welfare or Medicaid benefits if someone doesn't consent.
Explaining alternative methods of birth control and the risks, side effects, and irreversibility of sterilization, orally and in writing, also in a person's language.
Waiting at least 30 days after a person signs the consent form before sterilization (except for premature delivery and emergency abdominal surgery).
Prohibiting obtaining consent while someone is in labor, before or after an abortion, or while the person is under the influence of alcohol or other drugs.
Prohibiting hysterectomies for sterilization in federally funded programs.
Imposing a moratorium on federally funded sterilizations of people under 21 who have been declared

legally incompetent or are involuntarily institutionalized.
Auditing sterilization programs in the ten states where most federally funded sterilizations are performed.[28]

The government usually does not monitor or enforce these regulations, but it does appear that they have reduced the amount of sterilization abuse. If you are considering sterilization, make sure that the clinic or hospital performing it complies with these regulations. If you suspect that it doesn't, contact your local women's health group or one of the following organizations: American Civil Liberties Union Reproductive Freedom Project (address in Resources), National Black Women's Health Project, National Latina Health Organization/Organizacion Nacional de la Salud de la Mujer Latina, National Women's Health Network, Native American Women's Health Education Resource Center (addresses in chapter 27 Resources).

Tubal Ligation

Female sterilization is effective immediately. It can be done under general, spinal, or local anesthesia, and women usually go home the same day. In the first year after the operation, female sterilization is almost 100% effective. A recent U.S. study of its long-term use[29] found that over time, the risk of failure increased. By five years after sterilization, more than 1% of women had become pregnant, and by ten years, the failure rate rose to 1.8%. The higher failure rates were associated with the use of spring clips or bipolar coagulation. Also, rates were higher for some women than others: Black, non-Hispanic women experienced a higher failure rate than white, non-Hispanic women; and younger women had higher failure rates than older women. Although this study confirms that female sterilization is an extremely effective method of birth control, it also reminds us of the importance of being fully informed about the technique a practitioner plans to use and of taking into consideration our own individual circumstances.[30]

Laparoscopy, or "Band-Aid" surgery, is the most common surgical technique for sterilization in the U.S. Although a laparoscopy can be done under local, general, or spinal anesthesia, usually local anesthesia with a light sedative is adequate. The actual procedure takes about 30 minutes. First, the practitioner makes a small incision in the woman's belly button. The woman is tilted back, head down, allowing her intestines to move away from her fallopian tubes. The tubes are moved into view by inserting a clamp (tenaculum) onto the cervix and an instrument (sound or intrauterine cannula) through the vagina and then manipulating the uterus and tubes. Next, her belly is inflated with gas (carbon dioxide, nitrous oxide, or room air) to make the tubes visible. A laparoscope (a thin tube containing a viewing instrument and a light) is inserted through the incision to enable viewing of the tubes. An instrument to block the tubes is introduced through

sterilization abuse involving many Chicana women with low incomes. (See "A Health Research Group Study on Surgical Sterilization: Present Abuses and Proposed Regulations," Health Research Group, 1973.) GAO reports (single copy) are free. Write to U.S. GAO, Distribution Section, Room 1518, 401 G Street NW, Washington, DC 20548. Indicate the report number and date. Health Research Group reports are available from HRG, 2000 P Street NW, Washington, DC 20036.

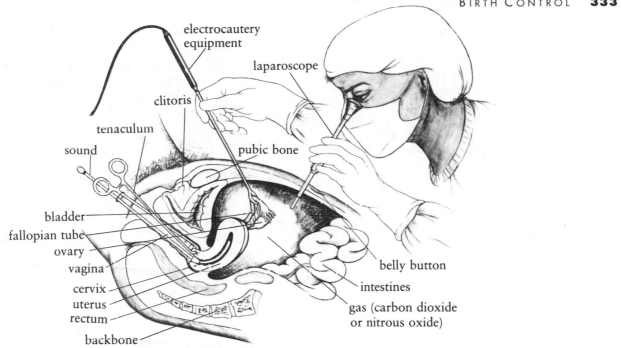

electrocautery
equipment

laparoscope

clitoris

tenaculum

sound

pubic bone

bladder

fallopian tube

ovary

vagina

cervix

uterus

rectum

backbone

belly button

intestines

gas (carbon dioxide
or nitrous oxide)

A *tubal ligation* (side view)/Christine Bondante

the laparoscope or through a second tiny incision below the belly button. The tubes can be blocked by burning (electrocoagulation or cautery) or cutting them, clipping them shut, or applying rings to them. The incisions are sewn closed. Afterward, some women feel pain in their shoulders from the gas as it rises up and is absorbed by the body.

The *minilaparotomy,* or minilap, involves making a small incision just above a woman's pubic bone, moving the tubes into view with a tenaculum and ultrasound (see illustration above), pulling the fallopian tubes up through the incision, and blocking them with rings or clips or by tying and cutting them. The incision is sewn shut. Women seem to have more cramping and pain afterward than with a laparoscopy, sometimes lasting a few days.

Sterilization by *laparotomy* involves major surgery (see "Laparoscopy," chapter 24, Selected Medical Practices, Problems, and Procedures, p. 596). Sterilization through a woman's vagina *(colpotomy* or *culdoscopy)* or cervix *(bysteroscopy)* have an increased risk of infection and failure, so these techniques are generally not recommended.

Sterilization probably does not affect a woman's hormone secretions, ovaries, uterus, or vagina. Her menstrual cycle continues but may become irregular. An egg ripens and is released from an ovary every month but stops part way down the tube and is reabsorbed by her body.

Complications and Negative Effects

Whenever surgery involving an anesthetic is performed, certain complications are possible. Major complications happen relatively rarely and depend a great deal on the skill and experience of the practitioner performing the sterilization. Cardiac irregularity, cardiac arrest, infection, internal bleeding, and perforation of a major blood vessel are a few of the potential hazards.

Laparoscopic techniques may involve specific problems such as internal burn injuries or punctures to other organs or tissue, skin burns, puncturing of the intestine, perforation of the uterus, and carbon dioxide embolism (which may cause immediate death).

Some women experience a post-tubal sterilization syndrome (post-TS syndrome), consisting of irregular menstrual cycles, painful periods, midcycle bleeding or no periods; this may create the need for repeated dilation and curettages or, in some cases, complete hysterectomies.

Reversibility

No woman should undergo sterilization with the hope that the procedure can be reversed. If you think there is any chance you may want to have children someday, use a reversible form of birth control.

Nonetheless, recent advances in microsurgery have increased the possibility of reversing tubal ligation, called *reanastomosis.* It is major surgery, requiring extreme skill on the part of the surgeon, highly specialized and expensive equipment, and a woman in good health. The operation can cost $10,000 to $15,000 or more. This means that only women with substantial resources will be able to have plastic surgery to repair the tube(s), and even then success is not guaranteed.

Before undergoing reanastomosis, a woman and her partner should be tested for fertility potential. Also, the woman should have a laparoscopic examination to

Quinacrine, a drug used to treat malaria, has been studied as a nonsurgical form of sterilization in Chile, Texas, and Vietnam (see chapter 26, The Global Politics of Women and Health, p. 734). Because recent animal studies have demonstrated toxic effects, scientists and the World Health Organization recommend that its use be discontinued for this purpose. Women's health activists are campaigning against its use for sterilization purposes, because a few well-funded individuals continue to promote quinacrine in developing countries. For more information on this campaign, contact the Boston Women's Health Book Collective.

determine whether her tubes are too damaged to be repaired. Cauterization tends to destroy a significant amount of the tube. Clips and rings seem to destroy much less of the tube but still make reversal highly unlikely.

New Techniques in Female Sterilization

Possible new techniques involve injecting substances into the fallopian tubes, inserting pellets or plugs, modifying surgical procedures, and using new types of clips or rings. We have also heard of experiments using methyl cyanoacrylate, also known as Krazy Glue or Superglue; and silicone plugs. The negative and long-term effects of these substances are unknown.

Male Sterilization—Vasectomy

Male sterilization is a much simpler process than female sterilization. Usually done in a doctor's office or in a clinic, the operation takes about half an hour. The practitioner applies a local anesthetic (such as lidocaine), makes one or two small incisions in the scrotum, locates the two vasa deferentia (singular: vas deferens, tubes that carry sperm from the testes to the penis), removes a piece of each, and ties off the ends. Men are not sterile immediately because sperm are already in the vasa deferentia. For this reason, use another method of birth control for two months or until the man has had two negative sperm counts.

"No-scalpel" vasectomy is used increasingly throughout the world. It was developed in China, where it is now the standard technique used for vasectomies. In no-scalpel vasectomy, a practitioner uses an instrument that punctures a tiny hole in the scrotum, lifts the vas deferens out through the hole, removes a piece of it, and then ties off the ends. No-scalpel vasectomy appears to be as effective as the scalpel method but has a lower complication rate.

Vasectomy leaves the man's genital system basically unchanged. His sexual hormones remain operative, and there is no noticeable difference in his ejaculate

RESEARCH AND DEVELOPMENT OF ANTIFERTILITY "VACCINES"
by Judith Richter

Probably the most heated debate in the field of contraceptive research today concerns the development of immunological birth control methods, more commonly known as antifertility "vaccines." Several research institutions have been developing this totally new class of contraceptives for the past three decades.

Immuno-contraceptives aim to trick the immune system into generating a temporary immune reaction against components that are indispensable to reproduction—namely, the hormones that trigger the monthly ripening and release of the egg cells in women or the production of sperm cells in men, the egg or sperm cells themselves, or pregnancy-related hormones. To do so, part of the chosen reproductive cell or molecule is linked to a "carrier" such as diphtheria toxoid, so that the immune system perceives it as "foreign" to the body and thus to be eliminated. Theoretically, immuno-contraceptives can be developed for both men and women. However, most of the international research so far has focused on methods for women, and more particularly on the development of various immuno-contraceptives against human chorionic gonadotropin (HCG), a hormone produced in a woman's body shortly after fertilization of the egg cell. The research community argues that a long-acting, systemic method that allows for regular menstrual bleeding without hormonal effects would represent a valuable new option. If this so-called pregnancy hormone is effectively intercepted by antibodies, the early embryo cannot implant (and the woman has menstrual-like bleeding).

Since the 1970s, more than 400 people have been enrolled into clinical trials in at least seven countries: Australia, Brazil, Chile, Dominican Republic, Finland, India, and Sweden. There have been difficulties with generating and maintaining an immune response, as well as with adverse effects. For example, the product of the Indian developer, the National Institute of Immunology, was effective for only 80% of the women, for an average of three months. In Sweden, the World Health Organization's Special Programme of Research in Human Reproduction (WHO/HRP) had to suspend its phase II clinical trial because of unacceptable adverse effects.

Since 1993, a decentralized international campaign, currently coordinated by the Women's Global Network for Reproductive Rights (WGNRR), has been challenging the development of immunologically based birth control methods. By spring 1997, nearly 500 women's, Third World solidarity, consumer action, human rights, development, and medical groups and organizations from 41 countries had signed a Call for a Stop of Research on Antifertility "Vaccines" (Immunological Contraceptives). They claim that the risks to the health and well-being of users and potential fetuses from the manipulation of the immune system for contraceptive purposes cannot be justified by any advantage over existing contraceptives.

Immuno-contraception is likely to be a rather unreliable form of birth control because of the very nature of the immune system. Our immune responses are known to vary, depending on a host of factors internal and external to our bodies. Also, as yet there is no acceptable way to interrupt an ongoing immune reaction, so the product cannot be "switched off" at will. This compounds the critics' concerns about potentially serious adverse effects, such as the induction of autoimmune diseases and allergies. They warn that because of their technology-inherent features, antifertility "vaccines" will have a higher potential for abuse than any existing contraceptive method: Depending on the particular type, the action may last from one year to life, they cannot be discontinued at will, and they are easy to administer on a mass scale, even without the knowledge of the woman or man.

References:

Ada, G. L., and David Griffin, eds. *Vaccines for Fertility Regulation: The assessment of their safety and efficacy.* Proceedings of a symposium convened by WHO/HRP. Cambridge, England: Cambridge University Press, 1991.

"Call for a Stop of Research on Antifertility 'Vaccines' (Immunological Contraceptives)," 1993. Reproduced in Richter, Judith, *Vaccination against Pregnancy: Miracle or Menace?* London and Atlantic Highlands, NJ: Zed Books Ltd.; Australia and New Zealand: Spinifex Press, 1996.

Richter. *Vaccination against Pregnancy.*

Talwar, G. Pran, et al. "A vaccine that prevents pregnancy in women." *Proceedings of the National Academy of Science, USA* 91 (August 1994): 8532–536.

WHO/HRP. "Anti-HCG vaccine phase II trial status report," *Progress in Human Reproduction* no. 30 (1994): 8

because sperm make up only a small part of the semen. Some men, although they know these facts, are still anxious about what a vasectomy will do to their sexual performance. Talking with someone who has had a vasectomy can help allay such anxieties.

In some men, antibodies to their own sperm can be found after a vasectomy. Some research suggests that these antibodies may lead to certain diseases of the immune system, yet many fully fertile men also have such antibodies, and so far this suggestion is without support.

Men who have undergone vasectomy may have an increased risk of prostate cancer.[31] A 1980 report indicating that vasectomy may induce atherosclerosis (hardening of the arteries) has not been supported by other studies.[32]

Experimental operations have placed plastic plugs or injectable chemicals into the tube to plug it up temporarily, so that if the man later wants to have a child he can have the plug taken out. These methods appear to be reversible but not quite as effective as vasectomy. Researchers are also exploring ways to produce temporary sterility by increasing the temperature of a man's testicles through hot, shallow baths or ultrasound.[33]

Vasectomy should be considered irreversible.

ABSTINENCE

There is nothing wrong with abstinence. In fact, sometimes it may be just what we want. Abstinence means making love without having intercourse. It is the most effective form of birth control, has been used for centuries, and is still very common. It has no physical side effects, but many women feel better if prolonged sexual arousal is followed by orgasm (see sections on masturbation or oral sex in chapter 11, Sexuality).

Long before ejaculation, a man's penis may discharge a few drops of fluid. This pre-ejaculatory fluid does not contain sperm; however, it can transmit diseases, including HIV. Do not have any unprotected vagina-to-penis contact, mouth-to-penis contact, or penis-to-anus contact if you or your partner currently has HIV or any other STD or if you are not in a mutually monogamous relationship.

NONMETHODS

Douching

Some women douche with water or other special solutions immediately after intercourse in an attempt to remove semen from the vagina before sperm enter the uterus.

Douching is the least effective of all methods. The force of ejaculation propels sperm through the cervical opening. Some will reach your uterus before you've reached the bathroom, and the douche, which is liquid squirted into your vagina under pressure, will push some sperm up into your uterus even as it is washing others away.

Douching also puts the burden of birth control exclusively on the woman, who must hop up and run to the bathroom immediately. Don't use it!

Avoidance of Orgasm by the Woman

Some people think that in order to conceive, a woman must have an orgasm. This is false. One of the major differences between men and women in reproduction is that a man must have an erection and ejaculation to cause a pregnancy, whereas a woman can conceive without any sexual arousal.

NOTES

1. In 1996, a report by the Institute of Medicine in the U.S. recommended (pp. 10, 2) "that priorities for new research be assessed against . . . a new 'woman-centered' agenda." This agenda "reflects a more expansive view of contraception that attempts to integrate concerns for contraceptive efficacy into concerns for the overall reproductive health and general well-being of . . . women." Polly F. Harrison and Allan Rosenfield, eds., *Contraceptive Research and Development: Looking to the Future.* Committee on Contraceptive Research and Development, Division of Health Sciences Policy, Institute of Medicine (National Academy Press, 1996). The IOM was chartered in 1970 by the National Academy of Sciences to conduct research and to advise the federal government about medical care, research, and education.

2. WHAM and the Population Council (PC) sponsored two international meetings which brought together women's health advocates, social and biomedical scientists, and policy makers from around the world to discuss the development of microbicides (May 1994) and the key practical and ethical dilemmas raised by clinical testing of new microbicides (April 1997). (The Population Council, "Partnership for Prevention: A Report of a Meeting Between Women's Health Advocates, Program Planners, and Scientists," 1994; WHAM/Population Council "Symposium on Practical and Ethical Dilemmas in the Clinical Testing of Microbicides," forthcoming 1998. Both reports are available from the International Women's Health Coalition, 24 East 21 Street, New York, NY 10010.) Following the 1997 meeting, WHAM decided to end as a formal entity but to continue to work as part of a wider, more flexible network in pursuit of its original goals: to "help ensure that the scientific community's commitment to microbicide research results in the availability of vaginal products that are safe, effective, and meet women's needs"; and to "help develop an approach to reproductive technology development that engages women as active partners in all aspects of the process, including the setting of research agendas and all stages of testing and introducing new products." Statement of Group Principles, WHAM, May 18, 1995, pp. 1, 4, 5. Available from International Women's Health Coalition. The partnership between WHAM and the PC broke new ground and proceeded slowly and cautiously. Some of the women's

groups to which individuals in WHAM belonged had an oppositional relationship with research agencies including the PC. The Population Council has historically been identified with the population control establishment; thus, in its "Statement of Group Principles," WHAM warned that its work with the PC on microbicides did not constitute an unconditional endorsement of the PC. WHAM reserved the right "to independently evaluate and interpret the implications of research findings for women's lives." The WHAM effort was an extremely important step in the history of dialogue among women's health advocates, social scientists, and biomedical researchers. It was the first time that staff of an organization like the PC asked women's health advocates to offer their views on the research and development process from the outset. Nonetheless, in all of the partnerships like this one that we know about, there remains a fundamental power imbalance between the agencies controlling the funds and the feminist activists whose voices are heard only at the agencies' discretion. Until new strategies appear, women's health advocates should continue to look for new ways to make our voices heard. Increased dialogue can help clarify the terms of conflict and reveal areas of commonality on which to build.

3. Sandra D. Lane, "From Population Control to Reproductive Health: An Emerging Policy Agenda," *Social Science and Medicine* 39, no. 9 (1994): 1303–314.

4. On Lea's Shield, see Christine Mauck et al., "Lea's Shield: A Study of the Safety and Efficacy of a New Vaginal Barrier Contraceptive Used With and Without Spermicide," *Contraception* 53 (1996): 329–35. The global strategy to prevent STDs and HIV/AIDS has been to encourage people to reduce the number of sexual partners and to use male condoms. This strategy does not address the power imbalances that exist between women and men that make it virtually impossible for some women to refuse unwanted or unprotected sex. This strategy also does not acknowledge that in many cultures a woman's social status depends on her ability to bear children. Research on microbicides and monoclonal antibodies does take these political and cultural circumstances into account. On microbicides, see Christopher J. Elias and Lori L. Heise, "Challenges for the Development of Female-Controlled Vaginal Microbicides," *AIDS* 8 (1994): 1–9; Christopher Elias and Christina Coggins, "Female-controlled Methods to Prevent Sexual Transmission of HIV," *AIDS* 10, suppl. 3 (1996): 543–51. On monoclonal antibodies, see Richard A. Cone and Kevin J. Whaley, "Monoclonal Antibodies for Reproductive Health: Part I. Preventing Sexual Transmission of Disease and Pregnancy with Topically Applied Antibodies," *American Journal of Reproductive Immunology* 32 (1994): 114–31.

5. Jane Cottingham and Suman Mehta, "Medical Barriers to Contraceptive Use," *Reproductive Health Matters* 1 (May 1993): 97.

6. James Trussell et al. "Contraceptive Failure in the United States: An Update," *Studies in Family Planning* 21 (1990): 51–54. For a further discussion of our decision, see S. E. Bell, "Translating Science to the People: Updating The New Our Bodies, Ourselves," *Women's Studies International Forum* 17, no. 1 (1994): 9–18.

7. According to one survey conducted periodically by the National Center for Health Statistics, in 1995, 18.9% of U.S. women at risk of pregnancy reported using male condoms as their method of birth control. Condom use increased between 1988 and 1995, especially among women under the age of 30. (In 1995, 29.7% of women aged 15–19 were using condoms, 24% of women aged 20–24 were using them, and 22.8% of women aged 25–29 were using them.) James Trussell and Debbie Kowal, "The Essentials of Contraception: Efficacy, Safety, & Personal Considerations," chapter 9 in R. Hatcher et al. *Contraceptive Technology,* 17th rev. ed. New York: Irvington, 1998.

8. The evidence of a link between damaged vaginal tissue and HIV infection comes from several studies of commercial sex workers and is reviewed in Willard Cates, Jr., and Katherine M. Stone, "Family Planning, Sexually Transmitted Diseases and Contraceptive Choice: A Literature Update—Part I," *Family Planning Perspectives* 24, no. 2 (1992): 75–84. For more on this controversial topic, see U.S. Department of Health and Human Services, "Update: Barrier Protection Against HIV Infection and Other Sexually Transmitted Disease," *Morbidity and Mortality Weekly Report* 42, no. 30 (August 6, 1993): 589–91; Pamela Stratton and Nancy J. Alexander, "Prevention of Sexually Transmitted Infections: Physical and Chemical Barrier Methods," *Infectious Disease Clinics of North America* 7, no. 4 (1993): 841–59; Robert Hatcher et al., *Contraceptive Technology,* 16th ed. (New York: Irvington, 1994), 183–86.

9. Stratton and Alexander, "Prevention of Sexually Transmitted Infections," 850; Cates and Stone, "Family Planning," 80–81.

10. See Hatcher et al., *Contraceptive Technology,* 16th ed., 235–36; American College of Obstetricians and Gynecologists, "Hormonal Contraception," *Technical Bulletin* no. 198 (October 1994): 3–4; J. E. Buring, "Low-dose Oral Contraceptives and Stroke," *New England Journal of Medicine* 335, no. 1 (1996): 53–54.

11. N. Weiss, "Third Generation Oral Contraceptives: How Risky?" [Commentary]. *The Lancet* 346, no. 8990 (December 16, 1995): 1570; D. Carnall, H. Karcher, L. Gunnar Lie et al., "Third Generation Oral Contraceptives—The Controversy," *British Medical Journal* 311 (December 16, 1995): 1589–590; J. P. Vandenbroucke and F. R. Rosendaal, "End of the Line for 'Third-Generation Pill' Controversy?" [Commentary]. *The Lancet* 349 (April 19, 1997): 1113–114.

12. Hatcher et al, *Contraceptive Technology,* 16th ed., 236; see also L. Chasan-Taber, W. C. Willett, J. E. Manson, et al., "Prospective Study of Oral Contraceptives and Hypertension among Women in the United States," *Circulation* 94, no. 3 (August 1996): 483–89.

13. American College of Obstetricians and Gynecologists, "Hormonal Contraception."

14. R. Turner, "No Overall Pill and Breast Cancer Link, but Young Users' Risk May be Higher," *Family Planning Perspectives* 27, no. 1 (January/February 1995): 45–46.

15. R. Hatcher et al., *Contraceptive Technology,* 16th ed., 240; American College of Obstetricians and Gynecologists, "Hormonal Contraception."

16. R. Hatcher et al., *Contraceptive Technology,* 16th ed., 243.

17. R. Hatcher et al. *Contraceptive Technology,* 16th ed., Table 10-6; A. Kubba, "Drug Interactions with Hormonal Contraceptives," *International Planned Parenthood Foundation Medical Bulletin* 30, no. 3 (June 1996): 3–4.

18. In a recent study of Norplant's effectiveness, no pregnancies occurred and body weight did not make a difference in the effectiveness of Norplant. One thousand one hundred ninety-eight women from clinics in the U.S., Egypt, Chile, Finland, Thailand, and Singapore participated in the three-year clinical trial. See Irving Sivin et al., "Clinical Performance of a New Two-Rod Levonorgestrel Contraceptive Implant: A Three-Year Randomized Study with Norplant Implants As Controls," *Contraception* 55, no. 2 (1997): 73–80.

19. For the effects of DMPA on seizures and sickle-cell anemia, see American College of Obstetricians and Gynecologists, "Hormonal Contraception"; M. Klitsch, "Injectable Hormones and Regulatory Controversy: An End to the Long-Running Story?" *Family Planning Perspectives* 25, no. 1 (January/February 1995): 37; "New Era for Injectables," Supplement to *Population Reports* K-5, 23, no. 2 (August 1995).

20. Cates and Stone, "Family Planning," 76. See also James Trussell and Charlotte Ellertson, "Efficacy of Emergency Contraception, *Fertility Control Reviews* 4, no. 2 (1995): 8–11.

21. K. Treiman, L. Liskin, A. Kols, and W. Rinehart, "IUDs—an Update." *Population Reports,* Series B, no. 6. Baltimore, MD: Johns Hopkins School of Public Health, Population Information Program, December 1995. Available from Population Information Program, Johns Hopkins School of Public Health, 111 Market Place, Suite 310, Baltimore, MD 21202. Multiple copies are $2 each; free to developing countries. E-mail: PopRepts@welchlink.welch.jhu.edu

22. There is no consistent system of classification used to specify conditions that do not absolutely contraindicate IUD use but warrant caution and careful monitoring. We have decided to use three classes ("do not use," "risks outweigh advantages," and "advantages outweigh risks"), as we have in the past, because we believe that this provides women with more guidance in deciding for themselves.

23. According to a press release from the Population Council, "International Scientific Conference Hears Evidence Supporting Safety, Effectiveness, and Reversibility of Modern Intrauterine Devices," 20 April 1992, "currently available information indicates that PID in IUD users" is not related to the string. There is still controversy about the short-term use of antibiotics at the time of insertion. According to Treiman, Liskin, Kols, and Rinehart, "IUDs—An Update" (p. 13), "no benefit has been demonstrated in routine use of antibiotics at the time of IUD insertion. When the IUD is inserted correctly, using proper infection-prevention techniques, there is little risk of infection for healthy women."

24. Hatcher et al., *Contraceptive Technology,* 16th ed., 352; *Population Reports,* December 1995, 16–17. There seems to be consensus that pregnancies with IUDs, other

than the Dalkon Shield, are not likely to result in a septic abortion.

25. Trieman, Liskin, Kols, and Rinehart, "IUDs—an Update," 10.

26. Deborah Rogow and Sonya Horowitz, "Withdrawal: A Review of the Literature and an Agenda for Research," *Studies in Family Planning* 26, no. 3 (May/June 1995): 140–53; Gerard Ilaria et al., "Detection of HIV-1 DNA Sequences in Pre-ejaculatory Fluid" [Letter], *The Lancet* 340, no. 8833 (December 12, 1992): 1469; J. Pudney et al., "Pre-ejaculatory Fluid as Potential Vector for Sexual Transmission of HIV-1" [Letter], *The Lancet* 340, no. 8833 (December 12, 1992): 1470.

27. Rahemah Amur et al. "Sterilization Rights Abuses and Remedies," *A Sourcebook for the 11th National Women and the Law Conference,* Spring 1980. See also "WHO Eligibility Criteria for Contraceptive Use: Combined Injectables and Sterilization," *Outlook, Program for Appropriate Health* (PATH), 14, no. 1 (May 1996): 5.

28. R. P. Petchesky. "Reproduction, Ethics and Public Policy: The Federal Sterilization Regulations," *Hastings Center Report* 9, no. 5 (October 1979): 29–41.

29. See H. B. Peterson et al. (For the U.S. Collaborative Review of Sterilization Working Group), "The Risk of Pregnancy after Tubal Sterilization: Findings from the U.S. Collaborative Review of Sterilization," *American Journal of Obstetrics and Gynecology* 174 (1996): 1161–170.

30. According to the authors of the study, it isn't clear why black women experienced a higher failure rate than white women: "although black women were more likely than white women to experience sterilization failure after adjustment for other known factors, black race may have served as a marker for other unmeasured determinants of risk." H. B. Peterson et al., "The Risk of Pregnancy after Tubal Sterilization."

31. C. Mettlin, N. Natarajan, and R. Huben. "Vasectomy and Prostate Cancer Risk," *American Journal of Epidemiology* 132, no. 6 (1990): 1056–61.; L. Rosenberg et al. "Vasectomy and the Risk of Prostate Cancer," *American Journal of Epidemiology* 132, no. 6 (1990): 1051–55 (discussion, pp. 1062–65).

32. H. B. Petersen, D. H. Huber, and A. M. Belker. "Vasectomy: An Appraisal for the Obstetrician Gynecologist," *Obstetrics and Gynecology* 76, no. 3 (1990): 568–72.

33. E. A. Lissner, "Frontiers in Nonhormonal Male Contraception: A Call for Research," March 8, 1994. Available from Boston Women's Health Book Collective, 240A Elm Street, Somerville, MA 02144.

RESOURCES

General

American Civil Liberties Union/Reproductive Freedom Project
125 Broad Street, 17th floor; New York, NY 10004
E-mail: aclu@aclu.org
Web site: http://www.aclu.org
Publishes *Reproductive Rights Update.*

Center for Reproductive Law and Policy
120 Wall Street, 18th floor; New York, NY 10005
Publishes *Reproductive Freedom News.*

Cottingham, Jane, and Suman Mehta. "Medical Barriers to Contraceptive Use." *Reproductive Health Matters* no. 1 (May 1993): 97–100.

Davis, Angela. "Racism, Birth Control and Reproductive Rights." In M. G. Fried, ed., *From Abortion to Reproductive Freedom: Transforming a Movement.* Boston: South End Press, 1990.

Gordon, Linda. *Woman's Body, Woman's Right: A Social History of Birth Control in America,* rev. ed. New York: Penguin Books, 1990.

Hartmann, Betsy. *Reproductive Rights and Wrongs: The Global Politics of Population Control and Contraceptive Choice,* rev. ed. Boston: South End Press, 1995.

Hatcher, Robert, et al. *Contraceptive Technology,* 17th rev. ed. New York: Irvington, 1998. A comprehensive handbook on birth control methods.

Institute of Medicine. Polly F. Harrison and Allan Rosenfield, eds. *Contraceptive Research and Development: Looking to the Future.* Washington, DC: National Academy Press, 1996.

International Women's Health Coalition (IWHC)
24 East 21st Street; New York, NY 10010; (212) 979-8500
E-mail: iwhc@igc.apc.org
Web site: http://iwhc.org
Promotes women's reproductive health and rights by providing support to colleagues in eight countries of Asia, Africa, and Latin America; builds local organizational capacity and facilitates contact within and across countries and regions.

Mintzes, Barbara, ed. *A Question of Control: Women's Perspectives on the Development and Use of Contraceptive Technologies.* Amsterdam: WEMOS; HAI; Women's Health Action Foundation, 1992.

Seaman, Barbara, and Gideon Seaman. *Women and the Crisis in Sex Hormones.* New York: Bantam Books, 1979.

Trussell, James, and Kathryn Kost. "Contraceptive Failure in the United States: A Critical Review of the Literature." *Studies in Family Planning* 18 (September/October 1987): 237–83.

Yanoshik, Kim, and Judy Norsigian. "Contraception, Control, and Choice: International Perspectives." in K. S. Ratcliff, ed., *Healing Technology: Feminist Perspectives.* Ann Arbor: University of Michigan Press, 1989.

Barrier Methods

Chalker, Rebecca. *The Complete Cervical Cap Guide.* New York: Harper & Row, 1987. This is an excellent resource, not only for its clear and concise information about the cap, but for information about birth control more generally.

Gollub, Erica L., and Zena A. Stein. "Commentary: The New Female Condom—Item 1 on a Women's AIDS Prevention Agenda." *American Journal of Public Health* 83, no. 4 (April 1993): 498–500.

Hooton, T. M., et al. "A Prospective Study of Risk Factors for Symptomatic Urinary Tract Infection in Young Women." *New England Journal of Medicine* 335 (August 15, 1996): 468–74.

Lane, M. E., et al. "Successful Use of the Diaphragm and Jelly by a Young Population: Report of a Clinical Study." *Family Planning Perspectives* 8, no. 2 (1976): 81–86.

Liskin, L., et al. "Condoms—Now More than Ever." *Population Reports,* Series H, no. 8 (September 1990). Available from Population Information Programs, Johns Hopkins University, 327 St. Paul Street, Baltimore, MD 21208.

Mauck, Christine K., et al., eds. *Barrier Contraceptives: Current Status and Future Prospects.* New York: Wiley-Liss, 1994.

Trussell, James, et al. "Comparative Contraceptive Efficacy of The Female Condom and Other Barrier Methods." *Family Planning Perspectives* 26, no. 2 (March/April 1994): 66–72.

———, et al. "Contraceptive Failure in the United States: An Update." *Studies in Family Planning* 21, no. 1 (January/February 1990): 51–54.

Natural Birth Control

Note: These are some of the publications or resources currently available. Please understand that they are not meant to take the place of a group in which these skills are shared on a women-to-woman basis. We do not recommend that you use the information for contraception until you have participated in such a group.

Billings, Evelyn, and Ann Westmore. *The Billings Method.* New York: Ballantine, 1986. A popularized introduction to the ovulation method.

Doyle, Suzannah Cooper. "Fertility Awareness: Reclaiming Reproductive Control," *WomenWise* 14, no. 2 (summer 1991): 6.

———. *A Fertility Awareness Self-Instruction Course,* 1995. $65.50 postpaid (includes follow-up counseling). Available from Fertility Awareness Services, Box 986, Corvallis, OR 97339, USA.

———. *The Ovulation Method Charting Booklet,* 4th rev. ed., 1997. Three years of mucus/BBT/cervix charts with guidelines, $17.50 postpaid from Fertility Awareness Services, Box 986, Corvallis, OR 97339, USA.

Guren, Denise J., and Nealy Gillette. *The Ovulation Method—Cycles of Fertility.* Bellingham, WA: Ovulation Method Teachers Association, 1983.

Kass-Annese, Barbara, and Hal Danzer. *The Fertility Awareness Handbook.* Alameda, CA: Hunter House, 1992.

Labbok, M.H., et al. "The Lactational Amenorrhea Method (LAM): A Postpartum Introductory Family Planning Method with Policy and Program Implications," *Advances in Contraception* 10, no. 2 (June 1994): 93–109.

Rogow, Debbie. "Teaching Fertility Awareness: How a Government Family Planning Program Got Involved in Sexuality." In Sondra Zeidenstein and Kirsten Moore, eds., *Learning About Sexuality.* New York: Population Council and International Women's Health Coalition, 1996, 180–92.

Trussell, James, and Laurence Grummer-Strawn. "Contraceptive Failure of the Ovulation Method of Periodic Abstinence." *Family Planning Perspectives* 22, no. 2 (1990): 65–75.

Weschler, Toni. *Taking Charge of Your Fertility: The Definitive Guide to Natural Birth Control and Pregnancy Achievement.* New York: HarperCollins, 1995. A comprehensive guide to natural birth control, well researched and documented.

Winstein, Merryl. *Your Fertility Signals: How to Read Them to Achieve or Avoid Pregnancy Naturally.* St. Louis, MO: Smooth Stone Press, 1994.

The Pill and Other Hormones

Cannold, Leslie. "The New Progestogen 'Third Generation' Oral Contraceptive Pills: How Safe Are They?" *Healthsharing Women* 6, nos. 3 & 4 (December 1995–March 1996): 14–19.

"Consensus Statement on Emergency Contraception." *Contraception* 52, (1995): 211–13.

Ellertson, Charlotte. "History and Efficacy of Emergency Contraception: Beyond Coca-Cola." *Family Planning Perspectives* 28, no. 2 (March/April 1996): 44–48.

Gill, Sarah, "Discrimination, Historical Abuse, and the New Norplant Problem." *Women's Rights Law Reporter* 16, no. 1 (fall 1994): 43–51.

International Planned Parenthood Federation. International Medical Advisory Panel (IMAP), "IMAP Statement on Breast Feeding, Fertility and Post-Partum Contraception." *International Planned Parenthood Federation Medical Bulletin* 30, no. 3 (June 1996): 1–3.

Lewry, Natasha, and Charon Asetoyer, "The Impact of Norplant in the Native American Community," June 1992. Available for $5.00 from Native American Women's Health Education Resource Center (see chapter 27 Resources).

Samuels, Sarah E., and Mark D. Smith, eds., *Dimensions of New Contraceptives: Norplant and Poor Women.* Menlo Park, CA: Henry J. Kaiser Family Foundation, 1992.

Seaman, Barbara. *The Doctors' Case against the Pill,* 25th anniversary ed. Alameda, CA: Hunter House, 1995.

IUDs

Bardin, C. Wayne, and Daniel R. Mishell, eds. *Proceedings from the Fourth International Conference on IUDs.* Boston: Butterworth-Heinemann, 1994.

Geyelin, Milo. "Dalkon Shield Trust Hailed as Innovative, Stirs a Lot of Discord." *The Wall Street Journal* (June 3, 1991): pp. 1, 5.

Mintz, Morton. *At Any Cost: Corporate Greed, Women, and the Dalkon Shield.* New York: Pantheon, 1985.

Treiman, K., L. Liskin, A. Kols, and W. Rinehart. "IUDs—An Update." *Population Reports,* Series B, no. 6 (December 1995). Available from Population Information Program, Johns Hopkins University, 327 St. Paul Street, Baltimore MD 21208.

Sterilization

Chi, I-Cheng, and D. B. Jones, "Incidence, Risk Factors, and Prevention of Poststerilization Regret in Women: An Updated International Review From an Epidemiological Perspective." *Obstetrical and Gynecological Survey* 49, no. 10 (1994): 722–32.

Lissner, E. A. "Frontiers in Nonhormonal Male Contraception: A Call for Research," updated version (March 8, 1994) available from the Boston Women's Health Book Collective, 240A Elm Street, Somerville, MA 02144.

Petchesky, Rosalind Pollack. *Abortion and Woman's Choice: The State, Sexuality, and Reproductive Freedom,* rev. ed. Boston: Northeastern University Press, 1990.

Peterson, H. B., et al. (for the U.S. Collaborative Review of Sterilization Working Group), "The Risk of Ectopic Pregnancy After Tubal Sterilization." *New England Journal of Medicine* 336 (March 13, 1997): 762–67.

———. "The Risk of Pregnancy after Tubal Sterilization: Findings from the U.S. Collaborative Review of Sterilization." *American Journal of Obstetrics and Gynecology* 174 (1996): 1161–170.

Wilcox, L. S., et al., "Risk Factors for Regret After Tubal Sterilization: Five Years of Follow-up in a Prospective Study," *Fertility and Sterility* 55, no. 5 (May 1991): 927–33.

Additional Online Resources *

About Go Ask Alice!
http://www.columbia.edu/cu/healthwise/about.html

Ann Rose's Ultimate Birth Control Links Page
http://gynpages.com/ultimate

Planned Parenthood: Your Contraceptive Choices
http://www.igc.apc.org/ppfa/contraception/choices_main.html

Reproline
http://www.reproline.jhu.edu

Teen Health Web Site
http://chebucto.ns.ca/Health/TeenHealth/index.html

* For more information and listings of online resources, please see Introduction to Online Women's Health Resources, p. 25.

By Christie Burke with Sylvie Ratelle,
based on earlier work by Mary Crowe
with Judy Norsigian

WITH SPECIAL THANKS TO Katherine M. Stone
of the Centers for Disease Control and
Prevention and Catherine Liu of the
American Social Health Association *

Chapter 14

Sexually Transmitted Diseases

* Thanks also to the following for their help with the 1998 version of this chapter: Judith Wasserheit and Wanda Jones, both of the Centers for Disease Control and Prevention, Deborah Anderson, Ann Rampolo, Liza Rankow, Margaret Warwick, and Cheryl Young. Over the years since 1969, the following people have contributed to the many versions of this chapter: Esther Rome and Fran Ansley with Hilde Armour, William McCormick, Michelle Topal, Pam White, and Paul Wiesner.

Many people, including medical providers, still believe that "nice" girls don't get sexually transmitted diseases (STDs). When we do, we may be labeled "promiscuous" if we are single or "unfaithful" if we are in a monogamous relationship. Worst of all, we may not get medical help and/or counseling when we are sick and need it most. As long as our society continues to look upon STDs as punishment for people who have casual sex, the problem will be hard to talk about, much less eradicate.

It is a woman's right to enjoy and be proud of her sexuality, without fear of disease. That means learning how to prevent STDs, which are infections, before they happen, as well as how to get cured after the fact, whenever this is possible. We can help prevent the spread of infection without giving up our sex lives.

Because STD is hard to talk about, it can be difficult to find the information we need. Sometimes it seems easier to avoid the issue and forget about prevention, especially when our sexual partners are uncooperative or even hostile to the idea of "safer sex." But the recent epidemic of human immunodeficiency virus (HIV) infection and AIDS (see chapter 15, HIV, AIDS, and Women) has raised public awareness about the need to practice prevention to avoid getting a deadly virus for which there is no cure. More people are now willing to talk about using condoms—a primary means of STD prevention—although many still don't. Changing our attitudes and behavior remains a major challenge.

I've been so upset these last few days. My husband told me he'd slept with someone else and might have gotten an STD. I didn't know what to do. How could I call up my regular doctor and expose myself? If I asked any of my friends what to do, they would be mortified. I saw an ad yesterday for an STD hot line, and after a

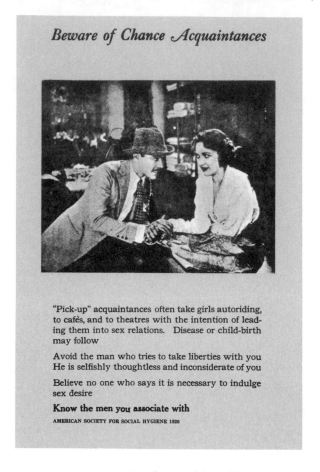

Beware of Chance Acquaintances

"Pick-up" acquaintances often take girls autoriding, to cafés, and to theatres with the intention of leading them into sex relations. Disease or child-birth may follow

Avoid the man who tries to take liberties with you
He is selfishly thoughtless and inconsiderate of you

Believe no one who says it is necessary to indulge sex desire

Know the men you associate with
AMERICAN SOCIETY FOR SOCIAL HYGIENE 1926

American Social Health Association

lot of hesitation I called. It was a relief to get information without anyone knowing who I was.

Having an STD can affect the way we feel about ourselves, our sexuality, and our relationships. We may feel victimized, angry, or depressed and may even blame ourselves unfairly.

If one person in a supposedly monogamous couple gets an STD, it often serves as a dramatic focus for other problems the couple might have.

When we returned home from our summer vacation, I started having a vaginal itch. Then I noticed my husband was itching, too. I asked him if he had slept with anyone else recently. He admitted to me he had slept with the baby-sitter.

Every year, more than 12 million new cases of STDs are diagnosed in the U.S. Until recently, all STDs were considered to be a problem of epidemic proportions. Today's picture is more mixed. Some STDs, like syphilis, have been greatly reduced, and public health policy is aimed at eradicating this disease. However, cases of other STDs are increasing—including human papillomavirus infection (HPV, or genital warts), which has been linked to cervical cancer, and HIV, which almost always develops into acquired immunodeficiency syndrome (AIDS).

STDs interact with each other in the body, and many STDs appear to increase the risk of catching HIV. On a positive note, recent international studies show that when STD prevention programs are put in place, HIV infection rates can drop by as much as 40%.

Women are more likely than men to develop serious medical conditions as a result of STDs and to suffer from chronic conditions caused by these infections. Often women don't have symptoms, so we may not be aware we have an STD until it becomes serious. When such diseases go untreated, we are likely to develop medical conditions such as pelvic inflammatory disease (PID). PID can result in infertility, chronic pelvic pain, an increased risk of ectopic pregnancy, and, rarely, death. (See chapter 24, Selected Medical Practices, Problems, and Procedures, for more on PID.)

WHAT ARE STDs?

"STD" is a term applied to more than two dozen diseases that are transmitted primarily through anal, oral, or vaginal sex. Their effects are not limited to the reproductive organs, and they do not always have to involve sexual activity, but most often they do. In most cases, the organisms that cause STDs enter the body through the mucous membranes: the warm, moist surfaces of the vagina, urethra, anus, and mouth. However, in some instances, exposure to sores or other types of skin-to-skin contact may be sufficient to transmit infection (see description of each disease). In addition, any cuts or lesions that allow germs to get into the bloodstream may increase the risk of transmission, particularly for blood-borne infections such as HIV and hepatitis B.

Most STDs that are caused by bacteria, protozoa, and other small organisms can usually be cured with antibiotics or topical creams and lotions. Among the most common STDs are two bacterial infections known since ancient times: syphilis and gonorrhea (the "clap"). A third, chlamydia, is becoming alarmingly widespread today. All three may be cured with antibiotics, but they can cause serious complications if left untreated.

Viral infections, however, while treatable, are not curable. These include herpes; human papillomavirus (HPV), which causes genital warts; and human immunodeficiency virus (HIV), which produces AIDS. Treatment may help relieve the symptoms and/or slow the progression of the disease.

Hepatitis is the only STD for which a vaccine exists.

Some other common STDs include trichomoniasis, which is caused by protozoa and is treated by a simple oral antibiotic, and scabies and crabs, which are tiny organisms that infest the skin or pubic hair and can be treated by the application of topical creams and lotions. Bacterial vaginosis may or may not be sexually transmitted, because changes in vaginal flora (the organisms that naturally live in a healthy vagina) may occur without sexual contact. There are over 24 STDs, more than we will be able to cover in this chapter. For additional descriptions of STDs, read chapters 15, HIV, AIDS, and Women, and 24, Selected Medical Practices, Problems, and Procedures, or the *STD Handbook* (Montreal Health Press). See the Resource section for a complete listing.

HOW LIKELY AM I TO GET AN STD?

The most likely way to get an STD is to engage in unprotected vaginal, anal, or oral sex, although the diseases described in this chapter can also be transmitted through other intimate sexual and skin-to-skin contact and through donor insemination.

In general, any physical activity that allows blood or other infected body fluid or tissue to come in contact with the mucous membrane, or to enter the body through cuts or lesions, could transmit an STD. Oral sex, penetration with fingers, and sharing infected and unsterilized sex toys, as well as touching open sores and then other parts of the body, may all be potential ways to transmit diseases. If any of your sexual partners (or their partners) has an STD, you are likely to become infected unless you practice prevention consistently. Although it is rare for STDs to be transmitted on inanimate objects, contagion is possible when fresh body fluids are on the object (such as a shared sex toy). Toilet seats or towels are possible but unlikely routes of transmission.

Statistically, if you are young (between 15 and 24), are sexually active with more than one partner, and live in an urban setting, where the number of people with STDs is greater and other risk factors are multiplied, you are at highest risk. Unprotected sex with a new partner, or with anyone whose sexual history you do not know, may put you at risk. For many women, poverty may contribute to a higher risk of STD. Not having enough money can mean lack of access to prevention and treatment, engaging in commercial sex work, economic dependence on a partner who may be exposing you to infection, or just being preoccupied with day-to-day survival, so that STD prevention may not be your highest priority.

Some biological factors may also affect risk for certain groups of women. In young girls, the cervix is not yet fully developed and is more vulnerable to infection. Older women are more likely to get small abrasions in the vagina during sexual activity as a result of thinning of the membrane and, possibly, dryness. Women who already have an infection, particularly one with genital lesions, are more likely to get or transmit another STD, including HIV.

If you are a woman who has sex exclusively with other women, your chances of getting an STD are significantly lower. However, since many women who consider themselves lesbian may also, currently or in the past, have been involved with men, it is more difficult to determine the risk of transmission exclusively from woman to woman. More research is needed in this area.

BRIEF SUMMARY OF PRECAUTIONS

1. STDs are very common. If you are sexually active in anything but a totally monogamous relationship with someone who is having sex only with you and does not have an STD, you have a high risk of getting an STD. If your partner is not monogamous, you may be exposed to STDs, including HIV, from your partner's partners.

2. The best way to deal with STD is to avoid getting it in the first place. Practice prevention wherever possible. See the box on p. 344 for more information.

3. If you think there is the slightest possibility that you or your partners have an STD, get medical attention as soon as you can. **Remember, you might not have any symptoms.** In the meantime, try to find out whether the person you had sex with has been exposed to an STD.

4. Don't have sex until you and all your current partners (and their partners) have been tested, treated, and cured (check with your health care provider).

5. If you do have an STD, inform all your recent partners personally. Even an anonymous letter will do. The partner notification services available at local Department of Health offices will inform people anonymously, without revealing your identity.

6. Before accepting treatment, make sure you understand what you are taking and for how long, the side effects, and any followup tests or treatment required. Don't be embarrassed about asking questions. It's your life, not theirs.

7. Remember, even if you are cured you can get the same STD again. Also, having one STD doesn't protect you from getting others. Viral STDs—such as herpes, HPV (genital warts), and HIV—cannot be cured. Specific treatment and management strategies are covered later in this chapter and in chapters 15, HIV, AIDS, and Women, and 24, Selected Medical Practices, Problems, and Procedures.

BIRTH CONTROL AND STDs

The Pill, Norplant, and the IUD **do not** protect against STDs. Birth control pills are linked to changes in the cervix that may increase the risk for certain STDs, particularly chlamydial infection (see chapter 13, Birth Control), and possibly for HIV infection as well

PREVENTING SEXUALLY TRANSMITTED DISEASES

Using any of the prevention methods described below should reduce your chances of catching an STD. Consider using more than one method since no method, including condoms, is 100% effective.

1. Latex condoms (rubbers) used during vaginal, oral, and anal intercourse are the best-known preventive method. The man or you must put the condom on his penis before it touches your vulva, mouth, or anus. If you or your partner experiences irritation or other adverse reactions to latex condoms, try another brand, a polyurethane condom, or condoms without spermicide. Condoms without nonoxynol-9 are available for oral sex, in flavors that may make them more pleasant to use. Latex condoms have been more widely tested and found effective for disease prevention, but polyurethane condoms also provide protection. **Never use an oil-based lubricant—such as Vaseline—with latex, as it will break down the rubber and destroy its protection.** (See chapters 13, Birth Control, and 15, HIV, AIDS, and Women.)

2. Use the new female condom (Reality®, Femidom®, Femy®). This could be useful if your male partner(s) can't or won't use condoms. Small amounts of any lubricant, including oil-based ones, may be used inside the pouch or on the penis. Using a spermicide containing nonoxynol-9 with the female condom may irritate the vaginal surface. (See chapter 13, Birth Control, for more information on the female condom.)

3. Use vaginal spermicides (contraceptive foams, films, creams and jellies).* You can purchase them in a drugstore without a prescription and use them with or without a diaphragm or condom. Using a barrier contraceptive—condom or diaphragm—with spermicide may increase your protection. When using a condom, put an applicatorful of spermicide inside the vagina before sexual intercourse.

    Using nonoxynol-9 can irritate the vaginal mucosa. Whether this increases the risk of HIV transmission is still uncertain. The question is controversial because much of the research indicating increased risk was based on very frequent use among sex workers.

4. A diaphragm (with spermicide) gives better protection against STDs that affect the cervix, such as gonorrhea and chlamydial infection. Other cervical barrier contraceptives, such as caps and the sponge, have not proved to be as effective for STD prevention. Cervical barriers do not protect you from infection in other parts of the body, such as the vulva, vagina, or rectum, by organisms such as herpes, warts, or syphilis.

5. Washing the genitals before and right after sex may not help much. Douching, in most cases, does not prevent STD, as it washes away the normal vaginal secretions that help our bodies fight off infection and may even push infections higher up in your reproductive system. Men should wash their testicles and penis, particularly after anal sex and before going on to vaginal or oral sex.

6. Barrier methods can be used for mouth-to-vagina or mouth-to-anus contact. Dental dams (squares of latex used by dentists) can be used as a barrier for oral sex. Some people now place household plastic wrap over the area before contact, then discard it after one-time use. If nothing else is available, you can cut up a latex glove and use that as a barrier.

    Remember: Barriers don't protect you from an infection on parts of the body that they do not cover.

7. Avoid sharing sex toys. Body secretions on sex toys may transmit STDs. Some people soak sex toys in hydrogen peroxide for 15 minutes. Also, be very careful in any sexual activities that involve blood, including bondage and discipline. Direct contact with the blood—including menstrual blood—of an infected person can transmit HIV or hepatitis.

8. **Talk to your lover about STD before having sex.** Ask if she or he has been exposed to an STD. This is especially important if you are pregnant! Look carefully at your body and your lover's, checking for a bad smell, an unusual discharge, sores, bumps, itching, or redness. If you think you or your partner may have an infection, don't touch the sores or have sex. Also, remember that a person may be infected with an STD, such as herpes or HIV, and look completely healthy.

It's one thing to talk about "being responsible about STD" and a much harder thing to do it at the moment. It's just plain hard to say to someone I am feeling very erotic with, "Oh, yes, before we go any further, can we have a conversation about STD?" It is hard to imagine murmuring into someone's ear at a time of passion, "Would you mind slipping on this condom just in case one of us has an STD?" Yet, it seems awkward to bring it up any sooner if it's not clear between us that we want to make love.

For some ideas on how to talk about sex more comfortably with a lover, see chapter 11, Sexuality.

9. *We do not recommend morning-after antibiotics for STDs.* Taken just before or within nine hours after exposure to an infected person, these antibiotic pills contain enough drug to prevent these diseases, but not enough to cure an established infection. Taking antibiotics frequently or in less than the optimal dosage may encourage the development of resistant strains of bacteria.

* Many creams, films, foams, and jellies have been shown in the laboratory to kill organisms that cause gonorrhea, syphilis, trichomoniasis, candidiasis, chlamydial infection, HIV infection, and herpes. In actual use, they have been shown to be effective only against chlamydial infection and gonorrhea. Test your sensitivity to these products on your body before using them during sex. Try latex separately from nonoxynol-9, and experiment with different brands of condom or spermicide. These products have not been tested for use in anal sex.

(see chapter 15, HIV, AIDS, and Women). Most evidence indicates that IUDs may actually increase the chance that gonorrhea and chlamydial infection will lead to pelvic inflammatory disease.

Barrier methods of contraception, however, help to prevent STDs (see the box on pp. 344–45). Women who have had either a hysterectomy or a tubal ligation, or who have gone through menopause, still need to use barrier methods of protection (usually contraceptives) to reduce their risk of STD infection. See chapter 13, Birth Control, pp. 294–303, for illustrations and discussion of barrier methods.

WHY PREVENTION MATTERS

Preventing infection is more urgent today than ever before, because of the increase in viral and incurable STDs. Infection with most STDs increases your chances of contracting and possibly transmitting another STD, including HIV. Also, if you have more than one STD, they may be interactive. For example, in a woman infected with HIV, the symptoms of a second STD, such as herpes, will be more serious and debilitating.

If you are sexually active, you may be at risk for STDs. It's important to stop the chain of transmission whenever you can, and to seek a cure when you know you are infected. Routine gynecological care, including Pap smears, is necessary to maintain your sexual health, but you must understand that a Pap smear is a test for cancer, not for STDs. There are specific tests for

each STD (see pp. 348–56). You should also consider regular screening for "silent" STDs such as chlamydial infection.

SOCIAL PROBLEMS

Medical Care and the Morality Issue

The social stigma attached to STDs often affects the quality of the medical care we receive.

Until recently, medical schools virtually ignored STDs. As a result, physicians who received their training prior to the past few years may not know much about diagnosing and treating STDs, especially when there are no symptoms, or when the symptoms are characteristic of other infections. This lack of training in medical school reflects the values of a larger society that considers STD an appropriate punishment for "immoral" sex. Women, especially, are more readily accused of being "promiscuous" than men. Women living in poverty and women of color are more often stigmatized than white middle-class women.

People at all levels of responsibility, too moralistic or too ashamed about sex, have slowed down research into improved methods of prevention and have curtailed the spread of information about available methods of prevention and cure.

With the advent of widespread birth control, which reduced the fear of pregnancy, fear of STD became the last deterrent to sex outside of marriage. Despite our recognition of the need to prevent STDs, moralistic attitudes continue to block access to information and contraceptive devices that help prevent STDs, especially for teenagers.

A recent report from the Institute of Medicine entitled *The Hidden Epidemic: Confronting Sexually Transmitted Disease* calls for a national system of STD prevention, using four major strategies: a change in social attitudes, strong leadership, innovative education, and access to care.

Money and Politics

Apart from AIDS, treatment of STDs and their complications costs over $10 billion a year. Yet, funding for research, clinical training, public education, screening, and treatment programs for other STDs remains inadequate. In addition to alarming increases in the number of people with STDs and related medical conditions, the link between HIV transmission and other STDs is another compelling reason to support STD prevention.

Passage of the Infertility Prevention Act of 1992—developed in part through the leadership of the Congressional Caucus for Women's Issues—led to a program to screen and treat women in family-planning and other community clinics for chlamydial infection and gonorrhea, the two leading causes of preventable infertility. Where fully implemented, the Infertility Prevention Program has reduced infection rates by as much as 60%. However, the program still reflects restrictive attitudes toward women's sexuality. While very effective, it still focuses only on women's reproductive health rather than on healthy sexuality.

More outreach workers should be involved in running community screening programs to make tests, screening, and treatment available to people of all economic and social groups. We can also ask for routine screening tests for STD when we go for medical care; medical workers will be more apt to include tests if a large number of clients request them.

The Need for Education

The incidence of many STDs has been reduced in this country through the work of agencies funded to provide primary and secondary prevention, as well as by the personal behavior change of people at risk. However, because of public attitudes, changes have been slow to occur. Several European countries and China have reduced their STD rates through education and prevention. Sweden, by more freely promoting the condom, has reduced the incidence of STDs without restricting sexual activity.

Education and prevention campaigns for women must be developed that are culturally relevant and that provide the support we need to protect ourselves against infection. We must initiate more effective public education programs without moral overtones in our schools and communities.

Some nonjudgmental films, pamphlets, and brochures (see Resources) are already available that we can distribute in public places such as libraries, schools, movie houses, social centers, and health facilities. We can talk with friends, parents, and children to make sure they have as much accurate information as possible. We can support women's centers and other STD educators as they work for more complete sex and health education. When our society accepts sexuality it will be more likely to encourage STD prevention.

WOMEN-CONTROLLED PREVENTION

One of the most exciting changes in recent years is an increased focus on STD prevention methods that women can control. Development of the female condom (see chapter 13, Birth Control) was a breakthrough in this area. Studies of usage and acceptability that have been done so far show that this device is likely to require the cooperation of both partners—which is often a problem if the female partner has no control in the relationship—but is generally well liked by those who try it: as many as 50 to 70% of women from different population groups in 27 countries, and a comparable percentage of men. An extensive, federally funded study indicates that the female condom becomes easier to use when women learn more about it through counseling and have had more experience using it. However, the need to obtain men's cooperation may limit its use.

Several advocacy projects are trying to ensure that women's needs and perspectives are integrated into all phases of microbicide development. The Microbicide Research Advocacy Project, sponsored jointly by the Center for Women Policy Studies and the Reproductive Health Technologies Project, has garnered wide medical and political support for taking consumer acceptability into account in clinical trials of new microbicides. The Health Development Policy Project and Women's Health Advocates for Microbicides are working internationally to encourage development of disease prevention methods that are safe and effective and that meet the needs of women.

In addition, other approaches to woman-controlled protection are being explored, including creams that may keep viruses from attaching to the vagina or moving farther inside the body, and products that change the vagina's Ph (acidity), so that viruses will be less likely to survive and grow there.

Some people believe that the development and use of home testing kits would also allow women more control over preventing and dealing with infection. Others are concerned that home testing for STDs could be misleading and emotionally distressing without proper education, counseling, and, in the event of a positive test result, referral to support and/or treatment.

TREATMENT—CONVENTIONAL VS. ALTERNATIVE AND SELF-HELP

In most cases, treatments for STDs caused by bacteria involve high doses of antibiotics, which kill the bacteria. Antibiotics are not effective against viral infections like herpes. Some people are allergic to penicillin or related drugs, while others suffer unwanted side effects from other antibiotics. Sometimes antibiotics just don't work. (Information on antibiotics is listed under each infection.) Most herbalists do not recommend treating serious infections like gonorrhea, chlamydial infection, or syphilis with natural remedies—at least not without first trying antibiotics.

No matter what treatment you use, **remember that curing a sexually transmitted disease does not make you immune to future infection.**

What to Do If You Think You Have an STD

Get a diagnosis as early as possible. Most STDs are easy to cure, though it can be difficult to wade through the medical system to get care. Women who think they may have an STD can get medical treatment in various places. Some of the advantages and disadvantages of each are listed in this section.

The ASHA, an excellent source of information on all STDs, operates several hot lines (see Resources), including the National AIDS Hot Line: (800) 342-AIDS. Call them for more information or addresses of places to get treated.

Local Hospital, Managed Care Plan, Primary Care Physician, or Gynecologist

You may want to discuss STD risks and/or treatment with a provider with whom you feel comfortable, and who feels comfortable talking about sexuality and STDs. However, while the AMA has developed guidelines for sexual history-taking, many providers do not have the time or inclination to do this if you have no symptoms. Not all physicians have the equipment necessary to do routine STD testing, nor are they necessarily well informed about these diseases. If you receive treatment, you may want to ask whether your provider is following the most recent Centers for Disease Control and Prevention guidelines. The 1997 treatment guidelines are now available via computer. (See the Resource section for information.)

Unless you are severely ill and in true need of emergency care, a hospital emergency room is not likely to give you the time, expertise, and sensitivity required in treating STD symptoms.

Any kind of discrimination in the medical system makes it more difficult to discuss such intimate matters as sexual behavior, STD risk, and infections. Many medical providers still exhibit a negative attitude toward women's sexuality, as well as racism and homophobia. They may not bother to test a white, middle-class woman or an older woman, even when she has symptoms. For lesbians, "coming out" to a health care provider may be necessary to make sure appropriate information, tests, and treatment are given for STD symptoms.

The first time I asked a gynecologist for a routine gonorrhea culture, he smiled with a comradely look in his eye. "But I'm sure no man you'd be involved with would have gonorrhea."

On the other hand, they may be overly suspicious about the possibility of STD in women of color and women with low incomes.

Feminist Health Centers and Family Planning Providers

Women's health centers often offer the most sympathetic care for women with STD. If they lack the necessary diagnostic equipment for your STD, they will refer you to a sympathetic doctor or clinic. For a list of feminist health clinics, write to the National Women's Health Network, 1325 G Street NW, Washington, DC 20005.

Some family-planning providers also offer STD counseling and testing or referral. If you have a long-established relationship with your family-planning provider, that may be the best person to ask for STD counseling, risk assessment, or a referral for treatment if necessary.

Public Health STD Clinics

STD clinics are free to teens and provide services regardless of ability to pay.

Some women may want a more anonymous setting for information about, or the diagnosis and treatment of, STDs. STD clinic personnel are likely to have the most expertise in testing, diagnosing, and treating such diseases. You may be able to find a walk-in public health clinic in your area. To find the most conveniently located public health facility, call the National STD Hot Line: (800) 227-8922.

Going for Treatment

Before going to a physician or clinic, it's a good idea to call ahead to get an idea of the services offered and the charges. Tests are often free, but there may be a fee for the visit. If you are a minor and don't want your parents notified or sent the bill, ask about the policy on this.

If you are a minor, you can receive examination and treatment without your parents' permission in every state. The law, however, does not *prevent* the physician from telling your parents. You may want to ask your practitioner what her or his policy is before going for services.

Wherever you decide to go for care, you have a right to courteous and thorough treatment. Expect to have a medical history taken and to undergo a pelvic exam. (See chapter 24, Selected Medical Practices, Problems, and Procedures, p. 591) The health care practitioner should explain any test, treatment, and negative side effects. Before leaving, know what your followup care will be. If your doctor or medical care worker is too busy to answer your questions, ask to speak to someone else. It's always a good idea to take someone with you. Don't leave before your questions have been answered. Even then, however, you may still feel uncertain about your treatment. Sometimes tests are not accurate; sometimes treatments don't work. That can mean more medical visits, time, and money. Treatment can be painful: two big shots in the buttocks for syphilis, for example. But the alternative —not getting treatment—is worse.

STD and Female Circumcision

If you have been circumcised, you may be at higher risk of catching an STD from an infected partner. This is because some circumcised women are more likely to have small wounds resulting from intercourse, and others may have unhealed ulcers or inflamed vulval membranes. Infibulated women or women whose vaginal outlet has been altered from the scar of the circumcision may have difficulty in getting rid of the infection, even with treatment, because of inadequate drainage of vaginal secretions. In some cases, surgical opening of the scar may be necessary before the infection can be cleared completely. For further advice, talk to a gynecologist or to a support group that helps circumcised women with their physical and emotional needs: (See "RAINB♀" in chapter 24 Resources.)

STDS and the Law

Physicians and clinics are required by law to report all cases of gonorrhea and syphilis to the state or local health officer. Chancroid, granuloma inguinale, and lymphogranuloma venereum are also reportable in most states. Chlamydial infection is reportable in some states.

If you have gonorrhea or syphilis, a social worker may interview you and ask for the names of your sexual contacts/partners (people you may have caught the disease from or given it to). Partners should be notified anonymously—your name is not mentioned. If you do not wish to give their names, say you will contact them yourself. Then it is your responsibility to contact each person you've had sex with and ask him or her to seek treatment. Remember, you may be saving their fertility or even their lives.

SYMPTOMS AND TREATMENT

Gonorrhea

Gonorrhea is caused by the gonococcus, a bacterium shaped like a coffee bean, which works its way gradually along the warm, moist passageways of the genital and urinary organs and affects the cervix, urethra, and anus. It can be passed to another person through genital, genital-oral (which exposes the throat), and genital-anal sex. You can get a gonorrhea infection in your eye when you touch it with a hand that is moist with infected discharge. A mother can pass it to her baby during birth. Children with gonorrhea who were not infected at birth are generally found to have been sexually abused.

Untreated gonorrhea can lead to serious and painful infection of the pelvic area, PID, which can lead to sterility and, less commonly, to disseminated gonococcal infection (DGI) when the disease spreads throughout the body.

Remember, it is important to use preventive measures, because a woman often does not have early symptoms. By the time pain prompts her to see a doctor, the infection has usually spread considerably. A woman who has had a hysterectomy can be infected in the cervix (if it is left) and in other parts of the body, in the same way as women who have not had their uterus removed.

Symptoms

At least 50% of women infected with gonorrhea may have no symptoms at first. Women who develop symptoms usually do so within ten days of infection. The cervix is the most common site of infection. In cervical gonorrhea, a discharge develops that is caused by an irritant released by the gonococci when they die. If you examine yourself with a speculum, you may

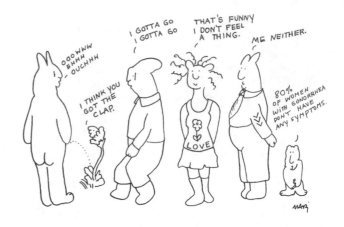

Mari Stein

see a thick discharge, redness, and sometimes small bumps or signs of erosion on the cervix—or you may not see anything abnormal. You may at first attribute your symptoms to other routine gynecological problems or to the use of birth control methods like the Pill. The urethra may also become infected, possibly causing painful urination and burning. As the infection spreads, it can affect the Skene's glands (on each side of the urinary opening) and the Bartholin's glands (on each side of the vaginal opening; see diagrams of the female pelvic organs in chapter 12, Understanding Our Bodies). If the disease spreads to the uterus and fallopian tubes, you may have pain on one or both sides of your lower abdomen, vomiting, fever, and/or irregular menstrual periods, or you may feel pain during intercourse. The more severe the infection, the more severe the pain and other symptoms are likely to be. These symptoms may indicate PID.

Gonorrhea can also be spread from a man's penis to a woman's throat (pharyngeal gonorrhea) or rectum. You may have no symptoms. If you do, depending on the area infected you may have a sore throat, swollen glands, rectal pain or inflammation (proctitis), discharge, or bleeding.

If the eyes become infected by gonococcal discharge (gonococcal conjunctivitis), blindness can result if the eyes are not treated (or if preventive treatment is not given to newborns). Disseminated gonococcal infection, rare but serious, occurs when bacteria travel through the bloodstream, causing pustular skin rash and painful, swollen joints or, rarely, infection of the heart valves, arthritis, or meningitis. Gonorrhea can be treated and cured with antibiotics at any stage to prevent further damage, but damage already done usually cannot be repaired.

Men's Symptoms

A man will usually have a thick, pus-like discharge from his penis, which may be red and inflamed, and will usually feel pain or burning when he urinates. He may have to urinate frequently and/or find blood in his urine. Some men have no symptoms.

Gonorrhea in a man is often confused with similar

symptoms of another infection, such as chlamydial infection. An inflammation not caused by gonorrhea is called nongonococcal urethritis (NGU). This term does not mean that the cause of the infection has been found; it only means it is not caused by gonorrhea. If you have had sex with a man who has a discharge from his penis, get him to go for a test right away. You may be able to obtain a diagnosis the same day, and treatment for both of you could begin immediately. If the cause of the infection is not identified by the first test, it is a good idea to insist on further testing.

Testing and Diagnosis

It is important to be tested for gonorrhea before taking medication, because a test done while treatment is being given is not accurate. Don't douche right before a test, because you can wash away the accessible bacteria, giving a false negative test result. Also, douching may push bacteria farther up into your reproductive tract and increase your risk of more serious infection.

Of the different tests available for detecting gonorrhea, the Gram stain is not commonly used outside of STD clinics and may miss up to 50% of cervical infections. The Gram stain cannot detect infections of the throat. It detects 98% of the gonorrhea cases in men who have a urethral discharge, but only 70% in men who have no symptoms.

The culture test is more reliable, but it takes longer. It involves taking a swab of the discharge, rolling it onto a special culture plate, and incubating it under special laboratory conditions for 24 to 72 hours to let the gonorrhea bacteria multiply. The swab from the cervix is the best single test: it is about 86 to 96% accurate. However, even the culture test can be inaccurate, primarily because it is difficult to maintain specimens in good condition during transportation to the lab. Test accuracy also depends greatly on which sites are chosen for testing. If you have the most commonly affected sites (cervix and anal canal) cultured, there is about a 90% chance of finding any existing infection. (Many women with gonorrhea also have trichomoniasis and/or chlamydial infection.) About 50% of women with an infected cervix also have infection in the anal canal. If you have had a hysterectomy, ask for a urethral culture, too. If you have had oral-genital sex, ask for a gonococcal throat culture. Ask what kind of medium is used for culturing. Thayer-Martin or Transgrow media are best.

Some women have the Gram stain for initial screening and the culture test to confirm the diagnosis. If the stain is negative but you have definitely been exposed to gonorrhea, you may want to be treated anyway while waiting for the results of the culture to come back.

The DNA probe (Gen-Probe), which is sent to specially equipped laboratories to be processed, detects a particular sequence of DNA that is specific for gonorrhea, in the bacteria tested. It can detect over 90% of gonorrhea cases in the cervix, and in the urethra of infected men. It has not been approved to detect gonorrhea in the throat or anus.

One of these tests should be available in physicians' offices and clinics. If you have any doubts about the accuracy of your test results, you may want to repeat the test if the result was negative, or confirm a positive test result with a culture. If your sexual partner's test result is positive, you may want to be treated at the same time, regardless of your test results.

Other Tests

The Food and Drug Administration (FDA) has recently licensed two new tests for gonorrhea. The ELISA technique (trade name, Gonozyme) detects antigens to the gonorrhea bacteria in cervical, anal, or urethral specimens in one or two hours, but the technology is complicated and expensive. Rapid gonorrhea tests (30 minutes to several hours) may give a positive result when you are not infected (false positive) or a negative result when you are infected (false negative). These tests are not as reliable as the culture tests. Medical practitioners still prefer the culture test.

Treatment

Many physicians prescribe medication before the culture test result is back or diagnosis is certain for three reasons: Tests are not always accurate; the physician is not sure you will come back; and the sooner the gonorrhea is treated, the easier it is to cure. Ask about medication for your partner.

On the other hand, some places refuse to treat you, even when you are certain of infection, until a positive diagnosis is made. One argument in favor of waiting for test results is that you should not take antibiotics unnecessarily. Another argument is that you may not have gonorrhea but another infection that should be treated differently. See, for example, "Chlamydial Infection" on p. 350.

An IUD may make cure more difficult because it helps spread infection and increases the chances of getting PID. The IUD should be removed after you have been on medication for at least 24 hours.

The CDC recommend one dose of ceftriaxone as the preferred initial treatment for gonorrhea. Because chlamydial infection frequently coexists with gonorrhea, the CDC also recommend ongoing treatment with doxycycline (seven days) to treat it. However, if it is possible to test for chlamydial infection (see p. 350), you should do this first in order to avoid a possibly unnecessary use of antibiotics. Doxycycline, which is taken twice a day, is preferable to tetracycline, which has more side effects. Neither should be used by a pregnant woman, who should take erythromycin instead (this is just as effective if taken correctly).

Followup

With ceftriaxone, a followup culture to test for cure is not necessary.

Gonorrhea and Pregnancy

Pregnant women should receive at least one routine gonorrhea culture during pregnancy. A pregnant woman with untreated gonorrhea can infect her baby as it passes through her birth canal. In the past, many babies went blind from gonococcal conjunctivitis. All states now require the eyes of newborns to be treated with silver nitrate drops or antibiotic drops to prevent this disease, even when the mother is sure she does not have gonorrhea and knows the treatment is unnecessary.

Chlamydial Infection

Chlamydial infection, caused by the bacterium *Chlamydia trachomatis,* is the most common bacterial STD in the U.S. today. It can cause very serious problems for women, including urethral infection, cervicitis (inflammation of the cervix), pelvic inflammation, and infertility as well as dangerous complications during pregnancy and birth (see p. 351). In men it can cause NGU, an inflammation of the urethra. This organism can also cause proctitis (inflammation of the rectum).

Chlamydial infection is transmitted during vaginal or anal sex with someone who already has it, or through cervical secretions on sex toys shared by partners. It can also be passed to the eye by a hand moistened with infected secretions and from mother to baby during delivery. It is possible but unlikely for chlamydial infection to pass to the throat if you perform oral sex on an infected man.

Symptoms

Four-fifths of women with chlamydial infection have no symptoms. The most common symptom among women is increased vaginal discharge, which usually develops seven to 14 days after exposure to the chlamydia bacterium. Painful urination, unusual vaginal bleeding, bleeding after sex, and low abdominal pain are other signs. The cervix may or may not appear inflamed on examination. If you have no symptoms, you must rely on your partner to tell you whether she or he has symptoms or has been diagnosed for NGU. It is important to get regular screening for chlamydial infection if you are sexually active.

Men's Symptoms

When infected, men usually have a burning sensation upon urination and a urethral discharge that appears one to three weeks after exposure. The symptoms may be similar to those of gonorrhea but are usually milder. The incubation period is also generally longer—at least seven days. Up to 25% of men have no symptoms, even though they can still transmit the disease. Frequently, only one member of a couple will have symptoms, while the other carries the infec-

tion. Both partners must be treated to prevent passing it back and forth.

Some health care practitioners are not aware enough of the dangers of chlamydial infection. In addition, because chlamydial infection is so easy to confuse with gonorrhea and other diseases, practitioners often misdiagnose it. They also overlook women's symptoms or attribute them to other causes.

It started out as cystitis. A few months later I started having fever, chills, and a lot of pain in my lower abdomen. The doctor never said anything about the possibility of chlamydial infection or PID. Instead, they did tests for gonorrhea, which were negative. After six months of being really sick, I was given ampicillin, which didn't help. They kept saying, "There's nothing wrong with you. You must be having emotional problems." After nine months I had a good case of PID, which they called "a little pelvic infection." It wasn't until my husband came down with symptoms of NGU that they took me seriously and treated us both with the right drugs.

Remember, the usual treatment for gonorrhea is *not* effective against these organisms. If you think you have been exposed to chlamydial infection and not gonorrhea, wait for the results of a test before accepting treatment for gonorrhea.

Testing and Diagnosis

At present there are many tests for chlamydial infection. In most cases, if you or your partner has a discharge, you will be tested for gonorrhea. You should also be tested for chlamydial infection. If the results of both tests are negative, you may be told that the problem is nongonococcal urethritis (NGU) and/or mucopurulent cervicitis (MPC). (See the section on NGU and chlamydial infection, p. 351.)

Certain tests for chlamydial infection (such as the monoclonal antibody test, the immunoenzyme test, and the DNA probe) have become less expensive, more rapid, and more widely available than traditional culture tests. They are less reliable than culture tests but offer a valuable aid to diagnosis.

There are also several new, FDA-approved tests for chlamydial infection, one of which also tests for gonorrhea. These tests (trade names Amplicor, LCX), which use DNA amplification technology, have a much higher rate of accuracy. However, they are relatively expensive and are not yet widely available.

Treatment

Doxycycline has been the standard treatment for chlamydial infections. The CDC now recommend doxycycline for seven days or azithromycin in one dose as the treatment of choice. Erythromycin is often prescribed when doxycycline cannot be given, such as during pregnancy. Azithromycin is often given during pregnancy. However, if you are allergic to erythromycin, you should not take azithromycin. Many of the other antibiotics commonly used for STD infections, including penicillin, are not effective. People with chlamydial eye infections are treated with oral antibiotics.

Take all the medication prescribed, or the infection may come back later, cause more trouble, and be harder to get rid of. Usually it clears up within three weeks. If not, go back to the health care practitioner, who will prescribe a different antibiotic or a longer treatment time. Regular sexual partners should take doxycycline or azithromycin whether or not they have symptoms.

Before taking any antibiotics, check with your doctor about possible undesirable effects. Pregnant women should not take tetracycline or doxycycline. Avoid alcohol until the infection has been cured, as it may irritate the urethra. Have no sexual contact involving the genitals until you and your partner are cured. If you seem to keep having recurrent episodes of chlamydial infection and antibiotics have not cleared it up, you may have another bacterial infection or possibly a stubborn case of PID.

Chlamydial Infection and Pregnancy

Studies indicate that 8 to 10% of all pregnant women may have a chlamydial infection which, if untreated, can then be transmitted to the baby during birth. A pregnant woman with a chlamydial infection has a 70% chance of passing it to her newborn baby. Infected babies may develop conjunctivitis or pneumonia. The disease has also been linked to miscarriage, ectopic pregnancy, premature delivery and postpartum infections. Because of these risks, testing for chlamydial infection may soon be recommended for all pregnant women.

Nongonococcal Urethritis (NGU) and Chlamydial Infection

NGU is a term used for any discharge from the urethra that is found *not* to be caused by gonorrhea. It is not a real diagnosis, and it does not rule out several other causes. The infection may be caused by chlamydia. It may also be caused by an organism known as *Ureaplasma urealyticum,* which can be found in the genital tracts of many apparently healthy people with no symptoms. Nonetheless, ureaplasma and a related organism called *Mycoplasma genitalium* are associated with some cases of urethritis.

Because *Ureaplasma* and some mycoplasmas are possible causes of cervicitis, PID, infertility, miscarriage, and premature birth, some researchers think that a woman with infertility or a history of repeated miscarriages should be tested for these organisms, as well as for chlamydia.

Herpes *

Herpes (from the Greek word meaning "to creep") is caused by the herpes simplex virus, a tiny primitive organism studied considerably in recent years. The virus enters the body through the skin and mucous membranes of the mouth and genitals and travels along the nerve endings to the base of the spine, where it sets up permanent residence, feeding off nutrients produced by the body cells. There are two types of herpes simplex virus (HSV). Type I (HSV I) usually is characterized by cold sores or fever blisters on the lips, face, and mouth, while Type II (HSV II) most often involves sores in the genital area. While HSV I is usually found above the waist and HSV II below, there is some crossover, primarily caused by the increasing practice of oral-genital sex. In this chapter we will be concerned with genital herpes.

You can get herpes by direct skin-to-skin contact during vaginal, anal, or oral sex with someone who has an active infection. It may also be possible to spread it from mouth to genitals (or eyes) via the fingers, or to transmit it on shared sex toys. Although the disease is most contagious from the time the skin reddens until the sores crust over, herpes can be transmitted when no symptoms are present. Most transmission occurs when people are asymptomatic.

Be careful at all times to wash your hands after contact with sores. Be especially careful not to touch your eyes if your hands might have any fluid from the sores on them.

Symptoms

Symptoms usually occur two to 20 days after infection, although most people may not have symptoms or may not be aware of them until much later. An outbreak of herpes usually begins with a tingling or itching sensation of the skin in the genital area. This is called the *prodromal* period and may occur several hours to several days before the sores erupt, or it may not occur at all. You may also experience burning sensations; pains in your legs, buttocks, or genitals; and/or a feeling of pressure in the area. Sores then appear, starting as one or more red bumps and changing to watery blisters within a day or two. Blisters are most likely to occur on the labia majora and minora, clitoris, vaginal opening, perineum, and occasionally the vaginal wall, buttocks, thighs, anus, and navel. Women can also have sores on their cervix, which usually cause no discernible symptoms. Many women have sores on both the vulva and the cervix during a first infection. Within a few days, the blisters rupture, leaving shallow ulcers that may ooze, weep, or bleed.

* The Herpes Resource Center (HRC), an organization run by the American Social Health Association (ASHA), provides support, information, and self-help groups for people with herpes. It also publishes an informative quarterly journal, *The Helper,* and operates The National Herpes Hot Line: (919) 361-8488 (see Resources).

Usually, after three or four days a scab forms and the sores heal themselves without treatment.

While the sores are active you may find it painful to urinate, and you may have a dull ache or a sharp burning pain in your entire genital area. Sometimes the pain radiates into the legs. You may also have an urge to urinate frequently and/or a vaginal discharge. You may also have vulvitis (painful inflammation of the vulva). During the first outbreak, you may also experience fever, headache, and swelling of the lymph nodes in the groin. Some women with severe outbreaks may develop urinary retention. If urination does not start after you follow suggestions in the self-help section (see p. 353), seek a clinician's help. The initial outbreak is usually the most painful and takes the longest time to heal (two to three weeks).

Men's Symptoms

Men may experience pain in the testicles during the prodromal period, followed by sores that usually appear on the head and shaft of the penis but can also appear on the scrotum, perineum, buttocks, anus, and thighs. Men can also have sores in the urethra without knowing it. There may also be a watery discharge from the urethra.

Recurrences

Some people never experience a second outbreak of herpes, but many do, usually within three to 12 months after the initial episode and often (though not necessarily) in the same area of the body. The more severe the first episode of HSV, the more likely it is that herpes will recur. Recurrent episodes are usually milder, last from three days to two weeks, and do not involve the cervix. They often seem to be triggered by stress, illness, trauma to the skin, menstruation or pregnancy, and certain foods. Most people find that the number of yearly recurrences decreases with time. Recurrent herpes is associated with lowered resistance. People who are deficient in B vitamins or who are unusually tense seem to get more frequent recurrences. Studies show that HSV II in the genital area is much more likely to recur than HSV I.

Testing and Diagnosis

You and your health care practitioner can usually diagnose herpes by sight when the sores are present, although herpes is occasionally confused with chancroid, syphilis, or genital warts. Several lab tests confirm the diagnosis or indicate the presence of herpes, although few tests can distinguish between HSV I and II, except for those performed on active genital lesions. Since so many people have been exposed to some kind of herpes in their lifetime, tests that do not distinguish Type I from Type II may be of little value in determining whether you have genital herpes. If you have a genital sore, have it checked right away, while it is still active.

The Tzanck Test

This test is similar to a Pap smear. A scraping is taken from the edge of an active sore, smeared on a slide, air-dried, and sent to a lab for evaluation. Although it detects infection less accurately than a culture, it can be used for both men and women and is inexpensive. It cannot differentiate between HSV I and HSV II.

Viral Culture

A viral tissue culture can be made that uses living cells to grow the virus. This test has an advantage in that it can distinguish between HSV I and HSV II, but it is expensive, and not all laboratories or doctors are equipped to perform it. The test is more accurate than the smear and should be done when the sores first appear. This is considered the most accurate method.

Other Tests

You can get a blood test to measure the level of herpes antibodies in the blood. (Once you have been exposed to the virus, your body manufactures antibodies to fight off the infection.) For this test, two ampules of blood are drawn, one during the initial attack and the second four to six weeks later. If you have herpes, the second sample will show a much higher antibody level. (It takes about two weeks to build antibodies.) This test is effective only when performed during the initial infection of herpes in persons who do not have oral herpes, because this test cannot distinguish HSV I from HSV II. Because most people with a first herpes infection are asymptomatic, this test is not generally helpful.

Newer blood tests may soon be available.

Treatment

At present there is no medical cure for herpes, although researchers are investigating vaccines, antiviral therapy, and immune-system stimulants. In the meantime, keep the sores clean and dry. If they are very painful, you may want to get a prescription for xylocaine cream or ethyl chloride. If you are having an outbreak of genital herpes, your health care practitioner may prescribe an oral antiviral drug called acyclovir (trade name, Zovirax), valacyclovir hydrochloride (Valtrex), or famcyclovir (Famvir). The earlier these drugs are taken (within 72 hours of the appearance of sores), the better they work. (Acyclovir ointment is also available to treat the sores, but it is less effective.) These drugs, taken at the onset of an outbreak, can reduce its severity and duration. Taken daily, they reduce the frequency of outbreaks. They also decrease the frequency of "shedding" (transmitting the virus without having symptoms). If recurrences are frequent (six or more a year), the drugs can be taken daily to prevent them.

Some evidence suggests that early application of topical 15% idoxuridine (IDU) in dimethyl sulfoxide (DMSO) reduces the severity of lesions on the labia and shortens the healing time. Homeopathic treatments have also been helpful (see chapter 5, Holistic Health and Healing).

However, none of these treatments can cure herpes. People who have it learn to live with it.

Self-Help and Alternative Treatment

Maintaining a healthy lifestyle, including good diet, sufficient rest, and exercise, is recommended as a means of reducing the number and severity of outbreaks, although you will probably not be able to prevent recurrences entirely. However, if you follow some of the self-help suggestions provided here, you may be able to prevent some episodes and limit or alleviate symptoms when they do appear. (If you are pregnant, you need to be especially careful, and you may wish to consult your doctor before using the alternative treatments listed here.)

When sores first appear, take warm sitz baths with baking soda three to five times a day. In between, keep sores clean and dry. A hair dryer helps to dry sores. Sores heal faster when exposed to air, so wear cotton underpants or none at all. If it hurts to urinate, do it in the shower or bathtub or spray water over your genitals while urinating (using any plastic squeeze bottle). When the sores break, apply drying agents, such as hydrogen peroxide or Domeboro, which is available in drugstores. For pain relief, take acetaminophen (e.g., Tylenol) or aspirin.

Many women have found the following alternative treatments very helpful for herpes. They may or may not work for you. Because some of the products mentioned below must be purchased at a health food store, they may be expensive. We suggest that you pick one or two. Remember, all are most effective when combined with good nutrition and rest.

1. Echinacea capsules are available at health food stores. Take two capsules every three hours, make a tincture and apply (1 teaspoon every two hours for three to four days), or make a soothing tea (4 cups a day).

2. Some people take as much as 2,000 milligrams of vitamin C. If you experience gastric distress or diarrhea, take less and then increase the dose gradually until you experience problems again, then take the next lower dose. Vitamin B complex, vitamin E, and vitamin A help somewhat in preventing recurrences, particularly in times of stress. Because vitamin A is stored in the body, be cautious about taking more than 10,000 international units (much higher doses can be toxic). Beta-carotene, a source of vitamin A, is often recommended because it does not accumulate in the same way and is considered safer.

3. Chlorophyll (in powder form) and wheatgrass are described as antiviral herbs. Drink them with warm water. Also, eating blue-green algae (3,000 milligrams daily) may be helpful.

4. Lysine is an amino acid that many women find very effective in suppressing early symptoms. If you stop using it, symptoms may reappear. Take 750 to 1,000 milligrams a day until the sores have disappeared. Thereafter, take 500 milligrams a day. Lysine seems to work by counteracting the effects of arginine (a substance found in foods such as nuts —especially peanuts—chocolate, and cola), which may stimulate a herpes infection. During any herpes episode, it is wise to avoid arginine-rich foods.

5. Take 5 to 60 milligrams of zinc daily.

6. Grape skins may be antiviral. Some women recommend eating red grapes.

7. Acupuncture treatments administered at the first signs of an episode sometimes prevent recurrences. Fingertip stimulation of acupressure points in the feet may also prevent outbreaks (three thumbs forward of the ankle bulge, along the line between the ankle bulge and little toe). It is important to apply acupressure accurately, using a detailed chart.

8. Many people apply aloe vera gel to sores to dry and heal them. Neosporin, Campho-Phenique, and povidone-iodine (Betadine) can also aid in healing.

Relief of Symptoms

Herpes can be very uncomfortable. The remedies described below are intended to relieve the symptoms. However, treatments that keep the sores moist may also prevent healing. Also, the open lesions may allow the infection to spread to new sites on the body.

For symptomatic relief, you might try compresses made of clove tea, black tea bags soaked in water (tannin is anesthetic), or sitz baths with uva ursi (also called kinnikinnick/bearberry). You can also apply poultices made of pulverized calcium tablets, powdered slippery elm, goldenseal, myrrh, comfrey root, or cold milk. Make a paste of any of these and apply to the sores. After applying the paste, keep it moistened with warm water.

Herpes and Pregnancy

Studies show that women who get primary herpes while pregnant have an increased risk of miscarriage and premature delivery. Equally important, when a mother is shedding virus at the time of delivery, herpes can be transmitted to the baby during passage through the birth canal and may cause brain damage, blindness, and death. Scary as this sounds, it is important to know that this is rare, occurring only in one out of every 5,000 normal births. The risk is much higher when mothers have a primary (first) outbreak at the time of delivery; when they have sores, their babies have at least a 50% chance of contracting herpes during a vaginal birth. For a mother with recurrent sores, the risk goes down to less than 4% because she has passed antibodies on to the baby through the amniotic fluid and the baby's blood.

Pregnant women who don't have herpes should avoid unprotected sex with partners who have herpes. If you are pregnant and have recurrent herpes, tell your physician or midwife. If you have prodromal symptoms or active sores at the time of delivery, you will usually have a cesarean section within four to six hours of the time the waters break. After birth, take care not to infect the infant. Always wash your hands before touching the baby, and avoid touching the sores if you have any.

Prevention

Efforts to develop a vaccine against herpes have been unsuccessful so far. Researchers continue to pursue the possibility of a genetically engineered vaccine. Because there is no cure for herpes, it seems especially worthwhile to protect yourself from getting it. That does *not* mean that you should never have sex with someone who has the virus in a latent stage; it simply means using your common sense in evaluating the risk and taking simple precautions when possible. At least 30 million Americans are infected, but only one-quarter to one-third of them know they are. The following suggestions (along with the general methods outlined on p. 344) may also reduce your chances of getting herpes.

1. **Question partners carefully about their history of STDs before you begin a sexual relationship.** If your partner has herpes, it may be a good idea to take the precautions listed on p. 344, even if no symptoms are present. This is because herpes can be shed and transmitted even when a person does not have any symptoms.

2. Avoid sex with someone who has active sores.

3. Because herpes can be spread by skin contact from one part of the body to another, try to avoid touching an open sore. Wash your hands after examining yourself or touching the genital area. Always wash your hands before inserting contact lenses.

Protecting Others (If You Have Herpes)

1. If you have active sores, do not have sex. Consider using barrier protection such as condoms for intercourse and dental dams or plastic wrap for oral sex, even when no sores are present (in between outbreaks).

2. Do not donate blood during an initial outbreak.

3. Men should not donate sperm during an active outbreak of herpes.

4. Avoid performing oral sex if you have active oral-labial lesions (fever blisters, cold sores).

Preventing Recurrences

1. Herpes attacks seem to be triggered by stress. If possible, figure out what precipitated your attacks and try to eliminate or reduce tension in your life.

2. Limit the use of stimulants such as coffee, tea, colas, and chocolate.

3. Increase your intake of vitamins A, B, and C and pantothenic acid as well as zinc, iron, and calcium to help prevent recurrences.

4. Avoid foods that have a lot of arginine (such as nuts, chocolate, cola, rice, and cottonseed meal). Instead, eat foods high in lysine: potatoes, meats, milk, brewer's yeast, fish, liver, and eggs.

5. If your outbreaks are very severe or frequent, ask your health care provider about taking oral acyclovir for prevention. This is expensive but effective.

Living with Herpes

Accepting herpes as a permanent part of your life may be difficult. You may feel shocked when you discover that you have herpes and it cannot be cured. You may feel isolated, lonely, and angry, especially toward the person who gave you the infection. You may become anxious about staying in long-term relationships or having children. Not everybody experiences herpes in these ways, nor do these responses necessarily last forever.

After the first big episode of herpes, I felt distant from my body. When we began lovemaking again, I had a hard time having orgasms or trusting the rhythm of my responses. I shed some tears over that. I felt my body had been invaded. My body feels riddled with it; I'm somehow contaminated. And there is always that lingering anxiety: Is my baby okay? It's unjust that the birth of my child may be affected.

If you are in a close relationship with someone who doesn't have herpes, it can affect you both in subtle ways.

Sometimes it bothers both of us. My lover feels she has to protect me from stress because I'm about to get a herpes attack. Then she neglects to ask me for attention, time, or comfort when she needs them.

How much herpes affects your relationships can depend a lot on how much you trust each other and how comfortable you feel about sharing your concerns.

The way we experience herpes may have a lot to do with our attitudes about disease. For example, people who see herpes as a symptom of stress, illness, or other problems rather than as a medical disaster seem to have a much easier time finding their own ways of coping with it.

Herpes is an inconvenience and a pain, but it's something you learn to live with. I think of it as an imbalance, because I know it's related to stress, I keep myself in as good physical condition as possible and try not to get too upset about it.

The one good thing I can say about herpes is that it keeps me honest in taking care of myself. When I feel my vulva start to tingle and ache, it's immediately a reminder to me to slow down. I take long, hot baths. I try to think relaxing, releasing thoughts and send healing, calming energy to that area. Sometimes I meditate.

Humor is the best way of coping with herpes. There is so much serious, scary stuff about it. You've got to recognize that it's just one of the bad tricks people have to live with.

Herpes may be easier to cope with if you feel comfortable enough to talk about it openly. Some people manage to talk themselves out of recurrences.

Syphilis

Syphilis is caused by a small spiral-shaped bacterium called a spirochete. You can get syphilis through sexual or skin contact with someone who is in an infectious (primary or secondary and possibly the beginning of the latent) stage when symptoms are present (see below). A pregnant woman with syphilis can also pass the disease to her unborn child, whether she has symptoms or not.

Syphilis spreads via open sores or rashes anywhere on the body containing bacteria that can penetrate the mucous membranes of the genitals, mouth, and anus. It can enter via broken skin on other parts of the body, but the disease is not usually transmitted through nonsexual contact.

Symptoms

Once the bacteria have entered the body, the disease may go through four stages, depending on when a person is treated. However, it may remain asymptomatic for a long time.

Primary

The first sign is usually a painless sore called a *chancre* (pronounced "shanker"), which may look like a pimple, a blister, or an open sore and shows up nine to 90 days after the bacteria enter the body. The sore usually appears on the genitals at or near the place where the bacteria entered the body, including the fingertips, lips, breast, anus, or mouth. Sometimes the chancre never develops or is hidden inside the vagina or the folds of the labia, giving no evidence of the disease. Only about 10% of women who get these chancres notice them. If you examine yourself regularly with a speculum, you are more likely to see one if it develops. At the primary stage, the chancre is very infectious. The preventive methods outlined on p. 344 work only if the physical barrier covers the infectious sore. With or without treatment, the sore will heal, usually in one to five weeks, but the bacteria, still in the body, increase and spread.

Secondary

The next stage occurs anywhere from one week to six months later. By this time, the bacteria have spread all through the body. This stage usually lasts weeks or months, but symptoms can come and go for several years. They may include a rash (over the entire body or just on the palms of the hands and soles of the feet), a sore in the mouth, or flu-like symptoms. You may lose some hair or discover a raised area around the genitals and anus. During the secondary stage, syphilis can be spread through mucus patches or condylomalata, raised areas that may resemble genital warts.

Latent

During this stage, which may last ten to 20 years, there are no outward signs. However, the bacteria may be invading the inner organs, including the heart and brain. The disease is not infectious after the first few years of the latent stage, when no symptoms of the second stage are present.

Tertiary (Late)

In this stage, the serious effects of the latent stage appear. Depending on which organs the bacteria have attacked, a person may develop serious heart disease, crippling, blindness, and/or mental incapacity. With our present ability to diagnose and treat syphilis, no one should reach this stage. Syphilis in this stage is not infectious.

Men's Symptoms

Men's symptoms are similar to women's. Men, however, notice chancres more readily than women do, and they more frequently seek treatment during the primary stage of the disease. The most common places for the chancre to appear are the penis and the scrotum. It may be hidden in the folds under the foreskin, under the scrotum, or where the penis meets the rest of the body. In the primary stages, men are more likely than women to develop swollen lymph nodes in the groin.

Diagnosis and Treatment

Syphilis can be diagnosed and treated at any time. Syphilis can be confused with several other STDs, including chancroid, herpes, and lymphogranuloma venereum (LGV).

Early in the primary stages, a health care practitioner can look for subtle symptoms like swollen lymph glands around the groin and examine some of the discharge from the chancre, if one has developed, under a microscope (a dark-field test). Do not put any kind of medication, cream, or ointment on the sore until a clinician examines it, because the syphilis bacteria on the surface are likely to be killed, making the test less accurate. Antibodies to the spirochetes can be detected in the bloodstream one or two weeks after the chancre has formed. Two blood tests are used to diagnose syphilis. One is a screening test called the VDRL or RPR. The second (FTA-ABS or MHA-TP) confirms it. If you suspect that you have been exposed to syphilis, you should get prophylactic (preventive) treatment as indicated by your health care provider. Because the incubation period of syphilis can be as long as 90 days, the baseline initial test, if the result is negative, should be repeated monthly for a total of four times if you do not receive treatment. If you are sexually active with more than one partner, or if your sexual partner is, request a syphilis blood test during regular health checkups.

Penicillin by injection, or a substitute such as doxycycline or tetracycline pills for those allergic to penicillin, is the treatment for syphilis. Because people sometimes have relapses or mistakes are made, it is important to have at least two followup blood tests to be sure the treatment is complete. Depending on what stage the disease has reached, the tests should be done three to six months and one year later. The first three stages of syphilis can be completely cured with no permanent damage, and even in late syphilis the destructive effects can be stopped from going any further.

Syphilis and Pregnancy

A pregnant woman with syphilis can pass the bacteria on to her fetus, especially during the first few years of the disease. The bacteria attack the fetus just as they do an adult, and the child may be born dead or with important tissues deformed or diseased. The mother should get treated as soon as possible. If she does so before the 16th week of pregnancy, the fetus will probably not be affected. (Even after the fetus has gotten syphilis, penicillin will stop the disease, although it cannot repair damage already done.) Every pregnant woman should get a blood test for syphilis as soon as she knows she is pregnant, again before she delivers, and anytime she thinks she may have been exposed. If she has the disease, she can be treated for it before she gives it to her fetus.

Genital Warts and Human Papillomavirus Infections *

Genital warts are caused by the human papillomavirus (HPV), similar to the type that causes common skin warts. Over 70 types of HPV cause invisible infections, warts, or flat lesions in the genital area. HPV usually spreads during sexual contact with an infected partner, male or female. Some HPV-caused lesions on the cervix are associated with an increased risk of cervical cancer, particularly those associated with HPV Types 16 and 18. Unfortunately, these cervical lesions are often not visible to either the health care practitioner or the women who have them.

Genital warts usually appear from three weeks to eight months after exposure. Warts, like invisible HPV infections, are contagious, so it is advisable for your male partners to use condoms if either of you has been exposed to the virus. The visible genital warts look like regular warts, starting as small, painless, hard spots or flaky lesions that often appear on the bottom of the vaginal opening. Warts also occur on the labia, on the vulva, inside the vagina, on the cervix, or around the anus, where they can be mistaken for hemorrhoids. Warmth and moisture encourage the growth of warts, which often develop a cauliflower-like appearance as they grow larger. Cervical lesions, though more prevalent than the visible warts, cannot be seen by the naked eye and produce no symptoms.

Men's Symptoms

Warts occur on the head of the penis (often under the foreskin), on the shaft of the penis, or occasionally on the scrotum. Using a condom can help prevent the spread of warts.

Diagnosis and Treatment

Diagnosis of warts is usually made visually, on clinical examination. An abnormal Pap smear may indicate the presence of HPV, and a colposcopy, which uses magnification to examine the vagina and cervix, will usually be done to look for warts and lesions. If lesions are found, a biopsy (analysis of a small sample of tissue) may be done to look for cervical cancer or precancerous conditions. If you have cervical warts or lesions, Pap smears (for early detection of unusual cell changes) should be done more often: every three to six months. A colposcopy may also be needed more regularly. (See chapter 24, Selected Medical Practices, Problems, and Procedures, for more information on colposcopy and biopsy.) Because HPV proliferates when the immune system is impaired, it has become one of the markers for diagnosing HIV in women. (See chapter 15, HIV, AIDS, and Women, p. 371, for more information on HPV and HIV.)

---

* See "Who Is at Risk of CIN (Dysplasia) or Cervical Cancer?," chapter 24, Selected Medical Practices, Problems, and Procedures, p. 655.

There are several treatments for warts.

1. *Podophyllin* solution is often applied to the warts. You need to wash it off two to four hours later to avoid chemical burns. Protect the surrounding skin with petroleum jelly (e.g., Vaseline). Sometimes several treatments are necessary, and they are not always successful. A safer self-treatment is also now available by prescription: Podofilox.

2. *Trichloracetic acid* (TCA) is also often used by medical practitioners and appears to be better than podophyllin in several respects. It is usually equally effective. The strength of TCA is more easily controlled; it works on first contact with the skin and then stops in about five minutes, reducing the danger of scarring. It does not seem to provoke severe reactions, as podophyllin occasionally does. TCA can be used during pregnancy.

3. *Cryotherapy* (freezing) can remove small warts. This hurts briefly and sometimes causes scarring. You may want a local anesthetic.

4. *Surgery or electrodesiccation* (using an electric current to destroy tissue) becomes necessary for very large warts that fail to respond to other treatments. This procedure requires an anesthetic. If you have a cardiac pacemaker, be sure to tell your practitioner, as the electric current may disturb it.

5. Recent studies suggest that *laser beams* applied to warts are an effective treatment that does not affect normal tissue or cause scarring. Some practitioners recommend it particularly for HPV infections of the cervix (warts and other lesions). Local or general anesthesia may be necessary, depending on the number and size of the warts. Only physicians specially trained to do laser therapy should perform this treatment.

No matter what treatment you get, it is important to remove warts to reduce spreading of the virus. Sexual partners also should be treated. However, warts may reappear after any treatment, and you may need to have them removed more than once. Once you have been infected, HPV can be transmitted even if you have no warts. Your partners should also be examined and treated for HPV.

Prevention

HPV is highly contagious. The best way to prevent HPV infection and the warts it causes is to use barrier methods when you have sex involving genital contact.

Genital Warts and Pregnancy

Warts tend to grow larger during pregnancy, probably because of the increasing levels of progesterone. If the warts are on the vaginal wall and become very large or numerous, the vagina may become less elastic, making delivery difficult. Do *not* use podophyllin to remove warts, as it is absorbed by the skin and can cause birth defects or fetal death. ASHA maintains a program of support services for those infected with HPV (see Resources).

Other Sexually Transmitted Diseases

There are many more STDs than we can cover in this chapter. See chapter 24, Selected Medical Practices, Problems, and Procedures, for information on common infections that can be transmitted nonsexually as well as sexually. See chapter 15, HIV, AIDS, and Women, for information on HIV/AIDS. Hepatitis B and STDs that are rare or that tend to affect men more than women (such as chancroid, lymphogranuloma venereum, granuloma inguinale, and intestinal STDs) are discussed in the *STD Handbook* (see the Resource section).

RESOURCES

Bell, Ruth, et al. *Changing Bodies, Changing Lives: A Book for Teens on Sex and Relationships,* rev. ed. New York: Vintage, due Spring, 1998. An *Our Bodies, Ourselves* for teens.

Campaign for Women's Health and the American Medical Women's Association. *Women and Sexually Transmitted Diseases: The Dangers of Denial.* 1994. Available from Glaxo-Wellcome's publications department, (919) 483-2697.

Centers for Disease Control and Prevention. "1993 Sexually Transmitted Diseases Treatment Guidelines." *Morbidity and Mortality Weekly Report* 42, no. RR-14 (1993). This report is updated regularly. It outlines treatments for each STD as well as special recommendations for pregnant women, adolescents, and persons with HIV.

Cherniak, Donna. *STD Handbook.* 1997. Available from Montreal Health Press, P.O. Box 1000, Station Place du Parc, Montreal, PQ Canada H2W 2N1. Also available in French as *Les maladies transmissibles sexuellement.* Excellent overall discussion of STDs for nonclinicians. Covers prevention and treatment.

Division of Sexually Transmitted Disease Prevention, Massachusetts Department of Public Health; Ratelle S., C. Burke, and C. Keenan. *Women and Sexually Transmitted Disease: The Social Context* (1994) and its companion piece *STD and Women: Trend Analysis 1985–1994.* Overview of epidemiological as well as psychosocial issues. Periodically updated. Available in limited quantity through MDPH/STD, State Laboratory Institute, 305 South Street, Jamaica Plain, MA 02130.

Ebel, Charles. *Managing Herpes: How to Live and Love with a Chronic STD.* Available from the American Social Health Association, P.O. Box 13827, Research Triangle Park, NC 27709.

Eng, Thomas R., and William T. Butler, eds. *The Hidden*

Epidemic: Confronting Sexually Transmitted Diseases. Washington DC: National Academy Press, 1997.

Holmes K. K., et al., eds. *Sexually Transmitted Diseases,* 2nd ed. New York: McGraw-Hill, 1990.

Rosebury, Theodore. *Microbes and Morals: The Strange Story of Venereal Disease.* New York: Ballantine Books, 1973. An excellent historical look at STDs, including an examination of their origin and spread.

Santa Cruz Women's Health Center. *Herpes.* 1986. Available from Santa Cruz Women's Health Center, 250 Locust Street, Santa Cruz, CA 95060; (408) 427-3500. This is a comprehensive 30-page booklet on prevention, symptoms, and traditional and nontraditional treatment.

Talking About STDs with Health Professionals: Women's Experiences is available from the Kaiser Family Foundation. A questionnaire assessing whether women were asked adequate questions to assess their risk of STDs was conducted for the Foundation with *Glamour* magazine and analyzed by health experts. Call the Foundation's request line: (800) 656-4533. Ask for package #1313.

Wade, Burwell. "Can Alternative Medicine Work?" *The Helper,* American Social Health Association (winter 1991).

World Health Organization. *Management of Patients with Sexually Transmitted Diseases: Report of a WHO Study Group.* Technical Report Series, No. 810. 1991. Available from World Health Publications, 49 Sheridan Avenue, Albany, NY 12210; or call (518) 436-9686.

Organizations

American Social Health Association (ASHA)
P.O. Box 13827; Research Triangle Park, NC 27709
Web site: http://sunsite.unc.edu/ASHA

An excellent resource, which operates hot lines and publishes numerous materials. ASHA's National Herpes Resource Center publishes a special herpes newsletter. Single copies of ASHA's many publications, including the following, are available for free:

"Some Questions and Answers about NGU"
"Protect Yourself and Your Baby from Sexually Transmitted Disease (STD)"
"Some Questions and Answers about Chlamydia"
"Some Questions and Answers about PID"
"Herpes: Questions and Answers"
"Some Questions and Answers: HPV and Genital Warts"

Write or call (919) 361-8400 and ask for the Distribution Department.

Centers for Disease Control
National Center for HIV/STD and TB Prevention; Division of STD Prevention; Atlanta, GA 30333
Web site: http://www.cdc.gov/nchstp/od/nchstp.html

Herpes Resource Center
Free service (but not a free call). Independently operated by the American Social Health Association, (919) 361-8488, Monday through Friday, 9 A.M. to 7 P.M., EST.

National Herpes Hot Line
(919) 361-8488
Open Monday through Friday, 9 A.M. to 7 P.M., EST.

National Sexually Transmitted Disease (STD) Hot Line
(800) 227-8922
Open Monday through Friday, 8 A.M. to 11 P.M., EST.

Planned Parenthood
Your local office is listed in the white and yellow pages of your phone book.

Public Health Department
STD Division (state level)
Your local office is listed in your phone book.

Additional Online Resources *

About Go Ask Alice!
http://www.columbia.edu/cu/healthwise/about.html

Sexually Transmitted Infections: The Facts
http://www.igc.apc.org/ppfa/stis/sti_facts_main.html

The STD Homepage
http://med-www.bu.edu/people/sycamore/std/std.htm

Welcome To The Safer Sex Page!
http://www.safersex.org

* For more information and listings of online resources, please see Introduction to Online Women's Health Resources, p. 25.

Chapter 15

HIV, AIDS, and Women

By Michele Russell and Wendy Sanford, with Maria Jobin-Leeds, based on earlier work by Mary Ide

With special thanks to Mary Guinan, Wanda Allen, the Women of Color AIDS Council (especially Karen McManus, Malkia Kendricks, and Charlotte, Colleen, Jackie, Shirley and Yolani), Patricia O. Loftman, Peggy Lynch, Lucia Ortiz-Ortiz, Belynda Dunn, Anna Forbes, Sophie Godley, and Laura Whitehorn*

Acceptance was the key for me. I had to accept that I had this virus and there was nothing I could do to make it go away. . . . My worst day with HIV is ten times better than my best day in active addiction.[1]

Having AIDS is like continually having to put out brush fires in my body.

We must advocate for ourselves. You are not alone. . . . We have no reason to be ashamed. It is time we run our lives.[2]

* Thanks also to the following for their help with the 1998 version of this chapter: Linda Evans, Linda King, Regina Maclean, Janet L. Mitchell, Liza Rankow, Susan Rosenberg, and Tracy Walton. Over the years since 1991, the following women have contributed to the many versions of this chapter: Amy Alpern, Marion Banzhaf, Laurie Cotter of ACT/UP New York, Deborah Cotton, Risa Denenberg, Liz Galst, Jenny Keller, Vicky Legion, the Chicago Women and AIDS Project, Patricia O. Loftman, Janet L. Mitchell, Jamie Penney, Lindsey Rosen, and Susan Rosenberg.

INTRODUCTION†

Many different women have a stake in understanding HIV infection and AIDS: those of us who are HIV positive and want to live as well and as long as we can; those who don't have HIV and want to protect ourselves, or want to support family and friends who have the infection; activists and advocates for women's health; teachers of young people; and health care providers who want to give the best care possible. It is the goal of this chapter to be useful to each of these groups, to help us find our common ground, and to offer further resources. Information about HIV and AIDS changes rapidly. Please use this chapter as a springboard for locating the most current information you can find about treatments, prevention, and living with AIDS.

† For a definition of HIV infection and AIDS, as well as many of the terms that will be used in this chapter, please see the box on p. 361.

WOMEN AND HIV/AIDS IN THE U.S. —AN OVERVIEW

The AIDS epidemic in the U.S. began in the 1980s. As we approach the turn of the century, there is finally some good news. People are living longer with AIDS. For those with access to the new combination treatments, HIV infection is becoming a manageable chronic disease. Women are being included in more clinical trials. Health care providers recognize the gynecological symptoms of HIV/AIDS more readily than they did ten years ago, and a female-specific diagnosis for AIDS (invasive cervical cancer) has been recognized since 1993. More researchers are asking what puts lesbians at risk for infection. New treatments have reduced the number of babies born with HIV infection. In many communities, women with HIV infection and AIDS are supporting each other, doing outreach, teaching prevention, getting into recovery from substance abuse, and finding hope.

Yet there is bad news, too, and much of it is for women. While the death rate for some groups of white men with AIDS decreased for the first time in 1996, it increased for women, primarily in the African-American, Latino, Native American, and immigrant communities, and white communities where incomes are low. Of all the women in the U.S. who have had AIDS, 75% have been African-American and Latina, even though they account for only 21% of the U.S. population. In 1995, AIDS was the leading killer of African-American women in the U.S. aged 25 to 44. In 1994, AIDS was the third leading cause of death for young women in the U.S.

Behind these statistics are racism, economic injustice (e.g., lack of jobs, housing, and good child care), and sexism, which have determined the direction of the disease, putting some of us at risk more than others. Here are examples:

- Unequal male-female power relationships get in the way of our using protection in sex. Many men pressure or even force women into unprotected sex, whether we are wives, girlfriends, or paid sex workers. Because HIV is more efficiently transmitted sexually from a man to a woman, we are more at risk than men are from these acts. Even when "force" is not present, we may be unwilling to bring up the issue of safer sex because we fear being hurt or abandoned by our partners. For example, "A recent study among African-American women in Los Angeles showed that condoms were less likely to be used by couples in which the woman was dependent upon her male partner for rent money."[3]
- Substance use, both through shared needles and through unprotected sex with male users, is now the most significant contributing factor for women in the U.S. who are infected with HIV. Of all cases reported in women through 1995, 43% occurred in injection drug users and 17% in sex partners of injection drug users. Substance use has been a major factor in the destruction of communities of color for decades. It can be traced to racism and its impact on communities of color through poverty, lack of educational and meaningful employment opportunities, substandardized housing, high levels of violence, and inadequate health care. Substance use has been allowed to continue in communities of color unabated because it has a minimal effect on the larger middle-class white community and, in fact, provides economic support for segments of that white community. Treatment programs are especially inaccessible to those of us who live in poverty, who are of color, and/or who are pregnant or have dependent children.

- Research on what will protect women from HIV has been slow. For instance, a woman who wants to get pregnant must have unprotected sex or insemination. This puts her at risk if her partner or donor has HIV. Women need a dependable noncontraceptive vaginal microbicide—a substance that will prevent HIV transmission without preventing pregnancy. Yet, research in this area of critical interest to women is only in the early stages.
- There is often more focus on women as "infectors" of children and men than as people deserving of prevention and treatment in our own right. Some of us finally achieved access to treatment only when our children were found to be infected.
- Because of the myriad insensitivities of health and medical institutions to women, especially to women of color and lesbians, many of us seek care for HIV or AIDS only at the later stages of illness. Or we may go without treatment for STDs or vaginal irritations, which can increase our risk of being infected by HIV if we are exposed.
- Women are still taught to put others' well-being before our own. Family responsibilities are expected to—and often do—take precedence over our seeking health care for ourselves. We are the major caregivers for those who are ill with AIDS, and there is little support for us in this role. Caring for ourselves comes last on the list.
- Women make less money than men, and often as single parents have financial responsibility for more family members, so we usually have fewer financial resources with which to care for ourselves. Too often, public support for the things that would help us fight HIV/AIDS are lacking: drug treatment programs, housing, adequate nutrition, jobs with health insurance, and child care.
- While the new combination therapies (see p. 361) allow many people to live longer with HIV or AIDS, these therapies are expensive and often have complex dietary requirements that make them hard to use if we live in poverty, are homeless, or use drugs.

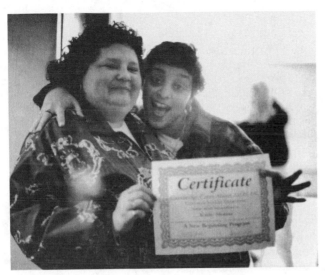

A woman receiving a certificate from Cambridge Cares About AIDS/Terri Ruth Unger

Women are often blamed for getting HIV, whether from unsafe sex or shared needles: our behavior, it is said, puts us at risk of HIV/AIDS. This is part of the story, but it's not that simple. Racism, sexism, poverty, and economic discrimination set up a situation in which some of us may make choices that put us at risk for HIV in order to save ourselves or our children from other kinds of harm like being raped, or going hungry, or losing a place to live. Are we therefore to blame for getting HIV? Not exactly! On the other hand, simply citing the role of poverty and other oppressions in the spread of HIV can give the impression that women are victims of forces beyond our control. It doesn't help to see ourselves as victims. We are women living in a context of high risk caused by social injustices that are beyond our individual control. Within that context, we seek to help each other make the best decisions we can—about survival, about protection, about treatment, and about living with the disease.

Many courageous women live with AIDS, care and plan for our children, support each other in recovery from substance abuse, and share the spiritual strength that can grow as we come out of isolation. Activist women in prison are becoming AIDS educators and fighting for better medical care for inmates. Some major AIDS organizations have developed powerful programs for women, some explicitly including lesbians. As more and more children are orphaned by AIDS, women activists are developing creative approaches to guardianship that give mothers maximum input and control. Many dedicated health care providers are teaching other providers to treat women with HIV infection or AIDS with respect and to give us the information we need to be able to participate in the difficult decisions that will affect the course of the illness.

Women's experiences with HIV/AIDS in the U.S. over the next decade will depend on fundamental so-

GLOSSARY: SOME TERMS THAT HELP IN UNDERSTANDING HIV/AIDS

AIDS: The abbreviation for aquired immune deficiency syndrome. AIDS is a viral syndrome (a group of diseases) resulting from the weakening of the immune system brought about by advanced HIV infection. It is diagnosed by the presence of an AIDS-defined opportunistic infection or malignancy, or a CD4 lymphocyte count of less than 200 cells per microliter.

ANTIBODY: A special protein that is created by our body's immune system and used to fight specific agents that cause infection. Most HIV screening tests test for this antibody. Unlike antibodies to many other viruses, antibodies to HIV do not destroy the infecting virus.

ANTIRETROVIRAL DRUGS: Drugs—AZT (zidovudine, or ZVD), 3TC, ddI, ddC, d4T—that act at a certain stage of the viral replication, preventing the virus from reproducing any further and infecting new cells. These drugs do not work on already infected cells.

ASYMPTOMATIC: Has HIV but shows no signs or symptoms of the infection. It is possible to infect others even if you are asymptomatic.

COMBINATION   THERAPY/"COCKTAIL": New treatment therapies that involve combining two to three drugs, usually two antiretroviral drugs with one protease inhibitor. Combination therapy has been shown to be more effective than one drug alone to reduce the amount of HIV in the body: the virus often becomes resistant to single drugs quickly, and the combination therapy seems to prevent resistance and to be more effective in decreasing the "viral load."

HIGH-RISK OR UNSAFE BEHAVIOR: Activities that can transmit HIV by allowing the exchange of blood (inlcuding menstrual blood) or semen between two people. (Other bodily fluids that can carry risky levels of HIV are vaginal fluids and breast milk; tears and saliva do not.) The two most high-risk activities are having anal or vaginal sex without condoms, and sharing needles for injecting drugs, hormones, vitamins, or for tattooing.

HIV: The abbreviation for human immunodeficiency virus, believed to be the underlying cause of AIDS. The virus infects and destroys the CD4 lymphocytes, also known as T cells, which are central to keeping the immune system healthy. As the immune system is weakened, the body becomes vulnerable to opportunistic infections and diseases.

continued on next page

HIV POSITIVE (HIV+)/HIV-INFECTED/ SEROPOSITIVE: Infected with HIV.

IMMUNE SYSTEM: The system that protects the body from infection and tumors. In this system, specialized cells and proteins in the blood and other bodily fluids work together to eliminate disease-producing agents and other toxic foreign substances.

IMMUNOSUPPRESSION: The term indicating that the immune system has been weakened, whether in response to HIV infection or to other factors.

OPPORTUNISTIC INFECTIONS (OIs): Infections or malignancies that occur in people with severely weakened immune systems resulting from chemotherapy or advanced HIV disease. People with healthy immune systems are usually able to fight off these diseases. Some examples include *Pneumocystis carinii* pneumonia (PCP), *Mycobacterium avium* complex (MAC), Kaposi's sarcoma (KS), and invasive cervical cancer.

PERSON LIVING WITH AIDS (PLWA): A positive term for someone who has AIDS. Using PLWA (or PWA) helps avoid negative and judgmental terms such as AIDS victim, innocent victim, or AIDS carrier.

PROPHYLAXIS: Treatments to prevent the occurrence or recurrence of opportunistic infections. For example, Bactrim is prescribed to prevent the occurrence of the pneumonia called PCP.

PROTEASE INHIBITORS: Drugs that act at another stage of viral reproduction than the one where antiviral agents act. These drugs block the protease enzyme that allows the virus to reproduce itself. Some examples are Saquinavir, Crixivan, and Ritonavir. In combination with other drugs, protease inhibitors seem to be very effective in reducing viral loads in most people.

SAFER SEX: Practices that reduce the chance of exchanging blood and semen during sexual encounters.

SEROCONVERSION: Change in a person's blood from having no HIV antibodies (seronegative) to having HIV antibodies (seropositive). This usually happens within six weeks to six months of exposure.

T CELL OR CD4 CELL: A type of white blood cell (lymphocyte) that is critical to maintaining the body's immune system. Because HIV destroys these cells, this count is used as a marker of the severity of HIV infection and the strength of the immune system.

VIRAL LOAD (HIV RNA): The amount of HIV measured in the bloodstream. A viral load test is used to indicate the need for and response to treatment and is the most accurate predictor of disease progression.

cial changes that address poverty, racism, and sexism. Also critical will be the work of AIDS activists: dedicated women and men willing to organize public pressure for women-centered research, treatment, and support, and for access by all women to treatment, basic nutrition, housing, and health care. This work, in turn, depends on all of us believing in our inherent right to feel well, to enjoy sex without risking our health, to take good care of ourselves and each other, and to get the health and medical care we need.

THE GLOBAL PICTURE

Some eight to ten million adults and one million children are infected with HIV worldwide. Nearly half of them are women, 93% are in developing countries, and nearly all are infected through unprotected heterosexual intercourse. Please see Resources for sources of information on the complex global HIV/ AIDS picture.

SPECIAL ISSUES

Sex Workers/Prostitutes

The U.S. public, media, police, and courts tend to blame sex workers, not male clients, for the buying and selling of sex. In the same way, sex workers have been accused of spreading HIV when, in fact, a woman sex worker is far more likely to contract HIV from a male client than she is to give it to him. Laws in many states require mandatory HIV testing of sex workers who are arrested, with no similar move toward testing their clients. Sex workers ask for protection and decent health care rather than harassment and mandatory testing.

Sex workers in poorer sections of the sex industry are the ones who are most vulnerable to HIV. Many men will pay more for unprotected sex. Believing that younger women are infection-free, some men seek out the youngest and most vulnerable among us. Women who work on the street, who are trading sex for drugs, or who are very young may not have the money for condoms and may fear that insisting on condom use would make a client take his business elsewhere, or even commit rape. Some sex workers who do use condoms in sex for pay do not use protection with a lover, even if he or she may put us at risk; some may want sex with a lover to feel different, others may find it harder to set our own terms when it's not a business proposition. Yet women sex workers in the U.S. have built on years of experience in using condoms as protection from STDs and provide some of the most successful examples of women making changes to safer practices. Sex workers in some communities have helped to train AIDS educators to teach effectively about safer sex.

Lesbians and HIV

Lesbians have been told we're a low-risk group, yet defining risk in terms of groups rather than behavior is fatal.

Lesbianism is not a condom.[4]

Although the risk of woman-to-woman sexual transmission of HIV is low, lesbians are still very much at risk for HIV infection through injectable drug use and through unprotected intercourse with a man. Our risk for HIV infection depends on what we *do,* not who we are. Some of us have sex with men, some use IV drugs, some are sex workers, some are raped, some seek donor insemination in order to become pregnant, and some use risky practices, like sharing sex toys, with women partners.

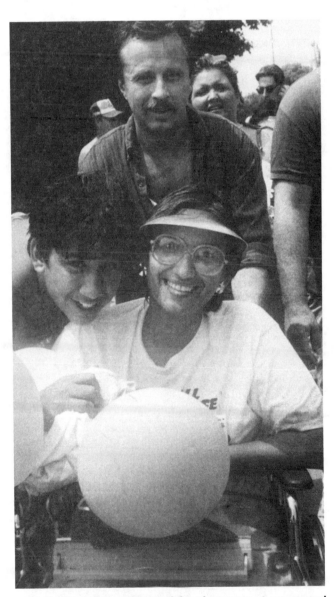

HIV-positive Latina AIDS activist Liz Ramos at an annual fund-raising walk in Boston/Ellen Shub

There are added "risk" factors for lesbians. Many health care providers have negative attitudes toward lesbians that make us reluctant to seek care. Especially if we are not having children or don't need birth control, we may delay going for gynecological care. Some providers are ignorant about HIV risk factors for lesbians and may fail to caution us about risky behaviors or explore possible symptoms. Many lesbians have jobs without health insurance and are almost never covered by a partner's health insurance.

For lesbians with HIV infection or AIDS, it helps greatly if we can find health care providers who are comfortable with lesbians. When programs and services provide environments that are safe and supportive, displaying information and resources specific to lesbians, we may feel more comfortable going for treatment and even identifying ourselves. The successful programs take into account the fact that many lesbians with HIV are lesbians of color, or live in poverty, or are injection drug users. One example of a successful program for lesbians infected and affected is the Lesbian AIDS Project in New York City (see Resources).

The lack of reported cases of woman-to-woman sexual transmission can make it tempting to not protect ourselves when we have sex with a woman. Yet, there are risky woman-to-woman activities with an HIV-infected partner, like sharing sex toys or penetrating each other's anus or vagina manually with fingers that have cuts or bleeding hangnails. Please see "Safer Sex Guidelines," p. 366.

Women in Prison[5]

Women in prison who are HIV positive or who have AIDS are the front line of this crisis. We live isolated, enclosed, and in a particular form of hell.

Women in prison are simply incarcerated members of the community who could be one's mother, sister, or friend. Without community support to those inside, the fight for our lives is almost overwhelming.

It helps a lot if an HIV-positive prisoner stops smoking, develops an exercise program, cuts out pills and junk food, etc. But that's very hard in an atmosphere where collective wellness programs don't exist—no smoke-enders program to turn to—and where the self-respect and self-value necessary are under daily bombardment by the entire prison system.

Women living with AIDS in prison may die more quickly of the disease than women on the outside. We contend with living conditions that are most often unhealthy and a health care system that is dramatically inadequate: most prison systems do not have an infectious diseases specialist on staff, and it is a struggle even to get the twice-a-year Pap test that is part of good care for many women with HIV. It's also hard for HIV-positive women in prison to feel the self-esteem and pride that are basic to the ability to fight for health and life. That's why a major goal of HIV/AIDS work in prison is to create an atmosphere in which it's safe to be public about being HIV-positive.

Sisterhood and empowerment have become motivating concepts for women in prison to advocate for our own health needs and to build self-help programs. Please see chapter 27, Organizing for Change, for a discussion of the important HIV/AIDS work being done by prisoners. Activists on the outside can make a big difference by supporting the demands of incarcerated women for decent health care, participation in clinical trials with neutral group monitoring (that is, with no prison staff present), support for communication with our children about HIV and AIDS, community participation in AIDS education in prisons, and compassionate release for women who are ill.

TRANSMISSION: HOW HIV IS PASSED FROM ONE PERSON TO ANOTHER

Two conditions must be met for HIV to pass from one person to another.

1. *The virus must be present, and in sufficient quantity* in at least one of the people involved. Blood, semen, vaginal fluid, and breast milk of a person with HIV carry a sufficient quantity of the virus to cause infection. The fluid that comes out of a penis before the man ejaculates (pre-cum) might have enough virus to infect you. Unless they have blood in them, other fluids do not have enough virus to infect you (like saliva, tears, sweat, urine, feces, and vomit.) Gay sex, anal sex, or IV drug use do not themselves create HIV infection.

2. *The virus must get into your bloodstream.* The virus can enter your body through the mucous membrane that lines the vagina and rectum; directly into the blood via a needle; through the skin via any open cut, wound, or scratch; or through the mucous membrane in the eyes, the nose, and the inside of a man's penis.

The virus can enter mucous membranes more easily if there are tiny tears or inflammation from vigorous penetration during sex, or sores from a sexually transmitted disease or untreated vaginal infection. Thus, if you are exposed to HIV through unprotected sex, your risk of becoming HIV-infected is increased if you have any sexually transmitted disease (STD)—like genital herpes, chancroid ulcers, or syphilis—or if you have vaginal irritation due to yeast (candida), trichomoniasis, or bacterial vaginosis.

Here are the ways that HIV can be transmitted:

- Through sharing needles that contain blood, including works for IV drugs (heroin, cocaine, speed) or needles shared for tattooing or body piercing.
- Through penis-in-vagina and penis-in-anus sex ("butt-fucking"). There is also some risk with other sexual activities: fisting, finger fucking, rimming, sharing uncleaned sex toys such as dildos and vibrators, and oral sex. Contact

between your mouth and a man's penis is more risky if he ejaculates, and should be avoided. Deep kissing is low risk, though it could be risky if both people had bleeding gums or mouth sores, allowing for blood-to-blood transmission.

- Through receiving a transfusion of HIV-infected blood and blood products (these are now fully screened in the U.S.).
- Through donor insemination with HIV-infected semen.
- For infants, through pregnancy, childbirth, and breast-feeding. (See "HIV and Pregnancy," p. 373.)

HIV *cannot* be transmitted by insects or through food preparation, drinking out of the same glass, handshakes, or toilet seats. You can't get HIV from donating blood through the Red Cross or other agency.

PROTECTING OURSELVES FROM HIV

HIV can live in the body for ten to fifteen years, often without creating symptoms. We cannot look at someone and tell whether they have the virus, so it's very possible to get infected, or to infect someone else, without knowing it. If we have unprotected sex or share needles with someone today, we expose ourselves to everyone she or he has exchanged body fluids with in the past decade. Even in monogamous long-term relationships, our lovers may be having sex with other women and/or men and not telling us, or using drugs and not telling us. Or they may have been infected by something they did long before they met us. *The only answer is to act as though one or both partners is HIV positive and to use protection.*

Obstacles

There are barriers that are known to stop HIV transmission: latex condoms and gloves, dental dams, plastic wrap. Yet, many of us are not protecting ourselves, or we do so sometimes and not others. Why aren't we building safer sex into our lives?

Our Own Attitudes

Who, me??? I'm not a gay man or a junkie, so I'm safe. . . . I have good taste in men . . . or women. . . . I can tell who's infected. . . . If he had HIV he'd have oily hair and broken skin. . . . I love him so much—he'd never do anything to hurt me. . . . If I bring a condom, he'll think I'm a sleaze. . . . It's not romantic. . . . I'm a lesbian and we're supposedly low risk. . . . I'm afraid he'll refuse. . . . He's too important to risk losing. . . . I need the drugs and he won't give them to me if I make trouble. . . . I can't carry condoms around —my mother would find them. . . . He'll get mad. . . . I'm not worth protecting. . . . Talking about sex is too embarrassing. . . . I just can't deal. . . .

With thoughts like those, who's going to pull a condom or a roll of plastic wrap out of her pocketbook?

That condom seems to pour cold water on the romance by saying, "OK, to be brutally honest, we've both slept with other people." The condom seems like a statement of distrust: "You could give me a disease; you could kill me."

If we have been sexually abused at some time in our lives, and if we haven't had help dealing with the pain from that, it can be extra hard to insist on safer sex.

Our Partner's Attitudes

Some men complain that condoms ruin sex. Some are afraid that they won't keep an erection while putting on a condom. Or they think it's not really sex without penetration and insist on intercourse even if there's no protection. If they are used to being in charge sexually, they may resent it when we initate safer sex. They may feel that we're accusing them of sleeping around or of using injectible drugs. A lesbian lover may believe there's no HIV risk for lesbians, or resist cleaning sex toys. Many sex workers' clients refuse to pay for protected sex, or pay more for sex without condoms. Or there are cultural reasons. A woman's group from Chicago wrote:

If you're "poor" and Latina, sexuality is one area over which men still feel like they have some control in their lives. If the women bring home the safer sex message, we may become lightning rods for the frustration and anger the men feel as a result of racism, unemployment, and poverty. The educational strategy has to be developed by the community itself.

Whatever the reason, our suggesting safer sex can provoke a response we didn't look for.

Ann's partner poked a pencil through the six condoms she brought home from the clinic, snarling, "I'll show you what I think of this shit."

The choice may seem to be unsafe sex or no sex.

A lot of these guys would rather dump you than use a condom.

Other Factors

You may want to have a baby, which means you don't want to use a condom or any birth control method.

You and your partner may already be HIV-positive, so you may think there's no reason to continue to use protection. (This isn't true—see p. 373.)

Safer sex supplies may be too expensive or too hard to get. One large Chicago clinic serving eight housing projects receives a state allotment of less than one-fifth of a condom per client each month.

TEENS AND PROTECTION FROM HIV

Teen women are vulnerable to HIV and other sexually transmitted diseases. Do you feel "immune" to HIV? Are you a risk taker? Is your boyfriend older and more powerful than you? Are you afraid to ask him to use a condom? Talking to a trusted woman friend or mentor, or calling an AIDS hot line, may help you find the information and examples you need to negotiate safer sex. If you have been sexually abused, it may feel harder to establish a sexual life that is healthy, happy and protected from HIV, but it's possible. There are many teen women who, on their own and with the support of adult women or a program, have made the commitment to avoid HIV: some by staying virgin, some by using protection. Serving as a peer educator about safer sex and substance abuse can help. Unfortunately, conservative religious and political groups in many areas of the country have fought against AIDS education and condom distribution in the schools. If condoms aren't available in your school, and you can't afford to buy them, try a Planned Parenthood office or an STD clinic.

Overcoming the Obstacles

From a group of women friends around a kitchen table getting down to basics about safer sex, to the pioneering prison-based ACE peer education project, to some of the great hot lines listed in the Resources, we can help each other protect ourselves. Here are some things that different women have found effective: Read everything you can about condom use and practice putting one on a banana or a cucumber; practice with your friends what you are going to say with a partner; talk with your partner about how to make using condoms sexy; put the condom on together; put it on with your mouth; explore lovemaking that doesn't include penetration—more women have orgasm that way (see chapter 11, Sexuality); make some rules for yourself about what you will and will not do, like "Safer sex until we test"; don't get so high or drunk that you can't stick to your beliefs; get some therapy to help you deal with a history of sexual abuse.

Don't fool yourself. Challenge the myths. Remember that you can't tell by looking at someone whether he or she is infected. Love does not protect you from HIV. Having only one sex partner doesn't protect you. Having him pull his penis out of your vagina before coming may reduce the risk but doesn't fully protect you. Birth control pills and diaphragms protect you from pregnancy but not from HIV. (HIV can get through the wall of the vagina anywhere, so a diaphragm is not an adequate barrier.)

If a man resists using a condom, you could try a sexy approach like "I'm so hot for you, and a condom keeps you hard longer." If he cares about having a family, try telling him that you don't want to get an infection that will hurt his ability to have children with you. When men won't cooperate, we need protection methods we can control as women. Some women have been glad to have the female condom (see chapter 13, Birth Control, p. 298). However, no data exist on whether it protects against HIV infection. It is not fully woman-controlled, because your partner can feel the rim and must cooperate. The female condom is also too noisy or too costly for some, and it is not available in stores in many communities of color. Unfortunately, a vaginal microbicide, which women could insert vaginally before sex to kill the virus, is still in the research stage. When possible, consider ending a relationship in which a partner resists your efforts to protect yourself.

Risk Reduction

If you can't use a condom, you can reduce your risk by using *something*. Sometimes it's good to know we can take little steps that will help to protect us even if we can't do as much as we'd like to. Here are "risk reduction" steps we can take with vaginal and anal sex, starting from the smallest:

- Make sure you don't have any STDs or untreated vaginal infections.
- Have the kind of sex with your hands, mouth, and body that avoids penetration by his penis.
- If you have penetration, but no condoms, try to get him to come (ejaculate) outside your body.
- Put in some spermicide with nonoxynol-9 or, better, use a diaphragm with spermicide. These have not been proved to be effective against HIV but may be better protection than nothing.
- Have him wear condoms at least during penetration and ejaculation.
- Try the following step that some women have: put the female condom inside your vagina before you and your partner begin to be sexual; this way he may be less likely to object.

For women, safer sex is about power: power to feel worthwhile, having enough self-esteem to want to protect ourselves. Power to hold our ground and persuade a sex partner to use protection. Power to support ourselves and our children financially if we leave a partner who won't use protection. Power to feel proud of our sexuality and to speak openly about sex, even when it is hard to talk about. Drugs and alcohol weaken our power to protect ourselves; if we are addicted, the power we need depends on access to affordable treatment. All women deserve the power to keep ourselves and our loved ones healthy.

NONOXYNOL-9 AND RISK REDUCTION

Nonoxynol-9 (or N-9, a sperm-killing ingredient in many widely available contraceptive creams, foams, jellies, films, and sponges) has killed HIV in some laboratory tests. However, it has never been conclusively proved to be effective against HIV in use with a partner. Some AIDS prevention programs, including that of the New York State Health Department, advise women to use N-9—preferably with a diaphragm, or by itself—as a "risk reduction" measure when a male partner refuses to use a condom. Experts at the Federal Centers for Disease Control disagree with this advice, citing the lack of proof of N-9's effectiveness in preventing HIV transmission. They fear that women who use N-9 might have a false sense of security and be less careful about using condoms, thus putting themselves at more risk for HIV. In addition, high or frequent doses of N-9 (more than once a day) can cause irritations in the vaginal lining, which could actually increase the risk of HIV transmission. Until this debate is settled, and until there are other, more dependable woman-controlled methods of protection, each woman will have to make her own decision about N-9.

Safer Sex Guidelines

Safer sex boils down to four guidelines:

1. Think and talk about the prevention of HIV and other STDs long before having sex.

2. Know that safer sex can be fun, imaginative, and intimate. Get creative. Try lots of things that are low risk.

3. Use barriers to protect yourself from potentially infected blood, semen, or vaginal fluids.

4. Avoid drugs and alcohol that could get in the way of your protecting yourself.

The two sexual acts that present the highest risk for HIV are vaginal intercourse and anal intercourse. There are also many other risky behaviors for heterosexual or same-sex couples. The following suggestions are some ways to enjoy sex while reducing the risk of infection with HIV. These methods are effective only if the condom or other barrier is in place *before* sexual contact.

- *Penis-vagina intercourse.* For the best protection, the man uses a latex (not lambskin) condom, lubricated to avoid tearing. (See chapter 13, Birth

Control, p. 299, for guidelines on condom use.) Use a water-based lubricant like K-Y Jelly, Astroglide, or Probe. Do not use oil-based lubricants like Vaseline, butter, or Crisco, which will damage condoms within minutes. You can also hold the condom rim while you're having sex, visually check the condom during sex, change the condom when changing activities or if the sex lasts a long time, use your own condom and not the man's, so you'll know it was stored correctly and wasn't damaged by heat or light. If a man resists using a condom, see above.

No other method of protection—neither the female condom nor spermicide containing nonoxynol-9—has been conclusively proved to prevent HIV transmission during penis-in-vagina intercourse.

- *Penis-anus intercourse.* This is a high-risk activity because the fragile tissue in the rectum tears easily and thus can let HIV directly into the bloodstream. If you do it, the man should use a strong latex condom with lots of water-based lubricant. Some sources suggest using two condoms at once (put one condom on, add lubricant, and put a second one over it), but others say that the condoms may tear.

- *Oral sex on a man.* Oral sex is not as risky as vaginal or anal sex, especially if you do not take semen into your mouth. For maximum protection, use unlubricated latex condoms as soon as he is erect, since the pre-cum (drops of fluid that come out of the penis before he comes) can contain HIV. Use a new condom each time. If semen gets into your mouth, don't swallow it.

- *Oral sex on a woman.* This also carries some risk, especially if the woman has her period or a vaginal infection, as both can transmit HIV. For protection, cover your partner's vulva and anus with nonmicrowavable plastic wrap, a dental dam, or a cut-open latex glove or nonlubricated condom. Try lubricating the side that touches your partner. Be sure to keep the same side against her vulva. Dental dams used by dentists are small and thick, but some sex boutiques carry ones that are larger, thinner, and flavored. To turn a latex glove into a barrier with a tongue condom, wash the powder out, cut off the four fingers, slit it up the side, leaving the thumb intact, and enjoy.

- *Fisting and finger play.* Fisting (putting a hand or fist into the rectum or vagina) or finger play (playing with the vagina or labia or touching your partner's anus) carry some risk because the internal tissue can be easily bruised or torn. HIV can travel into the bloodstream through cuts on your fingers, or vice versa. For protection, use latex gloves (or finger cots for finger play), and change them with each use.

- *Rimming (mouth-anus contact).* Rimming has some risk of HIV transmission if there is blood in the partners' feces or saliva. Rimming can also spread hepatitis and intestinal parasites. For protection, use nonmicrowavable plastic wrap or dental dams (see "Oral sex on a woman" earlier).

- *Water sports* (sex partners urinate on each other). Can be risky if there is blood in the urine. Wear goggles for this to protect your eyes, and avoid any broken skin or cuts.

- *Dildos, sex toys, vibrators.* If shared, they can transmit HIV from one partner to the other. Use a dildo with a condom, and do not share a dildo without washing it clean of any body fluids and putting on a new condom. Do not share sex toys and vibrators. Clean dildos and sex toys thoroughly with hydrogen peroxide or bleach after each use.

- *Bondage or S/M (sado/masochism).* Negotiate first with your sex partner(s) that no blood, semen, or vaginal fluids will get inside you or onto irritated or cut skin. If an abrasion or cut results from an S/M scene, clean it well, cover it with a bandage, and keep it away from body fluids. Clean any S/M gear after use (see dildo cleaning above).

- *Least risky sexual activities* include kissing (unless you have cuts in your mouth, gum disease, or bleeding cuts in your gums from flossing), hugging, rubbing, hand jobs, mutual masturbation (avoid getting the ejaculate or vaginal fluids of your partner on your skin if you have small cuts or sores), fantasizing, and massage.

Safer Sex Supplies

Condoms (for men and women), lubricants, and spermicides are available from most drugstores, health clinics, and sex boutiques. For latex gloves, finger cots, and dental dams, check with a local hospital, health

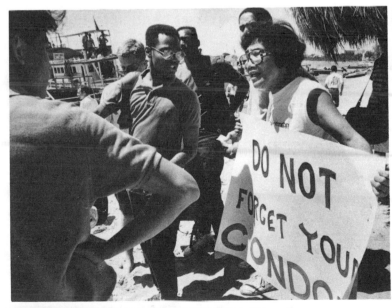

A nurse-midwife teaching safer sex to U.S. GIs on Pataya, an island that the military has used for "R and R" /S. Asabe

clinic, or sex boutique. Planned Parenthood or STD clinics, Title X family planning clinics, and some high schools give free supplies of condoms.

HIV-Safe IV Needle Use

Sharing needles in injection drug use is extremely risky for HIV transmission. If you inject drugs, think about changing to a non-IV drug (sniffing or smoking), or stopping. Drug treatment centers can help you evaluate your drug use and decrease your need or stop (see chapter 3, Alcohol, Tobacco, and Other Mood-Altering Drugs, for more information.) If you continue to use IV drugs, don't share needles or works with anyone. Try not to reuse needles or syringes, and if you do, clean them and the cooker with full-strength household bleach (three rinses of bleach is best, then three rinses of clean water). In an emergency, rubbing alcohol, vodka, or wine can also be used, but they are not as good as bleach. Use fresh cotton and water each time.

Take advantage of needle exchange programs that exist in some areas; such programs have been highly successful in decreasing HIV transmission among injection drug users.

Donor Insemination and HIV Prevention

If you are considering getting pregnant through donor insemination, be aware that if the donor has HIV infection, you are vulnerable to being infected by the semen. See the section on donor insemination in chapter 18, Assisted Low-Tech and High-Tech Reproductive Technologies, for more.

HIV SYMPTOMS AND TESTING

Symptoms of HIV Infection

It is frightening to notice symptoms of HIV infection. Many of us might want to ignore them as long as we can. Yet, the earlier we can get treatment, the more

"MORNING AFTER" TREATMENT

If you have been raped, had a condom break, or engaged in unprotected sex with someone whom you know to be HIV infected, you may be able to obtain treatment immediately, without waiting for tests to show the presence of HIV antibodies. Those who have accidental needle sticks in health care settings have access to such treatment. The treatments have potentially serious side effects and can cost up to $1,000, but you and your health care provider may decide that the protection is worth it.

HIV TESTING

Finding out that you are HIV-positive is life changing and traumatic; finding that you are not HIV-positive is challenging in its own way. Check to see if there are support groups or counselors in your area to help you with testing decisions, and/or look for a testing site where good counseling is provided.

What Is the HIV Antibody Test?

It is a blood test for antibodies to HIV, the virus believed to cause AIDS. When a person is infected with HIV, the body's immune system produces antibodies in an attempt to fight HIV. A small sample of blood will detect the presence of these antibodies. The test is often inaccurately called an "AIDS test," but it does not tell you whether you have AIDS.

What Are Reasons to Take the Test?

1. You want to know whether you are infected so that you can consider getting medical help (including early intervention therapies, which can help a person live longer and better with HIV), enrolling in drug trials, or pursuing holistic, nonbiomedical treatments.

2. You think that knowing your antibody status may help keep you from having unsafe sex and/or sharing needles.

3. You are thinking about having a baby or breast-feeding your baby.

4. You would feel less stress if you knew for certain whether or not you are infected.

Are There Reasons Not to Take the Test?

You may choose not to be tested if you have never done anything to put yourself at risk for HIV infection, or if you are being pressured by a healthcare provider or other advisor to have the test in a setting where the results will not be anonymous (see below) or where you don't feel safe.

When Should the Test Be Taken?

Take the test a minimum of six weeks after your last possible exposure to HIV. Ninety-eight percent of infected people show antibodies within two months of exposure.

chance we have of living longer and better with HIV. Keep in mind that we can have the infection for ten years or more without having any noticable symptoms, and that early HIV symptoms are similar to those of common illnesses like the flu. If you or your partner(s) pursue any activities that are high risk for HIV transmission, watch for a flu-like illness.

The symptoms of early infection can include weight loss, fatigue, swollen glands (lumps in the neck, armpits or groin), persistent dry cough, and skin rashes. Later on in the illness, there can be night sweats, fevers, thrush, headaches, diarrhea, and loss of appetite.

Recurrent vaginal yeast infections, chronic pelvic inflammatory disease, and frequently recurring, severe genital herpes, do not necessarily mean that you have HIV but they can be symptoms of HIV in women. Most women with a well-functioning immune system will recover with standard treatment for a gynecological condition, but a woman who is HIV-positive may require more intensive treatment or may experience a more rapid progression of infection. Among women with HIV infection, there is also a high incidence of human papillomavirus (HPV), the virus that causes venereal warts (condyloma). If you have one or more of these conditions, you may want to ask a health care provider about HIV.

LIVING WITH HIV/AIDS

Most important, at least for me, is learning to live with the AIDS virus—learning how to put myself first.[6]

We all have to die from something, but why die before you're dead? Life is what you make of it. The feeling of wellness comes from within—your spirituality—one's belief in self, and a desire to live. . . . Personally, I do not consider HIV as a death sentence. I know that as long as I take care of myself through good nutrition, proper sleep, attending support groups, visiting my physician, and keeping my recovery [from drug use] up front, I will be all right.... I was so convinced I was going to die that I didn't pay taxes for four years. Now the IRS is saying, "You're gonna live and you're gonna pay us."[7]

If your test result is positive for HIV, remember that this does not mean you have or will ever get AIDS. It is a time to take particularly good care of your health, if you can, by eating better, resting more, and protecting yourself from other STDs. There are promising new combination treatments, or "cocktails" (see p. 361), which may make a difference in whether you develop AIDS or not. Finding health care is a crucial step, especially finding a health care provider experienced in treating HIV infection. So is negotiating whatever insurance or disability benefits might be available to you. Finding emotional support is important, too: Without support you may feel too frightened to act or too angry to proceed. Seek out groups in your community for women who are HIV-positive. In groups you can give and get support, share ideas, and learn. A newsletter for women with HIV may give you support and information as well (see Resources).

We must continue to take care of ourselves and our partners medically, physically, emotionally, and sexually. Women from the Women of Color AIDS Council in Boston offered the following advice:

- For your primary health care, find a health care provider with a background in infectious diseases or obstetrics and gynecology, who knows and understands HIV disease. In this era of managed care, access to specialists may be limited.
- Remember that your provider works for you, and you must be comfortable with him or her. If not, do not be afraid to find a different provider.
- Learn all you can about HIV so that you can advocate for yourself. READ. Stay up to date with the newest information and treatments (see Resources).
- Learn to listen to and know your body, so that you will be aware of changes.
- Create a network among women in your community. Take advantage of existing resources and services. The support of others often can give us the strength to deal with the stresses and challenges we face in life.
- Be open to counseling, therapy, and self-reflection. HIV can cause depression and feelings of hopelessness. It is very important to seek help and not isolate yourself.
- Never give up. If there is no answer at one number or if the resources are not available, call the next number.
- If you are thinking about getting pregnant, make sure you have preconceptual care. There are treatments that can increase the possibility of your child being born without HIV.
- If you are using drugs or alcohol, enroll in drug treatment or seek out Narcotics Anonymous or Alcoholics Anonymous resources.

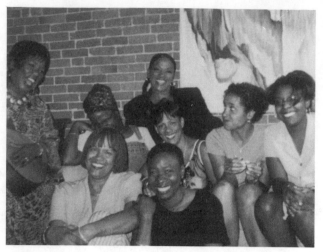

Members of the Women of Color AIDS Council in Boston, spring 1997/Michele Russell

- Take life one day at a time.
- Practice safer sex: *"You can only be responsible for your own safety. Proceed with caution at all times."* Use protection even if your partner isn't HIV-positive, because avoiding STDs can keep you healthy longer.

Getting the Best Health Care Possible

I strongly believe that you must feel comfortable with your care providers. Deciding what approach to take in your treatment should be a team effort between you and your providers.

Here are some questions that might be helpful to ask when you choose a health care provider for HIV care:

- What kind of holistic alternatives do you have experience with (e.g., acupuncture)?
- What is your attitude toward people in recovery or actively using drugs?
- Are you up to date on the very latest HIV care? (Protease inhibitors? Viral load testing?) Are you familiar with how the different drugs affect women?
- How would you react if I chose to become pregnant?
- What other HIV care services are part of the practice?
- Are you planning to be around for a long time?
- Are you willing to do regular viral load testing even if I don't have the money or insurance to cover it? Will you advocate for me in getting medications?
- Is child care available for me during health care appointments if I need it?
- What are the attitudes and practices of the nursing and support staff at the hospitals where you might send me for inpatient care?

An ugly thing about the U.S. health care system is that we are likely to receive worse care for HIV and AIDS if we are women of color or "poor," or undocumented. There are some highly dedicated health care providers at every level of the system, but those in poorer facilities are working against immense obstacles to provide adequate care. Even nonmedical factors have an impact: As simple a matter as child care can make the difference in whether the mothers among us can come for treatment. An AIDS hot line or agency may be able to help you find the best care possible in your area (see Resources).

The best health care means frequent visits for physical exams and laboratory tests. What follows is what should be the basic, minimal standard of care for all people with HIV or AIDS:

1. Frequent CD4 (or T) cell monitoring and viral load testing to help you plan and assess treatment. T cell monitoring will show how well your immune system is doing, and viral load testing will show how much virus is in your body at a given time.

2. Vaccinations. Vaccinations should be brought up to date, especially for pneumonia, tetanus, and flu.

3. Treatment. HIV can be treated in three ways: treating the virus itself with antiviral medications, treating or preventing the opportunistic infections, and boosting the immune system (through self-care and nonmedical alternatives). See "Options for Care," below.

4. Support for our emotional well-being is important, as are nutritional advice and the assistance of a social worker.

5. Finally, HIV-positive women often have chronic vaginitis, pelvic infections, vaginal and cervical diseases, or bacterial lung infections. There is a high incidence of human papillomavirus (HPV), which causes cell changes that can lead to cervical cancer. Unless these underlying problems are adequately treated, even the standard care regimen may fail to improve our health or extend our lives. A Pap smear every six months is part of good care.

Options for Care

Decisions about the kind of care we want for HIV infection or AIDS are important. Usually we want to be the ones to make these decisions at every stage along the way, using input and advice from our health care providers and from a support group if one is available to us. Many AIDS service organizations hold strategy sessions for treatment issues, and there are some great treatment hot lines (see Re-

> With self-care, and paying attention to our own health and our own needs—maybe for the first time ever—some women with HIV feel better than we ever have. Being HIV-positive or having AIDS, we may qualify for government aid and have access to financial support for the first time in our lives. Those of us who find a support group, or an AIDS activist group, often find that we are less alone than ever before. Helping other women avoid getting HIV can make us feel better: there's more to live for. Many of us who have found treatment for drug or alcohol addiction find that life looks better than it ever did. More than one woman has said, "The virus gave me my life."

sources).* No one should be forced into taking medications she doesn't feel comfortable with, nor should anyone be denied what she thinks is appropriate treatment for her.

Self-Care

Staying as well as we can physically and emotionally is extremely important. To maintain physical and emotional health, proper nutrition, hygiene, exercise, and enough rest are all necessary. If you smoke, consider stopping: smoking has been shown to damage the immune system, and those of us with HIV are especially vulnerable to upper respiratory infections. If you drink alcohol, consider drinking in moderation or stopping entirely. If you are concerned about a problem with alcohol and or drugs, contact your local AA chapter or speak to your health care provider.

HIV infection, and some of the drugs used in treating it, can deplete us physically. Proper nutrition—good, varied, healthy food—helps strengthen our immune system. A nutritionist may be a good resource for information about diet and vitamins. Sometimes nutritional supplements such as "instant breakfast" can provide energy and weight gain.

Because people with HIV are vulnerable to microbial and fungal infections, we have to avoid exposure to microbes. We must be very careful with food preparation, making sure food is clean and well prepared. Raw fish and shellfish, and rare or undercooked meats and poultry, should be avoided. It is also suggested that people with HIV not clean cat litter boxes, bird cages, or fish tanks (or do so with gloves) to prevent toxoplasmosis, an opportunistic infection. Finally, practicing safer sex, whether our partners are HIV-positive or not, is critical: it not only protects our partners but also protects us from microbes that might weaken us or make us sicker.

* For systematic reviews of the effectiveness of different forms of care relating to HIV/AIDS, you can contact the Cochrane Collaboration HIV/AIDS Group, in Resources. Chapter 25, The Politics of Women's Health and Medical Care, has more on the Cochrane Collaboration.

Nonbiomedical (Holistic, Nonallopathic) Care

Alternative treatments, used in conjunction with more common, allopathic medical treatments like drugs, may reduce the severity of symptoms associated with HIV disease and bolster the immune system, although there is no documented proof. The use of Chinese medicine—both acupuncture and Chinese herbs—may sometimes improve CD4 cell counts and immune system functioning, abate some drug side effects, and also relieve some symptoms, such as night sweats, nausea, diarrhea, and neuropathies (pain or lack of feeling in the extremities).

Several mind/body medical practices have helped to improve immune system functioning and enhance a person's sense of quality of life. Such practices include visualization, relaxation, physical exercise, and cognitive therapy. Both acupuncture and chiropractic care can reduce stress and muscle tension and may be successful in treating insomnia, neuropathies, and headaches.

Some AIDS service organizations, hospitals, and clinics provide alternative therapies regardless of an individual's ability to pay. If you have health insurance, some alternative treatments may be covered. Please see chapter 5, Holistic Health and Healing, for more on alternative health care.

Medical ("Allopathic") Treatment

The medical system has earned our mistrust. It has mistreated women and neglected women of color. And yet those of us living with HIV know we cannot beat this disease without medical assistance. How do we put aside our very healthy skepticism and participate in medical trials, take their medications even though they are not entirely sure they can help us, and trust in a system which has so let us down? I say we do it with our eyes wide open. We learn all we can and become as educated consumers as possible.

Here is a brief summary of some of the options and issues in deciding about medication for HIV or AIDS.

1. Preventing growth of the virus through antiviral therapy.

Antiviral therapy incudes the traditional antiviral drugs like AZT (known now as ZDV), 3TC and ddI, and now includes the new class of drugs called protease inhibitors, which can radically lower viral load (see Glossary.) There are now drug combinations, or "HIV cocktails," that put together two or three drugs so that the virus won't become drug-resistant so easily. These have stopped or dramatically reduced the replication of HIV in the human body, resulting in a drop in death rates and improvement in quality of life. For the first time in the epidemic, even the most critical, discouraged skeptics have hope. While we still don't have a cure for HIV, we can say that HIV will become a manageable, long-term illness for many.

Yet many of us have serious questions about these new medications. Much of the news regarding protease inhibitors is based on the experiences of middle-class gay white men. Many women of color and women living in poverty find these drugs difficult to get or to use. Protease inhibitors are very expensive, ranging from $6,000 to $16,000 per year. They have to be taken at just the right time of day, often with food or even special diets, and in some cases the drug must be refrigerated. If you don't take the drugs in exactly the right way, you may develop HIV strains that are drug-resistant, and you may not be able to use the drugs again later in the course of the illness. For some, the requirements of the drugs seem unappealing, or impossible to meet. *"How many people do you know eat three full meals a day? On my budget let's be realistic."* The "HIV cocktail" combination therapies don't work for everyone, especially those who have a history of taking AZT. There are side effects, including nausea, severe diarrhea, and fatigue, and potentially life-threatening effects, including a small risk of liver failure. Some of the protease inhibitors react negatively with certain drugs—for example, asthma medications—and can result in possible liver disease.

Yet, the combination therapies are the first potentially good news in a long time. Every woman who wants to use them should have access to them. Many women with low incomes, who are homeless, or who use IV drugs worry that doctors may not offer the "cocktails" because they think we might be "noncompliant" and thus poor risks. *"You know people look at you, see you're black or Latina and think you must be a welfare mom, or an addict and stupid."* AIDS activists need to focus on access to these new medications for all women.

2. Preventing opportunistic infections via prophylactic treatment.

Using medications prophylactically (for prevention) against PCP, the devastating pneumonia that people with AIDS often get, is essential. Bactrim, which is commonly used, should be monitored closely by a health care provider. There are preventive drug treatments to be considered, as well, for toxoplasmosis, tuberculosis, cryptococcal disease, frequent or severe recurrences of herpes simplex virus or yeast infections, and other opportunistic infections.

Clinical drug trials. If new drugs are being tested for AIDS treatment, you may want to try them. Participating in a clinical drug trial, which tests new treatments on humans in an effort to prove drug safety, efficacy, and appropriate dose levels, is one way to benefit from the newest research and to receive free medicine and medical attention. It involves risks, but many PLWAs prefer the risk of taking a new drug that might help to the near-certainty of suffering without it, especially if they have a virus that is resistant to approved treatments. You can contact the National Institutes of Health (NIH) at (800) TRIALS A about trials.

HIV and Pregnancy

I have had patients with HIV infection who were not so gently pushed to have tubal ligations that they have come to regret, since the chances of having an infected baby have decreased in this country over the years.

—A nurse

If either we or our partner have HIV, the decision about whether to get pregnant or to continue a pregnancy is loaded with questions: Will my child be infected? If I become ill, is there someone in my life who would care for my child?

It is possible for HIV to pass from a pregnant woman to her fetus during pregnancy and childbirth. Without intervention, it will happen about 25 to 33% of the time in the U.S. Some AIDS policymakers have actively discouraged all HIV-positive women from becoming pregnant and have encouraged pregnant HIV-positive women to terminate their pregnancies. However, recent research has proved that mother-to-infant HIV transmission (often called vertical transmission) can be greatly decreased with antiviral treatment. In clinical trials, a two-thirds reduction in mother-to-infant transmission of HIV was observed in women who received oral ZDV (popularly known as AZT) during pregnancy and intravenous ZDV during delivery, and whose infants received oral ZDV for six weeks after delivery. There seemed to be no adverse effects on the pregnant women or their babies, although the long-term effects of ZDV and other antiviral drugs, protease inhibitors, or combination therapies on pregnant women and the fetus or the grown child are unknown.

This option offers increased choice and hope for those of us who are HIV-infected and want to bear children—and a good reason to be tested when we wish to become pregnant. The Federal Centers for Disease Control (CDC) has recommended routine counseling and voluntary testing of all pregnant women. Some people have suggested *mandatory* testing of pregnant women, but this is controversial. The likelihood of being tested against our will could make women decide not to seek prenatal care at all, which would be a great loss.

Studies are being undertaken to explore other ways to lower the risk of transmission, including delivery by cesarean section and treatment of HIV-infected women with ZDV in combination with HIV immune globulin. After the birth, since HIV can pass to the infant through the mother's milk, it is considered best for a woman with HIV infection not to breast-feed.

Taking care of our health both before and during pregnancy, in terms of food, sleep, exercise, and STD prevention, is a key to our well-being and that of the baby, and may actually reduce the risk of giving birth to an HIV-positive baby. Current research suggests that pregnancy will not accelerate HIV disease, bring on symptoms, or complicate pregnancy for a woman who is asymptomatic or shows no signs of sickness. However, pregnancy in women with advanced stages of HIV disease does appear to worsen symptoms. A low CD4 cell count (below 300), anemia, inflammation of the placenta, the presence of other infections, and advanced AIDS may each increase the risk of transmission to the fetus and affect our health and the progress of a pregnancy.

Every infant born to an HIV-positive woman will have its mother's antibodies in its blood and may test positive for HIV antibodies for a year or so even if it is not infected. The PCR test can determine quickly if the infant is infected. (PCR, or polymerase chain reaction test, is a highly sensitive test that can detect fragments of genetic material of viruses or other organisms in blood and tissue.) Some policymakers advocate routine or mandatory testing of all newborns for HIV as a means of assessing the percentage of reproductive-age women who are infected with HIV. Many of us who are concerned with women's rights strenuously oppose any testing that is done without the informed consent of the mother. The time and money involved in widespread newborn screening would better be spent on maternal and child health services, as well as on prevention, education, and treatment of HIV disease.

Ironically, if you are HIV-positive and pregnant and wish to terminate your pregnancy, you may find that abortion clinics will refuse to take you or will charge extra. This reflects some providers' ignorance and fear regarding HIV transmission. Advocates are fighting to preserve the reproductive rights of HIV-positive women, including access to nondiscriminatory health care, whether we choose to become pregnant and carry a pregnancy to term or terminate it.

Personal Issues in Living with HIV or AIDS

The list of personal dilemmas and questions for women with HIV or AIDS and our families is long. The hot lines, organizations, newsletters, and books at the end of the chapter will offer support for dealing with questions like these: What about my sex life as a PLWA? Who will care for my children if I get too sick? Do I want to tell my family and friends I have HIV? My co-workers? My children? What if people find out? How do I deal with health care providers who don't respect me because I use drugs or sell sex, or because they think I do? How do I get on public assistance? What legal protections are there for me if I feel I am being discriminated against because of HIV? How do I face the possibility of my death? Would planning for my funeral help me feel empowered? What if I get on the new treatments and suddenly realize I'm not going to die anytime soon—how do I adjust?

Preparing for our children's care in the case of incapacitating illness or death. Although more people are now living longer with HIV, it remains a life-threatening disease. If we are mothers, the thought of getting too sick to care for our children, or dying while they are young, is often the hardest thing to bear. Many states have enacted important "standby guardianship" laws that allow us to decide in advance who will become guardians of our children, while still caring for them ourselves for as long as we are able.

Getting involved. Many women have found that getting active in the community helps us feel better emotionally and spiritually while living with HIV or AIDS. During the periods when we're not feeling sick, we might join a group to pressure a hospital to improve its treatment of PLWAs, to lobby the city council or Congress for better AIDS legislation, or to convince a church or other religious group to open up about HIV. Many women become peer counselors, educating people in our communities about preventing HIV. Or we can get involved in recovery programs, become a sponsor, encourage other women in their recovery from drug or alcohol use. As one woman from the AIDS Action Committee in Massachusetts said, "If I can save one more person, it's worth it."

....

NOTES

....

1. Belynda Dunn, AIDS Action Committee of Massachusetts African-American education specialist, in personal conversation, March 1997.
2. Elizabeth Banks, "Living with HIV," *Sojourner: The Women's Forum* 22, no. 7 (March 1997): 20.
3. Gail Elizabeth Wyatt, "Transaction Sex and HIV Risks: A Women's Choice?" *HIV Infection in Women: Setting a New Agenda,* Washington, DC (February 22–24, 1995): S2. Abstract Number WA1–1.
4. Amber Hollibaugh of the Lesbian AIDS Project in New York City.
5. This section is based on writings by Susan Rosenburg, Laura Whitehorn, and Linda Evans, political prisoners in the federal prison system who are HIV/AIDS educators and activists. See box in chapter 27, Organizing for Change.
6. Elizabeth Banks, "Living with HIV."
7. Belynda Dunn, see note 1, conversation.

....

RESOURCES

....

Books and Articles

ACT UP/New York Women and AIDS Book Group. *Women, AIDS and Activism.* Boston: South End Press, 1990. Essays on the health and policy issues of concern to women affected in any way by HIV and AIDS.

Banzhaf, Marion D., ed. *Pregnancy, HIV and You: A Handbook for Women with HIV.* New Brunswick, NJ: New Jersey Women and AIDS Network, 1997. (908) 846-4462.

Brown, Treeby Williamson, and Barbara Aliza. *A Changing Epidemic: How State Title V Programs Are Addressing the Spread of HIV/AIDS in Women, Children and Youth.* McLean, VA: Association of Maternal and Child Health Programs, 1995. Special section on Title V involvement in comprehensive school health programs and HIV prevention education.

Center for Disease Control and National AIDS Clearinghouse. *Hispanics and HIV/AIDS: A Guide to Selected Resources.* Rockville, MD: Centers for Disease Control and Prevention, 1995.

Chicago Women's AIDS Project. *Girls Night Out: A Safer Sex Workshop for Women: Manual for Peer Leaders.* Chicago: Chicago Women's AIDS Project, circa 1990. Available from the Chicago Women's AIDS Project, 5249 North Kenmore, Chicago, IL 60640; (773) 271-2242.

Corea, Gena. *The Invisible Epidemic: The Story of Women and AIDS.* New York: HarperCollins, 1992. An important classic.

Faden, Ruth R., and Nancy E. Kass, eds. *HIV, AIDS and Childbearing: Public Policy, Private Lives.* New York: Oxford University Press, 1996.

Farmer, Paul, Margaret Connors, and Janie Simmons, eds. *Women, Poverty and AIDS: Sex, Drugs and Structural Violence.* Monroe, ME: Common Courage Press, 1996.

Goldstein, Nancy, and Jennifer L. Manlowe, eds. *The Gender Politics of HIV/AIDS in Women: Perspectives on the Pandemic in the United States.* New York and London: New York University Press, 1997.

Harris, A. "The Invisibility of Lesbians with AIDS," in Vida, Ginny, et al., eds. *The New Our Right to Love: A Lesbian Resource Book.* New York: Touchstone, 1996, 108–11.

Harrison, Michelle. *The Preteen's First Book About Love, Sex, and AIDS.* Washington, DC: American Psychiatric Press, 1995.

Kloser, Patricia, and Jane MacLean Craig. *The Woman's HIV Sourcebook: A Guide to Better Health and Well-Being.* Dallas: Taylor Publishing Co., 1994.

Kurth, Ann, ed. *Until the Cure: Caring for Women with HIV.* New Haven: Yale University Press, 1993.

Lyon-Martin Women's Health Services. *National Lesbian/Bisexual HIV Prevention Network HIV Prevention Manual.* San Francisco: Lyon-Martin Women's Health Services, 1991.

Mann, Jonathan M., and Daniel J.M. Tarantola, eds. *AIDS in the World II: Global Dimensions, Social Roots, and Responses.* New York: Oxford University Press, 1996.

Minkoff, Howard, Jack DeHovitz, and Ann Duerr, eds. *HIV Infection in Women.* New York: Raven Press, 1995. By professors and physicians, experts in their specialties.

National Women's Health Network. *Women and HIV/AIDS Packet.* Washington, DC: NWHN, 1997. Full of up-to-date articles. Available from the National Women's Health Network Clearinghouse, 514 10th Street NW, Suite 400, Washington, DC 20004; (202) 628-7814.

Patton, Cindy. *Last Served? Gendering the HIV Pandemic.* Bristol, PA: Taylor and Francis, 1994. Dense, academic, thought-provoking.

Rudd, Andrea, and Darien Taylor, eds. *Positive Women: Voices of Women Living with AIDS.* Toronto: Second Story Press, 1992.

Schneider, Beth, and Nancy Stoller, eds. *Women Re-*

sisting *AIDS: Feminist Strategies of Empowerment*. Philadelphia: Temple University Press, 1994.

Siegal, Diana Laskin, and Christie Burke. "Midlife and Older Women and HIV/AIDS: My (Grand)mother Wouldn't Do That," in Goldstein and Manlowe, op. cit., 155–67.

Wilton, Tamsin, Lesley Doyall, and Jennie Naidoo, eds. *AIDS: Setting a Feminist Agenda*. Bristol, PA: Taylor and Francis, 1994.

World Health Organization. *Women and AIDS: Agenda for Action*. Geneva: WHO, 1994.

Newsletters and Magazines

Positively Aware. A monthly publication primarily by men, which has some useful articles for women. Test Positive Aware Network, Inc., 1258 West Belmont Avenue, Chicago, IL 60657-3292; (773) 404-8726; E-mail: tpanet@aol.com; Web site: http://www.tpan.com.

POZ Magazine. Well balanced between women and men, white people and people of color; has updated medical information and good columns on sex. Published in Spanish four times a year. POZ Publishing, 349 West 12th Street, New York, NY 10014-1721; (800) 973-2376; Web site: http://www.poz.com

World Newsletter, published by WORLD—Women Organized to Respond to Life-Threatening Diseases, 3958 Webster Street, Oakland, CA 94609; (510) 658-6930. For and by women infected or affected by HIV/AIDS. Includes articles on lesbians, bisexual women. WORLD also conducts educational programs and retreats for women with HIV.

Organizations

National Organizations

ACT UP (AIDS Coalition to Unleash Power)
332 Bleecker Street, Suite G5; New York, NY 10014; (212) 966-4873
E-mail: actupny@panix.com
Web site: http://www.actupny.org
    AIDS activist organization.

Centers for Disease Control and Prevention
P.O. Box 6003; Rockville, MD 20849-6003; (800) 458-5231
E-mail: aidsinfo@cdcnac.aspensys.org
Web site: http://www.cdcnac.org
    U.S. government agency that has many good publications as well as the latest in treatment information.

Cochrane Collaboration HIV/AIDS Group
Contact: Gail E. Kennedy
Cochrane HIV/AIDS Group; San Francisco Cochrane Center; Institute for Health Policy Studies; University of California; 1388 Sutter, 11th Floor; San Francisco, CA 94109
E-mail: sfcc@sirus.com
    For updated information on research results from high-quality studies. (See chapter 25, The Politics of Women's Health and Medical Care, p. 710.)

National AIDS Hot Line
(800) 342-AIDS; Spanish: (800) 344-7432; TTY: (800) 243-7889
    Information, education, and national and local referral. English-language line is open 24 hours a day, 365 days a year; Spanish-language line is open seven days a week from 8:00 A.M. to 2:00 P.M., EST; TTY line is open Monday through Friday, 10:00 A.M. to 10:00 P.M., EST.

National Association of People with AIDS
1413 K Street, NW, 7th floor; Washington, DC 20005; (202) 898-0414
E-mail: napwa@thecure.org
Web site: http://www.thecure.org/nap.main.html
    Operates a clearinghouse of HIV/AIDS information.

National Lesbian and Gay Health Association (formerly National Gay and Lesbian Health Foundation)
1407 S Street NW; Washington, DC 20009; (202) 939-7880
    Health care advocacy; directory of U.S. lesbian/gay health services; national conferences.

National Minority AIDS Council (NMAC)
1931 13th Street, NW; Washington, DC 20009-4432; (202) 483-6622
    National education and advocacy group addressing impact of AIDS on communities of color.

Teens and AIDS Hotline
(800) 234-TEEN
    Nationwide referral service.

Women of color organizations: Several women-of-color activist groups provide information and support for women with HIV/AIDS. These include the National Latina Health Organization, the National Black Women's Health Project, the Native American Women's Health Education Resource Center, and the Asian American Women's Health Organization. For contacting information, please see Resources in chapter 27, Organizing for Change.

A Few Local and Regional Organizations

To find the AIDS organization nearest you, call the CDC National AIDS Clearing House at (800) 458-5231. Not all AIDS organizations focus equally on women. The groups listed below focus well on women's issues; most offer support groups, education, referrals. One of these groups may be able to advise you on choosing the organization nearest you that has the best approach to women and HIV/AIDS.

Adolescent AIDS Program
Montefiore Medical Center; 111 East 210th Street; Bronx, NY 10467; (718) 882-0023
    HIV testing/counseling, clinical services, support groups, case management, referral, safer sex education.

AIDS Action Committee of Massachusetts
131 Clarendon Street; Boston, MA 02116; (617) 437-6200; Hot line: (800) 235-2331; Youth Hot line: (800) 788-1234; TTY: (617) 450-1427

Chicago Women's AIDS Project
5249 North Kenmore; Chicago, IL 60640; (312) 271-2242

Lesbian AIDS Project, GMHC (Gay Men's Health Crisis)
129 W. 20th Street, 2nd floor; New York, NY 10011; (212) 807-6664
Web site: http://www.gmhc.org

Lyon-Martin Women's Health Services
Lesbian HIV/AIDS Program; 1748 Market Street, Suite 201; San Francisco, CA 94102; (415) 565-7674

New Jersey Women and AIDS Network
5 Elm Row, Suite 112; New Brunswick, NJ 08901; (908) 846-4462

People of Color Against AIDS Network
607 19th Avenue East; Seattle, WA 98112; (206) 322-7061
   Prevention, outreach, and educational materials.

PROTOTYPES—W.A.R.N. (Women and AIDS Risk Network)
5601 West Slauson Avenue, Suite 200; Culver City, CA 90230; (213) 641-7795
   Many services, including court referral for sex workers.

San Francisco AIDS Foundation (including Women and AIDS Network)
P.O. Box 426182; San Francisco, CA 94142-6182; (415) 864-4376; Hot line: (800) 863-AIDS; Hot line (in North Carolina): (800) FOR-AIDS

Sisterlove Women's AIDS Project
1132 West Peachtree Street, Room 111; Atlanta, GA 30309; (404) 872-0600
   Safer sex education, advocacy, workshops, women of color.

Whitman-Walker Clinic
1407 S Street NW; Washington, DC 20009; (202) 797-3500
   Has innovative workshop for the lesbian community on sexuality, safer sex, and communication.

Legal Resources

AIDS Law Project, Gay and Lesbian Advocates and Defenders
P.O. Box 218; Boston, MA 02112; (617) 426-1350; (800) 455-GLAD; TTY: (617) 426-6156
E-mail: gladlaw@aol.com
Web site: http://www.glad.org
   Legal advocacy on issues of discrimination, confidentiality, and access to health and medical care.

American Civil Liberties Union AIDS Project
132 West 43rd Street; New York, NY 10036; (212) 944-9800, ext. 545
E-mail: aidsinfo@aol.com
Web site: http://www.aclu.org
   Litigation and educational materials.

Treatment Resources

AIDS Treatment Data Network
611 Broadway, Suite 613; New York, NY 10012; (212) 268-4196; (800) 734-7104
   Information on research and treatment, educational materials, access to AIDS-related clinical drug trials.

Project Inform
1965 Market Street; San Francisco, CA 94103; (415) 558-8669; Treatment Hot line: (800) 822-7422
Web site: http://www.projinfo.org
   Nationwide referral to treatment centers, information on the latest studies.

Prison Resources

AIDS Counseling and Education (ACE)
Bedford Hills Correctional Facility; 247 Harris Road; Bedford Hills, NY 10507; (914) 241-3100, ext. 260
   Nationwide model for peer education for prisons, created by and for women prisoners. Peer counseling, education groups, peer support, health advocacy, inmate and worker education, workshops for general public.

National Prison Project
1875 Connecticut Avenue NW, Suite 410; Washington, DC 20009; (202) 331-0500
   Information, studies, referral.

Social Justice for Women
MCI Framingham Women and AIDS Project; 108 Lincoln Street, 6th Floor; Boston, MA 02111; (617) 482-0747
   Monitors medical care, treatment, and aftercare services for HIV-positive women at MCI Framingham; group education programs; individual counseling.

Family Resources

Life Force: Women Fighting AIDS
165 Camdan Plaza East, no. 310; Brooklyn, NY 11201; (718) 797-0937

Make-a-Wish Foundation
100 West Clarendon, Suite 2200; Phoenix, AZ 85013-3518; (800) 722-WISH
Web site: http://www.wish.org

Sunburst National AIDS Project
P.O. Box 2824; Petaluma, CA 95953; (707) 769-0169
   Week-long camp.

Adoption Programs

Families and Children's AIDS Network
53 West Jackson Boulevard, Suite 409; Chicago, IL 60604; (312) 786-9255

"Just Kids"
P.O. Box 42; New York, NY 10014; (212) 627-3390

Positively Pediatrics and Adolescents
P.O. Box 4512; Queensbury, NY 12804; (518) 798-8940

Additional Online Resources *

AIDS Education Global Information System
http://www.aegis.com

AIDS Treatment News Internet Directory
http://www.aidsnews.org

HIV/AIDS Treatment Information Service
http://www.hivatis.org/atishome.html

HIV Positive: Women and Children
http://www.hivpositive.com/f-Women/
WoChildMenu.html

The Journal of the American Medical Association:
HIV/AIDS Information Center
http://www.ama-assn.org/special/hiv/hivhome.htm

Welcome To The Safer Sex Page!
http://www.safersex.org

* For more information and listings of online resources, please see
Introduction to Online Women's Health Resources, p. 25.

By Catherine Harris-Vincent, with Jennifer Yanco and Linda King, based on earlier work by Jane Pincus and Jill Wolhandler

WITH SPECIAL THANKS TO Denise Bergman, Paula Harris-Vincent, Joyce Maguire Pavao, Carolyn Rudin, Kay Schlozman, Dianne Weiss, and all those who contributed their knowledge, thoughts, and experience *

Chapter 16

....

Unplanned Pregnancies: Finding Out You're Pregnant and Deciding What to Do

You think you are pregnant, and you're not sure that you want to be. Whether you are 15 or 45, already have children or have never been pregnant before, you may feel alone with a huge decision on your hands. Many women find it very useful at this time to reach out to someone equipped to give us the support we need, even if we are not inclined to talk about our personal life with others. One of the benefits of talking and being listened to can be the discovery of inner strengths that you weren't aware of. Often it helps to hear your thoughts out loud. There *is* help to guide you through this time. We hope that this chapter will be one step in helping you find the support and information that you need.

Women are the ones who conceive, and therefore the presumption of responsibility for decisions surrounding an unexpected pregnancy falls on us. Often we are left on our own to find our way through this

* Thanks also to the following for their help with the 1998 version of this chapter: Joan Ditzion, Paula Doress-Worters, Mary Howell, Leslie Linson, Carol Lynch, Leslie Panton, Ellen Rollins, Norma Meras Swenson, and Vernette Allen Williams.

difficult time. As we make our way through this process, we have the right to receive whatever support and advice we need and the right to make our own decisions. We have the legal right to terminate the pregnancy, as well as the right to carry it to term.

More than any other time in a woman's life, being pregnant requires that you be conscious of how you are situated in the world—how valued, safe, and comfortable you are. Our race, class, religion, disability, age, sexual orientation, and marital status can influence how we are perceived by the professionals we come into contact with, and the kind of advice they give us. You may be up against an invisible bottom line: Is the life you are carrying perceived as a burden or as an asset to the world? If you do not feel respected and valued during all aspects of the decision-making process, including counseling and medical care, perhaps you need to get moral support in one place and medical advice elsewhere.

Most of us feel vulnerable while talking with a health care practitioner. The relationship is unbalanced; the practitioner is presumed to be the expert. Many health care practitioners have been taught to

EMERGENCY CONTRACEPTION

If you have had unprotected sex (vaginal intercourse) or a contraceptive failure within the last 72 hours, emergency contraception is an option. If you have been forced to have sex against your will, emergency contraception may be the last thing on your mind, but being pregnant may be the last thing you would want. **For the names of providers in your area who offer emergency contraception services, call the hot line at (800) 584-9911.** For more information, see chapter 13, Birth Control, p. 324.

provide care for, and are oriented toward, a white, middle-class, heterosexual population. If you feel pressured to make a decision that does not reflect your needs, remember that this may have more to do with the prejudices of the practitioner than with what is best for your actual circumstances. Some women are urged to carry their pregnancies to term; others are not

only urged to have an abortion, but also to consider sterilization. These are *your* decisions to make, and you deserve counseling and support that help you arrive at the best decisions for *you*. Remember, no matter how much expertise a practitioner has, she or he is not living your life.

FIRST STEPS

First you need to find out whether or not you are in fact pregnant. If you suspect pregnancy but haven't had a test yet, don't assume that you are pregnant. Use birth control if you continue to have sex and don't want to get pregnant. If you had sex without "going all the way" (without penetration), it is still possible that you are pregnant, if sperm from the man you had sex with got near the entrance of your vagina.

Signs of Pregnancy

Some women suspect they are pregnant prior to a missed period. Other women need one or more of the pregnancy signs to tune them in to the fact that their bodies feel different. Some women need to wait for confirmation by a health care practitioner. Keep in mind that the signs of pregnancy vary from woman to woman and from pregnancy to pregnancy.

Early Signs of Pregnancy

Early signs of pregnancy may include, but are not limited to, the following:

- A missed menstrual period
- A period that is lighter or shorter than usual
- Breast tenderness or enlargement, nipple sensitivity
- Frequent urination
- Tiredness
- Nausea and/or vomiting
- Feeling bloated or crampy
- Increased or decreased appetite
- Feeling more emotional or moody

If you suspect you are pregnant, we suggest that within the next 24 hours you make arrangements to have a pregnancy test. Early confirmation of pregnancy will provide you with the greatest number of options. You will have more time to make thoughtful decisions, make use of services, and choose supportive people to discuss this with.

Pregnancy Testing [1]

Where to Get a Pregnancy Test

Pregnancy tests are available through many clinics and health care providers such as doctors, midwives, nurse-practitioners, and physician assistants. In many places, family-planning organizations (Planned Parenthood, for example), women's health centers, and

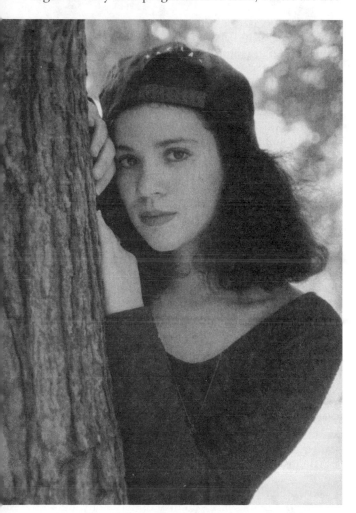

Sandra Lopez/The Boston Photo Collaborative

abortion clinics offer pregnancy testing services. You can also purchase a home pregnancy test in most drugstores. When choosing where to take a pregnancy test, consider the cost and timing, the confidentiality of the results, and the respect you will receive.

Think about possible costs in addition to the cost of the test itself. Will you have to take time off work, find child care, or travel to get the test? You will need to be tested as soon as possible so as to have the maximum time available for decision making. Be aware that some places offer free services as a way to promote something else. For example, groups like Birthright advertise free pregnancy testing and counseling. But these groups give out antiabortion propaganda, hoping to frighten you and convince you not to consider abortion even if you do not want to have a baby. Avoid people who tell you what to do, and stay with people who help you clarify what is best for you.

You may be concerned about others finding out that you are getting a pregnancy test. Will you have greater control over this if you do a home test or go to the clinic? Wherever you go to be tested, be prepared for the possibility of hearing well-intentioned but insensitive remarks. The person who tells you the result of your test may make assumptions about you and tell you about abortion, but not about prenatal care, having a baby, or adoption. She or he may assume it is okay to tell your partner or parents without your permission, may act as if you are in a crisis situation and feeling terrible, or may congratulate you on the "happy news."

Types of Pregnancy Tests

All pregnancy tests are designed to detect the presence of the hormone called human chorionic gonadotropin (HCG). During pregnancy, HCG is first secreted into the woman's bloodstream; a little later, it can also be detected in her urine. There are several tests which determine whether you are pregnant; they are based on the detection of HCG in either your blood or your urine. Most clinics now use urine tests that can detect HCG as early as ten days and almost always by 14 days after conception.

If you have the privacy you need, you may choose to do a home pregnancy test. At this writing, a single test generally costs under $10, and a double test $12 or more. Look for a home test kit with clear, easy-to-follow instructions. It is crucial that you follow the instructions precisely in order to get an accurate result. This includes careful timing of the steps that require a specified waiting time; you may want to have someone help you with the timing of the test. You are wise to buy a two-test pack because you will probably want to repeat the test immediately to confirm a positive result, or repeat it a few days to a week later if the first test result was negative or unclear. Be cautious about assuming that a negative result means you aren't pregnant. Test results can be negative because the test wasn't performed correctly or because it was too early in the pregnancy for HCG levels to be detectable. If your pregnancy test results are negative but you have no menstrual periods, see a health care practitioner.

Pelvic Exam

For many women, the next step will be a pelvic exam, which will confirm whether you are pregnant and, if so, give an estimate of just how far along the pregnancy is. Along with an enlarged and softened uterus, there are other pregnancy signs that you or your health care practitioner may recognize, such as your cervix becoming softer and changing from a pale pink to a bluish color because of the increased blood circulation. (You can see this yourself if you have a speculum and a mirror.)

The pelvic exam can be upsetting; if you would be more comfortable having a woman examine you, you should request this. If your pregnancy is a result of forced sex, a pelvic exam may feel like another violation. In such cases, it is advisable to alert your health care practitioner to your situation and to bring along a support person. The pelvic exam will indicate how much time you have to decide what to do next. (For more information on having a pelvic exam, see chapter 24, Selected Medical Practices, Problems, and Procedures, p. 591.)

If there's reason to suspect an ectopic pregnancy or multiple births, your health care practitioner may suggest an ultrasound/sonogram to confirm, locate, and size your pregnancy. There is debate about the safety and usefulness of ultrasound. If you are advised to have ultrasound, learn why it is being recommended. Then decide for yourself whether you really need it. (See "Fetal Ultrasound," chapter 19, Pregnancy, p. 462.)

NOW YOU KNOW YOU'RE PREGNANT

Once your pregnancy has been confirmed, you will need time to adjust to the news. Pregnancy is a powerful, life-changing time for most women. You may not feel the way you imagined you would, or the way people expect a pregnant woman to feel. You may feel emotionally and spiritually unequipped to handle the physical fact of pregnancy. But trust yourself and any feelings you may have. You can discover what is best for yourself. Quiet reflection, talking with trusted friends or family, talking with a counselor, writing, music—there are many ways to think this through.

Some people may try to make you feel irresponsible for taking time to thoughtfully consider what is best for you and those you care about. But the opposite is true —it is a highly responsible and moral act to clarify the right course of action for yourself. Some women know what they need to do right away; others find that with contemplation they change their minds. Many women find themselves emotionally torn for a long time before they see their way clear to the next step.

Depending on your relationship with the man you become pregnant with, you may or may not want him involved in this decision. Remember that you are the one who is pregnant, and you must feel confident that your decision is the best one for you. Your age; your marital status; your sexual orientation; your cultural, religious, and community ties; and the circumstances under which you became pregnant are some of the factors that will affect how you approach your decision and the steps you take. You may discover that even considering not wanting to be pregnant is contrary to society's norm of woman-as-mother. Take time to listen to your instincts and your needs, and don't be pressured by others—but don't put this decision off.

Making Decisions

Your next step is to decide whether to have an abortion, or to continue the pregnancy and either raise the child yourself or have your child parented by someone else. At this point, you may be feeling social pressures, and you may be grieving because your pregnancy is not what you imagined it should or could be. In addition, your body is going through hormonal changes that affect your outlook.

Some women find that they do their best decision making on their own; however, most women find that talking with others helps them to understand and clarify how they are feeling. While you may choose to talk to someone you already know, many women find it helpful to seek counseling from an experienced professional. If you need help finding a counselor, you can call your local family-planning clinic or Planned Parenthood; they often either provide these services or can refer you to other places in your area. Whomever you decide to speak with should be supportive, nonjudgmental, and unbiased. Beware of agencies listed in the yellow pages that state that they offer decision counseling, but are actually part of antiabortion organizations and will try to pressure you into continuing your pregnancy. Remember, no one should be telling you what to do. If friends, family members, or counselors have their own strong opinions about what you should do, you may want to wait until you have made your own decisions before talking with them. Sometimes doing what your heart says is the right thing means going against what your friends, family, partner, religion, and/or community feel you should do. You may need support to stand against the opinions of others.

Give yourself plenty of opportunity for deep thought and honest evaluation of *your* needs. Perhaps you already have a child or children whom you celebrate having in your life, but you still need to make the decision about parenting another child. Perhaps you anticipated sharing parenting, but your partner is unwilling to parent at this time, and you are unsure whether you want to become a single mother. You may be involved in an abusive relationship, and having a child, or another child, may make it harder for you to leave. You may feel a strong need to finish school and establish yourself in the workplace, and now you have to decide whether you want to revise that plan in order to raise a child. You are not alone.

I was the mother of three little boys. Being a mother and having children has always been very important to me, and this made the decision that much more difficult. Loving children as I do, I also knew that having the baby and then giving it up for adoption would not be an option for me.

My lover was opposed to having the child [as a team] and I didn't want another child without his help, so I decided on abortion. I was not happy with this because I wanted the child and was in love with the father.

Before I made the decision to have the abortion, I cried a lot. I would wake up around 4:30 in the morning and think about what to do, and cry. I'm sure experiencing the loss of a potential child was part of it.

An abortion would have destroyed me because of my own moral sense. I was 15 and I had a lot of hopelessness then. The baby was symbolic of hope for me. . . . I was praying for a miscarriage but it was wishful thinking. I knew another girl who had gone to a maternity home and gave her baby up for adoption, and that seemed most viable. It occurred fleetingly to me that I might parent, but I wanted the rest of my life.

Some women find that they have enough support and stability to welcome a child into their lives even though their pregnancy wasn't planned.

Abortion

In the U.S., abortion is a safe and legal option, which many women choose, although finances and geography may limit its accessibility. The safest, easiest, and most affordable time to have an abortion is within the first three months of pregnancy. If you're considering having an abortion, you can find detailed information in chapter 17, Abortion.

Carrying Your Pregnancy to Term

If you have decided to carry your pregnancy to term, you may choose to parent your child yourself, to have your child adopted by another family, or to have your child fostered while you decide how to proceed further. Whichever option you choose you may want to read about pregnancy and childbirth in chapters 19 and 20.

Parenting

If you are wondering whether you want to be a parent, please see the introduction to Part Three, Sexual Health and Controlling Our Fertility, p. 263, and chapter 21, Postpartum. Parenting is a life-changing decision.

Informal Foster Care

Throughout history, shared child-rearing in extended families and among networks of friends has ensured that all the children in a community have a chance to thrive. Based on the belief that children belong to all of us and that we are all responsible for their well-being, informal foster care relies on those best able to care for children to step in and help those least able. This system is common throughout the world and in many communities in the U.S.

In this type of foster care, you choose to give your baby to someone you know and trust—one of your own family members, a friend, a member of the birth father's family—to care for and raise temporarily or permanently.

In my family we call this word-of-mouth adoption. My grandmother did this a lot; she took in children from family members. Although there was no legal status, cousins became siblings and some of my family who I consider to be aunts are actually only distantly related to me.

Although this kind of arrangement is not legally binding, it may give your child a better chance of receiving the consistent care, love, and support that is so important to his or her developmental process. In the formal foster care system, it is rare for a child to remain in a stable home for any length of time. If you decide to have a friend or family member foster your child, it is advisable to create a temporary guardianship that will allow her or him to make medical decisions in your absence. In some states, this guardianship will require you to sever your parental rights; in other states, there are provisions for guardianship without the loss of parental rights.

Formal Foster Care

If you are considering formal foster care as an option, you should be aware that being part of a large, impersonal system presents risks to yourself and your child. The goal of foster care should be to provide you time to resolve your problems and make decisions about your parenting ability. It is not in the best interest of your child for him or her to remain in the foster care system for an extended time. Children who spend many years in foster care often end up going from one placement to another. If you are considering foster care, you need to ask whether you will have any control over who fosters your child once you enter the system. Find out what process you will have to go through if you try to regain custody of your child.

While many people become foster parents out of a true concern for children's well-being, it is important to survey the changing landscape of foster care. Increasingly, the motivation for fostering is an economic one. Ask how foster parents in your state are recruited and screened. Think about the family's motivation for fostering, and how public policies influence this.

From a legal perspective, you put yourself at risk of losing your parental rights when you give your child into another's custody, whether this is a formal or an informal placement. The law sees this as a rejection of the child, and if the family or state petitions to sever your parental rights, you will be at a disadvantage. Some legal systems view the choice of foster care as abandonment, and it may be difficult or impossible to regain custody of your own child. In some state systems, it will be up to your child's social worker to determine if you are a "good" parent and deserve another chance to parent your child.

Adoption

You might decide to carry your pregnancy to term and have your child adopted by another family. A thoughtful adoption plan worked out with an adoption counselor—along with a strong, ongoing support system—can make this an experience you can look back on with peace, knowing that it was the best option for you and your child. Your life will go on after the adoption, although your subsequent family life may be affected by the adoption decision.

Adoption is an upwardly mobile institution. Agencies and adoptive parents point to the improved economic, educational, and social advantages when instituting and encouraging adoption. This perpetuates the wrongful assumption that people living in poverty make less effective and less desirable parents than those with financial resources. You may feel pressured to opt for adoption because you don't feel financially set up to provide for a child. But remember, the important things for a child are a comfortable, safe, and stable environment. Babies and young children are remarkably resilient and adaptable when they have a consistent, emotionally nurturing caretaker. The external conditions do not all have to be "ideal."

Historically, adoption has often served as a tool of racial and class discrimination in the U.S., and a form of social control over women's sexuality. It has given many white families with resources the opportunity to adopt healthy white children (or any other children they wished). As late as the 1970s, it was also common practice in white middle-class families to hide the children of "unacceptable" relationships: women who became pregnant "out of wedlock" or by men of a different race or class were often sent away during pregnancy and expected to surrender their babies for adoption. Often, the birth mother never knew what happened to her child and the child was given, at best, only sketchy information about her or his birth parents. This was the dominant society's way of denying women's sexuality and the possibility of legitimate loving relationships across race and class.

The harm that was done to women through coercion and the closed adoption process has been recognized, resulting in more open adoptions that protect the birth mothers' rights. These changes can make adoption a more humane and sensitive process for both the birth mother and her child; but adoption remains a difficult choice.

Counseling

Counseling plays an important part in the creation of a thoughtful adoption plan. You should seek out a trained adoption counselor who understands all the issues that are unique to adoption. Whether you have found your own counselor or are working with someone through an adoption agency, her role is to help you understand and explore the choices you have. You will then be able to clarify whether you want to continue the adoption process and, if so, which adoption plan is best for you. A counselor should explain the various levels of open adoption and their emotional impact for you and your child. There have been many changes over the last ten years in multiracial and biracial adoption. Be sure your counselor is well versed and up to date on these issues.

A good counselor will also be emotionally supportive and will share her knowledge in a way that encourages you to ask questions. She will know that although she may be giving the same general information to all of her clients, each one will be affected differently. She is willing to reflect *with* you, and not *for* you, on the choices that are most suitable for your life. Ideally, your counselor will also spend time helping you explore your vision of how you'd like your life to be. Whether or not you ultimately decide on adoption, you will be facing a new direction.

Other people such as the birth father, your parents, or others may also become involved with the counselor. If your decision is emotionally difficult for them, she can help them come to terms with it, and with their own grief over the loss of this child in their lives. If necessary, she can help them understand that this is your decision and their interference could be harmful. The time after you release your child might be easier for you if your family and community accept your decision.

For African-American women, adoption may open an unexpected wound inherited from slavery when women were not able to keep their children. The impact of this loss is often unacknowledged, and it may create situations where others are not supportive of your decisions. A counselor who has a deeply held regard for the African-American experience in the U.S. can be most helpful.

Counseling and support are important throughout the adoption process. Even after the adoption is complete, you may find it helpful to talk with someone who is familiar with your situation.

Sometimes I get calls from birth mothers on the birthday of their child. They just need to touch base with someone who understands what they've been through.

Developing an Adoption Plan

Reputable adoption agencies are often your best option. They provide legal services and counseling—and it is you who are the client, not the adoptive family. You can ask about agencies at the clinic where you had your pregnancy test, or perhaps your health care practitioner can provide some leads. Agencies are also listed in the yellow pages. (To avoid using a less desirable agency, call your state's office for children to get a list of the agencies that have had complaints lodged against them.) It is advisable to hire your own lawyer so that your rights are clearly protected throughout the adoption process. A reputable agency will cover that cost. You might ask an agency what counseling and legal services it offers, how it finds adoptive families, what kind of evaluations it requires, what its policy is on interracial adoption, and any other questions you have. No agency should offer you money to give up a baby.

Some women find an adoptive family through a newspaper ad, an independent adoption facilitator, a medical practitioner, or a lawyer, and make an adoption plan directly with them. If you take this route, be cautious—you will need to be your own advocate. Make sure you have your own lawyer. Most states require that adoptive families undergo an evaluation. Find out what criteria are being used in this evaluation and whether important criteria are missing. If your state does not require an evaluation, you may have certain conditions you want the adoptive family to fulfill. If the adoption takes place through a lawyer, keep in mind that she or he is working for the adoptive family and not for you and will have the client's best interests at heart, not yours. This may also be the case if your medical practitioner has matched you up with a family. In this instance, it may be better for you to seek prenatal care from another health care practitioner whose first concern is looking after you. Keep in mind that families and people do change over time, and you cannot pin your hopes on how things appear at the moment of adoption.

Adoption is now a much more open process than it once was. In many agencies, it is now standard practice for the birth mother to choose the adoptive family from a pool of applicants. It may be easier for you to release your child if you feel some connection with the adoptive family. If this choice is not offered to you, find another agency to work with. The secretive nature of closed adoptions is now considered to be psychologically unhealthy for both you and your child. Today, almost all agencies require the birth mother to provide a complete medical history and to update it if any significant illnesses occur.

Many agencies also require the adoptive families to provide yearly updates of their child's growth. These are placed in the child's file for the birth mother to read whenever she wishes. Often, birth mothers write letters to their child and have them placed in the file so the child will have access to them. It is also possible for the birth mother to decide whether she wishes the adoption to be more open than this. Open adoptions can range from only choosing the family to having ongoing visitations with the child. In all cases, the birth parents terminate their parental rights and the adoptive parents become the "parenting" parents.[2]

Some birth mothers choose to meet with the family they are considering to determine how comfortable they would be having their child raised in this family. All of the decisions concerning involvement with the adoptive family and your child should be made with your adoption counselor. Together you can explore the emotional effect each choice might have, and determine what is best for you. The adoptive families that you are considering will also have their own preferences for how open they wish an adoption to be.

People choose to adopt children for lots of different reasons. Among them are not being able to have their own children, preferring to adopt a child because of genetic risks to biological children, wanting a larger family but not wanting or being able to bear more children, or wanting to care for children who might otherwise be underserved by adoption agencies. Some African-American families, for example, are choosing to complete their families by adopting children of color rather than giving birth to more of their own. Some families may adopt because they have the emotional and physical resources to care for a child with special needs; however, if your child has a disability, it may take longer to find a family who will welcome your child into its home.

In choosing a family, you will want to consider the kind of family atmosphere you want your child to grow up in. Children do best when living with a family and in a community they can feel part of. Because we live in a society highly segregated along racial and ethnic lines, it can be especially hard for a child of color to grow up in a community where she or he is bombarded with stereotypes of people of color. This has been especially hard for children of color adopted into white communities. Even though the laws that prohibited white families from adopting children of color have changed, if you are giving birth to a child of color and want a multiracial family for that child, you may be able to find an agency that will act on your preferences. A good agency will have made strong efforts to ensure it has a good recruitment process for attracting multiracial and multiethnic families, and it will make matching the child's background with the adoptive parents' a priority. But you may not have an option of placing your child with a family of similar background. In this case, it is best to look for a family with connections to your community, such as those living in an integrated neighborhood. This may provide better support systems for your child and decrease the psychological isolation that she or he may experience.

If you or the birth father are of Native American descent and are, or could be, registered with a tribe, then your adoption options will probably be determined by the Indian Child Welfare Act of 1978. This law requires that "in the absence of good cause to the contrary" a child's extended family be given preference for adoption, followed by members of the same tribe and then by other Indian groups. A tribe has the right to bar its children from being adopted by families outside of the Indian Nation. This means that if a child registered to a tribe is adopted by a white family without the tribe's consent, the adoption can be revoked at any time and the child will be returned to the tribe. If you think your child might be subject to this law, you will need to contact the social services of your tribal administration or the American Indian Urban Center.[3]

Preparing for the Birth

In choosing the kind of care you will get through pregnancy, we urge you to consider a midwife, as she is usually able to give you the emotional support and nurturing you will need, as well as providing continuous prenatal and birthing care (see chapter 19, Pregnancy, p. 451). As you approach the time when you will give birth, it is important to think about how you want this experience to be. If you give birth in the hospital, some of the things you might consider include the following:

- Do you want to stay in the maternity ward, or elsewhere where your contact with other mothers and babies will be limited?
- Do you want your baby to room-in with you, where you will be responsible for care and feeding, or do you want the nursery staff to do the majority of the care? You can choose to do as much or as little as you wish.
- How much access to your baby do you want the adoptive parent/s to have while you are in the hospital? This will be your opportunity to be with your baby and to start saying your good-byes. This process may be complicated by the presence of the adoptive family, as they will be in a very different frame of mind than you are. You should be cautious about letting them have the third ID bracelet, which would allow unlimited access to your baby.
- Will you breast-feed or bottle-feed your baby? While the colostrum (first milk) is important for your baby, breast-feeding may be emotionally painful for you. It may also make your physical recovery more difficult once your milk comes in and you do not have your baby with you to nurse.
- If you have a son, you may want to consider the pros and cons of circumcision. You have the right to make this and any other medical decisions until such time as you relinquish that right. This change will occur when you sign the adoption papers, which is determined by the laws of the state in which you give birth to your baby.

- Are there mementos of your child that you wish to keep, such as a copy of your baby's footprint, photos, a lock of hair, the ID bracelet?
- Some adoption agencies will give you the option of giving your child directly to the adoptive family. Pictures of this event can be saved so that everyone can see how much a process of love this was.
- You will be responsible for filling out the parental birth certificate and for giving your baby a name.

After you have released your child and returned home, you will experience the normal physiological and emotional readjustments to a nonpregnant state, as all women do. However, these changes may be more difficult because you may also be grieving the loss of your child. You may also experience depression after the birth. This is a time when you should call upon the people in your support system. Your counselor, people at the adoption agency, or other birth mothers will understand the decisions that you made and their impact. It is important to not isolate yourself, and to look after your emotional and physical well-being as you recover.

Now That You've Made Your Choice

Once you've committed yourself to taking one route over others, it's important to be gentle with yourself. You have gone through an arduous journey to reach this decision, one that you will live with for the rest of your life. Whatever route you decided to follow, you may feel grief at the path you didn't take. For most women, part of the decision-making process is grieving. Grief about your decision doesn't necessarily mean you've made the wrong decision but rather that you are feeling your loss, whether it's loss of the pregnancy and its potential, loss of the child you are giving to another family to parent, or loss of the life you had before you became a parent. Remember that you need support during this time.

The most important message to take away from this chapter is that you need to take time to feel all your emotions, reflect on your situation, and find the course of action that is best for you. You're not the same woman that you were before you found out you were pregnant; it will take some time to get to know the new woman you've become.

Notes

1. Factual information from Robert A. Hatcher et al., *Contraceptive Technology* (New York: Irvington Publishers, 1994).
2. Quoted from Center for Family Connections brochure.
3. Jeanne Warren Lindsay, *Pregnant? Adoption Is an Option* (Buena Park, CA: Morning Glory Press, 1997), p. 118.

RESOURCES

For resources on abortion, see chapter 17. For resources on parenting, see Introduction to Part Three, Sexual Health and Controlling Our Fertility.

Books

Aigner, Hal. *Adoption in America: Coming of Age.* Greenbrae, CA: Paradigm Press, 1986.

Andersen, R. *Second Choice: Growing up Adopted.* Chesterfield, MD: Badger Hill, 1993.

Arms, S. *Adoption: A Handful of Hope.* Berkeley, CA: Celestial Arts, 1990.

Arthur, S. *Surviving Teen Pregnancy: Your Choices, Dreams and Decisions.* Buena Park, CA: Morning Glory Press, 1991.

Baker, N. *Babyselling: The Scandal of Black Market Adoption.* New York: Vanguard Press, 1978.

Colgrove, M., et al. *How to Survive the Loss of a Love.* Los Angeles, CA: Prelude Press, 1993.

Gediman, J., and L. Brown. *Birthbond: Reunions Between Birthparents and Adoptees: What Happens After.* Far Hills, NJ: New Horizon Press, 1989.

Gilligan, C. *In a Different Voice.* Cambridge: Harvard University Press, 1993.

Krementz, J. *How It Feels to Be Adopted.* New York: Knopf, 1988.

Lifton, B. J. *Lost and Found: The Adoption Experience.* New York: HarperCollins, 1988.

———, and J. Robert. *Journey of the Adopted Self: A Quest for Wholeness.* New York: Basic Books, 1994.

Lindsay, J. W. *Pregnant? Adoption Is an Option.* Buena Park, CA: Morning Glory Press, 1997.

Lopez, Charlotte. *Lost in the System.* New York: Simon & Schuster, 1996.

Panuthos, C., and C. Romeo. *Ended Beginnings: Healing Childbearing Losses.* South Hadley, MA: Bergin and Garvey, 1984.

Riben, M. *The Dark Side of Adoption.* New York: Harlo Press, 1988.

Rillera, M. J. *Adoption Searchbook: Techniques for Tracing People.* Westminster, CA: Pure, Inc., 1991.

Roles, P. *Saying Goodbye to a Baby: A Book About Loss and Grief in Adoption.* Washington, DC: Child Welfare League of America, 1989.

Schaefer, C. *The Other Mother: A Woman's Love for the Child She Gave up for Adoption.* New York: Soho Press, 1992.

Silber, K., and P. Dorner. *Children of Open Adoption.* San Antonio, TX: Corona Publications, 1990.

Simon, R. J., and H. Alstein. *Transracial Adoptees and Their Families: A Study of Identity and Commitment.* New York: Greenwood, 1987.

Solinger, R. *Wake Up Little Susie: Single Pregnancy and Race before* Roe vs. Wade. New York: Routledge, 1994.

Sorosky, A., et al. *The Adoption Triangle: The Sealed Or Opened Records: How They Affect Adoptees, Birthparents, and Adoptive Parents,* 2nd ed. San Antonio, TX: Corona Publications, 1989.

Stiffler, L. V. *Synchronicity and Reunion: The Genetic Connection of Adoptees and Birthparents.* Hobe Sound, FL: FEA Publishing, 1992.

Triseliotis, J. *In Search of Origins.* Boston: Beacon Press, 1975.

Verrier, N. *Primal Wound: Understanding the Adopted Child.* Lafayette, CA: Nancy Verrier, 1993.

Wadia-Ells, S., ed. *The Adoption Reader: Birth Mothers, Adoptive Mothers and Adopted Daughters Tell Their Stories.* Seattle: Seal Press, 1995.

Waldron, J. *Giving Away Simone.* New York: Anchor Books, 1997.

Periodicals

Adoption Therapist
Hope Cottage Adoption Center; 4209 McKinney Avenue, Suite 200; Dallas, TX 75205; (214) 526-8721
E-mail: adoption@hopecottage.org
Web site: http://www.hopecottage.org

Chain of Life
Janine Baer
P.O. Box 8081; Berkeley, CA 94707
E-mail: jabaer@pacbell.net
This newsletter offers feminist, gay, and lesbian perspectives.

Compact
Center for Family Connections; 2326 Massachusetts Avenue; Cambridge, MA 02140
Newsletter on adoption, foster care, guardianship.

Open Adoption Birthparent
R-Squared Press; 721 Hawthorne Street; Royal Oak, MI 48067

Readers Guide to Adoption-Related Literature
William L. Gage
2300 Ocean Avenue; Brooklyn, NY 11229
This guide is updated periodically.

Reunions
Edith Wagner
P.O. Box 11727; Milwaukee, WI 53211-1727

Organizations

Adoption Connection, Happenings
11 Peabody Square, Room 6; Peabody, MA 01960; (508) 532-1261

Adoption Crossroads
Choices, Education, Search, Support (ACCESS); 356 East 74th Street, Suite 2; New York, NY 10021-3925; (212) 988-0110
E-mail: cera@idt.net
Web site: http://www.adoptioncrossroads.org

Adoption Resource Center
P.O. Box 383246; Cambridge, MA 02238-3246

Adoptive Family (formerly OURS)
3333 Highway 100 N.; Minneapolis, MN 55422; (612) 535-4829

ALMA (Adoptees Liberty Movement Association)
727 Radio City Station; New York, NY 10101-0727; (212) 581-1568
Web site: http://almanet.com
This organization offers a databank service. There are local chapters.

American Adoption Congress
1000 Connecticut Avenue NW, Suite 9; Washington, DC 20036; (202) 483-3399; (800) 274-6736
Web site: http://rdz.stjohns.edu/amer-adopt-congress
There are local chapters.

Center for Family Connections
350 Cambridge Street; East Cambridge, MA 02139; (617) 547-0909; and 301 East 21st Street; New York, NY 10010; (212) 253-6902
E-mail: kinnect@aol.com
Servicing the community of adoption, foster care, guardianship, kinship, and alternative reproductive technologies through training, education, consulting, and therapy.

Child Welfare League of America, Adoption Report
440 First Street NW; Washington, DC 20001; (202) 638-2952
Web site: http://www.cwla/org

CUB (Concerned United Birthparents)
2000 Walker Street; Des Moines, IA 50317; (800) 822-2777; or P.O. Box 396; Harvard Square; Cambridge, MA 02138
This organization offers an extensive list of publications. There are local branches.

FACT (Family Connections Training Institute)
2326 Massachusetts Avenue; Cambridge, MA 02240
Comprehensive family systems training program for work with complex blended families. Training for parents and professionals, internships, and supervision of postgraduate studies.

International Soundex Reunion Registry (ISSR)
P.O. Box 2312; Carson City, NV 89702; (702) 882-7755
This organization offers the best adoption registry.

National Adoption Information Clearinghouse
P.O. Box 1182; Washington, DC 20013-1182; (703) 352-3488; (888) 251-0075
E-mail: naic@calib.com
Web site: http://www.calib.com/naic/index.htm

Orphan Voyage of Alabama
1610 Pinehurst Boulevard; Sheffield, AL 35660; (205) 383-7377
Adoptee support and a clearinghouse service are offered.

PACER (Post Adoption Center for Research and Education)
P.O. Box 309; Orinda, CA 94563; (510) 935-6622
This organization offers regional adoptee support and resources.

Truth Quest
P.O. Box 638; Westminster, CA 92684; (714) 892-4098
Write for referrals and publication lists.

By Marlene Gerber Fried, with
Maureen Paul, based on earlier work by
Jill Wolhandler and Trude Bennett,
with Ruth Weber and Dana Gallagher

WITH SPECIAL THANKS TO Centre de Sante des
Femmes de Montreal, Carol Franzblau,
Suzanne Hendrick, Martha Katz, Luita
Spangler, and Laurie Williams *

Chapter 17

Abortion

* Over the years since 1969, the following people have contributed
to the many versions of this chapter: Vickie Alexander, Diane
Balser, Pamela Berger, Sarah Buttenweiser, Helen Caulton, Concord
Feminist Health Center, Terry Courtney, Debra Drassner, Carol
Driscoll, Margie Fine, Marlene Gerber Fried, Linda Gordon, Nancy
Miriam Hawley, Liz Hill, Debra Krassner, Elizabeth McGee, Judy
Norsigian, Ana Ortiz, Jane Pincus, Stephanie Poggi, Loretta Ross,
Wendy Sanford, Kira Sarpard, Meredith Tax, and Susan Yanow.

Unless women can decide whether and when to have children, it is difficult for us to control our lives or to participate fully in society. For this reason women have always used abortion as a means of fertility control. Legal, safe, and affordable abortions are an important part of having that control. Information about and access to all methods of fertility control are unevenly distributed, within the U.S. and worldwide. Moreover, no birth control method is 100% effective. Without safe, legal, and affordable abortions, women can never be assured full control over our fertility. (Please see later in this chapter for the history and current status of the right to abortion in the U.S.)

Women of various ages, races, religions; from all economic classes; whether married, single, or lesbian;

and in committed relationships or not have abortions for many reasons. You may not be able to afford a child. You may want to finish school. You may have decided not to have children. The pregnancy might pose a threat to your health or sometimes even your life. You may have become pregnant through rape, incest, or another type of coerced sexual encounter.

Even a planned pregnancy may become unwanted if economic or personal circumstances change. In addition, a woman may not feel capable of parenting a child that she learns, through amniocentesis, will have a potentially serious genetic disability. (In this case, support and information are critical to making a decision. See also the box on "Abortion, Amniocentesis, and Disability," p. 403.)

Deciding whether to have a baby or an abortion is always a serious choice. No one should be forced to stay pregnant or to become a mother against her will. You have to decide what you believe is responsible, moral, and best for yourself and the important people in your life, depending on your needs, resources, commitments, and hopes (see chapter 16, Unplanned Pregnancy).

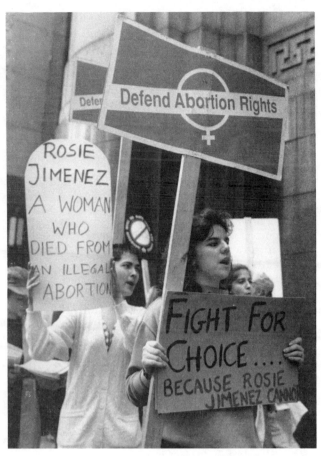

Ellen Shub

As black women we have never been able to say clearly that we support abortion. But being able to control our reproduction directly affects the quality of our lives and, in some cases, whether we even have lives. It is very hard for women to say that when the deal goes down, we choose ourselves.

I was 16, pregnant, and couldn't tell my parents. It's not that they would hurt me or anything like that —but I didn't want to hurt them. Because I wasn't getting my parents' permission, I had to go in front of a judge. It made me angry. This judge doesn't even know me. Even though he let me do what I wanted to do—have an abortion—I'm still mad about the judge. The abortion itself was fine. I feel good that I was able to do all of this.

Opponents of abortion tell us that no woman ever wants to have an abortion and that abortion is always traumatic, but sometimes women are forced by economic necessity or psychological desperation to have them. When I was young and unwillingly pregnant and afraid I wouldn't find an illegal abortion in time, that was traumatic. My desperation consisted of not wanting to be a mother at that time. I did want to be sexually active. Having an abortion produced great relief, the end of my trauma.

HOW PREGNANT ARE YOU?

In pregnancy, a tiny ball of cells attaches itself to the lining of the uterus about one week after conception. A mass of tissue called the *placenta* develops in the uterine lining to nourish the *embryo*. By the end of the second month, the embryo, now called a *fetus,* is surrounded by a protective fluid-filled sac, the *amniotic sac.* At about 20 weeks, the woman begins to feel the fetus move. Sometime between the 24th and 28th weeks, the fetus reaches the point at which it may live outside the mother for at least a short while under intensive hospital care.

The length of a pregnancy is usually counted from the first day of the last normal menstrual period (LMP)* and not from the day of conception (fertilization). Pregnancy is divided into three parts, called trimesters. The *first trimester* is the first 13 weeks after the LMP; the *second trimester* is the 14th through the 24th weeks after LMP; 25 weeks from the LMP and later is the *third trimester.* Abortion is safer, easier, and less expensive in the first trimester. It may be difficult to find a facility that provides second-trimester abortions and impossible to get a third-trimester abortion unless your life is endangered by your pregnancy.

The first day of the last menstrual period is the most common way to date a pregnancy, but you must consider whether that period was normal for you. If it came at an unexpected time or was lighter than usual, conception may have happened *before* that bleeding.

If you chart your body changes with a fertility awareness method (see chapter 13, Birth Control, p. 305), you will have a written record of ovulation and will be able to recognize pregnancy quite early. If you do cervical self-examination, you may notice that your cervix has changed color and become bluish purple, which happens early in pregnancy. Signs of pregnancy can help confirm the date of conception (see chapter 16, Unplanned Pregnancy, p. 379).

An experienced health care worker or medical practitioner can estimate the length of a pregnancy by feeling the size of the uterus during a pelvic exam. This is usually accurate within a two-week range. Ultrasound, another method for determining the length of a pregnancy, is accurate within three to seven days during the first trimester, but it has a similar two-week margin of error later in the pregnancy. The practitioner doing the abortion makes the final decision about how far advanced the pregnancy is and whether she or he is willing to perform the abor-

continued on next page

tion. If the practitioner refuses to do the abortion, you may have to find someone else.

Some women want to remove a pregnancy as soon as possible and/or prefer not to know whether they actually are pregnant. However, having an abortion before you know for sure that you are pregnant does not necessarily mean that you won't have any feelings about pregnancy and abortion to deal with. One drawback is that you may indeed not be pregnant; there are many reasons for a period to be late, including anxiety about being pregnant! Most providers will want to confirm the pregnancy, by blood or urine test or by ultrasound, before doing the abortion procedure.

* LMP dating can be inaccurate, particularly for women with irregular menstrual cycles. Some women may need a pelvic exam or an ultrasound to confirm the duration of pregnancy.

It seemed like a punishment. I used birth control and got pregnant anyway. I no longer trusted my diaphragm, my lover, my body. My guilt about being pregnant turned into anger when I learned that no method of birth control is 100% effective! I took all the precautions and still needed an abortion.

Deciding to have an abortion wasn't a difficult decision or a big deal. From the way everyone I told reacted, though, I started wondering if something was wrong with me for not being upset.

I became pregnant the first time just after I graduated from a Christian university. I had the baby and gave it up for adoption. Three months later I was pregnant again. I couldn't go through another adoption. I had an abortion, and God was with me as much on that table as earlier on the delivery table. [People need] to understand the horror of being pregnant when you don't have the resources or emotional strength to have a child.[1]

ABORTION METHODS

When you are considering an abortion or choosing where to have an abortion, you have a right and a need to know the procedures used at each stage of pregnancy, the risks and possible complications, and the cost.

There are many kinds of abortion procedures. They are generally divided into two main categories: *surgical* and *drug-induced.* In a surgical abortion, the contents of the uterus (embryo or fetus, placenta, and built-up lining of the uterus) are removed. Different methods are used, depending on how large the pregnancy tissue has grown, the training of the person performing the abortion, the approaches favored by the local medical community, and the equipment

available. The other category of procedures is drug-induced abortions. Until recently, these abortions were performed only during the second or third trimesters. In 1996, however, drugs became available to induce abortion early in a pregnancy. While doctors call these "medical abortions," we refer to them here as "drug-induced" abortions, since all abortions are medical procedures.

The chart on p. 393 summarizes the various abortion methods. The numbers in this section refer back to the chart. These procedures may not all be available in your area, or different names may be used for some of them. Ask for explanations of words and terms you don't understand.

1. *Vacuum aspiration* is the most common abortion procedure. Done during the first three months of pregnancy, it carries the least chance of complications and considerably less risk than pregnancy, labor, and delivery. In fact, it is now the safest of all operations, safer than tonsillectomies or circumcisions. It takes only a short time (five to 15 minutes) and can be done by trained practitioners as easily and safely as by doctors.* Vacuum aspiration abortions are now available throughout the U.S. though some women have to travel many hours to get to an abortion facility. Improvements in ultrasound technology, coupled with early pregnancy detection tests, now make it possible to perform aspiration procedures as early as three to four weeks LMP (sometimes even before your period is due) and to know for sure that the abortion is complete.

During a vacuum aspiration procedure, the contents of the uterus are removed through a straw-like tube that is passed through the cervix into the uterus. The tube, called a *cannula,* is attached to a source of gentle suction—an electric pump or a syringe—which draws out the tissue. When a syringe is used instead of an electric pump, the procedure is referred to as *manual vacuum aspiration.*

Abortions by manual vacuum aspiration done later in the first trimester may require some cervical dilation and a larger cannula. This technique has been exported to many Third World countries because it is easy to train laypersons to do it, and it does not require a motorized suction pump or much equipment. In many of these countries, manual vacuum aspiration is used to abort pregnancies up to 12 to 14 weeks after

* Unfortunately, in most states it is illegal for nonphysicians to perform abortions. In Vermont, however, women trained as physician assistants (PAs) have performed one-third of the abortions for years, with an excellent safety record. However, antiabortion politicians have been trying to change Vermont laws to restrict the performance of abortions to physicians only. This would make abortions harder and more expensive to obtain, prevent women from turning to other skilled women for abortions, and reinforce the power of doctors.

In Montana, the right of PAs to provide abortions is being challenged in court. In New York, a statuatory ruling in 1996 enabled PAs to begin training for and performing abortions. Strategies are being explored in other states. For more information, contact the National Abortion Federation or the Abortion Access Project of Massachusetts (see Resources).

ABORTION 391

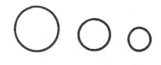

Cannulas
6-, 8-, 12-mm diameters

Robbie Pfeufer

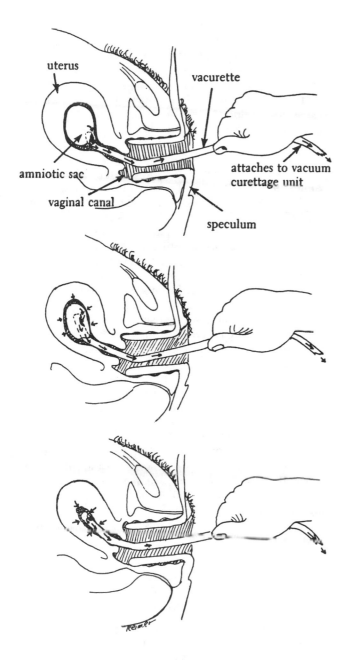

Vacuum suction abortion/Nina Reimer

MENSTRUAL EXTRACTION

In the early 1970s, self-help groups at the Feminist Women's Health Center in Los Angeles and elsewhere developed a technique using a small flexible plastic cannula to remove the lining of the uterus at about the time that the menstrual period is due. Women practiced on each other in order to develop safe instruments and techniques. Menstrual extraction is done on an experimental research basis by women in advanced self-help groups; it cannot be obtained at a medical facility.

Menstrual extraction also helps women avoid the discomfort of a menstrual period, provides information about menstruation, and enables women to learn basic health care skills. A very early pregnancy, if present, would probably be removed along with the lining of the uterus.

We need to do more research before we can know whether frequent extraction of the uterine lining creates any long-term or delayed health problems, although there is no evidence of any so far. Several aspects of the techniques developed for menstrual extraction have been incorporated into medical practice for early abortion with flexible cannulas.

Internationally, a similar technique, called menstrual regulation (MR), is used in developing countries—throughout Latin America, in Asia, in many African countries, and on a limited basis in the Middle East. MR has dramatically reduced the complication rate in countries in which abortion is unsafe because it is either inaccessible or illegal.

Women in the U.S. who do ME consider it to be legal—a home health care technique. They do not see themselves as performing abortions, since no medical diagnosis of pregnancy has been made. ME has not been challenged in court, and it is difficult to say what would happen if a suit were to be brought under current abortion laws or those governing the practice of medicine.

Menstrual extraction is a powerful example of medical research done by women on and for ourselves.

the LMP, though in the U.S., this procedure is generally limited to very early pregnancies.

In the U.S., most clinics perform vacuum aspiration abortions (also known as *suction curettage*) using an electrically powered aspirator as the source of suction. There are several variations of this method. Some clients, especially woman-owned and woman-controlled feminist health centers, have trained practitioners to use minimal dilation and small flexible cannulas, which reduce the chance of tearing or perforating the uterus or cervix. *Curettage,* or scraping the inside of the uterus with a metal loop called a *curette,* is not routinely necessary. Experiences at these clinics and others show that this approach is more comfortable for women than that of most conventionally trained providers, who use larger, rigid cannulas (which require more dilation) and a curette after the suction.

2. In an *early drug-induced abortion,* the provider gives either an oral dose of *mifepristone* (better known by its French name, RU-486, or the "abortion pill") or an injection of *methotrexate.* Both drugs are taken in conjunction with *misoprostol,* a prostaglandin. With mifepristone, you return to the clinic within 36 to 48 hours for misoprostol, which is generally given as a vaginal suppository (some clinics may use oral prostaglandin). With methotrexate, the misoprostol suppository is often administered at home, five to seven days following the methotrexate injection.

Mifepristone interrupts pregnancy by blocking the action of the hormone progesterone, which prepares the lining of the uterus for a fertilized egg and thus maintains the pregnancy. It can prevent implantation of a fertilized egg in the uterus or can bring on menses even if implantation has already taken place.

Methotrexate is used for abortion because it stops a pregnancy from growing and interferes with the attachment of the placenta to the uterine wall. Both methotrexate and mifepristone are most effective when taken in conjunction with a prostaglandin, which causes contractions of the uterus, helping to expel the lining and the fertilized egg and thereby ending the pregnancy.

Although an early drug-induced abortion may be performed as soon as a woman knows she is pregnant, most providers like to wait until the amniotic sac is visible on an ultrasound (usually 30 to 35 days after the LMP).

3. *Dilation* (sometimes referred to as *dilatation*) *and evacuation (D&E)* is used for abortions between 14 and 24 weeks. The cervix is dilated with laminaria (small reeds left in the cervix for several hours or overnight to gently stretch the cervix open). The doctor removes the pregnancy tissue from the uterus using vacuum aspiration techniques along with forceps. Because the fetal tissue is larger and the uterus is softer and easier to injure than in the first trimester, a D&E is more complicated and requires a high level of skill on the part of the person performing the abortion.

4. *Dilation and extraction (D&X),* also known as *intact D&E,* is a procedure that allows the removal of the fetus intact. It is most commonly used from 14 to 24 weeks, but it may be used later if serious medical conditions warrant termination of the pregnancy. The cervix is progressively dilated over many hours with laminaria and mechanical dilators; then, the fetus is removed intact, often with forceps. A needle may be inserted to collapse the fetal skull so that it can pass through the cervix. Aspiration and curettage are often used to remove the placenta.

This procedure is sometimes used when there are serious medical or fetal problems, because it allows the doctor to retain intact tissue necessary for determining what went wrong. In addition, a D&X allows a woman to abort without going through labor. She and her family may also prefer the D&X because they do not want the fetus dismembered or because the procedure allows them to see the fetus and say good-bye.

Few physicians are trained to do this procedure; thus, it may not be available in your area. Nor is it likely to become more widely available in the near future. In 1996, in response to a campaign by the antiabortion movement, Congress voted to outlaw this procedure.* While President Clinton vetoed the legislation, and other efforts by state legislatures to pass similar legislation have been struck down as unconstitutional, bans are in effect in some states and the issue is still in the forefront of the antiabortion movement's agenda.†

5. A drug-induced abortion used during the second trimester is referred to as *labor induction*—drugs are used to induce labor and delivery of the fetus. One procedure used for labor induction is *instillation.* The doctor injects (instills) an abortion-causing solution (saline, urea, and/or prostaglandin) through the abdomen into the amniotic sac, which surrounds the fetus. (Before 16 weeks after the LMP, this sac is not large enough to be located accurately, so the induction procedure cannot be used until this time.) Hours later, contractions cause the cervix to dilate and the fetus and placenta to be expelled. After the abortion, a D&C is often performed to remove any remaining tissue. A hospital stay of 12 to 48 hours is involved in this procedure, which is expensive.

Today, *prostaglandin vaginal suppositories* are often used to induce abortion in the second trimester. The suppositories are placed in the vagina to cause uterine contractions strong enough to expel the fetus. Prostaglandin suppositories are FDA-approved for pregnancy termination from 12 to 20 weeks after the LMP, and for termination up to 28 weeks after the LMP if the fetus has died.

6. In a *hysterotomy,* the surgeon removes the fetus and placenta through an incision into the abdomen and uterus, like a small cesarean section. The incidence of serious complications for this kind of major surgery is considerably higher than for other methods of abortion. You may need a hysterotomy if induction methods have been repeatedly unsuccessful or can't be used for medical reasons.

POSSIBLE COMPLICATIONS OF SURGICAL ABORTIONS

As with any medical procedure, having an abortion involves risks and possible complications. However, serious complications arising from surgical abortions before 13 weeks are quite unusual: 97% of women

---

* Antiabortionists refer to the D&X with the misleading and emotionally charged phrase "partial-birth abortion."
† This legislation passed the House of Representatives again in 1997, and as of this writing, appeared likely to be signed into law.

Abortion Methods

PROCEDURE	TECHNIQUES	WEEKS AFTER LMP	WHERE PERFORMED	COMMON ANESTHESIA
1. Vacuum aspiration	Dilation (in some cases), suction, curettage (in some cases)	3–6	Clinic, MD office	None, local, conscious sedation, (general)*
2. Early drug-induced "medical"	Mifepristone/ methotrexate plus prostaglandin	4–7	Clinic, MD office, outside of medical setting	None
3. Dilation and evacuation (D&E)	Dilation, suction, curettage, use of forceps	14–24	Clinic, MD office, (hospital)*	Local, conscious sedation, (general)*
4. Dilation and extraction (D&X) Intact D&E	Dilation, use of instruments to remove fetus, suction to remove placenta	14–24 (later if there are serious medical complications)	Clinic, hospital	Local, conscious sedation, general
5. Labor induction A. Instillation abortion (urea, saline, prostaglandin, or combination)	Injecton of liquid through the abdomen into amniotic sac	16–24	Hospital	Medication to dull the pain of labor and delivery, epidural
B. Prostaglandin suppositories	Drug inserted into the vagina to cause labor and miscarriage	13–20 (28 if there is fetal death)	Hospital	Medication to dull the pain of labor and delivery, epidural
6. Hysterotomy	Uterus cut open to remove fetus	16–24 or later, if woman's life is in danger	Hospital	General

* Parentheses indicate a less common practice.

LMP: Last normal menstrual period.
Dilation: Enlarging the cervical opening by stretching it with instruments called dilators or with laminaria (see p. 392). Many medical technicians use the word "dilatation" to mean the same thing.
Suction: Drawing out the contents of the uterus through a narrow tube attached to a gentle vacuum source.
Curettage: Scraping the inside of the uterus with a metal loop, called a curette, to loosen and remove tissue.
Forceps: Grasping instrument used to remove tissue.
Amniotic sac: Sac of fluid surrounding the fetus.
Prostaglandin: Hormone-like substance that causes uterine contractions.
Saline: Salt water.

report none, 2.5% have minor complications that can be handled at the doctor's office or clinic; less than 0.5% require some additional surgical procedure and/or hospitalization. Complication rates are somewhat higher for abortions performed between 13 and 24 weeks. Overall, the D&E procedure is safer than instillation methods; however, this is partly because women can have D&E's earlier in the second trimester than instillation procedures. After 16 weeks, these methods carry about the same complication rates. Death rates are quite low: one for every 160,000 women who have legal abortions. A woman's risk of death in carrying a pregnancy to term is ten times greater. The later the abortion, the more chance of complications. Signs of a complication will generally appear within a few days after the abortion. Listed in this section are the possible risks and complications of surgical abortions, their symptoms, and treatments (see p. 401 for risks and complications of early drug-induced abortions; see p. 404 for additional risks and complications of second-trimester drug-induced abortions).

Infection

Infections occur in less than 3% of cases. Most are easily identified and treated if followup instructions are clear and are observed. Signs of an infection are fever of 100.5°F or higher, bad cramping, excessive bleeding, and/or vaginal discharge with a foul odor. Infections are treated with antibiotics. It is important to have an exam after finishing the medication to make

Possible Complications of Abortion Procedures

PROCEDURES	POSSIBLE COMPLICATIONS
Vacuum aspiration	Infection
Dilation and evacuaton	Retained tissue
Dilation and extraction	Perforation
	Hemorrhage
	Continuing pregnancy (missed abortion)
	Cervical tearing
	Uterine perforation
	Reaction to anesthesia
	Postabortal syndrome (blood in uterus)
Early drug-induced	Uterine bleeding
	Nausea
	Headache
	Weakness
	Fatigue
	Cramps, abdominal pain
	Vomiting
	Diarrhea
	Incomplete abortion
Labor induction	
A. Instillation	Infection
	Retained tissue
	Hemorrhage
	Cervical tearing
	Drug reaction
	and others (see p. 404)
B. Prostaglandin	Severe gastrointestinal side effects
	Fever
Hysterotomy	Risks of major surgery (see p. 392)

sure the infection is gone. Left untreated, an infection can cause serious illness, sterility, or even death.

If the provider suspects that the fetus has died before the abortion procedure, antibiotics may be ordered to prevent infection.

Retained Tissue

Since the practitioner can't actually see inside the uterus during the abortion, occasionally she or he leaves some tissue behind. Signs of retained tissue include very heavy bleeding, passage of large blood clots, strong cramps, bleeding for longer than three weeks, or signs of pregnancy (for instance, sore breasts, nausea, tiredness) lasting more than a week. Tissue remaining inside the uterus may become infected. Sometimes drugs are given to stimulate the uterus to contract and push out the retained tissue. The other treatment is to remove the tissue by an aspiration procedure similar to a vacuum aspiration abortion. Retained tissue occurs in 1 to 2% of vacuum aspiration and D&E abortions; rates can be higher with induction abortion.

Perforation

Perforation of the uterus occurs if a surgical instrument goes through the uterine wall. Perforation happens in only approximately .1% of cases. It is more serious in a D&E than in a first-trimester abortion because of the larger instruments used. If you are awake, you are likely to feel a sharp pain or cramp. If perforation occurs, the medical staff will monitor your pulse, blood pressure, cramping, and bleeding very closely. If there are any indications that a large blood vessel or another organ has been injured, you will need hospitalization and possibly surgery. If the abortion has not been completed when the perforation occurs, it is usually finished in a hospital. The perforation may heal itself, or it may require surgical repair. Very rarely (less than one in 10,000 cases), hysterectomy is required.

Hemorrhage

Uterine hemorrhage (excessive bleeding), which is most often caused by failure of the uterus to contract and may require a blood transfusion, occurs in less than 1% of cases. It is more likely to occur in second-trimester abortions. Excessive bleeding can sometimes be a sign of retained tissue or perforation. Drugs may be given to stimulate contraction of the uterus, or an aspiration procedure may be done to slow down the bleeding. Check to see how much you are bleeding before you leave the clinic, and inform the recovery room staff.

Cervical Laceration (Tear), Continued Pregnancy, and Postabortal Syndrome

Other complications include a tear in the cervix, continued pregnancy, and postabortal syndrome (blood in the uterus). Cervical tears generally heal on their own; in less than 1% of cases, stitches are required.

Postabortal syndrome (blood in the uterus), which occurs in less than half a percent of cases, happens when the uterus doesn't contract properly or when a blood clot blocks the cervical opening and prevents blood from leaving the uterus. As blood accumulates, pain, cramping, and sometimes nausea increase. Sometimes you can push the clots out by deep massage (pressing hard with your fingers just above the pubic bone). If this doesn't work, the clots need to be removed by reaspiration of the uterus.

A continued pregnancy after a surgical abortion occurs in less than 0.5% of all cases. It happens most often when you have a very early abortion (less than six weeks after the LMP), but it may also happen if you have a multiple pregnancy. If a pregnancy is not removed, signs of pregnancy are likely to continue, and the abortion will have to be repeated a week or so later.

Possible Effect on Future Pregnancies

Having an abortion does not decrease the chances of having a healthy baby in the future. There is some indication that having several abortions may slightly increase the chances of miscarriage or premature birth, but not enough good research on this issue has been done. (Dilating the cervix should be done as little and as gently as possible in order to minimize the chances of weakening it.)

CONTROLLING PAIN AND ANXIETY

In an abortion, there are two primary ways to reduce pain and anxiety: *nonpharmacological methods* such as deep breathing, meditation, visualization, and massage, and *anesthesia* (pain- and anxiety-reducing drugs). Each method is described below.

Nonpharmacological Methods

Although it is not widely available in clinics at this point, some women prefer a nonpharmacological approach to controlling pain and anxiety. A clinic in Texas has successfully used relaxation techniques, in-cluding guided imagery and deep breathing. The counselors there take an individual approach to pain management and discuss the woman's prior experiences with pain during the first phone contact. They are trained to work with women who want medication, those who do not, and those who want to pursue some combination of pharmacological and nonpharmacological methods. This approach requires more training on the part of counselors, but it offers women genuine choices in abortion care. Even if the clinic doesn't offer this, you may be able to do relaxation and visualization on your own (see chapter 5, Holistic Health and Healing).

Anesthesia

If you are going to have an abortion by a suction method, you may have the choice of using anesthesia (pain- and anxiety-reducing drugs). If you understand what your options are and how they may affect you, you can decide which type of anesthesia you prefer, or decide not to have any at all.

Three basic types of anesthesia are used for surgical abortions: *general anesthesia,* which makes you unconscious ("asleep"); *local anesthesia,* which affects only the cervix; and *conscious sedation,* the use of analgesic or antianxiety drugs to create a state of "depressed consciousness." Conscious sedation is often used in combination with local anesthesia.

General anesthesia is usually given intravenously (IV, injected into a vein in the arm). It causes unconsciousness and a loss of protective reflexes; you won't see what's happening or feel pain, but you may well hear what is being said. General anesthesia carries the highest risk and usually is not necessary.

Local anesthesia is injected into the cervix (neck of the uterus). It numbs the cervical muscle, easing cramps that may occur when instruments such as dilators are passed through the cervix. Cramps caused by contractions of the uterus as it is emptied are not lessened by this method, however.

Local anesthesia is often combined with conscious sedation. In many clinic settings, an IV is used to inject drugs such as fentanyl (a pain reliever) and/or Versed (an antianxiety drug), which provides relaxation without loss of consciousness. You can still respond to verbal and physical stimuli and can maintain your own airway and other protective reflexes. Usually patients remain alert during the procedure and recover quickly.

Any anesthetic drug has risks and complications, in addition to the risks of the abortion. With a local you may briefly experience ringing in your ears, or tingling or numbness in your lips or mouth. Seizures or serious allergic reactions are rare. With the addition of conscious sedation, you may experience some dizziness or nausea.

If you have general anesthesia, you may feel groggy, nauseated, and disoriented after you wake up; some people do not feel well even a couple of days later. You may wake up with cramps. These cramps may not be different from cramping after an abortion with local or no anesthesia, but they can be much harder to deal with when you wake up mentally affected by the anesthetic drugs. A serious reaction, though rare, may damage the liver or other organs. In addition, general anesthesia increases some of the risks of the abortion itself. For example, there is more bleeding because the uterine muscle is more relaxed.

For a first-trimester abortion, general anesthesia is not medically necessary. For a second-trimester D&E, which takes longer and may be more uncomfortable, general anesthesia is sometimes used. Some women, for their own reasons, choose not to be awake during a first-trimester abortion. Most women, however, find the cramps quite bearable.

I felt real good about my decision not to be put to sleep for my abortion. I found out that I have the strength to face my fear of pain. My cramps were bad for a few minutes, but I concentrated on deep breathing and held my counselor's hand. Ten minutes later I felt fine and ready to go home.

Each woman's abortion experience is a unique one, within a known range of possibilities. No one can predict whether you will find the cramping painful or mild, or how the anesthesia will affect you. Try to find out what drugs are used in the facility you plan to go to. Information about drug effects and risks should be a part of your preparation for an abortion and will help you make the best choices if decisions are left up to you. Some facilities have a set way of doing things, and they may or may not respond to your requests.

Sometimes abortion facilities have their own reasons for using general anesthesia or conscious sedation for first-trimester abortions. A nurse-counselor at one abortion facility said:

Black and Hispanic women are all screamers. We try to give them general anesthesia so that they don't upset the other patients or the staff. Teenagers and Medicaid patients also should have a general.

This is an example of racist stereotyping as well as value judgment by a woman whose culture forbids loud noises to express emotions. Why should women of a certain race, culture, economic status, or age automatically be subjected to the health risks of general anesthesia, while white middle-class women have the choice of local anesthesia?

ABORTION FACILITIES

As part of an overall strategy aimed at decreasing women's access to abortion, the antiabortion movement has been targeting abortion facilities and providers (see p. 415 for more information on abortion politics). Since the early 1980s, there has been a tremendous decline in services, in the number of abortion providers, and in training. In 1996, 84% of U.S. counties had no abortion services at all. Services are concentrated in urban areas, but even in cities, few facilities offer abortions beyond 13 weeks. How much choice you have about where your abortion takes place depends on where you live, how much money you have or what your insurance will cover, how old you are, how far along you are in your pregnancy, and which referral sources are available to you.

Agencies That Can Help You Get an Abortion

If you need an abortion, there are a variety of responsible sources of information.

For reliable information, contact abortion providers (may be listed in the yellow pages), gynecology clinics at non-Catholic hospitals, neighborhood health centers, family-planning clinics, women's centers, and feminist health centers (listed in phone books, local newspapers, and college campus directories). Planned Parenthood has offices in almost every state, providing referrals and, in some areas, operating reproductive health clinics that provide abortions. You can also get information from the National Abortion Federation Hotline, the National Women's Health Network, or other national organizations (see Resources for names and numbers). These organizations will also have information about Medicaid funding and funds for women with low incomes who seek abortions.

Some antiabortion groups masquerade as referral agencies and try to "persuade" women not to have abortions. These are often listed as "problem" or "crisis" pregnancy centers in the phone book. If you're not getting the information you want, feel free to leave or hang up the phone. If you can, take someone you trust with you.

What to Look for in Choosing a Facility

Most first-trimester abortions, and many second-trimester procedures as well, are done in freestanding clinics that are not part of hospitals. Abortions are also done in doctors' offices, hospital outpatient clinics, and in hospitals, sometimes with an overnight stay. Second-trimester D&E abortions can also be performed safely in a properly equipped clinic or doctor's office.

Legalization has meant safe facilities, but how we feel after an abortion can also be influenced by the quality of counseling and treatment by the staff, which vary with the motivations of those who run or own a facility and with abortion politics. Antiabortion propaganda is pervasive in our society. Messages that abortion is wrong, that women who have abortions are selfish or irresponsible about sex and birth control, that abortion is murder, and that abortion is an emotionally traumatic experience have created a climate in which abortion is cloaked in guilt, shame, and fear. Even many supporters of abortion rights portray abortion as a necessary evil. Unfortunately, some counselors and medical staff at clinics express these views. Unsupportive, insensitive treatment by clinic staff is especially problematic and can make an abortion unpleasant or worse. You are entitled to be treated with respect. A staff member at a feminist clinic says how it should and can be:

At our clinic, counselors are trained to help each woman sort out her feelings. We do not invade anyone's privacy if she tells us that her decision is clear and not coerced, and that she does not want to discuss her reasons or feelings. Women talk with each other, not just with the counselor. We provide very detailed and accurate information about the abortion procedure. A woman can have a friend stay with her during the abortion. When there is a decision to be made, the woman herself is an active participant.

Racial and cultural barriers also shape our experience.

Just because they give you a white woman to talk to don't mean you got counseled. She was nice; she gave me good information. I'm explaining to her how I feel about this whole thing. She tells me that she thinks that I'm not ready to have an abortion and she's going to send me home. Well, I hit the roof! "You're going to send me home? Do you know how hard it is to get here?" She didn't understand what I was saying to her. I was saying, "Yeah, if I had a baby I could deal with it. I have to deal with anything that comes up. This is how my life has been, how my mother's life, all the people I knows life has been. You deal with whatever shit happens. But if I had a choice, I would prefer not to have this baby. And since I do have this choice, this is what I want to do."
I think that a lot of the problem was she was white and I was black. She didn't understand what it meant to me, a black woman, and I guess to black women, period, to have a baby.

An African-American counselor says:

I am the only woman of color working at the clinic. It is important for me to be there for women of color who come to have abortions, otherwise all they see are white faces. I became a counselor because I knew I could make a difference—I wanted to help all women.

The antiabortion movement has made abortion and family planning clinics, their clients, and their personnel targets for harassment and violence. Although large antiabortion demonstrations, pickets, and blockades outside clinics have decreased, it is not uncommon for antiabortionists to demonstrate there or try to prevent women from entering. Many clinics have escorts who will meet you outside and accompany you for your appointment. Some clinics have alternative entrances to avoid protesters. Sometimes, abortion rights advocates are at the clinics to support and protect women going in.

After the murder of several doctors and clinic workers, most clinics instituted new safety precautions.

WHAT YOU NEED TO KNOW

Whether you have to search to find one abortion service or you can choose among several facilities, ask questions beforehand. Not only can you get an idea of what to expect, but you can also prepare yourself to negotiate for options that may not be part of the standard procedures.

1. What are my options for procedures? Is any type of drug-induced ("medical") abortion offered? What are the differences in terms of numbers of visits, costs, restrictions?

2. Is there a mandatory waiting period that will require me to visit the clinic before I come for the abortion?

3. Cost? Must the fee be paid all at once? Will Medicaid or health insurance cover any of it? Is everything included, or may there be additional charges (for example, for a Pap smear or for RhoGAM)?

4. Are there age requirements or special consent requirements? Do I have to tell my parents, get their consent, and/or bring proof of age? Will my parent or guardian need to visit the clinic?

5. How long should I expect to be at the facility? Will everything be done in one visit?

6. Will child care be provided for my child(ren)?

7. What do I need to bring with me?

8. Is there anything in my medical history that would interfere with my getting an abortion at that facility?

9. Can I bring someone else with me? Can she or he stay with me throughout the counseling and the abortion procedure if that's what I want?

10. Will there be a counselor or nurse with me to provide information and support before, during, and after the abortion?

11. Will there be staff people who speak my native language? If not, will the facility provide an interpreter?

12. Can the facility accommodate any special needs I have (for example, wheelchair accessibility)?

13. What type of abortion procedure will be done?

continued on next page

14. What anesthesia and other medications are available? What choices do I have? Are there extra costs?

15. Will the facility be responsible for routine followup care? For treating complications? What type of backup services are available in case of emergency?

16. Will a breast exam, Pap smear, or culture for chlamydial infection and gonorrhea be done?

17. Will birth control be available if I want it?

18. Are abortions performed if women are HIV-positive?

19. Could there be antiabortionists picketing or blocking me from entering the clinic? If so, what arrangements are there to deal with this?

Ask about *anything* that concerns you. Often, the way the staff answers questions indicates their attitude toward women coming for abortions. Trust your feelings about the way you are treated on the phone as well as in person.

When you go to the clinic, heightened security may feel frightening. However, these measures have been put in place to make clinics safer for workers and clients. At the clinic, you may have to be buzzed in, your bags may be searched, the receptionist may sit behind bullet-proof glass, and a security guard or policeman may be at the door. Some women like to have their partner with them during the abortion procedure, but because of increased security, several clinics have stopped this practice.

Many women feel upset and angry at having to deal with protesters and security measures at clinics. Some want to confront protesters; others prefer to avoid or ignore them. Antichoice protests at abortion clinics constitute harassment, and clinic violence is a form of terrorism. No one but you has the right to decide whether you will have an abortion. No one has the right to try to interfere with that decision.

HAVING A FIRST-TRIMESTER ABORTION

Of the one and a half million abortions performed each year in the U.S., almost 90% take place in the first trimester. The majority of first-trimester abortions are vacuum aspiration procedures, while the remaining first-trimester procedures are early drug-induced abortions.

Having a Vacuum Aspiration Abortion

Vacuum aspiration procedures are performed in outpatient clinics. Clinics vary a great deal, and your experience may be very different from another woman's, even at the same clinic. If your state requires a waiting period before an abortion, you may have to visit the clinic twice. During the first visit, state law may require that you watch a videotape or listen to a lecture designed to discourage you from having an abortion.

The Preliminaries

After arriving at the clinic, you will fill out a medical history form. A health worker will draw blood to check for anemia and the Rh factor,* do another pregnancy test, and check your pulse, blood pressure, and temperature (vital signs). Most clinics will then provide individual and/or group counseling. The counselor explains the abortion procedure and what to expect afterward. She may also talk about birth control options. The counseling session is a time for you to ask questions and express any fears or concerns, especially about the pregnancy or the abortion. Being in a group provides an opportunity to talk with other women who are having abortions. Discussing your experiences together can help you feel clearer, stronger, and less alone.

The two rooms where the abortions were done opened on to the porch where the six of us were waiting. One girl from the group, who had said she never had a pelvic examination in her life, was just coming out of the abortion room. She had just had her abortion and looked okay. That was comforting. A 17-year-old girl came in. She was very scared. I held her hand and comforted her. I hadn't had my abortion yet and was scared, too (although I'd had one operation, two children and a D&C with a spinal). Something amazing happened when I held her hand. Any fear I'd had disappeared as if it were drawn out of me. We were all such different women who for varying reasons were having the identical physical thing done to us.

The Abortion

The counselor will take you to the exam room after you go to the bathroom. Before the abortion itself, the provider performs a bimanual exam to feel the size and position of your uterus, confirming the stage of pregnancy. She or he needs this information to decide how large a cannula to use and the angle at which to insert instruments safely. If you've never had a pelvic exam, tell your counselor. Whether this is your first

---

* Blood is either Rh positive or Rh negative. When an Rh-negative woman carries an Rh-positive fetus, antibodies against the Rh factor in the fetal blood cells can build up in her blood. In a subsequent pregnancy, these antibodies can react against an Rh-positive fetus, causing serious harm and even endangering its survival. An injection of a blood derivative (one brand name is RhoGAM) within 72 hours after the end of every pregnancy usually prevents antibody formation. If you are Rh negative, be sure to get the injection before you leave the clinic.

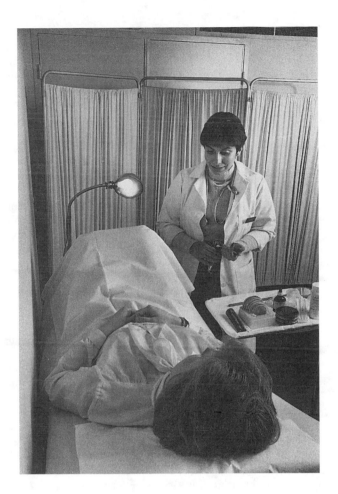

or stronger menstrual cramps. Two to eight dilators may be used. Dilating usually takes less than two minutes.

A sterile straw-like tube is inserted through the cervix into the uterus. Cannulas are made in different diameters, from the size of a small drinking straw to the size of a large pen (5 to 12 millimeters). The later the pregnancy, the larger the cannula needed to remove it. Tubing connects the cannula to a bottle. The *aspirator,* a motorized suction machine, creates a vacuum in the bottle. As the cannula is moved along the uterine walls, gentle suction draws pregnancy tissue out through the cannula and tubing into the bottle. The aspiration usually takes no more than a few minutes.

Forceps may also be used to remove tissue. Some practitioners insert a curette and scrape the inside of the uterus to make absolutely sure there is no retained tissue. Others think that this additional step is unnecessary.

As the uterus is emptied, it starts to contract to its nonpregnant size. These contractions can range from hardly noticeable to painful cramps—each woman is different. Breathing deeply and in a regular pattern, especially with the help of a counselor or friend, can help you to relax your body, "riding through" the cramps. It is also important to keep your stomach muscles as relaxed as possible and not to move around.

exam or you have had others, make sure that the practitioner goes slowly, is gentle, explains what is happening, and allows you to have some control over the procedure.

Next, the medical provider inserts a speculum into your vagina, separating the vaginal walls to see the cervix. You may feel pressure, but this should not hurt. Have the practitioner readjust the speculum if it pinches. A culture specimen to test for chlamydial infection and gonorrhea may be taken, and a Pap smear may be done if you haven't had one recently.

The medical provider thoroughly wipes your vagina with antiseptic solution to help prevent infection. If you are having a local anesthetic, it is injected into the cervix. Since the cervix has very few nerve endings, you may not feel this at all, or it may feel like a pinch or pressure. Next, a tenaculum is attached to the cervix to keep the cervix steady. You may feel a pinch, a cramp, or nothing at all. Some practitioners then measure the inside of the uterus with a thin rod called a *sound;* others believe that this is not necessary. Sounding may cause a short cramp. The cervical opening is gradually stretched by the insertion and removal of dilators of increasingly larger sizes. You will probably feel some kind of cramping, perhaps similar to mild

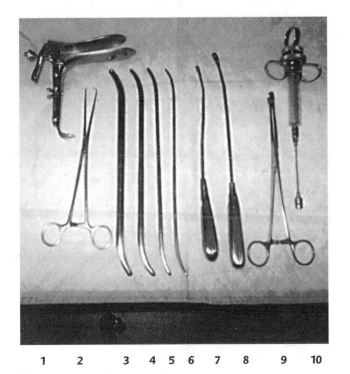

| 1 | 2 | 3 | 4 | 5 | 6 | 7 | 8 | 9 | 10 |

Left to right: 1. speculum; 2. tenaculum; 3., 4., 5., 6. dilators; 7., 8. curettes; 9. forceps; 10. syringe/Amy Jacques/ *Planned Parenthood League of Massachusetts*

Cramps should lessen immediately after the cannula is removed or within the next ten minutes or so.

After the Abortion

After wiping out your vagina and checking for bleeding, the practitioner will remove the speculum. Then you can move into a more comfortable room to sit or lie down for a while. You may feel weak, tired, crampy, or nauseated for a while, or you may be ready to get up immediately. Some clinics will require that you stay for a certain amount of time after the procedure. If you need pain medication, you can request it, and it should be provided if needed. Before you leave, your vital signs, cramping, and bleeding should be checked, and a counselor should explain aftercare instructions (what to expect and watch for).

The abortion itself was amazingly quick and painless (considering the propaganda to the contrary). I spent an hour lying down to recover. I remember being elated—it was over and it had been so simple!

It hurt so much. It was incredible. The people at the clinic were really sweet and helpful, but they should have told me how much it was going to hurt. What hurt the most was that I could feel when they were scraping around inside. I've talked to a lot of girls who said the same thing happened to them when they were really far along. That's why it pays to have an abortion as early as possible.

I experienced some pain with the procedure, but mostly it was just a series of new sensations. I had never been so aware of my uterus.

Having an Early Drug-Induced Abortion

Early drug-induced abortions (also known as "medical" abortions) are new in the U.S. and, in 1997, not widely available. However, in other parts of the world, they are rapidly becoming a common means of having an early abortion (before seven weeks). As described on p. 392, an early induced abortion combines one of two drugs—mifepristone (RU-486) or methotrexate—with the prostaglandin misoprostol.

The Procedure

The protocols are somewhat different for mifepristone and methotrexate. They are also new and are therefore still subject to change. At this point, an early drug-induced abortion involves several visits to a doctor or clinic, beginning with thorough counseling, a physical examination, and a determination of the length of pregnancy by vaginal ultrasound.

If the abortion is done with mifepristone, at the first visit you take 600 milligrams of mifepristone and remain under observation for at least half an hour. At the second visit, 36 to 48 hours after the first, you are given

400 micrograms of the prostaglandin misoprostol by vaginal suppository. You may be asked to remain at the clinic for four hours after taking the misoprostol. In France, about two-thirds of the women have their abortions during this period.

A methotrexate abortion begins with an injection at the clinic. You are given the misoprostol to take home and insert intravaginally five to seven days later. Some clinics require you to return to the clinic 24 to 48 hours after the misoprostol insertion for an ultrasound to see if the abortion has occurred. If the abortion hasn't occurred, you are given a second dose of misoprostol to insert, and asked to return to the clinic in about a week for another ultrasound. (Since administering misoprostol at home has been done with methotrexate, it is likely that a similar protocol will be developed for mifepristone abortions.)

You may, initially, be given both doses of misoprostol to take home. In this case, you will have to determine for yourself whether the abortion has occurred after the first dose. If you are not sure, err on the side of taking the second dose, as it won't hurt you. About 40% of women need the second dose to abort.

After inserting the misoprostol, you can expect cramping to begin within two to four hours. Bleeding will start within one-half to ten hours after cramping. Bleeding at the start will be like a heavy period and may include blood clots, some quite large. You may also see light pink or gray tissue, as in a first-trimester miscarriage. The bleeding decreases after a few days to a light flow, then spotting, which may continue for a few weeks. Bleeding that is never more than a light flow means you probably need the second dose of misoprostol.

If you have taken mifepristone, you are likely to abort within 24 hours after you take the misoprostol. Methotrexate abortions are not always as predictable: Most women abort within a few days after the misoprostol, but in 25% of cases, women have a "delayed response" and don't abort for about three weeks.

Severe lower abdominal cramps often mean that pregnancy tissue is passing down the cervix. This may occur in waves. Generally, cramping will be mild after the tissue passes (about four hours). Remember, when you will abort is not completely predictable, and you may pass the pregnancy tissue at an unexpected time or place.

With both mifepristone and methotrexate, you will be asked to return to the clinic about ten days to two weeks after your initial visit for an ultrasound. This is done to confirm that the pregnancy has been terminated. You should not try to make this determination yourself. (In the case of methotrexate, if termination was confirmed after the first dose of misoprostol, you will not have to make another followup visit.) If the abortion is not complete, it is very important to complete the abortion with a vacuum aspiration abortion. Methotrexate, in particular, has been associated with serious birth defects.

The failure rate for mifepristone is 4 to 6%. Although methotrexate has been studied much less, this experience suggests that it may not be as effective as mifepristone (the failure rate may be closer to 10%). Women are advised to avoid sexual intercourse until their followup exam determines whether the abortion is complete.

Side Effects Associated with Early Drug-Induced Abortion

You are likely to experience cramping and light bleeding after the oral dose of mifepristone. With mifepristone or methotrexate, women report feelings similar to "morning sickness": fatigue, nausea, headaches, dizziness, hot flashes, or, in rare cases, transient fever or mouth sores (methotrexate only). In 80% of all women, the uterine contracting activity produced by the prostaglandin causes side effects of stronger cramping, diarrhea, and vomiting. In some cases, women require mild painkillers. Bleeding can last anywhere from four to 40 days; the average is ten days.

Risks and Complications

French statistics indicate that one out of every 1,000 women taking mifepristone will hemorrhage and need a blood transfusion. This is 20 times the risk of a vacuum aspiration abortion. *You should call your health care provider if you experience any of the following:*

- Excessive bleeding: soaking one maxi pad per hour for more than three hours in a row, or two maxi pads per hour for more than two hours in a row.
- Severe pain that is not reduced by rest, pain medication, heating pad, or hot water bottle.
- Continued vomiting: inability to keep anything down for more than four to six hours.
- Fever greater than 100.5°F.

It is important to understand that misoprostol, by itself, will not cause an abortion. If you receive two doses of misoprostol at the clinic, but use only one, don't pass the remaining dose on to desperate friends. *The use of misoprostol alone is not likely to cause an abortion and may harm the developing fetus.*

The Experience of Women with Early Drug-Induced Abortion

France has had the most extensive experience with mifepristone (RU-486). About 70% of eligible women (those whose pregnancies are 49 days or less past their LMP) have selected early drug-induced abortion over surgical abortion. Overall, this is 30% of all abortions in France. In the largest study, the vast majority of women who aborted with RU-486 were satisfied with the procedure. The main reasons women cited for preferring early drug-induced abortion included the fact that they could avoid a surgical procedure (in France, D&Cs are more common than vacuum aspiration abortions), that it takes place earlier, that it seemed more "natural," and that the procedure seemed less medical and more in the hands of the woman than the doctor. Some women feel that the experience is more private, and they like the fact that the actual abortion may take place outside the clinic setting, while others prefer to be in the clinic with other women going through a similar experience.

Some women in the U.S. have described the experience similarly: "It feels more natural." "It gave me more control." "It ended up feeling like what I imagined a miscarriage to feel like."

Other women have been disappointed with the experience. Lots of women have the idea that an early drug-induced abortion is much simpler than it is—a matter of taking a couple of pills. Women talk about the experience being painful. Others, especially women with busy schedules, find that it is too inconvenient: too many visits to the clinic and too much uncertainty about when the actual abortion will happen.

Those who have experienced early drug-induced abortion, especially with methotrexate, suggest that women must be counseled carefully about the pain, the amount of bleeding, and the emotional consequences of essentially "miscarrying" at home.

Is Early Drug-Induced Abortion Safe and Effective?

Mifepristone has been tested in over a dozen countries in Europe and in the U.S. More than 200,000 women in Europe have used it over 11 years, and its efficacy and short-term safety is well documented. Its introduction in the U.S. was delayed because of political threats and intimidation from the antiabortion movement. The drug causes few side effects, exposure is brief, the dosage is small, and most of the drug is eliminated from the body within two or three days. Although women of color were not well represented in the French trials, they made up approximately one-third of women in the U.S. trials of 2,100 women at 17 sites. Women of color described their experience in exactly the same way as did white women.

Because methotrexate has been widely used in the U.S. for over 40 years to treat arthritis, psoriasis, and ectopic pregnancy, its long-term safety and side effects are well documented. Like many other drugs, methotrexate acts differently in the body when used in a short-term low dose than when used at higher levels over the long term. The side effects, such as hair loss, that result from the higher doses given to cancer patients do not occur in the comparatively smaller doses used for ectopic pregnancy and early abortion. Methotrexate clears the body quickly, having a half-life of ten hours, and appears to have no long-term side effects. It has no known detrimental effect on future fertility.

During tests of RU-486 in France, a few serious cardiovascular complications, including one fatal heart attack, occurred following injection of a prostaglandin called suprastol. This prostaglandin is no longer used. Cardiovascular complications were most often associated with patients who were heavy smokers. There is no evidence that the prostaglandin misoprostol, which is now prescribed, is associated with any such cardiovascular side effects. However, because the long-term effects are unknown, the National Women's Health Network recommends that the FDA require studies with long-term followup monitoring of women who have early drug-induced abortions.

Women with the following conditions are advised *not* to choose early drug-induced abortion (U.S. protocols would exclude women with these conditions):

Pregnancy over 49 days
Suspected ectopic pregnancy
Long-term steroid use
Chronic adrenal failure
Kidney and liver disorders
Smokers over the age of 35
Severe asthma or hypertension
Blood clotting disorders
Anemia

Early Drug-Induced Abortion in the Developing World

Both those who favor early drug-induced abortion and those who oppose it agree that approval in the Northern Hemisphere will lead to its use in the Southern Hemisphere. Women in so-called developing countries have expressed interest in mifepristone, especially in countries where abortion is illegal or inaccessible. Various international organizations have estimated that between 70,000 and 200,000 women die each year from unsafe or poorly performed abortions, or self-abortions. Many more women become seriously ill and permanently impaired or infertile through inserting unsterile objects and caustic solutions into the uterus.

There is no question that women desperately need safe abortion procedures, especially in countries where abortion is illegal. In Brazil, for example, thousands of women have used an easily available oral prostaglandin—alone—to attempt an early self-abortion. Most often this does not bring on a successful abortion, and it is dangerous to the developing embryo. But many women, following the oral prostaglandin, go to a hospital for treatment of their bleeding—usually a D&C—that completes the abortion.

Even without proper medical backup, some women argue, the use of mifepristone would provide a safer overall situation, because the risk of infection would be greatly reduced by avoiding the use of unclean instruments. At the same time, women's health advocates are concerned about the distribution of drugs that require careful supervision and medical backup in countries without adequate medical facilities. The fact that early drug-induced abortion involves heavy bleeding is also a serious concern, given the large numbers of women in developing countries who suffer from malnutrition and severe anemia. Extra precautionary screening would be required, since these women would be at high risk for hemorrhage.

Early Drug-Induced Abortion and the Politics of Abortion Rights

Many advocates see early drug-induced abortion as a way around the antiabortion movement. They believe that increasing the sites at which abortions are provided makes it difficult for antiabortionists intent on harassment and violence to locate their targets. Early drug-induced abortion will expand abortion services, because doctors who do not do surgical abortions are more likely to provide this service. It is also possible that other providers such as physician assistants, nurse-midwives, and nurse-practitioners will be able to provide the service, which is primarily a matter of prescribing the medications. Finally, some advocates project a future in which early drug-induced abortion will be private and will take place outside of a medical setting.

The authors of this chapter can't stress the continued need for surgical abortion enough. Early drug-induced abortion is effective only in the very beginning of a pregnancy. Those women who face the greatest barriers in access to abortion—women with limited funds, of whom a disproportionate number are women of color, and young women—typically have abortions later. Advocates must also resist efforts to use early drug-induced abortion to legitimize further restrictions on abortion rights (such as pushing back the time after which abortion will become impermissible) or to further stigmatize and marginalize surgical abortion. Surgical abortion is necessary, not only as a back up to failed early drug-induced abortion, but as the safest and best method for the vast majority of women who do not make their decisions until after the seventh week of pregnancy.

While the expansion of abortion procedures is welcome, early drug-induced abortion is not the solution to the political battle. The antiabortion movement is dedicated to outlawing all abortions—including early drug-induced abortions. While it may be more difficult for antiabortion activists to fight on more fronts, new technologies will not stop the disturbing trend toward deadlier violence against abortion providers and clients. The antiabortion movement must be defeated politically.

HAVING A SECOND-TRIMESTER ABORTION

Of the 11% of abortions that take place after the first trimester: 6% occur between 13 to 15 weeks, 4% at 16 to 20 weeks, 1% after 21 weeks, and .04% (about 600 per year) after 26 weeks.

Most often, women have second-trimester abortions because they were unable to get the money together in time to have first-trimester abortions. Ironically, a later abortion is an additional financial drain: it costs more, requires more time off from work, and may involve extra expenses for travel to an appropriate facility. Other reasons for second-trimester abortions may include errors in pregnancy detection: false-negative pregnancy test results or inaccurate uterine sizing by medical practitioners. Women who were pregnant when they started taking birth control pills or who were not told that it is possible to get pregnant with an IUD in place sometimes do not even suspect pregnancy for several months.

Occasionally, a woman (especially a teenager) may not admit the possibility of pregnancy. If you lack support, money, or information, you may feel afraid, overwhelmed, and unprepared to deal with pregnancy, so you may deny it, hoping it will somehow go away on its own. In addition, teenagers sometimes must deal with parental notification and consent laws—getting legal permission to have an abortion from a parent or judge may take weeks or even months.

Given these all-too-common situations, a woman may come to the experience of a later abortion already emotionally exhausted. A large percentage of these women who bear the brunt of attitudes that "blame the victim" have few financial resources, are young, and/or are women of color. Women seeking second-trimester abortions are often treated as though they are stupid and/or irresponsible and deserve to be "punished." The unsupportive atmosphere can make an already emotionally difficult and painful experience that much worse.

Most doctors and hospitals do not perform second-trimester abortions, and few OB/GYNs are trained to do them. In 1975, Dr. Kenneth Edelin was convicted for manslaughter for performing a routine hysterotomy on a woman whose pregnancy was between 20 and 28 weeks after the LMP. Although a higher court overturned the conviction and acquitted him of all charges, hospitals around the country, never enthusiastic about second-trimester abortions, reacted by closing down these services or by bringing in costly equipment to try to keep alive fetuses that show signs of life when expelled.

Since 1995, the antiabortion movement has been attempting to outlaw the D&X procedure (see p. 392). They are using this issue to challenge all abortions after 24 weeks—and to continue to chip away at women's reproductive rights.

The vast majority of second-trimester abortions performed are D&E or labor induction procedures.

Having a D&E Procedure

Having a dilation and evacuation (D&E) is similar to vacuum aspiration (see "Having a Vacuum Aspiration Abortion," p. 398). However, because the pregnancy is further along, the cervix needs to be dilated more. Often dilation is begun ahead of time, either using a synthetic dilator (Lamicel is the most common) several hours before the procedure or by placing one or more *Laminaria* sticks into the cervical opening the day before the procedure. (If this extra visit is inconvenient or impossible for you, you may consider requesting the synthetic dilator.) *Laminaria* is a sterilized seaweed that absorbs moisture and expands, gradually stretching the cervix. Some women feel pressure or cramping with *Laminaria* in place. There is a small risk of infection, and occasionally, the *Laminaria* itself starts to bring on a miscarriage.

The *Laminaria* is removed at the time of the abortion. Dilators are used to enlarge the cervical opening further, if necessary. Then the doctor uses forceps, a curette, and vacuum suction to loosen and remove the uterine lining, placental tissue, and fetal tissue. Drugs may be given to help the uterus contract, which slows down the bleeding that normally occurs.

The D&E has several advantages over second-trimester induction procedures, which induce labor and delivery of the fetus. Not only is the D&E safer, but it is physically and emotionally easier for a woman. D&E is much quicker (ten to 45 minutes, in contrast to

ABORTION, AMNIOCENTESIS, AND DISABILITY

The availability of amniocentesis (see chapter 19, Pregnancy, p. 462), with the option for abortion if serious genetic impairments are found, should not conflict with our commitment to build a better world for people with disabilities. The disability rights movement has pointed out the danger in equating the presence of a genetic impairment with the notion of a life not worth living. A woman should have the right to bear a child with a disability and not be punished by lack of support for that choice. All of us can reach out and create networks of information so that a woman confronting the diagnosis of Down syndrome or any other potentially serious disability in her fetus can meet other parents and children living with these conditions and learn realistically about the quality, cost, and availability of the services that make such lives better.

The antiabortion movement has tried to make an alliance with disability rights groups by claiming that pro-choice organizations advocate abortion in all cases of a fetus with disabilities. Abortion rights supporters must clearly distance themselves from eugenicist groups and arguments (see below and p. 412 on eugenics). Support for disability rights is an important aspect of reproductive freedom.

many hours with an overnight stay in a hospital for induction abortion), and complications are less likely. D&E can be done in a properly equipped doctor's office or clinic with local anesthetic and perhaps also conscious sedation.

The biggest problem with D&E is that it is not widely available. There are not enough people trained to do this procedure, especially after 18 weeks past the LMP. Only 7% of OB/GYN residency training programs routinely offer training in second-trimester abortion. We need more doctors to learn this procedure, which, compared with a second-trimester induction, *is both safer and less upsetting for women.*

Having a Second-Trimester Induction Abortion

Abortion by labor induction from 16 to 24 weeks of pregnancy is a more difficult experience than a first-trimester abortion or a second-trimester D&E. There may be hours of uncomfortable labor as the uterus contracts to open the cervix and expel the fetus. The complication and mortality rates, though no higher than for full-term pregnancy and delivery, are higher than for earlier abortions or either the D&E or D&X procedure performed by a skilled doctor. Emotionally, too, it can be a hard experience. If this is a wanted pregnancy, and the fetus has a severe anomaly (a potentially severely disabling condition), the decision to abort may be especially difficult. Even when you are very sure you do not want to have a baby, the pain and/or discomfort, the length of time, the similarity of the experience to delivery of a baby, an intimidating or unsupportive hospital atmosphere, and the influence of a very vocal part of society that says that later abortions are "bad"—all these factors can make abortion by labor induction upsetting. None the less, women decide to have an induction abortion for a variety of reasons, including fear of surgery, unavailability of other procedures, the familiarity for some of going through labor, and a wish to deliver the fetus intact and say goodbye.

When choosing a facility, pay attention to both your emotional and physical needs. (Unfortunately, it may be difficult to find *any* medical facility near you where second-trimester abortions are performed.) Doctors usually do second-trimester induction abortions in general hospitals, where the quality of care and degree of personal attention vary greatly. A few small hospitals and clinics specializing in abortion try to make late abortion as comfortable as possible. Some hospitals have a separate second-trimester abortion unit with counseling and special staff. They avoid insensitive treatment such as placing abortion patients in rooms with women who are having babies. In any hospital, you may be left alone a lot, not told clearly what is being done to you, not offered enough pain medication (if you want it). Unfortunately, if you do not have the time and money to travel for an abortion, you may have to accept whatever kind of care you can find. Talk with

SECOND-TRIMESTER LABOR INDUCTION PROCEDURES: A COMPARISON OF SALINE, UREA, AND PROSTAGLANDIN ABORTIONS

Fewer than 1% of all abortions are performed by the labor induction method, and they are almost always done in a hospital. Most second-trimester abortions are now D&E procedures.

There are various means of inducing a miscarriage, and several new methods are being explored. One traditional method is instillation. In this procedure, the medical provider injects a miscarriage-causing solution through the abdomen into the amniotic sac, and uterine contractions expel the fetus. Two commonly used solutions are a saline (salt) solution and urea. These are often combined with prostaglandins to cause labor contractions and abortion. In some hospitals, you will have a choice of methods if you are firm about requesting it.

Compared with urea, saline solution has a higher serious complication rate, but a lower rate of incomplete abortion and consequent D&C. Prostaglandins are often given with these solutions to hasten the abortion process; however, they may cause gastrointestinal side effects such as vomiting and diarrhea. Saline carries a greater risk of serious emergency, such as shock, and even death if careless instillation allows salt to enter a blood vessel. For this reason, saline instillation is becoming less common. Liver or kidney problems, heart failure, high blood pressure, and sickle-cell anemia are medical reasons not to have a saline abortion.

Prostaglandin vaginal suppositories are now also available to induce abortion in the second trimester. They are relatively safer than instillation methods, but they have a higher rate of incomplete abortion. Nausea, vomiting, and fever are common side effects. (Refer back to the table of complications on p. 394, for risks associated with saline and urea instillations and prostaglandin suppositories.)

the doctor beforehand, as well as with staff at the hospital, about the type of care you want to receive. Try to bring a friend who can give you support and help see that your needs are respected and responded to.

The Preliminaries

Read the box (p. 397) for suggestions of questions to ask when you set up an appointment. Plan to be at the hospital overnight. If you are having an out-of-town abortion, make sure before you go that you have the name and phone number of a doctor or clinic at home to call in case of questions or complications after the abortion.

The same tests and examinations are necessary as for surgical abortion. In taking your medical history, the medical staff should check for conditions that would contraindicate the use of saline or prostaglandin methods. If you are going to have a prostaglandin abortion, the hospital may ask you to come in the day before for insertion of *Luminaria*.

The Procedure

For an instillation procedure, the medical provider cleans your abdomen, numbs a small area below your navel with a local anesthetic, and then inserts a needle through the skin into your uterus. This may sound scary, but you will probably feel only a slight cramp when the needle enters your uterus. The miscarriage-inducing solution is slowly injected into the amniotic sac. You may experience pressure or a bloated feeling. If you are having saline and feel waves of heat, dizziness, backache, extreme dryness, or thirst, tell the doctor right away; this may indicate that the salt is entering a blood vessel, which is dangerous.

With prostaglandin suppositories, there is no injection. The suppositories are inserted directly into the vagina. It will take hours before the labor contractions begin: from eight to 24 hours or more with saline, less with prostaglandin. Medication can relieve nausea and diarrhea caused by prostaglandin. If labor contractions don't begin within the expected time, you may be given oxytocin or other medication to stimulate contractions. This carries a risk of rupture of the uterus if the contractions are too strong. Sometimes an instillation is done a second time.

At first, the contractions will probably feel like mild cramps. Later you may feel a lot of pressure in the rectal area and then a gushing of liquid from the vagina—this is the breaking of the amniotic sac (bag of waters). Each woman's labor is different in terms of how long it takes and how it feels.

As a rule, the contractions are not as strong as those of full-term labor and delivery, but they can be painful. Relaxation, deep breathing, or panting can help make the later contractions easier to tolerate. Sitting or squatting may be the most comfortable, though hospital staff may want you to lie down. Support and comfort from a friend can help, too. No general anesthesia is given, but you may be given an epidural (regional anesthesia commonly used in childbirth). Tranquilizers and pain medication should be offered if they won't slow down the labor.

Eventually the contractions will expel the fetus and the placenta. If the placenta is not expelled within an hour or two after the fetus, most physicians will do a D&C to remove the retained tissue.

You will probably stay in the hospital for several hours after the abortion. Aftercare is the same as for a suction abortion.

AFTER AN ABORTION

Aftercare

Women have a variety of experiences after an abortion. Most of us feel fine and do not have any problems, but some feel tired or have cramps for several days. Bleeding ranges from none at all to two or three weeks of light to moderate flow, which may stop and then start again. The signs of pregnancy may last up to a week. Some women experience a variety of changes four to seven days after an abortion, when there is a drop in hormone levels. The hormonal change may cause bleeding, cramping, breast soreness, and/or feelings of depression to increase or appear if they have not been present.

Here is a list of ways to take care of yourself after an abortion:

1. Try to follow what your body needs. Rest for a day or so if you feel tired. (If you can't rest because you have no one to help take care of your children or you have to go to work to keep from losing your job, you may recover more slowly.) Avoid heavy lifting or strenuous exercise in the next few days, as it may increase your bleeding. Drinking alcohol may also have this effect. Sometimes a medical provider will prescribe drugs that stimulate the uterus to contract on the theory that this contraction may keep bleeding to a minimum and help expel any tissue retained in the uterus.

2. To help prevent infection, don't put anything into your vagina. This will avoid introducing germs that may travel up into your uterus before it has had a chance to heal completely. Don't use tampons, douche, or have intercourse for two to three weeks. It is okay to take tub baths or swim, unless you are bleeding.

   You may have been given antibiotics. Studies have shown that prophylactic antibiotics (used for prevention) decrease the risk of postabortal infection. However, some people think you should never take unnecessary antibiotics because (a) overuse can lead to developing resistance and (b) antibiotics kill both the good and the bad bacteria in our bodies (consequently, women often develop yeast infections from antibiotics). They may also mask the signs of infection. If you decide to take antibiotics, be sure to take them according to directions.

3. Watch for signs of complications (see p. 394). If you have a fever of 100.5°F or higher, severe cramping or pain, foul-smelling vaginal discharge, vomiting, fainting, excessive bleeding, or signs of pregnancy that last longer than a week, report this to the clinic or doctor immediately. Remember that complications are rare, but they do happen. It is not your fault if you have a complication. If a complication is not taken care of as soon as possible, it

406 Our Bodies, Ourselves for the New Century

might turn into a serious situation, so don't ignore the possible warning signs. Often a call to the clinic will reassure you that what is happening to you is not a complication after all, but within a range of normal experience. Getting high on alcohol or drugs during this time may impede your ability to recognize the warning signs of a possible complication.

After the abortion, I had retained tissue. I needed a reaspiration [basically, a second abortion] to prevent an infection and remove the remaining tissue. Although the national rate of complications is very low, I was enraged to be a statistic. I had decided to terminate my pregnancy, but I didn't expect another abortion one week later. I didn't have any choice but to see it through and get my body back to normal.

4. Often the place where you had the abortion is the best source of information or care in case of a possible complication. Call the staff there if anything is bothering you, even if you cannot go back there for care. If you need followup medical attention, try to consult people who are experienced in treating women who have had legal abortions. Stay away from hospitals, clinics, and practitioners who are against abortion. They may try to make you feel that you "deserve" the complication as "punishment" for having had an abortion, and they may not be well informed about proper treatment for postabortion problems.

5. It is important to get a checkup in two to three weeks. A pelvic exam gives information about the small possibility of retained tissue or infection that may not be causing any symptoms yet, and it assures that the cervix is closed. Also, you can get any routine gynecological care that was not done at the time of the abortion.

   This is often a good time to discuss birth control, which may have been difficult to talk about at the time of the abortion. At a feminist health center you may have a chance to learn more about your body, including breast and cervical self-examination techniques. You may also be asked to talk about what's been happening since your abortion—both body changes and feelings. It can be especially helpful to talk with other women who have had abortions recently. Many of us are reassured by learning that our experiences are shared by other women. If you are one of the few women who has a continuing problem or complication, you need good information and medical help until the problem is over.

6. Think about birth control. Your next period will probably start four to six weeks after your abortion. If you do not get your period in six weeks, contact your health care provider. *You can get pregnant immediately after an abortion, even before your next period, so you need to use reliable birth control if you have intercourse and don't want another pregnancy.* You may say and believe, "I'll never have intercourse again, so I don't need birth control," but later you may change your mind. A reliable method of birth control is the only way to prevent pregnancy if you have intercourse again.

Choosing a birth control method is a very individual matter (see chapter 13, Birth Control). Some facilities will encourage you to use certain birth control methods, especially pills, which you can start taking the day of a first-trimester abortion. If you do this, you will be protected after the first cycle of pills, four weeks later. However, the hormone-like drugs in the pills affect your whole body and can cause changes that are similar to the signs of pregnancy, which can be confusing right after an abortion. It is probably not a good idea to have an IUD inserted at the time of an abortion, because of the greater risks of infection and perforation. Also, the IUD effects of cramping and bleeding may mask the symptoms of an abortion-related infection. A diaphragm or cervical cap can be fitted or refitted at the postabortion checkup. You can start a natural birth control class after an abortion, or obtain foam and condoms from a drugstore without a prescription. If the clinic or health care practitioner encourages you to use "the shot" (Depo-Provera) or Norplant, or to be sterilized, be sure to find out about the risks involved. (See chapter 13, Birth Control, for discussion of the reversibility of various methods of birth control.)

Regardless of the method of birth control you choose, it is important to understand that while you may be protected against pregnancy, you may still be vulnerable to sexually transmitted disease, including HIV (see chapters 14, Sexually Transmitted Diseases, and 15, HIV, AIDS, and Women, on STDs and HIV). To protect yourself from AIDS and other diseases, use condoms, even if you are using another form of birth control.

Feelings After an Abortion

There is no single way in which women experience abortion. Positive, negative, or mixed feelings are all natural. Women often feel new strength in having made and carried out an important, often difficult decision.

I feel proud of myself that I made the choice to have an abortion and finish college. I never made a decision before that said I was the most important person. Choosing abortion is about empowerment. It's about making a choice in favor of myself and my own future. It was giving myself a vote of confidence.

My unwanted pregnancy and my abortion led me to explore and gain a full understanding of my fertility cycle and my body. This knowledge has helped me feel whole. I have always been pro-choice, but now I feel able to face antichoice propaganda with the power of my own personal experience. I feel good that I can use my experience to help my sisters, my women friends, and, possibly someday, my daughter.

I am a 15-year-old Latina. When I got pregnant, I couldn't tell my mother. In my family, my pregnancy would be considered a disgrace and an insult to the family. I would have to leave the house. My boyfriend thought I should have an abortion, and so did I. I didn't really feel that I had a choice. We did not have the time or money to bring a child into this world. I know what I did was right. I also know that after the abortion I wept tears of sadness and tears of satisfaction.

The escorts took me and my boyfriend through the crowd. The demonstrators held pictures of bloody fetuses and yelled at me not to murder my baby. The whole thing really stirred me up. After the abortion I was so angry. Who do they think they are, trying to tell me what to do?

Sometimes women feel guilty about having an abortion. This is not surprising because our society still doesn't particularly accept the choice of abortion. So much emphasis is put on motherhood and fetal rights that many people act as though a fetus is more important than a woman.

The antiabortion movement, playing on women's fears, has portrayed abortion as a traumatic and dangerous procedure. They talk about "postabortion syndrome," claiming that women experience long-term psychological effects and diminished fertility. These claims are not true. Legal abortion does not hinder fertility; dangerous illegal abortions do. Severe depression after an abortion is extremely rare. In fact, many women experience relief. Others experience sadness or a sense of loss.

Negative feelings about sex, or intercourse in particular, after an abortion are not uncommon. Some of us, however, have the chance to choose a reliable method of birth control for the first time after the abortion and are more relaxed about sex. Sometimes the abortion provokes other changes. Relationships may end. The whole experience may strengthen a relationship or enable us to make other positive changes in our lives. Whatever our feelings, we can support each other by breaking the silence and isolation surrounding abortion.

I had an abortion in 1970, yet I find it difficult to write about abortion. I have escorted friends to get abortions, yet I find it difficult to talk with them about abortion. They felt they needed to be secretive about their experience. They did not hear voices validating their decision, so they questioned their choice. It is not easy for black women to talk about abortion. It is not easy for black women to have abortions. But we have spoken silently with our actions, having abortions at twice the rate of white women . . . and without com-munity support because of the conspiracy of silence surrounding abortion. A silent community cannot support sisters doing what they need and choose to do.

We need to start telling our stories about how illegal abortion killed our mothers and how legal abortion saved our lives. We have to talk to each other as black women, sister to sister.

Some of us, following our abortions, are angry and bitter because we did not have the resources—decent jobs, child care, education, food—to raise a child. We may be angry that Medicaid did not pay for the abortion and we had to spend money needed for food, rent, and clothes.

Taking away Medicaid funding says to poor women, "you don't deserve this." With Medicaid abortion, poor women had a little bit of control. They don't seem to get it—for poor women, abortion is a matter of survival. If I have this one more child, it etches away my margin of survival.

Whatever our feelings, being able to talk about them with a sympathetic and objective friend, relative, counselor, or group is often helpful. Talking helps some women feel better, resolve difficulties, and move on.

My conflicts about the abortion were resolved about a year and a half later, when I found the courage to speak of it in a women's group. The calmness and caring the other women shared with me, as well as some of their own experiences with abortion, helped me resolve my own feelings.

If you would like help from someone with special training, the facility where you had the abortion or any of the groups listed earlier in this chapter can refer you to someone to talk with: social worker, counselor, clergyperson. There are also a few postabortion support groups run by pro-choice women. If there is no such group near you, consider a women's support group, a therapy group, or individual therapy. You may be able to find a support group that is free or inexpensive through a women's center or clinic in your area.

Some of us may have other ways besides talking to resolve difficult feelings: yelling, crying, prayer, music, meditation, art, athletics, or other physical activity. Some of us block our feelings rather than feel them, joke about them, put them away to deal with later, or take pride in getting through something on our own without expressing our feelings. We must respect the different ways women deal with feelings.

Some of us choose to translate our feelings into action: do political work to keep abortion legal, work for improvements in abortion services, demand child care and jobs, fight against restrictions that prevent Medicaid or insurance from paying for abortions, educate our daughters about sex, help a friend who is dealing with an unwanted pregnancy.

When I was 15 and pregnant, abortion was illegal. I was denied any choice—I had a baby that I gave up for adoption. This experience has been a driving force in my life. I became an OB/GYN; I do abortions because I am totally committed to making sure that other women have the options that I didn't have.

HISTORY OF ABORTION

Over several centuries and in different cultures, there is a rich history of women helping each other to abort. Until the late 1800s, women healers in Western Europe and the U.S. provided abortions and trained other women to do so, without legal prohibitions.

The State didn't prohibit abortion until the 19th century, nor did the Church lead in this new repression. In 1803, Britain first passed antiabortion laws, which then became stricter throughout the century. The U.S. followed as individual states began to outlaw abortion. By 1880, most abortions were illegal in the U.S., except those "necessary to save the life of the woman." But the tradition of women's right to early abortion was rooted in U.S. society by then; abortionists continued to practice openly with public support, and juries refused to convict them.

Abortion became a crime and a sin for several reasons. A trend of humanitarian reform in the mid-19th century broadened liberal support for criminalization, because at that time abortion was a dangerous procedure done with crude methods, few antiseptics, and high mortality rates. But this alone cannot explain the attack on abortion. For instance, other risky surgical techniques were considered necessary for people's health and welfare and were not prohibited. "Protecting" women from the dangers of abortion was actually meant to control them and restrict them to their traditional child-bearing role. Antiabortion legislation was part of an antifeminist backlash to the growing movements for suffrage, voluntary motherhood, and other women's rights in the 19th century.*

At the same time, male doctors were tightening their control over the medical profession. Doctors considered midwives, who attended births and performed abortions as part of their regular practice, a threat to their own economic and social power. The medical establishment actively took up the antiabortion cause in the second half of the 19th century as part of its effort to eliminate midwives.

Finally, with the declining birth rate among whites in the late 1800s, the U.S. government and the eugenics movement warned against the danger of "race suicide" and urged white, native-born women to reproduce. Budding industrial capitalism relied on women to be unpaid household workers, low-paid menial workers, reproducers, and socializers of the next generation of workers. Without legal abortion, women found it more difficult to resist the limitations of these roles.

---

* For more information, see Linda Gordon's *Woman's Body, Woman's Right,* rev. ed. (New York: Penguin Books, 1990).

Then, as now, making abortion illegal neither eliminated the need for abortion nor prevented its practice. In the 1890s, doctors estimated that there were two million abortions a year in the U.S. (compared with one and a half million today). Women who are determined not to carry an unwanted pregnancy have always found some way to try to abort. All too often, they have resorted to dangerous, sometimes deadly methods, such as inserting knitting needles or coat hangers into the vagina and uterus, douching with dangerous solutions like lye, or swallowing strong drugs or chemicals. The coat hanger has become a symbol of the desperation of millions of women who have risked death to end a pregnancy. When these attempts harmed them, it was hard for women to obtain medical treatment; when these methods failed, women still had to find an abortionist.

Illegal Abortion

Many of us do not know what it was like to need an abortion before legalization. Women who could afford to pay skilled doctors or go to another country had the safest and easiest abortions. Most women found it difficult if not impossible to arrange and pay for abortions in medical settings.

With one exception, the doctors whom I asked for an abortion treated me with contempt, their attitudes ranging from hostile to insulting. One said to me, "You tramps like to break the rules, but when you get caught you all come crawling for help in the same way."

The secret world of illegal abortion was mostly frightening and expensive. Although there were skilled and dedicated laywomen and doctors who performed safe, illegal abortions, most illegal abortionists, doctors, and those who claimed to be doctors cared only about being well rewarded for their trouble. In the 1960s, abortionists often turned women away if they could not pay $1,000 or more in cash. Some male abortionists insisted on having sexual relations before the abortion.

Abortionists emphasized speed and their own protection. They often didn't use anesthesia because it took too long for women to recover, and they wanted women out of the office as quickly as possible. Some abortionists were rough and sadistic. Almost no one took adequate precautions against hemorrhage or infection.

Typically, the abortionist would forbid the woman to contact him or her again. Often she wouldn't know his or her real name. If a complication occurred, harassment by the law was a frightening possibility. The need for secrecy isolated women having abortions and those providing them.

In the 1950s, about a million illegal abortions a year were performed in the U.S., and over a thousand women died each year as a result. Women who were victims of botched or unsanitary abortions came in

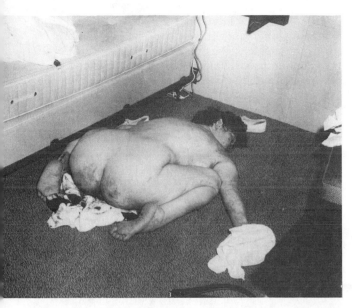

This controversial photograph first came to widespread notice when it appeared in *Ms. Magazine* in the early 1970s. It was later incorporated into *The New Our Bodies, Ourselves* as a depiction of an anonymous victim of an illegal abortion. We now know that the photo is of Geraldine Santoro. The story of her life and tragic death from an illegal abortion is told in the documentary film *Leona's Sister Gerri* (see Resources)./(Files of Dr. Milton Halpern, former medical examiner, New York City)

desperation to hospital emergency wards, where some died of widespread abdominal infections. Many women who recovered from such infections found themselves sterile or chronically and painfully ill. The enormous emotional stress often lasted a long time.

Poor women and women of color ran the greatest risks with illegal abortions. In 1969, 75% of the women who died from abortions (most of them illegal) were women of color. Of all legal abortions in that year, 90% were performed on white private patients.

Attempts to Make Illegal Abortion Less Dangerous

Many communities had informal networks of people who knew where women could obtain abortions. In the 1960s, clergy groups and feminist groups set up their own referral services to help women find safer illegal abortions. Some groups found that they needed to learn more about women's bodies and about abortion techniques in order to evaluate abortionists and help women avoid dangerous procedures. As they learned, they began to seek and create better, safer alternatives.

In Chicago, a group of women formed the Jane Collective, which provided safe, effective, and supportive illegal abortions. When they discovered that one of the skilled abortionists they used was not a doctor, Jane women realized that they could learn to perform the abortions with adequate training, and they did. Over a

four-year period, the Jane Collective was able to help more than 11,000 women get illegal first- and second-trimester abortions with a safety record comparable to that of legal abortions done in medical facilities. They also reduced the cost, charging only $50 and refusing to turn away any woman because of inability to pay the fee. In this way, they put many of Chicago's expensive and unsafe illegal abortionists out of business.

Groups like the Jane Collective demonstrated that determined and dedicated laywomen with no formal medical training can, with careful instruction and practice, perform abortions competently and humanely. Laura Kaplan, a former Jane member and author of *The Story of Jane*, says:

> We were ordinary women who, working together, accomplished something extraordinary. Our actions, which we saw as potentially transforming for other women, changed us, too. By taking responsibility, we became responsible. Most of us grew stronger, more self-assured, confident in our own abilities. In picking up the tools of our own liberation, in our case medical instruments, we broke a powerful taboo. That act was terrifying, but it was also exhilarating. We ourselves felt exactly the same powerfulness that we wanted other women to feel.

Throughout the world, whenever abortion has been illegal and unsafe, committed individuals have provided safe abortions clandestinely, treated women with complications, and helped women find safe providers. Jane and others doing similar work insisted that women who came to them always receive emotional support, reassurance, and kindness. However, illegality is a major barrier to safety and accessibility. Even Jane had to set up security measures to protect the identities and safety of those involved. They could not discuss their activities over the phone or in writing. They could not speak publicly and encourage other women to join them.

Some women have written about learning how to do abortions using "alternative" methods and claim to have had good results, especially within one to four weeks after conception. Yet, information about many of these abortion techniques, especially herbal ones, is incomplete, vague, or even inaccurate. While attempting to induce an early abortion with acupuncture, acupressure, or vitamin C may not be successful, it is not likely to involve serious risks. Taking herbal preparations, however, may be dangerous, sometimes even deadly, when women do not have extensive knowledge of herbs and cannot recognize the signs of complications. Pennyroyal is a potent herb listed in many books and articles as an abortion-causing substance (abortifacient). However, without clear instructions about safe dosages, the dangers of overdose, and the differences between the oil and a tea brewed from the leaves, trying pennyroyal may be dangerous. In fact, some experts report that pennyroyal poisoning occurs regularly and is potentially deadly. They also say that it fails to induce abortion in most cases.[2]

The Push for Legal Abortion

In the 1960s, inspired by the civil rights and antiwar movements, women began to fight more actively for their rights. The fast-growing women's movement took the taboo subject of abortion to the public. Rage, pain, and fear burst out in demonstrations and speakouts as women burdened by years of secrecy got up in front of strangers to talk about their illegal abortions. Women marched and rallied and lobbied for abortion on demand. Civil liberties groups and liberal clergy joined in these efforts to support women.

Reform came gradually. A few states liberalized abortion laws, allowing women abortions in certain circumstances (e.g., pregnancy resulting from rape or incest, being under 15 years of age) but leaving the decision up to doctors and hospitals. Costs were still high and few women actually benefited.

In 1970, New York State went further, with a law that allowed abortion on demand through the 24th week from the LMP if it was done in a medical facility by a doctor. A few other states passed similar laws. Women who could afford it flocked to the few places where abortions were legal. Feminist networks offered support, loans, and referrals and fought to keep prices down. But for every woman who managed to get to New York, many others with limited financial resources or mobility did not. Illegal abortion was still common. The fight continued; several cases before the Supreme Court urged the repeal of all restrictive state laws.

On January 22, 1973, the U.S. Supreme Court, in the famous *Roe v. Wade* decision, stated that the "right of privacy . . . founded in the Fourteenth Amendment's concept of personal liberty . . . is broad enough to encompass a woman's decision whether or not to terminate her pregnancy." The Court held that through the end of the first trimester of pregnancy, only a pregnant woman and her doctor have the legal right to make the decision about an abortion. States can restrict second-trimester abortions only in the interest of the woman's safety. Protection of a "viable fetus" (able to survive outside the womb) is allowed only during the third trimester. If a pregnant woman's life or health is endangered, she cannot be forced to continue the pregnancy.

Abortion After Legalization

Though *Roe v. Wade* left a lot of power to doctors and to government, it was an important victory for women. Although the decision did not guarantee that women would be able to get abortions when they wanted to, legalization and the growing consciousness of women's needs brought better, safer abortion services. For the women who had access to legal abortions, severe infections, fever, and hemorrhaging from illegal or self-induced abortions became a thing of the past. Women health care workers improved their abortion techniques. Some commercial clinics hired feminist abortion activists to do counseling. Local women's

groups set up public referral services, and women in some areas organized women-controlled nonprofit abortion facilities. These efforts turned out to be just the beginning of a longer struggle to preserve legal abortion and to make it accessible to all women.

Although legalization greatly lowered the cost of abortion, it still left millions of women in the U.S., especially women of color and young, rural women, and/or women with low incomes, without access to safe, affordable abortions. State regulations and funding have varied widely, and second-trimester abortions are costly. Even when federal Medicaid funds paid for abortions, fewer than 20% of all public county and city hospitals actually provided them. This meant that about 40% of U.S. women never benefited from liberalized abortion laws.

During the late 1970s and early 1980s, feminist health centers around the country provided low-cost abortions that emphasized quality of care, and they maintained political involvement in the reproductive rights movement. Competition from other abortion providers, harassment by the IRS, and a profit-oriented economy made their survival difficult. By the early 1990s, only 20 to 30 of these centers remained.

Eroding Abortion Rights: After Roe v. Wade

When the Supreme Court legalized abortion in 1973, the antiabortion forces, led initially by the Catholic Church hierarchy, began a serious mobilization using a variety of political tactics including pastoral plans, political lobbying, campaigning, public relations, papal encyclicals, and picketing abortion clinics. The Church hierarchy does not truly represent the views of U.S. Catholics on this issue or the practice of Catholic women, who have abortions at a rate slightly higher than the national average for all women.

Other religious groups, like the Mormons and some representatives of Jewish orthodoxy, have traditionally opposed abortion. In the 1980s, rapidly growing fundamentalist Christian groups, which overlap with the New Right and "right-to-life" organizations, were among the most visible boosters of the antiabortion movement. These antiabortion groups talk as if all truly religious and moral people disapprove of abortion. This is not true now and never has been.*

The long-range goal of the antiabortion movement is to outlaw abortion. Their short-range strategy has been to attack access to abortion, and they have had successes. The most vulnerable women—young women; women with low incomes, of whom a disproportionate number are women of color; all women who depend on the government for their health care —have borne the brunt of these attacks on abortion rights.

The antiabortion movement's first victory, a major setback to abortion rights, came in July 1976, when

---

* For pro-choice religious perspectives, write to RCRC: the Religious Coalition for Reproductive Choice (see Resources).

Congress passed the Hyde Amendment banning Medicaid funding for abortion unless a woman's life was in danger. Following the federal government, many states stopped funding "medically unnecessary" abortions. The result was immediate in terms of harm and discrimination against women living in poverty. In October 1977, Rosie Jiménez, a Texas woman, died from an illegal abortion in Mexico, after Texas stopped funding Medicaid abortions.

It is impossible to count the number of women who have been harmed by the Hyde Amendment, but before Hyde, one-third of all abortions were Medicaid funded: 294,000 women per year. (Another 133,000 Medicaid-eligible women who needed abortions were unable to gain access to public funding for the procedure.) Without state funding, many women with unwanted pregnancies are forced to have babies, be sterilized, or have abortions using money needed for food, rent, clothing, and other necessities.

Although a broad spectrum of groups fought against the Hyde Amendment, countering this attack on women who lack financial resources was not a priority of the pro-choice movement. There was no mass mobilization or public outcry. In the long run, this hurt the pro-choice movement, as the attack on Medicaid funding was the first victory in the antiabortion movement's campaign to deny access to abortion for all women.

Young women's rights have been a particular target of the antiabortion movement. About 40% of the one million teens who become pregnant annually choose abortion. Parental involvement laws, requiring that minors seeking abortions either notify their parents or receive parental consent, affect millions of young women. As of early 1997, 35 states have these laws; 23 states enforce them. In some states, a physician is required to notify at least one parent either in person, by phone, or in writing. Health care providers face loss of license and sometimes criminal penalties for failure to comply.

Antiabortion forces have also used illegal and increasingly violent tactics, including harassment, terrorism, violence, and murder. Since the early 1980s, clinics and providers have been targets of violence. Over 80% of all abortion providers have been picketed or seriously harassed. Doctors and other workers have been the object of death threats, and clinics have been subject to chemical attacks (for example, butyric acid), arson, bomb threats, invasions, and blockades. In the late 1980s, a group called Operation Rescue initiated a strategy of civil disobedience by blockading clinic entrances and getting arrested. There were thousands of arrests nationwide as clinics increasingly became political battlefields.

In the 1990s, antiabortionists increasingly turned to harassment of individual doctors and their families, picketing their homes, following them, and circulating "Wanted" posters. Over 200 clinics have been bombed. After 1992, the violence became deadly. The murder of two doctors and an escort at a clinic in Pensacola, Florida, was followed by the murder two

WEAKENING THE CONSTITUTIONAL PROTECTION FOR ABORTION

When in 1980 the Supreme Court upheld the Hyde Amendment, it began eroding the constitutional protection for abortion rights. Since then, there have been other severe blows. In *Webster v. Reproductive Health Services* (1989), the Court opened the door to new state restrictions on abortion. In *Hodgson v. Minnesota* (1990), the Court upheld one of the strictest parental notification laws in the country.

These trends were further codified in *Planned Parenthood v. Casey,* a 1992 decision upholding a highly restrictive Pennsylvania law that included mandatory waiting periods and mandatory biased counseling. Two frightening themes emerged in the *Casey* decision. First, the Court sanctioned the view that government may regulate the health care of pregnant women to protect fetal life from the moment of conception so long as it does not "unduly burden" access to an abortion. Second, the Court showed little concern for the severe impact of state restrictions on women with few financial resources.

In the aftermath of *Casey,* many states have passed similar restrictions, which have the effect of limiting access to abortion, especially for women with low incomes, teenage women, and women of color.

These infringements on abortion access have curtailed the abortion rights of millions of women. In the face of the unrelenting efforts of the antiabortion movement, those of us who believe that women should make their own reproductive decisions will have to become involved in the ongoing struggle to preserve and expand abortion rights.

women receptionists at clinics in Brookline, Massachusetts. A health care provider spoke about the impact of the violence:

*The fear of violence has become part of the lives of every abortion provider in the country. As doctors, we are being warned not to open big envelopes with no return addresses in case a mail bomb is enclosed. I know colleagues who have had their homes picketed and their children threatened. Some wear bullet-proof vests and have remote starters for their cars. Even going to work and facing the disapproving looks from co-workers—isolation and marginalization from colleagues is part of it.**

* To find out more about violence at clinics and how to respond, contact the National Abortion Federation, NOW, or The Feminist Majority Foundation (see Resources).

The antiabortion movement continues to mount new campaigns on many fronts. Most recently, it has aggressively put out the idea that abortion increases the risk of breast cancer. In January 1997, the results of a Danish study, the largest to date (involving one and a half million women), showed that there is no connection.[3] Unlike previous studies, this one did not rely on interviews and women's reports but instead used data obtained from population registries about both abortion and breast cancer. Despite the lack of medical evidence and the fact that the scientific community does not recognize any link, the antiabortion movement continues to stir up fears about abortion and breast cancer.

Legal but Out of Reach for Many Women

We have learned that legalization is not enough to ensure that abortions will be available to all women who want and need them. In addition to a lack of facilities and trained providers, burdensome legal restrictions, including parental consent or notification laws for minors and mandatory waiting periods, create significant obstacles. A minor who has been refused consent by a parent may have to go through an intimidating and time-consuming judicial hearing. Mandatory waiting periods may require a woman to miss extra days of work because she must go to the clinic not once, but twice, to obtain an abortion. If travel is required, this can make the whole procedure unaffordable. In other words, for millions of women, youth, race, and economic circumstances together with the lack of accessible services—especially for later abortions—translate into daunting barriers, forcing some women to resort to unsafe and illegal abortions and self-abortions.

REPRODUCTIVE FREEDOM VS. POPULATION CONTROL

While most women's health groups see the fight for abortion rights in the context of defending the rights of all women to make their own decisions about reproduction, not all advocates of abortion rights share this understanding. Some view legal abortion and contraception as tools of population control.

Advocates of population control blame overpopulation for a range of problems, from global poverty to ethnic conflict and environmental degradation. Historically, this type of thinking has led to a range of coercive fertility control policies that target Third World women. These include sterilization without a woman's knowledge or consent; the use of economic incentives to "encourage" sterilization, a practice that undermines the very notion of reproductive choice; the distribution and sometimes coercive or unsafe use of contraceptive methods, often without appropriate information; the denial of abortion services; and sometimes coercive abortion. For example, HIV-positive women in the U.S. (who are overwhelmingly women of color) are often pressured to have abortions, though only 20 to 25% of their children will be HIV-positive

---

ABORTION ACCESS IN THE U.S.

- It is conservatively estimated that one in five Medicaid-eligible women who want an abortion cannot obtain one.[4]
- In the U.S., 84% of all counties have no abortion services; of rural counties, 95% have no services.[5]
- Nine in ten abortion providers are located in metropolitan areas.[6]
- Only 17 states fund abortions.[7]
- Only 12% of OB/GYN residency programs train in first-trimester abortions; only 7% in second-trimester abortions.[8]
- Abortion is the most common OB/GYN surgical procedure; yet, almost half of graduating OB/GYN residents have never performed a first-trimester abortion.[9]
- Thirty-nine states have parental involvement laws requiring minors to notify and/or obtain the consent of their parents in order to obtain an abortion.[10]
- Twenty-one states require state-directed counseling before a woman may obtain an abortion.[11] (This is often called "informed consent"; some critics call it a "biased information requirement.")
- Many states require women seeking abortions to receive scripted lectures on fetal development, prenatal care, and adoption.[12]
- Twelve states currently enforce mandatory waiting periods following state-directed counseling; this can result in long delays and higher costs.[13] (Seven more states have delay laws which are enjoined—i.e., not enforced due to court action at the federal or state level.)

---

and new treatments during pregnancy have reduced the likelihood even further.

Women with few economic resources, especially women of color in the U.S. and throughout the world, have been the primary targets of population control policies. For example, although abortion has become increasingly less accessible in the U.S., sterilization remains all too available for women of color. The federal government stopped funding abortions in 1977, but it continues to pay for sterilizations. During the 1970s, women's health activists exposed various forms of sterilization abuse (see section on sterilization in chapter 13, Birth Control). Since the 1980s, advocates have fought against new policies that coerce women with low incomes into using Norplant, a long-term hormonal contraceptive.

In the Third World, in addition to the widespread unavailability of desired contraceptives, there is a long history of coercive fertility control, primarily funded and inspired by developed countries, especially the

U.S. (see chapter 26, The Global Politics of Women and Health, for the international dimensions of population control).

The right to abortion is part of every woman's right to control her reproductive choices and her own life. We must reject all efforts to coerce women's reproductive decisions. The goals of reproductive rights activists must encompass the right to have children as well as the right not to.

ABORTION WORLDWIDE

Unsafe abortion is a major cause of death and health complications for women of child-bearing age. Whether or not an abortion is safe is determined in part by the legal status and restrictions, but also by medical practice, administrative requirements, the availability of trained practitioners, and facilities, funding, and public attitudes.

While it is difficult to get reliable data on illegal and unsafe abortion, several well-known organizations and researchers, including the World Health Organization, the Alan Guttmacher Institute, and Family Health International, make the following estimates:

- Worldwide, 20 million unsafe abortions are performed annually. This equals one unsafe abortion for every ten pregnancies and one unsafe abortion for every seven births.
- Ninety percent of unsafe abortions are in developing countries.
- One-third of all abortions worldwide are illegal.
- More than two-thirds of countries in the Southern Hemisphere have no access to safe, legal abortion.
- Estimates of the number of women who die worldwide from unsafe abortions each year range from 70,000 to 200,000. This means that between 13 and 20% of all maternal deaths are due to unsafe abortion—in some areas of the world, half of all maternal deaths. Of these deaths, 99% are in the developing world, and most are preventable.
- Half of all abortions take place outside the health care system.
- One-third of women seeking care for abortion complications are under the age of 20.
- About 40% of the world's population has access to legal abortion (almost all in Europe, the former Soviet Union, and North America), although laws often require the consent of parents, state committees, or physicians.
- Worldwide, 21% of women may obtain legal abortions for social or economic reasons.
- Sixteen percent of women have access only when a woman's health is at risk or in cases of rape, incest, or fetal defects.
- Five percent have access only in cases of rape, incest, or life endangerment.
- Eighteen percent have access only for life endangerment.

AFRICAN-AMERICAN WOMEN FOR REPRODUCTIVE FREEDOM

Choice is the essence of freedom. It's what we African Americans have struggled for all these years. The right to choose where we would sit on a bus. The right to vote. The right for each of us to select our own paths, to dream and reach for our dreams. The right to choose how we would or would not live our lives.

This freedom—to choose and to exercise our choices—is what we've fought and died for. Brought here in chains, worked like mules, bred like beasts, whipped one day, sold the next—244 years we were held in bondage. Somebody said that we were less than human and not fit for freedom. Somebody said we were like children and could not be trusted to think for ourselves. Somebody owned our flesh and decided if and when and with whom and how our bodies were to be used. Somebody said that black women could be raped, held in concubinage, forced to bear children year in and year out, but often not raise them. Oh, yes, we have known how painful it is to be without choice in this land.

Those of us who remember the bad old days when Jim Crow rules and segregation were the way of things know the hardships and indignities we faced. We were free, but few or none were our choices. Somebody said where we could live and couldn't, where we could work, what schools we could go to, where we could eat, how we could travel. Somebody prevented us from voting. Somebody said we could be paid less than other workers. Somebody burned crosses, harassed and terrorized us in order to keep us down.

Now once again, somebody is trying to say that we can't handle the freedom of choice. Only this time they're saying African-American women can't think for themselves and, therefore, can't be allowed to make serious decisions. Somebody's saying that we should not have the freedom to take charge of our personal lives and protect our health, that we only have limited rights over our bodies. Somebody's once again forcing women to acts of desperation, because somebody's saying that if women have unintended pregnancies, it's too bad, but they must pay the price.

Somebody's saying that we must have babies whether we choose to or not. Doesn't matter what we say, doesn't matter how we feel. Some say that abortion under any circumstance is wrong, others say that rape and incest and danger to the life of the woman are the only exceptions. Doesn't matter that nobody's saying who

continued on next page

decides if it was rape or incest, if a woman's word is good enough, if she must go into court and prove it. Doesn't matter that she may not be able to take care of a baby, that the problem also affects girls barely out of adolescence, that our children are having children. Doesn't matter if you're poor and pregnant—go on welfare or walk away.

What does matter is that we know abortions will still be done, legal or not. We know the consequences when women are forced to make choices without protection—the coat hangers and knitting needles that punctured the wombs of women forced to seek back-alley abortions on kitchen tables at the hands of butchers. The women who died screaming in agony, awash in their own blood. The women who were made sterile. All the women who endured the pain of makeshift surgery with no anesthetics and risked fatal infection.

We understand why African-American women risked their lives then and why they seek safe, legal abortion now. It's been a matter of survival. Hunger and homelessness. Inadequate housing and income to properly provide for themselves and their children. Family instability. Rape. Incest. Abuse. Too young, too old, too sick, too tired. Emotional, physical, mental, economic, social—the reasons for not carrying a pregnancy to term are endless and varied, personal, urgent and private. And for all these pressing reasons, African-American women once again will be among the first forced to risk their lives if abortion is made illegal.

There have always been those who have stood in the way of our exercising our rights, who tried to restrict our choices. There probably always will be. But we who have been oppressed should not be swayed in our opposition to tyranny of any kind, especially attempts to take away our reproductive freedom. You may believe abortion is wrong. We respect your belief and we will do all in our power to protect that choice for you. You may decide that abortion is not an option you would choose. Reproductive freedom guarantees your right not to. All that we ask is that no one deny another human being the right to make her own choice. That no one condemn her to exercising her choices in ways that endanger her health, her life. And that no one prevent others from creating safe, affordable, legal conditions to accommodate women, whatever the choices they make. Reproductive freedom gives each of us the right to make our own choices and guarantees us a safe, legal, affordable support system. It's the right to choose.

We are still an embattled people beset with life-and-death issues. Black America is under siege. Drugs, the scourge of our community, are wiping out one, two, three generations. We are killing ourselves and each other. Rape and other unspeakable acts of violence are becoming sickeningly commonplace. Babies linger on death's door, at risk at birth: born addicted to crack and cocaine, born underweight and undernourished, born AIDS infected. An ever-growing number of our children are being abandoned, being mentally, physically, spiritually abused. Homelessness, hunger, unemployment run rife. Poverty grows. Our people cry out in desperation, anger, and need.

Meanwhile, those somebodies who claim they're "pro-life" aren't moved to help the living. They're not out there fighting to break the stranglehold of drugs and violence in our communities, trying to save our children or moving to provide infant and maternal nutrition and health programs. Eradicating poverty isn't on their agenda. No—somebody's too busy picketing, vandalizing, and sometimes bombing family-planning clinics, harassing women and denying funds to poor women seeking abortions.

So when somebody denouncing abortion claims that they're "pro-life," remind them of an old saying that our grandmothers often used: "It's not important what people say, it's what they do." And remember who we are, remember our history, our continuing struggle for freedom. Remember to tell them that we remember!

Original Signers:
Byllye Avery (National Black Women's Health Project)
Rev. Willie Barrow (Operation Push)
Donna Brazile (Housing Now)
Shirley Chisholm (National Political Congress of Black Women)
Representative Cardiss Collins (U.S. Congress)
Romona Edelin (National Urban Coalition)
Jacqui Gates (National Association of Negro Business and Professional Women's Clubs, Inc.)
Marcia Ann Gillespie (Ms. Magazine)
Dorothy Height (National Council of Negro Women)
Jewel Jackson McCabe (National Coalition of 100 Black Women)
Julianne Malveaux (San Francisco Black Leadership Forum)
Eleanor Holmes Norton (Georgetown University Law School)
C. Delores Tucker (DNC Black Caucus)
Patricia Tyson (Religious Coalition for Abortion Rights)
Maxine Waters (Black Women's Forum)
Faye Wattleton (Planned Parenthood Federation of America)

Additional Signers in 1994:
Tony M. Bond
Sen. Carol Moseley-Braun (D-IL)

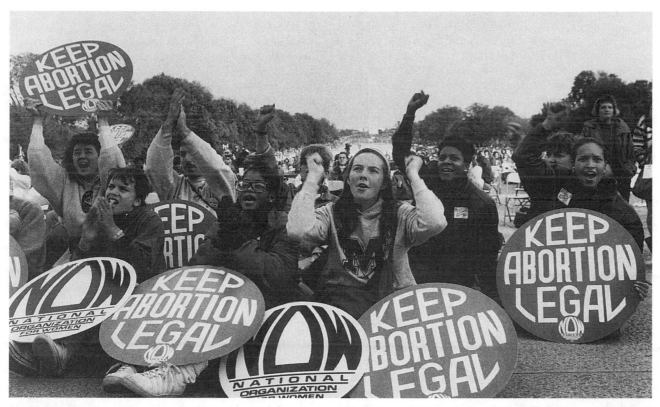

Ellen Shub

Rep. Corrine Brown (D-FL)
Rep. Eva Clayton (D-NC)
Rep. Barbara-Rose Collins (D-MI)
Rev. Alma Crawford
Evelyn S. Field
Rev. Catherine Godbolte
Rev. Dr. Claudia Highbaugh
Beverly Hunter
Rev. Elenora Giddings Ivory
Bernice Powell Jackson
Terri James
Rep. Eddie Bernice Johnson (D-TX)
Bisola Marignay
The Rev. Dr. Joan Martin
Cassandra McConnell
Rep. Cynthia McKinney (D-GA)
Rep. Carrie P. Meek (D-FL)
Mary F. Morten
Cynthia Newbille
Mary Jane Patterson
Loretta Ross
Jerald Lillian Scott
Beverly W. Stripling
Elizabeth Terry
Mable Thomas
Winnette P. Willis
Kim Youngblood

Note: Organizations are given for identification purposes only.

TAKING ACTION

To the antiabortion movement and to religious fundamentalists, abortion, reproductive rights, and sexual rights all symbolize women's independence and sexual freedom and the consequent breakdown of the male-dominated family. Those who oppose the basic right of women to control our bodies have come to fear women's ever-bolder demands as workers, as mothers, and as human beings. They have responded by trying to control women's sexuality and fertility. They have created an atmosphere that is volatile, stigmatizing, irrational, and too often violent, so that even being vocally pro-choice can feel risky.

Even so, women have stood up against these forces. Abortion rights activists have responded to the attacks on *Roe v. Wade* and to antiabortion violence by organizing large national demonstrations, clinic defense, intensified public education campaigns, and other forms of political activism. Unfortunately, the attack on abortion rights continues. Activists have learned that securing these rights is an ongoing struggle, requiring continued action.

In the late 1970s and 1980s, new reproductive rights groups and organizations of women of color emerged outside the mainstream pro-choice movement. They took the lead in promoting a broader understanding of women's reproductive rights and health. This organizing has been energized through alliances with women's organizing worldwide. The series of United Nations conferences that took place during the 1990s

—the Earth Summit in Rio de Janeiro (1992), the International Conference on Population and Development (ICPD) in Cairo (1994), the Economic Summit in Copenhagen (1995), and the Fourth World Conference on Women in Beijing (1995)—have given women's organizations and activists throughout the world unprecedented opportunities for interaction. The fight for abortion rights is indeed part of a global struggle.

At the 1995 Fourth World Conference on Women in Beijing, nongovernmental organizations (NGOs) worked to include abortion rights in the Platform for Action, without allowing the antiabortionists to use abortion to eclipse other issues of importance to women. Despite the efforts of conservative Islamic and Catholic delegations to condemn abortion, the Platform for Action includes a statement of sexual rights and calls on countries to consider reviewing punitive laws on illegal abortions. Although this was a compromise for abortion rights advocates who seek the affirmation of abortion rights for all women, it was a major step forward.

The U.S. movement has much to learn from our sisters in other countries. Internationally, especially in the developing world, the women's agenda integrates a wide range of issues. Advocates for women's rights and health place abortion in a broad framework that includes concerns about maternal and infant mortality, population control, economic justice, violence against women, and environmental destruction. Women's groups from the developing world bring a broadened understanding of women's oppression, one that focuses on the rights of the least privileged women in the world and is committed to resisting fundamentalism, militarism, and the drain of economic resources from the developing world.

In the U.S., activists must also place abortion in the context of the larger fight for women's rights. We need a new movement that will fight for all of the rights all women need to make reproductive freedom a reality. While we work for abortion rights we need to make connections with women opposing racist abuse of sterilization and those demanding welfare rights, disability rights, gay and lesbian liberation, economic rights, child care, and health care. Reproductive freedom is part of the fight for human rights.

NOTES

1. From Anne Eggebroten, ed., *Abortion—My Choice, God's Grace: Christian Women Tell Their Stories* (Pasadena CA: Hope Publishing House, 1994).
2. *American Medical News* (Dec. 16, 1996).
3. M. Melbye et al., "Induced Abortion and the Risk of Breast Cancer," *New England Journal of Medicine* 336, no. 2 (1997).
4. S. Henshaw, "Factors Hindering Access to Abortion Services," *Family Planning Perspectives* 27, no. 2 (1995): 54–59, 87.
5. Henshaw, op. cit.
6. Henshaw, op. cit.
7. Center for Reproductive Law and Policy, "Portrait of Injustice: Abortion Coverage Under the Medicaid Program," (Jan. 1997).
8. C. Westhoff, "Abortion Training in Residency Programs," *Journal of the American Medical Women's Association* 49, no. 5 (1994): 159–62, 164.
9. Westhoff, op. cit.
10. Center for Reproductive Law and Policy, "Restrictions on Young Women's Access to Abortion Services," (Nov. 1997).
11. Personal conversation with Alan Guttmacher Institute staff based on their November 1997 figures.
12. Center for Reproductive Law and Policy, "Reproductive Freedom in the States: Mandatory Delays and Biased Information Requirements," (Nov. 1997).
13. See Note 11.

RESOURCES

Books

Baehr, Ninia. *Abortion Without Apology: A Radical History for the 1990s*. Boston: South End Press, 1990.

Cohen, Sherrill, and Nadine Taub, eds. *Reproductive Laws for the 1990s*. Clifton, NJ: Humana Press, 1989.

Davis, Susan E., ed. *Women Under Attack—Victories, Backlash and the Fight for Reproductive Freedom*. Boston: South End Press, 1988 (originally published by CARASA, Committee for Abortion Rights and Against Sterilization Abuse, New York).

Faux, Marian. *Crusaders: Voices from the Abortion Front*. New York: Carol Publishing Group, 1990.

———. Roe v. Wade: *The Untold Story of the Landmark Supreme Court Decision That Made Abortion Legal*. New York: New American Library, 1988.

Federation of Feminist Women's Health Centers. *A New View of a Woman's Body*. Los Angeles: Feminist Health Press, 1981.

Ferraro, Barbara, and Patricia Hussey with Jane O'Reilly. *No Turning Back: Two Nuns' Battle with the Vatican over Women's Right to Choose*. New York: Poseidon Press, 1990.

Frankfort, Ellen, and Frances Kissling. *Rosie, the Investigation of a Wrongful Death*. New York: Dial Press, 1979.

Fried, Marlene Gerber, ed. *From Abortion to Reproductive Freedom: Transforming a Movement*. Boston: South End Press, 1990.

Ginsburg, Faye D. *Contested Lives: The Abortion Debate in an American Community*. Berkeley: University of California Press, 1989.

Gordon, Linda. *Woman's Body, Woman's Right: Birth Control in America,* rev. ed. New York: Penguin, 1990.

Harrison, Beverly Wildung. *Our Right to Choose: Toward a New Ethic of Abortion*. Boston: Beacon Press, 1983.

Hartmann, Betsy. *Reproductive Rights and Wrongs:*

The Global Politics of Population Control. Boston: South End Press, 1995.

Joffe, Carole. *Doctors of Conscience: The Struggle to Provide Abortions Before and After* Roe v. Wade. Boston: Beacon, 1995.

Kaplan, Laura. *The Story of Jane: The Legendary Underground Feminist Abortion Service.* New York: Pantheon, 1995.

Kaufmann, K. *The Abortion Resource Handbook.* New York: Simon & Schuster, 1997.

Lader, Lawrence. *RU-486: The Pill That Could End the Abortion Wars and Why American Women Don't Have It.* Reading, MA: Addison-Wesley, 1991.

Luker, Kristin. *Abortion and the Politics of Motherhood.* Berkeley: University of California Press, 1984.

Messer, Ellen, and Kathryn E. May. *Back Rooms: Voices from the Illegal Abortion Era.* New York: Simon & Schuster, 1988.

Petchesky, Rosalind Pollack. *Abortion and Woman's Choice: The State, Sexuality, and Reproductive Freedom,* rev. ed. Boston: Northeastern University Press, 1990.

Raymond, Janice, et al. *RU-486: Misconceptions, Myths and Morals.* Cambridge, MA: Institute on Women and Technology (Department of Urban Studies and Planning, MIT), 1991. (Cottingham, Jane, and Paul Van Look. "RU-486: Misconceptions, myths and morals: A critique," June 1992. Available for $2.00 from the Boston Women's Health Book Collective, Box 192, West Somerville, MA 02144.)

Periodicals

The Fight for Abortion Rights and Reproductive Freedom Newsletter
Civil Liberties and Public Policy Program
Hampshire College

ProChoice IDEA
ProChoice Resource Center

Reproductive Freedom News
Center for Reproductive Law and Policy

Reproductive Rights Update, A Quarterly Report
American Civil Liberties Union

The Washington Memo (twice monthly) and *Family Planning Perspectives* (bimonthly)
The Alan Guttmacher Institute

Audiovisual Materials

Abortion Denied: Shattering Young Women's Lives, 1990, color, a video about the devastating effect of parental consent/notification laws. Available from The Feminist Majority Foundation, 1600 Wilson Boulevard, Arlington, VA 22209.

Abortion: Stories from North and South, a 16-mm 1984 color film/video. An historical and cross-cultural documentary that is quite powerful; however, international family-planning programs are presented uncritically.

Available from Cinema Guild, 1697 Broadway, New York, NY 10019; (212) 246-5522; E-mail: cinemag@aol.com

Back-Alley Detroit: Abortion Before Roe v. Wade, 1992, 45-minute color video by Daniel Friedman and Sharon Grimberg. This excellent documentary exposes the underworld that criminalization of abortion created, and tells the stories of those who defied abortion laws. Available from Filmmakers Library, 124 East 40th Street Suite 900, New York, NY 10016; (212) 808-4980; (800) 555-9815.

Casting the First Stone: Portraits of Women and Men on Both Sides of the Abortion Controversy, one-hour 1991 video. Tells the story of six women and spans three decades. Available from Women Make Movies, 462 Broadway, Room 500, New York, NY 10013; (212) 925-0606; E-mail: rnso@wmm.com

Concentric Media Video Trilogy. The following three films were directed by Dorothy Fadiman. The film company can provide speakers and a guide to organizing a screening. P.O. Box 1414, Menlo Park, CA 94026; (415) 974-5881; E-mail: staff@concentric.org

When Abortion Was Illegal: Untold Stories, 1993 color video giving personal accounts that reveal the medical and legal consequences during the era of criminal abortion. (See Concentric Media above.)

From Danger to Dignity: The Fight for Safe Abortion, 1995 57-minute video that contains interviews and rare archival footage of the activists, doctors, clergy, and legislators whose work together led to *Roe v. Wade.* (See Concentric Media above.)

The Fragile Promise of Choice: Abortion in the United States Today, 1996, 57-minute video that traces the erosion of access to safe abortions, the shortage of trained providers, the threat of violence, and legislative restrictions. (See Concentric Media above.)

Holy Terror, a 16-mm 1986 color film/video. A documentary presenting the rise of antiabortion efforts of the religious New Right. Available from Cinema Guild (see *Abortion: Stories . . .* above).

Jane: An Abortion Service, 1994, 60-minute color video about a Chicago-based women's group that performed nearly 11,000 safe illegal abortions. Informative, inspiring, good for teaching and outreach. Filmmakers Kate Kirtz and Nell Lundy are available to speak. Available from Juicy Productions, Inc., P.O. Box 268581, Chicago, IL 60626; (312) 409-8394.

Leona's Sister Gerri, directed by Jane Gillooly, 1995, a 37-minute documentary about Gerri Santoro, who died in 1964 from an illegal abortion. (See photo on p. 409.) Available from New Day Films, 22D Hollywood Avenue, Hohokus, NJ 07423; (201) 652-6590; Fax: (201) 652-1973; E-mail: tmcndy@aol.com

Motherless, 1993, 27-minute documentary about illegal abortion, inspired by Linn Duvall Harwell's story of the death of her mother in 1929 from complications of a self-induced abortion. Filmmakers Janet Goldwater, Barbara Attie, and Diane Pontius have created a powerful educational tool. Available from Filmmakers Library. (See *Back-Alley Detroit* above.)

No Going Back. This 1988 video presents menstrual

extraction as an abortion method that can be used by women in self-help health groups. Available from the Federation of Feminist Women's Health Centers, 633 E. 11th Avenue, Eugene OR 97401; (541) 344-0966.

On Becoming a Woman, a 1989 color video about mothers and daughters working to communicate honestly with each other. Full of candid, emotional conversations about menstruation, sexuality, birth control, teen pregnancy, and relationships. Available from National Black Women's Health Project, 514 10th St. NW, Suite 400, Washington, DC 20004.

Silent No More, a 1989 color video. Four white women talk about their illegal abortions. Available from Civil Liberties and Public Policy Program, Hampshire College, Amherst, MA 01002.

Organizations

Abortion Access Project of Massachusetts
P.O. Box 686; Boston, MA 02130; (617) 661-1161
E-mail: rcaap@aol.com
Works on access issues, especially hospitals and training; available for technical assistance.

Alan Guttmacher Institute
1120 Connecticut Avenue NW, Suite 460; Washington, DC 20036; (202) 296-4012
E-mail: policyinfo@agi-usa-org
Web site: http://www.agi-usa.org
Nonprofit research and policy institute that studies reproductive health issues.

American Civil Liberties Union (ACLU)
Reproductive Freedom Project; 125 Broad Street; New York, NY 10004; (212) 549-2500
E-mail: rspaclu@aol.com
Web site: http://www.aclu.org/issues/reproduction/hmrr.html
Involved in litigation relevant to abortion rights.

American Medical Women's Association (AMWA)
801 N. Fairfax Street, Suite 400; Alexandria, VA 22314; (703) 838-0500; Fax: (703) 549-3864
Web site: http://www.amwa-doc.org
Promotes women's health and works to increase the influence of women in medicine.

Catholics for a Free Choice (CFFC)
1436 U Street NW, Suite 301; Washington, DC 20009; (202) 986-6093; Fax: (202) 332-7995
E-mail: cffc@igc.apc.org
A national educational organization that supports the right to family planning and abortion.

The Center for Reproductive Law and Policy
120 Wall Street, 18th floor; New York, NY 10005; (212) 514-5534 and 1146 19th Street NW; Washington DC 20036; (202) 530-2975; Fax: (202) 530-2976
Involved in reproductive rights policy and litigation worldwide.

The Civil Liberties and Public Policy Program (CLPP)
Hampshire College; Amherst, MA 01002-5001; (413) 582-5645
E-mail: clpp@hampshire.edu
Web site: http://hampshire.edu/~clpp
Resource for campus and community reproductive rights and health organizations. Newsletter, conferences, speakout videos.

The Federation of Feminist Women's Health Centers
633 E. 11th Avenue; Eugene, OR 97401; (541) 344-0966; Fax: (541) 344-1993
A nonprofit association of women's health projects that provides health services to women, including abortion, well-women care, and birth control.

The Feminist Majority Foundation
1600 Wilson Boulevard, Suite 801; Arlington, VA 22209; (703) 522-2214; Fax: (703) 522-2219
E-mail: femmaj@feminist.org
Web site: http://www.feminist.org
An advocacy and research group that aims to get women into positions of leadership throughout society and to promote a national feminist agenda.

International Women's Health Coalition
24 East 21st Street; New York, NY 10010; (212) 979-8500
E-mail: iwhc@igc.apc.org
A private, nonprofit organization dedicated to improving women's reproductive health in less industrialized countries.

Medical Students for Choice
2484 Shattuck Avenue, Suite 250; Berkeley, CA 94704; (510) 540-1195
E-mail: msfc@ms4c.org
Web site: http://www.ms4c.org
Organizes pro-choice medical students.

The National Abortion and Reproductive Rights Action League (NARAL)
1156 15th Street NW, Suite 700; Washington, DC 20005; (202) 973-3000
E-mail: naral@naral.org
Web site: http://www.naral.org
Works to elect pro-choice officials to all levels of government and to protect the right to choose in the legislatures, the courts, and at the clinics. Its Campus Organizing Project assists young activists.

The National Abortion Federation (NAF)
1755 Massachusetts Avenue NW, Suite 600; Washington, DC 20036; (202) 667-5881
E-mail: naf@prochoice.org
Web site: http://www.prochoice.org/naf
An association of abortion providers, individuals, and organizations working in reproductive health and abortion rights. NAF's toll-free hot line gives referrals for abortion services and funding. Hot line: (800) 772-9100, Monday through Friday, 9:30–5:30 EST; in Canada, (800) 424-2280.

The National Black Women's Health Project (NBWHP)
1211 Connecticut Avenue NW, Suite 310; Washington, DC 20036; (202) 835-0117
E-mail: NBWHPDC@aol.com
   Advocacy organization addressing health issues facing black women and their families.

The National Latina Health Organization (NLHO)
P.O. Box 7567; Oakland, CA 94601; (510) 534-1362; (800) 971-5358
Web site: http://clnet.ucr/edu/women/nhol
   Promotes self-help methods and self-empowerment processses. Latinas for Reproductive Choice, part of NLHO, takes public stands on reproductive issues and is involved in education and advocacy work.

The National Network of Abortion Funds
c/o CLPP; Hampshire College; Amherst, MA 01002-5001; (413) 582-5645; Fax: (413) 582-5620
E-mail: clpp@hamp.hampshire.edu
Web site: http://hamp.hampshire.edu/~clpp/nnaf
   An association of 41 grassroots abortion funds that provide funding and other support for low-income women seeking abortions. Publishes "Legal but Out of Reach," a booklet of women's stories.

The National Organization for Women (NOW)
1000 16th Street NW, Suite 700; Washington, DC 20036; (202) 331-0066
E-mail: now@now.org
Web site: http://www.now.org
   Works on a range of issues, including reproductive rights, welfare rights, and affirmative action.

The National Women's Health Network (NWHN)
514 10th Street NW, Suite 400; Washington, DC 20005; (202) 347-1140
   Works for abortion rights and other women's health issues. Maintains national communications about anti-abortion legislation, RU-486, and harassment of feminist abortion providers.

Native American Women's Health Education Resource Center
P.O. Box 572; Lake Andes, SD 57356; (605) 487-7072
   Has organized a Native American reproductive rights coalition.

The ProChoice Resource Center
174 E. Boston Post Road; Mamaroneck, NY 10543; (914) 381-3792; (800) 733-1973; Fax: (914) 381-3876
   A national group advising and training grassroots groups and a clearinghouse for information.

The Religious Coalition for Reproductive Choice (RCRC)
1025 Vermont Avenue NW, Suite 1130; Washington, DC 20002; (202) 628-7700; Fax: (202) 628-7716
E-mail: info@rcrc.org
Web site: http://www.rcrc.org
   An ecumenical coalition of 36 religious denominations and organizations. Has many publications on positions of religious organizations with regard to abortion rights.

The Reproductive Health Technologies Project
1818 N Street NW, Suite 450; Washington, DC 20036; (202) 530-2900; Fax: (202) 530-2901
E-mail: rhtp@basshowes.com
   Promotes public education and dialogue about drug-induced abortions.

The Women of Color Partnership Program (WOCPP)
c/o Religious Coalition for Reproductive Choice
(see above for address)
   Created by RCRC as a way for women of color to become actively involved in the reproductive choice movement.

Additional Online Resources *

Abortion and Reproductive Rights Internet Resources
http://www.caral.org/abortion.html

Abortion Clinics OnLine
http://www.gynpages.com

The Abortion Rights Activist
http://www.cais.com/agm/index.html

National Network of Abortion Funds
http://hamp.hampshire.edu/~clpp/nnaf/index.html

National Women's Health Organization: Abortion Information
http://gynpages.com/nwho/index.html

Planned Parenthood
http://www.ciserv.com/PlannedParenthood2

---

* For more information and listings of online resources, please see Introduction to Women's Health Online Resources, p. 25.

By Ruth Hubbard and Ami Jaeger, with
Jane Pincus and Wendy Sanford

WITH SPECIAL THANKS TO Lori Andrews,
Geri Ferber, Barbara Katz Rothman,
and Nancy Reame*

Note: This chapter covers donor
insemination, in vitro fertilization and
related technologies, surrogate motherhood,
and sex preselection. If you are facing
infertility, you might want to start with
chapter 22, Child-bearing Loss, Infertility,
and Adoption, which addresses the emotional
issues and step-by-step decisions surrounding
infertility, as well as the choice of adoption

Chapter 18

Assisted Low-Tech and High-Tech Reproductive Technologies

* Thanks also to the following for their help with the 1998 version
of this chapter: Lisa Angeraime, Diane Clapp, Jenifer Firestone,
Janna Jacobs, Linda King, Lynne Millican, Shannon Minter, Judy
Norsigian, Abha Sur, and the National Center for Lesbian Rights.
Over the years since 1982, the following also contributed to this
chapter: Gena Corea.

Imagine a group of women in a heated discussion about assisted reproductive technologies (ARTs). One woman who is experiencing infertility, and who powerfully wants to give birth, would like to make use of all the available diagnostic and treatment options, but she has no money and no insurance. Another, who also wants to bear a child, can afford to try everything possible to become pregnant. A third has not wanted to use technology to have a baby; instead, she has adopted a child. A fourth woman, who is strapped for money and wants to be of use, has had another couple's embryo implanted in her womb and wonders whether she will be able to give the baby up. A fifth, with three daughters, is trying to have a son. The sixth woman works in an underfunded public hospital; as she struggles to give adequate prenatal care to women in poverty, she questions the use of so many resources to develop ARTs.

From in vitro fertilization and embryo transfer to genetic diagnosis of an embryo before implantation, and even perhaps cloning, research scientists and physicians are devising technologies that can drastically change our relationship to child-bearing. Such technologies pose a dilemma for the authors of this book. On one hand, it is clear that some technologies help, or have the potential to help, some of us who badly want biological children and would otherwise be unable to have them. Scientific breakthroughs now offer reproductive alternatives to some infertile couples, single persons, lesbian or gay couples, postmenopausal women, women who have had chemotherapy, and fertile couples at risk of passing on a genetic disorder that they don't want their child to inherit. However, we are concerned about serious issues ranging from who does (and doesn't) get to use ARTs, to the risks they pose for women.

The authors of *Our Bodies, Ourselves for the New*

Century are aware of strongly competing needs and values regarding the more invasive and costly of the ARTs. We want to give accurate and useful information to women who are considering, or using, the technologies in an effort to have children. We want to honor the pain and frustration of women who struggle with infertility. We know that some readers have taken our previous critique of ARTs as an insensitive attack on their own needs and choices. Yet, at a time when the media and medical worlds seem to be entranced by the new technologies, and when ARTs are becoming a business, the voice of caution is often too silent. We want, therefore, to offer a careful critique not only of these technologies but also of the political and social contexts in which they are being used.

CONCERNS ABOUT THE MORE INVASIVE AND COSTLY OF THE ARTs

Some of the questions are economic. Who owns these technologies, and who profits from them? Who has access to them and who doesn't? How else might the money—and the talent—be used? Most of the money that goes into developing medical technology might be more wisely spent on preventive health measures to avoid some causes of infertilty like sexually transmitted diseases, and on basic maternal and infant health care services that are unavailable to many who live in poverty. It could go into cleaning up the increasingly toxic workplaces and neighborhoods, which also contribute to infertility. It could help make existing technologies accessible to all women, irrespective of race, ethnicity, financial resources, or insurance coverage.

Many of the new technologies involve an alarming degree of invasiveness and medical manipulation of women's bodies. Despite claims that these technologies "serve" women, our experiences with other medical technologies have taught us to be suspicious. (For instance, physicians and hospitals almost always pressure us to submit to birthing technologies that are clearly unnecessary and possibly harmful.) The long-term effects of many of the ARTs—on us and on our children—are not yet known.

As technologies proliferate, ethical challenges increase. No other generation has had to deal with the complex problems raised by the conflicting ethical principles in this particular arena. For instance, what should be done with the extra eggs and sperm (gametes), fertilized eggs (embryos), or frozen embryos that have not been implanted? Should a mother be forced against her will to give up her baby after birth if she decides she wants to keep it, even if she earlier contracted to have the baby for another woman or couple? What about the practice of aborting some fetuses during a multiple pregnancy so that one will thrive? Or, how about the potential for selecting which embryo to implant according to sex or genetic or physical constitution (including disability), or in order to produce a child who will be able to supply a needed organ or bone marrow transplant to a parent or sibling? And should children be told about the various technologies by which they came to be; does silence about these matters help or hurt the children?

The many possibilities of gestational surrogacy illustrate the kinds of dilemmas that can be raised. Gestational surrogacy, in which one woman is implanted with an egg from another woman after it has been fertilized, allows postmenopausal women to be pregnant even though they are no longer producing eggs. Should there be an age limit? In the U.S., the limit has been age 55; yet, in at least one case a 60-year-old woman falsified her medical records and conceived through egg donation. In Italy, there has been no age limit. The American Civil Liberties Union sees the age restriction in the U.S. as a form of age discrimination. Even more controversial is the use of gestational surrogacy to create children with eggs from women who have died, for either partners or grandparents to parent (called postmortem reproduction). In addition, a case has been reported in Italy of the use of a gestational surrogate to carry two unrelated embryos simultaneously for parenting by different couples. Can public policies be developed to address such possibilities adequately or fairly?

The compensation of participants raises further ethical questions about ART. Gamete donors, sperm banks, surrogates, health care professionals, lawyers, brokers, and adoption agencies are all compensated for their contributions to the process. Does compensation induce women to participate in a process they might not otherwise consider while allowing third parties (i.e., doctors and lawyers) to profit? Is procreation being reshaped as a manufacturing process?

The commercialization of in vitro fertilization treatments has resulted in the emergence of questionable ethical practices among infertility specialists, such as money-back guarantees if pregnancy is not achieved, and the option of reduced treatment costs for egg sharing with other women. One of the most appalling events has been the deliberate theft of embryos by physicians at the University of California at Irvine in 1994 for use by other infertile women.

What is the final goal of those who carry on reproductive engineering? Proponents talk about goals like "the ultimate manufacture of a human being to exact specifications." Who will decide these specifications? In a society where women have less power than men, and women of color have less power than white women, will these technologies be a means of further controlling our freedom to make choices about our bodies, exposing us to yet more exploitation and abuse? Will they be used to create more white babies for affluent families, while babies of color worldwide suffer from high infant mortality rates?

The scientists who research these technologies, the physicians who apply them, the legislators who approve and fund the research, and the pharmaceutical company directors who translate them into products to be profited from are usually well paid, white, and male. To what extent are these people motivated to address the needs of diverse women? Reseachers, for example, may be more interested in the fame and funding that come from achieving scientific break-throughs than in the well-being of women.

This society, like so many others, judges our worth as women by our fertility. As if wanting a baby and being unable to bear one isn't painful enough, family, friends and even people we don't know well heap an extra load of guilt on us by making us feel inadequate or unwomanly if, in the face of all the new resources, we still can't bear children "of our own." The mother of the first test-tube baby expressed the guilt she had felt:

"I'm not a normal woman," I told John. . . . "I wouldn't even blame you now if you went off with someone else." . . . It wasn't John's fault. He could have as many children as he liked with another woman. A whole football team.[1]

These pressures may explain why some of us pursue time-consuming, painful, and at times degrading tests and medical manipulations to have a child. Even when we are exhausted and drained of almost every cent we possess, each new technological intervention offers yet another possibility of success, hooking us into continued involvement.

*It is an emotional roller coaster because every month your hopes rise and you think "Oh, **this** treatment will work," and then it all falls apart. Then you reconstruct all that hope and you go through it again.*

Some infertility specialists may play upon a woman's or couple's intense desire to have a child. You may feel that you have lost control and that you are manipulated by the succession of procedures: Isn't there always something more that you can do? How can you bring this process of attempted conception to closure? As one woman said,

If there's always something more that you can do, it becomes a situation where you don't even have control over when is enough.

Even the less invasive infertility techniques can expose a very private corner of our lives and open us to endless questions and advice from relatives, friends, and physicians, who may recommend surgery, drugs, or other risky and invasive procedures. Our partners often share our sense of violation and our increased uncertainty.

There is no inner recess of me left unexplored, unprobed, unmolested. It occurs to me when I have sex that what used to be beautiful and very private is now degraded and terribly public. I bring my menstrual cycle charts to the doctor like a child bringing home a report card. Tell me, did I do well? Did I ovulate? Did I have sex at the right times as you instructed me?

If you are deciding whether or not to use ART, or how far to go, it may help to talk with friends and other women and families who have used these technologies, and those who have chosen not to. Be on the lookout for knowledgeable, compassionate support. Such guidance will enable you to be the best judge of what you need, what pressures you are feeling, and what decisions will serve you best in the long run.

There will always be those of us with a fierce desire to bear children. Even under optimal social and economic circumstances worldwide, there will always be children whose biological parents cannot care for them. Once we connect ourselves to the larger community, we may feel less pressure to give birth to our "own" children, and be more apt to adopt or to become foster parents, or to love, nurture, and be loved by our neighbors', friends', or relatives' children. (For more on adoption as an alternative, see chapter 22.)

DONOR INSEMINATION (DI) *

The simplest, most widely used, and least invasive of the technologies we are considering, DI does not require professional help, and you can do it at home. This kind of insemination is often called "artificial insemination by donor" or "alternative insemination." It can be used by women (lesbian and otherwise) who wish to get pregnant without having a male partner. It can be used by women with male partners when the man has fertility problems or risks passing on a hereditary disease the couple wants to avoid, or if the couple experiences structural or psychological barriers to intercourse. At present, women in the U.S. are conceiving more than 30,000 babies a year by this method.

To use DI on your own, you should have no fertility problems and your menstrual cycle should be fairly regular, although you can check your fertile time even when your cycle is irregular. To find out when you are likely to ovulate, you can chart your basal body temperature and mucus consistency for a few months (see "Fertility Observation," chapter 13, Birth Control, p. 305). A urine test kit purchasable in a drug store can help you time the insemination by detecting the hormone burst that precedes ovulation by about 24 hours. The kits contain detailed instructions and are relatively simple to use. There are several brands, all of which work on the same principle.

Fresh Sperm vs. Frozen Sperm: Protecting Your Health

To protect your health, the American Society for Reproductive Medicine (formerly the American Fertility Society) has issued guidelines strongly advising

---

* An excellent resource for anyone choosing DI is *Lesbians Choosing Motherhood: Legal Implications of Alternative Insemination and Reproductive Technologies,* edited by Kate Kendell and Robin Haaland, 1996 (see Resources).

women to use only frozen, not fresh, semen. You can use semen from a sperm bank or bring your donor's semen to a sperm bank. It will be tested for infectious diseases, including HIV/AIDS, and then frozen and held in quarantine from three to six (some say nine) months. At that point, the donor should be tested again. Only if *that* test result is also negative should the semen be used. Some physicians have the facilities to screen and store frozen semen correctly. Sperm banks do *not* screen for genetic anomalies; donors are asked for their history, but they may not know that problems exist, or they may not mention some they know about.

Unfortunately, using frozen semen takes more time and usually costs more money: about $130 per vial of semen. DI through a physician costs about $140 a month at two inseminations per cycle with fresh semen and $200 to $300 if frozen semen is used. This does not usually include practitioners' fees. Sadly, insurance covers DI in only a few states, and then usually only for heterosexual couples for "medical reasons," i.e., if the man's sperm is inadequate.

It takes longer to become pregnant with frozen semen because sperm motility (capability for movement) is decreased upon thawing; thawed sperm cells also have a shorter life span than fresh sperm, and a reduced ability to penetrate cervical mucus. This may mean that you will need to attempt more inseminations in order to become pregnant.

Women who cannot afford frozen semen or clinic and physician fees, and who use fresh semen, are at a greater risk for HIV and other infections. The donor may not be aware of an infection himself, or he may neglect to tell you. If you must use fresh sperm, it's safest if your donor is celibate or at least monogamous, if he's practiced safer sex for at least six months before the insemination, if he's sober, and if both he and his sexual partner(s) can show you the negative results of two or more recent HIV antibody tests. (See chapter 15, HIV, AIDS, and Women, for more.)

Choosing a Sperm Donor

There are several ways of obtaining semen. You may ask a male friend or acquaintance to donate sperm. If you want anonymity, you may ask friends to find someone for you. You can get inseminated with the help of a health care practitioner or clinic with access to a sperm bank. You can also negotiate directly with a sperm bank, which will send you a catalog of unidentified potential donors with basic information about their size, eye and hair color, race, and ethnicity. Once you narrow the choice down to a few, you will see the "long file" on each, which will include family medical history and short essays by the donor about his personality and about his reasons for donating semen. Once you choose among the donors, you can negotiate with the sperm bank about how and when each "straw" containing semen will be delivered, and how much each will cost. Some sperm banks offer the DI children a choice of finding out who the donor is,

although usually not until the child reaches adolescence or later. It is important to think through whether this is an option you want for your child. (See the book *Lethal Secrets,* in Resources.)

You can inseminate at home, or go to a clinic to be inseminated. Ask other women what they decided to do and why. You can learn a great deal from their experiences.

As a single woman doing donor insemination, I found it very difficult to get support from medical staff, support groups, and even my own friends. It was a lonely experience. Everything in the patient education materials talked about "husbands." Well, I didn't have one, and that didn't make it any easier!

If you are not using semen from a sperm bank, you might want to have your donor's fertility checked by a fertility clinic before attempting an insemination. Sperm analysis is relatively cheap, and male infertility is fairly common. If the semen comes from a sperm bank, you can ask your health care practitioner to examine it for sperm number and motility after it thaws. If it is of inferior quality, you can get a replacement straw.

Insemination

When you inseminate, the semen should be at body temperature. When you know that you are about to ovulate, thaw the semen from the sperm bank for a few hours at room temperature, or ask the sperm donor to ejaculate into a clean (preferably boiled, but always cooled) container. (Frozen sperm is preferable healthwise—see above.) Semen should be used as quickly as possible, but surely within 30 minutes of ejaculation or thawing; you or your partner can maintain the semen's temperature by placing the container in your armpit, cleavage, or crotch. Suck up the semen with a needleless hypodermic syringe, an eye dropper, or a turkey baster. You (or your partner or friend) then gently insert the syringe into your vagina while you lie flat on your back with your rear up on a pillow. Empty the syringe into your vagina to deposit the semen as close to your cervix as possible. Continue lying down comfortably for ten minutes or so, so that semen doesn't leak from your vagina.

Even if you do not have a partner to assist you in this process, it can help to have loving friends with you while you inseminate.

One of the few humorous aspects of becoming a single mom was getting pregnant. After a miscarriage it took several insemination attempts for me to get pregnant. In the absence of a significant other to do the inseminating, I asked various friends to do the honors. When I needed to inseminate over a long holiday weekend on the Cape with friends, everyone wanted a piece of the action. I inserted the speculum while the three of them crowded between my legs, squinting through the flashlight, and ogling my textbook-perfect cervix. As if being initiated into a revered secret society, each one enthusiastically took her turn drawing the specimen into the catheter and dribbling it into my mucus-covered os. We just laughed and laughed at this insemination by committee.

It is a good idea to inseminate every other day over the five days just before, during, and after you ovulate. Most women under 35 become pregnant after doing DI for three to five cycles. However, this varies depending on the quality of the sperm, whether it's been frozen, and your own fertility. Health care professionals don't yet understand all the factors involved.

An increasing number of women are choosing to become inseminated at health centers or clinics. You may feel more secure doing so. Health care practitioners are there to assist you, but it also turns the experience into a more medical and initially more expensive event. Some clinics try to increase pregnancy rates by adding ovulatory enhancement drugs to trigger more eggs to be released (also increasing the chance of a multiple pregnancy). Some may even suggest intrauterine insemination (in which the sperm is specially prepared by removing prostaglandins, which can cause cramping, and inserted directly into your uterus via a tiny catheter). These more invasive approaches to insemination may or may not be what you want. Remember that it is up to you whether or not to accept any drugs or technical interventions that are offered.

Knowing Your Donor vs. Anonymity *

Mutual anonymity between you and the man who donates the sperm may be important for both of you and can forestall legal and emotional complications. A known donor may later decide that he wants to have custody and visitation rights. Problems have arisen when a man who gave his sperm had a change of feelings and sued for visitation or wanted to give the child his surname. Single and lesbian women especially have to guard against this kind of harassment. The sperm donor, too, may need protection, because a court may later assert a *known* donor's responsibility for child support.

There are also arguments *against* anonymity. Sometimes unmarried women, both heterosexual and lesbian, want the donor to be a friend who wants to be involved in the child's life. Also, just as adopted children are making increasing efforts to locate their biological parents, some children conceived by DI may later be disturbed and angry if they cannot find out who their biological father is. In addition, health problems may arise that may make us or our children want to have access to the sperm donor's medical history. (Most sperm banks will contact the donor when a medical need arises.)

* See also "Legal Issues" in chapter 10, Relationships with Women.

Legal Issues

The legal status of DI differs in different states and is sometimes unclear. It is a good idea to be aware of the laws in your state.

There is an automatic assumption in every state that the biological father of a child is the legal father. Every state has its own regulations for how the donor can legally relinquish his parental rights; many states require a physician's involvement for this. If you don't want the donor to be considered the legal father of the child, be sure to comply with whatever steps your state requires. In some states, the lesbian partner of a woman who has a child by DI can adopt that child, so that both can be legal parents. (This is called co-parent adoption; see the section on legal issues in chapter 10, Relationships with Women.)

If you have a known donor, you may want to create a written agreement with the donor (and preferably also with his partner, if he has one), to clarify everyone's intentions. The agreement could spell out specifically that you do (or don't) want him considered to be the child's parent, what his role is expected to be (if any), how much contact he is to have with the child, etc. However, there is no state where a written agreement like this is legally enforceable.

Is DI for You?

DI isn't right for everybody. It raises different questions for different people. Some married women have said that they felt as though they were committing adultery. (The Roman Catholic and Orthodox Jewish religions do consider DI to be adultery.) A partner may not feel as involved in the pregnancy or parenthood as you had hoped, because the baby isn't his or her biological child. If you value genetic continuity and family resemblances highly, then DI is not for you. Think about what you will tell close friends and family, and—most important—what you will tell your child. Many heterosexual parents in the past have kept DI a secret, perhaps to protect the man from the embarrassment of having people know he is infertile. (Fertility and sexual potency—particularly in the sense of the ability to achieve erection and ejaculation—are often mistakenly linked.) Don't assume from the start that you must be secretive or, conversely, tell all.

There is a growing body of work on the psychosocial adjustment and development of children conceived via DI. The bottom line is that these children are well adjusted and high on the development charts in some variables. However, most studies so far have been done on children of heterosexual couples who have not told the children about their origin.[2]

Many women have used DI happily and successfully. Two lesbian partners, who plan to raise children together, told about the bond it created between them for one to help the other with her insemination. Another woman, more ambivalent, said:

Our daughter is really extraordinary—enormous energy, very strong-willed, and totally different-looking from either of us. I am reminded constantly that her father was a stranger.

And one wrote:

My husband and I had more than our share of doubts right up until the moment of our daughter's birth. When we saw our baby girl, all our doubts disappeared.

As with all ARTs, even with this most low-tech version, it is important to know that we can stop trying when the effort no longer feels right.

I decided to try one last time to inseminate, but this cycle was different in that I did not feel the enormous pressure to succeed. Marie and I now had decided upon adoption as another option, which felt like a tremendous relief. As it turned out, I became pregnant . . . When I look at my daughter, I am so aware of what a miracle it is to have her in our lives.

IN VITRO FERTILIZATION (IVF) AND RELATED TECHNOLOGIES

In vitro is Latin for "in glass." In vitro fertilization (IVF) involves extracting ripe eggs from your ovary, fertilizing them with sperm in a glass dish, and placing the embryo back in your, or another woman's, womb. IVF is a biologically and technically complicated procedure that is still experimental in many respects and poses risks for women. It is intended primarily for women whose ovaries and uterus appear to function normally, but whose fallopian tubes are blocked or don't function properly so the egg cannot get to the uterus. (Ironically, many who seek IVF might not need it at all if the medical and public health community had provided information and regular screening for preventable diseases that can lead to infertility in the first place, like pelvic inflammatory disease, endometriosis, and sexually transmitted diseases.) IVF will cost from $10,000 to $15,000 in addition to the medical expenses associated with pregnancy and birth. Despite the high cost in money, time, and emotional wear and tear, many women decide to be screened, via infertility testing, for the procedure, and then decide to try it. Every year in the U.S., about 20,000 women undergo some 40,000 cycles of IVF, and about 6,000 IVF babies were born in 1994.[3]

While the authors of this book have many concerns about the use of IVF and its related technologies (please see the introduction to this chapter for more on this), we also feel it is important that if you have made the decision to undergo IVF, you get accurate and useful information. We hope the following discussion will help you keep as much control as possible in an enterprise that is so highly technical, and so commercialized, that it tends to be controlled by the providers and technicians rather than by the women who are trying to have children.

IVF is an expensive and rigorous experience, with risks. If you choose to undergo IVF, try to surround yourself with support. You might want to supplement the medical routines you will have to follow with help from friends, family, other women who have gone through the procedures, infertility support groups, and a therapist, if necessary.

Making the decision to do IVF was a difficult one. Everything felt so clinical. I had to carry my husband's sperm to the lab, and have my eggs taken from me and my embryos put back into me in a treatment room in a clinic. It was a far cry from making our baby at home. When the clinic called to say that my eggs had fertilized, I started to feel bonded to them. When they didn't implant, and I got my period, I really grieved for what we almost had.

It is important to select a physician with whom you feel comfortable, who will take the time to listen to all your hopes and fears and answer all your questions. You may want to look for a clinic that provides counseling for you, and jointly for you and your partner. Discuss with your health care practitioner the time frame in which you will be trying to become pregnant; implantation usually occurs after four to six cycles. You might think in advance about how long you want to undergo IVF and, if it isn't working, what will help you recognize when it's right for you to stop, then discuss this with your partner or supportive friends as well as your health care practitioner. This may help you respect your own limits in a process that can take on a momentum of its own.

In choosing a clinic, be aware that it is in each clinic's interest to promise high success rates. Federal law requires clinics to report pregnancy rates. Ask what the live birth rate is, the live birth rate per stimulation cycle, and the pregnancy rate per embryo transfer for women of your age (success diminishes with age) and with your particular diagnosis. Check out the clinic's statistics with the American Society for Reproductive Medicine, or call Resolve for more specific information (see Resources for both). Despite promises that with more experience the success rates of IVF clinics will improve more than just a little, they remain just about what they were in the early 1990s.

It is also important to know the risks involved with IVF. Some of the risks are associated with the drugs, some with the procedure itself. Drug risks include ovarian hyperstimulation syndrome (OHSS), which is a shift or imbalance in the hormone system. In severe cases, OHSS results in swelling of the ovary and the collection of extra fluid in the pelvis. Hospitalization is rarely needed, but in rare cases OHSS can be fatal. The drugs are a suspected risk factor in ovarian cancer and in increased ovarian cyst formation. Risks suspected with GnRH (Lupron—see p. 426) include oversuppression with impaired ovarian reserve, and possibly memory impairment. Good studies are needed to determine the true risks of taking these drugs. The risks associated with egg retrieval and embryo transfer include infection, needle injuries, adverse reactions to anesthesia, and reduced uterine receptivity because of a thinner endometrium. With IVF there is an increased risk of ectopic pregnancy (pregnancy in the fallopian tube); miscarriage rates are as high as 20 to 24%; and you have a greater chance of multiple pregnancies, which put more stress on your body and on the babies, and tend to medicalize your pregnancy.

There are other issues, as well. A procedure that requires this much technical expertise is completely under professional control. We and our partners will never have much say about where or how we want it done. Because the pregnancies are so precious (emotionally, technically, and financially), we are under pressure to "manage" pregnancy and birth just as the physicians order, regardless of how we might wish to have our babies. Many women who become pregnant via IVF have a cesarean section, which always gives the doctor more control over the birth without necessarily improving birth outcomes. (Some women who use IVF may have medical complications, either from their infertility or the IVF pregnancy, that may make cesarean section necessary.)

Are there risks to the children born of IVF? Most IVF providers argue that if an egg or embryo is damaged, it simply won't develop. But we won't know whether that is true until thousands of babies conceived in vitro have had a chance to grow up. There is no doubt, however, that multiple pregnancies, especially those involving more than twins, bring greater risks to the babies than single pregnancies do.

IVF Procedure

Different physicians and clinics are developing their own methods and modifications, and the use of drugs depends on a woman's age. The procedure usually involves the following steps:

1. To trigger the development of viable follicles, you will be given combinations of various hormones. (See chapter 22, Child-bearing Loss, Infertility, and Adoption, for more on these hormones.) The most commonly used fertility drugs are injectable human menopausal gonadotropins (hMG), which contain follicle-stimulating hormone (FSH) and luteinizing hormone (LH). New brand names for hMG appear frequently; Humegon is a current one. Some drugs contain only FSH (one brand is Fertinex). Many centers combine hMG and FSH with so-called gonadotropin-releasing agonists (substances that enable changes to occur), such as GnRH (Lupron or Synarel). GnRH controls the rate of follicle development. During the first part of each of your cycles, you will have ultrasound monitoring of the follicles and frequent blood tests to check hormone levels. About 10 to 20% of women cannot continue beyond this point because of poor or limited follicle development.

2. A few hours before the egg would be naturally released if it were not retrieved, you will get a final injection of hCG, regardless of whether hMG, FSH, or GnRH was used to stimulate follicle growth. The hCG completes egg maturation. Your medical practitioner will retrieve the eggs from the ovary, using ultrasound-guided needle aspiration. While you are under light sedation, she or he will insert a thin needle into your vagina and through the vaginal wall into the body cavity in order to remove the mature eggs from the ovarian follicles. You are likely to receive local anesthesia, which numbs the upper vaginal wall. After they are removed, the eggs are inspected and brought to maturity in an incubator for two to 36 hours. Sperm and eggs are then mixed and incubated for 12 to 18 hours. (With this and all IVF-related procedures, make sure that any donated sperm or eggs are screened for transmissible diseases.)

3. If fertilization takes place, the embryos are transferred to your uterus after 24 to 60 hours, when they reach the four- to eight-cell stage. In order to increase implantation rates, frequently three or four embryos will be transferred.

    You should be aware that you can decide beforehand (and record your decision through an informed consent document, or an additional contract or directive) what you want done with the embryos that result from IVF. You may have them frozen for later implantation for yourself, so that if this IVF cycle fails, you can bypass steps 1 and 2 in a next attempt; about 50 to 70% of frozen embryos survive the thawing process, and, when implanted, 13 to 15% result in pregnancy. You may donate them for research, or to another woman for implantation. Or, you may have them discarded. Before donating them to another person, it is wise to consider the emotional effects of doing so, if you cannot achieve a pregnancy yourself. You might also want to prepare a directive about what should become of your embryos in the event that you are divorced or die.

4. Twelve to 14 days after the embryo transfer, you can have a pregnancy test done or do one yourself (kits are widely available in drugstores). If the result is positive, you will receive progesterone suppositories or shots for as long as ten to 12 weeks. Only 10 to 15% of women undergoing IVF get to this point.

It is inevitable that mistakes will be made, and these may cause women to believe that the process, or we ourselves, have "failed."

As more personnel become involved in handling gametes and embryos, the number of embryos lost be-

cause of negligent handling or accidents in the laboratory may increase. Often couples may not learn of these mishaps, but be told that "eggs did not fertilize," that "zygotes didn't cleave," or that "your embryos were not viable." Internal pressures to cover up errors should be resisted.[4]

As IVF clinics proliferate, it is clear that more regulation is needed.*

Techniques Related to IVF

Intercytoplastic sperm injection (ICSI) is a procedure in which sperm is injected into an egg in an attempt to achieve fertilization. However, using sperm cells that have not been able to fertilize an egg on their own might lead to as yet unknown problems in the future. In *gamete intrafallopian transfer* (GIFT), the egg is "harvested" by ultrasound-guided needle aspiration, as in IVF. Egg and sperm are mixed in the body cavity during a procedure using a laparascope (see chapter 24, Selected Medical Practices, Problems, and Procedures, p. 596) and placed back in the fallopian tube. GIFT has a higher success rate than IVF. (See note 3 for statistics on GIFT and ZIFT.) *Zygote intrafallopian transfer* (ZIFT) involves the laparoscopic "harvesting" of the egg, fertilization by sperm outside a woman's body, and then placement of the embryo, at an early stage of cell division, in the fallopian tubes. ZIFT has a slightly higher success rate than GIFT and IVF. *Micromanipulation of the egg* (making a small opening in the outer membrane of the egg wall) is another technique used to increase fertilization rates.

Donor egg IVF has become an option for women with early menopause (premature ovarian failure) or who have disorders that may be genetically transferred. In these instances, either a woman or a clinic finds another woman willing to donate her eggs. This donor will undergo the same hormone treatment to induce ovulation as do the women undergoing IVF, but once her eggs have been retrieved and fertilized, any resulting embryos will be placed in the uterus of the woman who is trying to become pregnant. Women who use this option have a 30 to 40% chance of becoming pregnant. They are not genetically related to the fetuses they carry. Donor egg IVF has been used by some lesbian couples; when one member of a couple donates the egg and the other is the birth mother, both have a biological connection to the child.

IVF can also be used for *preimplantation genetic diagnosis*. This procedure tests the DNA of an embryo (thus testing for certain transmissible characteristics of the child that would develop from that embryo) before it is placed in your uterus. If you know that a condition such as cystic fibrosis or Huntington's disease runs in your or your partner's family, this procedure makes it possible to avoid having a child inherit it, without terminating an already started pregnancy. In preimplantation genetic diagnosis, one of the cells is removed from each of the four- to eight-cell embryos, before the embryos are put into your uterus or frozen and stored for possible future use. The DNA of the removed cell is tested for the condition you wish to avoid, and only the embryos that pass this screen are implanted. This procedure does not guarantee a healthy baby, only one that will not develop the condition(s) for which the embryos have been tested.

This high-tech procedure, which can also be used for sex preselection, allows parents to make the decision not to implant an embryo that is of the "wrong" sex or "wrong" health status. These decisions have complicated social and ethical implications. (For a related discussion, please see the box on "Abortion, Amniocentesis, and Disability," in chapter 17, Abortion, p. 403.) Were such decision-making to pass out of the hands of parents and into the control of medical or government personnel, the procedure could easily become a form of social control. It raises many of the toughest social and ethical questions discussed in the introduction and elsewhere in this chapter.

CLONING

This term is used to describe two different procedures. One procedure depends on the fact that all the cells of an early embryo are equivalent. When implanted, each can develop into a complete organism that will be genetically identical to organisms developed from the other cells that came from that embryo. Such organisms would be "clones" of one another, and the procedure is sometimes called *artificial twinning*. So-called identical twins, who develop by one embryo splitting into two, are clones of each other in this sense. Researchers have been able for some time to produce animal clones for cattle breeding by splitting embryos in this way.

A newer and more specialized cloning procedure hit the headlines in early 1997, when researchers in Scotland who study livestock breeding discovered a way to produce a lamb without using sperm. They made a lamb by taking an egg from one sheep and removing its genetic material, then transferring into this egg the genetic material taken from a single mammary gland cell of another sheep, a six-year-old adult female. Normally, embryos originate only from the reproductive cells (eggs and sperm), because of these cells' capacity to undergo millions of cell divisions and further development into different cell types, each with a special function (e.g., hair, kidney, bone cells). Once the specialized body cells (*somatic cells*) are formed, they normally can only divide and produce more cells like themselves. Some body cells, like those of the spinal cord, lose even this ability. Scientists had believed it was impossible to make these specialized adult cells act like embryonic cells and produce an entire organism. Creating the sheep was an amazing scientific breakthrough because it showed for the first time that the genes of adult cells could be reprogrammed to retrieve their embryonic "memories" and

---

* For a copy of model legislation to regulate IVF services, send $3.00 to the BWHBC, 240A Elm Street, Somerville, MA 02144.

behave like the fertilized egg from which they arose many, many cell divisions ago. (That the reasearchers named the baby lamb "Dolly" after Dolly Parton, an entertainer who has been the target of jokes because of her large breasts, suggests the persistence of sexism and poor taste among even the finest research scientists.)

These techniques are of major interest to animal breeders, who are constantly looking for ways to avoid the element of chance in traditional animal breeding. It is not clear what, if any, relevance these techniques have for human reproduction. Few practical uses can be envisaged for human cloning, and those that have been put forward—extra copies of people for spare parts or to replace a dying loved one—are deeply problematic to most people. Great Britain, where "Dolly" originated, and the entire European community, have passed laws against human cloning. Some people argue against such legislation on the basis that no doors should be legally closed to free inquiry. To others, this is a weak argument against a technology that would turn people into objects, manufactured according to specifications.

CONTRACT (OR "SURROGATE") MOTHERHOOD

Contract, or "surrogate" motherhood—whereby a woman goes through pregnancy and gives birth to a baby destined for another person or couple—is a controversial practice made more widely available by the development of certain ARTs. It is called *surrogacy, AI (artificial insemination) surrogacy; surrogate motherhood;* and *contract motherhood.* (From time to time, this chapter will use the word "surrogate," in quotes, because the term implies that the woman who carries the baby is not its mother.) As surrogacy is most often practiced in the U.S., one woman—the *"surrogate" mother*—contracts with a man, or with a couple, to be inseminated with his sperm via *donor insemination* and to bear a child that she will turn over to him or them at birth. Typically, the man is married and his wife adopts the baby. They pay the "surrogate" mother her expenses and a fee (usually about $15,000). A mediating agency and/or a lawyer may require substantial additional fees. As of 1996, there had been about 6,000 such births in this country.

Gestational surrogacy (sometimes called being a *gestational carrier*) is similar to surrogacy, but it differs in that the egg used to create the embryo is not that of the woman who carries ("gestates"), and gives birth to, the baby. Thus, the gestational carrier has no genetic relationship to the child. The eggs and sperm of the contracting couple (called the donated *gametes*) or of others who have provided them, are brought together in a laboratory by *in vitro fertilization* techniques. The resulting embryo is implanted in the gestational surrogate mother.

Surrogacy may help some women who have a fertile male partner or sperm donor but cannot get pregnant or carry a fetus to term, or both. Gestational surrogacy can be used when a man and woman can conceive, but the woman cannot carry the fetus to term. Surrogacy also affords possibilities for men without female partners.

As you may imagine, this enterprise raises a host of social, legal, and financial questions. Can we, before we even become pregnant, contract to give up a baby (whether or not it is genetically related to us) and be sure that we will want to live with the decision once the baby has been born? Aren't the issues currently being raised by birth mothers who have given up children for adoption likely to surface for "surrogate" mothers? It is also far from obvious what the couple's obligations should be if they separate or change their minds during the pregnancy. If the baby they contracted for is born with an unanticipated health problem, formal surrogacy agreements spell out that the contracting couple must accept the child. A stickier issue is whether the contracting couple can require the "surrogate" mother to have amniocentesis (and, presumably, consider an abortion if a health problem is predicted or verified).

Not only do those of us who become surrogate mothers bear the stresses and risks of pregnancy and birth, but our life may be controlled in many ways. We may have to undergo certain kinds of testing or restrictions during pregnancy, for instance, which we might not normally choose for ourselves. For gestational "surrogates," there are additional physical and financial burdens: In order to gestate an embryo that is not our own, we must undergo repeated hormonal injections and blood sampling, and the invasive procedure of embryo transfer.

Another strong concern is that the surrogacy option puts pressure on some of us to "rent out" our bodies as a way to earn money. One woman said, "It's a business endeavor that satisfies monetary needs and emotional needs." But, in that case, what is a fair price? A $15,000 fee provides a "surrogate" mother with only $2.11 an hour. Some surrogate mothers have asked to be paid only for their expenses, saying that they want to give the child as a gift to a woman who cannot bear children. By contrast, some advocates of paid surrogacy argue that it enhances the choices for all parties involved and that "surrogate" mothers should be paid more money for their time and efforts. Some critics argue that neither surrogate mothers, lawyers, brokers, nor gamete donors should be paid for their services.

At least 16 states have enacted surrogacy legislation, addressing the tough issues of whether a contract signed before a baby's conception should be legally binding after birth, who the legal parents are, whether third parties should be involved, and whether payment should be allowed. The legislative approaches range from banning paid surrogacy contracts to legalizing them. Only a minority of state laws address parental rights for both the gestational mother and the potential parents—an issue that can become as complicated as there are personal situations to sort out.

The courts have tackled several surrogacy cases. So far, only a small number of women have changed their minds and sued the couple to keep their maternal rights. In the landmark "Baby M" decision, the court did not recognize the contract and did not require the surrogate mother to relinquish her parental rights; the court held that the man providing the sperm was the legal father, and the surrogate (who had both a pregnancy and a genetic link) was the legal mother. In cases involving surrogate gestational mothers, courts are adopting the position that the people who provided the gametes (sperm and egg) are the legal parents, and have not recognized the gestational surrogate (who has a pregnancy link but not a genetic link) as a legal mother. It becomes more complicated when the couple who provided the gametes divorces during the pregnancy. In one gestational surrogacy case, when the couple divorced, the wife was able to assert her parental rights and request shared custody because she had a genetic link to the baby. In another case, the court's award of parental rights relied not on genetic links, but on the intentions of the gamete-providing couple to rear the child.

The long-term impact on all the parties involved in a surrogacy arrangement is unknown. Are there "safeguards" that can protect any of them from harm? The child born of surrogacy arrangements is perhaps most at risk, and can be protected only by clearly establishing parental rights before birth and providing a stable, nurturing home for him or her. The surrogate mother is at physical, emotional, and financial risk. Whether, and how, she should be protected is being hotly debated. Whether a contract can protect her, or whether she should even be allowed to enter into a contract, is at the heart of such debate. The intended parents risk that the surrogate will change her mind and not turn the child over to them. State laws vary, but usually, so far, a contract cannot compel a woman to relinquish a child to whom she has given birth. Nor can the intended parents compel the surrogate to terminate the pregnancy, and in most states they must accept the child. The egg donors are at physical risk, which can best be reduced by safe medical practices. The egg donor, like sperm donors, should be able to decide whether she wants to permit the child to contact her later or maintain her privacy. Payment to sperm donors has never been questioned, although payment to egg donors is banned in some states. There is no logical reason for this disparity.

Concerned about the fine line between "gestational services" and the actual "purchasing" of a child, and about the potential problems for children of surrogacy arrangements, the National Women's Health Network issued the following critique in 1987 which remains compelling today:

1. Commercial surrogacy arrangements are contrary to public policy and existing laws, disregard the value of human life, exploit women, and should be prohibited by law.

2. Laws against commercial surrogacy arrangements should be directed against any party to such an arrangement including, but not limited to, the man

and/or woman who seek to purchase a child, the woman who carries and/or gives birth to the child, the agency or attorneys who are paid for the transaction, the physician or medical center which is paid for the medical testing and procedures, and any other brokers to the arrangement.

3. All surrogacy contracts or agreements should be unenforceable, because no woman should be forced to give up a child on the basis of a surrender signed prior to conception or birth. The gestational mother—the woman who gives birth to the child —is, and should continue to be, recognized as the mother for all legal purposes. Furthermore, surrogacy contracts violate existing laws and public policy.

Some feminists disagree, arguing that paid surrogacy enhances the choices for all parties involved. See Resources for fuller discussions of this controversial topic.

SEX PRESELECTION

Attempts to control the sex of a child span from low-tech approaches like restricting intercourse or insemination to specific times of the month, to the controversial method of selective abortion, to high-tech scenarios involving the selection of which embryos to introduce into a woman's womb. Some couples try to choose the sex of their child for medical reasons, because certain inherited diseases—for example, hemophilia and a type of muscular dystrophy—are much more likely to affect boys than girls. But some people just feel strongly that they want to have a child only if they can be sure it will be the gender they prefer.

The lower-tech methods for attempting to control the sex of a child before conception depend on the fact that a child's sex is determined by the father. The reason is as follows. All our cells contain 46 chromosomes, which come in 23 pairs. We get one member of each pair from our mother, the other from our father. One of the 23 pairs determines sex. They are the *sex chromosomes*, called X and Y. Women have two X chromosomes; men have one X and one Y. Mature eggs and sperm contain only one member of each chromosome pair and therefore only one sex chromosome. Since a woman has only X chromosomes, all her eggs contain an X. Since a man is XY, about half his sperm cells contain an X chromosome and half a Y. If an egg (which is always X) is fertilized by a sperm that contains an X, the child will be a girl (XX); if it is fertilized by a sperm that contains a Y, the child will be a boy (XY). (In rare instances, it is not clear whether a baby is a boy or a girl. Please see the introduction to Part Two for a brief discussion and resources about intersexuals and transsexualism.)

The low-tech methods of sex preselection try to favor the X- or the Y-bearing sperm, but none are very effective. They rely on observations that Y-bearing sperm tend to swim faster and would be more easily damaged by the acidic environment of the vagina than

X-bearing sperm, whereas X-bearing sperm appear to live longer and be more sensitive to the alkalinity in the cervix, uterus, and fallopian tubes. One recommendation is that to improve the likelihood of conceiving a girl, you should have intercourse or inseminate 36 to 48 hours before ovulation and, for a boy, try delaying intercourse or insemination until two to 24 hours before you ovulate (see "Fertility Observation," chapter 13, Birth Control, p. 305). Confusingly, other researchers have come up with the opposite recommendation: that intercourse/insemination a few days before ovulation weights the chances in favor of boys, and intercourse/insemination at the time of ovulation weights them very slightly in favor of girls.

Another recommended technique makes use mainly of the differences in the sensitivities of X and Y sperm to acid and alkali. Proponents suggest that to load the dice in favor of a girl, you use a mildly acidic douche (2 tablespoons of white vinegar in a quart of lukewarm water) before intercourse/insemination, deposit the semen close to the entrance of the vagina (so that the sperm must spend a longer time in the acidic environment of the vagina), be in a face-to-face position, and avoid your own orgasm, which increases the alkalinity of the vagina. If you prefer a boy, you use an alkaline douche (2 tablespoons of baking soda in a quart of water) and reverse the other conditions. Neither method guarantees success, but they may improve the odds.

Obviously, these methods deal only in probabilities. If your genetic history is such that a male child would have a 50:50 chance of inheriting a disease you wish to avoid, you may want to be more certain. In that case, have a health care provider determine the fetus's sex after you are pregnant. In addition to sex, increasing numbers of sex-linked diseases can now be diagnosed in a fetus. If you learn that the fetus is male, or if you learn that the disease you feared is, in fact, present, you can be more prepared for coping with the disease both emotionally and practically should you decide to continue the pregnancy. You can also make the difficult decision whether to end the pregnancy. (Please see the box on "Abortion, Amniocentesis, and Disability," in chapter 17, Abortion, p. 403.)

Fetal sex can be determined during IVF before the embryo is implanted (see p. 427). It can be determined during the first trimester of pregnancy by *chorionic villus sampling* (CVS). (Please see "Tests and Procedures," chapter 19, Pregnancy, p. 462, for description and risks.) Fetal sex can also be determined by amniocentesis, but this cannot be done until about the 14th week of pregnancy. Since it takes another three or four weeks to complete the chromosomal analysis, if you decide to abort, it means a second-trimester abortion—more painful, risky, and psychologically difficult than early abortion.

Members of the antiabortion movement have attempted to manipulate qualms about this practice into opposition to all abortions. By exaggerating the incidence of abortions for sex selection, they claim that this is further evidence of the callousness and selfishness of those who advocate choice.

Feminists in other countries, such as India, have protested sex selection for different reasons. Where there has been strong cultural pressure to bear male children, women have used abortion to avoid giving birth to female children. In India, for example, the usual sex ratio has been reversed, resulting in a significant demographic imbalance in favor of men. This reversal has been attributed primarily to willful neglect of female babies, but sex selection certainly adds to it. Indian feminists have called for an end to the widespread use of amniocentesis and chorionic villus tests for sex selection. Although this practice is now illegal in some places, it continues in a country where female infanticide is still practiced. Furthermore, the death rate for girls and women is higher than that for boys and men at every stage of their lives, because females have less access to essential resources, including food and medical care.

Studies have shown an almost universal preference for males, especially as first-born children. Because of this, population control advocates have supported sex selection as a way of limiting population growth. They argue that people often have more children than they really want because they keep trying for a boy. Preselecting will therefore lead to fewer children born; in addition, if fewer girls are born, there will be fewer women bearing children in the next generation.

Among feminists there is disagreement about how best to oppose this practice and change the conditions that give rise to it. In both China and India, women's groups are engaged in public education and other political campaigns to change the societal values and attitudes toward women that are the root causes for this destruction of female fetuses. Although some advocate banning the tests, arguing that they do not offer real choices, others distrust government intervention and believe that women must ultimately make their own decisions. Some oppose sex selection, seeing it as part of a growing trend to create "made-to-order" children. Still others see the effort to police sex selection as part of the effort to control and criminalize the behavior of pregnant women.

Thoughtful people may disagree about the morality of sex preselection or what to do about it. We must recognize the different realities in women's lives and the importance of supporting each woman's right to make her own reproductive decisions.

CONCLUSION

Many of us writing this book would not choose to use, and would not advise others to use, the high-tech and invasive ARTs. Many of us have experienced the powerful desire to have a biological child. Yet, many of these techniques involve so much social and medical manipulation of women and of our reproductive systems that we believe the risks and costs to be high enough to induce us to urge women seriously to consider the alternatives before going down this route.

For those who do pursue IVF and its derivatives, it is important to become fully informed of the physical, emotional, and financial burdens involved; to strengthen ourselves with information so that we can remain as much in charge as possible of the various decisions we will have to make; and to gather around us the support we will need for what is frequently an arduous path. It is important to allow ourselves to stop when we want to, despite the pressures to "succeed" and to bear children of "our own," and despite the pressures that arise from our culture's fascination with technologies and from the commercialization of ARTs. It is important to be aware as well of the wider societal balance of needs, and to put whatever pressure we can on our health care settings and governments to address the lack of basic prenatal and other health care for women and children. We need to create a social policy around these procedures that will work better for all women.

NOTES

1. Lesley and John Brown with Sue Freeman, *Our Miracle Called Louise* (London: Magnum Books, 1979), p. 83.
2. A. Brewaeys, "Donor Insemination: The Impact on Family and Child Development," *Journal of Psychosomatic Obstetrics and Gynocology* 17 no. 1 (1996): 1–13; also, S. Golombok et al., "The European Study of Assisted Reproduction Families: Family Functioning and Child Development," *Human Reproduction* 11, no. 10 (1996): 2324–331.
3. The Society for Assisted Reproductive Medicine (SART) gathers statistics on ART. Its most recent report (published in 1996, reporting figures as of 1994) provides the outcomes and success rates of 249 centers offering ART. SART reported a 21% live birth rate for IVF, 28% rate for GIFT (gamete intrafallopian transfer, see later in chapter), and 29% rate for ZIFT (zygote intrafallopian transfer, see later in chapter). Additionally, transfer of frozen embryos resulted in a 15% delivery rate, and a 57% birth rate for donated eggs. The miscarriage rate for IVF pregnancies was 13%, but for women over 40 the miscarriage rate was 30%. (Society for Assisted Reproductive Technology [SART] and the Society for Reproductive Medicine [ASRM], "Assisted Reproductive Technology in the United States and Canada: 1994 Results Generated from the ASRM/SART Registry," *Fertility and Sterility* 66, no. 5 (1996): 697–705.)
4. J. Robertson, "Legal Trouble Spots in Assisted Reproduction," *Fertility and Sterility* 65, no. 1 (Jan. 1996): 11–12. A zygote is an embryo in an early stage of cell division.

RESOURCES

For resources on Donor Insemination, please see chapter 10 Resources.

Books

Arditti, Rita, et al., eds. *Test Tube Women: What Future for Motherhood?* New York: Routledge, Chapman and Hall, 1989. A classic.

Baran, Annette, and Reuben Pannor. *Lethal Secrets: The Psychology of Donor Insemination*. New York: Amistad Press, 1993. Critique of secrecy about donor insemination.

Corea, Gena. *The Mother Machine: Reproductive Technologies from Artificial Insemination to Artificial Wombs*. New York: Harper & Row, 1985. A classic.

Field, Martha A. *Surrogate Motherhood: The Legal and Human Issues*. Cambridge: Harvard University Press, 1990.

Kendell, Kate, and Robin Haaland, eds. *Lesbians Choosing Motherhood: Legal Implications of Alternative Insemination and Co-parenting*. 3rd ed. San Francisco: National Center for Lesbian Rights, 1996.

Klein, Renate D. *Infertility: Women Speak Out About Their Experiences of Reproductive Medicine*. Boston: Pandora Press, 1989.

Macklin, Ruth. *Surrogates and Other Mothers: The Debates over Assisted Reproduction*. Philadelphia: Temple University Press, 1994.

Noble, Elizabeth. *Having Your Baby by Donor Insemination: A Complete Resource Guide*. Boston: Houghton Mifflin, 1987. Still a popular resource, and lesbian-friendly.

Rae, Scott B. *The Ethics of Commercial Surrogate Motherhood: Brave New Families?* Westport, CT: Praeger, 1994.

Ragon, Helena. *Surrogate Motherhood: Conception in the Heart*. Boulder, CO: Westview Press, 1994.

Raymond, Janice G. *Women as Wombs: Reproductive Technologies and the Battle over Women's Freedom*. San Francisco: Harper San Francisco, 1993.

Rothblatt, Martine. *Unzipped Genes: Taking Charge of Baby-Making in the New Millennium*. Philadelphia: Temple University Press, 1997. Critique of the Human Genome Project.

Rothman, Barbara Katz. *Re-creating Motherhood: Ideology and Technology in a Patriarchal Society*. New York: W. W. Norton, 1989.

———. *The Tentative Pregnancy: Prenatal Diagnosis and the Future of Motherhood*. New York: Penguin, 1987. A classic.

Rowland, Robyn. *Living Laboratories: Women and Reproductive Technologies*. Bloomington: Indiana University Press, 1992.

Seibel, Machelle, and Susan Crockin, eds. *Family Building Through Egg and Sperm Donation: Medical, Legal and Ethical Issues*. Boston: Jones and Bartlett, 1996.

Seibel, Machelle, et al., eds. *Technology and Infertility: Clinical, Psychological, Legal and Ethical Aspects*. New York: Springer-Verlag, 1993.

Spallone, Patricia. *Beyond Conception*. Granby, MA: Bergin & Garvey, 1989.

Stephenson, Patricia, and Marsden G. Wagner, eds. *Tough Choices: In Vitro Fertilization and the Reproductive Technologies*. Philadelphia: Temple University Press, 1993.

Articles

American Fertility Society. "Ethical Considerations of Assisted Reproductive Technologies." *Fertility and Sterility* 62, no. 5 (Supplement 1, 1994).

Baird, P. "Proceed with Care: New Reproductive Technologies and the Need for Boundaries." *Journal of Assisted Reproduction and Genetics* 12, no. 8 (1995): 491–98.

Macklin, R. "Ethics, Informed Consent, and Assisted Reproduction," *Journal of Assisted Reproduction and Genetics* 12, no. 8 (1995): 484–90.

Pollitt, Katha. "Checkbook Maternity: When Is a Mother Not a Mother?" *The Nation,* 251, no. 23 (Dec. 31, 1990): 825, 840–46.

Robertson, J. "Legal Trouble Spots in Assisted Reproduction." *Fertility and Sterility* 65, no. 1 (Jan. 1996): 11–12.

Sandelowski, Margarete. "Compelled to Try: The Never-Enough Quality of Conceptive Technology." *Medical Anthropology Quarterly* 5, no. 1 (March 1991).

Shushan, A. et al. "Human Menopausal Gonadotropin and the Risk of Epithelial Ovarian Cancer." *Fertility and Sterility* 65, no. 1 (1996): 13–18.

Periodicals

Fertility and Sterility. Published by American Society for Reproductive Medicine, Birmingham, Alabama. See Organizations.

Journal of Assisted Reproduction and Genetics. Published by Plenum Publishing, (212) 620-8000.

Organizations

American Society for Reproductive Medicine (ASRM)
1209 Montgomery Highway; Birmingham, AL 35216-2809; (205) 978-5000
E-mail: asrm@asrm.com
Web site: http://www.asrm.com

Council for Responsible Genetics
5 Upland Road, Suite 3; Cambridge, MA 02140; (617) 868-0870
E-mail: crg@essential.org
Web site: http://www.essential.org/crg

Resolve, Inc.
1310 Broadway; Somerville, MA 02144-1731; (617) 623-1156; Help line: (617) 623-0744
E-mail: resolveinc@aol.com
Web site: http://www.resolve.org

Audiovisual Resources

On The Eighth Day: Perfecting Mother Nature, 1992, Nicole Hubert, producer. Excellent two-video series discusses and critiques reproductive technologies. Part One, Making Babies, is about infertility treatments. Part Two, Making Perfect Babies, is about genetic manipulations in the quest for "perfect" babies; includes perspectives of people with disabilities. Available from Women Make Movies, 462 Broadway, Suite 500, New York, NY 10013; (212) 925-0606.

PART FOUR:

Child-bearing

Introduction

By Jane Pincus and Judy Luce

THE POWER OF BIRTH IN WOMEN'S LIVES

Pregnancy and birth are as ordinary as breathing, thinking, working, and loving, and as extraordinary as a spectacular adventure into a new world. Our lives expand in all dimensions. As we coordinate pregnancy, work, and family; as we labor, give birth, and raise our children, we use our abundant capacities for creativity, flexibility, resilience, determination, intuition, endurance, and humor.

As mothers and expectant mothers we are of all races and ethnicities. We are biological mothers, adoptive mothers, stepmothers, and guardians of each others' children. We are heterosexual, bisexual, and lesbian. We are teenagers, young, and middle-aged. We have partners, are married, and are single. We have disabilities. We have low, middle, and high incomes; we range from being homeless to being financially wealthy. We live in cities, suburbs, villages, and the countryside. We go to work and to school, and we work at home. Our pregnancies are planned and unplanned. We have good prenatal care and poor prenatal care. Some of us are unable to get any prenatal care at all. We give birth at home, in birth centers, and in hospitals. We welcome our babies alone and surrounded by family and friends. Whoever we are and however we become mothers, we deserve to have the means to care for ourselves and our babies well. We deserve to feel that we and our babies are welcome in our homes, our neighborhoods, and all the institutions of our society.[1]

When you are pregnant you need encouragement, love, and support from family and friends; knowledge about pregnancy; prenatal care; financial security; a safe work and home environment; appropriate resources, such as high-quality child care and transportation; enough time for child-bearing leave with assured job continuation; adequate food; time for rest and exercise; and a skilled, wise, trusted caregiver who respects you. You need continuity of care throughout the childbearing year, confidence in your ability to give birth, and people who are interested in you and care about you as well as your babies.

During labor you need to be in a reassuring nurturing environment, as close to home and to your own culture as possible, so that you can shape your labor as it unfolds. You need adequate food and drink to maintain strength and energy. You need attendants who believe in you and know how to patiently observe the natural process of labor; who sustain and guide you,

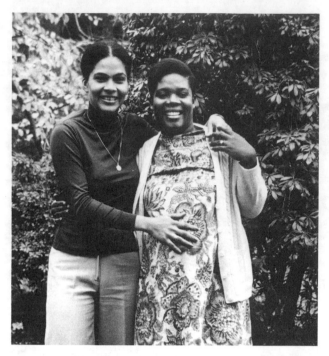

Peter Simon

helping you to relax and adopt comfortable labor positions. You need accessible medical resources in case of emergency.

After the birth, you need time to be with your baby. You may need a helping hand during the days and weeks after birth to help care for your family. You continue to need nourishment, rest, and exercise. With a first child you will want information, encouragement, and the influence of experienced parents to help you be a good mother. You may want access to family planning facilities that offer practical support and reinforcement, so that you can plan any future pregnancies.

In a more humane society we could achieve a *climate of confidence* by creating a maternity care system with women, babies, and families at its heart and midwives as its primary practitioners.[2] Policy makers and caregivers would pay careful attention to our language, culture, and experience, valuing our strengths and treating us with dignity. A just social and economic system would give us strength and confidence, banish ignorance, and minimize fear. It would allocate resources equitably, furnishing everyone with enough to eat, affordable housing, and effective prenatal care. Midwives would attend the majority of births, with physicians providing appropriate consultation and medical referral. We would give birth at home, in birth centers, or in hospitals, wherever and however we wanted, assured of skilled, compassionate assistance. National health insurance would guarantee care for everyone. Generous family leave policies and day care facilities would provide job security and enable us to stay with our babies and families for longer periods of time. In such a world, health care costs would plum-

met, women would flourish, birth would unfold naturally, and babies would thrive.

Such a vision counters the pervasive *climate of doubt* about child-bearing that exists in this country. Our obstetrical system is part of a larger medical-industrial complex that shapes our beliefs, expectations, and experiences. Medical schools train physicians to focus on risk and pathology; to view childbirth as a dangerous, unbearably painful, and messy process, "managed" only in hospital settings with the routine use of a wide array of tests, drugs, and technologies, most of which have never been proved to be safe or beneficial.[3] Obstetricians and hospital administrators purchase drugs and machines, thus sustaining wealthy and influential instrument and drug companies. Hospitals, modeled on factories, have rules and schedules of their own that interfere with the unique flow of each woman's labor. Interventions that "save time" are used to replace nursing staff. It can be a challenge to find a middle ground between acquiescence and rebellion. Within this system the sexual, social, and spiritual dimensions of pregnancy, birth, and motherhood are ignored, suppressed, or completely unknown.[4]

Indifferent to the circumstances of our lives, purely medical obstetrics applies inadequate solutions to problems caused by social and economic ills. Those of us with little money, lacking the resources to foster healthy pregnancies, already struggle with general health problems caused by poverty. Some of the basic provisions for care and support (such as Title V block grants and welfare payments), meager as they were, are now being eliminated. As women of color, we confront the built-in race and class biases of a flawed and unkind maternity care system.[5] Sometimes practitioners pit woman against child, treating us merely as "hostile environments"—containers for babies rather than loving mothers. Without private insurance, we become readily available "cases," serving as "learning material" for medical students. We commonly receive fragmented, hurried, disrespectful care during pregnancy. If we cease to seek prenatal care after undergoing one too many inconveniences or indignities, health problems may develop or go unrecognized until the last moment. Then, in the ensuing times of crisis, obstetricians and neonatologists "rescue" our babies by means of technology and costly medical surveillance.* Little if any provision is made for helping us nurture these tiny babies once we bring them home.

The prevalent system makes it difficult, if not impos-

---

* A 1989 Harvard Medical School Dean's report states that infant deaths are caused by "the relatively poor health status of poor women; inadequate provision of prenatal care services; the growing social systems based on insurance coverage; inadequate mechanisms for providing community-based care to high-risk infants after they leave the hospital; and most fundamental, the dramatic increase in the numbers of children being born into poverty, as this can always overwhelm what medical science can provide."

sible, to choose alternatives such as nurse-midwives, independent community midwives, freestanding birth centers, and home birth. Most physicians pay no attention to the overwhelming evidence in scientific and lay literature throughout the world (even in their own medical literature!) that midwifery alternatives to conventional obstetrics are better and safer for most women and babies. What's more, they actively harass and persecute not only alternative practitioners, such as midwives, but those physicians who support midwifery care and women's choices in childbirth. In many cases, health insurers do not pay for midwifery care.

In response to the passionate efforts of childbirth activists and midwives, many hospitals have become more woman- and family-oriented, extending their programs beyond birth into the postpartum period. Some enlightened physicians appreciate midwifery skills and are genuinely committed to new models of care.

Nonetheless, it is not women's needs that alter hospital policies but budget priorities dictated by a for-profit health care system and programs such as "managed care." Economically threatened hospitals compete for clients, initiating expensive marketing campaigns to attract us. Obstetrics is big business; giving birth in a particular hospital is the first point of entry into that institution for a significant number of women and families.[6]

All women benefit from the elimination of restrictive practices and the provision of space and resources for family-centered care. It is crucial, however, to distinguish real changes from merely cosmetic ones. At teaching hospitals and associated prenatal clinics, the training of medical students and residents still takes priority over empathetic care for women.[7] The imposition of arbitrary time limits on labor, the inappropriate use of interventions, and the perception of childbirth as illness prevail. A "normal standard vaginal delivery" involves the use of a wide range of interventions. The more a labor deviates from an elusive "norm," the more interventions are brought into play to make it conform. Women who behave "unacceptably" by questioning obstetrical routines or asserting their wishes may be labeled as "difficult" and treated with hostility. Nurse-midwives practicing in some hospitals must perform a delicate balancing act so as not to encounter resistance or lose their jobs, meeting excessively restrictive protocols for "normal" birth.

In the late 1960s and early 1970s, many of us experienced natural physiological childbirth as a creative and empowering event. During this era, nurse-midwives expanded their practices, and the new independent midwife movement was born. Optimistically, we believed that we could give birth as we desired simply by preparing ourselves and informing our practitioners about what we wanted. Naively, we believed that we could change obstetrical education, practice, and philosophy.

But the last two decades have seen obstetrical power and practice firmly entrenched, with physicians educated and trained as narrowly as ever. These obstetrical procedures—described by some as rituals learned by both physicians and childbearing women—control and distort the transformative process of birth.

[these procedures] are patterned and repetitive . . . profoundly symbolic, communicating messages through the body and the emotions concerning our culture's deepest beliefs about the necessity for cultural control of natural processes, the untrustworthiness of nature and the associated weakness and inferiority of the female body, the validity of patriarchy, the superiority of science and technology, and the importance of institutions and machines.[8]

Since we rarely if ever see other women giving birth, naturally or otherwise, we fear the act of giving birth, and the pain. Caregivers become "handlers," pushing us into institutional frameworks. Medical language itself can destroy self-confidence, with ourselves as "patients"; doctors "managing labors," "monitoring high-risk pregnancies," and "delivering babies"; and with disempowering descriptions such as "failure to progress," "inadequate pelvis," and "incompetent cervix."

Tests and technologies proliferate, becoming the norm simply because they exist, their risks often undisclosed and benefits unproven. Wanting to feel informed and in control, eager for knowledge, and worried about not doing "everything possible," we think that medical technology will guarantee a healthy pregnancy and a perfect baby. Sometimes, with luck and support, we can choose only those procedures that relieve worry and enhance confidence, and avoid the rest. But all too often, fearing that something will go wrong that could have been prevented, we feel selfish or guilty questioning routine experimental or invasive procedures. The deceptively simple "Don't you care about your baby?" leads to capitulation. We consent to a process of medicalization that makes us mistrust our healthy bodies, our deepest selves. "I feel so overwhelmed," says one woman; "I am consumed with deciding what tests to have. I can hardly enjoy being pregnant or cherish the changes in my body."

Our prime task as authors, then, is bring to light stories about truly natural births and to describe pregnancy, labor, and birth as the flowing, organic events they can be. In this way, we hope to preserve women's knowledge about midwifery and childbirth, to counteract the technological bias of the present generation, and to add to the wealth of knowledge that enhances women's experiences *wherever* they give birth. We describe and keep alive traditional midwifery beliefs and techniques for attending women in the most positive, joyous, and respectful manner possible.

The language of midwifery is our "mother tongue," which replaces words like "management" and "monitoring" with "attentiveness" and "tuning into all that is happening, expecting the best and prepared to assist and intervene when necessary." We resist the imposition of the clock and other management concepts on a process whose rhythm and fragility is akin to the opening of a bud and whose power is that of the flower that miraculously pushes its way up through the pavement. We maintain this culture by retelling those birth stories in which women have felt healthy, vital, powerfully strong and creative.[9]

As we work and fight for social and economic justice we create vital models of community care.

The Childbearing Center of Morris Heights in the Bronx, New York, is one example of what women can do when given access to resources, education, and policy. The center provides teenagers with a nurturing four-month parenting program that helps them gain confidence and competence. In addition, midwives offer "grandmother brunches" for the older women, during which they describe their practice of combining the best of the midwifery tradition with access to medical care, if needed. Community women fully participate in the running of the birthing center.[10]

What's unique about [being] the community midwife is that when I see the mother at her home and help her, I'm going to see her again—we go to the same foodstore and we know the same people, so there's that continuity. . . . A midwife doesn't just catch babies. A midwife is an educator as well. What I see as the most powerful aspect of [the Traditional Childbearing Group] is that we teach Black empowerment. We want you to know that you're somebody. You have to love yourself, you have to love your unborn baby and that your baby's being born Black. It already has something against it. You're all it's got and you have to get yourself empowered to keep this baby alive, so that he or she can make and be the great spirit that's meant to be. Go back to our history. Start with someone in your family who knows the power of your family line. You have to honor yourself and be proud so that you can maintain your pregnancy and do it with dignity by taking care of yourself. You can read. You can eat right. Things you can control, let's start with that and then we can challenge the system.[11]

We encourage you to join the dedicated individuals and the local and national groups active in childbirth reform (see Resources for a partial listing), in challenging the medical appropriation of our bodies and souls. We assert that a just society must be the basis of high-quality maternity care. We celebrate pregnancy, birth, and motherhood as natural, joyous, strengthening events of life, and we honor the mothers who are bringing our children into this world.

NOTES

1. Based on Alice LoCicero's written communication, February 1997.
2. Women's Institute for Childbearing Policy, The National Black Women's Health Project, The National Women's Health Network, Boston Women's Health Book Collective, *Childbearing Policy Within a National Health Program: An Evolving Consensus for New Directions* (Women's Institute for Childbearing Policy, P.O. Box 72, Roxbury, VT 05669, 1994).
3. See M. Enkin et al. *A Guide to Effective Care in Pregnancy and Childbirth* (Oxford: Oxford University Press, 1995). Also see The Cochrane Pregnancy and Childbirth Database (listed in chapters 19 and 20 Resources), *Care in Normal Birth,* World Health Organization, 1996 (Maternal and Newborn Health/Safe Motherhood Unit, WHO, 1211 Geneva 27, Switzerland).
4. Susan L. Diamond, *Hard Labor* (New York: Tom Doherty Associates, Inc., 1996), an honest appraisal by a former labor and delivery nurse, who gives us an inside view of hospital practices. More convincing than any polemic, her experiences make a strong case that midwives, not obstetricians, should attend women in labor.
5. See Evelyn White, ed., *The Black Women's Health Book* (Seattle: Seal Press, 1994).
6. Ruthie H. Dearing, Helen A. Gordon, Dorolyn M. Sohner, and Lynne C. Weidel, *Marketing Women's Health Care* (Rockville, MD: Aspen Publishers, Inc., 1987).
7. Council on Resident Education in Obstetrics and Gynecology, "A Design for Resident Education in Obstetrics and Gynecology" (Washington, DC: The Council, 1986). This official document makes explicit on the opening page that patient care should be subordinated to educational objectives; it "establishes the program's primary responsibility for education, secondarily providing clinical services."
8. Robbie E. Davis-Floyd, *Birth as an American Rite of Passage* (Berkeley: University of California Press, 1992), 152.
9. Judy Luce, "Midwifery and Home Birth: Honoring the Power of Women," *Vermont Alternative Medicine Newsletter #5* (Amvita, Middlebury, VT) February 1997.
10. Jennifer Dohrn, selections from an interview in *The Birth Gazette* 7, no. 4 (Fall 1991): 16.
11. Shafia Monroe, midwife, interviewed in *Sojourner,* March 1991, p. 2H.

By Jane Pincus and Judy Luce, with
Audrey Levine, Robin J. Blatt, Linda
Holmes, and Marsha Saxton

WITH SPECIAL THANKS TO Carol Sakala,
Denise Bergman, Esther Entin*

Chapter 19

Pregnancy

I sit here on the porch as if in a deep sleep, waiting for this unknown child. I keep hearing this far flight of strange birds going on in the mysterious air about me. How can it be explained? . . . Suddenly everything becomes alive . . . like an anemone opening itself, disclosing itself, and the very stones themselves break open like bread.[1]

Events unfold simultaneously when you become pregnant. This is a time of transition. You are becoming a mother, beginning a new relationship, creating a larger family. Your body and feelings are changing. Your baby is growing within you. Pregnancy gives you

* Thanks also to the following for their help with the 1998 version of this chapter: Loreta Cavicchi, Jennifer Colby, Sally Dames, Robbie Davis-Floyd, Joan Ditzion, Jenifer Firestone, Kathleen Hearn, Rick Hearn, Mirza Lugardo, Edith Maxwell, Sharon Nobles, Mamie Ramey, Peggy Thurston, Laurie Williams, and Jennifer Yanco. Over the years since 1969, the following people have contributed to the many versions of this chapter: Ruth Bell, Robin Blatt, Jenny Fleming, Linda Holmes, Judy Luce, Jane Pincus, Bebe Poor, Judi Rogers, Becky Sarah, and Norma Swenson.

a special opportunity for expansion, change, and transformation. Your pregnancy will have much in common with those of other women. Yet, it is yours, and unique. Our society tends to treat pregnancy matter-of-factly, medically, mechanically. But it is much more: a profoundly personal and social event, significant for you and all the people in your life.

TIME OF YOUR BABY'S BIRTH

Now that you know you're pregnant, you will want to know approximately when your baby will be born. Normal gestation can range from 37 weeks to 43 weeks, with most births occurring between 39 weeks and 41 weeks. The "due date" is merely the center of that "window." Only a small percent of women give birth on their projected due date. If you know the length of your menstrual cycle and the date of your last period, you are often the best judge of when you conceived.

Nowadays, almost all practitioners in a medical setting use ultrasound to "date" fetal maturity. Routinely performed at a time when the embryo is most vulnerable to outside influences, it is costly and unnecessary. Its findings are often inaccurate and can be alarmist, suggesting problems that don't exist. Also, its long-term effects are unknown. Ultrasound devalues and bypasses what we know about our own menstrual cycles, and often it is no better a predictor of the time of birth than your own prediction and/or the information gleaned from your physical exams from month to month. Ultrasound may help you determine when you conceived if you are not having regular periods, or if you have become pregnant while taking birth control pills. In these cases, having an estimate based on ultrasound may reduce the chances that your health care practitioner will induce labor before you are ready. (For more on fetal ultrasound, see p. 462.)

CARING FOR YOURSELF

First Trimester (First to 12th Week)

Note: In this chapter we use the words "embryo" and "fetus" for the first trimester, and "baby" for the rest of pregnancy, labor, and birth.

Physical Changes

During these first 12 weeks, the embryo miraculously grows from two cells into a fully developed fetus. You may have none, some, or many of the following early signs of pregnancy. If your periods occur regularly, you will probably notice that you've missed one. (Some women do bleed for the first two or three months even when pregnant, but it usually lasts a short time, and the bleeding is scanty.) About seven days after conception, the tiny group of cells that becomes the embryo (blastocyst) attaches itself to the uterine wall, sometimes causing slight vaginal spotting (called implantation bleeding), while new blood vessels are being formed. You can confirm your pregnancy with a home pregnancy test and/or a visit to your health care practitioner for a pelvic exam.

Increased hormonal changes cause you to urinate more often. Your enlarging uterus begins to press on your bladder. Your breasts swell and become tender as the milk glands begin to develop. Because the blood supply to your breasts increases, veins become more prominent. Your nipples and the area around them (areola) may darken and become larger.

You may feel nauseated, mildly or enough to vomit, because of physiological changes. Even if you can't eat much during the first few months, your growing fetus is taking from you what it needs. Eat lightly throughout the day, and try food high in protein. Munching crackers or dry toast early in the morning can help. Avoid greasy, spiced food. Don't worry if you can't eat a lot, but don't try to fast, and at least drink juice. Apricot nectar helps some women, as does powdered ginger, ginger tea, mint tea, vitamin B_6, or acupuncture. Nausea can tire you out. It usually disappears after the first trimester, although it can continue

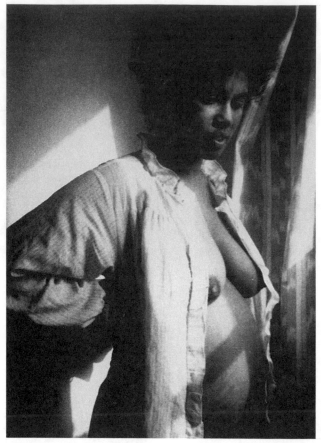

Jenny McKenzie

throughout the pregnancy. If you consider it extreme, check with your health care practitioner.

It is absolutely normal to feel very tired, even exhausted. You are working hard, growing a baby.

Some women have an increase in clear, nonirritating vaginal secretions. As hormones cause vaginal changes, women are more susceptible to yeast infections. You can treat them with herbs or over-the-counter preparations. If the discharge is itchy, thick, or yellowish, check with your health care practitioner. The joints between your pelvic bones begin to loosen because of the pregnancy hormone relaxin, and they become more movable about the tenth or 11th week.

To maintain bowel regularity, eat foods high in fiber content and fresh fruits, and drink a lot of water. Eat healthy, nutritious foods. You will begin to gain weight.

Your Feelings About Yourself and Your Pregnancy

At the beginning of pregnancy, whether it is your first or your fifth, your feelings can shift from delirious joy to deep sadness, with a whole range of possibilities in between. They will depend on whether your pregnancy is planned or unplanned, whether you want to be pregnant, the state of your health, the physical and economic demands on your life, the support you have at work and at home, and how your family and friends respond to you. Creating and deepening bonds with people who make you feel special can be a source of strength.

You may feel increased sensuality, a sensual opening out toward the world, and a traveling inward. You may have heightened perceptions; new energy; a feeling of being in love, really special, fertile, potent, creative. You may sense expectation, harmony, peace.

I'd been wanting a baby so much for three years, had had ovarian cysts and had almost given up trying. Pregnancy came as a surprise. Even before I actually knew about it I felt ecstatic, in love, full of emotion, feeling everything intensely! During my second pregnancy—I wanted to see if I could do it again! —I loved resting my arms upon my big belly.

We inseminated at home and were amazed at how easy it was to get pregnant. Just a few hours afterwards, Annie said, "I feel kind of sleepy and want to relax. I want to lie down and be by myself." When she didn't get her period in the next few weeks, and the pregnancy test showed just a little pink, we were so excited!

You may ask yourself: What's going to happen to me? How will being pregnant change me? Will I be able to cope well? What supports do I have? Can I physically handle birth? How long can I keep working? Will I be laid off? Do we have enough money? How will this affect my relationship with my partner? Will my baby be healthy? Will I be a good parent?

And you may have surprisingly strong negative feelings: Shock. I'm losing my individuality. I'm not sure I want to be a mother. I can't feel anything. I'm ambivalent about this baby growing in me. I'm angry, scared, worried. I don't know what's going to happen. I'm tired. I'm sick every morning. I'm not ready to be pregnant once again. I feel so alone; I have no one with whom to share this intimate time.

Sometimes it seemed like I had gotten pregnant on a whim—and it was a hell of a responsibility to take on a whim. Sometimes I was overwhelmed by what I'd done. A lot of that came from realizing that I had chosen to have the baby without the support of a man. I was scared up until the third trimester that I wasn't going to make it.

Negative feelings are natural. They may be plentiful or rare, depending on your circumstances. By dealing with them and not avoiding them you come to know yourself better. Feelings may change toward the positive as you get used to the fact of pregnancy, become attached to your growing baby, and prepare to labor and give birth.

Seeming Absence of Feelings

Because of your particular personality or your background, you may not let yourself feel much connection with your baby until after it is born. In some cultures, for superstitious or practical reasons, women do not buy baby clothes or furniture beforehand. Once the suspense is over and you know you have weathered the storm, you can celebrate the fact that your baby has arrived, is real, and is safe in your arms.

Second Trimester (13th to 26th Week)

Physical Changes

This is usually the most comfortable part of pregnancy. Many women have a lot of energy and sleep well. At about the fourth month, your growing baby begins to take up much more space. Your womb begins to swell, your waist expands, and your clothes fit more tightly. For the first time you will feel the baby move (light movements called "quickening"), often while you are waiting to fall asleep at night. You are gaining more weight. Your blood volume is increasing by 40 to 60% to enable your placenta (the organ nourishing your baby) to function efficiently. Your uterus is growing, its weight increasing 20 times, stretching the skin.

In some women, the line from the navel to the pubic region darkens too. Sometimes pigment in the face becomes darker, making a kind of mask. It disappears afterward. The increased color around your nipples and in the line on your abdomen will fade, but it may not disappear completely.

You may salivate more or sweat a lot. Some women get cramps in their legs and feet. When this happens, pull your toes toward your knees. Regular exercise and good nutrition will minimize their occurrence.

By midpregnancy your breasts, stimulated by hormones, become larger and heavier. You are just about ready to begin nursing. If your nipples are turned in (inverted), talk with your health care practitioner, a La Leche League member (see Resources, pp. 496–501), or a lactation consultant about the ways in which you can prepare them for breast-feeding.

Eating well in frequent small amounts, drinking lots of healthy fluids including water, and exercising will stimulate your bowels if they have slowed down, thus preventing constipation. Don't use laxatives. If heartburn bothers you, try fresh or dried papaya, or papaya tablets (not seeds, however) available at health food stores. You may use antacids that don't contain aluminum.

Women prone to varicose veins may get them at this point. It's helpful to wear support stockings a half size larger than usual. Alternate resting with walking or mild exercise. Mild swelling (edema) of the hands and feet is normal. However, if you have headaches, nausea, dizziness, or high blood pressure, contact your health care practitioner.

Wear loose, comfortable clothing. Borrow clothes from friends. Browse yard sales, shop in used clothes stores or stores for larger women. You can modify your pants by piecing in an elastic stretch panel. Unbelted smocks are useful as dresses, and large men's shirts are great. Get as much rest as you can. Try to set aside small segments of time for total relaxation.

Your Feelings About Yourself and Your Pregnancy

I was excited and delighted. I really got into eating well, caring for myself, getting enough sleep. I liked walking through the streets and having people notice me.

I don't like being pregnant. I feel like a big toad. I'm a dancer, used to being slim, and I can't believe what I look like from the side. I avoid mirrors.

The first movements you feel can be amazing:

I was lying on my stomach and felt something, like someone lightly touching my deep insides. Then I just sat very still and for an alive moment felt the hugeness of having something living growing in me. Then I said, "No, it's not possible, it's too early yet," and then I started to cry. . . . That one moment was my first body awareness of another living thing inside me.

After the first movement you may wait days for another sign. Soon the movements become frequent, familiar, and welcome. The baby begins to feel real. You can feel from the outside the firmer shape of your uterus.

Each of my pregnancies was different from the others. With my first baby, I felt him to be very much a part of me. His movements were slow, dreamy, and wavelike. My second child felt very separate, from early on very different from me, kicking hard and in a hurry to be born.

When I could feel the baby move and Jenny couldn't yet, she'd say, "Wait a minute! I'm doing all the housework in this joint and where are my perks?" Then every night after dinner we'd sit on the couch together and listen to music. She would put her hand on my womb to feel the baby dance and move around. We sat together for hours and never got bored.

A midwife reflects: *Your baby lives within you. You are closer now than you will ever be again, though you have never seen or touched him or her. Talk to your baby. Listen to your baby. Your experience in being pregnant and giving birth and your baby's experience are intertwined. Walk in oneness with your baby everyday. Listen, really listen.*

You may be surprised, nevertheless, by the unpredictability of your thoughts and feelings.

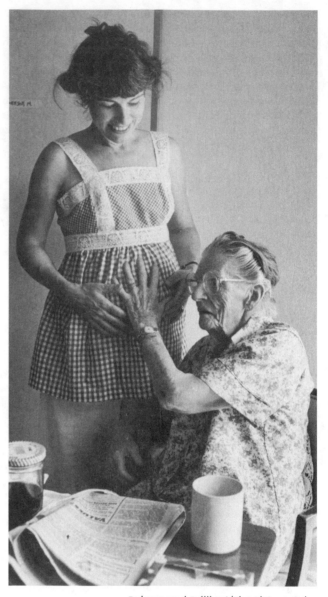

Palmer and Brilliant/The Picture Cube

Last night its kicking made me dizzy and gave me a terrible feeling of solitude. I wanted to tell it, "Stop, stop, stop, let me alone." I want to lie still and whole and all single, catch my breath. But I have no control over this new part of my being, and this lack of control scares me. I feel as if I were rushing downhill at such a great speed that I'd never be able to stop.

Even during the most positive pregnancies you may have moments, hours, and days of anxiety, confusion, and feeling blue. Try talking with intimate friends or your partner (who may have concerns of his or her own). It may help to make a list, or to write in a journal if you don't already do so. Take this opportunity as a time to learn more about yourself.

It seems that my feelings about my pregnancy, my body, the coming of the baby, were inextricably wound into my feelings, problems, hopes, and fears for our relationship. . . . It's hard to separate which feelings were a result of my unhappiness about us . . . which ones were my own negative feelings about having a less functional body (I wanted to keep working and active, but my body was so cumbersome that I was always worn-out and tired), and which ones were just moods caused by pregnancy.

Throughout most of my many solo years I have managed to remain sexually active. This is no small feat for a single lesbian. But for some reason, throughout most of my pregnancy I had no sexual suitors. It made me very sad to experience my wanting pregnant body in, what was for me, a once-in-a-lifetime extraordinary state, alone. I think my pregnancy was actually the loneliest time of my life.

During these weeks many women have vivid, sometimes unsettling, dreams.

For two nights now my falling asleep has given rise to that old childhood dream-image of falling down a deep, dark, square hole ever diminishing in size.

I'm in a hospital in a room all alone, a cold room. The nurse gives me a shot. I have my baby and don't feel a thing. I look up and see my baby floating in a beaker, alive. I can't go to her. I'm sad and frustrated.

The hopefulness of pregnancy can contrast sharply with a harsh world.

In the supermarket a woman was screaming at her child, and then she hit him in the face. I know that if I hadn't been pregnant I would have done something. But all I could do was stand there, immobilized and speechless, tears running down my face.

I remember feeling overwhelmed by sad things I saw, and by things that could happen to innocence. I'd wake in the night and think people were going to come in and take things, take the baby from me. I was beginning to be out of control, I was terribly afraid of chance. I've always been afraid of irrationality, of fate.

You may fear miscarriage, or worry that your baby will be born unhealthy or even die. It's important to acknowledge these fears, but don't dwell upon them. If they continue to disturb you, talk with family, friends, or a trusted counselor.

Sometimes, during your pregnancy, someone you know will miscarry, or her baby will die. It may be hard for you to reach out to her when you are feeling vulnerable and a bit fearful yourself, but showing your love and empathy can lessen her sense of isolation and help relieve her feelings of disappointment, sadness, and loss. We are all interconnected.

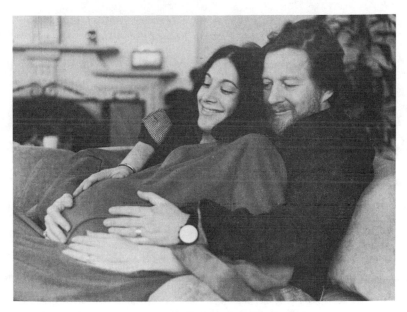

Jim Harrison/Stock, Boston

Your Partner's Feelings About You and Pregnancy

If you have a partner, his or her feelings are probably as complex as your own, depending upon his or her family background, treatment when growing up, attitudes toward self, and ideas about beauty and slimness. She or he can reflect back to you the ways in which you are changing and help you to care for yourself and to receive the best possible care from others.

It surprised us and took us a while to understand that we had different visions about how we'd go about being pregnant. I had a more holistic approach. But finally I realized that it was her pregnancy this time; she knew what she wanted. So I had to make a conscious decision to suspend my own ideas and visions until I could be pregnant myself. After I separated my desires from hers, everything became easier.

From a father-to-be:

We were so excited about Ruth's pregnancy. Then, when she was four months along, I was in a serious car accident. Ruth was amazingly strong. She negotiated among the always busy, sometimes unsympathetic specialists patching me up. She saw that I got the best care. She showed me what a fantastic mother/protector she would be for our child. I felt guilty because I couldn't be taking care of her. Once when I was swamped with drugs and pain, I saw Ruth nodding her head that it was all right to sign something, telling me with her eyes that it was OK, that everything would be fine. All my apprehension and fear disappeared. I knew I could trust her completely. I hope during her labor and delivery I can give her my strength to draw on. There are some lingering effects of the accident, but it is all behind us. I am ecstatic

*about the birth, scared, happy, more emotions than I
thought I could feel at any time. The personality, emotions, mind, life-force of Ruth and I are in this growing child, a magical combination of the two of us that
I can't wait to meet!*

Your partner may find it hard to support you, feeling
tired, left out, or neglected. Try to involve him or her
in your pregnancy, to prepare, plan, and learn together. If she or he cannot provide the support you
need, or if you are without a partner, seek out a friend
or family member who will give you what you need.

Third Trimester (27th Week to Beginning of Labor)

Physical Changes

Your womb is becoming very large. It may push
your navel inside out. It is made up of strong muscle
groups and will contract more and more often. You
will feel it tighten and release. These are practice contractions (called Braxton-Hicks) that prepare your
womb for eventual labor. Your belly can feel fairly
hard to the touch, or soft and jelly-like.

You can feel and see movements from the outside
now as the baby changes position, turns somersaults,
and hiccups. Sometimes it presses on your bladder,
making you want to urinate. You'll urinate more often;
tell your health care practitioner if you feel pain, burning, or tenderness. Sometimes toward the end of your
pregnancy the baby's weight will press on the nerves
at the top of your legs. Occasionally the sciatic nerve,
which runs from your buttocks down your legs, may
also get pinched and be painful.

Until 32 to 34 weeks, the baby will change position

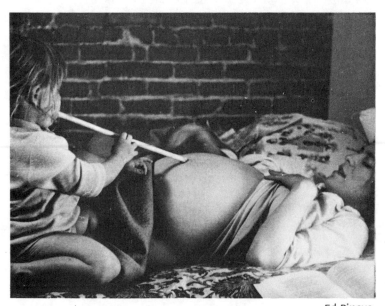

Ed Pincus

often. Then it tends to settle into a head-down position, but it still can move around. It wakes and sleeps,
and is more active at certain times of day. If there's a
change or a decrease in the level of its activity and you
are concerned, call your health care practitioner. Keep
in mind that as its body is now larger, there is less
room for it to move, and its movements are less
sharply defined.

Your center of gravity will change noticeably during
this trimester. You'll walk and balance yourself differently. Rather than leaning back to counteract the
weight and bulk, tuck your pelvis in. Your pelvic joints
continue to widen.

Pink, reddish, or darker lines may appear on your
belly. Drinking lots of fluids helps keep your skin moist.
If it becomes dry, use oil in your bath or after a shower.

It becomes increasingly uncomfortable to lie on
your stomach. Sleep on your side. Some women find
long body pillows comforting. Toward the very end of
pregnancy, sleeping on your back can cut down the
blood supply to your uterus. You may also experience
shortness of breath. Propping yourself up with pillows
behind your back can lessen the pressure on your
diaphragm. Since your chest has widened, you are still
breathing in more air when you are pregnant than
when you are not.

You continue to gain weight. If you have varicose
veins, try to avoid standing for long periods at a time.
Find occasions to raise your feet.

Your stomach is being squeezed. Once again, eat
small amounts of food at a time, often, to forestall or
relieve indigestion. If you have heartburn, sleep with
your head and shoulders raised. Mild swollen hands
and ankles are normal, but be sure to report any dizziness, nausea, elevated blood pressure, or headaches
to your health care practitioner.

Sometimes the increasing weight presses the veins
in your rectum and they dilate, becoming painful
(hemorrhoids). If so, lie down, elevate the bottom half
of your body, and apply ice packs or heat—whichever
feels most comfortable. Tucks pads, herbal remedies,
or Preparation H may be helpful. Also take warm baths
and apply soothing ointments designed for this purpose. Eat vegetables and bran, cut back on spices, and
continue to exercise when you can.

A good diet will help keep you healthy and your
baby growing. In the third trimester of pregnancy,
some women, especially malnourished women (teens
are often malnourished), develop a combination of
high blood pressure; swelling of face, hands, and feet
(edema); elevated amounts of protein in the urine; and
abnormalities in liver function. While these conditions
can occur separately and even together for other reasons, they may also be symptoms of preeclampsia.
Often headaches that accompany swelling are the first
sign. If you have these symptoms, get them checked
immediately. Mild symptoms, when detected early,
can be treated at home with rest and good nutrition
and often eliminated. If undiagnosed and untreated
they can develop into full-blown eclampsia with con-

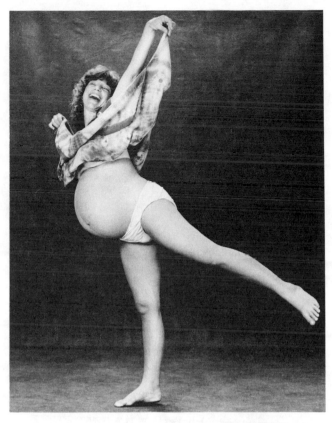

David Alexander

vulsions and fetal death. All serious preeclamptic conditions must be treated in the hospital.

If you aren't sleeping well because the baby's movements demand your attention or make you uncomfortable, take walks and soothing baths. Drink warm milk, valerian root tea, or raspberry tea. Brisk exercise during the day helps you sleep better. Never take sleeping pills.

I think there is a reason for this non-sleeping: there's work getting done. That restlessness needs to happen. Your energy builds up for the coming event. I remember pacing my house at midnight, burning with energy, finally finding the tiny sandals my first child had worn as a toddler. I carefully cleaned and polished them for the new baby. Then I slept fine.

About two to four weeks before birth, and sometimes as early as the seventh month, the baby's head settles into your pelvis. This is called "lightening" or "dropping," as the uterine ligaments relax, giving you more room to breathe and to eat.

Just Before Labor Begins

I had a feeling of being at the end, of nothing else being terrifically important.

I thought it would never end. I was enormous. I couldn't bend over and wash my feet. And it was incredibly hot.

I started to feel it was too long. Dick took pictures of me during the eighth month. I saw my face as faraway and sad.

The relationship of mother carrying child is most beautiful and simple. I pity a baby who must come out of the womb.

I wonder what it looks like. How fantastic that it only has to travel one-and-a-half feet down to get born.

My kid is dancing under my heart.

WHAT YOU CAN DO TO PUT YOURSELF AT EASE DURING PREGNANCY AND MAINTAIN YOUR HEALTH

Preparation for Pregnancy, Labor, and Birth

Considering pregnancy or becoming pregnant gives you the opportunity to develop new patterns for taking care of yourself. At this time, when you may be more sensitive to impressions and influences, seek out the most supportive people possible. You have the best reason in the world for eating well; quitting smoking, drinking, and substance use; and avoiding workplace toxins. Before pregnancy, preparation also includes taking folic acid supplements to reduce the incidence of neural tube defects such as spina bifida (see p. 444) and seeing a genetic counselor if you have a family history of genetic vulnerabilities, such as sickle-cell anemia or Tay-Sachs disease.

Prenatal Care

Prenatal care consists of three interrelated "programs": the care you give yourself, the care you receive from friends and family, and regular visits to your midwife or doctor. You will visit your health care practitioner monthly until the eighth month, biweekly until the ninth month, then weekly until labor begins. Your health care practitioner will follow the progress of your pregnancy, provide guidance and information about your care, and screen you for potential problems. At each visit, she or he will check gestational growth, heart tones, and, later in pregnancy, the baby's activity. He or she will provide information about the changes in your body, take your blood pressure, note your weight gain and diet, and check your urine for protein and sugar. A thorough health care practitioner will also ask how you are feeling and address any problems, concerns, and emotional and social issues you might have.

Sometimes it may be difficult to get to your prenatal visits. Try to arrange transportation, child care, or time off from work in advance. Be prepared to wait when you go for your appointment. Bring someone along with you if you can. Make a list of all the questions, concerns, and developments you want to tell your health care practitioner about. Taking good care of your pregnancy and yourself means that your good mothering has already begun.

Nutrition (see also chapter 2, Food)

It is essential to eat well. By doing so, you enable all the systems that support pregnancy to function at their best. You expand your blood volume to meet pregnancy's increased demands on your body; you create an efficient placenta; you help your baby achieve a healthy birthweight; you decrease the likelihood of labor complications; you lower your baby's risk of infections, anemia, prematurity, low birthweight, stillbirth, and brain damage; and you store the fats and fluids needed for breast-feeding. You will need to continue to eat and drink healthy foods and fluids after your baby is born, to keep up your strength and nourish your baby, especially if you are breast-feeding. This can be the perfect time to learn about healthy foods and good nutrition. Do not deprive yourself to feed other family members. You may be eligible for the WIC (Women, Infants and Children) program, a supplemental food program sponsored by the government. Designed for pregnant and breast-feeding women as well as for children up to five years old, WIC provides milk, fruit, cereal, juice, cheese, and eggs, and it offers some prenatal and breast-feeding education. If you are on public assistance you are automatically eligible for WIC. Many women well above the poverty level are eligible as well. Ask your health care practitioner, or contact a prenatal clinic or your local health department to find out how to sign up.

Instead of large meals, eat a wide variety of fruits, vegetables, and grains (whole-grain bread, cereals, pasta, tortillas, brown rice) in small amounts often. This advice comes in handy during early pregnancy if you are nauseated, or toward the end, when your baby takes up a lot of room and you feel so full already. Select low-fat foods. In the second half of pregnancy your nutritional needs increase significantly.

Special Nutritional Needs Before and During Pregnancy

Folic Acid. Folic acid is essential for protein synthesis in early pregnancy and also for the formation of blood and new cells. It is found in green leafy vegetables; citrus fruits and juice; dried peas, beans, and lentils; asparagus; broccoli; liver; beef; and fish. The U.S. Public Health Service recommends getting .4 mg daily, either through food or supplements.

Iron. Iron is a main component of hemoglobin, which carries oxygen throughout your body and to

EATING WELL EACH DAY

Eat as wide a variety of foods as you can, high in complex carbohydrates (not the simple carbohydrates found in white flour and sugar) and low in fat. Use fats and oils sparingly.

Dairy / Calcium: Three Servings a Day

Skim milk; low-fat yogurt; cheeses such as ricotta, mozzarella, parmesan, romano, cheddar, cottage cheese. Use dry milk powder when cooking foods. Seaweed, calcium-fortified soymilk, sesame seeds, butter, molasses, shellfish, and green leafy vegetables contain calcium. Some tofu is made with calcium lactate.

Protein: Three Servings a Day

Poultry, fish, lean beef or lamb; dry beans; eggs; nuts; seeds; peanut butter (two tablespoons count as one serving); tofu; nut-grain-bean combinations.

Vegetables: Four Servings a Day of Green and Yellow Vegetables

Spinach; lettuce; broccoli; cabbage; Swiss chard; kale; collard, mustard, and beet greens; alfalfa sprouts; carrots; potatoes; green peppers; cabbage.

Fruits: Three Servings a Day

Fresh and dried fruits; oranges; grapefruit; apples; bananas.

Complex Carbohydrates: Nine Servings a Day

Grains, cereals, pasta, rice, corn (cornbread, tortillas, pancakes). Fortify food with wheat germ and brewer's yeast.

Drink six to eight glasses of liquid a day—water, herb teas, fruit and vegetable juices. Avoid sugar-sweetened juices and sodas.

Salt to Taste

your baby. It is obtained from prune juice, dried fruits, legumes, blackstrap molasses, lean meat, liver, egg yolk, and food cooked in iron pans. Your body has an amazing capacity to absorb iron, and your fetus will also take from you the iron it needs for the first six months. Most women have adequate amounts of iron and there is no reason to take a supplement. In the middle trimester, iron levels tend to drop as the increased fluids from blood volume expansion dilute your blood. This is perfectly normal; they will rise in the last trimester. If you go into your pregnancy anemic, you will need to increase your intake of iron through diet, herbs and teas high in iron, and sometimes iron supplements. Routine prenatal care assesses your blood iron levels.

Weight Gain

Women's bodies grow and flourish in pregnancy. Enjoy your pregnancy and the beauty of your changing body. You are beautiful even if it is difficult to feel so, brainwashed as we are by countless images of skinny models and movie stars and by unhealthy, unreasonable cultural norms of thinness. Some partners and family members may find it hard to accept your expanding body. Don't let anyone deter you from gaining an appropriate amount of weight.

When you eat well, your weight will take care of itself. Pregnancy is not the time to diet. Gaining 25 to 35 pounds and even more is normal and healthy. Every woman's metabolism is different.

In the not-so-distant past, most physicians restricted weight gain and salt intake during pregnancy, going so far as to prescribe diet pills (amphetamines) and diuretics, which eliminate crucial fluids and minerals from the body. They erroneously believed that they were preventing preeclampsia, or toxemia (which involves liver malfunction). Although amphetamines and diuretics are no longer used, some physicians still advise or scare women into limiting their salt intake and gaining only a little bit of weight, which can endanger their health and their pregnancies. Instead, the fact is that eating well, salting to taste, and including lots of protein in your diet maintains health.[2] Midwives, nurse-practitioners, and family practitioners emphasize eating well more often than do the vast majority of obstetricians. Some physicians may make derogatory comments about your weight gain. Find a health care practitioner who emphasizes good nutrition and who encourages you to feel comfortable gaining weight and to be happy with your changing looks and growing sense of self.

Preparation for Breast-feeding
(see also "Breast-feeding Your Baby," chapter 21, Postpartum, p. 507)

Nursing is the best thing for mothers, and mother's milk is the best thing for babies. Those first few days of colostrum (first milk: a clear, thin liquid) provide your baby with invaluable antibodies. Nursing just after birth and for at least the first few months will connect you with your baby immediately and intimately. If you are undecided, take time to talk with midwives, childbirth educators, and mothers who have happily breast-fed their babies and to read available books. La Leche League has been a useful resource for decades.

INFORMING YOURSELF ABOUT DRUGS, ALCOHOL, AND OTHER POSSIBLY HARMFUL SUBSTANCES

Good nutrition and good health practices will help you have a healthy baby. Poor maternal health and nutrition, certain environmental and occupational exposures, smoking, the use of recreational drugs and alcohol, some medications (prescription, over-the-counter, and herbal), and some vitamins or nutritional supplements are a few of the things that may have an unwanted effect on the developing baby.

Fetal vulnerability begins at the start of pregnancy, often long before you know you are pregnant or seek prenatal care and counseling. When you contemplate pregnancy, think about the way you live and your health practices for the risks they may pose to the growth of a healthy infant. You can affect your pregnancy in a variety of ways. Some substances or exposures may pose an immediate risk to the pregnancy or to the baby, such as those drugs that increase the risk of bleeding. Certain substances might cause fetal malformations that are evident prenatally or at the time of birth. Sometimes negative effects may not be immediately obvious: You may not be able to identify behavior disorders, learning disabilities, or delayed development and growth for the first few months or years. Some effects are not noticed until adulthood (for example, increased vaginal cancer in women whose mothers took DES during pregnancy). Refer to the Cochrane Collaboration of Drugs (see chapter 25, The Politics of Women's Health and Medical Care, p. 710) for a database of regularly updated reviews of common substances and drugs.

The following substances have predictable negative effects:

Alcohol

No safe limit has been established for alcohol consumption during pregnancy. The consumption of as little as one or two ounces daily during the first trimester is associated with infants born with features of fetal alcohol syndrome (FAS). This syndrome includes abnormalities in growth, in the formation of internal organs, and in the neurosensory system. FAS is one of the leading causes of mental retardation.[3] The Surgeon General advises pregnant women to consume no alcohol.

continued on next page

Smoking (Including Marijuana)

Smoking is associated with abnormalities of the placenta (placental abruption, placenta previa), miscarriage, premature delivery, and low-birthweight babies. In addition, tobacco use during pregnancy has been implicated in as many as 2,200 infant deaths a year from sudden infant death syndrome.[4]

Prescription and Over-the-Counter Medications

Some of these medications are known to cause fetal malformations. For example, isotretinoin (Accutane), a treatment for severe acne, causes malformations in as many as 23% of infants born to mothers using this product.[5] Vitamin use may cause problems—for example, evidence suggests that more than 10,000 IUs a day of vitamin A poses a risk to the central nervous system of the growing baby.[6]

Cocaine, Heroin, and Other Illegal Drugs

Illegal drugs have been associated with miscarriage, premature delivery, and poor fetal growth. Additional concerns have been raised about organ formation and neurodevelopment in prenatally exposed infants. When a pregnant woman uses addictive drugs, including heroin and methadone, her infant may be born addicted and may experience prolonged symptoms of drug withdrawal, including extreme irritabilty and poor feeding ability. Cocaine use has also been implicated in placental separation. Using several drugs at once increases the risk of negative affects. Additionally, impurities and dilutants are present in illegal drugs, such as herbicides, arsenic, coumadin (a blood thinner), and many other substances that can harm both mother and fetus.

Diagnostic Procedures, Including X Rays

Avoid elective procedures during pregnancy. If you must have certain procedures done, your health care provider and all technicians involved should be aware of your pregnancy. Take all appropriate precautions, and obtain guidelines for followup care from your practitioners.

You must weigh the risks of any particular practice against its benefits and the alternatives. Make choices that are as safe as possible for your pregnancy. Often, you can find out about and avoid workplace dangers (see chapter 7, Environmental and Occupational Health). If you use illegal drugs, or alcohol, you can seek available substance abuse counseling (see chapter 3, Alcohol, Tobacco, and Other Mood-Altering Drugs, and p. 459). If you need help to quit smoking, many local hospitals, clinics, HMOs, and community groups sponsor free or low-cost smoking cessation workshops and clinics. If your health care requires the use of medications, discuss safer alternatives with your health care practitioner rather than stopping the medications on your own. Pharmacists can provide information regarding over-the-counter medications and their potential dangers to pregnancy. Many drug package labels and inserts give this information as well.

You can also get information regarding drug safety, environmental exposures, and lifestyle practices during pregnancy from health care providers, from books, and from the Internet.

Making Love During Pregnancy

I wanted to make love more than ever.

I remember feeling very sexy. We were trying all these different positions. Now that we were having a baby, I felt a lot looser. I used to feel uptight about sex for its own sake, but when I was pregnant I felt a lot freer.

I felt very ambivalent about making love. I had miscarried several times. I wanted to make love and I was scared. As a single woman it was hard to find men who found me attractive with my belly so big. I had no sexual contact at all during the last two months.

You may feel more open, giving, and sensuous than ever before, or you may want to turn inward. With each month, each trimester, you may feel different. Be assured that intercourse and other forms of making love will not hurt the pregnancy. Enjoy pregnancy as a time to experiment with many different ways of loving, from massage and touching to exploring a range of lovemaking positions. You'll find that certain positions are more comfortable than others (see chapter 11, Sexuality).

If you have an orgasm, your uterine contractions may continue afterward, your uterus tightening and relaxing. Lovemaking can bring on labor toward the end of pregnancy only if labor is about to begin anyway. The prostaglandins concentrated in semen do soften the cervix.

You should not have penetrative sex if you experience vaginal or abdominal pain or any uterine bleeding, if your membranes have ruptured (waters have broken) because then there is danger of infection, or if you have reason to think that a miscarriage may occur. If either you or your partner has herpes sores, avoid any contact with the sores. Continue to protect yourself against HIV/AIDS.

Moving Around and Becoming Comfortable (see also chapter 4, Women in Motion)

Physical activity and exercise are important for good health. Continue doing what makes you happy, gives you energy, and creates a sense of well-being. It makes pregnancy easier. Check out the resources in your community, from swimming to yoga, and see Resources, pp. 496–501, for specific exercise books. You can practice labor positions, such as squatting, a position that opens your pelvis and facilitates labor. Meditation and relaxation techniques may also calm and center you, and you can draw upon them during labor.

Perineal Exercises

These exercises (popularly known as Kegels) consist of contracting and releasing your pelvic floor muscles and are simple to do. They help you prepare for childbirth by increasing your muscle tone so that you will consciously be able to let go of tension in your pelvic area during labor. See chapter 12, Understanding Our Bodies, p. 274, for instruction on how to do perineal exercises.

CARE DURING PREGNANCY: TIMING AND CONTENT OF EXAMS

Your first checkup can be with an independent (lay, community) midwife, a nurse midwife–staffed birthing center, a family practitioner, or an obstetrician in a clinic, private practice, or group practice. During your first few visits, the health care practitioner will take a complete history, including menstrual history, previous pregnancies and births, operations, abortions, illnesses, drugs taken, and family illnesses and conditions, such as high blood pressure or heart disease. Visits to health care practitioners will be one of your sources for learning about pregnancy. They provide you with information, answer your questions, and can help you feel good about yourself. Ask for information about the purposes and results of any tests recommended, and the results of the tests you receive. If you are not comfortable with your health care practitioner and if you have a choice of another, then find someone else. Trust your intuition. Your peace of mind is important. (See "Choosing a Health Care Practitioner," p. 451).

Most midwives, especially those in a noninstitutional setting, spend a great deal of time with you. They will take a complete medical and social history and discuss at length your and your partner's wishes and plans for pregnancy and birth. Obstetricians' exams may be much more cursory. The quality of prenatal visits is as important as the number.

At your initial visit, your weight and blood pressure will be checked. Usually, but not always, you will have a breast exam. Pelvic exams are often done to determine signs of pregnancy, such as the softening of the tip of your cervix and of your uterus. Many health care practitioners and women consider these exams to be invasive and unnecessary. (Pelvimetry, the outdated, so-called scientific measuring of the size of your pelvis, is a useless tool. It not only makes women feel inadequate but has led uninformed physicians to plan cesareans rather than let a woman give birth naturally.) You may have a Pap smear. The most common blood test includes a complete blood count; blood type; determination of Rh+ or Rh−; an antibody screen; and tests for syphilis, hepatitis B, and rubella immunity. You may also be tested for STDs in addition to syphilis if you have not been tested recently. (See chapter 14, Sexually Transmitted Diseases, for a description of the effects of untreated STDs upon newborns and "HIV and Pregnancy," chapter 15, AIDS, HIV, and Women, p. 373. If you have HIV, treatments now exist that greatly reduce the risk of passing it on to your baby.) Discrimination exists in that women with low incomes and women of color are often tested excessively. A urinalysis will check for protein and glucose, and a urine culture will reveal any urinary tract infections. If you are at special risk for diabetes (family history, extra-large babies, stillbirths) you will want to check your blood sugar level and receive nutritional counseling.

Some health care practitioners ask you to chart what you eat over a three-day period and then discuss it with you.

If you or your partner has a history of herpes or genital warts, be aware of outbreaks and use condoms during lovemaking. Eat foods rich in lysine, an amino acid, such as fish and potatoes. Avoid nuts and chocolate. Your health care practitioner may also prescribe lysine supplements, if necessary. You may be able to reduce outbreaks by eating well and minimizing stress.

Be sure to tell your health care practitioner if, at any time, you have pain, bleeding, or any other symptoms that worry you.

The baby's heartbeat is not audible with the fetoscope until 18 to 20 weeks, usually after you yourself have felt movement. You may choose whether to have the Doppler (ultrasound) device used for that purpose or a simple fetoscope (practitioners in most hospitals and clinics use the Doppler device). In general, internal exams are not usually necessary and are invasive.

It is critical that you seek out prenatal care, in addition to the care you give yourself. Many of us in rural areas or in cities find it hard to see a nurse or physician regularly; we go to the hospital only after labor begins. Sometimes it is possible to find an experienced independent midwife nearby. Although some clinics are staffed by nurse-midwives, many clinics and hospitals are not easily accessible by public transportation. Depressing, even hostile conditions include crowded waiting rooms, long waits (from two hours to a whole day), lack of privacy, and overworked, exhausted, or careless staff. Continuity of care does not exist. Scheduling and staffing patterns are frequently designed to

A BREECH BABY

If at some point after the 34th week of pregnancy you or your health care practitioner discover that your baby is in the breech position (presenting buttocks or feet first) try the following exercise. While lying on your back on a flat surface, raise your pelvis with pillows to a level nine to 12 inches higher than your head. Your stomach should be empty. Lying head down on a collapsed ironing board with one end propped on a couch or chair can be more comfortable. Perform this posture three times a day for ten minutes each time, and visualize your baby turning, turning. Practice this until the baby shifts position or labor begins.

CARING FOR OUR FUTURE

Our goal: to have excellent services available to *all* pregnant women, especially those of us who experience more problems because we lack needed physical, social, and economic support. (Other countries, such as France, offer financial incentives for women to make prenatal visits.) Such services would cover the entire childbearing year from pregnancy to the months after the baby is born, and include home care. They would be woman-and-family oriented, culturally appropriate, nonjudgmental, skilled, and compassionate. In the long run, this humane, preventive care would significantly decrease the appallingly expensive medical costs of "rescuing" low-birthweight and premature babies in intensive care nurseries, those tiny babies born "incompletely formed, to be attached to electronic monitors and infusions . . . the survivors too frequently develop blindness, hearing loss, infections, and permanent handicaps."[8]

Some important figures:[9] Infant mortality (deaths of infants under one year) is an important measure of a nation's health. The United States ranks 24th in infant mortality rate compared with other industrialized nations, with 8.5 per 1,000 infant deaths in 1992. More than twice as many African-American babies die as white babies. The statistics for Native American births are close behind. Among Hispanics, Puerto Ricans have the highest rate. Mortality rates among low-birthweight and very-low-birthweight babies have increased, largely because of the steady increase in preterm births. The 1997 Welfare Reform Law is sure to affect families adversely, forcing more women further into poverty, cutting essential services, and leading to more illness and death.[10] (On the positive side, severe complications of delivery have decreased, and more women breast-feed for at least four months.)

It is intolerable that in this wealthy country, access to high-quality health care is not a *fundamental human right.* "Improvements," while desirable, of course, are usually due to "rescues" of premature and low-birthweight babies rather than to a nationally planned program of health promotion and education. Various groups are fighting for this to happen. We join them in this seemingly endless struggle.

meet practitioners' training needs, not ours. Too often, the differences in class and racial and cultural backgrounds between practitioners and clients prevent rapport and understanding. There's often a lack of respect for women and families who come from other countries and cultures, as is shown by the dearth of translators for those of us who don't speak English, and ignorance about our beliefs and practices. It is no wonder that so many women become discouraged from going for appointments.

What I hated most about City Hospital was the "cattle run." There was always a mad rush for the elevator before clinic was about to begin. When we arrived, every patient was assigned a number. We waited, seated in rows on long, hard benches. The bathroom stank. The rooms were dirty, drab, and overheated. The medical staff were often overworked and overwhelmed; the nurses and the doctors were impersonal. I rarely saw the same doctor twice. Another concern was: Why didn't I ever see any physicians of color?

Continuity of care throughout pregnancy, emotional support, and education are all-important. They enhance our well-being and our health. "The effects of warmth and kindness on measurable outcomes of pregnancy may be difficult to demonstrate, but these qualities are simply good in themselves. Many things that really count cannot be counted."[7] This common-sense remark cannot be repeated too often.

LEARNING ABOUT PREGNANCY AND BIRTH

Seek out other child-bearing women. Talk with your partner and with family or friends you enjoy. Have a good time. Don't isolate yourself. Imagine how you want the birth to be. A wise midwife reminds us:

As you read, study, go to classes—whatever you are doing to prepare for your birth, remember that in the *deepest sense you already know everything you need to know to give birth. Sometimes you'll have to learn to trust your body, to open yourself to the process, and to dispel the cultural attitudes and fear that interfere with the process. All you need is the willingness to do so.*

Classes

You will meet other women and families in childbirth classes. You may have a choice of classes where you live. Large cities often hold classes at community clinics, health centers, birth centers, and hospitals that are taught by nurses, midwives, or physicians. HMOs, home birth groups, and independent teachers also frequently hold classes. If no classes exist, get together with other pregnant women.

Community-based classes are likely to be smaller and more personal than hospital classes, and much richer in content, as you will meet women planning to use different kinds of caregivers and birthplaces. The people you meet in classes may become good friends over the coming years.

A local gay and lesbian health center helped us form a lesbian pregnancy group. We met every month, rotated houses, and ate dinner. None of us had known each other before, but we were all at just about the same place in our pregnancies. We talked about common pregnancy concerns, how it was changing our relationships, what it means to our families, and about issues for the nonpregnant moms like feeling left out of the process at times. Now our babies are about one year old and we are still meeting together.

Home birth classes can often give you the most positive and complete information about normal labor and birth. Women planning to give birth in places other than home attend them also. They touch on a wide range of concerns: the physiology of labor and birth; visualization; relaxation; discussions of fantasies, feelings, and fears; information about hospitals' use of routine drugs and interventions and their risks and occasional benefits; breast-feeding; parenting. Couples visit with their new babies to describe their experiences and answer your questions.

Watching a film shown during one class was the first time I'd ever seen anything be born. Hearing the deep sounds some women make as they give birth, hearing them talk, made it real. I see that it's a lot of work; people are working hard to make the birth happen. A person can go through all that and be fine!

Most hospital and health plan classes tend to focus on labor and delivery by preparing you to accept their particular "management" of birth, presenting obstetrical procedures and techniques as if they were a normal and inevitable part of childbirth—basically, socializing you into hospital routines. Hospital-affiliated childbirth educators often feel constrained by their jobs in what they can say and how they can encourage you. Occasionally in hospitals you will find instructors strongly dedicated to your having the best possible experience. Independent childbirth instructors offer information about the widest array of alternatives.

A number of communities now have special swimming and exercise classes for pregnant women, which can also lead to sharing information and building friendships.

Childbirth Preparation Methods

Childbirth preparation and classes came about as a result of the efforts of dedicated childbirth activists (Margaret Gamper, Dr. Grantley Dick-Read, Marjorie Karmel, Elisabeth Bing, Lester Hazell, Niles Newton, Doris Haire, Norma Swenson, and Sheila Kitzinger, to mention just a few) who succeeded in reforming some obstetrical practices and educating us all. Their efforts have spanned at least seven decades.[11] In the 1960s, many of them fought for women to be awake and conscious during birth—an important advance, since many in the previous generation of women had been drugged and unconscious.

The Lamaze and Bradley methods of childbirth preparation, sponsored by organizations of the same name, are now the most popular. They help hundreds of women to go through labor and birth with more joy, control, and dignity than they would have without such preparation, knowledge, and support. Lamaze teachers, who used to focus mainly on breathing and relaxation, have expanded their scope to include a wide range of issues, as have teachers of the Bradley method (formerly called the "husband-coached method of birth"). Both organizations sponsor Mother and Baby Friendly Childbirth Initiatives, realizing now more than ever the need to counter the excessive medicalization of birth.

For those of us who choose to or must give birth in hospitals, these methods enhance our labors. Coexisting with some or many forms of intervention, they do not always stave off hospital practices. You can be mentally active and physically inactive, breathing deeply and trying to relax as you are hooked up to an IV, drugged by an epidural, your labor "augmented" with Pitocin. Some labors don't adapt themselves easily to methods too rigidly enforced; instead, you may have to adapt what you have learned to the rhythm of your own labor. Actually, we don't have to learn complicated breathing techniques—we can breathe in a rhythm that matches our labors. In the words of one midwife: "Teach women how to breathe? Why, we *know* how to breathe, honey—we've been doing it all our lives!"

Books About Childbirth

Almost every childbirth book contains useful bits of knowledge. One simple sentence will confirm in a flash your own intuition and insights, or give you courage where you were once afraid. Some books are reissued year after year and serve as reliable, inspiring guides. But remarkably few books describe the childbearing year in a consistently positive way. Too many seemingly pro-woman books contain conflicting comments; the most attractive layouts veil insidious mes-

CHOICE AND LIMITS TO CHOICE

The alternatives of choices available in childbirth may not address parents' . . . concerns about maternity care adequately because the choices offered are limited, and because parents are not really free to choose. Obstetric care is organized in ways that limit choices, being a hierarchical system dominated by an engineering model of birth, in which caregivers contact parents very briefly and are themselves interchangeable, where efficiency is paramount, and where the technology that has been adopted is confining rather than freeing.[12]

In those parts of the country where women and health care practitioners have succeeded in expanding alternatives, you may be able to choose both practitioner and birthplace. The options available in some institutions now include the presence of families and friends during labor and birth, doulas (labor attendants), and tubs for relaxing and easing pain and for water births.

However, your town, or the city nearest you, may have only one clinic, hospital, and physician. Physicians' groups may maintain standards of practice that conflict with your wishes and values. Current economic pressures and the resulting health organizations and insurance policies reduce access to choice. Managed care and HMOs restrict you to just a few health care practitioners. Practitioners and birthplaces are linked. Most physicians will not attend you at home, and most independent midwives cannot or will not attend you in hospitals. Laws in most states limit nurse-midwives to attending women in hospitals or birthing centers; some states permit them to attend home births. Most women with low incomes have access only to clinics. Many doctors won't accept Medicaid clients. Regulations may limit malpractice insurance and medical backup for independent midwives.

The fact that the medical establishment is the dominant system curtails your choices. Books and childbirth classes generate the illusion that you can make choices that run counter to the system. But once you are in the hospital, despite all you have learned and all you have done to prepare yourself, the power and practices of the institution limit your control over the environment.

Chance and luck play a huge role in what happens during labor in the hospital. A wonderfully encouraging nurse may be on duty, or your nurse may have never seen a normal labor and won't understand or respect your wishes. Your physician, whom you trust, may be busy with another birth or on vacation, and a doctor you've never met before thinks your ideas absurd and does things his or her own way. In addition, the presence of drugs and equipment, with personnel trained (or needing training) and eager to use them, can alter your determination if you don't have enough support when labor becomes intense.

Learn what is available in your area. Get names of health care practitioners from people you trust. Contact the Midwives Alliance of North America (MANA), the American College of Nurse-Midwives (ACNM), the National Association of Childbearing Centers (NACC), or Doulas of North America (DONA) as well as any nearby regional or community groups (see Resources, pp. 496–501).

When you interview health care practitioners, be clear about the kind of experience you want. Bring your partner or a family member with you for company and support and to help you remember what you want to say. Trust your instincts. If you are not treated with respect, find someone else. If you want a high level of decision making and choice, you may do better to select a midwife rather than an obstetrician, and a birth center or your home, rather than a hospital, as birthplace. If you are wondering whether your insurance policy covers the care you seek, ask; and if you get a no, pursue it—you may get what you want.

Choices may not always be clear and simple. Try to build in flexibility, and keep your options open as long as you can so that you can change your mind if you wish.

I'd planned to leave all my care and my decisions to my doctor. He seemed nice enough. I didn't know very much about childbirth. The big change happened after a few months. I told him that I wanted a doula with me during labor. "What book are you reading?" His tone of voice was so scornful and angry. "If it's not written by a doctor I can't comment on it." Wanting to check out his attitude, I asked Annette, my doula, to come to my fourth-month checkup. My doctor ignored her completely; she was invisible to him. He told me not to do Kegel exercises, and listed things I wasn't supposed to do. I realized then that he wasn't thinking of me but of what would make things easy for him. So I decided to leave. Now my labor had become my own responsibility. I wasn't ready for that. So I began to learn about nutrition, everything! What is hard to express is the endurance—I spent five months of pregnancy asking questions. I found a wonderful nurse-midwife practicing in a hospital birth center. My beautiful labor and the birth of my daughter were the culmination of a lot of decisions I'm happy with. I experienced the strength I always knew I had.

sages. Many authors individualize your struggle. They ask you to fight against attitudes and practices you intuitively know are not for you, or to adapt yourself to them without an analysis that places them in a broader context. Most often, these authors, who may spend their lives working for maternity care reform, end up by echoing the madness of our obstetrical system; they adopt medical language and undercut positive information with negative content. For instance, they may urge you to choose the kind of health care practitioner, labor, and birth you desire, and then direct you to the very institutions that limit these choices. They might encourage you to choose health care practitioners and then mention only obstetricians, as if midwives didn't exist. Or, in recommending midwives, they tell you of nurse-midwives and ignore independent midwives. One popular book builds you up for "Dr. Right" before warning you that he [sic] may be on vacation when you are ready to give birth! Another vastly popular book bases its content on worry, offering only medical, not midwifery, information. A book's organization is revealing: for instance, if a description of a cesarean section occurs within a chapter concerning the eighth month of pregnancy, such a juxtaposition subtly directs your thinking towards the possibility—nay, probability—of having a cesarean section.

Choose books that give you comfort. Check them out for content and organization if you have the time. Make sure they make sense to you. Discuss them with friends.

The Internet is another source of information. Use it wisely, and critically (see p. 501).

CHOOSING A HEALTH CARE PRACTITIONER

Since health care practitioners vary in their approaches to pregnancy and birth, don't make any assumptions until you have had a chance to talk to her or him and observe how you are treated and how your concerns are addressed.

When women go to practitioners for checkups, they should walk out from every visit feeling ten feet tall! Every site of care and style of care, no matter who gives it, ought not only to give surveillance but should educate and empower, should enhance every woman's feeling of her ability to do what she's doing well.
—A nurse-midwife

Choose your birth attendants carefully. They are an outward reflection of your state of consciousness. They will become your intellectual interpreters of your pregnancy and birth, and often your emotional support. The letters after their name and their gender don't tell you very much about them. There are some doctors who are more like midwives, and midwives who are more like doctors. How you feel about them and how they feel about birth are just as important as how skillful they are in their practices.
—An independent midwife

Midwives

Women have cared for child-bearing women for thousands of years. In many communities they were (and still are) recognized as "wisewomen" and consulted not only about child-bearing but about illness, abortion, and child health.

When midwives are free to practice as they choose, they offer us continuous care during pregnancy, labor, and birth, and after the baby is born. Midwife-attended births often mean fewer complications and fewer interventions.[13]

Midwives, at their best,

pay attention to you within your family context and care about your family dynamics, helping you sort out feelings and deal with practicalities.

bring to their work a strong combination of practicality and spirituality, being concerned with your well-being and satisfaction as well as your and your baby's safety.

encourage you to take charge of your care, to believe you are equal to the responsibility, and to feel in control of your experience.

are knowledgeable about normal pregnancy, labor, and birth.

respect the process of birth, trust the unique course of each labor, patiently watch it unfold, sustain and guide you, encourage you to find comfortable efficient labor positions and deal with contractions and pain, and help you ease the baby out.

bring you through difficult moments, sometimes turning what seems like a complicated labor into a normal one.

recognize complications that require a doctor's attention and call upon doctors for help when necessary.

In the U.S. today, there are two main types of midwives: certified nurse-midwives and independent (lay, direct-entry) midwives. They share similar philosophies about child-bearing, although their education, training, and practice may differ widely.

Certified Nurse-Midwives (CNMs)

More and more community clinics and hospitals are staffed by CNMs, nurses educated in graduate or certificate programs as specialists in normal birth and in well-woman care. They follow an organized program of study designed to meet the present standards of knowledge, skill, and judgment established by the American College of Nurse-Midwives (ACNM). Graduates are evaluated and certified after passing examinations, and each state licenses nurse-midwives to practice under its own regulations.

CNMs work in their own private practices, in private physician practices, freestanding birth centers, hospitals, health departments, and sometimes homes. They always practice in collaboration with physicians, referring women who have problem pregnancies to them and calling upon them in situations and emergencies

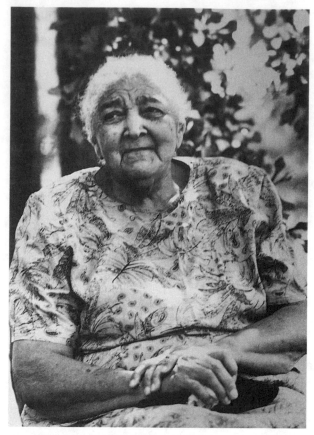

Mrs. Margaret Charles Smith, midwife (see box at right)
/William F. Dickey

that require medical advice and care, or surgical attention.

CNMs in the United States got their start in the 1920s, when nurses associated with the Frontier Nursing Service and Maternity Center Association began attending women living in poverty in Appalachia and New York City. CNMs worked in and out of hospitals for the next 50 to 60 years. Not until 1971 did the American College of Obstetricians and Gynecologists (ACOG) recognize their existence officially.

Nurse-midwives have been instrumental in creating out-of-hospital birth centers and in-hospital alternative maternity care programs in response to parents' complaints about conventional hospital care. They often attend women with low incomes when physicians will not, and they fight along with clinic clients for simple changes in obstetrical routines. Said one nurse-midwife: "It is a victory for us to enable clinic women to labor upright. Otherwise they'd be flat on their backs the whole time."

While some physicians appreciate the high-quality care that nurse-midwives offer, many others, especially obstetricians, consider nurse-midwifery to be an economic threat as well as a challenge to their competence as clinicians. As a result, they may refuse to develop the necessary cooperative relationship, attempt to prevent other physicians from doing so, or punish them when they do. Also, the increasingly

SOUTHERN BLACK MIDWIVES— A PROUD TRADITION

by Linda Janet Holmes *

I'm worth millions of dollars for what I've done. I thought I was doing a big thing. I was proud of it. The lives that I've saved going to deliver all of these babies, 'til I got something to be thankful for.
—Mrs. Margaret Charles Smith, midwife, Eutaw, Alabama

Mrs. Smith and other southern black midwives supported generations of birthing families, black and white, long before the emergence of today's independent midwife. Many southern black midwives trace their midwifery heritage to great-grandmothers who were midwives during slave times. These midwives "made a way out of no way" when hospitals and doctors refused to provide care to poor women and women of color. Southern black, Native American, and Latina midwives continued their widespread midwifery practices much longer than other ethnic groups because of the prevailing racist noncaring attitude among the dominant white medical establishment.

Although discrimination and a lack of access to medical care presented problems, midwives were good news for most families. Black families in the South can truthfully say, "Midwives got us here." In fact, until 1950, midwives attended the majority of all black babies born in the South. This continued to be the case in some small and rural isolated towns until the 1970s. But the anti-black-midwife laws that swept across the South about that time put an end to the legal practice of lay midwifery. With the advent of Medicaid and civil rights legislation, physicians suddenly found an economic incentive for extending hospital-based obstetric services to black women. In order for doctors to take full economic advantage of this situation, midwives had to be displaced. No "grandmother" clause for senior experienced midwives to continue their practices was provided, and few mechanisms existed for midwives to fight the laws. Thus they were forced to abandon their midwife calling. Today, states like Alabama have no independent midwives emanating from the southern black midwifery tradition.

As access to quality prenatal care continues to be lacking and choices in alternative birthing practitioners and sites remain limited, the loss of midwives is a pity. In addition to their profound sense of spirituality, midwives were particularly sensitive in understanding the emotional, social, and physical needs of families. For example, they cooked food, made beds, and took care of children, as well as waiting on babies ("waited on" is an expression used by many southern black midwives to define their childbirth attendant roles). Other aspects of their community roles included counselor for baby ills, advisor for women's health problems, community herbologist, and general healer. Most active and experienced midwives never lost a mother and rarely lost a baby.

Midwives who maintained culturally based expressions about the birth event were recognized ritual specialists. They supported mothers in carrying out rituals such as burial of the afterbirth and the "taking up" ceremony, a special ceremony for bringing mother and baby out into the world on a specific day following birth. Many of these traditions paralleled practices in African cultures.

As for actual midwifery practices, southern black midwives shared a philosophy and practice common to midwives around the world. They believed in keeping their mammas stirring, as they say, during labor. They were masters of various massage techniques that they applied during pregnancy and birth. They assisted mothers in using the traditional birthing positions taught to them by their mothers or the community's elder midwives, recognizing the wisdom of stooping, kneeling, or squatting to make birthing much easier. In the normal birthing process, they did not long for drugs and technology, but encouraged women in labor to drink teas and use other home remedies to gently urge the birthing process along.

Past midwives acquired their skills through apprenticeships with other experienced midwives. They also gained knowledge from their personal childbirth experiences, and some learned partially from local physicians through observation and by attending special classes held by public health clinics and black hospitals.

Although traditional southern black midwives are no longer the community champions of birthing care that they once were, efforts are being made to recognize their dignity and wisdom. Newly published oral histories, photographic exhibits, videos, films, and other historical records preserve the past and link these women with contemporary midwives practicing today.

But there is still much work to be done in reclaiming the midwifery history of women of color. If you are black and were born in the South before 1950, there is a good chance that you had a healthy birth at home and were guided into the world by the hands of a midwife. Join us in honoring midwives and their contributions. Their valuable work inspires all of us who champion midwifery knowledge and practice today.

* Co-author of *Listen to Me Good* (with M. Smith, see Resources, pp. 496–501).

technological approach to birth makes it difficult to adopt a midwifery approach.

Nurse-midwives, embedded in the medical system, have access to an array of resources, including physician backup. But this same system imposes constraints upon them. For instance, under the aegis of "managed care," clinic rules mandate brief prenatal visits, which affects the quality of care offered. And hospitals require baseline monitoring strips for women in labor, using a machine called a fetal monitor; this means that not only is labor interfered with (women have to lie down), but all concerned become dependent on electronic tools that are unnecessary for normal labor. Thus, restrictions on CNM practice are often due to practice norms, physician pressures, and lack of backup.

Despite their excellent record, and although they are increasingly in high demand (most women attended by nurse-midwives would choose them again), there are simply not enough CNMs. Too few training programs exist. For several years, many state laws restricted or prohibited nurse-midwifery practice. Nurse-midwifery is a collaborative profession, and nurse-midwives may find it difficult to link up with physicians. It is still the case in some places that CNMs cannot provide full-scale birthing care. For example, in Alabama they are relegated primarily to prenatal care and do little actual birth care.

Most nurse-midwives are now covered by insurance policies.

Independent Midwives (Also Called Direct-Entry, Lay, or Community Midwives)

Over the past 25 years, a new group of independent midwives has come into being. They are rooted in their communities and attend those women who choose to give birth at home. Some acquire their skills through apprenticeship with other midwives and (sometimes) supportive physicians as well as through reading and study. Others combine apprenticeship with attendance at one or several of the midwifery schools that have emerged over the past 15 years in Texas, Florida, New Mexico, Washington, and elsewhere. They become specialists in normal pregnancy, labor, and birth. Increasingly, they are the most skilled, knowledgeable, competent birth attendants in their communities. They screen pregnant women for risks and encourage them to obtain physician backup when needed. They know how to recognize labor complications, and they call for assistance when necessary.

Just as nurse-midwives are meeting standards and offering peer support, so women in the independent midwifery community keep in constant communication about their work. Both groups of midwives have joined forces to create the new Certified Professional Midwife (CPM). The North American Registry of Midwives (NARM), an organization created by the Midwives' Alliance of North America (MANA), together with a certification task force of midwife representatives from 40 states, has established criteria for validating the knowledge, skills, and experience of the CPM.

Independent midwives are also actively engaged in developing and maintaining communication with the medical community so that women will have adequate backup care. They try to educate physicians, nurses and medical personnel about the competency of midwives and the benefits and limits of midwifery care.

Midwives differ in personality and practice, in levels of experience, and in the manner in which they acquire their skills. The degree of cooperative backup varies, and some of them must depend on the emergency room rather than a specific physician. When you interview a midwife, look for competence, flexibility, and empathy. Ask her about her practice, experience, and commitments to see if she can meet your needs and wishes.

Some insurance pays independent midwives. Other midwives have a sliding scale or offer individuals different ways to pay. The care they provide begins with long, in-depth sessions with women and their families during pregnancy and continues through the days and weeks following birth.

I want to be where women are. I want to be where women want to be. I am fascinated to watch them be powerful. I see them emerge from their birth experiences and make changes in their own lives.

At the heart of midwifery lies the belief that the passage through the birth canal is a healthy experience for mother and baby. The midwife believes in the ability of a woman's body to move toward health, to compensate for irregularities, and to overcome pain. She sees birth as an expression of spirit in a physical act [and] believes that the baby benefits from this creative expression and actually likes being born.[14]

When a new client comes to me and asks about what kind of instruments or tools I use, I smile and hold up my hands. After 20 years and some 2,500 births, I am grateful for my hands and for the knowledge that they have all by themselves. My hands are used to soothe a brow, to massage a back, to pour water on a laboring tummy, to assure with a gentle touch that all is well, to lift a new baby onto Mom's tummy. And yes, to lift a stubborn cervical lip, to massage away an adhesion caused by prior forceps, to support a perineum with a wicked old episiotomy scar. When I die, I want my only grave marker to be two beautiful hands, folded in prayer.[15]

Physicians

Physicians assist at 95% of births in the U.S. Obstetrician/gynecologists, trained primarily as surgeons, see women for brief, periodic checkups; are usually in and out of your room during labor; and often arrive just before delivery. Often they practice in groups, and they may control childbirth practices in one hospital or throughout the region. In most suburban and metropolitan areas, only ob/gyns have delivery room privileges in hospitals. In teaching hospitals and medical centers, all of the MDs who attend you will be ob/gyns or ob/gyn residents in training. Though most obstetricians are not trained to deal with normal labor (see chapter 20, Childbirth, p. 469), their surgical skills are invaluable in real emergencies.

Family practitioners (MDs and DOs, or osteopaths) are "primary care" physicians trained in family medicine, which means that they can give basic, comprehensive care to any person of any age. They are more likely to know your family personally. Most of them have obstetrical experience, and some specialize in obstetrics. They have delivery room privileges in most community hospitals.

Those family practitioners and obstetricians who have our interests at heart listen to what we want, teach us a lot, learn from us, and alter their practices as they learn. Such physicians are rare.

In my relationship with families I get as much as I give. I see women doing marvelous jobs: During labor and birth they are autonomous, assertive, really pleased with themselves. To be part of their birth experiences is exciting for me in turn. My presence helps them to feel safe having their babies at home.
—A family practitioner

Dr. E. checked me out during my pregnancy because I had a particular medical problem. (Otherwise the midwives he worked with would have seen me.) Though he stayed with me during labor, Bonnie, my labor coach, acted as midwife, suggesting what to do, applying hot compresses. Dr. E showed her a lot of respect, the respect she deserved to have. It tickled me to overhear him say to the medical student present, "Now here's birth with dignity! I certainly don't need to be here."
—A mother describing her labor in a hospital birthing room

For a description of doulas, see chapter 20, Childbirth, p. 474.

PLACES OF BIRTH

Where to have your baby is one of the most important decisions you will make. If you plan to have your baby at home, you will be able to labor and give birth freely, without restriction. If you choose a birthing center or hospital, seek out "mother-friendly" practices, policies, and attitudes (see also chapter 20, Childbirth).

Mother-Friendly Practices [16]

A mother-friendly birth center or hospital:

welcomes the birth companions you choose, including partner, family members, and/or friends, and your

QUESTIONS FOR HEALTH CARE PRACTITIONERS—Midwives, Nurse-Midwives, Physicians

(As you ask your questions, you can get a good idea about a health care practitioner's beliefs, attitudes, and practices. Is she or he really listening to you?)

What is your philosophy of childbirth? What was your training? Where did you train? How long have you been in practice? How many births have you attended? How many have you been responsible for? Were they in hospitals, birthing centers, or homes? Do you practice alone or with other people? What is their experience? Do they share your beliefs and manner of practice? Who takes your place when you cannot be at the labor and birth? Will you be easy to reach when I need you?

What kind of prenatal care do you offer? Do you consider good nutrition, exercise, and breast-feeding important? What kind of childbirth preparation do you recommend? What kind of tests do you advise during pregnancy, and why?

What kind of labor support do you provide? Do you stay with women throughout labor? Do you appear just before birth? What do you think of having doulas or other labor assistants present? Of family and friends being present? What is your advice about moving around during labor, adopting the positions I choose, eating and drinking as needed? Will I hold my baby right after birth and breast-feed? How often will I see you after my baby is born?

What procedures do you do routinely? Under what circumstances and with how many women do you use drugs and interventions? What kind? IVs? Amniotomy? Electronic fetal monitors? Epidurals? Pitocin to speed up labor? Forceps or vacuum extractors? Episiotomy? What is your protocol for twins and breech births? Do you attend VBACs (vaginal births after cesareans)? How many of your clients have them?

Can you give me the names of some women who have used your services? How much do you charge? Are you covered by insurance?

Additional Questions for Midwives Who Attend Birth at Home

How often will you visit? Where will I go for any lab work? What kind of childbirth preparation do you recommend? Are you in communication with other midwives in the area? How do you define and handle complications? What drugs and equipment do you use in the home?

When and why? Who does your medical backup and where does it take place? Under what conditions would we go to the hospital? What experience do you have? Would you stay with me if we had to transfer? What has been your training in newborn resuscitation? How many times do you visit after the baby is born?

Additional Questions for Nurse-Midwives Who Give Care in Private Offices, Clinics, or Hospitals

What percentage of your clients require a physician's care? Under what circumstances do you call in a doctor to assist you? Who has the power to make decisions? Will you stay with me if I am transferred to a physician's care in an emergency?

And for Nurse-Midwives and Physicians Practicing in Freestanding Birth Centers

What are your requirements for admission? What percentage of your clients transfer to the hospital? Why? What are your backup arrangements? When do you advise women to go into the hospital?

labor support person (a friend, doula, or labor support professional); encourages you to walk around during labor, to move about and choose the positions you want and need during labor and birth; offers access to water (tubs and/or showers).

provides care that addresses and respects your beliefs, values, and customs.

encourages all mothers to breast-feed (there should be lactation consultants on staff) and care directly for their babies as often as possible, and all families to touch and hold their new babies, including babies who are premature, are sick, or have other problems.

has clear policies and procedures for consulting and collaborating with other maternity services and links you up after birth to appropriate community resources, including follow-up calls and home visits.

gives you an accurate description of its practices and procedures, including rates of interventions and outcomes.

educates staff in nondrug methods of pain relief and does not promote the use of analgesic or anesthetic drugs unless required to correct a specific complication.

does not routinely perform practices and procedures that scientific evidence shows to be useless or harmful, such as shaving, enemas, IVs, early rupture of membranes, electronic fetal monitoring, episiotomies; has low rates of cesareans (for hospitals, 10 to 15% and for birth center transfers, much lower).

provides for, in the event of (rare) complications, an anesthesiologist on 24-hour call, a practitioner trained in neonatal resuscitation, and a neonatal intensive care unit.

Women have all sorts of complicated concerns and restrictions, wishes, apprehensions, and convictions about where to have their babies.

I chose the hospital because I wanted the whole experience to be separate from the rest of my life and I felt safest there.

Jordan was born at home. For several months I couldn't decide where to give birth. The birthing center near the hospital is run by nurse-midwives. Some of them are nice, but their protocols are pretty strict and made me nervous. I wanted peace and calm, with no time limits, no interruptions, and an attendant who believes in me completely, as Anita, my midwife does.

I was aware of the home birth movement, but for me I couldn't do it comfortably. If anything happened, I'd never forgive myself. My parents would never forgive me. But I know childbirth is a fairly normal process so I didn't want to go to the Boston centers. I wanted a labor coach because I wanted to stay home as long as possible during labor. I chose Dr. M and the birthing room of the small hospital he worked at.

It would freak out our landlords if we gave birth in our apartment. I don't feel at home there anyway, and have no special attachment to it. I'm also a little nervous. So we're planning to use the hospital birthing room. Our doctor is a family practitioner.

After Noah was born at home I know what a truly good experience is. I felt rested, healthy, ready to have a baby. My husband was as involved, eager, and interested as he could be. My friends were all around me. It's incredible to think about doing the hardest, most concentrated, intense work you will ever do in your life in an unfamiliar place—the most intimate experience and you are sharing it with strangers.

Freestanding Birth Centers

Freestanding birth centers are homelike primary care centers with access to specialist consultation and hospital acute-care services as needed. Although nurse-midwives operate or staff 75% of the 145 centers in the U.S., obstetricians and family physicians who have a more natural approach to birth are increasingly interested in them. The birth center philosophy is simple—that pregnancy and birth are normal until proved otherwise. Programs focus on safe and sensitive care, promoting family health and enhancing your confidence in your body and your ability to give birth and nurture your newborn. Practitioners encourage families to become involved and participate in the care and the celebration of a new life. However, many free-

standing birth centers are being taken over by nearby hospitals because of "managed care" and must abide by hospital protocols, which can limit the practice of their original philosophy.

A 1989 study of almost 12,000 women in freestanding birth centers concluded that they offer a cost savings of 30 to 50% as compared with hospitals, and they minimize the cesarean rate (4.4% compared with 24% nationally).[17] There are 100 birth centers currently being developed throughout the country. Some centers are owned by hospitals, and others have contracts with HMOs, as they have proved to be so cost-effective. Most insurers pay for birth center services. This innovation is receiving increasing international attention as nations struggle to provide affordable, continuous, high-quality care to child-bearing women and families. Look for centers licensed by the state and/or accredited by the Commission for Accreditation of Freestanding Birth Centers. Call the National Association of Childbearing Centers (NACC) to find a birth center near you (see Resources, pp. 496–501).

Home Birth

A growing number of women, attended by midwives and physicians, are giving birth at home. Although home births make up only a small percentage of overall births in this country, they teach us how labor and birth can flow outside of an institutional setting and offer an inspiring, safe alternative.[18] Many women who have had powerful home birth experiences have become midwives, childbirth educators, doulas, and community activists, working for truly woman-centered care.

At home you shape your birth experience as you labor and give birth in familiar surroundings. Labor usually unfolds harmoniously, over a period of hours or sometimes days. Your birth attendants respect and support you. You may invite family and friends to

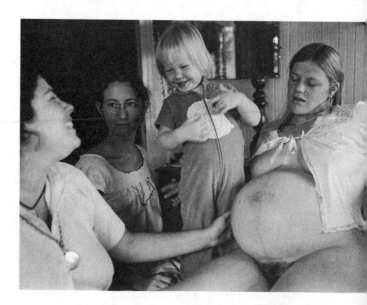

Suzanne Arms

share the wonder of birth and welcome the new baby. You can do so many things that help you labor well. After the birth you can relax, eat, be cared for, and get to know your baby. You have all the time in the world.

It was a really beautiful thing to do—not only to be freed from the atmosphere and personnel of the hospital (and who knows what it means for a newborn to see wood walls and carpeted floor, to smell real human smells, to feel wool and cotton and flannel clothes instead of starchy, white, deodorized . . .) but also to know that my body and her body knew what to do, and probably did it better than any doctors could. She was crying before the push that sent her into the world had faded and was wide awake from the start.

If you choose to give birth at home in this country, you are swimming against the mainstream and you will have to take the initiative. Institutional opposition is strong. Women who plan home births are often denied prenatal care or backup emergency care by local obstetricians who are openly hostile and say they "can't afford the risk."

Most physicians oppose home birth outright. They might try to frighten you with tales of what might happen, ignoring data and studies that demonstrate the safety of home births.[19] It is inconvenient and frightening for them to be away from the hospital technology upon which they so depend, for they have learned of no other way to help women during labor. It is psychologically threatening for them to be the invited guest in your home, where you set the tone and they are not in control. Fear of malpractice suits and condemnation by peers make most physicians unwilling to attend.

Most complications of childbirth can be handled without difficulty by a health care practitioner experienced in normal births at home. Birth is not risk-free anywhere. However, it is rare that hospital care unexpectedly becomes instantaneously necessary. A well-known matched controlled study comparing the outcomes of 1,046 home births with those of 1,046 hospital births found no significant differences in maternal or infant mortality or morbidity.

Many families planning home births make preliminary backup arrangements with local hospitals. Birth attendants have differing criteria for transferring a birth to the hospital. Their decisions may vary depending on the nature of the problem, their experience, the available equipment, their agreements with supporting physicians, and the nature of the backup facility as well as its distance.

Hospital Birthing Rooms

Many hospitals now offer labor and delivery rooms (LDRs) or labor, delivery, recovery, and postpartum rooms (LDRPs), where you can labor and give birth in the same room. In the best of these institutions, the philosophy will center on you and your needs and be family-oriented, flexible, respectful, and as noninter-ventionist as possible. A midwife describes the birthing room at her local hospital:

It's a really casual place. I went over and sat on the rug. The woman and her husband were dancing together . . . they were cheek to cheek . . . just lost in their own worlds. After a while he opened his eyes . . . and gave me this incredible smile. He said, "Oh, this is the prom we never had." It was as if we were watching a ballet of lovers. She would pull herself away from him and . . . undulate and wriggle and boogie . . . and he'd come to her and massage her . . . When the woman would look at us—you know how they're so far out there, they need a tether—she'd look and all we had to do was smile and nod our heads . . . then, all of a sudden she said, "Oh damn! unnh! I'm pushing already! I was having such a great time!"[20]

However, the mere existence of these rooms does not always guarantee you an autonomous labor and delivery. In some places, regulations are restrictive, and if your labor deviates from a mythical "norm" you may find yourself hooked up to a fetal monitor and subjected to an array of interventions. Under these circumstances, you may feel that you have to prove yourself—a stress that can make you tense and slow your labor.

Some hospitals still have separate rooms for labor, giving birth, and staying in after the birth.

Preparing for Birth and Beyond: A Personal Care Plan (Especially If You Plan to Have Your Baby in a Hospital)

Envision your birth. Don't plan it. You can no more plan the birth of your child than you can plan for the rest of your life. But you can plan the kind of care you want and whom you'll want to attend you. Stating your wishes in writing helps you focus your ideas. Express yourself diplomatically and firmly. Send copies to your health care practitioner, his or her associates, the hospital administrator, and the head of nursing. Bring a copy with you when you go to the hospital. Decide what your bottom line is—what you absolutely won't give up. Such a "plan" works sometimes, but not always.

PREGNANT WOMEN: SOME SPECIAL CONSIDERATIONS

In Your Teens and Pregnant

Becoming pregnant as a teenager will present you with many challenges. Because of our society's negative attitudes toward teen pregnancy, we forget that in earlier times, and presently in many countries around the world, women often have several children before the age of 20. Be assured that with support you can have a healthy pregnancy and give birth with ease. If you don't feel ready to be a parent, you have other options (see chapter 16, Unplanned Pregnancies, p. 381).

In your early teens, you yourself are still growing physically, and you need to eat a lot more healthy, nutritious food than usual. You have a lot of preparing to do—getting good prenatal care, learning about pregnancy and birth, making sure you know where you and the baby will live, figuring out how to stay in school or at your job, getting health insurance, lining up baby-sitters and child care, being sure you will have enough money. It can seem overwhelming, but don't forget that in order to nurture your baby, you must be nurtured yourself. Take advantage of any support systems available to you. The more helpful the people (family, friends, the baby's father, school counselors, public health nurses) you can surround yourself with, the better. They can help you to stay healthy and feel positive about pregnancy and birth, to plan for your and your baby's future, and to care for your new family. See also Ruth Bell's *Changing Bodies, Changing Lives* for invaluable information about teenage pregnancy.

If You Are in Your Late 30s or 40s

Many more women are becoming pregnant for the first time in their late 30s and early, middle, and late 40s.[21] Although you may feel more ready to have a child, both emotionally and physically, than you did in your twenties, the medical establishment, by virtue of your age alone, may consider your pregnancy "high-risk." They may label you as an "elderly primagravida" and view your baby as a "premium baby" requiring extensive inventions. They share our society's stereotype that women in their mid-30s and in their 40s are past their prime and aging fast. This belief gives them "reasons" to intervene.

In reality, the elevated risks with age are limited. There may be some genetic risks and risks associated with conditions that may develop with age, such as diabetes and hypertension. Create for yourself a climate of confidence, and be sure to find a satisfactory support system.

Child-bearing and Sexual Abuse

If you have a history of sexual abuse, the effects of that abuse may surface during your child-bearing year. Whether you remember the specifics of your abuse or not, unsettling memories, dreams, and/or feelings may occur or recur. For example, you may have flashbacks during prenatal checkups or while nursing or bathing your baby. Try to find a health care practitioner with whom you feel comfortable enough to tell at least part of your story. A therapist may also be helpful during this time. Switch practitioners if you are dissatisfied or uncomfortable. Also, find people to talk to among your friends and family. Though having a history of sexual abuse may raise difficult issues, keep in mind that pregnancy, birth, and motherhood—some of the

deepest experiences of body and soul—can be immensely empowering and healing, both physically and emotionally.

If You Are Experiencing Abuse or Violence [22]

If you are being hurt verbally, emotionally, or physically, and you trust your health care practitioner with personal confidences, your prenatal visits may provide you with an opportunity to seek help. Although prenatal screening for certain medical considerations is routine, violence is more common and dangerous than many other medical problems. It can hurt not only you but your unborn baby, causing miscarriage or putting you and your baby at risk during labor and birth. Some studies find that one in 15 women are battered during pregnancy, and it's highly probable that this figure is misleadingly low. Many physicians attending pregnant women do not notice or recognize the marks of abuse (bruises, depression, drinking to cope), or they fail to address or report it. Service providers in battered women's programs were the first to publicize the fact that many pregnant women experience violence.[23]

Intimate partners, former partners, or parents and other family members are the usual assailants. If you are abused, look in the phone book and/or call a local woman's center to locate battered women's shelter offering refuge and help (see chapter 8, Violence Against Women). **There is NO justification for abuse.**

He became jealous and possessive. He'd ask me, "Why spend money on baby clothes when we need it for food? Why are you reading all those books; they're filling your head with garbage." He'd want more sex and say, "Don't make excuses." He wouldn't let me see my family or friends and isolated me. Because I was large and clumsy I was no longer the "showpiece." I became the butt of jokes. He made a lot of comparisons with animals. I was the "heifer." He whittled away my self-esteem. Then he started pushing and shoving me to see if I would fall, and ended up elbowing my stomach or letting the door fall back into my stomach. That was the pattern. I couldn't talk to anyone about it. I lost four out of eight pregnancies. I left him after 14 years.

I have always wondered if this "capacity-to-give-birth-envy" were not a major force behind the subjugation and abuse of women from the beginning of time.

Pregnancy, idealized as a state that must be respected by others, may in fact increase your risk of being beaten. Some women don't experience abuse until they are pregnant. Too many men subordinate women with verbal or physical abuse, or both. They may use alcohol and other drugs to excuse their lack of control. Your partner may feel powerless, becoming angry and jealous because you are slipping out of his control. The family dynamic is changing. You look and act different. Your body is changing; you focus inward. You are tired; you don't want to make love. The specter of future financial and emotional pressures, such as unemployment, insufficient income, and sharing your attention with someone new all increase the possibility of violence. You are indeed more defenseless and often economically dependent, which makes it very difficult to take action against violence.

If your partner's remarks change from loving to degrading, take notice. If you are isolated, do everything you can to end your isolation. Find other women to talk with. Exchange experiences, insights, and solutions. Try to get out of your situation, to protect yourself and your baby.[24]

Drug and Alcohol Treatment: Protecting Our Rights as Pregnant Women

Recently, there have been instances of pregnant women who use alcohol or drugs being charged with civil and criminal child abuse or with delivering illegal substances to minors. Though courts dismissed most of these charges, many of us are afraid to seek treatment for substance abuse because we do not know whom to trust. There *are* safe places to turn to.

You may find a local treatment program that addresses the needs of pregnant women. If none are available, or if you don't feel safe in any that exist, you can attend a local AA (Alcoholics Anonymous) or NA (Narcotics Anonymous) meeting. Both guarantee anonymity, and you may find someone there who can provide trustworthy contacts. Women's health centers, state health departments, and health care providers you trust may give you more leads.

Federal law (42USC Section 290dd2, and its implementing regulations 42CFR, part 2) makes it illegal for drug or alcohol treatment programs to disclose information about you without your consent. However, other health care providers are not covered by these restrictions; if they suspect that someone will harm herself or others, or suspect child or elder abuse, they are legally required to report it. The best way to ensure confidentiality is to ask for it directly.

If you experience discrimination in trying to find treatment, or believe that your rights to confidentiality have been violated, contact the Center for Reproductive Law and Policy (see chapter 13 Resources), or the Legal Action Center (see chapter 3 Resources).

If You Have a Disability [25]

As women with disabilities, we share with all women the right to be in control of our own bodies, to give birth, and to parent our children. We need to assert these rights while educating ourselves about what having a child will mean for us and our families. Asking these questions beforehand can help you clarify your thoughts and wishes: Will pregnancy and birth put my health at risk? If so, how? Are there ways to lessen the risk? Would I want to have a baby despite the risk? Will I pass on my disability to my baby?

Be prepared for people to try to talk you out of having a baby. Others often can't imagine how we cope with life and therefore can't understand how we could possibly be mothers. Women with disabilities can be good mothers: We do it all the time—and always have! Even mothers who are not disabled can become disabled at any time. Don't let other people's ignorance make your decision for you. Learn whether your disability is genetic—most are not (see p. 460). Your health care provider or a genetic counselor may be able to provide you with the information you'll need.

Many women with disabilities encounter inaccessible facilities, insensitive practitioners, ignorance, and discrimination when they attempt to get adequate medical care. Be prepared to advocate for yourself and educate your health care practitioner about your disability, or find an advocate who can help. Arrange in advance for the accommodations you'll need when you phone for appointments. Health care providers are legally obligated to make reasonable accommodations for you.

Ask about how pregnancy will affect your disability, and about the possible effects of medication on you and your baby. Opinions may differ. Don't hesitate to get opinions from other specialists. Find out what to expect in the final months of pregnancy. Some women find that advanced pregnancy limits their mobility or exacerbates other health problems. Many doctors and midwives simply have had no experience dealing with pregnant women with disabilities, as research, data, and training about pregnancy for women with disabilities is very limited. Use all the resources at your disposal if your practitioner doesn't know. Try to find other women with your disability who have had babies. Contact organizations that deal with your specific disability. The Internet may be helpful.

Ask your health care practitioner how your disability will affect labor and birth, and consider possible complications and pain. Decide ahead of time who you want to be with you during labor and birth and where you want to have your baby. If your health plan doesn't allow you to make these decisions, try to meet all of the members of the health "team" who might be with you when you give birth. It can help to tour the hospital or birth center in advance. You might want to include a brief biographical statement about yourself and a paragraph telling people how you want to be treated (e.g., "Don't talk to me through my attendant/interpreter; talk to me directly"). Bring copies to hand out to everyone. It may prevent you from having to answer the same questions over and over.

Unlike your home, hospitals are rarely set up for the convenience of people with disabilities. Because you can't control your environment and accommodations, your stay there often feels disabling in itself. Many women with disabilities need to remain longer in the hospital after childbirth than women usually do. Ask your health care practitioner to deal with the hospital and insurance company about your length of stay. Before you go into labor, also ask your health care practitioner to advocate for you if necessary.

Being in the hospital and experiencing the intense physical changes of labor can make you feel as helpless as when you first dealt with your disability. These feelings can be overwhelming. Remind yourself that you are the expert on your own care and needs. Trust yourself to handle difficult situations and people. Also make sure that someone accompanies you to act as your advocate whenever you are unable to communicate or if you are not getting what you want, and for general, loving support.

For Information on Pregnancy and AIDS, See chapter 15, HIV, AIDS, and Women.

If You Have Been Circumcised (see also chapter 24 for further discussion)

As more women who have undergone circumcision live in the U.S., it is important that health care providers learn about this issue and approach it with sensitivity.

If you have undergone circumcision, you may be concerned about your ability to give birth and fearful of negative and judgmental reactions from health care providers. These concerns are often compounded by language barriers. If you have had a clitoridectomy, or clitoridectomy and removal of labia, you may need no medical intervention in order to have a normal vaginal delivery. The most severe type of circumcision, called infibulation, or scarring that has altered the vaginal opening, may require some surgical intervention before or during the second stage of labor. In most cases, a simple defibulation using local anaesthetic to cut open the skin covering the vagina is sufficient. This procedure is preferably done before or during pregnancy so that the wound heals before the birth.

GENETIC SCREENING AND DIAGNOSTIC TESTING DURING PREGNANCY [26]

Many physicians routinely recommend genetic and diagnostic testing during pregnancy to screen for various medical problems. While these tests can sometimes provide useful information, the routine use of certain blood tests, ultrasound, and amniocentesis can medicalize your pregnancy; pose risks to you and your baby; erode your ability to choose the kind of pregnancy, labor, and birth that you want; and generate tension, fear, and costs. In addition, test results may be inaccurate or misleading, may tell you little about the severity of a potential disability, and can lead to a "cascade" of further testing and interventions.

Genetic screening and prenatal testing raise complex issues. Your decision to have a test or not depends upon many considerations such as your family situation, your attitudes toward medical procedures and risks, what the test results would mean to you, your beliefs about abortion, and your feelings about the possiblity of having a child with a disability.

In addition, many people have great concerns about the social and political implications of routine screening for conditions such as Down syndrome and spina bifida. Because some people assume that a child with a disability would necessarily have a unhappy life or be too much of a burden, women with positive test results may face pressure to have an abortion. Getting to know children (and adults) with disabilities and their parents can help you learn more about what it might be like to parent a child with a disability.

At 27 I gave birth to a baby girl with Down syndrome. Three years later when I became pregnant my family, doctor, and friends pressured me to have an amnio, since I was at higher risk for another Down child. I refused because I simply would not have an abortion at five months and more importantly, I knew with all my heart that had I known my Ellie was Down syndrome before she was born, it would have told me NOTHING about who she was and who she is becoming.

Because I was 37, the doctor with whom my midwife consulted strongly advised "Triple Marker" (enhanced MSAFP) testing, stressing the noninvasive nature of the procedure. The results suggested my child was at higher risk than average for both spina bifida and Down syndrome. Although I had definitely decided against amniocentesis because of the risk of losing the baby, I agreed to an ultrasound. It "eliminated" spina bifida, but not the risk of Down and showed cysts on my baby's brain that I was told are usually absorbed, but not always. All that information I'd been given inadvertently, the expense, testing and waiting, and I spent the next four months wondering and waiting uncertainly for the birth of my daughter. She was born at home, a lovely, perfectly healthy 7-pound baby. But the testing had altered my whole pregnancy experience.

After the terrible loss of my first child at age three from Tay-Sachs [a fatal genetic disease] my husband and I agreed to have Tay-Sachs screening for our second pregnancy. We were devastated to find out that that baby also had Tay-Sachs. We had to decide whether to abort this baby. It was such a wrenching decision because I felt like it somehow negated my first child's life as well as this baby's. But . . . we could not go through the loss of another child. We did abort. Finally we had another baby without Tay-Sachs. She is fine.

Since the mid-1980s, both nonprofit and commercial genetic laboratories have introduced new genetic tests into the "market." These lucrative tests have often been introduced prematurely and overused. Physicians may persuade you to undergo such tests not for your own good or the good of your baby, but to acquire experience in performing them, and then to produce studies assessing the results. They may also be protecting themselves, "doing everything possible" in case something goes wrong. You are much more likely to be subjected to a barrage of tests if your doctor is technologically oriented or if you plan to have your baby in a large teaching hospital. Many midwives, especially those working outside of institutions, believe these tests are unnecessary, and they are less likely to suggest that they be routinely performed. Instead, they carefully discuss with you the implications of testing. Often the very existence of these tests pressures us into having them done.

My doctor insisted I should have amniocentesis and downplayed any risks. "Well, when are you going to do it?" he kept asking. Finally, during one checkup, he got me when I was feeling very vulnerable. Yet even when I got up on the table to have it done, I hadn't really made up my mind about it.

I was 37, healthy, had had two children and was pregnant again after 17 years. I just knew I didn't want a needle poking into my womb.

My son was born 14 years ago. In the past three years I had an abortion and a miscarriage. Once again I became pregnant. Though I had planned to have an amniocentesis done that last pregnancy, the miscarriage changed my mind: When the medical center sent out an informational pamphlet about amniocentesis which said that there was a 1.5% chance of miscarriage or fetal damage, and after Steven and I had done a lot of reading, I realized that if I had to go through another loss I'd be a basket case. So I decided not to have it done.

Then came the enormous pressure. Here I was, 38. My doctor urged me; so did my father, my husband's parents; my sister had had one and so had all my friends, without questioning. I even knew abstractly that I'd rather have a miscarriage than a Down syndrome baby.

For three weeks I was a wreck. Then one of my friends asked me, "What would be the worst thing?" I said, "The worst thing would be if the baby were healthy and amniocentesis caused a miscarriage." That did it: no amniocentesis. I'd really made the decision. We lived with it fine. And Sarah is wonderful and healthy. There is no easy answer.

Deciding About Tests

Before making decisions about testing, we need to ask what information will be obtained, what can be done with it, and what will we do with it.

Consider the following: You have the right and responsibility to ask for and to receive information about the reason for the test; an up-to-date description of the test, including the type of preparation necessary, the kind of equipment used, the issues to be confronted,

and the ensuing laboratory procedures; an unbiased description of the health conditions being assessed as well as the range of expression and possible treatments; the information yielded by the test; where to get additional information; the best medical facility for the test you are considering; the best practitioner; the accuracy of the test, stated as either a quoted range ("96 to 98%") or a percentage ("98%"); the possibility of error or contamination; and a clear statement of the physical risks for you and your baby, with their incidences noted (as in a 1.5% risk of miscarriage). Be aware that it may not be possible to keep test results confidential.

Detailed informed consent forms can also provide a framework for your questions and answers. Informed consent must be a process involving the exchange of information between you and your health care provider about tests, treatment, and research. Neither the informing nor the consenting is meaningful unless it is part of an ongoing dialogue.

An increasing number of health care practitioners are now requiring "informed refusals" (relatively new in health care), which state that a test has been recommended and refused. Informed refusal can be as important as informed consent. It confirms that information was provided and tests were knowingly and willingly declined. Many women experience informed refusal processes as forms of coercion that shift the burden of proof from the health care provider to present valid reasons for the testing, to the woman who is being asked to refuse the dominant forms of care assumed to be routine. One woman described it as being dragged on to a moving train and then asked if she wanted to jump off as the train continued on.

Consent forms provide a record of information consciously exchanged. They safeguard your rights and your freedom of choice and autonomy. Make sure that the consent forms also include, in addition to the items in the earlier paragraph, a statement indicating that you have spoken with your health care practitioner, have read the consent document, and have been given a chance to ask questions. You must provide a signature; the form must be dated.

Think about why you want the test or tests. Talk it over with your physician, family, and friends, and other women who have made these decisions.

Think about what decisions you will make based on the test results. In the rare instances when the results reveal a potential fetal disability, knowing about certain conditions beforehand may enable you and your family to prepare for the special needs of a new baby, for fetal surgery or organ donation, for putting a newborn up for adoption, or for ending the pregnancy with an abortion. Explore your attitudes and presumptions about disability and what makes a life "worth living." Talk with people who have had direct experience with the conditions or disabilities being tested for.

While a genetic screening test provides a signal or alert to the possible existence of a genetic condition, by itself it cannot give any definite information, nor can it "fix" a condition. It can only suggest which individuals might be offered further diagnostic tests to confirm the presence or absence of a specific condition. Having a baby always involves unknowns, and even the available tests can't identify all problems. They do not magically "prevent" disease and disability.

The Tests and Procedures

Maternal Serum Alpha-Fetoprotein (MSAFP) Screening

This blood screening test, performed at 16 weeks of pregnancy, is used to identify women who may have a higher than usual chance of carrying a fetus with a neural tube condition, such as spina bifida (an open lesion along the backbone—a condition that can vary from mild to severe)[27] or anencephaly (the tube remains open at the top—a fatal condition). These conditions occur in two of 1,000 babies. Researchers have found that women carrying an affected fetus have higher than normal levels of alpha-fetoprotein (AFP). Women with elevated AFP levels are usually advised to have further testing. Ultrasound and amniocentesis increase the accuracy of diagnosis. However, increased AFP levels can be difficult to interpret. These tests often yield false-positive results, caused by certain other rare disorders, a multiple pregnancy (carrying twins or more), or an incorrect estimate of fetal age.

Medical personnel and laypeople have raised questions about routine AFP screening, which subjects so many women to tests when so few will actually have any problems. Inadequate counseling, lack of cultural and linguistically appropriate information, and the procedures themselves can cause extreme stress.

Enhanced MSAFP (Fetoscreen, Downscreen, Triple Screen, and AFP Plus)

This relatively new blood screening test measures levels of alpha-fetoprotein (AFP) in addition to one or two other biochemical markers (unconjugated estriol and human chorionic gonadotropin) to determine the probability of the presence of fetal Down syndrome, with a 60 to 65% accuracy, which needs to be further confirmed by amniocentesis.

Fetal Ultrasound (Sonography)

Ultrasound is often used throughout pregnancy, although the place, if any, for routine ultrasound has not been convincingly established, and we don't know enough about its long-term effects on babies. Many studies conclude that its routine use is not appropriate for most pregnancies. It is used for many reasons: to confirm or date a pregnancy, to check for multiple births, to examine the baby at different stages of development, to find out the location of the placenta and other organs, and as an adjunct to other genetic reproductive procedures. The procedure is done by placing a probe (transducer) on the mother's abdomen or in-

serting it into her vagina (some women feel more comfortable inserting it themselves). It uses intermittent high-frequency sound waves to create pictures of the inner organs by recording their echoes, much as sonar determines shapes in the water. A technician or physician moves the probe around, and a computer translates the echoes into pictures on a video screen. These days it has become very common for families to show their ultrasound photo or video to family and friends, which makes the pregnancy "more real" for others but which can incline some women to discount their own sense of how their pregnancies are progressing. When practitioners insist upon using it to confirm the date of conception, rather than trusting a woman's knowledge of her cycle, they are often just plain wrong. It can become one of the first medical instruments of control of your pregnancy.

Chorionic Villus Sampling (CVS)

This relatively new and still experimental test is performed under ultrasound guidance between ten and 12 weeks of pregnancy. It involves undergoing ultrasound, and the insertion of a suction catheter into your vagina or a needle into your abdomen to remove a piece of the chorion (the chorionic villi, finger-like projections of tissue that later become the placenta), the outer tissue of the sac surrounding the embryo. The test is used for chromosomal analysis and for biochemical and DNA studies. Its safety, accuracy, and long-term effects are mainly unknown. It is, however, known that a significant number of babies are harmed by the test: they are born with complications such as limb deficiencies. Other risks are infection of the mother, bleeding, cervical lacerations, and miscarriage. Two percent to 2.5% of fetuses die as a result of this procedure.[28]

Fetal Cell Sorting

This experimental procedure is being developed as a noninvasive form of prenatal testing, with the aim of making invasive techniques obsolete. It involves taking a small amount of blood from your arm in order to isolate and test fetal cells appearing in the maternal serum.

Amniocentesis ("Amnio" or "Tap")

This is an invasive surgical procedure requiring ultrasound. It is usually performed between 16 and 18 weeks of pregnancy, and it is now being offered in some settings as early as 12 weeks. It involves inserting a long thin needle through your abdominal wall into the womb and drawing off approximately four teaspoons of fluid into a syringe. The fluid contains cells and substances shed by the fetus that can be analyzed in specialized laboratories to determine the genetic status of the fetus. Tests other than routine chromosome analysis and AFP screening will be performed only if your physician indicates that they are necessary. Ordinarily, you would not consider any of them unless you have specific reasons to believe that your baby is at risk. More specific tests may be done to determine the presence or absence of approximately 80 rare conditions, such as Down syndrome, cystic fibrosis, neural tube defects, or sickle-cell anemia (done only in a few specialized centers). It is also used to determine the sex of your baby. The complications, although rare, include bleeding and infection. The miscarriage rate is estimated at 0.5 to 1.5%.

Some physicians use a local anesthetic to numb the skin; others don't. On rare occasions the physician will have to try a second time to get enough fluid. You may have some or all of the following sensations during the procedure: pricking or stinging of your skin, cramping when the needle enters the uterus, and pressure when the fluid is withdrawn. These reactions are normal and don't mean that anything is amiss, but they should diminish and disappear within a day. If they don't, call your physician.

Many physicians urge us to have amniocentesis performed. It is standard medical practice to offer the procedure to women older than 35, because older women have a slightly increased chance of having babies with Down syndrome (trisomy 21). Increased paternal age may also contribute to the condition. But amniocentesis is being offered to younger and younger women, and it has become common to be asked by friends if we know the sex of our baby.

When I became unexpectedly pregnant at 43, my doctor told me about amniocentesis, but I told him that because of my religion I wouldn't consider having an abortion no matter what the results of the test. He then suggested I consider having the test just to find out the condition of the baby—that probably we would be reassured that it was all right. I talked it over with my husband and he thought this idea made sense. It was very upsetting when we first learned the baby had Down syndrome, but this didn't change our original feelings. Learning the baby's condition early made all the difference. I attended a clinic which helps parents care for children with Down syndrome and talked with many parents. As well as preparing ourselves, my husband and I were able to help our three teenage children know what to expect. We all picked out the baby's name together, and the children are waiting for him to come home so they can help take care of him.

Whereas some women find the procedure easy, others find it an unpleasant, upsetting experience.

I was nervous. But my obstetrician met us in the waiting room and told me that discomfort is unusual. First they showed it on the ultrasound screen and then made a pen mark on my stomach where the needle was to go in. The whole procedure turned out to be completely painless. My doctor talked his way through. "Now I'm going to do . . . Now you'll feel . . ." It was reassuring. Then he told me to take it easy for a day.

After, we spoke to a genetics counselor and asked a lot of questions.

The procedure itself wasn't bad. My husband went with me. I found it kind of creepy thinking of that long needle, so I didn't look. It took longer than I thought. Having my own doctor there made a difference; I would have been more nervous in a clinic in somebody else's hands. Afterwards, however, I had bad cramps and was in great pain. I found it traumatic to hear [from the counselor] about all the genetic disabilities that could not be picked up and why the test might have to be done again. I stayed in bed for two days because I had lost a baby a few years before and was afraid of miscarriage. When it became clear that things were all right, I felt better.

Percutaneous Umbilical Blood Sampling (PUBS)

This is a newer experimental method of fetal blood sampling, performed from the 18th week and throughout the pregnancy. Using ultrasound, the physician guides a needle through your abdomen and uterus into the umbilical vein. The test measures fetal blood components directly, clarifies findings of other tests, and is used for the delivery of medications. PUBS has a higher complication rate than either amniocentesis or CVS, and it is used only in very special situations.

Other Prenatal Screening Tests

Another set of tests exists, originally designed as screening and diagnostic tools for women with health problems (diabetes, heart or kidney disease, or excessively high blood pressure), for women who have had a previous problem such as a stillbirth, when there is concern that a baby is not developing properly (intrauterine growth retardation—IUGR), or when there is concern about the well-being of a post-dates baby (a pregnancy that has gone beyond 42 weeks). The goal of these tests is to discover whether the baby is healthy enough to remain in the uterus. While they are sometimes successful in reassuring worried women and health care practitioners, and they sometimes result in health-promoting and lifesaving interventions, these tests, like the tests previously discussed, do not guarantee a healthy baby. In addition, researchers have not performed enough randomized clinical trials to prove that testing and knowing the results actually do reduce perinatal death. The tests have high false-positive rates, and medical people disagree over which results constitute "normalcy" and which mean danger. Despite such cautions, many doctors have begun performing biophysical and biochemical tests routinely on healthy women. This practice does reassure some women. But tests cost money, further medicalize pregnancy, possibly leading to test after test, and worry many women excessively and needlessly. Once again, use your own judgment, and resist their availability and others' urging you to have them done. It is most important that you feel as calm as possible during pregnancy.

Screening for Gestational Diabetes— The Glucose Tolerance Test

At 28 weeks it has become routine in medical practice to screen for a condition labeled gestational diabetes—not to be confused with early-onset or juvenile diabetes, or late-onset diabetes, which are diseases. There is significant controversy over routinely screening all child-bearing women in the absence of specific indications (such as family history of diabetes, obesity, a large-for-dates baby, feelings of exhaustion, excessive thirst). The oral glucose tolerance test (OGTT), which is used to diagnose this condition, does not produce reliable, repeatable values. Failure to consume adequate amounts of carbohydrates for three days before the testing, bedrest, and many medications can cause false-positive results. (Some critics suggest that if testing is to happen, the diagnostic levels for true diabetes be used and not for just the lower levels.) The concern is that a woman with this condition is at greater risk of having a large baby with shoulder dystocia (shoulders that have difficulty fitting through the birth canal) or will be delivered prematurely. In fact, most women with this condition have normal-size babies, and most large babies are born to women without it. The meaning and value of this testing has been questioned: It leads to women being labeled as "high-risk" with all the stress, anxiety, and unpleasantness such diagnosis produces. It does not lead to an improvement in the health of mothers and babies beyond that achieved through exercise and a healthy pregnancy diet. This test can also lead to unnecessary, costly, and risky interventions, including induction of labor at or before 40 weeks and all the consequences of induction (prematurity and the possibility of an unnecessary cesarean section).[29]

Beta Strep Testing

Because a certain percentage of women carry beta Strep bacteria (*Streptococcus* B), and because there is a small risk that this bacteria can cause a newborn's death, the Centers for Disease Control recommend that vaginal culture specimens be taken from all women between 35 and 37 weeks of gestation.

Tests to Assess Fetal Well-Being

As your pregnancy progresses, you become aware of the pattern of your baby's activity. Babies vary in their activity levels. Some are more active than others, and most alternate between activity and resting. Your perception of the movements will vary according to what you are doing. You know about your baby's routine, and this knowledge can provide information about your baby's health. Toward the end of your pregnancy, or if you carry it beyond 41 or 42 weeks, your health care practitioner may ask you to pay close attention to your baby's movements. Often during a visit, he or she may observe how active your baby is and check to see whether its heart rate speeds up after each movement. Babies often slow down just before labor begins. If you notice a marked change in your baby's activity level, tell your practitioner. A practitioner concerned about your baby may ask you to undergo one or more of the following tests to check your baby's well-being and the sufficiency of your placenta's functioning.

Nonstress Test

The test takes 20 to 40 minutes and is usually performed in a hospital maternity ward or wherever an external fetal monitor is available. Go for the test when you know your baby is "awake," or have a glass of orange juice before or during the test. You are connected to a fetal monitor, and a probe is attached to your belly that records the fetal heart rate. Make sure that you are sitting up or lying on your left side. A baseline rate is established. The baby moves by itself or when prodded. The test is "reactive" when fetal heart tones accelerate 15 beats above baseline three times within a ten-minute period. However, not all health care practitioners have the same standards for a normal response, or they may misinterpret their own findings. Negative results don't necessarily mean that a baby is in danger. This test is almost always performed before the contraction stress test.

Contraction Stress Test

A further refinement of the nonstress test involves assessing the fetal heart rate during and after a contraction that has been produced by nipple stimulation or by the introduction of oxytocin via IV. Contractions begin within 20 to 40 minutes. Three moderate contractions within ten minutes, each lasting about 45 seconds, is considered adequate for assessing the baby's well-being. The aim of this test is to determine your baby's condition by seeing how the placenta responds to the stress of a contraction, as recorded by the monitor. This oxytocin challenge test (OCT) has a high false-positive rate; the results are difficult to interpret, and observers give different readings. It is an unnatural intervention in many ways, and it can lead to unnecessary artificial induction of labor, to cesarean section, and to hospital-caused prematurity—the birth of a baby simply not ready to be born.

For an extensive discussion of testing and the complex, social, emotional, and logistical issues raised, see Robin J. Blatt's work and Barbara Katz Rothman's book *Tentative Pregnancy.*

NOTES

1. Meridel LeSueur, "Annunciation," in Elaine Hedges, ed., *Ripening: Selected Work* (Old Westbury, NY: Feminist Press, 1982), 128.
2. For 12 years Dr. Tom Brewer ran a clinic for low-

income women in California and helped them eat well-balanced diets. In his retrospective study of 5,615 pregnancies, there was one instance of severe eclampsia and less than 1% mild toxemia. You can see his book *Metabolic Toxemia of Late Pregnancy: A Disease of Malnutrition* (New Canaan, CT: Keats Publishing, Inc., 1996, c. 1982).

3. K. R. Warren and R. J. Bast, "Alcohol-related Birth Defects: An Update," *Public Health Report* 103, no. 6 (1988): 638–42.

4. J. R. DiFranza and R. A. Lew, "Effect of Maternal Cigarette Smoking on Pregnancy Complications and Sudden Infant Death Syndrome," *Journal of Family Practice* 40, no. 2 (1995): 385–94.

5. Teratology Society, "Recommendations for Isotretinoin Use in Women of Childbearing Potential," *Teratology* 44, no. 1 (1991): 1–6.

6. K. J. Rothman et al., "Teratogenicity of High Vitamin A Intake," *New England Journal of Medicine* 333, no. 21 (1995): 1369–373.

7. Ellen S. Lazarus, quoting Enkin and Chalmers, "Poor Women, Poor Outcomes: Social Class and Reproductive Health," in Karen L. Michaelson, *Childbirth in America: Anthropological Perspectives* (South Hadley, MA: Bergin & Garvey, 1988), 53.

8. From Jane Hodgson's review of Margaret Boone's book *Capital Crime: Black Infant Mortality in America* (Newbury Park, CA: Sage, 1989), in *JAMA* 63, no. 22 (1990): 3090.

9. U.S. Department of Health and Human Services, Public Health Service, *Healthy People 2000: Midcourse Review and 1995 Revisions* (Hyattsville, MD: Public Health Services, 1995).

10. The Association of Maternal and Child Health Programs (AMCHP), *The New Welfare Reform Law and Its Potential Effects on Maternal and Child Health,* (Washington, DC: AMCHP, 1997). Available from AMCHP (202) 775-0436. Also see Deborah Wingard, "Patterns and Puzzles: The Distribution of Health and Illness among Women in the United States," pp. 41–42, and Nikki V. Franke, "African American Women's Health: The Effects of Disease and Chronic Life Stressors," pp. 361–62, in Sheryl Burt Ruzek, Virginia L. Olesen, and Adele E. Clarke, *Women's Health: Complexities and Differences* (Columbus, OH: Ohio State University Press, 1997).

11. Margot Edwards and Mary Waldorf, *Reclaiming Birth: History and Heroines of American Childbirth Reform* (Trumansburg, NY: The Crossing Press, 1984).

12. M. P. M. Richards, "The Trouble with 'Choice' in Childbirth," *Birth: Issues in Perinatal Care and Education* 9, no. 4 (winter 1982): 253.

13. R. A. Rosenblatt et al., "Interspecialty Differences in the Obstetric Care of Low-risk Women," *American Journal of Public Health* 87, no. 3 (March 1997): 344–51. Also see Sheila Harvey et al., "A Randomized Controlled Trial of Nurse-Midwifery Care," *Birth* 23 no. 3 (September 1996): 128–35.

14. Peggy Spindel, "Midwives and Physicians: Making Home Birth Work Together," in S. Sagov et al., eds., *A Practitioner's Guide to Birth Outside the Hospital* (Rockville, MD: Aspen Systems, 1994).

15. Midwife Valerie El Halta, quoted in *MANA News* 14, no. 5 (Nov. 1996): 23.

16. This list is inspired in part by the new Coalition for Improving Maternity Services (CIMS) "Mother-Friendly Childbirth Initiative." The Initiative document contains a set of ten steps so that providers can determine whether the care they offer is "mother-friendly," and consumers can find a "mother-friendly" birth service. There is also a Spanish version. For copies, contact ASPO/Lamaze at (800) 368-4404 or (202) 223-4579, or http://www.lamaze-childbirth.com. CIMS urges you to send copies to as many people and institutions as you can.

17. Judith Rooks et al., "Outcomes of Care in Birth Centers: The National Birth Center Study," *New England Journal of Medicine* 321, no. 26 (Dec. 28, 1989): 1804–811.

18. See Ole Olsen, "Meta-analysis of the Safety of Home Birth," *Birth* 24, no. 1 (March 1997) and four articles on home birth in *British Medical Journal*, 313, no. 7068, (Nov. 1996).

19. U. Waldenstrom and C. Nilsson, "A Randomized Controlled Study of Birth Center Care versus Standard Maternity Care: Effects on Women's Health," *Birth* 24, no. 1 (1997): 17–26.

20. Candace Whitridge, interviewed in *The Birth Gazette* 5, no. 3 (spring 1989): 8.

21. Phyllis Kernoff Mansfield and William McCool, "Toward a Better Understanding of the 'Advanced Maternal Age' Factor," *Health Care for Women International* 10, no. 4 (1989): 395–415. Also, Phyllis Kernoff Mansfield, "Re-evaluating the Medical Risks of Late Childbearing," *Women and Health* 11, no. 2 (summer 1986): 37–60.

22. Julie Gazmararian et al., "Prevalence of Violence Against Pregnant Women," *JAMA* 275, no. 24 (June 26, 1996): 1915–920. Summarizes the methods and findings of studies examining the prevalence of violence against pregnant women, and synthesizing the findings by comparing the studies' similar and dissimilar results.

23. Eileen Geil Moran, "Domestic Violence and Pregnancy," in Barbara Katz Rothman, *The Encyclopedia of Childbearing* (New York: Henry Holt, 1993), 110–12.

24. From conversations with Rick and Kathleen Hearn—thanks!

25. Notes written by Marsha Saxton and Cindy Blank Edelman.

26. Written with the enormous help of notes from Robin J. R. Blatt, author of *Prenatal Tests: What They Are, Their Benefits and Risks, and How to Decide Whether to Have Them or Not* (New York: Vintage Books, 1988).

27. Contact the Spina Bifida Association of America, 4590 MacArthur Boulevard NW, Suite 250, Washington, DC 20007; (202) 944-3285, for more information. Web site: http://www.sbaa.org

28. Robin J. R. Blatt, "Chorionic Villus Sampling: The DES of the 1990s?" *Mothering* (spring 1994), 73–77.

29. For a more thorough discussion of the controversy, see Henci Goer's *Obstetric Myths vs. Research Realities,* 157–78, as well as Anne Fry's *Understanding Lab Work in the Childbearing Year,* in the Resources section, pp. 496–501.

Resources for chapters 19 and 20 appear on pp. 496–501.

By Judy Luce and Jane Pincus, with
Audrey Levine; based on earlier work
by Jane Pincus, with Norma Swenson

WITH SPECIAL THANKS TO Carol Sakala*

Chapter 20

Childbirth

We bring to childbirth our histories, our relationships, our rituals, our needs and values that relate to intimacy, our sexuality, the quality and style of family life and community, and our deepest beliefs about life, birth, and death.[1]

CLIMATE OF CONFIDENCE

When we are taught to listen to our bodies and trust in our abilities to give birth; when we are attended by practitioners who affirm the naturalness of birth and both teach and guide us through the birthing process; when the people who surround us provide love and affirmation, we are in a *climate of confidence* that allows us to have a voice in and to shape our unique birthing experiences.

We begin this chapter with the stories of women who have given birth—at home, in birth centers, and in hospitals—with the support they need to have confidence in their own birthing powers.

I had a long, drawn-out labor. Each person there got a chance to rest. They switched on and off being with me. I could do what I wanted. I was standing most of the time and walking around. I was so pleased not to be in bed. They encouraged me to eat; I did drink some tea. Finally they convinced me to lie down and I got a little sleep.

Labor was painful. Pain isn't an adequate word. I was bowled over by the intensity of the physical experience. I remember thinking as labor got heavy, women are fantastic, *they get pregnant over and over again and are strong enough; people go through this all the time. Nobody could have prepared me for it in words.*

I could imagine myself understanding how I'd take drugs if someone urged them on me in a hospital.

* Thanks also to the following for their help with the 1998 version of this chapter: Denny Bergman, Rebecca Corliss, Robbie Davis-Floyd, Supriya Guha, Linda Holmes, Mirza Lugardo, Edith Maxwell, Joyce McNeil, Peggy Thurston, Laurie Williams. Over the years since 1969, the following women have contributed to the many versions of this chapter: Ruth Bell, Jenny Fleming, Nancy Miriam Hawley, Linda Holmes, Judy Luce, Jane Pincus, Becky Sarah, Gail Sullivan.

But here, because everyone was saying, "Everything is fine," it was easy to keep going.

Laura called Peter [the doctor]. He came over, sat in a corner reading a magazine, saying, "This could take up to two hours. Don't worry. You have plenty of time."

Then came the best time of all. Pushing wasn't at all painful. Mary was holding the mirror; each time I pushed I could see the effects. Laura: "Try breathing —blow out from really deep inside you. Let your cheeks puff out." It worked. I started squatting, then sitting up with Lewis behind me. My final delivery position was on my side, one leg up on Laura's shoulder. With every single push I could see Emma coming out, bigger and bigger. After every push Laura would massage my perineum. The little—no, the big—head came out. She was cooing. It was the sweetest thing I ever heard. Laura said to Lewis and me, "Reach down and pull out your baby." It was a big surprise to us! We did! We pulled her out! I brought her to my breast. We were enthralled. The afterbirth came out with no problem. Laura showed it to us.

The whole experience changed my life. It taught me how deeply physical life is, and connected me much more with my body. I'd learned a refined kind of Catholicism where nothing was earthy, nothing was said aloud. But there's nothing subtle about being pregnant and having a baby!

A new lesbian mother tells this story about labor at home and then in the hospital.

I had been waiting for Yancey for a long time at a restaurant. Finally she arrived. Her shirt was on backward. She said: "My waters broke! I'm in labor!" We dashed home and called Elaine, our labor support, a nurse-midwife (for her) and Melanie, a good friend who is also a midwife, a lesbian with three children (for both of us). They said, "Relax, eat, drink." The house became calm. Yancey called from her room, "Come! My back is killing me!" Then she said "Leave!" An hour later, through the door, "This is getting hard. Call Melanie." She wanted to be in the bathroom so we set up a little nest there. Melanie stayed with her for five hours; I tossed and turned in bed. Then I heard, "Get up! We have to go right now! She wants to push!" I had the presence of mind to hang a diaper out the window, our prearranged sign to our neighbors that we'd need their car. I drove faster and faster, with Yancey on all fours on the backseat. In the hospital Yancey knew what she wanted. She'd say, "Touch me here" or "Stay awhile." Finally we encouraged Yancey to push. She said, "I'm afraid I'll hurt myself," and then, "OK, let's do it." She pushed hard, popped the baby's head out, looked at his face, said, "It's a boy," and reached down to pull him out herself. I was weeping, she was laughing, she was feeling so exultant. I cut the cord, intensely moved. Then Yancey had to get stitched up because she had torn a bit. I spent a sweet hour with our beautiful son.

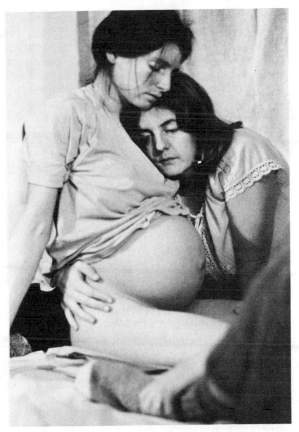

Suzanne Arms

Another woman and her husband created their own climate of confidence when they had their second baby in a large, busy city hospital where they were more or less left to themselves.

Labor really began at 12:30 A.M., on Monday. At 2 A.M. we went to the hospital. At 2 P.M. the next day I was working harder but still 4 centimeters dilated. The obstetrician wanted to give me morphine, saying, "This has gone on too long for a second labor. I'll put you to sleep for five hours and you'll wake up in active labor." Jack and I looked at each other and said, "This guy's really hot to trot." But we knew that when the baby's ready to be born, it would be born. We said we'd decide at 3 P.M. At 3 P.M. I was 5 centimeters dilated. Nurses were changing shifts. Though they were wonderful, there were never many of them around. I was sitting up. Jack and I used a lot of imagery. He helped me to breathe into the pain. We imagined wind and waves. I made sure the sensation would go down and through my cervix, and pictured my cervix opening, pictured myself being born. That helped a lot. Looking at Jack was best, or burying my face in his neck, or closing my eyes and going inside. If he hadn't been there, forget it. We were so concentrated on what we were doing. We knew it was our experience. He knew exactly what to do. He never left me.

At 3:30 they said they were thinking of breaking my

bag of waters, but because of the change in shifts, they never got around to do it. Then my waters broke by themselves and labor got harder. I felt pressure against my pubic bone, which was relieved by counterpressure and singing. Singing was exactly what I needed to do. All of a sudden I needed to push. "Don't push," they said. "I can't not," I said. I delivered my baby quickly. It was intense. I did my share of yelling. Her head came through while the doctor was still getting dressed, so I had no episiotomy. My baby nursed in the recovery room, just as I had dreamed about it last summer.

A midwife states:

All efforts are made to see birth as a continuum. I tell women who have prepared for home birth, who begin labor at home and then end up at the hospital, "Who you are never changes. Your planning, ideals, values, beliefs, principles never change just because you end up in the hospital, or with a cesarean. You are stronger than you would have been because you've gone through all those decisions and made the choices you did."

These women show us that giving birth can be richer than we ever imagined. They speak of excitement, doubt, determination, effort, learning about themselves; of momentary lapses and pulling themselves together; of hard work and giving in; of contentment, amazement, ecstasy, and exaltation. They listen to their bodies and remain open to their attendants' encouragement to relax and renew themselves. Their experiences make it vividly clear what birth can be and contrast sharply with the purely medical view of birth that focuses primarily on fear: fear of pain, fear that something will go wrong, fear that our bodies don't work.

CLIMATE OF DOUBT

The *climate of doubt*, with its overwhelming focus on worry and fear, has been in the making ever since obstetrics began in the U.S.

Brief History

More drugs and technologies are now used in "normal" births in America than anywhere else in the world. This reflects in part the desire to master, conquer, and control nature that was present among the colonists from the beginning.[2]

The present system was born in and shaped by the competition between male and female healers.[3]

In colonial America and the preindustrial U.S., midwives and community women attended child-bearing women, usually with excellent results. Sometimes, in extremely complicated situations, they called upon barber-surgeons, called "man-midwives." These men

used forceps and hooks, as few women did. Small wonder that the men regarded birth as deadly and dangerous, for they lacked the midwives' experience of hundreds of routine births that required no assistance.[4] Obstetrics became the first surgical specialty to be taught and practiced by male doctors in U.S. medical schools in the 18th century.

In the 1830s and 1840s, a strong grassroots popular health movement campaigned against a growing medical elitism, and many kinds of healing sects flourished. The medical "regulars"—upper-class and middle-class men—had nothing more to offer than lay practitioners; "they still couldn't claim to have any uniquely effective methods or special body of knowledge."[5] Nevertheless, they won out through political influence, and went on to found the American Medical Association in 1848.

About the same time, the profession of gynecology began to thrive. Some doctors performed cruel experimental surgery on many women, especially enslaved black women and poor women, in the name of science[6] (an experimentation that continues, in a milder form, in gynecology and obstetrics to this day).[7] Out of these devastating efforts grew "cures" for gynecological conditions, many of which were actually created by barbarous childbirth practices, although this connection was not recognized at the time. These procedures increased gynecologists' powers enormously, since the promise of cures and even of prevention lay with them.

The second half of the 19th century saw gynecologists and obstetricians gain even more control over women. This control represented political and economic triumph rather than scientific necessity. Admiring education and science, middle-class and upper-class women were able to afford doctors' fees. They continued to change their allegiance from midwives to "scientifically" trained doctors, who, as men of their own class, advised them in personal matters and judged their moral conduct—a role that continues today. Many upper-class and middle-class women wore tight corsets and were physically inactive. Some stayed in bed all day. Meanwhile, working-class women worked long hours in factories, fields, and upper-class households, attended by local midwives. Physicians looked upon these midwives as both economic threats and threats to the masculine medical order they were establishing. They waged a virulent campaign against them, stereotyping them as ignorant, dirty, and irresponsible. They deliberately lied about midwifery outcomes to convince legislators that states should outlaw them, when in fact midwives' safety records were often superior to those of physicians.[8] In addition, obstetricians campaigned to reverse the belief that birth was a healthy, natural process: "They set out to make mothers 'fear' the dangers of pregnancy and childbirth and think of 'no precaution as excessive,'"[9] all the while telling women of their right to be cared for by the only qualified providers: the obstetricians themselves. Doctors also deliberately excluded women from medical training,[10] fearing that if women were admitted to the profession, women patients would prefer physicians of their own sex, especially for childbirth.[11]

As medical boards and state legislators systematically suppressed midwifery, women had to move out of their homes into hospitals to give birth, which did not prove to be safer or better for them and their babies.[12] In 1900, 5% of babies in the U.S. were born in hospitals; by 1935, 75%;[13] and presently 98 to 99% are born in hospitals or birth centers. With the myth of safety grew other myths tied to obstetrical practices and technology (that only doctors can deliver babies; that labor is a process that needs to be "managed") that had no scientific basis. By giving birth in hospitals, women took the last step toward total dependence on the man-made, male-dominated obstetrical system. To this day, we struggle to change this de facto monopoly.

Institutions Contribute to the Climate of Doubt

Women experience the influence of the hospital setting long before labor begins. With the increasing routine use of pregnancy screening procedures, we are visiting hospitals earlier and earlier. When we enter these places for sick people, it is difficult not to view pregnancy, birth, and our bodies as unhealthy. From the very first ultrasound, hospital procedures bypass our maternal bodies, as family, technicians, and practitioners focus beyond ourselves on the blurry image of a fetus on a screen several feet away. Already, months before it is really born, the baby growing within seems to be outside our body. A process of continuous monitoring and surveillance has begun.

As we become "patients" and our experience is defined in medical terms, we become part of an impersonal production process. Upon entering the hospital in labor, we are often placed in wheelchairs. Our personal effects are removed. We are among strangers. We become anonymous. We are immobilized, hooked up to fetal monitors and IVs. Each "stage" of labor is allotted a certain amount of time, and no more.

During the 1950s and 1960s, operations research techniques used to expedite the manufacture of various forms of weaponry in WWII were applied to developing more effective obstetrical suites. Priorities were formulated to facilitate the efficient processing of as many women as possible rather than to allow for an adjustable tempo for each individual birth. The factory approach was soon incorporated into textbooks on hospital design: "The conveyor belt concept . . . emphasizes the repeated transference of a mother (as in motor-car assembly) from place to place, and also that unequal time periods at any station can render the process uneconomical."[14]

Such hospital routines debilitate us. We become passive, dependent. Until recently, routine enemas and shaving of the pubic area desexualized and in-

fantilized us. Even now, many hospitals do not allow food or liquids during labor, so that we become hungry, weak, our contractions slowed and our health endangered. The sterile hospital atmosphere caused one nurse-midwife to say regretfully, "The most natural aspects of birth—sexuality, blood, sweat, shit, movement, and sounds—have no place here."

Continuity of care, one of medicine's own standards for quality care, does not usually exist. Sometimes we are left completely alone for long periods of time—in no other culture are laboring women left so alone. Isolation and immobility during labor increase tension and fear, which increase pain, which causes more fear, which brings on more pain. In such surroundings, women end up "needing" pain relief, and obstetricians, anesthesiologists, researchers, and drug companies hasten to provide it in abundant variety. Those nurses who want to help us are overburdened with paperwork and have too many women to attend to at once.

At the other extreme, particularly in teaching hospitals, too many strangers—nurses, nursing and medical students, residents, lab technicians, and anesthesiologists—walk freely in and out of our room. The doctor—someone we may never have seen before—may appear briefly from time to time, or just before birth. After the baby is born, we meet a new set of nurses and a pediatrician. In large hospitals, a specialist in newborns (a neonatologist) may appear as well.

Medical Training Reinforces the Climate of Doubt

Nursing and medical students rarely, if ever, see a normal spontaneous labor and birth. To most of them, labor consists of a woman lying on her back, hooked up to a monitor and IV, her bag of waters broken artificially, her cervix ripened with prostaglandin gel, contractions "accelerated" with Pitocin, and her body immobilized by an epidural. The hierarchical nature of medical training, and the status our culture accords physicians, means that most of them never learn how to deal with a fully conscious, unanesthetized woman in labor. They don't sit through labor from beginning to end as midwives do, to find out how and what a woman feels, and to become acquainted with the unique rhythm of each labor.

Nor do medical students learn the midwifery skills of massage, physical assistance, and emotional support—those techniques providing comfort and facilitating labor that are so important to laboring women. Instead of "mastering the art of inactivity," most find it undramatic and boring to sit through labor (one obstetrician has a sign over his desk reading, "Birth is 95% boredom and 5% disaster"). Even if they want to, they don't have enough time. Instead, they learn to use technological interventions routinely to speed up labor. In addition, since obstetrics is a surgical specialty, students must meet a quota for procedures performed; in order to obtain experience, they have to practice on women whether procedures are indicated or not. They learn too that unless they have every available tool and instrument close at hand, they may be sued for malpractice at any moment.

Women trained as caregivers and practitioners within the medical system often adopt these practices and internalize the values inherent in the medical/technocratic approach to birth. Women obstetricians intervene in labor and utilize technology just as their male counterparts do. Even certified nurse-midwives working within large medical centers often use technology.

After such an education, it is no wonder that physicians genuinely believe we cannot and should not give birth without medical interventions.

Physicians' Attitudes Create and Sustain a Climate of Doubt *

Trained in a system where male bodies are the norm, most doctors believe womens' bodies and the birth process to be abnormal and dysfunctional. Among the most influential 20th-century obstetricians' writings, we find appalling descriptions of labor and birth—Joseph B. DeLee's, for example, who in 1920 compared labor to a crushing door, and birth to falling on a pitchfork, its handle driven through the perineum.

In both cases, the cause of the damage, the fall on the pitchfork and the crushing of the door, is pathogenic, that is, disease provoking, and anything pathogenic is pathologic and abnormal.[15]

The well-known author of *Birth Without Violence*, Dr. Frederick Leboyer, says:

One day, the baby finds itself a prisoner . . . the prison comes to life . . . begins, like some octopus, to hug and crush . . . stifle . . . assault . . . the prison has gone berserk with its heart bursting, the infant sinks into this hell . . . the mother . . . she is driving the baby out. At the same time she is holding it in, preventing its passage. It is she who is the enemy. She who stands between the child and life. Only one of them can prevail. It is mortal combat not satisfied with crushing, the monster . . . twists it in a refinement of cruelty.[16]

Women Internalize the Medical Model of Birth †

Childbirth has always involved perfectly natural fears of something going wrong, of the unknown, of pain, and of the risk of death. Birth is as safe as life

---

* Obstetric myths without scientific basis continue to influence practice in modern obstetrics. See Henci Goer, *Obstetric Myths vs. Research Realities: A Guide to the Medical Literature,* as well as Enkin et al., *A Guide to Effective Care in Pregnancy.*
† Ann Oakley's *Subject Women* (New York: Schocken Books, 1980) has an excellent discussion of women's attitudes about themselves and professionals' attitudes toward them. Diana Scully's *Men Who*

....

LABOR

....

Embracing Your Labor: Creating a Nurturing Birth Environment Wherever You Give Birth

For many women, labor is the most powerful experience of their lives and the hardest, most intense work they've ever done. There are many ways you can prepare to meet this challenge.

Surroundings and People

Familiar people help you feel comfortable. Some women give birth at home, where they feel most free to be themselves. Freestanding birth centers are home-like; you can cook, use the living room, spend time with children and friends. In a hospital, you can bring "home" along with you—clothes, personal objects, tapes for music. The reassuring touch of loved ones provides comfort and strength and adds to your confidence. Even if you want to labor alone at times, nearby support is reassuring.

The pain was like a hurricane shaking me apart. I yelled a lot and walked around and took showers. I remember looking at Paul and thinking, What are you so happy about? This is terrible. Yet I know that the grin on his face sustained me. I needed his touch and his joy, and I needed—very differently—the midwife's words and knowledge and reassurance.

Choose people who understand your wishes, who focus on your needs, and who won't be hurt if you are irritable or demanding or if you ask them to leave.

---

gets, yet we can never be completely certain of the outcome wherever and however we give birth. We are assaulted by assumptions about our inability to give birth without interventions. We are presumed unable and unwilling to handle the pain and intensity of labor. Inevitably, most of us internalize these powerful negative attitudes. Medical practice thrives on our fears. One mother says:

Control Women's Health describes obstetrical residents' attitudes toward the women they see in hospitals. Gayle Peterson, in *Birthing Normally*, details some of the ways in which our beliefs and attitudes can affect pregnancy and labor, and Robbie Davis-Floyd, in *Birth as an American Rite of Passage,* chronicles the deep cultural and historical roots underlying the medical model of birth, physician's attitudes and practices, and the way women adopt them. She describes the belief in technological progress that is central to our society and analyzes the many ways in which hospital birth expresses this ideology.

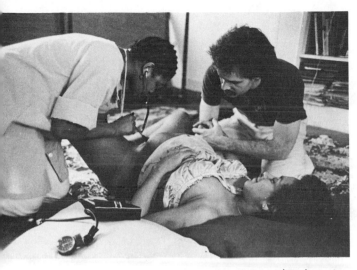

Ann McQueen/Stock, Boston

It is as if our confidence is a large, bright piece of fabric. When little pinprick holes of fear and doubt appear, the medical mentality makes them larger and larger until the once-beautiful cloth is nothing but gaping holes.

When we do not have experienced, empathetic women by our side during labor, listening, encouraging, providing information, and enhancing our confi-

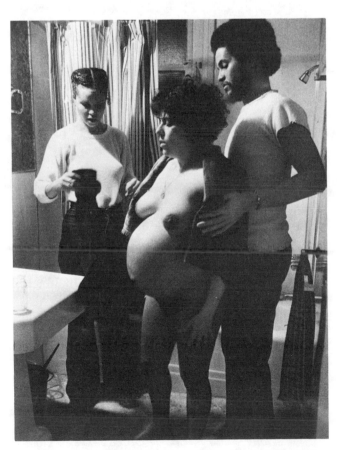

Suzanne Arms

SIMPLE AND EFFECTIVE WAYS TO HELP WITH THE PAIN AND INTENSITY OF LABOR

Activity

Stay home as long as you can during early labor. If you are still in early labor (less than 5 centimeters dilated) when you go to the birthing facility, walk around or return home instead of being admitted. Move around and change positions. Being upright, as when you are walking or rocking, can help you relax, can alleviate pain, and can make contractions work more effectively. Being on hands and knees also helps, especially with back labor. You can rock back and forth, dance slowly and rhythmically, and move in ways you'd never dream possible.

Nourishment

Drink and eat light foods. If you don't feel like eating you can sip juices, tea with honey, or soup. (Warm beverages tend to relax you and help you open.) This helps strengthen you, prevents dehydration, facilitates labor, and makes you better able to handle contractions. It keeps your baby vigorous. Labor requires great energy, equal to that required for running a marathon or long-distance swimming.

Breathing

You know how to breathe—don't stop! Deep breathing relaxes you, dissipates tension, helps you focus and get inside your labor. Imagine your breath carrying oxygen to every part of your body. Open your mouth and throat. Relax into any tenseness Smile, laugh, sing, chant.

Some women who have practiced special techniques may become too tense.

I was with a woman doing rigid strong labor breathing she had learned in a childbirth class. She was tight, exhausted. I said, "You don't have to do that." "What will I do?" "Just see what happens." She began to relax. When she let go trying to keep her control, her energy started to flow. Over the next few hours she started doing little sighs which became moans at the end. On the floor, kneeling, she breathed into her husband's lap and rocked her pelvis. He started to breathe and rock with her.

continued on next page

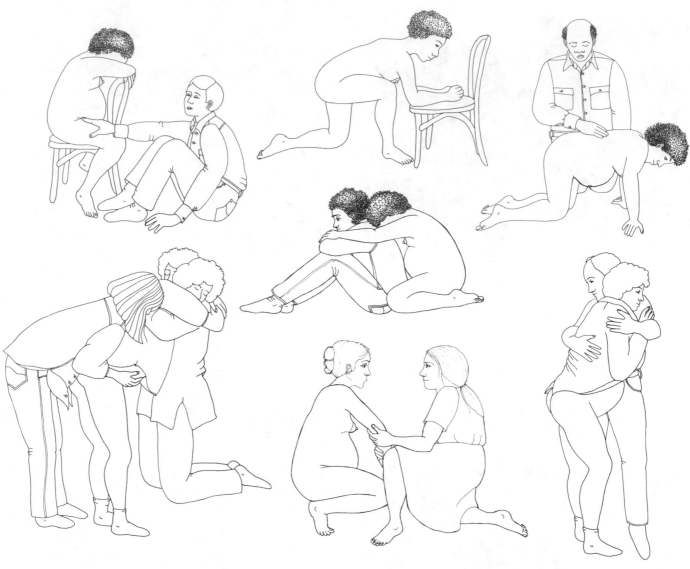

Dana Sibley

Endorphins

When you relax, your body produces its own substances for pain relief, called *endorphins*. They actually block pain reception.[17] They help you feel exhilarated during labor, and mellow and peaceful between contractions. Fear, on the other hand, causes you to secrete adrenaline into your bloodstream, which tenses you up, slows your labor, makes it more painful, and inhibits the secretion of endorphins. By relaxing, you enable endorphins to flow again. Endorphins won't make labor painless, but they make it bearable, particularly if you are surrounded by empathetic and supportive attendants.

Expressing Emotions

In labor you may run the gamut of emotions; so much is happening in your body. Birth is a time of transition and transcendence. Some women need to retreat. Others express anger, exaltation, fear, and pain; and some of us need encouragement to do so. Do what feels best for you; it may change from hour to hour.

Rocking, breathing, groaning, mouthing circles of distress, laughing, whistling, pounding, waving, digging, pulling, pushing—labor is the most involuntary work we do. My body gallops to these rhythms . . . labor is a drama in which the body stars . . .[18]

Enjoying Water

Baths and showers are relaxing. Some women stay in the shower for hours. One midwife says, "It's better than Pitocin for getting contractions going!" Deep water lifts your uterus up and away from your spine, which can reduce the intensity of contractions, especially back labor.

Receiving Supportive Assistance

Many women appreciate physical support, touch, and massage. Ask others to help you when you squat, stand, or kneel; to lean against you; to hold you under your arms; to let you hang from their shoulders; to hold you however you want to be held. "Drink in" touch. Companionship and contact can make you feel at ease, sustained, and loved. Or you may not want to be touched at all; this is all right. You may simply want the presence of others. Your support people may know exactly what to do without being asked. Or they may not. If it doesn't feel right, speak up.

I asked my two friends to massage deeply and hard, putting a lot of pressure on my lower back muscles to counter all that force. I liked feeling their hands supporting my belly at the same time.

Imagining

In south India, birth attendants place a flower near the laboring woman; as its petals unfold, her cervix opens, and when the flower is in full bloom, they know it is time to push. Opening is a ceremony, a celebration. Imagine being in a place you love the best, where you are most happy. Open your mind to images. Imagine your baby hugged by your uterus, pushing down, opening you, ready to be born. Imagine your muscles letting go; your cervix stretching, opening, open . . . open . . . OPEN. Imagine you are a flower opening, a light exploding. Think ever-widening circles, ripples formed by raindrops on a pond. A woman, in labor after two previous cesareans, dreamed of a doughnut hole getting larger and larger. When she awoke, her baby was moving through her pelvis and she was pushing.

These ideas and activities can help you cope with the sensations and pain of labor.

A Word to Family and Friends

Be present. Be quiet. Be in tune. Focus your attention on the woman in labor. Be joyful, encouraging, positive, uplifting. Be calm. Don't communicate anxiety or fear. Don't focus on time. Leave the room if you feel uncomfortable. Don't expect a laboring woman to be stoic or polite or patient with you. She may not want you to touch her at all or she may not want you to stop, even for a second. If she tells you to go away, don't take it personally. Allow her space to be alone, if that is what she needs. Don't feel sorry for her; show your belief in her strength. If she says, "I can't stand this anymore," encourage her, affirm her, tell her she can. She is doing it. Suggest a walk, a shower, a bath, a change of position. Help her concentrate and keep focused on the present. Hold her, sing, chant, laugh, moan, rock with her. Breathe along with her, if this helps. Provide hot compresses, cool cloths or a hand fan, liquids, and light nourishment. Let her lean against or on you. Help her be free to go deep inside herself and be in touch with her body and follow its rhythms. (Special thanks to Becky Sarah.)

dence; when we put our faith only in people who don't believe in our ability to give birth; when we depend, as they do, on their medical tools and techniques, then we reinforce their belief that we can't do without them.

MAKING A BIRTH CARE PLAN

You can envision your labor and birth, imagine it, prepare for it—but you can't plan it, nor plan when it will happen. However, you can plan the kind of care you want. We encourage you to draw up a birth care plan well before you go into labor, laying out clearly where you plan to give birth, who will attend you, whom you want for labor support, and what kind of care you want. Make informed, reflective choices about interventions, drugs, and anesthesia. Negotiate ahead of time with your hospital or birth center and your practitioner, and visit the birth site to familiarize yourself with the routines and be better able to state your preferences. Plan to have your partner and/or advocate with you at all times during the birth. Such planning will prepare you to deal with any onslaught of institutional routines and medical procedures.

You will want to prepare your children for birth and make plans for their care whether you birth at home or in an institution. Children, even very young children, often do well at birth. For many women it is important that their children be part of the experience, or at least be present for the actual birth.

Laboring in water and giving birth in water are possible at home and in some hospital settings. You may want to research this and make certain your caregiver is comfortable with this choice and that the institution you choose is equipped with birth tubs.

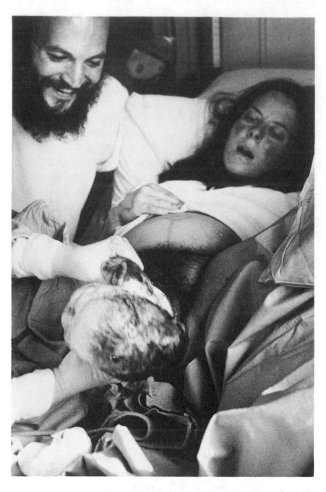

Vaughn Sills

WOMEN IN LABOR

Your Body Prepares for Labor

Labor continues the process begun at conception. It marks a significant transition for you and for your baby. Like pregnancy, labor is a total experience involving your body, mind, emotions, and spirit. It is important to remember that while we focus on what is happening to your uterus, it is *you* who are in labor. During labor, your uterine muscles will gradually stretch the cervix open for the baby to pass through, and push your baby through your vagina. This dance in which you and your baby participate has many intricate steps. You know how to give birth; the process is genetically encoded in your body, and it links you to thousands of generations of women giving birth.

Throughout pregnancy your uterus has been contracting in preparation for labor. Uterine muscles, tightening then loosening, exercise the uterus and prepare it to work efficiently during labor. Toward the end of pregnancy you may feel painless contractions (called Braxton-Hicks) more frequently, pulling and stretching more intensely; occasionally they are uncomfortable. Your cervix may begin to soften and thin

(ripen). Both effacement (thinning and drawing up of the cervix) and dilation (opening of the cervix) can occur before you feel regular, painful contractions. Some women efface and dilate for weeks before labor begins and yet progress very slowly once it starts; this dilation does not predict when labor will actually begin or how long it will last. Other women go into labor before starting to dilate and give birth a few hours afterward.

When you feel stronger contractions that are very regular, more like menstrual cramps, you may think you are in early labor (and sometimes you are), but often you are not. These warming-up contractions, misleadingly called "false labor," play a role in initial dilation and effacement. They usually stop after a while, though they can last for hours. When they occur, walk around and see whether they continue and whether the intervals between contractions become longer or shorter.

DOULAS: PROFESSIONAL LABOR SUPPORT

It can be extremely helpful to have a doula if you are planning to give birth in a birth center or hospital. Doulas are female caregivers, often members of your community, who have basic training and experience in, and will accompany you throughout, labor and birth. Mothering the mother, they focus on you, providing comfort and relieving pain, offering emotional support and reassurance. They can see to it that your labor is not interfered with. Studies demonstrate the benefits of such support; they include shorter labors, less medication and epidural anesthesia, fewer cesareans, less use of Pitocin, fewer instrument deliveries (forceps, vacuum extractor), and more alert newborns. Just as important is that supported women breast-feed more easily, have less depression following birth, and express more satisfaction with their birth experiences.[19]

Despite the broad range of differences in training among the support people, women in a wide variety of settings who receive such support report improved self-esteem and find the transition to mothering easier.

In response to the need for such caregivers, doula organizations have been formed in the past several years: DONA (Doulas of North America), ALACE (Association of Labor Assistants and Childbirth Educators), and NACA (National Association of Childbirth Assistants). Some hospitals are hiring doulas and making them available to women, and some HMOs are covering the cost of doulas.

What Causes Labor?

We don't know exactly what causes labor to begin. The size and maturity of the baby, physical changes in the placenta, and changes in the mother's hormonal levels help influence the start of labor. The mother's emotional readiness also seems to play a role. Labor begins when everything is ready, and usually it responds unkindly to being forced or rushed. Natural hormones called prostaglandins ripen or soften the cervix, and natural oxytocin (also a hormone) causes regular rhythmic contractions that dilate the cervix. Each labor has its own unique rhythm with periods of intense activity and restful plateaus. You need to respect your body's wisdom and the rhythm of your unique labor.

Some First Signs of Labor

More frequent and intense contractions signal approaching labor. Often diarrhea precedes labor for a few days, as your body's way of emptying itself in preparation for birth. You may feel an extraordinary burst of energy and a kind of nesting instinct. You may want to cook, clean house, and organize. You may suddenly want to sleep. You may experience the following:

Bloody Show

As your cervix begins to open, pink blood-tinged mucus that sealed the cervix begins to come out. Many women never have this *bloody show*. Others have it all through early and active labor. Although "losing your mucus plug" is often listed as the first sign of labor, it's not uncommon for the mucus plug to come out right before the baby.

Waters Leaking or Rupture of the Amniotic Sac ("Waters Breaking")

The membranes containing amniotic fluid may rupture as your baby's head presses down against them. (In 75% of women, membranes remain intact until full dilation.) Amniotic fluid, usually clear and odorless or milky, may gush or just trickle out. Some women think they are wetting their pants. If you can't stop the flow by holding it back, it is probably amniotic fluid. No matter how much fluid comes out, your body replaces it every few hours. There is no such thing as a "dry birth." After your membranes rupture, labor will probably begin within 12 to 24 hours (80% of women go into labor within 48 hours), though some women trickle for a few days or even weeks. Ruptured membranes increase the risk of infection. For this reason, it is important that you don't take tub baths (until your labor has clearly started), put anything into your vagina (no pelvic exams), or have sexual intercourse, and that you remain well-rested and drink often. If you do these things the chance of infection is minimal.

When your waters break or you begin to leak, notice the color of the fluid. Let your practitioner know if you see any brown or green staining, as it means that meconium (the tarry substance in your baby's bowels) has been squeezed out—a common occurrence, but occasionally an indication of fetal distress. After your membranes rupture, your caregiver may want to check the baby's heart rate and the baby's position.

Although physicians often request that you come to the hospital even if labor has not begun, your home environment is a safer place to be. Evidence supports a policy of watchful waiting in the first 48 hours, without any vaginal exams. There is no justification for routinely inducing labor after 12 to 24 hours, since induction carries the risk of failure, producing a cascade of interventions often resulting in a cesarean, because your body is not ready. While you wait for labor to begin, your practitioner may advise you to check your temperature to make sure there is no infection. Midwives are more likely to tell you to relax and that labor will begin soon. After 48 hours, practitioners may suggest various ways to stimulate labor such as castor oil, herbs, and nipple stimulation.

Contractions

Your uterus will begin to contract regularly and/or strongly after a while. At first it may feel like gas pains, menstrual cramps, backache, or a pulling and stretching in your pubic region. In early labor, contractions may be as regular as clockwork (perhaps ten minutes apart) or they may be irregular, inconsistent, and widely spaced but short. Sometimes, especially with a first baby, contractions come regularly, last for a long time, and are painful but don't cause dilation beyond 3 centimeters. Taking time to relax, rest, get support, and eat can get you through this "prolonged latent phase." Don't get discouraged.

If labor begins during the day, go about your daily routine, especially if this is your first baby, when labor usually takes longer. More often, labor begins at night when you are relaxed. Get as much sleep as you can. Sometimes a hot bath or shower will slow things down enough to allow you to sleep. If contractions get stronger, longer, and closer together, you usually are in labor.

At five A.M. I felt period cramps, was really excited. They weren't particularly painful. I knew something was happening! I waited for other signs. Had "bloody show." Beryl, my birth attendant, examined me. I was fully effaced and not dilated at all. Rick and I thought about what we wanted to do with the day. I baked a birthday cake, we took naps, had a quiet day together. I ate lightly all day, had spaghetti for dinner. We went to sleep; I woke up at 11:30 P.M. truly in labor.

An unplanned home birth:

I was probably in labor all day and didn't realize it. I went to take a shower, to wash my hair and shave my legs to be presentable. Lo and behold, my son was born then and there. The three of us went to the hospital, my head covered with shampoo.

Some women actively invite labor to begin.

My body felt different the night before, as if I'd become lighter and the baby had shifted position. I went into labor with my second child very consciously because I needed to. I don't believe in trying to control a process like labor, but it was wonderful to know I could invite it/allow it to start. My blood pressure had been climbing the last weeks of the pregnancy because of overwork and extreme stress. The midwife said to me firmly, "You must have the baby," so I went home to try. I thought about it, we made love, I let go of the reasons why it wasn't a good day, and in two hours my water broke with mild contractions starting up soon.

The Process of Labor

While labor is more akin to a bud opening than anything that can be charted or measured, we can describe how the process of labor might unfold for you and what you can do.

In early labor, moving around, walking, taking long baths, or making love if your waters haven't broken, showering, hugging, and kissing can help the labor process and relax you.

When we went for a walk we ran into friends. "What are you doing up? I thought you were in labor." It was fun changing people's image of a woman in labor.

We made love while I was in labor. We went to bed and had a wonderful time. I was happy to be giving —to him and to myself—and not just concentrating on contractions.

When you rest or go to bed, contractions may slow down. That's fine. Resting is important.

If you plan a hospital birth, remain at home until contractions are frequent and strong. The longer you stay out of the hospital, the less likely you are to have labor interventions. Many practitioners will not admit you until you are 4 to 5 centimeters dilated and active labor has begun. When labor becomes active, contractions are strong and rhythmic, and they dilate your cervix. You feel them building like a wave, pulling and tightening first in one place then expanding throughout your uterus, into your back or your groin, and then lessening. In between you can rest, sleep, walk, or talk. Urinate regularly. Deep relaxation between contractions renews your energy, helps reduce pain, and allows contractions to work effectively.

Contractions when most intense felt like a belt around my lower back and abdomen. Most of the feeling was in my lower back. Contractions had a curve:

strong at the beginning and then slowing down. You get to know them. What surprised me was that you're in two worlds. You have to concentrate on them when they happen, but when they stop, you're just regular. I've never felt so lucid, so clear, as in between contractions.

Language was really important, and I didn't like the word "contraction." I found when I was having my babies that if I thought "contraction" it meant making something tight. It's true the uterine muscles are contracting, but if everything's working right, at the same time the cervix is expanding. It's much more useful to think of the expansion . . .[20]

Giving Birth

Some signs indicate that your cervix has completely dilated and you are getting ready to move your baby down through your vagina (birth canal) and give birth: a powerful "opening up" feeling; more rapid, intense contractions; more rectal pressure. The more relaxed you are now, the better you'll feel. You may need encouragement to help you breathe deeply and focus your energies. Some women become quiet and inward. Others find it helpful to match this intensity with their voices or by changing positions.

Some women kneel, rock on hands and knees, lie on their side, stand in a shower, squat, or submerge in a tub of water. As the birth energy intensifies you may experience nausea, shaking, trembling thighs and legs, chills, and irritability. If you have these experiences at this point you can be comforted by knowing that this part of labor is almost complete.

When your cervix is fully open (dilated), labor often slows down. Contractions space out as if to give your body a rest. This plateau can last for a brief time or up to two hours. You may begin to feel more rectal pressure as the baby's head settles more deeply into your pelvis. Some women will feel no urge to bear down and will just want to sleep. For others, contractions may come so close together that it seems like one long one, and you may scarcely have time to take a breath before you feel an overwhelming urge to push.

The pushing stage can be a great relief because you become active, in contrast to the relaxed yielding and letting go necessary for opening the cervix. However, some women never feel that strong urge to push, and they move the baby down with contractions that feel no different from earlier ones. You are more in tune with the natural process of your labor when you wait to bear down until the urge becomes overwhelming; then, moving into the rhythm, you bear down only when the urge is there.

Sometimes, depending on the baby's position, pushing can be very painful, which may shock and disappoint you if you have been told how exhilarating pushing is. Breath-holding; strenuous active pushing; and sustained, directed bearing-down efforts, often taught in childbirth classes and advocated in hospitals, may result in a shorter "second stage," but they can deprive the baby of oxygen and result in lower Apgar scores.[21] (Apgar scores measure the newborn's well-being. See p. 479.)

Try different positions, choosing what is most comfortable. Being upright is of advantage to you and your baby; many women experience less pain and backache in this position.[22] Shorter, spontaneous pushing efforts are better for mother and baby. Breathe deeply and rest between contractions.

It is an amazing force that moves your baby through your vagina. Your uterus contracts involuntarily and will push the baby out when you work with it and give it time.

Some push, some don't push at all, some push in pleasure, some not, and some, like me, for hours. We wreak havoc, make animal faces . . . go red, go darker, whiter, stranger, turn to bears. . . . It is our work, our body's work that is involved in its own goodness.[23]

Some women utter deep, guttural, almost animal-like sounds, and feel that they and their babies are riding a powerful wave carrying them downward. Some women simply "breathe" their babies out.

It may take from twenty minutes to five hours to birth your baby. There is no justification for limiting this phase of labor to two hours or less, as some physicians do, as long as mother and baby are doing fine and the baby is descending.[24] Relaxing between contractions and only pushing with the rhythm of each one helps conserve your energy. Like active labor, pushing has a rhythm. It is often a slow, gradual process as the baby's head moves down with a contraction, then retreats a little, down during the next one, and then back again. This to-and-fro gently molds the bones of the baby's head and causes your pelvis to

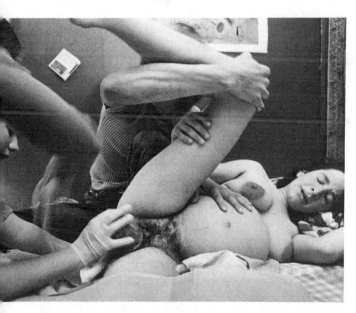

Suzanne Arms

The lithotomy position—lying on your back, feet up in stirrups—is the worst, most dangerous, and most ineffective position for labor. It is still used in many hospitals out of habit or for the convenience of the doctor. Insist on not being in this position.

open up slowly. Imagine your whole pelvis opening like the petals of a flower in sunlight.

You can be in any position when the baby emerges. Squatting opens your pelvis. Sitting on the toilet might help. Hands and knees, semi-reclining or side-lying with one leg supported are other options. In some places you can use birthing stools and squatting bars; midwives often bring stools with them. Some women squat in the shower and push while holding on to the handles or bars. You can push while sitting or squatting in a tub, submerged in water, which can feel almost effortless and soothing as you stretch and open wide to slip your baby out.

Direct your energy downward, outward, maintaining the gentle, rocking rhythm. Once your baby's head reaches the bottom of your birth canal and advances under the pubic arch, your perineum stretches slowly around its head, protecting it and your soft tissues, which have a great capacity to stretch and open for your baby's passage. Your attendant may ask you to breathe lightly so as not to push at all as she or he gently massages the area around the baby's head with oil and hot compresses. Relax your face and gently open your mouth and drop your jaw. When your mouth is open, your vagina opens and your perineum relaxes. Watching in a mirror or reaching down and touching your baby's head makes you smile, which also relaxes you.

I was holding back. This thought raced into my mind and out the other side: If I push hard enough, I'm going to become a mother. Ann said, "Next time you have a contraction, push a little bit; think open, you'll feel better." Amazing—I could feel her coming down; it did feel better.

Pushing was the strangest and in some ways the nicest sensation I've ever had. I could actually feel the shape of the baby, feel myself sitting on the head as it moved down . . . the thought of moving, especially from a good, comfortable, well-supported seated position, to flat-out on a bed seemed ridiculous. So there I was on my rocking chair, with my feet up on two little kitchen chairs, with Hersch on one side and the doctor on the other . . . it was like moving a grand piano across a room: that hard, but that satisfying.[25]

Your baby's head emerges first, unless the baby is in breech position (see p. 481). Before or during the next contraction your baby will rotate a quarter of a turn, unless it slips out quickly. Some babies are born in one continuous motion, and others seem to emerge inch by inch. Your attendant may check to see whether the cord is around the baby's neck and whether it is loose; quite often (60% of the time) the cord is there but presents no problem. While you wait for the baby to rotate and for the next contraction, your attendant may ask you to relax your face and perhaps blow gently, and to reach down and touch the baby's head. You'll want to breathe the baby out. Unless meconium has been present in the fluid, there is no need to suction the baby's mouth and nose at this time.

Within a few minutes, the baby was coming. I knelt on the bed, leaning forward against Thomas. It was a wonderful position, very solid and stable, yet my hands were free to reach down and feel her head. My older daughter was ready with a blanket to wrap the baby, and I will never forget the feeling of the little body sliding out and into my hands just as the sun came up. It's a great moment—the baby is there, it doesn't hurt anymore, both in the same instant. The room was full of light.

Nothing was happening on the bed; it seemed so much easier in the water. Everything I needed was there at the time. I said, "I feel kind of open!" Then I saw my son float out. It was great. He was so peaceful and calm. His eyes were open under the water.

Some babies breathe as they are being born and look pink immediately. Others look very still and bluish, almost purple, until breathing becomes regular and sustained. Occasionally a baby born with a lot of mucus in the mouth and nose will need to be gently suctioned. Not all newborns cry. Some cry for a moment, then stop. They may just breathe, blink, and look around, snuffle, or sneeze. Your baby will look wet and may be covered with a waxy substance called vernix. The baby's head may be temporarily oddly shaped, having become molded during the passage through your birth canal.

Some women feel that time stops and all their energy leaves them as they gaze in wonder at their newborn. When you feel ready, hold your baby close. Your baby belongs next to you. Cover your baby with blankets for warmth, and hold her or him naked against your breasts and belly so that the baby may touch your skin, smell you, feel you, hear you, look at you and the people next to you. Touch and talk to your baby. Enjoy this slow time.

Much has been written about this particular moment, but birth is the continuation of a process that began with conception. Your connection is already intimate. Newborns recognize their mother's scent, their parents' voices, and familiar sounds. When birth occurs at home, there is no interference during this period. Hospital attendants still must learn to respect how crucial it is that families be close to their babies at this time. One mother fighting separation from her baby was told, "You're bonded to her now, so what's the problem?" The issue isn't "bonding" but our *right* to enjoy the

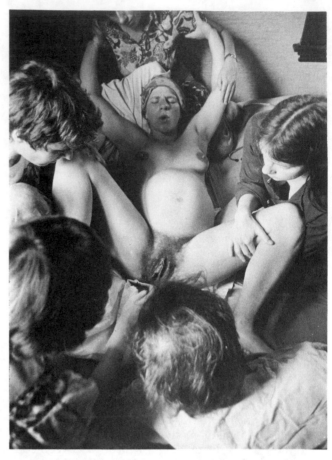

Jim Harrison/Stock, Boston

mutual pleasure of continuous contact, which takes time. Babies simply belong with their mothers.

If for some reason the first moments after birth don't turn out the way you want, and your baby has to be taken away for special care, you will still have many ways of becoming attached to each other. Bonding in humans is an ongoing process.

The first few hours of life are a time of heightened awareness for your baby. Both of you need peace, quiet, and no interruptions. Your baby will nurse; she or he may have already been sucking on hands and fingers in the womb before birth. Babies have an instinctive sucking reflex but show varying degrees of interest and take different amounts of time to nurse. Some latch on immediately, others more gradually over a period of a couple of hours. Smelling and licking and exploring your breast are part of the process. If you have received drugs, your baby may be too sedated to nurse well. Breast-feeding is facilitated if your baby nurses within the first hour or two. Let your baby suckle even if you don't plan to breast-feed, for babies receive important antibodies and nutrients from your colostrum, the first "milk." Suckling is important for you, too. It stimulates oxytocin, which enables your uterus to contract to expel the placenta and to stay contracted afterward, thus slowing down any bleeding. (See "Breast-feeding Your Baby," chapter 21, Postpartum, p. 507.)

Practitioners can unobtrusively evaluate your baby's well-being. Their conclusions are often expressed in the one- and five-minute Apgar score (from one to ten), which assesses color, muscle tone, reflexes, respiratory efficiency, and heart rate. Most infants score between seven and ten. Wherever you are, your attendant has oxygen and suctioning equipment at hand in case your baby needs help breathing. Gentle suctioning of the nose and throat is done if needed.

Your baby is still attached by the umbilical cord to its placenta inside of you. It is quite amazing to think that the placenta developed from the embryo and belongs to the baby. There is no rush to cut the cord (some placentas birth before the cord is even cut). When you wait until the cord stops pulsating before cutting it, your baby receives up to 50 milligrams of iron to add to his or her reserves for the first six months of life. Many physicians cut the cord as soon as the baby breathes. Let your practitioners know your wishes in this regard. The cord is clamped or tied off a short distance from the navel. You may want your partner or some family member to cut the cord. The bit of cord left on the baby's navel dries up and usually falls off within a week.

Birth of the Placenta

The birth of the placenta completes the birthing cycle. After a certain interval—five to 30 minutes or longer—the cord lengthens, you may feel a contraction, and you have a rush of blood and expel your placenta. Contractions usually come sooner when you are sitting up or squatting and the baby is suckling. It is extremely important that the placenta be totally out and that no fragments remain inside your uterus. This is best achieved by allowing the placenta to come out spontaneously. Until this happens, blood vessels remain open and can hemorrhage. Retained fragments can also lead to infection. Once the entire placenta is born, blood vessels close off. Your uterus clamps down and begins to shrink. Breast-feeding helps this process. Usually the placenta comes out by itself, helped along by your baby suckling or by stimulating your nipples. Midwives sometimes use herbs to facilitate separation of the placenta. If no bleeding occurs and all else is normal, wait patiently. Most placentas come out within an hour; some take longer. Hospital practitioners tend to rush this stage and actively assist the delivery of the placenta. Your attendant may give you a shot of Pitocin (synthetic oxytocin) to stimulate contractions, apply controlled contraction to the cord, or remove the placenta manually (if, for example, there is hemorrhage, and it must come out quickly). The placenta is a beautiful organ; make sure you get a chance to see it. The pattern of blood vessels resembles a "tree of life." Many cultures have rituals surrounding the afterbirth, including burying the placenta and planting trees or flowering shrubs over it.

We were married under a majestic oak tree. After Leah and Jonah were born, we took their placentas to that place and buried them there where they could continue to nurture. It felt like a sacred ceremony that bound us all together even more tightly.

THE FIRST HOURS AFTER THE BABY IS BORN

Mother and Baby

It is best if your baby stays with you for as long as you like after birth. Mother and baby can sleep and wake together and get to know each other, and the baby can nurse whenever desired.

Although at home and in freestanding birth centers mother and baby stay together, in hospitals you may have to insist on your right to remain together all the time. Make your wishes known ahead of time. *There is no medical reason to separate healthy mothers and babies after birth.* All babies benefit from being close to their families, even when they need medical observation or treatments at the same time.

Supportive Surroundings Following Birth

Where you are and who is with you matters as you begin mothering. It is best to be in a place where you are comfortable and can get to know your baby and gain confidence in your ability to care for him or her. This confidence grows with contact and with experience. While it may be helpful to receive guidance, no one will ever be more attentive and observant than you.

After a normal birth in a freestanding birth center, most women go home within six to 24 hours. The usual stay in a hospital lasts from four hours to three days, or three to five days after a cesarean. If you want to leave soon after the birth, make arrangements with your practitioner. Healthy mothers who have prepared for mothering, and babies who have adequate support and follow-up care available, even by phone, can go home within a few hours after birth. Many mothers are more relaxed at home, get more rest, and are more comfortable learning their mothering roles. There is less risk of infection.

Megan was born that day at noon, and by 5 P.M. I was back at home taking a much-needed shower, while Peter and my mother and his parents prepared supper and admired the baby. Then we all sat down to a celebration birthday supper, complete with cake and champagne and Megan in the middle of the table in her basket. By 9 P.M. Peter and I were asleep in bed with Megan snuggled between us. The next day, the

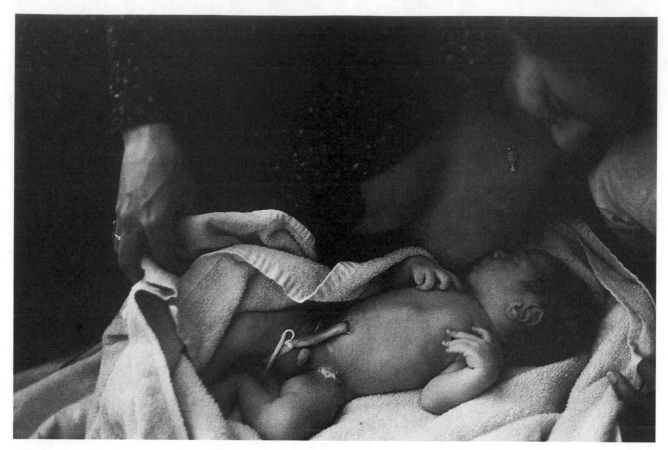

Ann McQueen/Stock, Boston

midwife came, checked me and the baby, and answered my barrage of questions. Later in the day, friends came bringing food and baby presents. I remember those days as among the happiest in my life.

You may want to stay in the hospital a few days, especially if you have other children at home or no household help, although most insurance companies will not pay for more than 48 hours. Some states now require insurance companies to pay for 48 hours of hospital care. Unfortunately, more cost-effective mother care (well-baby and mother care, and help with household and child care responsibilities) is seldom covered. Some women need and value the assistance and education they receive in caring for their newborn during their hospital stay. This assistance should empower you and not make you feel incompetent.

I have five kids at home. I look on this as my only vacation this year!

With *rooming-in,* your baby stays with you all the time. With *modified rooming-in,* your baby will be with you whenever you like, or just during the day, returning to the central nursery when you are tired. If you are breast-feeding, insist that no water or formula be fed to your baby. (See "Breast-feeding Your Baby," chapter 21, Postpartum, p. 507.)

Childbirth activists fought long and hard to get hospitals to implement rooming-in policies and early discharge. Demand to have your wishes met. Early and frequent contact will enhance your confidence, sharpen your mothering skills, and make you more adept at detecting problems. With rooming-in, your baby may cry less, nurse more often, and sleep better. Newborns and mothers often find it difficult to adapt to hospital routines.

In the ongoing debate about length of hospital stay, no one really addresses the critical problem that in this country we abandon new mothers when they leave the hospital, whether after 12 or 48 hours, in a way that no other industrialized country does. The Dutch government, for example, provides every woman with home care and guidance for at least two weeks following the birth; similar arrangements exist in other countries. We must demand that health care coverage include such services.

Hospital Routines for Newborns

Practitioners will perform a complete physical exam of your baby shortly after birth. Unless there is a problem, the exam does not need to be done right away. There is no reason it cannot be done in your presence. Feel free to ask questions.

Physicians recommend that babies' eyes be treated

with a substance that can prevent gonococcal infection. Traditionally, silver nitrate was used, but now there is widespread use of erythromycin, an antibiotic that is less irritating to the baby's eyes. Parents can sign a waiver and refuse the treatment. The gonococcal organism is treatable and clearly manifests itself when present, but if left untreated it can lead to blindness. If you refuse the treatment, pay close attention to your baby's eyes during the first week or so to make sure that they remain clear. If they do become runny and/or swollen, with lashes stuck together, consult with your pediatrician or practitioner. Even babies who have been treated with erythromycin may develop "newborn conjunctivitis."

Pediatricians recommend that babies receive vitamin K injections after birth to prevent a rare disorder (1 in 2,000) known as hemorrhagic disease of the newborn (when the blood doesn't have enough clotting factor). Twenty-five years ago, these injections became mandatory in hospitals to counteract the anticlotting effects of many drugs. In out-of-hospital births, most attendants will not use vitamin K unless there has been trauma. If the birth has been traumatic with excessive head-molding, or a face or breech presentation with lots of bruising, vitamin K is advisable. You can give vitamin K orally to the baby, but it has a bad taste. Discuss erythromycin and vitamin K with your practitioner. You have a legal right to refuse both treatments.

SPECIAL CONSIDERATIONS

Less Usual Presentations

The most efficient position for a baby's moving into the birth canal and through the pelvis is head down with the back of its head toward the mother's front. Another position is head first, but with the baby's face toward the mother's front (posterior presentation). This position sometimes causes a longer labor, and you often feel the contractions in your back, since the baby usually has to rotate into a more favorable position. Sometimes the baby doesn't rotate and is born face up. Walking up and down stairs, squatting, rocking on hands and knees, having someone press on your back, hot compresses, baths, and lots of encouragement can all help with a back labor.

Some babies (3 to 4%) present in a breech position at term, which means buttocks or feet first (footling breech). Sometimes you can help a breech baby turn after the 34th week of pregnancy (see chapter 19, Pregnancy, p.448). During labor the baby may or may not turn. A skilled practitioner may be able to turn your baby from the outside (external version).[26] There is no reason why you cannot birth a breech baby vaginally as long as you have a skilled, confident practitioner and as long as the labor progresses smoothly, the breech descends through the pelvis, and you do not actively push until the breech (presenting part) reaches the pelvic floor. Squatting widens your pelvis significantly.

Some physicians and midwives will attend a frank breech (buttocks first, with legs extended) or a complete breech (feet and legs curled beneath buttocks), but not a footling breech, which is usually delivered by cesarean (unless the baby is the second of twins, when the cervix has opened wide enough). Some skilled practitioners see no reason not to attempt a footling breech if the baby is of average size and the woman has a large pelvis. Attending breech births is a lost art in obstetrics;* presently, 95% of breech babies are delivered by cesarean. Most obstetricians rarely if ever learn version skills or attempt to turn babies, even though this practice could considerably reduce the number of breech babies at term. They don't help deliver breech babies vaginally, either.[27]

Very rarely, babies lie horizontally (transverse lie) and their heads never engage. They must be born by cesarean.

Premature Labor and Birth

A premature baby is one who is born before the 37th week of pregnancy. Until recently, a baby of 5½ pounds or less was considered premature, but we now know that maturity and functional development of the baby are more important than birthweight.

Poor health, inadequate nutrition, stress, and heavy smoking all increase the chance of premature birth. Specific causes of premature labor include infectious diseases, preeclampsia, diabetes, placenta previa (a placenta that lies very low in the uterus, covering the cervix), placenta abruptio (premature separation of the placenta), thyroid disturbances, fetal abnormalties, or, sometimes, multiple pregnancies. Young teens whose bodies are not yet completely developed and who also may have poor nutrition often give birth prematurely, which is why they need accessible birth control, education, and adequate social support when they become pregnant. Many problems can be avoided through good nutrition and detected by prenatal medical care and screening. However, in nearly half the instances of prematurity, the cause is not clear.

Premature labor proceeds like a normal, full-term labor. It may be a little slower owing to weaker contractions, or more rapid because the baby is smaller. Premature babies are extremely susceptible to the dangerous effects of the drugs used during labor, so giving birth without drugs will be of great benefit to your baby.

The smaller and more vulnerable the baby is, the more she or he needs immediate care and needs you. It is advisable that before 36 or 37 weeks, babies be born in a hospital or a well-equipped birth center. In the U.S., most premature babies are placed in oxygen-, temperature-, and humidity-controlled units, kept in intensive-care nurseries, and protected from every possible source of infection, which is common in hospitals. Increasingly, mothers are spending more time

---

* Midwives like Ina May Gaskin have revived this lost art. See Resources for her book, *Spiritual Midwifery*.

with their babies in these nurseries, most of which are set up for parents. Even the smallest premature babies thrive on "kangaroo care" (skin-to-skin contact). Be assertive about staying with your baby as much as possible—your presence, your voice, your touch, and your love will help her or him thrive.

You may sometimes need to remind hospital staff that this is *your* baby. Some hospitals are exploring the advantages of keeping older or larger premature babies in units close to their mothers' bedsides, to be cuddled and held close. These babies develop much more quickly than those left more to themselves. Parents are the most watchful and attentive caregivers. They notice changes that could signal problems, and alert nurses and doctors immediately. It is best to feed your premature baby breast milk.[28] The antibodies in colostrum fight the very infections to which the premature baby can succumb. The composition of your milk is right even for your premature baby. You can pump your own milk with an electric or hand breast pump (hospitals should supply them) if your baby is not able to nurse at first, and then feed it to the baby (see "Breastfeeding Your Baby," chapter 21, Postpartum, p. 507).

You may not be prepared yet for birth and motherhood, and may feel uncertain, anxious, and constantly worried about your baby. Find people to talk to. Hospital staff should be aware of your feelings, encourage you to spend as much time with your baby as possible, explain the reasons for all hospital procedures, and answer all your questions. You have the right to obtain accurate information about your baby's health status and prognosis, to participate in informed decision-making, and to decide about providing aggressive treatment for very ill infants.[29]

Concerned mothers have played an important role in searching out the latest information for the care of premature infants and in changing hospital policies.

I had been feeling contractions for several days, but since I was only 27 weeks I assumed these were Braxton-Hicks. After rising one morning I felt warm water pouring down my legs; I was in labor. Several hours later I gave birth to a baby boy weighing 1 lb. 12 oz. From the moment of birth he was alert and vigorous, much to the surprise of doctors (the contractions helped his lungs mature). I felt like I spent 13 weeks telling nurses and doctors that this was my baby, not theirs, and that he would not become exhausted if I held him to my breast and let him lick and sniff, even though he couldn't suck well yet. I spent a lot of time at the library and found a study that showed that sucking actually helped babies to thrive and gain weight, not lose weight, and that a pacifier would be helpful when I could not be there. I actually convinced the staff to change some of their practices.

Problems During Labor

During labor it is important that you tell your caregiver what you are experiencing, especially if you have sudden pain or uterine tenderness, if you feel feverish, or if you notice bleeding. Your caregiver will interpret what is happening and will be on the alert and prepared for any of the rare complications of labor such as an unusual presentation, a prolapsed cord (exceedingly rare), or excessive bleeding. She or he will be attentive to you and your baby's well-being, keeping track of your baby's heart rate and responding to any abnormalities. When appropriate, your caregiver will check your blood pressure or for the presence of fever. If severe nausea prevents you from keeping anything down, or if you have become extremely dehydrated, you may be given IV solutions. If so, request an IV pole on wheels so you can continue to move around, remaining as active as possible, and even showering if you wish. Even in high-tech settings where interventions have been deemed necessary, your birth can remain an emotionally and physically empowering event and a positive and affirming transition to motherhood.

"Problem Labors"

Your practitioners will determine whether your labor is progressing and whether contractions are effectively dilating your cervix. Sometimes contractions that are experienced as very strong, long, and regular over a long time do not open the cervix and may exhaust the mother and stress the baby. This kind of labor is called "dysfunctional" in obstetrical texts. Medical practitioners often respond with drugs to induce sleep, Pitocin to correct and augment the labor, or rupturing the membranes—all practices that can lead to a cascade of interventions (see p. 487) and create an atmosphere of crisis that further interferes with labor. Midwives often regard this kind of labor as a variation of normal labor, attributing a slow start to your uterus learning to contract efficiently or your baby moving into a more favorable position. They also recognize the role that fear can play in this kind of labor. They make sure that women eat well and drink enough, and respond with calm encouragement and supportive, noninterventive techniques, such as herbs, which often correct the situation.

Birth by Cesarean Section

Cesarean section, while at times a life-saving intervention for both mother and child, can be a cause of significant harm to mothers and provides no additional benefits to infants when performed outside of certain well-defined medical situations. We are beginning the long road back from an epidemic of unnecessary surgery.[30]

Having a healthy baby is everyone's goal. Cesarean sections are lifesaving operations when women have certain problems before or during labor: severe diabetes, transverse lie of the baby, failure of the baby to descend at all, cord prolapse, placenta previa, or placental dysfunction producing fetal distress.

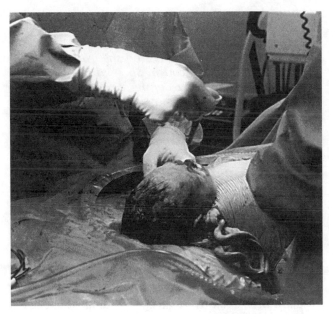

A cesarean birth/C. P. Oakes

I'd always dreamed of having a home birth, and if that weren't possible, to give birth in a birth center with a midwife. At 32 weeks, I had some bright red spotting. My midwife came to the hospital with me for an ultrasound, which showed that my placenta was partially covering my cervical opening. The obstetrician held out the possibility that the placenta might still move away from the cervix, although he was doubtful. I returned home with directions to call immediately if there was any more bleeding. At 35 weeks I woke to find blood pouring. With a towel between my legs I called my midwife, jumped in the car and headed to the hospital, where my lovely five-pound daughter Chiara was delivered by cesarean section. It wasn't what I'd planned, but I was grateful to be alive and have such a healthy baby.

Please let women know that in regard to cesareans there is a "gray area" between the life-or-death emergency situation and the absolutely unnecessary operation. In my case, I had been in extremely painful labor for hours and hours, with back-to-back long-lasting contractions (unexpected because my first labor had been intense, but short and manageable) . . . I walked, stood, squatted, took baths. Now, I'm no martyr, but I think I could have stood it if there had been any progress, but there was very little. Most discouraging, the baby's head wasn't engaged. After nine hours I said to my doctor, "I need a cesarean." Not one to jump into a c-section, he didn't want to do it right away. Finally, I had an epidural. When it took effect, I could smile again. We waited awhile longer— no progress. When he finally did the cesarean, he was amazed by the size of the baby. She was a giant! I know that some people believe that women can birth just about any size baby vaginally. Perhaps I would have been able to do so, too, if I had done other things

and been willing to labor for 24 more hours. Maybe not. I wonder if the intense pain was my body's way of telling me that vaginal birth was impossible this time. I am glad I made the choice I did.

Cesareans must be performed in hospitals wth proper drugs and anesthesia techniques, antibiotics, and blood transfusion equipment. Your pubic hair will be partially shaved and a catheter inserted into your urethra to keep your bladder emptied. In most situations you'll be given regional (spinal or epidural) anesthesia, which allows you to be awake. In an emergency you may be given general anesthesia. If you are awake for the operation, a sterile cloth screen will be placed between your head and belly. Sometimes you can watch in a mirror. Your abdomen will be washed with an antiseptic solution. When your abdomen has become numb or when you are unconscious, the physician makes a horizontal cut in your abdominal wall, low down near the line of your pubic hair. (A vertical cut is rarely necessary to get the baby out quickly.) The physician then cuts horizontally through the uterine muscle and eases the baby out. The baby's nose and mouth are suctioned. When your baby is breathing well, you or your partner can hold him or her. The physician then removes the placenta and sews you up, layer by layer.

Almost every woman needs to believe that her cesarean was necessary. However, allowing for an optimal national cesarean rate of 12% (a number many consider high, and certainly higher than achieved by many midwives), at least 50% of cesareans performed are unnecessary.[31]

A childbirth educator tells a typical story:

A woman phoned me today. She had given birth to her first child eight weeks ago. After being in labor for only four hours she had dilated from 4 to 9 centimeters. Suddenly they transported her to the delivery room, and yelled at her to push even though she didn't feel the urge to push and told them so. But they pressured her and, half-sitting up, holding her legs (a typical Lamaze position), she pushed for 26 minutes—she has it on record. At the end of that time her cervix was swollen—of course it swells when you push like that—and they told her that she wouldn't be able to deliver vaginally. Within 15 minutes she'd had a cesarean. Reason given: "Failure to progress."

While cesarean sections can be lifesaving and health-enhancing, they are not simply another way of being born. They carry considerable risks to mother and baby that don't exist in vaginal births.[32] We stress this because the medical community has the widespread attitude that "cesareans are not that bad" and "not such a big deal." Studies conclude that cesareans, being major operations, carry a two to four times greater risk of death to the mother than vaginal deliveries. They cause postoperative infections in 33% of women. They frequently cause respiratory distress in both premature and full-term babies and psychologi-

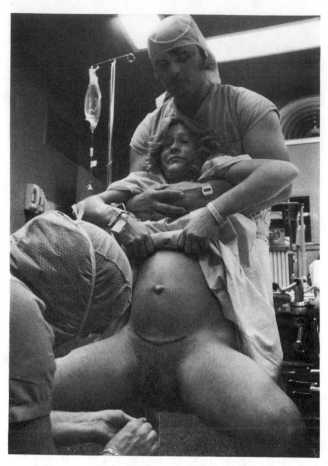

A vaginal birth after cesarean/Suzanne Arms

cal damage to the mother, if not to the family unit as a whole. The various types of anesthesia used can also have negative neurological effects on the baby.

What is happening, and why? Cesareans are the most common operation performed in the U.S.[33] In 1968, the national average cesarean rate was 5%. By 1987, the average had risen to 25% (in some hospitals 50% and higher). Today the rate is 20.8%.[34] Factors responsible for the high rate—some statistically measurable, others not—are many:

1. *"Once a cesarean, always a cesarean."* This dictum accounts for 30% of all cesareans. In fact, the majority of women can have vaginal births after cesareans (VBACs). They need information, encouragement, self-confidence, and support to do so.[35]

I had two cesareans, one because the doctor told me I had an "inadequate pelvis"; the second for "failure to progress" after only three hours of labor. That one was such a disappointment because I had searched long and hard to find a doctor who said he supported VBACs and I'd gotten hold of the X ray from my first birth that showed I had an adequate pelvis. [In my third pregnancy] I had lots of early labor; a few rounds of "false" labor. When my water began to leak and contractions began, I called the midwife who agreed

to attend me at home (I didn't think I'd ever have a vaginal birth in the hospital). My contractions were mild and it was late, so she suggested my husband and children go to bed; she said she would stay with me as I rested on the couch. She told me to imagine my cervix as an ever-widening circle, a ripple on a pond. I moved in and out of sleep, dreaming of a doughnut hole that grew larger and larger. Four hours later a huge, painful contraction woke me. My midwife, holding my feet, told me to expect more, but the very next contraction I was pushing and 45 minutes later my son was born into my waiting arms, a pound larger than my first two children. Yes, I slept right through my labor, and my pelvis was adequate. I knew I could do it, and I had!

Most often the condition that makes a cesarean necessary in one birth, if it had been necessary at all, will not exist in the next birth. In the past, physicians feared uterine rupture, which occurs very rarely and usually before labor begins. According to the 1994 VBAC guidelines from the American College of Obstetrics and Gynecology, almost all women with prior cesareans can plan a VBAC, including women with two or more low uterine incisions, women previously diagnosed with "cephalopelvic disproportion" (baby's head is too large for the pelvis), nondiabetic women expecting a baby larger than 8½ pounds, women who may need oxytocin to augment labor, and women considering using anesthesia, including the epidural. VBAC is safer in most cases than a scheduled repeat cesarean, and up to 80% of women with prior cesareans can deliver their subsequent babies vaginally (some midwifery services and birth centers have even higher rates).

2. *Obstetrical procedures and technology.* Fetal monitor use, elective induction, epidural anesthesia, early artificial rupture of membranes, immobilizing women while they labor on their backs, lack of skilled labor support—all these practices cause problems that can lead to interventions that result in cesareans.

3. *Obstetrical training and physicians' attitudes.* Physicians are not trained in normal birth, and often they don't learn skills such as external cephalic version for breech babies or how to deliver them vaginally, let alone the art of waiting patiently as a labor unfolds. At the same time that the birth rate in the U.S. has come down, obstetrics/gynecology is growing as a surgical specialty. Physicians-in-training need to perform a certain number of procedures as a requirement of their training.

Physicians' attitudes, while not statistically measurable, point to why cesareans are so dear to the medical heart. This discussion was heard among a group of doctors:

What's so great about delivery from below? . . . You want the baby squeezed out like toothpaste in a tube? . . . You might say we're helping women to do what nature hasn't evolved her to do for herself.

Physicians often believe that cesareans "make better babies." Infant mortality rates have declined over recent years, but not primarily because of cesarean sections. In fact, cesarean-section babies are often distressed. Mortality rates have improved because neonatal intensive care units keep alive low-birth-weight and premature babies who otherwise would die.

4. *Physicians' practice of defensive medicine.* It has long been argued that fear of lawsuits is one of the major causes for the increase in cesareans. In 1990, it was suggested in the *New England Journal of Medicine* that the most common cause of cesareans today is not fetal distress or maternal distress but obstetricians' distress.[36] Physicians believe that if they perform cesareans and the baby is born "less than perfect," they cover themselves legally. But recent studies show that more lawsuits have been instigated for malpractice associated with cesarean surgery than for failure to perform it, and that physicians don't change their practices in response to lawsuits.

5. *Changing indications for cesarean sections.* Women's bodies haven't changed, but physicians' eagerness to perform cesareans has led them to expand the meaning of dystocia ("difficult labor"). Physicians tell a woman that her pelvis is too small (*cephalopelvic disproportion*) or her labor too slow (*failure to progress in labor*)[37] and call both *dystocia,* whereas if she could instead labor naturally, moving around and squatting, she would give birth normally in most cases. Dystocia has been called a "wastebasket" term. Ninety-five percent of breech babies are unnecessarily delivered by cesarean section, and cesareans now replace forceps in many situations. The routine use of fetal monitors also increases the cesarean-section rate by suggesting fetal distress that is nonexistent.[38]

6. *Economic incentives.* Cesareans have been more lucrative for obstetricians, anesthesiologists, and hospitals, and to some they seem more convenient. This factor cannot be emphasized enough. As "managed care" becomes more the norm, however, there should be fewer incentives to perform cesareans, although presently, many HMOs function in the same manner as insurance companies, with little incentive to lower cesarean rates.

7. *The culture of fear surrounding birth.* Fear of labor and mistrust of our bodies and the birth process has contributed to the increase in cesareans. We are told that our babies are being "rescued." We need clear evidence of the need for a cesarean. We have a right to say no to fear.

By and large . . . American obstetrics has become so preoccupied with apparatus and with possible fetal injury that the mothers are increasingly being considered solely vehicles. In many cases small and uncertain gain for the infant is being purchased at the price of a small but grave risk to the mother.[39]

The International Cesarean Awareness Network, Inc. (ICAN) is an international organization founded

STANDING UP TO HOSPITAL ROUTINES

Hospitals can overwhelm you with their high-tech, impersonal settings. It may be difficult, but it is possible, to minimize, if not avoid altogether, routine and unnecessary interventions. To do this you can learn about the process of childbirth, the nature of your particular pregnancy, and the practices of the institution where you plan to give birth. Making a birth care plan, having an advocate with you, and negotiating ahead of time with your practitioner and the institution will help you navigate the medical system and achieve the kind of birth you want.

Either during preregistration or upon admittance, you will sign a patient consent form. The hospital must provide you with all the information necessary for you to make fully informed choices and thus give your "informed" consent, both for practices considered routine and in response to particular problems that may arise during labor and birth. Read any forms given to you. Ask questions. You can withdraw your consent at any time. Signing a form does not prevent you from taking legal action in the future.

Use a wheelchair only if you want to. A nurse or resident will ask about your pregnancy and labor. Hospital staff will listen to the fetal heartbeat with a fetoscope or doptone. The doptone is a form of ultrasound, so you may want to ask for a regular fetoscope instead. (Some nurses have never been trained to use regular fetoscopes, however.)

During all these procedures you can stand or sit. You don't have to get into bed or lie down, though you may be urged or expected to. A mother who gave birth twice lying flat on her back observed:

I've often thought that the best thing a woman can do for herself when she gets into the hospital is to stay upright, standing, sitting, kneeling, squatting. That way she remains active, in control.

When you lie on your back, your contractions change. In early labor they may slow down and even stop altogether. They may become more uncomfortable, making you tense up, which affects their efficacy.

In most hospitals and some birth centers, protocols require a 20-minute "test strip," using the external fetal monitor to check the course of the

continued on next page

baby's heartbeat during a series of contractions. There is no scientific evidence to support this routine: studies have demonstrated that it does not lead to improved fetal outcomes. On the other hand, it plays a powerful role in initiating you into routine hospital care and symbolizes the hospital's claim to authority over you. Ask for a human monitor instead! If the nurses aren't around and you have a birth attendant who knows how to listen to the baby's heartbeat, she can check the heart rate. You may have to lie down for a fetoscope but not for a doptone.

You will probably have an internal exam to check dilation and establish that labor has actually begun. In some hospitals nurses do them; in others, residents or doctors. This can feel invasive and uncomfortable.

I'd brought tapes and music, was walking and dancing. We'd created a wonderful mood. Then the resident came in and blew it. He examined me internally, causing more pain than ever in my life.

You have a right to insist that the person performing the exam be gentle, making sure you are comfortable and that you are not having a contraction at that time.

It is neither necessary nor beneficial for practitioners to perform repeated internal exams. They interrupt the flow of labor and lead to a focus on measurement and time.

You have the right to turn away residents and to say, "I want my own doctor or midwife." In teaching hospitals, residents are often the only doctors you get, and several of them may want to examine you. You have the right to say no. You can refuse to participate in teaching programs and to turn away bystanders and observers. Even in emergency situations, you have the right to ask questions and give informed consent or refusal. Focus on what you want and need. This is your labor and your birth. You may need a friend, family member, or birth attendant to help enforce your rights.

Nurses will be your most constant medical attendants if you have no midwife or doula. Even midwives may have to attend more than one laboring woman. Let the nurses know what you want. Many nurses are encouraging and helpful.

I was in labor for 36 hours altogether, most of them in the hospital. One nurse stayed in the room with me the whole time, sleeping in the other bed, keeping people from coming in. She'd tell them, "This is my patient; I'm in charge!" She helped me to have a beautiful vaginal delivery. Without her I would not have done it.

If you find yourself with a nurse who is not supportive or positive, ask for another. It may not be easy to ask, and another nurse may not be available, but it's worth a try. When you labor you are usually very sensitive to the energy around you; unsupportive staff can negatively affect you. Your partner and/or birth assistant can advocate for you. Look for a birthing place with arrangements for continuous care.

by concerned parents and professionals to support and inform women who have undergone cesareans, and to reform and humanize medical attitudes and policies. Its founders realized that their own cesareans had been medically unnecessary, and that, in ensuing pregnancies, most of them could labor naturally and deliver vaginally. The hundreds of women who contacted them reinforced these convictions. ICAN educates women and practitioners to decrease the number of women having a first (primary) cesarean and to increase the number of women having VBACS. They provide accurate information about pregnancy and birth through their quarterly newsletter, the *Clarion,* and promote legislation requiring hospitals and physicians to reveal statistical information so that women can make informed choices about where they wish to give birth. Throughout the country, local chapters provide VBAC groups and offer classes where women talk about their previous experiences, fears, and hopes, and learn concrete ways of preparing physically and emotionally for the births of their next babies (see Resources).

Our focus in pregnancy should be to grow healthy and confident and to give birth well and joyfully, not simply to prevent a medical procedure. Remember: this is your birth—a powerful physical, social, spiritual, and emotional event in your life. Do not let obstetrical practice define it for you.[40]

OBSTETRICAL PROCEDURES

The physiology of labor is both powerful and delicately balanced. Each element has a function in helping the baby to be born well. Attendants must honor this process as it unfolds with its varied rhythms and expressions. They should not interfere with the natural process without a valid reason. They must not interrupt it, hinder it, or arbitrarily attempt to speed it up. Labor opens the cervix and moves the baby through the birth canal. Labor is beneficial to the baby, not something to be bypassed. Amniotic fluid cushions the baby's head, and the bulging sac stretches the perineum slowly. As the baby passes over the perineum, excess fluid is squeezed from the baby's lungs. Like any other animal, we need a calm environment for labor to proceed at its own pace. Like elephants and dolphins, we labor best with empathetic females like ourselves nearby.

Occasionally things don't function properly and medical intervention is justified. However most obstetrical drugs and hospital procedures have never been scientifically proved to be beneficial for healthy mothers and infants. Obstetrical practice grew out of scientific dualism, mechanistic attitudes toward the body, and a view of the female body as abnormal, dysfunctional, and "dirty."* Interventions and drugs are now driven by the force of the medical-industrial complex: drug companies, researchers, insurance companies, the marriage of drug and equipment companies, health care institutions, and medical practitioners. Pregnancy is the leading "diagnosis" in this country, the leading reason for outpatient visits, and a lucrative market.[41]

It is a credit to our basic health and resilience that despite such assaults, attitudes, and forces, we and our babies emerge so healthy. It is sad that many of us "need" rescuing, expect intervention as the norm, and rely on it for safety and pain relief when it is not always safe and so many nonpharmacological methods of pain relief are available. Does it make sense to accept this tampering with our bodies, our strengths, and the safety of our children?

We recommend that you learn about routine interventions before choosing caregiver and birthing place. While information offers some protection, this careful selection of caregiver and place of birth may help ensure that you will use medical resources during labor only when you really need them, and that you will have a normal spontaneous labor and birth.†

Medical Procedures and Interventions During Labor and Birth

Like a snowball rolling down the hill, as one unphysiological practice is employed . . . another frequently becomes necessary to counteract some of the disadvantages, large or small, inherent in the previous procedure.[42]

In a normal labor there should be a valid reason to interfere with the birth process and evidence to support the safety and effectiveness of the interventions used.

If you are planning a hospital birth, find out about the procedures and drugs commonly used. You have a right to make choices about all procedures and interventions. Some institutions respect this right more than others, which is why it is useful to bring an advocate with you. Discuss your preferences beforehand, write

them down, and send copies to your physician or midwife, to the hospital, and to the head of nursing (see "Making a Birth Care Plan," p. 473). Once you arrive at the hospital, you have a right to know the names and risks of any drugs or treatments offered, and to accept or refuse them (see "Our Rights as Patients," chapter 25, The Politics of Women's Health and Medical Care, p. 713).

Pubic shaving and enemas, once routine, are totally unnecessary. No scientific or medical evidence supports their use; they do not, as was once believed, reduce infection or contribute to a "clean birth." You can request an enema if you think it will make you feel better or if feces in your rectum seem to be holding up labor. Enemas can stimulate labor, but you need a good reason to want to stimulate it. You often have a natural diarrhea that empties your bowel before labor begins. Why interfere with the natural process?

Immobility and lying down are more painful and increase the length of labor and the risk of distress to the baby while decreasing the strength and efficiency of contractions.[43] Instead, you can change position, walk, move your body, or take a shower or bath to relax, making labor less painful and contractions more efficient.

Rupturing the amniotic sac (amniotomy) early in labor is done routinely by many physicians as part of "active management of labor." Early amniotomy, more convenient for the doctor, does not usually benefit baby or mother.[44] The sac is punctured with a small plastic hook; it is painless but can feel invasive. Some physicians argue that this shortens the length of labor, but it interferes with the natural labor process and can cause decelerations in the fetal heart rate. It shouldn't be done in a normal labor. In 75% of women, the membranes remain intact until full dilation. Occasionally when a woman is in active labor with a bulging sac of water in front of a well-descended head, her practitioner may rupture the membranes to facilitate contractions or to speed up a prolonged labor. Some women experience this as a great relief. Some practitioners will rupture membranes earlier if they suspect meconium, but there is no evidence to support this practice.

Many hospitals continue to use **routine intravenous infusions (IVs)** for laboring women, along with restrictions about drinking and eating. No scientific evidence supports this practice or the claim that eating and drinking may cause aspiration of vomit if general anesthesia has to be used. IVs interfere with the natural process of labor, are often uncomfortable, and restrict our freedom to move about. In a normal labor they should not be used. To meet labor's enormous energy requirements, we should eat and/or drink as we wish throughout labor. IVs, used "just in case" something goes wrong, invite a "cascade of interventions"—drugs to correct low blood pressure caused by an epidural, a glucose solution to prevent you from becoming depleted and dehydrated because you are not eating or drinking, Pitocin to speed up labor, drugs to deaden the intensity of Pitocin-augmented contractions. In teaching hospitals, IVs are inserted simply for

---

* Michel Odent, throughout *Birth Reborn*, speaks of modern obstetric practice as "the systematic elimination of the mother from the childbearing process." Doris Haire wrote *The Cultural Warping of Childbirth* out of a concern that obstetric practices and drugs are causing retardation, brain dysfunction, and learning disabilities in our children.
† See Murray Enkin et al., *A Guide to Effective Care in Pregnancy,* 1995, for a summary of current research on maternity care practices, and the *Cochrane Pregnancy and Childbirth Database* (see box on p. 493) for updates.

instructional purposes. Both glucose and saline solutions can have harmful effects on mother and baby. If you must have an IV, ask for a *heparin lock* so that the line may be removed when not in use.

The Centers for Disease Control recommend that a woman whose culture was positive for Group B Strep at 35 to 37 weeks receive IV antibiotics during labor. If labor commences before 37 weeks, or if a mother has had a previous infant infected with Group B Strep, the same protocol is recommended, even without a positive culture. If membranes are ruptured for more than 18 hours or a mother develops a fever, antibiotics are also recommended. These are experimental strategies to prevent babies from being overwhelmed with Group B Strep.

Prostaglandin/Pitocin   induction/stripping membranes. Prostaglandins are now being used in hospitals to induce labor by ripening the cervix. A gel is inserted into your vagina either directly or via a diaphragm. Sometimes it begins to work in as little as an hour or two, but more often you will wait for six to 12 hours before being rechecked. Sometimes prostaglandins cause contractions to begin. If too much is used, your uterus can be overstimulated. Sometimes they cause nausea and headaches. This ripening is followed by induction with Pitocin (a synthetic oxytocin, the hormone that stimulates normal labor) given through an intravenous drip with a pump in order to control the dosage.

Since 1978, the FDA has opposed the practice of "elective" inductions—those carried out for the convenience of the mother or doctor—because of the attendant risks. They should not be done. If your cervix is ripe, your practitioner may attempt to hasten the onset of labor by "stripping" or "sweeping" your membranes, using fingers to separate the amniotic sac from the lower segment of your uterus. If there is a need to induce labor, this may work and is less invasive and carries less risk than Pitocin, although no evidence supports the reliability of this procedure. Induction carries the risk that a baby will be born prematurely, owing to inaccurate estimates of age. Artificially provoked uterine contractions can be much more violent, prolonged, and painful than natural ones, and they can cause high blood pressure. They may interfere with blood flow to the uterus and placenta, causing fetal distress. Uterine rupture, although rare, can occur. An induction's failure can result in a cesarean section.

Augmentation of labor with IV Pitocin is routinely done as part of the "active management of labor," adopted by many hospitals in the past few years. Its purpose is to speed up labor. There is no evidence that this practice benefits mothers or babies. In a normal labor, no need exists to speed things up. The negative side effects of IV Pitocin, one of which is increased pain, lead women to request drugs or anesthesia. This practice accompanies early amniotomy. As noted, both induction and acceleration of labor can involve considerable risks.[45]

Induction or acceleration may be appropriate when there is some question about the baby's survival and/or when the mother has preeclampsia, hemolytic disease (Rh factor), or maternal diabetes. In some of these situations, cesarean section is preferable when the use of Pitocin may further compromise the baby. If you and your physician agree upon the need to induce or augment your labor, your and your baby's heart rate must be constantly monitored. You will also need labor support to help you relax and cope with the pain of contractions in order to avoid drugs or epidural anesthesia and their attendant risks.

My doctor decided to induce my labor. At the hospital I was given Pitocin. My labor was very intense and unexpectedly short—four hours. My daughter had to be delivered by forceps because her heartbeat was slowing down and I couldn't push her out quickly enough. I was told her life had been endangered because my contractions were too strong and the placenta had separated from the uterine wall too early. My doctors were heroes! They had saved her life. Three years later, seven months pregnant, I asked my doctor a casual question about my first labor and delivery. He began reading my record to me. Amazed, I said, "That's someone else's record." It turns out that the Pitocin stimulated my labor too strongly so that indeed it wasn't natural and was dangerous, and then they gave me Demerol to slow everything down. I had never been told any of this. My strong contractions made the placenta separate early. I'm sure that the Demerol slowed my daughter's heartbeat and oxygen intake. It also explains why she was so sleepy the first three days and didn't immediately nurse. Now I know my doctors were responsible for the dangers to my daughter's life—if not completely, at least in great part. Induction complicated my labor and delivery.

This woman's experience is quite common. *Iatrogenesis* is the name given to problems that are caused by medical treatments or procedures.

Fetal monitors are machines that electronically record the baby's heart rate during labor. Used routinely without any evidence that they provide any benefit for low-risk women, they are of only questionable benefit for women with conditions that place them at risk. There are external and internal monitors. External monitors use electrodes strapped to the mother's belly after a gel has been applied to the skin; one picks up the fetal heart rate and records it on a strip of paper, while the other records intensity and duration of contractions. With internal fetal monitors, electrodes are connected to wires within a plastic tube, introduced into the woman's vagina, and attached directly to the baby's presenting part (usually the head) by means of metal clips or screws. These electrodes measure the baby's heartbeat. The woman's contractions are measured either by a pressure catheter introduced into her uterus through her vagina, or by an external tocodynamometer strap. A printout shows the baby's heartbeat, which is also audible. The woman will probably have a blood pressure cuff and often an IV.

Though these monitors may be useful in some truly high-risk situations, and necessary when labor is induced or accelerated or the woman is anesthetized, they entail many discomforts and risks to women and babies.[46] Ultrasound has never been proved safe in pregnancy. The straps and the pressure of the transducer may be uncomfortable. Ironically, fetal stress picked up by the monitor may be a product of invasive hospital routines and procedures, including the monitor itself. Since women with a monitor cannot move around much, if at all, labor may slow down or stop. Hospital personnel may interpret the machine data incorrectly. Incomplete understanding of the range and fluctuation in fetal heart rate during and between contractions has led to unnecessary forceps and, these days, unnecessary cesarean deliveries. A recent study demonstrated that 99.8% of the "abnormalities" picked up by fetal monitors are not indicators of distress.[47] Exemplifying the "cascade of interventions," a monitor is considered essential if a woman has epidural anesthesia, since the drugs used can cause the mother's blood pressure to drop significantly, thereby putting the baby into distress.

When monitors are used, hospital staff, partners, and attendants tend to focus on the machine, directing their attention and support away from you and your labor. In addition, women and babies run a greater risk of infection with the internal monitor and pressure catheter. The baby's scalp may bleed because of the way the electrode has been attached. Post-delivery rashes are common where the electrode was attached (85% in one study), and scalp abscess is not uncommon (20%).

The routine use of fetal monitors has not decreased the newborn death rate or the number of brain-damaged children. Several randomized controlled clinical trials demonstrated that the use of fetal monitoring, compared with listening to the baby's heart rate with a fetoscope, did not improve Apgar scores or decrease neonatal mortality.[48] Monitoring continues to contribute to the unacceptably high rate of cesarean sections in this country.

Two new developments in monitoring are the intrauterine pressure catheter and the fetal acoustic stimulator. The intrauterine pressure catheter is inserted vaginally into the uterus between the baby and the uterine wall. It is used to determine the intensity of contractions if a woman has received Pitocin and her labor is not progressing. In fetal acoustic stimulation, an instrument used abdominally emits sound waves to shock and "wake" a baby up. It creates a sudden, marked rise in the heart rate of a healthy baby. The efficacy and safety of these procedures have not been adequately assessed.

Routine episiotomy is the incision through skin and muscles in the perineum—the area between the vagina and the anus—to enlarge the opening through which the baby will pass. Many physicians perform it out of convenience, since it speeds up the birth, but it is rarely, if ever, justified.

Episiotomy is the most frequently performed obstetric operation in the West. It is one of the most intense and dramatic ways in which the territory of women's bodies is appropriated, the only operation performed on the body of a healthy woman without her consent. It represents obstetrical power: Babies can't get out unless they are cut out. It prevents women from experiencing birth as a sexual event, and is a form of ritual genital mutilation.[49]

Your perineum is designed to stretch and expand to accommodate your baby. Hormones cause your tissues to soften and stretch and your vagina to open. The baby's head slowly stretches these tissues as it moves back and forth, appearing and receding rhythmically, until finally, gradually, it emerges completely. Midwifery techniques—gentle guidance, touch, the use of oils and hot compresses for comfort; encouraging favorable positions such as being upright, sitting, or squatting; helping you breathe your baby out—work with this process and can prevent or minimize tearing. Most women do not tear at all.

The procedure is necessary *only* in rare cases of fetal distress when the baby must come out quickly, and perineal tissues won't stretch any more. If one is needed, ask for a *median cut* (in the middle), not a *mediolateral* (from the middle to one side), which is more painful and may interfere with sensation for a long time.

Doctors are taught that an episiotomy will prevent perineal tears extending to the anus (third-degree lacerations); that it will prevent damage to the baby's head; that it keeps the pelvic floor from becoming too stretched; that it is a safeguard against your uterus, bladder, or rectum prolapsing into your vagina; and that it prevents urinary incontinence later in life. No data support these arguments.[50] In practice, episiotomies are done simply to get the birth over with. Distressingly, some physicians claim they are performing a service to the woman's partner.

I saw my doctor at the checkup six weeks after my baby was born. Full of male pride, he told me during my pelvic exam, "I did a beautiful job sewing you up. You're as tight as a virgin. Your husband should thank me."

Many women find intercourse extremely painful after being stitched up too tightly. Stitches are often itchy and very painful for several weeks as they heal. Some women are allergic to the stitches; others have had stitches that didn't dissolve. Many women report permanently impaired sexual sensation after episiotomies.[51] You have a legal right to refuse episiotomy.

A vacuum extractor is often currently used in place of forceps to help push the baby out or to rotate the baby. It has a small suction cup that fits onto the baby's head. Its use can speed up birth if there is fetal distress during pushing, or shorten what physicians consider a long "second stage" of labor. The vacuum extractor is often used with epidurals, because the epidural often blocks pushing sensations. (If you have an epidural, allow it to wear off before pushing.) The use of the vacuum extractor can cause a blood-filled swelling on the baby's head, which can become infected.

Forceps may still be used in some situations, such as when the vacuum won't work because of a molded head or when a head needs to be rotated. Forceps resemble hinged salad tongs with long blades curved to fit the shape of the baby's head. Ideally they are used to widen the pelvis and guide the baby's head out of the vagina, not to pull on it. Doctors sometimes use them in uncomplicated labors to shorten pushing, which they mistakenly believe to exhaust the mother and pose a danger to the baby. Unless a mother is too tired to push effectively, or there is some indication that the baby is distressed or not advancing, forceps should not be used. Forceps have caused serious damage to babies when used inappropriately or by unskilled practitioners. As noted earlier, position changes, nourishment, and encouragement can help a mother push her baby out. Try midwifery approaches first.

For decades, cesarean sections have replaced forceps in most situations. In the 1990s, in the effort to lower the cesarean section rate, there has been a rise in vacuum extractor deliveries.[52] Here, as with other procedures, there must be a compelling reason to interfere with the natural birth process.

Pharmacological Methods of Pain Relief

In the hospital you may be offered, or you may request, "something" to relieve the pain and intensity of labor. This may happen near the end of active labor, from 8 to 10 centimeters of dilation—a period that presents a particularly difficult challenge, even though for most women this is the shortest part of labor.

We have presented an array of ways to make labor bearable that pose no risk to you or your baby, wherever you chose to give birth (see p. 471). Even if you have needed pain medication in a previous birth, every labor is different; and subsequent labors tend to go more quickly and smoothly. In hospital settings, practitioners use a variety of drugs and forms of anesthesia for pain relief and for operative procedures such as cesarean sections. Along with each drug often come two or three other procedures and, in addition, drugs designed to reduce the risk of the procedure or medication used. Interventions necessitate more interventions. They flow from attempts to "manage" birth and eliminate pain and often come at great cost to you and your baby.

Mothers often suffer more from the aftereffects of the drugs used in labor than from the labor itself. In addition, most drugs and anesthesia persist as you push your baby out, eliminating or altering sensation

and your experience of giving birth. Learn beforehand what the drugs and forms of anesthesia are, how they work, and their side effects in order to weigh their possible risks to you and your baby and their aftereffects against your ability to cope. New drugs and forms of anesthesia are being introduced (and sometimes reintroduced in different doses and in different ways) in the search for the magic solution to the "problem" of labor. We will present information on the more commonly used *analgesics,* which decrease our overall sensation of pain, and *anesthetics,* which remove our sensation of pain altogether by creating loss of consciousness, sleep, or a temporary loss of feeling in the specific area affected.

Every single drug given to the mother during labor crosses the placenta and reaches her baby, some in greater amounts and with greater rapidity than others. If the baby is premature, smaller than average, or in poor health, the consequences can be particularly dangerous. Even normal babies suffer from the effects of maternal medication.

No drug used for anesthesia has been proved safe for mothers and babies. Many obstetric drugs used routinely for labor and delivery have not been approved for that purpose by the FDA, and thus have the status of experimental drugs.[53] Some drugs approved by the FDA for use in labor have not been adequately studied for their delayed or long-term effects on infants. Some infants whose mothers received analgesia and anesthesia during labor and delivery have difficulty sucking and establishing breast-feeding and have delayed muscular, visual, and neural development in the first four to six weeks of life.[54] This doesn't mean that all babies will be so affected, or that the babies affected will be permanently delayed in development; but the first weeks of life *are* a critical time.

Anesthetized mothers often feel quite separate from their newborns:

I was really doped up when my baby was delivered and barely got to see that she was alive before she was whisked away to the nursery. When I finally woke up and she was able to be brought to me, I remember thinking, Is this really my baby? Do I really want to take her home with me? It took me a while to feel connected to her.

Do your research before labor begins, and go into labor with clear intentions about how you want to handle pain relief. Women have told us repeatedly that without this determination based on an understanding of the trade-offs, it becomes all too easy to say yes to drugs and anesthesia.

Analgesia: Tranquilizers and Narcotics

Tranquilizers
As soon as labor becomes intense, you may be offered a tranquilizer or a narcotic "to take the edge off your

contractions." Tranquilizers such as Vistaril are given primarily for anxiety; they are not painkillers. They can relax you in early labor or if you are exhausted and unable to rest. But once you have established a good pattern of labor, they can make you feel out of control and sharply reduce your ability to cope with your contractions. You may fall asleep until a contraction reaches its peak and then wake up, panic, and actually experience more pain than you would have without the drug, because panic and fear heighten pain. Tranquilizers may have a depressant effect on the newborn. For instance, Valium (diazepam) reduces a newborn's body temperature, muscle tone, and ability to suckle. Other tranquilizers may cause labor to slow down or even cease altogether.[55]

Narcotics

Narcotics such as Demerol, meperidine, Nubane, Stadol, and Nisentil provide relief from pain. Like all drugs, they cross the placenta and adversely affect you and your baby. Demerol in particular may impair the transfer of oxygen from the mother's circulation to that of the baby, resulting in oxygen depletion that can cause the brain to swell. It can also depress the respiratory and circulatory systems of the mother. All of these narcotics can depress the newborn's respiratory system as well as his or her psychophysiological functions after birth. At birth, infants whose mothers have been given narcotics may appear sleepy, dopey, and unresponsive to their environment. They may be less able to suckle, or reluctant to breast-feed at all. Narcotics can also make the mother drowsy and nauseated. Other drugs used for pain relief but not approved by the FDA for this use include Dilaudid, fentanyl (Sublimaze), and codeine. Phenergan is often used with Demerol to combat nausea and vomiting and to make Demerol work efficiently. Research has shown that this drug impairs the blood-clotting ability of newborns in a way that can cause bleeding within the brain.

Barbiturates

Barbiturates (Nembutal, Seconal), used to promote sleep, are known to be dangerous to the fetus, depressing respiration and responsiveness. They used to be given in combination with scopolamine (an amnesiac and a hallucinogen often referred to as "twilight sleep"), which had the nightmare effect of making women become physically violent during labor, talk uninhibitedly, or go into a stupor. Women felt the sensations but "forgot" what happened and later felt they had lived through some kind of torture.

When receiving analgesics, dizziness or lightheadedness can make it difficult to walk around during labor.

Anesthesia

Inhaled by the Mother

Once common, inhalation analgesia has been replaced in most hospitals by epidurals or systemic drugs. When inhalation analgesia is used, usually nitrous oxide combined with 50% oxygen is inhaled with each contraction and timed to work during the contraction's peak. These gases can slow labor and have potentially fatal complications if too much is inhaled. Nitrous oxide can delay the development of the baby's motor skills for months, frustrating the baby's attempts to sit, stand, and move around.

Regional Anesthesia

An **epidural** is a continuous regional anesthesia given to women during active labor. Drugs are re-administered until delivery. An epidural can be administered only by an anesthesiologist and requires his or her constant monitoring. Your blood pressure will be monitored with a blood pressure cuff usually attached to your arm at all times. Your heart rate will be monitored with an EKG. In many regional hospitals, an epidural is the most routinely used form of anesthesia, with more than 80% of women "choosing" it. So commonly used, it has made its way into comic strips and stand-up comedy shows.

During my prenatal visits my obstetrician encouraged me to have an epidural for labor. He told me there was no need to suffer as women had in the past. He assured me that epidurals were totally safe. I wasn't sure, but when he ended up inducing my labor with Pitocin because I was "late" [41 weeks], I found the contractions unbearable. My husband and I were left in the room alone except when a nurse came in to look at the monitor and check my blood pressure. I couldn't push well and my doctor used the "Mighty Vac" to pull my son out. He had such a hard time getting on to my breast; it was days before he really sucked well. I was upset when I found out that many babies born to women with epidurals have this difficulty. I've wondered what he meant by "safe."

Epidural anesthesia can be administered to laboring women at any time, but it should be started no earlier than 4 centimeters of dilation and no later than 9. The skin is anesthetized and an anesthetic, bupivacaine, is introduced through a tiny catheter placed in the woman's back through a needle. The catheter remains in place in the epidural space around, not in, the spinal column. A specially designed pump keeps the anesthetic dripping in measured doses. If a lot more is needed, the anesthesiologist will return and "top it off." When administered properly, epidurals will significantly diminish the sensations of labor in most cases and, unlike the standard spinal, numb only the area immediately around the perineum and lower uterus, belly to knees. Sometimes they just don't work effectively.

If you choose an epidural, you invite a number of interlocking procedures, most of which increase the risks of the method. An epidural requires an IV to administer fluids to offset the hypotension (low blood pressure) caused by the anesthetic; frequent monitoring of blood pressure, since the lowered blood pressure can cause distress to the baby as well as the mother; continuous monitoring of the baby's heart rate; and the use of a urinary catheter, since the epidural causes urinary retention. It also results in immobility. Epidurals frequently cause a slowing of labor that leads to the use of Pitocin for stimulating and strengthening labor and, following rupture of the membranes, the use of a pressure catheter to assess the strength of contractions. Often an internal fetal monitor is attached to the baby's head.

Many obstetricians and anesthesiologists would have us believe that the epidural is the answer to the "problem of labor." An epidural carries significant risks to mother and baby. Epidural anesthesia can cause disruptions in normal uterine function that cannot be completely corrected by the use of oxytocin. With epidural use there is a greater incidence of persistent malpresentations, such as posterior or transverse position of the baby's head, and a three to four times higher incidence of vacuum extractor or forceps delivery. There is also a tenfold increase in cesarean sections among women who have epidurals.[56]

Recent research has shown that the use of epidurals can lead to an array of unnecessary tests and procedures performed on newborns and a longer hospital stay than usual. Epidurals cause a rise in the body temperature of some women.[57] Since it is not possible to determine immediately whether the elevated temperature is the result of the epidural or of an infection, babies born to such mothers are often treated as if they have an infection or are at risk for one. They may be subjected to repeated cultures and blood tests, antibiotics administered by injection for 48 hours until culture results come back from the lab, chest X rays, and sometimes a spinal tap, a painful procedure that carries risks of its own. All this is done to rule out an infection suggested by an elevated temperature caused by the epidural. These procedures and the medical surveillance of the newborn produces fear and anxiety in the new mother that can affect her ability to rest and to nurse well and can undermine her confidence.

Some of the risks persist after birth. Women with epidurals have twice the rate of stress incontinence, which is the inability to control urine when coughing, sneezing, jumping, or moving quickly. Infants are often more profoundly affected. Research has shown that the epidural anesthesia (bupivacaine) can have prolonged adverse effects on the baby's development. Observed behavioral changes include decreased rooting activity (searching for the breast or food) and increased muscular floppiness.[58] Researchers note that these effects are less than those caused by high doses of labor medications or general anesthesia.

Epidural anesthesia can be useful in complicated and unusually difficult labor and delivery. When used for cesarean operations, it allows a mother to be awake and alert. Unlike a spinal, an epidural wears off quickly and does not ordinarily cause headaches.

Spinal anesthesia involves introducing an anesthetic agent into the space surrounding the spinal column, numbing the body completely from the waist down. It used to be frequently injected during pushing before the birth of the head, implying that this is the worst part of labor. Women, however, know that at this point the hardest work is over, and they describe the thrill and joy of pushing their babies out. The perineum usually becomes numb as it stretches to accommodate the head, producing a natural anesthesia. Spinals do not allow for this experience. Some aftereffects such as headache, stiff neck, or backache can be lessened if a small needle is used. A spinal is sometimes used for a cesarean following an ineffective epidural.

Intrathecal anesthesia ("walking epidural"), the latest in pain relief methods, combines the spinal as a pathway of entry with narcotic agents. This method, employed in the 1940s with higher dosages of narcotics, uses minute amounts of morphine with fentanyl, a very quick-acting drug not approved by the FDA for use in labor. Advocates for this method argue that it is effective for as long as eight hours, requires only tiny amounts of narcotics, allows women to walk around or rest, does not require the monitoring associated with epidurals, and does not interfere with pushing, since it does not alter pain sensations in the lower pelvis. These drugs can cause nausea, vomiting, and urinary retention necessitating a urinary catheter, as well as mild to severe itching. Like all drugs, they cross the placenta. After the birth, Narcan and Vistaril may be needed to counter the narcotic effects in the mother as well as the itching.

Nurses and midwives who observe women using this method describe a frequent slowing of labor, irritating and distracting itching, vomiting, and the discomfort of not being able to urinate and having a catheter. They have also observed that while babies appear responsive at birth, 24 hours later they exhibit uncoordinated movements and difficulty in nursing.

Caudals, once commonly used, require an injection into the sacral canal at the base of the back. For a continuous caudal (given from about 8 centimeters of dilation), a catheter is introduced into the lower back and the anesthetic is injected into the catheter in measured doses. A caudal requires a significantly larger dose of anesthetic than does either a spinal or an epidural and therefore carries a greater risk to both mother and baby. Furthermore, the failure rate for caudals is higher than for epidurals, owing to the greater chance of improper needle placement. Caudals carry the same risk of hypotension (drop in blood pressure) and subsequent lack of oxygen to the baby.

Pudendal blocks (*pudendum* is Latin for the external female genitalia, meaning "that of which one ought to be ashamed"!) anesthetize only the vulva and perineum with xylocaine and might be used when forceps are going to be used or episiotomies made. A pudendal block can cause the same neurological effect on the baby as an epidural injection of the same drug.

Paracervical blocks, administered by injecting anesthesia directly into the cervical area, once performed liberally, are now considered dangerous and should never be used.

EVALUATING OBSTETRICAL PRACTICES BY REVIEWING RANDOMIZED CONTROLLED TRIALS (RCTS):

The Cochrane Pregnancy and Childbirth Database (CCPC) (see also chapter 25, The Politics of Women's Health and Medical Care)

The CCPC offers high-quality information about the effectiveness of specific obstetrical tests, procedures, and interventions. Its systematic reviews and quarterly updates of findings about commonly utilized medical practices provide reliable information that can help us choose among practitioners and institutions, decide whether to use specific forms of care, and advocate for more appropriate maternity care. It tells us whether specific forms of care "work," "do not work," or are "experimental," not having been adequately studied. It also states whether they prevent risks, whether there are trade-offs between risks and benefits, and what side effects have been studied. A similar but smaller ongoing database that addresses neonatal care, focusing on problems of newborns, can be invaluable if your baby has serious problems.

The CCPC provides stark evidence, virtually impossible to ignore or disprove, of the degree to which current obstetrical practices are *not* based on the best available evidence and may indeed be harmful. It is the most reliable resource we have for questioning obstetrical routine. It identifies many effective low-tech and preventive practices not widely used, as well as practices that are effective when used appropriately, and ones that are unlikely to be beneficial but require more research, are of unknown effectiveness, or possess known benefits that must be weighed against the known risks.

The CCPC is limited in that by providing a "snapshot" of current medical practices, it represents only the medical view of child-bearing; the studies it evaluates reflect medical interests and perspectives. It contains little information about midwifery, practices that involve minimal risk, or the quality-of-life concerns so important to child-bearing women.

For a condensed version of a 1,500 page review of obstetrical studies, read *A Guide to Effective Care in Pregnancy and Childbirth* (see Resources). You can also access updates by subscribing to the service.

Thanks to Carol Sakala for preparing this information.

General Anesthesia

General anesthesia puts the woman completely to sleep and deadens her body to the point where she no longer perceives pain. It is usually only used for emergency cesareans when it would take too long to use regional anesthesia, or to perform surgical procedures after the birth such as removal of an abnormally adhered placenta, a very rare occurrence.

AFTERWORD *

Your baby is born. You have given her or him the healthiest and safest birth you could. You will become absorbed in your baby's daily unfolding and in the adventure and challenges of being a parent. You may feel fulfilled, ecstatic, and immensely close to your partner, your family, and your baby. You may have nagging doubts, emerging regrets, or fears that occasionally rise to the surface.

Birth is a powerful event. We relive the births of our children many times over during the following days, weeks, months, and years, thinking and talking about them, feeling them in our hearts. This reliving is a natural and sometimes essential means of understanding what has happened. When we have experienced birth in the setting of our choice with the support we needed, with few or no complications, we relive the event in a clear, happy way. But when unexpected complications and medical interventions alter the experience, we may have conflicting feelings—joy and disappointment, confidence and a sense of inadequacy—which can be confusing.

It can be difficult to find language adequate enough to express our wonder and sense of accomplishment, or our overwhelming feelings of frustration, anger, and outrage. It may not be enough to simply learn what happened. Powerful, ongoing feelings keep our memories alive. Unhappiness may be right on the surface, easily accessible, taking the form of grief, of anger, of having been violated. Or we may bury our strongest emotions, denying how terrible the experience was because to admit it would bring us to the edge of such deep anger. How to handle it? Whom to blame? We excuse and defend physicians and institutions, defensively describing bad experiences as good ones. We apologize for selfishly wanting more: "It doesn't matter. After all, my baby is healthy and that's all that counts. But why am I crying?" We feel ashamed of not having had that "natural" birth we'd prepared for. Other mothers may make us feel bad, too, by subtly implying that we were at fault. Or we feel distant from the baby.

My next memory was waking up the next morning. "You have a beautiful daughter," they said. "Where is she? Give her to me. She's mine!" They brought her. I wasn't even glad to see her. I wasn't sure she was mine.

---

* In extremely rare cases, a baby dies before, during, or just after delivery. The section on child-bearing loss in chapter 22, Child-bearing Loss, Infertility, and Adoption, may be helpful to women who face this rare and heartbreaking occurrence.

And worst of all, inappropriately, we blame ourselves—"My body just didn't work right"—instead of seeing clearly how the system might have undermined our knowledge and self-sufficiency. Too often we are subject to circumstances we cannot control. We always do the best we can at the time.

If you were dissatisfied with your experience, question what happened, talk about it, send for your hospital records, and check them against your memories of the event. Think about the choices you made, why you made them, and how strongly you feel about them. Your partner, a good friend, a counselor, or a women's group may help you. If you want to, write letters to those who have let you down: caregivers, facilities, or health plan administrators. The power of your words might help them become more respectful and responsive to other women.

After you explore your feelings and get your questions answered, you will then be better able to move on and to consider doing things differently next time if you plan to have more children. Sometimes it takes many years to understand fully what happened. This process of assimilation has propelled many of us into actively working to reform maternity care.

Even now, 17 years after my daughter's birth, I am still learning how dangerous the medical techniques used were for her. As for "natural" maternal feelings, *well, I just didn't have them. Move around during labor? I lay flat on my back, never dreaming another position was possible. Insist on keeping her with me after she was born? I held her for a moment, felt her breath on my hand, and let them take her away. (Though I kept repeating over and over, like a song to the white walls of the recovery room, "I have a daughter! A daughter! A daughter!" and I felt like a child at Christmas who had been given a marvelous present.) Sometimes I blame myself, but not for long. My tears still turn to anger as they have for years; both fuel my determination to help other women find alternatives to conventional obstetrical care. When I am lucky enough to be present at the births of my friends' children, the simplicity and joy of these births affirm and vindicate all of us who work toward loving and informed care for all child-bearing women.*

The second day was warm and sunny. We buried the placenta next to our house, and planted a yellow chrysanthemum over it to remind me always of the pain and joy that was Damara's birth, to remind me "Without a hurt the heart is hollow," to remind me of the oneness of life and creation (life is birth, but it is rebirth too), to remind me that for others as well, birth is one of the moments that is ours to live by, and it shouldn't be taken from anyone. In giving birth, we also give birth to ourselves.

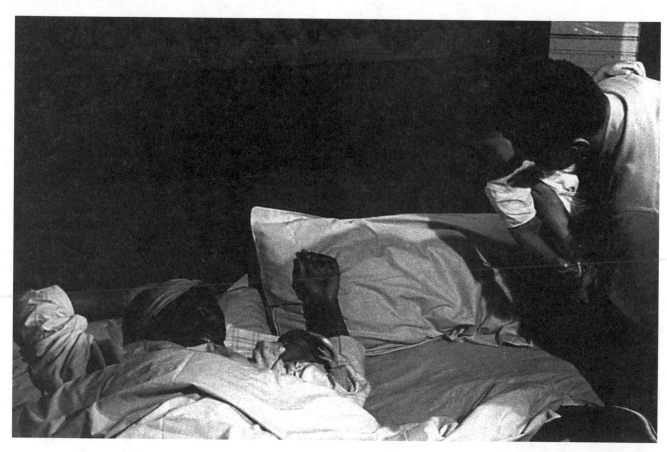

Robert Galbraith

If your childbirth experience was satisfying, empowering, and joyful, and if you were able to embrace your labor with the love and support and tender touch of others and give birth where you wanted, as you wanted, without interventions, then tell your stories to other women. Be a source of knowledge, wisdom, and support to them. Remind them that our bodies can work and we can birth well. Let them know we can shape our own birth experiences.

NOTES

1. Judith Dickson Luce, "Birthing Women and Midwife," in Helen B. Holmes, Betty Hoskins, and Michael Gross, eds., *Birth Control and Controlling Birth: Women-Centered Perspectives* (Clifton, NJ: The Humana Press, 1980), 240.

2. Dorothy Wertz, "Man-Midwifery," in *Birth Control and Controlling Birth*, 147.

3. Barbara Ehrenreich and Deirdre English, *Witches, Midwives and Nurses* (Old Westbury, NY: The Feminist Press, 1973), 41.

4. Wertz, "Man-Midwifery," 149.

5. Ehrenreich and English, *Witches, Midwives and Nurses*, 30.

6. G. J. Barker-Benfield, *The Horrors of the Half-Known Life: Male Attitudes Toward Women and Sexuality in 19th-Century America* (New York: Harper & Row, 1977).

7. Diana Scully, *Men Who Control Women's Health: The Miseducation of Obstetrician-Gynecologists* (New York: Teachers College Press, 1994). Gena Corea, *The Hidden Malpractice: How American Medicine Mistreats Women* (New York: Harper & Row, 1985).

8. Richard and Dorothy Wertz, *Lying-In: A History of Childbirth in America* (New Haven: Yale University Press, 1989), chapter 7. Neal Devitt, "Hospital Birth vs. Home Birth: The Scientific Facts, Past and Present," chapter 37 in D. Stewart and L. Stewart, eds., *Compulsory Hospitalization: Freedom of Choice in Childbirth*, vol. 2 (Marble Hill, MO: NAPSAC Publications, 1979).

9. Barker-Benfield, *The Horrors of the Half-Known Life*, 63.

10. Mary Roth Walsh, *Doctors Wanted—No Women Need Apply: Sexual Barriers in the Medical Profession 1835–1975* (New Haven: Yale University Press, 1977).

11. Wertz, "Man-Midwifery," 153.

12. Devitt, "Hospital Birth vs. Home Birth," 487–92.

13. ———, "Hospital Birth vs. Home Birth," 493–94.

14. Roslynn Lindheim, "Birthing Centers and Hospices: Reclaiming Birth and Death," *American Review of Public Health* 2 (1981): 1–29.

15. Joseph B. DeLee, "The Prophylactic Forceps Operation," *American Journal of Obstetrics and Gynecology* 1 (1920): 34–44.

16. Frederick Leboyer, *Birth Without Violence* (New York: Alfred A. Knopf, 1975), 24–26.

17. S. Jimenez, "Supportive Pain Management Strategies," in F. H. Nichols and S. S. Humenick, eds., *Childbirth Education: Practice, Research and Theory* (Philadelphia: W. B. Saunders, 1988).

18. Louise Erdrich, *The Blue Jay's Dance: A Birth Year* (New York: HarperCollins, 1995): 42.

19. M. H. Close, J. H. Kennell, et al., "Effects of Social Support During Parturition on Maternal and Infant Morbidity," *British Medical Journal* 293 (1986): 585–87. G. K. Hofmeyer et al., "Companionship to Modify the Clinical Birth Environment: Effects on Progress and Perceptions of Labour and Breastfeeding," *The British Journal of Obstetrics and Gynecology* 98, no. 8 (1991): 756–64.

20. Ina May Gaskin, "Practicing Midwifery—A Talk by Ina May Gaskin," *Childbirth Alternative Quarterly* (summer 1981): 4.

21. M. Enkin et al., *A Guide to Effective Care in Pregnancy and Childbirth* (New York: Oxford University Press, 1995): 227–28.

22. Ibid., 228–29.

23. Erdrich, op. cit., 47.

24. Enkin, op. cit., 239–40.

25. Barbara Katz Rothman, *In Labor: Women and Power in the Birthplace* (New York: Norton, 1991), 20.

26. Brigitte Jordan, "External Cephalic Version," *Women and Health* 7, nos. 3–4 (fall/winter 1982): 83–102, for a historical, cross-cultural, and physiological description of this procedure.

27. Mary Gabay and Sidney M. Wolfe, *Unnecessary Cesarean Sections: Curing a National Epidemic* (Washington, DC: Public Citizen's Health Research Group, 1994); and Henci Goer, *Obstetric Myths vs. Research Realities: A Guide to Medical Literature* (Westport, CT: Bergin & Garvey, 1995), 116–21.

28. La Leche League International, *Breastfeeding Your Premature Baby* (Shaumberg, IL: LLLI, 1990).

29. Helen Harrison, "The Principles for Family-Centered Neonatal Care," *Pediatrics* 92, no. 5 (Nov. 1993): 643–50.

30. M. Gabay and S. M. Wolfe, op. cit., 1.

31. Ibid.

32. Elizabeth L. Shearer, "Cesarean Section: Medical Benefits and Costs," *Social Science and Medicine* 37 (Nov. 10, 1993): 1223–231. Cynthia S. Mutryn, "Psychosocial Impact of Cesarean Section on the Family: A Literature Review," *Social Science and Medicine* 37 (Nov. 10, 1993): 1271–281.

33. M. Gabay and S. M. Wolfe, op. cit., vii.

34. S. J. Ventura et al. "Report of Final Natality Statistics, 1995." *Monthly Vital Statistics Report,* 45, no. 11, Supplement (Hyattsville, MD: National Center for Health Statistics, 1997).

35. Nancy Wainer Cohen and Lois Estner, *Silent Knife: Cesarean Prevention and Vaginal Birth After Cesarean* (South Hadley, MA: J. F. Bergin, 1983). B. L. Flamm, *Birth After Cesarean: The Medical Facts* (New York: Prentice-Hall, 1990). N. W. Cohen, *Open Season: A Survival Guide for Natural Childbirth and VBAC in the 90's* (New York: Bergin & Garvey, 1991). Enkin et al., *A Guide to Effective Care in Pregnancy and Childbirth,* 284–93. Henci Goer, *Obstetric Myths,* 284–93.

36. K. Kirkwood Shy et al. "Effects of Electronic Fetal-heart-rate Monitoring as Compared with Periodic Auscul-

tation on the Neurologic Development of Premature Infants" *New England Journal of Medicine* 322, no. 9 (March 1, 1990): 588–93.

37. D. Neuhoff, M. Burke, and R. Porreco, "Cesarean Birth for Failed Progress in Labor," *Obstetrics and Gynecology* 73, no. 6 (June 1989): 915–20.

38. In two articles in *Social Science and Medicine* 37, no. 10 (Nov. 1993), Carol Sakala presents overviews of the vast array of nonmedical variables that have been associated with cesareans in large multivariable studies.

39. Dr. I. Kaiser, quoted in National Institute of Child Health and Human Development et al., *Cesarean Childbirth: Report of a Consensus Development Conference* (Bethesda, MD: U.S. Department of Health and Human Services, 1982), NIH Publication No. 82-2067.

40. We want to acknowledge the contributions of April Kubachka, the present president of ICAN, and Lynn Richards to the discussion of cesareans and preventing them.

41. Edmund J. Graves and Maria F. Owings, "1995 Summary: National Hospital Discharge Summary." *Advance Data* no. 291. (Sept. 4, 1997).

42. Doris Haire, *The Cultural Warping of Childbirth* (Seattle: ICEA, 1972): 32. Available from ICEA (see Resources).

43. Enkin et al., op. cit., 204–7. R. Melzack et al., "Labor Pain, Effective Maternal Position on Front and Back Pain," *Journal of Pain Symptom Management* 6 (1991): 476–80.

44. Goer, op. cit., 239–47.

45. For critique of "Active Management of Labor" (AML), see Carol Sakala, "Medically Unnecessary Cesearean Section Births: Introduction to a Symposium," *Social Science & Medicine* 37, no. 10 (Nov. 1993): 1184–1185.

46. S. Thacker, "Lessons in Technology Diffusion: The Electronic Fetal Monitoring Experience," *Birth* 24, no. 1 (March 1997): 58–60. Goer, op. cit., 131–53.

47. Karin B. Nelson et al., "Uncertain Value of Electronic Fetal Monitoring in Predicting Cerebral Palsy," *New England Journal of Medicine* 334, no. 10 (March 7, 1996): 613–18. Dermot MacDonald, "Cerebral Palsy and Intrapartum Fetal Monitoring," *New England Journal of Medicine* 334, no. 10 (March 7, 1996): 659–60.

48. Enkin et al., op. cit., 210–16.

49. From a talk by Sheila Kitzinger, given at Boston College, Autumn 1981.

50. M. C. Klein et al., "Does Episiotomy Prevent Perineal Trauma in Pelvic Floor Relaxation?" *The Online Journal of Current Clinical Trials* 1 (July 1992), Document #10. Enkin et al., op. cit., 230–33. Goer, op. cit., 275–93.

51. R. J. Woolley, "Benefits and Risks of Episiotomy: A Review of the English Language Literature Since 1980," *Obstetrics and Gynecology Survey* 50 (1995): 806–20, 821–35.

52. S. J. Ventura, op. cit.

53. Doris Haire, "Update on Obstetric Drugs and Procedures: Their Effects on Maternal and Infant Outcome," *Birth Gazette* 13, no. 2 (1997): 33–36; and Carol Sepkowski et al., "The Effects of Maternal Epidural Anesthesia on Neonatal Behavior During the First Month," *Develop-mental Medicine and Child Neurology* 34, no. 12 (1992): 1072–89.

54. K. Dickerson, "Pharmacological Control of Pain During Labor," in Chalmers et al., eds., *Effective Care in Pregnancy and Childbirth* (two volumes) (Oxford: Oxford University Press, 1989).

55. Enkin et al., op. cit., 255–57.

56. Ibid., 257–59. Goer, op. cit., 249–73.

57. L. Fugi et al., "Maternal Pyrexia Associated with the Use of Epidural Analgesia in Labor," *Lancet* 1, no. 8649 (June 3, 1989): 1250–252.

58. Haire, 1997, op. cit., op. cit., and Goer, op. cit., 249–73.

....

RESOURCES FOR
CHAPTERS 19 AND 20

....

Each of these books contributes to an understanding of childbirth in the U.S. Many are recent; others—some of the most useful—are out of print and (we hope) available in libraries.

General Books About Child-bearing

Arms, Suzanne. *Immaculate Deception II: A Fresh Look at Childbirth*. Berkeley, CA: Celestial Arts, 1994. Update of the first and still powerful systematic exposure of the abuse of technology and intervention in normal childbirth. Angry, passionate. A beautiful tribute to midwives.

Armstrong, Penny, and Sheryl Feldman. *A Midwife's Story*. New York: Ivy Books, 1988. What a nurse-midwife learned about the beauty of birth while assisting Amish women at home.

———. *A Wise Birth: Bringing Together the Best of Natural Childbirth with Modern Medicine*. New York: William Morrow, 1990.

Barker-Benfield, G. J. *The Horrors of the Half-Known Life: Male Attitudes Toward Women and Sexuality in 19th-Century America*. New York: Harper & Row, 1976. Helps us understand the origins of current male attitudes toward women.

Cohen, Nancy Wainer. *Open Season: A Survival Guide for Natural Childbirth and VBAC in the 90s*. New York: Bergin & Garvey, 1991. Angrily, passionately criticizes an obstetrical system that does not change.

———, and Lois Estner. *Silent Knife: Cesarean Prevention and Vaginal Birth After Cesarean*. South Hadley, MA: Bergin & Garvey, 1983. How to prevent cesareans, have a vaginal birth after a cesarean, and to create positive attitudes toward child-bearing.

Davis-Floyd, Robbie. *Birth as an American Rite of Passage*. Berkeley: University of California Press, 1992. Anthropological perspective of obstetrical procedures as rituals of a technological, patriarchal society.

DeVries, Raymond G. *Making Midwives Legal: Childbirth, Medicine, and the Law,* 2nd ed. Columbus, OH: Ohio State University Press, 1996.

Edwards, Margot, and Mary Waldorf. *Reclaiming Birth:*

History and Heroines of American Childbirth Reform. Trumansburg, NY: The Crossing Press, 1984. The sole history of 20th-century women who worked for childbirth reform.

Ehrenreich, Barbara, and Deirdre English. *For Her Own Good: 150 Years of the Experts' Advice to Women.* New York: Doubleday, 1989. Indispensable classic exposes the unscientific basis of "scientific" expertise used to control women.

———. *Witches, Midwives, and Nurses.* Old Westbury, NY: The Feminist Press, 1973. How male doctors seized control of healing and birthing.

Frye, Anne. *Understanding Lab Work in the Childbearing Year,* 6th ed. New Haven, CT: Labrys Press, 1990. Available from Cascade Health Care Products, 141 Commercial NE, Salem OR 97301; (503) 371-4445. Accessible to child-bearing women and useful to midwives.

Goer, Henci. *Obstetric Myths Versus Research Realities: A Guide to the Medical Literature.* Westport, CT: Bergin & Garvey, 1995. This accessible critique of the clinical practices of modern obstetrics, and review of the scientific literature, demonstrates the lack of scientific evidence supporting these practices.

Haire, Doris. *The Cultural Warping of Childbirth.* Seattle: ICEA, 1972. Available from ICEA Bookcenter, P.O. Box 20048, Minneapolis, MN 55420. A classic pamphlet that reviews cross-cultural child-bearing practices and soundly criticizes our own.

Holmes, Helen B., Betty Hoskins, and Michael Gross, eds. *Birth Control and Controlling Birth: Women-Centered Perspectives.* Clifton, NJ: The Humana Press, 1980. Roundtable discussions of papers presented at the Ethical Issues in Human Reproduction Technology: Analysis by Women (EIRTAW) Conference, held in Amherst, MA. A classic.

Idarius, Betty. *The Homeopathic Childbirth Manual: A Practical Guide for Labor, Birth and the Immediate Postpartum Period.* Ukiah, CA: Idarius Press, 1996.

Jordan, Brigitte, revised and expanded by Robbie Davis-Floyd. *Birth in Four Cultures.* Prospect Heights, IL: Waveland Press, 1993. An anthropologist compares U.S. birth customs with those of Sweden, Holland, and the Yucatan, pointing out that those practices we label as "scientific" are actually a variety of birthing rituals.

Koehler, Nan. *Artemis Speaks: VBAC Stories and Natural Childbirth Information,* 2nd ed. Sebastopol, CA: Nan Ullrike Koehler, 1989.

Leavitt, Judith Walzer. *Brought to Bed: Childbearing in America 1750–1950.* New York: Oxford University Press, 1986. The history of childbirth in America and the intricacies of woman-physician interactions.

Logan, O., and K. Clark. *Motherwit: An Alabama Midwife's Story.* New York: E. P. Dutton, 1991. A wonderful account.

Martin, Emily. *The Woman in the Body: A Cultural Analysis of Reproduction* (new ed.). Boston: Beacon Press, 1992. Argues that medical texts depict birth through industrial production metaphors, with the uterus as the machine and the woman as laborer, under the efficient and coercive management of physicians.

Oakley, Ann. *The Captured Womb: A History of the Medical Care of Pregnant Women.* Oxford: Blackwell, 1984.

———. *Social Support and Motherhood: The Natural History of a Research Project.* Cambridge, MA: Blackwell, 1992. Raises questions about research on women, the meaning of "health," and the complex relations between social science research, academic "knowledge," and maternity care policy.

———. *Telling the Truth About Jerusalem,* New York: Basil Blackwell, 1986. Essays about pregnancy, the meaning of motherhood, and the significance of social support in pregnancy.

———. *Women Confined: Towards a Sociology of Childbirth.* New York: Schocken Books, 1980. Describes childbirth as a complex event in a woman's life; critiques the socialization of women and the medicalization of birth.

Pfeufer-Kahn, Robbie. *Bearing Meaning: The Language of Birth.* Urbana, IL: University of Illinois Press, 1995. Complex weave of sociological perspective and the author's own experience as a mother.

Rich, Adrienne. *Of Woman Born: Motherhood as Experience and Institution.* New York: W. W. Norton, 1976, 1995, 1996. Motherhood from a feminist viewpoint.

Rothenberg, Karen H., and Elizabeth J. Thomson, eds. *Women and Prenatal Testing: Facing the Challenges of Genetic Technology.* Columbus, OH: Ohio State University Press, 1994.

Rothman, Barbara Katz. *Encyclopedia of Childbearing: Critical Perspectives.* Phoenix, AZ: Oryx Press, 1993.

———. *In Labor: Women and Power in the Birthplace,* 2nd ed. New York: W. W. Norton, 1991. Compares the medical and midwifery models of birth.

———. *Re-creating Motherhood: Ideology and Technology in a Patriarchal Society.* New York: W. W. Norton, 1989. A discussion of the impingements on women's procreative lives.

———. *The Tentative Pregnancy: How Amniocentesis Changes the Experience of Motherhood.* New York: W. W. Norton, 1993.

Sagov, Stanley, et al. *Home Birth: A Practitioner's Guide to Birth Outside the Hospital,* Rockville, MD: Aspen Systems Corporation, 1984. Immensely useful.

Scully, Diana. *Men Who Control Women's Health: The Miseducation of Obstetrician-Gynecologists.* New York: Teachers College Press, 1994. Behind-the-scenes study of obstetrical training. Includes analyses of gynecology texts, observations of operating rooms and teaching hospital clinics, and interviews with medical students.

Smith, Margaret Charles, and Linda Janet Holmes. *Listen to Me Good: The Life Story of an Alabama Midwife.* Columbus, OH: Ohio State University Press, 1996. Highly recommended.

Tew, Marjorie. *Safer Childbirth? A Critical History of Maternity Care.* London: Chapman & Hall, 1990. Contains statistical, biological, and observational evidence that obstetrical care has made a negative contribution to safer childbirth. It concludes that safety in childbirth depends primarily upon women's good health.

Wertz, Richard, and Dorothy Wertz. *Lying-In: A History of Childbirth in America,* rev. ed. New Haven: Yale University Press, 1989. The most complete social, legal, and cultural history of childbirth in the U.S. up to and through the 1980s.

Planning for Pregnancy and Childbirth

Ashford, Janet Isaacs, ed. *The Whole Birth Catalog.* Trumansburg, NY: The Crossing Press, 1983. Fun to read. Gives an idea of women's child-bearing culture.

Balaskas, Janet. *Active Birth: The New Approach to Giving Birth Naturally.* Boston: Harvard Common Press, 1992.

———. *Natural Pregnancy.* New York: Interlink, 1990. Excellent resource for wellness and dealing with the discomforts of pregnancy.

Baldwin, Rahima. *Special Delivery: The Complete Guide to Informed Birth,* rev. ed. Berkeley, CA: Celestial Arts, 1986. Positive. Especially useful if you are planning a home birth.

Davis, Elizabeth. *Heart and Hands: A Midwife's Guide to Pregnancy and Birth,* rev. ed. Berkeley, CA: Celestial Arts, 1987. About setting up a midwifery practice. Pregnancy, labor, and birth from a midwife's point of view. Strong on the emotional aspects of child-bearing.

Dick-Read, Grantly. *Childbirth Without Fear,* rev. ed. New York: Harper & Row, 1994. The first book to speak of "natural childbirth." Stresses education and relaxation, and discusses the fear-tension-pain syndrome.

Gaskin, Ina May. *Spiritual Midwifery,* 3rd ed. Summertown, TN: The Book Publishing Co., 1990. Upbeat stories about childbirth from The Farm's midwifery service, followed by practical midwifery information.

Harper, Barbara, *Gentle Birth Choices: A Guide to Making Informed Decisions.* Rochester, VT: Healing Arts Press, 1994. Emphasizes the history and merits of waterbirth.

Hazell, Lester. *Commonsense Childbirth.* New York: G. P. Putnam, 1969. Conveys what it feels like to lose a child, critiques childbirth problems caused by the medical profession, and encourages home birth.

Kitzinger, Sheila. *The Experience of Childbirth.* New York: Viking Penguin, 1990. Psychological and physical aspects of child-bearing discussed in an informative, empathetic, broadminded manner.

Klaus, M., P. Klaus, and J. Kennell. *Mothering the Mother: How a Doula Can Help You Have a Shorter, Easier, and Healthier Birth.* Reading, MA: Addison-Wesley, 1993.

Lang, Raven. *Birth Book.* Palo Alto, CA: Genesis Press, 1972. Moving personal descriptions of birth by mothers and fathers. Vivid photographs.

Lichy, Roger, Eileen Herzberg. *The Waterbirth Handbook: The Gentle Art of Waterbirthing.* Lower Lake, CA: Atrium Publishers Group, 1993.

Limburg, Astrid, and Beatrijs Smulders. *Women Giving Birth.* Berkeley, CA: Celestial Arts, 1992. Written by Dutch midwives; warm photos of women giving birth at home and in hospitals. Interviews with mothers. Strong home birth emphasis.

McCutcheon, Susan. *Natural Childbirth the Bradley Way,* rev. ed. New York: Penguin, 1996.

Odent, Michel. *Birth Reborn,* "unrevised and unenlarged." Medford, NJ: Birth Works Press, 1994. Dr. Odent describes the evolution, practices, and philosophy of his maternity clinic in Pithiviers, France, a gentle, calm birth environment. Useful guide for practitioners trying to "demedicalize" their point of view.

Simkin, Penny. *The Birth Partner: Everything You Need to Know to Help a Woman Through Childbirth.* Boston: Harvard Common Press, 1989. Helpful for partners and other significant others who want to be involved and supportive during birth.

Preparing for Breast-feeding

Huggins, Kathleen. *The Nursing Mother's Companion.* Boston: The Harvard Common Press, 1990.

Kitzinger, Sheila. *Breastfeeding Your Baby.* New York: Alfred A. Knopf, 1989.

Articles, Booklets, and Technical Reports

Carty, E., et al., "Comprehensive Health Promotion for the Pregnant Woman Who Is Disabled," *Journal of Nurse-Midwifery* 35, no. 3 (1990): 133–42.

———, "Guidelines for Serving Disabled Women," *Midwifery Today* 27 (1993): 29–37.

Grant, A., et al. "Cerebral Palsy Among Children Born During the Dublin Randomised Trial of Intrapartum Monitoring." *The Lancet* (Nov. 25, 1989): 8674–880. Intensive internal electronic fetal monitoring during labor does not protect against cerebral palsy (all hospital births).

Mansfield, Phyllis Kernoff, "Re-evaluating the Medical Risks of Late Childbearing." *Women and Health* 11, no. 2 (summer 1986): 37–60. A critical review of the scientific literature relating to pregnancy and advanced maternal age suggests that delayed pregnancies do not pose a high risk for otherwise healthy women, and that it is the medical mismanagement of older women that creates problems, not maternal age.

———, and William McCool, "Toward a Better Understanding of the 'Advanced Maternal Age Factor.' " *Health Care for Women International* 10, no. 4 (1989): 395–415.

Mason, Jutta. "The Meaning of Birth Stories." *The Birth Gazette* 3, no. 3 (summer 1990): 14–19. How women's stories about birth surface when women give birth as they prefer, and disappear when obstetrical control intensifies.

Maternal and Newborn Health/Safe Motherhood Unit. *Care In Normal Birth: A Practical Guide, Report of a Technical Working Group.* Geneva: World Health Organization, 1996.

Pincus, Jane. "Advice Books for Childbearing Women: Choice or Coercion?" Available from the author at P.O. Box 72, Roxbury, VT 05669. A critical examination of ten modern childbirth books.

Sakala, Carol, "Midwifery Care and Out-of-Hospital Birth Settings: How Do They Reduce Unnecessary Cesarean Section Births?" *Social Science and Medicine* 37, no. 10 (1993): 1233–250.

Women's Institute for Childbearing Policy. "Childbearing Policy within a National Health Program: An Evolving

Consensus for New Directions," 1994. A collaborative paper, coordinated by Carol Sakala, of WICP, the National Women's Health Network, the National Black Women's Health Project, and the Boston Women's Health Book Collective. Available for $5 from Jane Pincus, Box 72, Roxbury, VT 05669. Calls for an approach to maternity care policy that combines women's health and public health perspectives and promotes midwives as the appropriate caregivers for child-bearing women.

Periodicals

The Birth Gazette
42, The Farm; Summertown, TN 38483

Birth: Issues in Perinatal Care and Education
Blackwell Scientific Publications; Three Cambridge Center, Suite 208; Cambridge, MA 02142

Journal of Nurse-Midwifery
Elsevier Science Publishing Co., Inc.; 655 Avenue of the Americas; New York, NY 10010

The Midwife Advocate
c/o MFOM
P.O. Box 3188; Boston, MA 02130

Midwifery Today
Box 2672-4; Eugene, OR 97402; (800) 743-0974

Mothering
P.O. Box 1690; Santa Fe, NM 87504; (505) 984-8116

Women and Health
The Haworth Press; 72 Griswold Street; Binghamton, NY 13904-1580

Catalogs

Send away for these five catalogs, and you will get an idea of just how many pamphlets, books, educational materials, and videos are out there!

Birth and Life Bookstore
(Now combined with Cascade, listed below)

Cascade Health Care Supplies
141 Commercial NE; P.O. Box 12203; Salem, OR 97301; (503) 371-4445
 Offers instruments and equipment for midwives as well as items and books for mothers and babies.

Childbirth in History
Janet Isaacs Ashford
327 North Glenmont Drive; Solana Beach, CA 92075
 Booklets and scripted slide shows with images and information concerning birth, midwifery, positions for labor, etc.

Informed Homebirth/Informed Birth and Parenting
P.O. Box 3675; Ann Arbor, MI 48106

ICEA Bookmarks
ICEA Bookcenter; P.O. Box 20048; Minneapolis, MN 55420; (800) 624-4934; Fax: (612) 854-8772

Organizations Concerned with Childbirth Education

American College of Nurse-Midwives (ACNM)
818 Connecticut Avenue NW, Suite 900; Washington, DC 20006; (202) 728-9860
Web site: http://www.midwife.org
 ACNM, founded in 1955, is the professional organization for nurse-midwives in the U.S. It administers national certification examinations, accredits nurse-midwifery educational programs, provides membership services, produces publications for its members and the public, and holds an annual convention.

American Foundation for Maternal and Child Health, Inc.
30 Beekman Place; New York, NY 10022; (212) 759-5510
 Provides scientific information to the public on obstetrical procedures and drugs that are potentially harmful to women, fetuses, infants, or children later in life.

Association of Labor Assistants and Childbirth Educators (ALACE)
P.O. Box 382-724; Cambridge, MA 02238; (617) 441-2500
Web site: http://www.alace.org

Birthworks
42 Tallwood Drive; Medford, NJ 08255; (609) 953-9380
 Offers childbirth education and national certification for childbirth educators.

Cesareans/Support, Education and Concern (C/SEC)
22 Forest Road; Framingham, MA 01701; (508) 877-8266
 Serves parents and professionals who want information and support in relation to cesarean childbirth, cesarean prevention, and VBACs.

Coalition for Improving Maternity Services (CIMS)
c/o Lamaze International (see below)
 A coalition of individuals and organizations that focuses on prevention and wellness as alternatives to high-cost screening, diagnosis, and treatment. It has produced an important consensus document, *The Mother Friendly Childbirth Initiative.*

Doulas of North America (DONA)
1100 23rd Avenue E; Seattle, WA 98112; (206) 324-5440
Web site: http://www.dona.com

Global Maternal/Child Health Association (GMHCA) and Waterbirth International
P.O. Box 366; West Linn, OR 97068; (800) 641-BABY or (503) 682-3600
 A membership organization. Provides the most complete resources for waterbirth.

Informed Homebirth, Inc.
P.O. Box 3675; Ann Arbor, MI 48106; (313) 662-6857
Founded by Rahima Baldwin, this organization offers classes to prepare parents for home birth, prepares certification for childbirth assistants and childbirth educators, and provides tapes for people planning a home birth. Sells books and videos.

International Association of Parents and Professionals for Safe Alternatives in Childbirth (NAPSAC)
Route 1, Box 646; Marble Hill, MO 63764; (573) 238-2010
Childbirth education that is openly antiabortion.

International Cesarean Awareness Network—ICAN (formerly Cesarean Prevention Movement)
1304 Kingsdale Avenue; Redondo Beach, CA 90278; (310) 542-6400; Fax: (310) 542-5368
Web site: http://www.childbirth.org/section/ICAN.html
Offers information and support for cesarean prevention and vaginal birth after cesarean (VBACs), as well as a feisty newsletter, *The Clarion;* conferences; and national training for childbirth educators.

International Childbirth Education Association (ICEA)
P.O. Box 20048; Minneapolis, MN 55240-0048; (612) 854-8660
Web site: http://www.icea.org
An interdisciplinary organization, founded in 1960, with regional chapters, that represents a federation of groups and individuals, both parents and professionals, who share an interest in childbirth education and family-centered maternity care. Has a training and certification program for doulas.

International Lactation Consultant Association (ILCA)
210 Brown Avenue; Evanston, IL 60202-3601; (708) 260-8874
Web site: http://www.erols.com/ilca
ILCA provides support and up-to-date material about breast-feeding.

La Leche League International, Inc. (LLLI)
9616 Minneapolis Avenue; Franklin Park, IL 60131; Hot line: (800) La Leche
Web site: http://www.lalecheleague.org
La Leche provides all kinds of information and support about breast-feeding. There are chapters in many cities.

Lamaze International
1200 19th Street NW, S-300; Washington, DC 20036; (800) 368-4404
Web site: http://www.lamaze-childbirth.com
Introduced Lamaze in the U.S., and offers classes and certification for childbirth educators.

Maternity Center Association
281 Park Avenue South; New York, NY 10128; (212) 777-5000
Founded in 1918, MCA began training public health nurses in midwifery in 1931. It established the MCA Childbearing Center in New York City in 1975, the coun-

try's first freestanding birth center. This organization offers excellent publications and conducts classes, conferences, and seminars.

Midwives Alliance of North America (MANA)
P.O. Box 175; Newton, KS 67114; (316) 283-4543
Web site: http://www.mana.org
Represents professional midwives on a regional, national, and international basis; promotes guidelines for midwifery education and training for basic competency of practicing midwives; promotes research as well as cooperation between midwives and other groups concerned with the health of women and their families. MANA encompasses both direct-entry community midwives as well as certified nurse-midwives.

Midwives Information and Resource Services (MIDIRS)
Institute of Child Health; Royal Hospital for Sick Children; St. Michael's Hill; Bristol, BS2 8BJ, U.K.; 011-44-272-251-791

National Association of Childbearing Centers (NACC)
3123 Gottschall Road; Perkiomenville, PA 18074; (215) 234-8068
Dedicated to developing closer ties within the rapidly growing national childbirth center movement and to promoting an understanding of the birth center concept.

National Association for Postpartum Care
P.O. Box 1012; Edmonds, WA 98020
Web site: http://orion.webspan.net/~callahan/napcsz. html

Traditional Midwife Center International
c/o Linda Holmes
64 Cambridge Street; East Orange, NJ 07018
A networking organization for individuals interested in collecting and preserving documents and artifacts pertaining to the practices of traditional southern granny midwives of African descent.

Cochrane Collaboration Child-bearing Resources

(See "Evidence-Based Practice . . . ," chapter 25, The Politics of Women's Health and Medical Care, p. 710, for background on the Cochrane Collaboration and for ordering information for *The Cochrane Library,* which contains the most recent version of Cochrane systematic reviews on the effectiveness of many obstetrical practices.)
Cochrane Pregnancy and Childbirth Group
Contact: Mrs. Sonja Henderson, Coordinator
Cochrane Pregnancy and Childbirth Group
Liverpool Women's Hospital NHS Trust
Crown Street Liverpool, U.K. L8 7SS
Web site: http://hiru.hirunet.mcmaster.ca/hirexd/hirexs. exe?JUMP=1765@cochrane
This is the administrative office for the Cochrane group that prepares systematic reviews of "randomized controlled trials of interventions involving the mother or

baby during and after pregnancy and childbirth (including lactation)."

Enkin, Murray W., et al. "Effective Care in Pregnancy and Childbirth: A Synopsis." *Birth: Issues in Perinatal Care* 22, no. 2 (June 1995): 101–10. Concise summary of Cochrane Pregnancy and Childbirth Database (CCPC) findings about the effectiveness of obstetrical practices.

Enkin, Murray, et al. *A Guide to Effective Care in Pregnancy and Childbirth,* 2nd ed. Oxford: Oxford University Press, 1995. Accessible overview of findings from the extensive Cochrane Pregnancy and Childbirth Database.

Sakala, Carol. "The Cochrane Pregnancy and Childbirth Database: Implications for Perinatal Care Policy and Practice in the United States." *Evaluation and the Health Professions* 18, no. 4 (1995): 428–66.

Additional Online Resources *

Childbirth.org
http://www.childbirth.org

The Homebirth Choice
http://www.efn.org/~djz/birth/homebirth.html

Lesbian Mothers Support Society
http://shell6.ba.best.com/~agoodloe/lesbian-moms

Midwifery, Pregnancy, Birth, Childbirth, Breast-feeding
http://www.efn.org/~djz/birth/birthindex.html

The Motherstuff Pages
http://www.teramonger.com/dwan/mother.htm

Pregnancy & Child Health Resource Centers
http://www.mayo.ivi.com/mayo/common/htm/pregpg.htm

WWW Pregnancy Ring
http://www.fensende.com/Users/swnymph/Ring.html

* For more information and listings of online resources, please see Introduction to Online Women's Health Resources, p. 25.

By Alice LoCicero and Deborah
Issokson, based on earlier work by
Dennie Wolf and Mary Crowe

With special thanks to Laurie Williams,
Helen Armstrong, Jane Honikman, Gail Levy,
Veronica Miletsky, Carol Sakala, and
Dianne Weiss *

BECOMING A MOTHER

The months after having a baby are a mix, a real mix. Some days you love it. Imagine having the chance and time to roll on the bed and drink in the smell of a baby and find the tiny daily changes in a body your body made. Other days you're on a bus with a wet baby and a stroller that's rolling down the aisle. You look at the neat, childless people in the other seats and you feel messy, clumsy, alone, and in the way. I remember Mondays when I could barely shuffle between my part-time job and the sitter's, with the baby wailing in the car seat. Then Wednesday would roll around, she'd wake up laughing with her arms out, we'd sail through the morning, and I'd come to work thinking, This isn't easy. But, God, does it matter!

* Thanks also to the following for their help with the 1998 version of this chapter: Betsy Bard, Kathy Behan, Ricky Carter, Joanne Chadwick, Karen Greene, Donal Grelotti, Pat Guthy, Ellen Lehn, Mirza Lugardo, Andrea Seek, and Lucie Viakinnou-Brinson. Over the years since 1969, the following women have contributed to the many versions of this chapter: Paula Doress-Worters, Esther Rome, Vilunya Diskin, Marty Reudi, and Robbie Pfeufer Kahn.

Celebration and change surround the birth of a baby. But the new life isn't just the baby's—it's yours, too. Being a mother can bring deep pleasure, intimacy, growth, and insight. Birth and nursing give us a new respect for our bodies. Caring for, playing with, and cuddling children, we discover new dimensions to loving.

I've never been as happy. I just seem calmer. I'm the same person. I've always been a worrier. I guess I worry about the same things that I've always worried about. But all those worries seem less important, because in the center of me, there's always Sam. And he's what's most important.

At the same time, all new mothers experience some degree of difficulty in the transition to parenthood. Many of us ignore our own physical and mental health and bury our needs for adult company, nurturance, and sexuality. Many women are under the chronic stress that comes from balancing the roles of mother, worker, and lover—even those of us who have the

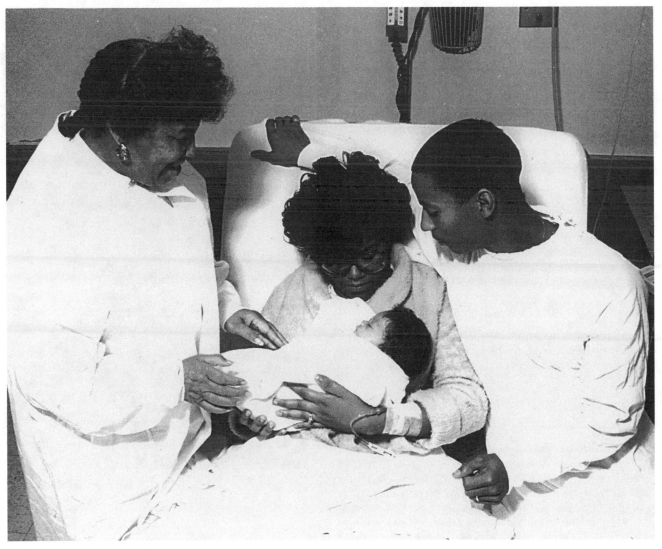

Robert Houston

protection of enough income, help, and closeness with friends or lovers. Added strain can come from being a young mother, having a low income or being homeless, having a physical or mental illness or disability, living in or trying to leave an abusive relationship, being isolated from family and friends, or having a baby who is ill.

Some of us worry about maintaining a home and providing our children with food and basic medical care. Many of us wake up, as never before, to the politics of being women and caregivers. As we move between our homes and workplaces, our own lives teach us about the changes in housing, health care, wages, and work structures that families need. The time we spend caring for our own babies makes us more concerned about all the world's children. The struggle against sexism, racism, violence, and global conflict takes on a new urgency.

THE POSTPARTUM EXPERIENCE

In this chapter we will discuss the postpartum period, which lasts about a year from the time of birth. We will describe the emotional and physical changes that occur after giving birth. We will consider what it means to become a mother, to adjust to life with a baby, and to face longer-term issues. The powerful feelings and experiences are not confined to this year alone. Whether you are a first-time mother or have had previous births, this is the beginning of a journey into a new phase of life.* We present the stories, wisdom, and strategies of many new mothers: women who had difficult and easy postpartum experiences, women who became mothers alone or with partners,

* In this chapter, we focus on the experience of birth mothers who are raising their children. We do not focus on adoptive mothers' or stepmothers' transition to motherhood. Some experiences of adoptive mothers and stepmothers are likely to be similar to those we describe; others may differ.

women with male and female partners, first- and many-time mothers, mothers who worked at home and mothers who chose or had to begin or continue outside work. When we move into the first year of motherhood prepared and aware, we can wrestle with the issues and take hold of the possibilities.

Immediate Postpartum Time

During the first few postpartum days, we make the transition from pregnancy to motherhood. This is a time of enormous change; physically, our bodies are recovering from birth. Emotionally, we may experience everything from exhilaration to exhaustion, uncertainty, and sadness. Many factors affect how we feel: our financial resources, our health, our readiness to become mothers, and the amount and kind of support we receive from partners, families, and friends.

Feelings About the Birth

If the birth has gone well and the baby is healthy, you may feel incredibly high, tremendously relieved, and proud of what you have just accomplished.

Even though I'd had a long and difficult labor, I felt ecstatic after the baby was born. I wanted to leap out of bed and run around the room to celebrate. Then, after a couple of hours, fatigue caught up with me and I began to feel utterly exhausted. Every muscle and bone ached. Still, I didn't mind somehow. It was a good kind of tiredness—the kind that comes when you've been pushed to the limits of your capabilities. Along with the weariness came new, quieter feelings of peace, happiness, tenderness for my baby, and a connection to all womankind!

But you may have other feelings, too, especially if the birth did not live up to your expectations or if you encountered unexpected interventions or complications.

We had planned a birth with no intervention, and I had an emergency cesarean instead. Even though I was relieved that everything was okay and thrilled with my baby, I had the nagging sense that I had failed somehow. Later I got over feeling that it was my fault, but I still felt cheated out of the birth experience we had hoped and planned for. Sometimes I still can't help feeling a little jealous when I hear women talk about their wonderful birth experiences.

In the days following delivery, you may think about the birth a lot, want to talk about it in detail, and try to resolve your feelings about it. You may relive it over and over, perhaps fantasizing different outcomes for parts you feel ambivalent about.

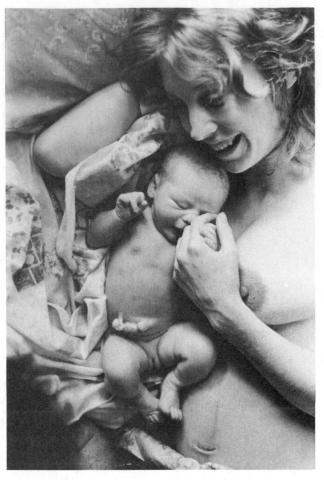

Jim Harrison/Stock, Boston

The Baby Blues

Within a few days after birth, you may experience the baby blues. This is very common: up to 80%[1] of new mothers report experiencing sadness, weepiness, moodiness, anxiety, tearfulness, tiredness, and fuzzy thinking. These feelings generally start on the third to fifth day after you give birth, and they resolve on their own a few days later. Although you may feel awful, generally a little support or nurturing, or a nap, can help you feel better. Talking with other mothers about fears and anxieties can help you feel less alone.

I was so emotional that I could hardly watch TV. I was set off immediately by anything the least bit sentimental, like stories about children or animals or even the news, especially if there were any problems that concerned a child. When my son was only days old, I watched a made-for-TV movie about babies who were switched at birth. I was weeping through the whole thing. I was so vulnerable to those feelings— like, Is this baby really mine? If my husband came home from work and didn't pay attention to me right away, I would cry. A friend told me that after you have a baby, you wear your heart on the outside, and it's so true.

Almost everyone has these feelings to some extent; postpartum blues often appear just as your milk comes in. Hormonal changes may be at least partly responsible for sudden shifts in mood, and depression can be heightened by being physically run down, anemic, or exhausted from being awakened repeatedly at night or by being alone or lacking support.

When depression lasts more than a few days, it is usually caused by a combination of social and physical factors. If you find that you don't feel better and in fact begin to feel worse, if others are concerned about you, or if you have more serious difficulties, you may be experiencing the beginning of something more severe than the blues. You need and deserve help in sorting out what's happening to you and to get treatment if needed. (See "Serious Postpartum Difficulties: When You Need Help," p. 514.)

Physical Changes After Birth: Taking Care of Ourselves

For me, physical recovery was no big deal. Because I had an easy birth and no episiotomy, I healed very fast and felt back to normal within a few days. The only thing that bothered me was sore nipples (for the first couple of days) and night sweats, which lasted about a week. Otherwise I felt terrific. Maybe I was just high from the birth, but I seemed to have a lot more energy then than I do now, several months later.

For at least two weeks after the birth I was very uncomfortable. In addition to feeling the episiotomy stitches, my whole pelvic area ached, and it hurt to stand for more than a few minutes. I couldn't sit for a week! Even after I got home, I found I couldn't do anything. I hated the feeling of being helpless. Because I was in so much pain, I was very touchy and found it hard to respond to my husband or to the visitors who came to see me and the baby.

Our bodies undergo enormous changes after birth —a pregnancy in reverse. Your uterus will become firm, contracting often and reducing in size so that by the tenth day after delivery you will no longer be able to feel it above the pubic bone. Breast-feeding your baby speeds up this process by releasing the hormones you need to trigger uterine contractions and keep them going. These contractions of the uterus are often strong, especially following a second or subsequent child. They may startle you, but they will ease within a few days. Drinking raspberry tea and resting with a heating pad on your belly may help.

As the uterine tissue breaks down it is expelled in a discharge called lochia, similar to a heavy menstrual flow, which usually lasts two to four weeks after birth. If bleeding is unusually heavy or suddenly resumes after this time, or if the lochia smells bad (a sign of infection), talk with your doctor or midwife. The immediate postpartum period is a time when infection can occur easily. Be on the lookout for signs—

excessive bleeding, fever—that something might be wrong.

Many women find that after delivery, their pelvic floor and abdominal walls are very slack. Perineal (Kegel) exercises (see chapter 12, Understanding Our Bodies, p. 274) immediately after birth, followed by gentle abdominal exercises and leg lifts, will help restore your muscle tone.

It may take a while for your bowels to resume regular functioning. Drinking a lot of liquids keeps bowel movements soft and helps prevent urinary tract infections as well. Eat bran and stewed prunes. Relax and let your body take over. As long as you don't strain, you won't dislodge your recovering organs (a common fear), tear your stitches, or aggravate hemorrhoids (varicose veins of the anus), which sometimes appear during pregnancy or labor. If you have hemorrhoids, wipe with toilet paper soaked in water or witch hazel after each bowel movement, and take frequent sitz baths (one and a half inches of warm water with a strong brew of comfrey tea) to promote healing.

During the first 24 hours after delivery, apply ice packs to your genital area (perineum, labia, anus) to reduce swelling. After 24 hours, try warm sitz baths (see above). We have heard many other recommendations for perineal care, including direct applications of witch hazel or a comfrey poultice to the perineum. Many women find these helpful for pain relief. However, there has not been sufficient research to determine the effectiveness of any of these applications. Your practitioner may recommend herbs, homeopathic remedies, or over-the-counter oral pain relievers. Make sure to tell your practitioner if you are breast-feeding, since everything you eat or drink is likely to reach your baby through the breast milk.

In another dramatic change, your blood volume is reduced by 30% during the first two weeks postpartum. Under any other conditions, this loss would be felt as exhaustion, but many women are exhilarated instead. If you feel very tired or weak, you may be anemic. Be sure to eat enough iron-rich foods (see nutrition chart, chapter 2, Food, p. 54). Check with your health care provider about the need for iron and vitamin supplements.

As your tissues rid themselves of excess fluids stored up during pregnancy, you may drink, urinate, and perspire more than usual. The sudden loss of estrogen can also cause night sweats, which may last for several weeks after birth. (These are similar to the night sweats of menopause.) Some women also experience "hot flashes" during nursing as their milk lets down.

For the first day or two of nursing, the baby is receiving colostrum, a pre-milk substance rich in antibodies. Some women experience a painful swelling in their breasts (engorgement) when the milk comes in. This can be quickly relieved, and you will not need to stop nursing. (See "Breast-feeding Your Baby," p. 507.)

If you are not going to breast-feed, you may be offered a drug to suppress your milk supply. We recommend that you refuse it. In the past, hospitals assumed that most women were not going to breast-feed, and they routinely gave new mothers shots of DES or androgen to suppress their milk supply. Those hormones were replaced by a drug called bromocriptine. Later, that too was found to be unsafe as a milk suppressant; in addition, women sometimes began to lactate again when they stopped taking it. There are safer alternative methods of suppressing your milk. Some practitioners recommend binding your breasts* or wearing tight clothing. Sage tea has been recommended as an herbal remedy.† You might try ice packs to relieve the pain which may occur when your milk comes in. Full relief with these methods may take two to three weeks.

After a vaginal delivery you will probably be out of bed within a few hours. Getting on your feet soon after birth means fewer bladder and bowel problems and a quicker recovery of energy. This doesn't mean, however, that you should resume normal activities right away. It is very important to take care of yourself during these early days after birth. Strenuous activity too soon can prolong the healing process and leave you feeling exhausted a week or two later. Even when you are feeling terrific, let other people take care of household chores and your other children. Keep visitors to a minimum. If you are alone at home, ask friends, relatives, or neighbors to run errands and bring in meals. Your hospital or insurance carrier may provide homemaker services or social services. For at least six weeks, you should set aside extra time for rest and exercise.

Our friends set up a great system. Each night for the first week they would bring over a pot of something to eat. But they liked to stay and eat with us. We had to be their hosts! Finally, we asked them just to bring the food and let us eat by ourselves. We were too tired for company.

Recovery After a Cesarean Birth

If you had a cesarean birth, the most important thing to note is that it is major abdominal surgery. You may feel sick and weak, as well as very sore around the incision. It may be very difficult to change positions and to get in and out of bed. Be sure to ask the nurses or midwives for helpful hints. You will probably have an intravenous feeding tube (IV) and a catheter (to drain the bladder) for 24 to 48 hours. The catheter may feel very uncomfortable; ask if it can be removed earlier. Also ask that the IV be placed so that it doesn't interfere with nursing the baby (see p. 508). If you had general anesthesia during the operation, your lungs will have accumulated fluid that must be coughed up. The "hut" or "chest" breathing exercises

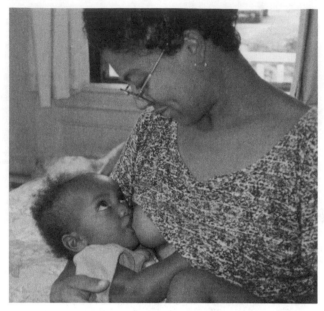

Judy Norsigian

you may have learned in childbirth classes can help you to do this without too much discomfort. The anesthesia you received temporarily interrupted your bowels. You may have gas pains or a constipated feeling as they begin to work again. You will not be able to eat solids until your bowels are working normally.

After a cesarean, you will be on your feet within a day. Walking may be painful, but it helps you to get your digestive system going and avoid blood clots in your legs (thrombosis). Within a few days you can begin exercises‡ that speed healing and restore muscle tone, but you should avoid heavy lifting and strenuous exercise for at least six weeks.

It is important that you feel cared for during your hospital stay, which may be for several days. Ask for whatever makes you feel better, whether it's frequent visits from your family and friends, food from home, or a massage when you're feeling tired and sore. Some hospitals allow partners to stay overnight (you may have to provide your own sleeping bag on the floor).

On the second day, I insisted on getting up and taking a shower. Washing my hair was a big step toward recuperation. It made me feel that I was taking charge of my body again. Exercising helped too—I started stretching my legs and doing ankle rotations immediately.

Hospitals often encourage a woman to stay several days following a cesarean. If you are feeling well enough and will have adequate help at home, you may choose to shorten your hospital stay. You can return as an outpatient to have your stitches removed.

---

* *A Guide to Effective Care in Pregnancy & Childbirth* (Enkin et al., 1995) notes that "there may be short-term disadvantages, but no long-term benefits, of nonpharmacological approaches to suppress lactation" (p. 372).
† See S. Weed's *Herbal for the Childbearing Year* in Resources.

‡ See E. Noble, *Essential Exercises for the Childbearing Years,* in Resources.

BREAST-FEEDING YOUR BABY

Breast milk is the best food for babies. It provides exactly the right balance of nutrients, adapting to your baby's changing requirements. Breast milk helps strengthen the infant's resistance to infection and disease—something no formula can do. Colostrum, the liquid in a mother's breasts before the milk actually comes in, is especially high in antibodies that protect the newborn against staphylococcus infections, polio virus, coxsackie B virus, infant diarrhea, and *Escherichia coli* infections, the very germs to which infants are usually most susceptible. Breast-feeding gives our babies a natural immunity to almost all common childhood diseases for at least six months and often until we stop breast-feeding completely.* In addition, babies who can tolerate no other food digest breast milk easily. The length of breast-feeding varies around the world and is determined by many factors, including cultural norms.

In general, breast-fed babies have fewer problems with allergies, constipation, indigestion, skin disorders, and future tooth decay than bottle-fed babies. Breast-feeding is even thought to encourage better development of the dental arch, preventing the need for orthodonture later on.[2] For all these reasons, the American Academy of Pediatrics officially endorses breast-feeding as the preferred way of feeding babies.†

There are other advantages to breast-feeding. Breast milk is economical. The milk supply adjusts to the baby's needs; the more the baby nurses, the more milk the breasts produce. As the baby weans, the breast milk supply tapers off.

Breast-feeding is an easy and convenient way to feed your baby. It is always available at the right temperature, and there are no bottles to carry around. (Formula must be prepared for each feeding in sterilized bottles or costly disposable bottle-bags.) If you are in the process of another life transition or have particular stresses, getting used to breast-feeding will be much easier than struggling with formula in new, unfamiliar, and sometimes inconvenient surroundings. Breast-feeding can provide you and your baby with relaxing and intimate moments together as you both go through these transitions.

Women who breast-feed tend to get back into shape earlier than those who don't. Beginning right after birth, breast-feeding helps your body expel excess fluids and tissue. Because the body burns about 1,000 calories a day to produce breast milk, nursing mothers tend to lose weight gained during pregnancy gradually during the first few months postpartum.

Breast-feeding can be relaxing, sensual, close, and satisfying. Some women become sexually aroused and even have orgasms while breast-feeding. This is because oxytocin, the hormone that triggers orgasm (and labor), is also responsible for the letdown of milk when stimulated by the baby's suckling. The breast-feeding mother and her baby have an intimate and interdependent relationship; many women feel extraordinarily close to their babies while nursing.

Not all women find breast-feeding instinctive and effortless.‡ New mothers are often denied the opportunity to learn by observing experienced nursing mothers because breast-feeding is often considered private. Some women find the first three weeks of breast-feeding challenging and frustrating. The postpartum hospital nurses, midwives, lactation consultants, La Leche League (see Resources), and other nursing mothers are excellent resources for help. If you don't feel comfortable with the advice you get from one of these sources, seek help from another. Getting advice and help early may lead to a more pleasurable nursing experience. While there are special nursing bras and clothing adapted for nursing, you may prefer to creatively adapt your own clothing in order to nurse comfortably.

Many myths attempt to discourage women from breast-feeding. As a result, women who choose to breast-feed may have trouble finding information and support for their decision, or may be pressured by family or doctors into stopping later on because they think that the baby isn't getting "enough" milk. If you are planning to breast-feed, make that clear to hospital nurses so they don't give the baby bottles. (If you're not sure whether you want to breast-feed, why not give it a try?) We may hear that nursing "spoils our figures" or ties us down so that we can't resume work or other activities. We may feel embarrassed or uncomfortable about using our breasts to feed our babies because society tells us (in subtle and not so subtle ways) that breasts are sex symbols and bodies are sex objects. In addition, formula manufacturers, the advertising industry, and hospitals continue to promote formula, even though research shows that breast milk is the best food for infants.

Some women choose formula so that other people can feed their babies. Occasionally, women who want to breast-feed have severe difficulties that lead them to switch to partial or complete bottle feeding at some point. If you decide to bottle feed, be assured that you can

continued on next page

still have a close relationship with your baby. Whether you feed babies by breast or bottle, they like to be held close and cuddled during feedings. This physical closeness is important to the baby's emotional health, for it satisfies her or his need for touching and sucking, which is especially strong in the early months.

Breast-feeding Under Special Circumstances

Women who have had cesarean births can also breast-feed their babies. It may be a little more difficult to get started if the mother is uncomfortable after surgery and/or the baby is sleepy from drugs used during delivery. The common position for breast-feeding (holding the baby on your abdomen) may be painful because of your incision. Ask for help finding a more comfortable position for nursing, such as lying on your side with your baby next to you. If you are concerned about pain-killing drugs passing through your milk to your baby, be sure your health care provider knows you are breast-feeding. If you need information about specific drugs and your provider doesn't seem knowledgeable, call La Leche League or consult the Cochrane Database (see chapter 20 Resources).

Mothers of premature babies and twins usually can and should nurse their babies.[5] If your baby is too small and weak to suck, you can express milk to be fed to the baby via a tube until she or he is strong enough to nurse. Even if you are separated from your baby by a prolonged hospitalization, you can usually make arrangements to breast-feed part-time (see below).

With few exceptions, mothers with illnesses requiring medication can and should continue to nurse. If you are taking drugs that will pass through your milk to the baby, you and your health care practitioner, together with a lactation consultant, can often make substitutions, lower the dosage, or eliminate the drug. Make it clear to your practitioner that you want to continue to breast-feed your baby. If you have HIV infection, breast-feeding is not advised, as the virus can be transmitted via breast milk.

Women who have had breast surgery for medical or cosmetic reasons should obtain advice and help from a knowledgeable lactation consultant. (See *The Nursing Mothers Companion* in Resources.)

If for some reason you must stop breast-feeding (or choose not to initially), you may be able to reactivate your milk supply later by allowing your baby to suckle frequently. It may take some time for your milk to come in, and the process can be frustrating and difficult. Some determined women have resumed nursing weeks or even months after stopping completely. Occasionally, mothers of adopted children have even managed to breast-feed their babies successfully.

La Leche League has documented examples of all the cases mentioned above and can provide invaluable information, advice, literature, and encouragement through what may be a difficult period.

Tips for Successful Breast-feeding

In order to establish and maintain a good milk supply, you must take care of yourself. This means eating high-protein foods—consuming a pregnancy diet (see chapter 19, Pregnancy, p. 444) plus 300 to 500 calories. Be sure to include foods rich in vitamins B and C, iron, and calcium.‖ If you have been taking prenatal supplements, keep taking them until your health care practitioner advises otherwise. Don't try to lose weight at this time. The ten or so extra pounds you retained after birth will help your body sustain milk production during the first few months. In addition, sudden weight loss can be harmful: If your body is forced to mobilize its fat supplies, your milk may contain higher amounts of some of the potentially hazardous chemicals found in our environment and food supplies.[3]

Be sure to drink plenty of liquids. A good rule of thumb is to drink a big glass of juice, milk, or water every time you nurse. Keep one by your bedside at night, too.

Getting enough rest is very important. It is difficult for your body to produce increasing amounts of milk when you are tired and run down.

Remember that whatever you eat or drink will be passed on to your baby via your milk. For this reason, it is wise to avoid caffeine and drugs (including over-the-counter remedies). Before taking any drugs, consult your health care practitioner to find out whether they are safe for nursing mothers. If your practitioner recommends an over-the-counter pain reliever, choose acetaminophen, such as Tylenol, if you can. Ibuprofen is also better than aspirin for this purpose.[4]

Contact La Leche League for a list of drugs to avoid while nursing. You may hear conflicting advice about alcohol consumption for breast-feeding mothers. In the absence of consensus on this, we recommend that you avoid any alcohol while breast-feeding.

Sharing Feedings

If you plan to return to work, want time for yourself, or feel it's important for your partner or other members of the family to feed the baby, it is possible to establish a part-time breast-feeding arrangement, especially after the first couple of months. You can express milk (by hand or breast pump), chill it (or freeze it if it is not used within a few hours), and leave it for others to give to the baby. You can get information, and usually lease or buy a breast pump, from La Leche League or lactation consultants.

If you choose to have another nursing mother breast-feed your baby in your absence, you will want to be sure that she is in good health and well nourished. Of special concern, you need to be sure she is not HIV-positive; does not have hepatitis; is not taking any drugs, including prescribed drugs; and does not drink alcohol.

If you must miss feedings on a regular basis, be sure to express milk at the appropriate feeding times to keep up your milk supply. Remember that breast-feeding is a matter of supply and demand. Some women find that expressing milk is a real inconvenience. Others have trouble expressing enough milk to keep up an adequate supply. In these cases, you may nurse only once or twice a day, giving your baby formula in between, or switch entirely to bottle feeding. The point is to reach a compromise that you feel good about for yourself and your baby.

Breast-feeding and Contraception

When you are totally breast-feeding your baby (i.e., not giving any supplementary formula or solid food), your menstrual periods usually do not return for seven to 15 months after birth, because the hormones that stimulate milk production also inhibit menstruation. However, many women begin to supplement breast milk with formula or solids by the time the baby is about six months old. Once you begin to supplement, you are more likely to ovulate. If you do not wish to become pregnant again, you will need to use birth control. Barrier methods are preferred for breast-feeding mothers (you may need to have your diaphram or cervical cap refitted). Avoid IUDs because of the increased risk of pelvic inflammatory disease. The long-term effects of birth control pills on breast-feeding mothers and babies have not yet been well researched. If you choose to take birth control pills, let your health care practitioner know you are breast-feeding. The progestin-only pill is less likely to adversely affect your milk supply.[5] We have serious reservations about oral contraceptives. Since steroids can get into the milk supply, there may be as yet undiscovered effects on the baby (see chapter 13, Birth Control). Remember that neither oral contraceptives nor total breast feeding provide any protection against STDs, such as HIV/AIDS, when you have sex.

Some Problems You May Encounter

Sore Nipples

Some women have sore nipples the first few days of breast-feeding. While hospitals often advise women to nurse only five minutes on each breast at three-hour intervals, many women find that nursing more frequently actually works better because the breasts don't become engorged (see below) and the baby sucks less vigorously at the nipple. If your nipples do become sore, exposing them to sunlight and air whenever possible will help. After each feeding, spread breast milk over the nipples and expose them to air as long as possible. Consult your health care practitioner or lactation consultant before using any other treatment. Some ointments may actually make nipple problems worse and may contain ingredients that could be toxic to the baby.

Engorgement

When your milk comes in on the second or third day, your breasts may feel full, heavy, and painful to the touch. In some cases, they are so full that you may have to express a little milk by hand before the baby can grasp the nipple. Frequent nursing on demand often prevents engorgement, but if it occurs, hot showers or hot compresses made with comfrey applied before nursing will usually remedy the situation within a day or so. By that time, your body will have adjusted its supply to the baby's demand for food. Massaging your breasts to promote circulation and letdown may also help. Some women also recommend ice packs for pain. Whatever you do, don't stop nursing!

Sore Breasts

If you have swelling, redness, or a painful lump in one area of your breast, you may have a plugged duct, which can be caused by poor letdown, engorgement, infrequent nursing, an ill-fitting bra, tight clothing, and/or stress and fatigue. Hot compresses, massaging the area, and increased nursing will usually ease the discomfort. If the swelling is accompanied by fever and a tired, run-down, achy feeling (like flu), you probably have a breast infection (mastitis). In that case, contact your health care practitioner or midwife, and make sure to get more rest. If the condition does not improve in 24 hours, you may need medication. Your health care provider should choose a medication that is safe for the baby. Continued nursing will also help the

continued on next page

infection to resolve itself. Rarely, a breast infection develops into an abscess that may have to be surgically drained. In most cases, however, early treatment will prevent this.

Concerns About the Adequacy of Your Milk Supply

You, or others, may become concerned about whether you are producing enough milk to meet your baby's needs. The concern may stem from any of several observations. For example, the baby may not be wetting the expected amount of diapers, the baby may be irritable between feedings, the baby may not be gaining weight at the expected rate, or your breasts may not feel as full as you think they should. Often, these concerns can be resolved easily through simple changes, such as increased rest, a change in diet, and/or a change in nursing patterns. It is important to seek advice promptly when these concerns arise, before the problems reach crisis proportions. Many successful breast-feeding mother-baby couples have faced similar challenges. Assistance with breast-feeding concerns can be obtained from La Leche League or lactation consultants.

If you are concerned that your milk supply is inadequate, try to cut down on outside activities and rest whenever possible. Some women also recommend supplemental brewers' yeast, which contains high amounts of B vitamins. You can also drink teas made from blessed thistle, chamomile, fennel, or fenugreek seed 30 minutes before nursing.

---

* Because of immunities in breast milk, some women whose babies are solely breast-fed may wish to delay having their babies inoculated against diseases. You might discuss this with your health care practitioner.

† There are serious disadvantages to formula. Despite the known disadvantages, some hospitals continue to promote its use. If you choose to breast-feed, be sure to make this known to your health care providers and any other hospital personnel involved in your or your baby's care.

‡ Some common problems include difficulty with letting down milk and maintaining an adequate milk supply when the baby grows quickly. If you do have problems, we recommend consulting nursing mothers or supportive groups (such as La Leche League) rather than relying on pediatricians for advice. Few physicians are experienced and/or supportive enough of breast-feeding to be really helpful; many of them discourage women from breast-feeding if the slightest problem arises.

§ Research shows that the milk of mothers of premature babies contains more protein and other nutrients than that of mothers with full-term babies. (La Leche Information Sheet no. 13, December 1980, available from La Leche League International. See Resources for address). Fortifiers are sometimes recommended to supplement breast milk for extremely tiny premature babies. These will be given in addition to breast milk, which is still the best food for your baby.

‖ If you are lactose intolerant, or do not wish to eat or cannot digest any dairy products, you can still successfully breast-feed. See other sources of calcium in chapter 2, Food, p. 55.

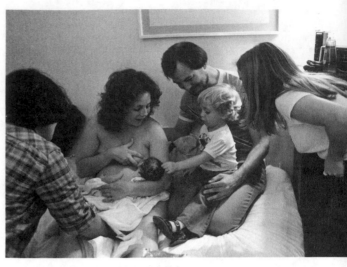

Suzanne Arms

ADJUSTING TO LIFE WITH A BABY

During the first few months after birth, we learn what it means to have a baby in our lives. Many women describe the early postpartum time as one of fragmentation and disorganization.

During those early weeks I felt like I was disappearing. I seemed to exist only in terms of other people's needs. Sometimes I wasn't sure where the baby ended and I began. I felt that I had lost my old self and was too tired, physically and emotionally, to find her again. But I was also discovering a new part of myself that I hadn't known about before: unexpectedly intense feelings for my new baby, a resurgence of love for my mother connection with other women. I went from despair, to overwhelming feelings of tenderness, all within the space of an hour.

Fatigue

Of all the stresses associated with the postpartum time, fatigue is the one mentioned by almost all parents. At some point, most of us "crash" under the pressure of night after night of interrupted sleep—some for only a short while, others for months—especially when there are other children at home and/or little outside help.

For the first week after the birth I was flying. I seemed to have plenty of energy for everything—my new baby, my husband, even the constant stream of visitors who filled the house. Then, one day, it just caught up with me. Suddenly I could hardly get through the day with two or three naps. By 9 A.M. I was exhausted. In addition, my perineum, which was nearly healed, suddenly began to ache and feel sore again. My body was clearly sending me a message. When I slowed down and began to take care of myself,

I felt better, but I never did recapture that initial high of those days after the birth.

The first six months of my third baby's life are a blur to me. Constantly tired and irritable, I somehow got through each day, but it certainly was no fun for us all. The older children (three and six) suffered from not getting enough attention. Because the baby was breast-feeding six times a day, there was almost no time to take the kids out or even get through the daily housekeeping. I still feel spread thin most of the time.

Some physical discomforts also contribute to fatigue. Common discomforts that last two to three weeks after birth are sweating (especially at night), loss of appetite, thirst (due to loss of fluids and nursing), and constipation. If you continue to lose sleep, you build up a backlog of REM* sleep loss, which can lead to emotional and physical disturbances. Your partner may also suffer the effects of sleep deprivation.

Some women get enough REM sleep even though the baby disrupts their usual sleep pattern. However, if you are someone who sleeps most soundly in your sixth or seventh hour of sleep, have someone else feed the baby during the night, early in the morning, or in the late afternoon, so that once a day you can sleep for a longer stretch than the few hours between feedings. If possible, nap whenever the baby naps.

Sexuality

Some of us have little or no interest in sex for a while after childbirth. Others resume sexual activity fairly quickly. We each need to set our own pace.

All that first year, our old forms of go-to-it sexuality were just too much. I was too tired and I'd fall asleep in the first five minutes, leaving Jack frustrated, even angry. Other times I'd have the nursing and holding of the baby on my mind and intercourse seemed rough and crude. Also, I think that by the end of a day I had had a lot of skin-to-skin rubbing and touching and didn't feel sexually hungry at all. But Jack hadn't had much at all. The unevenness was driving us nuts. After months and months of snarling, we just had to invent "middle ways" of being physical with one another. I think I picked it up from watching each of us with the baby—the nuzzling and snuggling that goes on with no expectation of orgasm, just affection.

Low sexual interest can result from having your life shaken up, feeling exhausted, or having to take care of your new baby, and possibly also other children and your partner. Some women find that breast-feeding and physical contact with the baby fulfill their desires for physical closeness.

Low sexual interest can have physical causes. If you had an episiotomy or tear in the perineum during birth, the area may be sore for several weeks. Your vagina may feel dry, lacking its normal lubrication because of lowered estrogen levels (more common in nursing mothers). Penetration—by a finger, penis, or dildo—may hurt, although other kinds of lovemaking that do not involve penetration may be just what you want (see chapter 11, Sexuality, p. 242).

If you feel physically and psychologically ready, and the bleeding (lochia) has stopped, there is no medical risk in lovemaking that includes penetration. If penetration is uncomfortable, you may want to use an unscented lubricant such as K-Y Jelly or a clear vegetable oil.† Some nursing mothers also experience painful cramps during and after intercourse. Women vary as to when they feel ready, emotionally and physically, to resume sexual activity.[6] If you are having heterosexual intercourse and want to use birth control, see chapter 13, Birth Control, for options. See also the box on breast-feeding, p. 504.

Learning How to Mother Your Baby

We may have grown up believing that because we are women, we are supposed to know how to care for a baby. Yet, it is really experience that teaches us to be good mothers, including our own experiences baby-sitting or watching our mothers care for younger brothers and sisters. In the beginning, we may be uneasy and afraid to trust our own good sense, especially with a first baby. Talking with other mothers about our feelings and fears can give us the confidence to try different things.

The first month was awful. I loved my baby but felt apprehensive about my ability to satisfy this totally dependent tiny creature. Every time she cried I could feel myself tense up and panic. What should I do? Can I make her stop—can I help her?

After the first month I got the hang of it, partly because I had such an easy child. She slept a lot, and when she was awake she was responsive—she'd look at me alertly and smile. Gradually my love for her overcame my panic. I relaxed, stopped thinking so much about my inadequacies, and was just myself. It was pretty clear from her responses that I was doing something right.

I didn't know how to change a diaper any more than my husband did. In fact, I may have been more nervous about it, since I was "supposed" to know how. I learned to do it because I had to learn, and my husband learned, too.

---

* REMs (rapid eye movements) are associated with dreaming, which occurs during the deepest phase of sleep and is believed to be necessary for physical and psychological replenishment.

† Avoid estrogen creams and/or pills recommended by some physicians, as the long-term effects of hormones on you and the baby are unknown.

Colic

Don't expect to love being a mother all the time. For instance, when your baby sleeps a lot, wakes up for feedings, smiles at you, and goes back to sleep again, the baby business is a breeze. But when a baby is colicky (a catchword to describe baby discomfort, fussiness, crankiness) and cries 16 hours out of 24, your physical and mental powers may be stretched to their limits. No amount of preparation can really equip you to withstand this calmly. There is nothing quite so jarring to the nerves as your own baby's cries. They can fill a new parent with feelings of impotence, guilt, and understandable impatience. Most babies are colicky for only a few hours each day—often in the late afternoon and evening—and usually outgrow it by about four months.

At around two weeks old she started crying from ten or 11 P.M. until six in the morning. We tried everything —walking, rocking, massage—but nothing seemed to help. Underneath I was sure it was my fault. One night, in desperation, Mark started dancing around the floor with her. I was so tired and they looked so funny that I started to laugh. Mark began to laugh, too, and the baby was so surprised that she stopped crying for a minute. It was enough to break the tension. After that, it seemed to get gradually better. I stopped blaming myself and realized that this was something she just had to go through, and all we could do was be there with her. After a few hard weeks she tapered off.

In many cases, colic is thought to be due to the immature digestive system of the baby.* Sometimes, however, an allergy to a protein in cow's milk is responsible. If you are breast-feeding, you can try to avoid dairy products for a week to see if that helps (see chapter 2, Food, p. 55, for alternative sources of calcium). Some vegetables (onions, garlic, cabbage, broccoli, cauliflower, Brussels sprouts) and occasionally wheat can also cause gas pains in breast-fed babies. It is a good idea to avoid any foods to which you are allergic, as the baby may also be sensitive to these substances. If you are bottle feeding and your baby has colic, there are several options you might try. Switching to a soy-based formula may help. You might consult your health care provider about special formulas for babies with colic. If you have been bottle feeding and wish to try breast-feeding your baby, you can build up a milk supply. For help with this process, call La Leche League or a lactation consultant (see Resources).

You can try massaging your colicky baby's tummy, getting in a warm bath with her or him (heat often has a soothing effect), and offering a very small amount of watered-down noncaffeinated chamomile or spearmint tea by cup or bottle. In very extreme cases, your health care practitioner may prescribe a medication for your baby. If you are uncomfortable giving medication to your baby, you may want to consult an alternative health care provider.

Mothering a colicky baby is a real challenge. It may help to remember that some babies adjust to life outside the womb more slowly than others. No one knows why some babies have colic. We do know, however, that colic goes away and babies who were once colicky grow into happy, cheerful babies and toddlers. In the meantime, love and nurture your baby as best you can. Seek help where you can. Family members or friends may be able to hold and walk your crying baby while you take a break. You may also get emotional support from family, friends, health care providers, or a parental stress hot line in your community.

Lifestyle Changes

Living with a new baby means changing our lives in many ways. We discover we are on 24-hour call.

I was used to getting out of the house in five minutes when I wanted to go somewhere. Now it can take me an hour to get organized for even a simple expedition. By the time I've gathered up the diapers, blankets, and rattles; fed and changed the baby; and put her in the Snugli, sometimes it's almost too late to go. And if I ever want to go out alone, I've learned I need to start phoning baby-sitters a week in advance.

Many babies are unpredictable in their sleeping and eating habits for the first few weeks. Some breast-fed babies continue to nurse frequently and wake at night for months. We may be overwhelmed by the constant demands of baby care and find it difficult to get on with the rest of our lives.

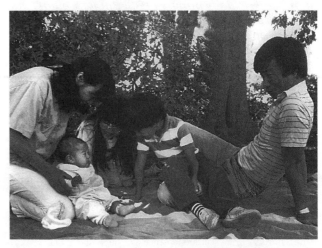

Elizabeth Crews/Stock, Boston

---

* During the 1950s, colic was usually thought to be caused by maternal hostility to the baby. Very few doctors still believe this. However, should you encounter a health care practitioner who seems to blame you for your baby's colic, consider switching to a different practitioner.

I had been told that most babies ate every three or four hours and slept the rest of the time. Not mine! She wanted to nurse every two hours and sometimes more often than that. Sometimes she would sleep for an hour, sometimes for 15 minutes. I loved her, but I also felt consumed by her needs. It was hard to adjust to the fact that I couldn't get anything finished, whether it was an article I was reading or folding the laundry. At the end of the day I would realize I hadn't accomplished anything. Once I accepted the fact that I was not going to function at my old efficient rate (at least for a while) and stopped feeling guilty about what I wasn't getting done, I felt freer to enjoy the time I was spending with my baby.

Some of us are reluctant or resentful about giving up activities we used to take for granted; for others, it's a holiday if we can stay at home for a while. Within a few months, when the baby is older and on a more predictable schedule, you'll have more flexibility.

For many of us, life with a new baby means coping with the monotony and isolation of long hours spent alone with an infant. There may be day after day without adult company.

After a week, I was going crazy being alone at home with the baby. So I borrowed a baby carrier and just took her every place with me. I learned how to nurse in public without being obtrusive and discovered she would sleep anywhere—in the carrier, on the floor of a friend's house, in a shopping cart, even in restaurants and movie theaters. Being mobile made me feel less confined and kept me in touch with the world.

It is only in Western, modernized societies that women are expected to "go it alone" with children. In many other cultures, postpartum mothers live among mothers, aunts, sisters, and cousins and are able to draw on their time, interest, and wisdom.

At home [in West Africa] it is different because you can stay at least a week in the hospital, and your family can sleep there with you. Here, I felt pushed out of the hospital after three days, and I was not ready to leave. I thought, "I don't know what to do with this little baby who is so helpless and so depending on me." In my country, when the child is born, you really have a network of women who come and help. They take care of the baby; they take care of you. You don't have to worry about who will take care of your child, because there's always somebody there with you. At home, you have all these traditional ways to do things—like how to bathe the mother and the child, how to help the abdominal muscles get back in shape, massage. There are beliefs about these things that are passed on. My mother bathed and massaged me and the baby for three months after he was born.

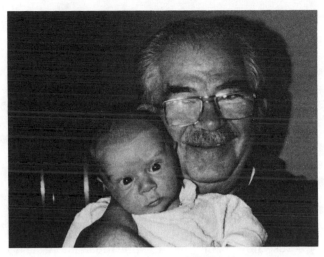

Nancy Miriam Hawley

Care and Support

New mothers need many different kinds of care: practical help, emotional support, financial support, nurturing, and guidance. As a new mother you may find yourself surrounded by interested and helpful family and friends. Or you may be isolated with no one to provide these kinds of care and no one to talk to.

I think it's very important for women to be able to talk to other mothers of young children. My image of motherhood was so far off from what it really is. I pictured everything being gauzy and clean and relaxing and peaceful, so I really thought I would be very happy just being at home and rocking my children and reading and cleaning. I had no idea it was going to feel so isolating. For me, the need for support was much, much greater than I anticipated, because I view myself as self-reliant and very independent. It was a bit of a surprise.

If you are fortunate, establishing new connections with others for mutual care and support may be as easy as joining an informal mother-baby group in your neighborhood.

When Willie was just a few months old, I joined a playgroup with several other mothers in the area. While the group was formed to get the babies together, its real function was as a support group for the mothers. It was reassuring to hear that someone else's baby was colicky and had been up all night and to trade information and suggestions as to what we could do. It was also a help to share some of my ambivalent feelings about motherhood and discover that I wasn't the only one. I came to look on the playgroup as an oasis in what was otherwise a somewhat lonely existence.

Some of us find it more challenging to overcome isolation. Lack of time, money, transportation, stable housing, or even safety may seem to stand in our way. Making contact with other mothers and finding sensitive role models and health care providers may be even more important under these circumstances. Local parks, playgrounds, churches, or community centers may be places to connect with people who can help decrease your isolation. You can bring your baby with you, and you may be surprised at the interest and attention you and the baby get.

Acknowledging Postpartum Feelings

Once the full impact of living with a baby hits us, we may feel pride, elation, love, attachment, and warmth. But many conflicting feelings, thoughts, and fears may also surface: I am supposed to be fulfilled because now I am a mother, but I feel ambivalent; I have to go back to work and I fear losing touch with my baby; I have to be around all the time just to meet my baby's needs, so I don't have time for my other interests; I've lost my independence; I feel scared and inadequate—I need mothering myself.

After the baby was born, she became the focus of everyone's attention, and I was reduced to the role of caretaker. People would come up and say, "What a lovely baby," and never even look me in the eye. I was proud of my baby, but I felt a nonperson myself. I wanted to say, "I'm the one who cleans up the messes and gets up at night. Pay attention to me, too!"

We may feel angry at ourselves, our partners, or our babies when we are particularly exhausted or isolated, or when we are not the perfect mothers we expected to be. Anger does not fit in with our fantasies about motherhood. Neither does grief, frustration, panic, or jealousy. But these feelings are there. Acknowledgment is the first step in dealing with our feelings.

SERIOUS POSTPARTUM DIFFICULTIES: WHEN YOU NEED HELP

Baby blues (see p. 504) are common, last only a short time, and go away by themselves. In this section we will discuss more serious postpartum difficulties. Their duration is not as predictable as baby blues, and you are very likely to need special attention and care. Health care practitioners frequently refer to these kind of difficulties as postpartum disorders. There are no official diagnoses for postpartum disorders; we will present information regarding depression, anxiety, and psychosis occurring during the first year after giving birth.

Postpartum Depression

Postpartum depression can range from mild to severe. You may feel any combination of the following: lonely, guilty, uncontrollably sad and weepy, unable to sleep, unable to eat, inconsolable, irritable, oversensitive, uninterested in affection or sex, anxious, exhausted, helpless, incompetent to care for your baby, suicidal, angry at your baby or others, resentful, frightened. You may have a pretty good idea about where the feelings are coming from (for example, troubles with your partner, or a crying baby who can't be comforted), or the feelings may seem to arise from nowhere. Postpartum depression can be disabling. If you or a woman you know suffers from these feelings, it is very important to seek help from someone you trust, such as your health care provider or clergy. Ask her or him to help you find a therapist, provider, or support person who is knowledgeable and experienced in helping women with postpartum depression. (See "Coping with Postpartum Depression" and "Treatment for Postpartum Difficulties," pp. 515 and 516.)

Causes of Postpartum Depression

Every new mother experiences some stress. Although no one can predict whether you will be affected by postpartum depression, we do know that certain stresses and the lack of certain supports can place you at risk. These include social isolation, such as the isolation that may occur after a move; problems in the relationship with your partner, including serious disappointment in your partner's ability to support you in the ways you need support; abandonment or the death of your partner; or abuse (if you are being abused, see chapter 19, Pregnancy, p. 458). Other factors may include recent job loss, housing problems, financial problems, illness, having had anxiety and/or depression during your pregnancy,* your memories of the birth experience as one in which you were helpless and disempowered, the burdens of being a single mother if family or friends are not coming through for you, having had past episodes of depression, having a baby with colic or with a difficult temperament, and a tendency to react strongly to hormonal changes—for example, if you have severe PMS.[7]

The six or eight months after Peter was born were hard. My physical energy started to return when he slept through the night and more when he stopped needing a 10 P.M. feeding. But my mental and emotional energy seemed to have disappeared for good. It was all I could do to get through a day. I took long naps and cried often. I got jealous about women my husband saw at work. I was out of touch with the me who had been an interesting, active, and humorous person. Love him as I did, in some moods I resented Peter for even existing. To most people I pretended to be a "happy, young mother," but I was quite depressed. I didn't know about postpartum depression, so I blamed what I was feeling on my own failure to be a good mother. I think I also blamed my husband, as though he could have made me feel better. He was worried about his job and resentful that I was too low to give

---

* In Ann Oakley's classic studies of postpartum mothers living in London, 98 of the 102 working-class women interviewed experienced recurrent depression.

him any comfort. He accused me of having a child and now "not wanting one." (He didn't know about postpartum depression either.)

Losses in New Motherhood That May Contribute to Postpartum Depression

In addition to the factors we mentioned earlier, there is a certain amount of normal loss involved in becoming a new mother. Not everyone becomes depressed as a result of these losses. If you find that you are grieving some losses, be assured that this is normal. Some women may experience overwhelming grief. If this happens to you, be sure to get support and help.

If your baby was premature or ill, had to remain in the hospital after you were discharged, or has ongoing health problems, depression may be a part of your process of grieving. Allowing yourself to mourn the image of a robust newborn may be helpful. Society tends to reward new mothers for being strong and "in control" when open expression of pain, disappointment, and sadness might at times be more helpful. Whether or not your baby has been ill, it may be helpful to allow yourself to mourn past losses that come to mind, such as past pregnancy losses through miscarriage or abortion, or giving a baby up for adoption, or the loss of your parents or loved ones. Also allow yourself to mourn the losses associated with becoming a mother, such as loss of freedom and autonomy and loss of your pregnant state. Your relationship with your partner is bound to change after your baby is born. You may experience that as a loss. If the birth itself did not measure up to your expectations, you may be grieving that loss as well. In the U.S., unlike other parts of the world, most women giving birth are anesthetized, cut (either for cesarean section or episiotomy), or both. Often, the experience of these interventions makes women vulnerable to depression following childbirth.* If you had planned to breastfeed and were unable to, or had to stop earlier than anticipated, this may also lead to feelings of sadness and loss. As your baby grows, becomes more interested in others and in toys, becomes mobile, and is weaned, you may also grieve the loss of the closeness you had with the baby as a newborn.

It can be helpful to talk with others about the sense of loss. Some mothers are reluctant to talk about this because it seems unacceptable to feel grief when you have a new baby. Be assured that loss and grief are normal parts of becoming a mother.

Preventing Postpartum Depression

We encourage all women to be active participants in caring for themselves physically and mentally. If you believe you are at risk for postpartum depression, there are some things you can do to prevent it, reduce

* K. Greene, "Birth, Trauma and Postpartum Depression." Paper presented at the Annual Meeting of the American Psychiatric Association, May 9, 1996, New York City.

its severity, or prepare for it so that you and your family can manage the situation if it occurs. Keep in mind that some women will be taken by surprise by postpartum depression, and some women will develop postpartum depression despite their best efforts at prevention.

Many women are encouraged to plan only for birth and do not receive adequate assistance in anticipating their postpartum needs and desires. Much of what you can do to prevent postpartum depression should be done before birth, and some can be done even before you get pregnant. Perhaps the most important thing you can do to prepare for your postpartum needs is to build up your support network in advance. Your support network could include your partner, family members, old and new friends, neighbors, co-workers, professional care providers, lactation consultants, other pregnant women, and new mothers. It can be very helpful to communicate your feelings and needs for various kinds of support. In order to do so, you have to accept that it is okay for you to have needs at this time, and to depend on others to help you. You may have to learn new ways to tell those in your network about the things you need and the ways they can help you. Talk to other new mothers and their partners about the changes that they have experienced and the ways they have coped.

If you had a difficult time following the birth of your first child, because of postpartum depression or other distress, you may find yourself worrying about whether it will happen again. There is no way to predict whether you will have difficulties again. Taking preventive measures before the baby is born will increase your chances of an easier time postpartum.

If you believe you may be at risk for postpartum depression, discuss it with your health care provider, and ask for help in finding suitable supportive resources, such as a knowledgeable therapist, who can help you assess your specific needs and find ways to meet them.

Coping with Postpartum Depression

Postpartum depression often feels debilitating—you feel as if you can hardly get out of bed in the morning, and the things you once did easily now seem to require massive effort. It may be helpful to remember that you are not alone (10 to 20% of new mothers experience postpartum depression) and you are not to blame.

Here are some suggestions that women have found helpful in coping with postpartum depression:

- Focus on goals for the day, rather than longer-term goals, which may seem insurmountable. Be sure that you have one thing to look forward to each day, such as a relaxing bath, time on the phone with a friend, a walk outdoors.
- Take advantage of free and low-cost activities. Libraries and churches often offer this kind of

information, as do local newspapers and parents' newspapers (often free).

- Look for opportunities to spend time with your partner and/or close friends. Time with adults (peers if you are a teenager) will help you feel like yourself.
- Ask for help! Do not be afraid to ask others for practical help as well as emotional support. This isn't a time to try to be completely self-sufficient.
- Allow yourself to accept a lot of help. Be a supportable person. You are entitled to get help at this time. For single mothers especially, family and friends are—as one woman put it— "better than vitamins, more than money."
- Use the people around you as resources to help you find professional help and support. You may need a therapist, a psychiatrist, a support group, an alternative practitioner, a nutritionist. (This may require you to explore your insurance options.)
- Evaluate (or re-evaluate) your plans regarding work outside the home. Explore, and try to expand, your options and choices. Do you need to get a job? Do you want to return to the same job? When will you be ready to return? Who can help you find a suitable job and child care? Do you need to take more time off, or cut down on your hours? If you need money to do this, you might ask for a loan or help from a family member or friend. If you have to return to (or start) work, and you are not feeling good about it, it may help to talk with a trusted friend.
- Join a support group for new mothers and babies. You may be able to find a support group for mothers with postpartum depression. You may find groups listed at your library, your church, or the office of your health care provider.*

Postpartum Anxiety

Anxiety is simply worry or nervousness without an easily understandable cause. You may feel jittery, or you may have difficulty concentrating, sleeping, or running your household. You may find yourself seeming overly concerned about your health, your baby's health, or the health of those around you. You may have physical symptoms such as rapid heartbeat, trembling, sweaty palms, or difficulty breathing. You may also have intensive, peculiar, frightening thoughts and/or feel compelled to perform common caretaking actions over and over again. Many new mothers experience some of these signs of anxiety, especially when they are fatigued. If, however, you find yourself experiencing anxiety so great that it disrupts your daily functioning, you should seek help (see below). Many of the suggestions for coping with postpartum depression are useful for coping with anxiety as well (see above).

* These suggestions are based on information obtained from Jan Honikman, founder and director of Postpartum Support International (see Resources).

Postpartum Psychosis

Although the incidence of postpartum psychosis is low (1 or 2 per thousand), it's a serious condition requiring immediate attention. Be assured that it can be successfully treated. Here are some of the signs and symptoms associated with postpartum psychosis: You may feel that you are being ordered by God or a power outside yourself to do things you normally wouldn't, such as harm yourself or your baby; you may feel confused or agitated; you may see or hear things that others don't; you may have extreme highs or lows of energy or mood; you may not be able to take care of your baby; you may experience your thoughts and feelings as being out of your control. If you are experiencing any of these symptoms, or any other extreme symptoms, or if those close to you are expressing concern, you deserve to receive treatment immediately. Ask someone to take you to a knowledgeable health care provider or to an emergency room and explain that you believe you are having a serious postpartum reaction and you need help from a provider who specializes in this condition. This condition is thought by many to be connected in some way to the massive hormonal changes that occur after childbirth, although no one yet knows why some mothers are more vulnerable to postpartum psychosis than others.

Treatment for Postpartum Difficulties

There are various options for treating postpartum difficulties. They include alternative treatments, such as acupuncture and homeopathic remedies, as well as focused (perinatal) psychotherapy, medication, and support groups. New information on research about treatment options is constantly becoming available. (For example, interpersonal psychotherapy currently seems to be a promising treatment for many women.[8] Also, researchers are investigating the safety of medication for breast-feeding mothers.) The therapist or support person you see should provide information about various treatment options, listen to your preferences, and work with you to devise a plan for your care. If you do not feel that the person you see is responsive to your preferences, we recommend seeking a second opinion. Remember that your well-being is crucial to your baby's healthy development; therefore, be open to considering a range of treatments, which may include some—such as psychotherapy or medication—that you might not otherwise have considered. If you're breast-feeding, be sure you discuss this with the person you consult. If you and your practitioner decide that the best treatment for you includes medication, this may require you to wean the baby. Depending on how long you need to take medication, it may be possible for you to relactate and resume breast-feeding when you stop taking medication. Discuss this with your health care practitioner, and get help from La Leche League.

Many practitioners believe that medication and hospitalization are necessary in the treatment of postpartum psychosis and severe postpartum depression. This is because these rare situations carry some risk to the well-being and even survival of mother and baby. Unfortunately, temporary weaning and separation of mother from baby may be necessitated by these treatments, because there are currently few units in the U.S. that accept mothers and babies together. (This kind of unit has proved successful in England, but lack of awareness and sensitivity to the needs of mothers and babies have led U.S. hospitals to allow cost and liability factors to dictate the types of care offered. Mutual support groups and women's groups should lobby hospitals to establish such units.) We can negotiate frequent, regular visits with our babies, with assistance and oversight by caregivers, during the short time when hospitalization is needed. Some very innovative, determined, energetic families, with considerable community support, may be able to arrange alternative forms of care for individual mothers. This should not be undertaken lightly, however. Ongoing therapy, monitoring, and consultation by experienced and knowledgeable caregivers must be a necessary part of such an alternative plan.*

While you are in the midst of postpartum difficulties, you may wonder whether having a baby was a good idea. You may believe that motherhood will always be associated with emotional distress. It may be hard to imagine that your feelings about yourself, your baby, or your family will ever be joyful and loving. Give yourself time to grow into the role of mother. You may take some time to explore what aspects of being a mother bring you pleasure and joy.

CELEBRATING THE PLEASURES

I had heard about the negatives—the fatigue, the loneliness, loss of self. But nobody told me about the wonderful parts: holding my baby close to me, seeing her first smile, watching her grow and become more responsive day by day. How can I describe the way I felt when she stroked my breast while nursing or looked into my eyes or arched her eyebrows like an opera singer? This was the deepest connection I'd felt to anybody. Sometimes the intensity almost frightened me. For the first time I cared about somebody else more than myself, and I would do anything to nurture and protect her.

We are surviving. Just. Why don't they give Croix de Guerres to people who can go without more than two hours total daily sleep for five weeks? I thought babies ate at six-ten-two-six-ten-two—mine does. He also eats at five-seven-nine-eleven and four-eight-twelve. I am getting rather used to going around with my breasts hanging out. They are either drying from the last feed or getting ready for the next one. But the love —I never knew, never imagined that I would love him

like this. This incredible feeling of boundless, endless love—a wish to protect his innocence from ever being hurt or wounded or scratched. And that awful, horrible, mad feeling in the first week that you'll never be able to keep anything so precious and so vulnerable alive.

They give me lots of joy; it gives me tremendous joy just looking at them. It's something I can't even measure.

LONG-TERM ISSUES

I was getting together all the stuff I needed to take Pablo out—you know, the blanket, the diapers, the toys. I did it very smoothly, thinking all the time about the different buses we had to take. "This is it," I said to myself. "Being a mother is under my skin, in my brain, part of the way I pick things up and put them down."

The period between six and 12 months after birth is often a time when chaos, fatigue, and uncertainty ebb away and a tide of confidence and energy washes in. This is partly because our babies begin to sleep through the night, eat solid food, take predictable naps in the morning and afternoon. But this return to normal also comes from our own practicing, experimenting, and learning during that first chaotic half-year. No matter how much smoother daily life becomes, parenthood alters practically all of our "old" ways.

Partnership

When I think back on it, adding a baby was like sending our relationship through a wringer and planting a garden smack in its middle—both at once.

Throughout the first year, adult caresses or conversations often lose out to a cry from the baby. Our partner becomes less a lover or a companion than "the other parent." Earlier in this chapter, we talked about practical issues in sexuality and child care that come up during the first months. Some deeper or more complicated issues arise as the people in a couple relationship undergo a gradual shift to parenthood. This is not an easy transition. Whether we have children at 18 or 38, we have to balance being a parent with all the other concerns of our lives, whether it's finishing high school, finding work, or caring for our own parents.

For both lesbian and heterosexual couples, one of the most difficult issues is jealousy, or competition for affection. Often there just isn't enough energy, time, and affection for everyone.

The baby is the important figure in both our lives right now. We still are partners, lovers, but . . . our primary nurturing and affection is with the baby.

When I nursed at night, the sight of me holding my full breast to this sleepy little baby used to drive Les

---

* We know of only one mother-baby unit in the U.S., which is in the Boston area.

nuts. When I'd get back into bed, he'd be wild to make love, fast and hard. It got to be quite a thing because I'd come back to bed feeling mild and sleepy. Les wanted to screw and I wanted to snuggle. We fought over it a lot until we realized we had to make time for some sex that was hard and fast and some that was cozy. A couple of months past the worst of it, we began to joke about "hard" and "soft" sex.

As we become parents, our roles in the relationship may become uncertain. What had been a smoothly functioning system with each person comfortably taking certain responsibilities may suddenly no longer work. For example, the woman who has given birth, who previously was the organizer of the household, may not be able to maintain that responsibility during the postpartum time. These changes may be very disruptive and disorienting, and they may create anxiety.

Changes in the partner relationship are frequently experienced as highly stressful.[9] If couples anticipate changes ahead of time and discuss their concerns, they will be better prepared to use this time as an opportunity to explore new roles and challenges. In partnerships where parenting and other responsibilities are shared, both partners are likely to be more satisfied, and the relationship is strengthened.

My husband got up at night to take care of the kids. He was very helpful, but I felt like I was the one doing everything. It was not 50–50, it was 75–25. He was gone all day and he was tired, but I was tired, too. I didn't have a break. So I thought he shouldn't have a break either. My mom helped me to be more relaxed and see things more objectively. I needed to accept things the way they were right then and enjoy my kids.

It's one of those "grass-is-greener" things—I envied, sometimes even hated Sam when he went out to work. I don't know what I was imagining—that he hung around talking, went out to lunch, did interesting things. One time he was watching me bathe Annie in the sink. He asked if he could do it—he stood there, soaping her back over and over like he couldn't get enough of it, and he talked about how he hated to leave us in the morning and how he worried he would be closed out, left looking in at what she and I had together.

When Laurie was born I was bound and determined to do it all—be a full-time mother, a full-time, perfect housekeeper. I spent that first year rushing like a madwoman from one duty to the next. I ended up feeling either like the good mother and the wicked wife or the wicked mother and the perfect wife. When I had Peter, my second, I said, "Hey, these kids are ending up with a six-thirty sweetheart, not a father, and I'm tired and lonely. There are two parents here; why am I in this alone?" When I asked Mike to help, he started taking Thursday afternoons off—out of back-vacation time. I still had the kids most of the time, but

the idea that he would do that made a big difference between us.

Realistically, not all partners can take time off. In those cases, the one who is away most can do whatever she or he can: bathe the baby in the evening, put the baby to bed, make dinner, keep the baby close at night, bring the baby for feeding if the baby is sleeping outside the parents' bed.

Postpartum: The Second Time Around

The postpartum time can be a very different experience the second time around. Some aspects are much easier; having been through it all before, you know what to expect and are comfortable with many of the practical issues of child care and parenthood. However, there are still unknowns that can make the postpartum time difficult with second and subsequent children. For example, your new baby may have a very different temperament than the first. Also, your relationship with your partner may be very different. In addition to all this, you now have two or more children, and have to find ways to balance their needs. You also have changed.

I started having children in my late 30s so I wanted them close together. My second child was born 17 months after the first. In some ways I enjoyed the whole experience more. As a second-time mother I was more relaxed and less anxious about every little thing, and my second baby was more easygoing than my first. But that first year was also very hard. I was exhausted just trying to take care of two babies in diapers. In addition, my oldest child was jealous and needed a lot of extra attention, which I couldn't always give. Having two babies on different feeding and nap schedules made life chaotic at times. I was much less mobile with two babies. Going to the grocery store could take all morning. What I found the hardest was having no time to myself. Someone always was wanting something. Unfortunately, my husband was not much help—his job required a lot of traveling and he was gone at least half of the time.

Now—a year and a half later—things are much easier. The kids go to family day care three days a week, and I've been able to go back to work part-time and resume some of the interests and friendships that I had given up. I finally feel like my life, which was out of whack for so long, is beginning to have a rhythm again. I feel like a survivor. I'm proud of my kids and myself for having made it through.

I had a really hard time emotionally after the birth of my first child. He had lots of problems right after birth, and we didn't know if he would make it. I remember crying constantly. Just sitting on the deck and crying. We almost lost this child that we wanted so desperately. How could I give my heart to him, when I was afraid I'd lose him? It took me a long time to let myself love him, but then I loved him so much. With my second child, it was very different. I had such an easy birth, and my daughter was a wonderful baby. I felt like a traitor to my son.

THE HEALTH AND WELL-BEING OF MOTHERS

There are plenty of manuals on health care for infants. But almost nowhere is there a discussion of the health problems women encounter because they are mothers. We who are writing this chapter firmly believe that every mother, for her own sake and the sake of her children, should do her best to attend to her basic needs, such as nutritious food, exercise, rest and sleep, intellectual stimulation, and contact with others. When you are absorbed in caring for your baby or children, you sometimes find that you have neglected yourself.

One day when I was leaning over to put Ben in the crib, I realized I had no idea what clothes I had on. I stayed there with my eyes half closed, not looking, trying to figure it out. I couldn't. I tried to remember brushing my teeth and I couldn't. I knew what shoes I had on, only because I only wore one pair ever.

Motherhood and Stress

Caring for infants and young children is rewarding but hard work. If you have a child between one and three, you are doing something for or with that child about every five minutes for as long as she or he is awake. While studies of stress have tended to ignore women at home with young children, research on factory workers shows that the result of routine work is fatigue, loss of concentration and appetite, and eventual loss of self-esteem. Besides neglecting yourself, it is almost inevitable that there will be times every day when you begin to feel that you have exhausted your resources and have a desperate need for a break. This is especially true for those of us who are on our own, whether by choice, through separation from a partner, or because our partners are uninvolved.* It is vital to pay attention to those feelings and find ways to take care of yourself. Continuous stress is not good for you —it puts you at risk for physical illness and psychological difficulties, such as depression. Taking care of your own needs is not only good for you but essential to your baby.

You might want to think about what kinds of things would help enable you to take a break. For example, you might ask a trusted friend or family member to take care of your baby for a short time while you

rest, exercise, read, take a relaxing bath or a walk, and/or enjoy social contacts. If there's no one around who can help in this way, you might take your baby or child along while visiting a neighbor or taking a walk.

When your baby or child is either napping or playing quietly, you may feel pressured to use that time to complete chores or work around the house. While this may feel satisfying in that it is productive and gets things done, there may be times when it would be better for you to rest or take care of your personal needs. (Dishes will get done later.)

MOTHERHOOD, WORK, AND CHILD CARE: CONFLICTING PRESSURES

All mothers have feelings—frequently mixed feelings—about spending time away from their babies. If we need to return to work (or school) soon after the baby's birth, we may feel relieved, or grief-stricken, or a combination of both. If we decide not to return to work for a while, or if we have never worked outside the home and don't plan to now, we may feel pleased because we are able to stay with our babies, or perhaps guilty about not contributing to the family income.

Besides dealing with your own and your family members' mixed and confusing feelings and messages regarding work and child care, you may also find yourself responding to changing and conflicting social pressures regarding these concerns. You may read conflicting points of view from highly regarded experts. In newspapers, you may read something about the horrors of poor day care one day, and the next day read about how well children in day care are doing (see "Child Care," p. 521).

If you can afford not to work outside the home for a while, and are trying to choose whether to return to work or stay at home for a time, it may be useful to talk to other mothers who have similar confused and mixed feelings, and to some who have made choices with which they are satisfied. It may also help to let family members know that such choices are not easy in a changing society, and that the best way they can help you is by listening and supporting your decision-making process—even if the ultimate decision is not the one they would have made.

If you have no choice but to return to work, you may find yourself feeling sad and/or angry at this situation. You may also worry about your baby and grieve the possibility of spending more time together when she or he is young. These feelings are normal, and accepting them may help you be able to seek resources and supports in choosing the best child care available for your baby. At work, you may find that you are not functioning as well as before maternity leave, or you are distracted by thoughts of your child or children. Try to establish ways of keeping connected with your baby while at work, such as a regular noontime phone call to the person caring for the baby.

* Many married women who are entirely responsible for the daily care of children live similar lives to those of single women, though they may have more money. Women who have distant or uninvolved partners may benefit from talking to single mothers about how they cope.

Even for women with good salaries, the transition is a challenge.

Going back, I told myself that I would be a new and better psychiatrist, because I have this new perspective on life . . . but that's also been hard, because I care so much about getting home. . . . It's probably going to be a year or so until I'm back to my old speed.

From a lesbian mother, whose partner gave birth:

Our daughter was born by emergency c-section at the start of a holiday weekend. I went back to work the very first working day. As the nonbiological mother, I was not permitted by my employer to take maternity leave. I felt lost and distracted. I normally saw my work role as a near total identity. But now, I had a daughter to care for. I was a mother with an infant sleeping in a cradle by my bed. I wanted nothing more than to sit and look at her and hold her. I had specifically read the chapters for new fathers in the books we had at home for new parents. Our baby slept in our room, so I was especially careful to get up quietly and shower and dress without noise. I was conscientious about straightening up, doing dishes, letting both members of my family sleep in, and washing bottles and making formula. The chapters all suggested that my partner needed my emotional support and help at home. I wanted to provide as much help as I could, but had to face the fact that I was away from them more than 40 hours each week. The chapters did not address the fact that I felt torn by the limits my work placed on my contact with my daughter. The chapters did not describe my sad feelings as I drove away from the house each morning. I really did not understand how men did it, leaving their partners and infants at home while they continued to interact with the world of work. I did not understand why men had not changed the work system to allow them to be home more with their families.

As it got closer to the time when I had to return to work, I kept wondering why no one had told me how hard it would be to leave my baby. I asked someone I thought of as wise, "Why didn't you tell me I would fall in love with my baby?" The wise person just shrugged, and said, "I thought you knew how you wanted to do things." There was no choice but to go back to work; I was earning most of the family income. But I just wasn't prepared for how wrenching it would be.

For some women, returning to work is a relief.

I loved my baby, but I was overwhelmed and distressed at home. My marriage was falling apart. I was desperate to go back to work, where I felt competent and in control. I counted the days till my maternity leave was over.

If you have chosen to stay at home, you may be worrying about whether your decision will be re-spected by others, whether you will be able to return to work at some future time, and whether you will continue to feel competent and capable in the world of work.

No matter what choices you make in a changing world, you are likely to have conflicting feelings or desires. There is no one best way to be a mother to your baby. Many different models lead to healthy babies and mothers. No one model is easy or perfect for every mother.

The real personal decisions and compromises involved in going to work while you have a baby at home are enough for any woman. Sometimes the baby is sick, some days she cries when you leave. But the tangle of guilts and shouldn'ts and dangers that have come to surround making that decision has just got to be cut away.

I'm a writer, and I've often done research for articles by tape-recording interviews on the telephone. When my son was about a month old, I thought I should be able to get back to my work during his naps. I began an interview with a well-known doctor, and my son immediately woke up and began to scream. I thought if I nursed him, he would quiet down. So there I was, trying to hold him and the phone and breast-feed and carry on the interview. The next thing I knew, the baby had thrown up on the tape recorder and shorted it out. Luckily, the doctor had seven kids and was very understanding.

I went back to work six weeks after my daughter was born. I remember the midwife saying to me, "You have your whole life to work; your baby will only be little for a short time. Why don't you just enjoy it and stay at home with her for a while?" She even suggested talking with my employer, but I was afraid of losing my job. I think now that I was overaccomodating. I wish I had waited longer before going back. Every morning when we are struggling to get out of the house by eight, I think, wouldn't it be wonderful to be able to stay home with my baby today? I really missed something by not waiting at least a few more weeks.

Designing Work Options

Most women work outside the home because they need to, in order to keep their families financially afloat. Many mothers of young babies are single, by choice or by circumstances they would not have chosen. Only a small percentage of women have partners whose incomes are sufficient to support a family. Additionally, half of us—one out of every two women—will be separated from a partner while we still have the responsibility for child support.* Single women and

* Only one in four noncustodial parents mandated by the court to pay child support is actually paying the full amount. (Arloc Sherman, *Wasting America's Future: The Children's Defense Fund Report on the Costs of Child Poverty.* Boston, MA: Beacon Press, 1994.)

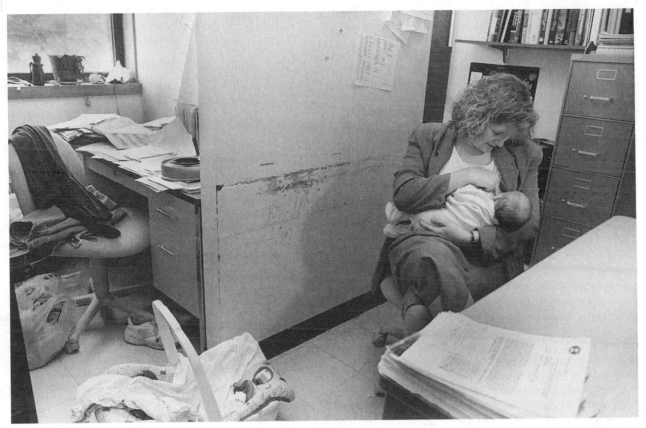

Linda Haas

lesbian couples have to face the fact that women earn only 76.4 cents* where men would earn one dollar. (For older women, the gap is greater; see chapter 23.) Most single mothers have no choice but to work or receive welfare.

Given the limits of the job market, women have been inventive when faced with the demands of wage-earning and child care. Some women have found jobs to do at home, such as computer programming, editing, catering, family day care, illustrating, typing. Some have learned to use existing work structures, such as working different shifts, so that they can share child care with a partner. Some women work part-time jobs that permit them to keep a foot "in both worlds." Women have taken the lead in developing workplace child care and demanding breast-feeding breaks (such

* "One of the reasons so many female-headed families with working mothers live in poverty is that, despite the substantial gains made by millions of women in the labor force, the ratio of women's medical weekly earnings to men's in 1994 was 76.4%. The majority of women still work in the lowest paid occupations—technical, clerical, service and sales jobs. In addition, ⅔ of all part-time workers are women, many holding more than one job. This frequently means they do not receive benefits from these jobs, no matter how many they hold." (Ruth Sidel, *Keeping Women and Children Last: America's War on the Poor.* New York: Penguin, 1996.)

breaks have been recommended by the International Lactation Organization for many years). Women have also helped in the design of newer employment options: flex-time, an arrangement that permits workers to come in quite early in the morning or much later in the day as long as they work their assigned number of hours; and job-sharing, which occurs when two people, both interested in part-time employment, share a single position.

Child Care

All mothers need to find child care sooner or later, whether it is for an afternoon off or for daily eight-to-six care. If you need child care, you have some choices about the kinds of arrangements to make. Depending on income and circumstances, you can call upon extended family, trade hours with other parents, form playgroups and parent cooperatives, or use private or publicly funded day care.

There is a big difference between what child care in this country could be and what it is, because it lacks financial support. The federal government has consistently refused to plan for or provide significant financial support to a national child care program. In addition, the meager financial support that was available under programs such as Aid to Families with Dependent Children is now contingent on parents being employed full-time, thus requiring the children to be cared for by others.

Research has shown that children can develop very well with more than one caregiver. Often, other caregivers can give them experiences that we could never offer. For example, children who have additional caregivers learn to turn to other adults, to get along with other children (if they are being cared for in group situations), to understand more fully the many roles women take on. Instead of asking "What do children lose when mothers work?" we must ask "What are the costs—to children, women, and society—when there is not enough good child care for all the families who seek it, and when most employers fail to respect or support the needs of mothers who are their employees."

Planning Ahead

To get a head start on child care, try to think during pregnancy what your child care needs are most likely to be during the first year: Will you be looking for occasional baby-sitting, part-time care, full-time care? If you work, find out from your employer or other workers about maternity leave (will it cost you seniority, vacation days, benefits?), taking sick days when your baby is sick, exemptions for working parents (some workplaces will give parents preference among shifts). Talk with your employer about your plans for returning to work.

Talk with other people you know who have children. Ask them what their child care needs were; how they met them; how they found good sitters, day care centers, or other forms of child care. Visit child care facilities: an infant day care center, a local baby-sitter, a family day care home. Talk to several people's favorite baby-sitters to find out what makes caring for someone else's child pleasant or difficult. These visits and conversations will give you a feel for the kind of child care you'll want to use. In addition, try to arrange friends or family members as reliable backup when you need to work and your child is sick, when your usual arrangements fall through, or in emergencies.

When to Start Day Care and How Often to Use It

Few women have the luxury of choosing when they return to work. Sadly, many women are under great pressure to arrange child care and prepare to return to work within six weeks of their baby's birth. This hardly allows time for mother and baby to establish routines and for mothers to master the new role. If you are fortunate enough to have a longer maternity leave, or to be able to choose the time of your return to work, we suggest staying at home for at least three to four months. This will let you get back on your feet and permit you to get to know your infant (babies begin to be much more responsive to faces, voices, and games about that time). If you are able to take a more ex-

QUESTIONS AND ANSWERS ABOUT LOOKING FOR CHILD CARE

What should I do if I need child care right away?

Even if you suddenly discover that you will need child care next week, don't panic. Try to visit a few providers and compare what you like and don't like about them. If you must, make temporary arrangements until you can find something permanent. Trust your instincts. If you choose child care in a hurry or decide on someone whom you feel uneasy about, there's a good chance it won't work out, and you'll have to start again.

How long in advance should I look for child care?

If at all possible, plan ahead. New parents can begin their child care search during pregnancy and make a final decision after the baby is born. Many child care programs enroll new children for September but are already filled up four to six months in advance. Year-round programs may also fill up fast. People who take care of children in their own homes may have waiting lists as well.

Will I find what I want?

Many communities just don't have enough child care to go around. Child care centers for infants and toddlers are especially hard to find, and they may have long waiting lists. Some types of care, such as family day care or playgroups, are not as "visible" or easy to find as centers. If you need financial assistance for child care, you may have to wait for an opening. A few forms of financial assistance are available to help eligible families pay for child care, including state-funded subsidy programs and tax credits. For more information, contact your local child care resource and referral agency.

You may also have to make some compromises: choosing a different type of care, looking outside your immediate neighborhood, paying more than you expected, or waiting awhile before you start using child care.

How do I know my child will be safe?

Many parents assume that because a child care center or family child care provider is licensed by the local or state licensing body, it must be good. You should always make sure that the program or provider you choose is licensed; however, licensing only sets minimum standards for health, safety, and the basic program. It is up to parents to make the final decisions about the quality of care and sensitivity shown to children.

Even if your best friend swears by a particular provider, it is not a guarantee that the provider is right for you and your child. Plan to visit and carefully check out all child care situations yourself. You know best what your child needs and enjoys.

Basic Questions

- Is the provider licensed? For what ages? For how many children?
- Is there an opening in your child's age group? If not, will an opening be available? Is there a waiting list?
- Is the location convenient for you to get to and from?
- What is the provider's fee? What does it include (e.g., meals, diapers, transportation, admission fee)? Will you have to pay tuition for days when your child is sick or on vacation?
- Does the provider offer any type of financial assistance for child care?
- Is the provider open during the hours you need child care? (Be sure to allow time for travel to and from the provider when deciding what hours you will need care.) If your schedule is unpredictable, is the provider flexible about drop-off and pick-up times?
- What is the yearly schedule? Is it a nine-month or a year-round program? Are there vacation weeks, holidays, and other times when the program will be closed? If the provider gets sick, is a backup person available?
- What is the policy for when your child is sick? Is the provider set up to care for sick children, or will you need to make your own arrangements? Will you need a doctor's okay for your child to be able to return to the program?

Once you have chosen a child care provider, your job isn't over. Both you and your child will need to develop and maintain a relationship with your provider. The provider will need your help to get to know your child and plan for your child's care. You will want to keep your child care provider updated on your child's home experiences and new achievements. In addition, you should try to be aware of your provider's needs and concerns. Remember, you and your provider are partners in helping your child learn and grow.

Once your child begins child care, visit often. Talk to your child's provider as often as possible. If you can, get involved in your child's center or home program. As a parent, you will probably visit your child care situation at least two times a day.

From *How to Select Child Care*, Child Care Resource Center, Inc., Cambridge, MA. Reprinted with permission.

tended leave and stay at home for a year or more, try to use child care at least occasionally before your baby is eight or nine months old: the age at which many infants become very frightened of strangers. Approach the task of finding child care with the understanding that children of different ages require different kinds of care. The quiet, calm care that was perfect for the first four months may be boring and frustrating for a child who is learning to walk.

There is the possibility of too much child care. Five days a week from 7 A.M. to 6 P.M. is a long time for anyone to be away from home. We believe that children need private time with people they know and love. Part of planning child care is providing time for parent and child to be together. If your schedule demands that you find care for such extended periods, plan times in the morning and evening when you can focus your attention and affection on your child. Alternatively, consider whether a family member or friend can pick up your child early on some days.

UNIVERSAL SUPPORT FOR MOTHERS AND BABIES

In this chapter, we have discussed many things: postpartum health care, breast-feeding, infant care, the transition to motherhood, coordinating work and motherhood and child care. Each woman and family should not have to face all the challenges and dilemmas of the postpartum time independently, as if there were no adequate models to follow or supports to guide the way. However, until there is universal, humane, high-quality care for mothers and babies, and until that care is a part of the fabric of everyday life, it will seem as if each family has to start from scratch. We conclude this chapter by proposing social changes that could make it easier for women to find their way through the transition to motherhood.

Major fundamental changes are needed before mothers and babies will be adequately nurtured and supported in the postpartum period. Such fundamental changes are unlikely to occur without loud and continuous protest from women and our advocates. We have to constantly recognize our rights and responsibilities to be proactive, to define our needs, and to ask questions in order to understand and evaluate the care offered to us. Society, in turn, must respond respectfully to women taking charge of our own care. The changes we are about to propose may seem to paint a picture of an unattainable ideal. But some of these changes have already affected scattered communities in the U.S., and in some parts of the world what we're working toward has become the norm.[10]

1. Communities must take responsibility for the provision of prevention-focused care, beginning with easy access to good health care and mental health care and effective health-focused education over the life span. Communities must provide easy access to prevention-focused health care and mental

health care, and health-focused education over the life span.

2. An effective social support network, providing both practical and emotional assistance, must be recognized as a critical preventive measure. This support should include assistance from family, friends, and neighbors, as well as from professional care providers and organized self-help groups.

3. Prevention-focused care and the social support network must become integral parts of a larger framework that will support women throughout the child-bearing period. This framework should include holistic perinatal care, exercise and nutritional guidance, options in childbirth education classes, humane childbirth practices, breast-feeding support, postpartum doulas, parenting education, new-mother-and-baby groups, and loss and grief groups.

4. The special needs of pregnant women and mothers with babies or young children must become a customary part of planning and design for parks, malls, libraries, airports, Laundromats, apartment buildings, shelters, and public transportation. For example, more public bathrooms should include facilities for changing babies' diapers. Malls should include areas for mothers to rest, breast-feed, and generally attend to their children's needs.

5. Employers must recognize that employees are also parents and enable them to fulfill both roles. This might require such measures as paid maternity and paternity leaves, flexible hours, equal pay for comparable work, and on-site child care (or assistance in arranging high-quality child care near the workplace), with encouragement for mothers to breast-feed and for parents to eat meals with their children during the day.

I don't find myself distracted [at work], except for the fact that I'm trying to pump milk for him during the daytime. During the morning, especially after a weekend together, I tend to get very engorged, and it's like having a full bladder. And it makes it very hard to think straight, and I get rushed, and a little irritable, and a little pressured. . . . I think that subtracts a little bit from my focus at work. . . . The bottom line is, you're making compromises and the thing that makes it possible is that my boss supports my doing that.

6. Child care must be subsidized and include enough spaces for families who want and need them. Child care workers must be respected as important professionals and paid as such. They should work only under the kinds of physical conditions, and for the number of hours, that permit them to be responsive and inventive caregivers.

Those of us who want to see all mothers and babies healthy, safe, and able to take on the responsibilities of our societies and our planet have much to do.

One day I thought about all the mothers in all the households: apartment buildings, one- and two-family houses, farmhouses, mobile homes, rented rooms. I thought of us at home alone with our children. I thought how if we were all to come out from inside those walls and see how many of us there were, talk about all we knew and what we needed, we would see how large the problem was and we would take action.

NOTES

1. Robin Lim, *After the Baby's Birth.* (See Resources, "Motherhood," below.)
2. La Leche League International, *The Womanly Art of Breastfeeding,* 5th ed. (New York: Plume, 1991).
3. Gail Brewer, ed., *The Pregnancy After Thirty Workbook* (Emmaus, PA: Rodale Press, 1978).
4. Murray Enkin et al., *A Guide to Effective Care in Pregnancy and Childbirth* (New York: Oxford University Press, 1995).
5. Jan Riordan and K. G. Auerbach, *Breastfeeding Human Lactation* (Boston: Jones and Bartlett, 1993).
6. Sheila Kitzinger, *The Year After Childbirth: Surviving the First Year of Motherhood* (New York: Charles Scribner's Sons, 1994).
7. Alice LoCicero, Dianne M. Weiss, and Deborah Issokson, "Postpartum Depression: Proposal for Prevention through an Integrated Care and Support Network," *Applied and Preventive Psychology* 6, no. 4 (fall 1997): 169–78; and Cheryl Tatano Beck, "A Meta-analysis of Predictors of Postpartum Depression," *Nursing Research* 45, no. 5 (Sept. 1996): 297.
8. Scott Stuart and Michael O'Hara, "Interpersonal Psychotherapy for Postpartum Depression: A Treatment Program," *Journal of Psychotherapy Practice and Research* 4, no. 1 (1995).
9. J. Belsky and J. Kelly, *The Transition to Parenthood: How a First Child Changes a Marriage, Which Couples Grow Closer or Apart, and Why* (New York: Dell, 1994).
10. Laurence D. Kruckman, "Rituals and Support: An Anthropological View of Postpartum Depression," in J. A. Hamilton and P. N. Harberger, eds., *Postpartum Psychiatric Illness: A Picture Puzzle* (Philadelphia: University of Pennsylvania Press, 1992), 137–48. Discussion of the kinds of supports for new mothers that have always been the norm in traditional societies. Some newer systems of community-wide supports have been instituted in cities, such as Seattle, Winnipeg, and Santa Barbara.

RESOURCES

(For more resources on parenthood and raising children, see the Introduction to Part Three, p. 266.)

Motherhood

Freidland, R., and L. Kort, eds. *The Mothers' Book: Shared Experiences*. Boston: Houghton Mifflin, 1981.

Kitzinger, Sheila. *The Year After Childbirth*. New York: Charles Scribner's Sons, 1994.

Lazarre, J. *The Mother Knot*. Boston: Beacon Press, 1986.

Lim, R. *After the Baby's Birth . . . A Woman's Way to Wellness*. Berkeley, CA: Celestial Arts, 1991.

Olds, Sally W. *The Working Parents' Survival Guide*. Rocklin, CA: Prima, 1989.

Exercise

Balaskas, J. *Active Birth: The New Approach to Giving Birth Naturally*. Boston: Harvard Common Press, 1992.

Noble, Elaine. *Essential Exercises for the Childbearing Year*. Harwich, MA: New Life Images, 1995.

Postpartum Disorders

Dix, C. *The New Mother Syndrome: Coping with Postpartum Stress and Depression*. New York: Pocket Books, 1985.

Dunnewold, A., and Sanford, D. *Postpartum Survival Guide*. Oakland, CA: New Harbinger Publications, 1994.

Kleima, K. R., and V. D. Raskin. *This Isn't What I Expected: Recognizing and Recovering from Depression and Anxiety After Childbirth*. New York: Bantam, 1994.

Panuthos, C., and C. Romeo. *Ended Beginnings*. South Hadley, MA: Bergin & Garvey, 1984. For an alternative spiritual approach, read the sections on postpartum issues.

Placksin, S. *Mothering the New Mother: Your Postpartum Resource Companion*. New York: Newmarket Press, 1994.

Romito, P. "Unhappiness After Childbirth," in I. Chalmers, M. Enkin, and M. J. N. C. Keirse, eds. *Effective Care in Pregnancy and Childbirth*. New York: Oxford University Press, 1989.

Breast-feeding

Eiger, Marvin S., and Sally Wendkos Olds. *The Complete Book of Breastfeeding*. New York: Workman Publishing, 1987.

Huggins, K. *The Nursing Mother's Companion*. Boston: Harvard Common Press, 1990.

Kitzinger, S. *The Experience of Breastfeeding*. New York: Viking Penguin, 1990.

La Leche League International. *The Womanly Art of Breastfeeding*, 5th ed. New York: Plume, 1991.

Pryor, K. *Nursing Your Baby*. New York: Pocket Books, 1991.

Raphael, D. *The Tender Gift: Breastfeeding*. New York: Schocken Books, 1976.

Baby and Child Care

Anderson, J. *The Single Mothers' Book: A Practical Guide to Managing Your Children, Career, Home Finances and Everything Else*. Atlanta: Peachtree Publishers, 1990.

Arthur, S. *Surviving Teen Pregnancy: Your Choices, Dreams and Decisions*. Bueno Park, CA: Morning Glory Press, 1991.

Brazelton, T. B. *Working and Caring*. Reading, MA: Addison-Wesley, 1992.

Comer, James P., and Alvin Pouissant. *Raising Black Children: Questions and Answers for Parents and Teachers*. New York: NAL/Dutton, 1992.

Sears, W., and Martha Sears. *The Baby Book: Everything You Need to Know about Your Baby from Birth to Age Two*. New York: Little, Brown, 1993.

Spock, B., and M. Rothenberg. *Dr. Spock's Baby and Child Care*. New York: NAL/Dutton, 1992.

Thevenin, T. *The Family Bed: An Age-old Concept in Child Rearing*. Wayne, NJ: Avery, 1987.

Weed, Susun. *Wise Woman Herbal for the Childbearing Year*. Woodstock, NY: Ash Tree Publishing, 1985.

Research and Policy-Oriented Resources

Murray, L., and P. J. Cooper. *Postpartum Depression and Child Development*. New York: Guilford Press, 1997.

Taylor, V. *Rock-a-by Baby*. New York: Routledge, 1996.

Women's Institute for Childbearing Policy. *Childbearing Policy within a National Health Program: An Evolving Consensus for New Directions*. Boston: Women's Institute for Childbearing Policy, 1994.

Organizations

Cochrane Neonatal Group
c/o Mrs. Diane Haughton, Coordinator
Dept. of Pediatrics; McMasters University;
1200 Main Street West; Hamilton, Ontario, Canada
L8N 3Z5
E-mail: <haughton@fhs.csu.mcmaster.ca>

This is the administrative office for the Cochrane group that prepares systematic reviews of "randomized controlled trials of interventions involving the baby during the first month after birth" and beyond "if they involve the later management of neonatal disease." (For more on Cochrane Collaboration, see box on "Evidence-Based Practice," chapter 25, The Politics of Women's Health and Medical Care, p. 710.)

The Marcé Society
Queen Margaret College; Clerwood Terrace, Edinburgh EH; 23-815 U.K.; (031) 339-0111, or c/o Michael O'Hara, Ph.D.; Dept. of Psychology; University of Iowa; Iowa City, IA 52242; (319) 355-2452

Write to them for organizations in other countries.

Postpartum Support International
927 North Kellogg Avenue; Santa Barbara, CA 93111;
(805) 967-7636
Web site: http://www.iup.edu/an/postpartum
  Write for a list of organizations dealing with postpartum in your area.

Additional Online Resources *

Family Q: The Internet Resource for Lesbian Moms and Gay Dads
http://www.studio8prod.com/familyq

Parentsplace: The Parenting Resource Center on the Web
http://www.parentsplace.com

Postpartum Education for Parents
http://www.marketmedia.com/pep

Pregnancy & Child Health Resource Centers
http://www.mayo.ivi.com/mayo/common/htm/pregpg.htm

* For more information and listings of online resources, please see Introduction to Online Women's Health Resources, p. 25.

Chapter 22

Child-bearing Loss, Infertility, and Adoption

By Catherine Romeo (Child-bearing Loss) and Diane Clapp (Infertility), with Mary Howell Raugust and Denise Bergman (Adoption), and Jane Pincus; based on earlier work by Norma Swenson (Adoption)

WITH SPECIAL THANKS TO Joan Rachlin, Ester Shapiro, Resolve, Inc., Joyce Maguire Pavao and Corinne Rayburn of the Center for Family Connection, and Marcie Richardson*

Many *of us* grow up dreaming of, playing at, and planning for the day when we will have and hold our own baby. The inner and outer forces that contribute to these dreams and desires are complex and powerful. For most women, wanting children feels like a primal need, and being unable to conceive or to carry a baby to term can be devastating. The death of a baby in or after childbirth is an immense and shocking loss. Other kinds of losses during pregnancy include miscarriage, the decision not to carry to term a baby with a fatal disease and, for many, conflicted feelings and sadness even after a chosen early abortion. These losses challenge us physically, psychologically, and spiritually. Cutting to the core of our identity as women, they challenge our assumptions about the course of our lives and our ability to control events, even about our capacities and worth.

* Thanks also to the following for their help with the 1998 version of this chapter: Libbi Campbell of Concerned United Birthparents, Deborah Issokson, Janna Zwerner Jacobs, and Kay Schlozman. Over the years since 1969, the following conributed to the many versions of this chapter: Barbara Eck Menning.

As a Cuban Jewish immigrant to the United States, I deeply transgressed my own family-based expectations that we would have our children in our early twenties, when I chose a professional path. Remarried at 40, I have since experienced five miscarriages, which I now view as caused by a history of chronic fatigue syndrome and an immunological reaction to the fetus. As part of my search both for fertility treatment and for a way of understanding the texture of my grief, I have explored the interwoven threads of emotional loss and of unyielding, accusing inner voices which tell me that, without my own baby, I will never prove that I am a "good woman" after all. This hard-won knowledge based on a profound sense of loss is a gift that has expanded my capacity to love and to give in the many relationships with children, students, and other loved ones which I cherish now more than ever.

Even the *threat* of loss has strong aftereffects:

I never comprehended what "powerless" or "vulnerable" really meant until I watched my tiny premie fighting for her life. The nightmare of those days casts a long shadow. I still struggle against trying to overprotect her, even though she's a sturdy four-year-old.

Community expectations and our particular cultural background affect the meaning of our experience of loss. For example, in some Latino communities, infertility—seen as only the *woman's* problem—is considered grounds for divorce.

After experiencing a terrible loss, we inevitably grieve, itself a first step in healing. Many people become crazed with grief and feel that it will never end; indeed, it can last for months and years, affecting us for the rest of our lives. Our society has few formal ways of dealing with losing a child. Planning some kind of ceremony may help acknowledge the occurrence. It is hoped that we will be able to use our energy, sorrow, anger, and determination to learn what happened, heal ourselves further, gain wisdom, and get on with life.

MISCARRIAGE

Miscarriage is the premature ending of a pregnancy, before the fetus or baby can live outside the womb. Even these days, many women have no idea that miscarriage is a fairly common event, occurring once in every five or six pregnancies—many before 12 weeks. **Early miscarriages can be nature's way of screening out future problems,** letting you know that something is preventing your pregnancy from developing as it should—that this pregnancy would not have been viable.

You cannot really prepare yourself for what happens until it occurs. A first miscarriage often comes as a cruel shock during the joyful time of early pregnancy.

When I found out I was pregnant, I danced around the house. My pregnancy was an easy one. My body was slowly and pleasantly changing. Because it was a conscious and well-thought-out decision to have a child, I felt free to revel in my pregnancy and motherhood. It was a special time. I mention all of this because it is partially by understanding the depth of the joy that one can understand the depth of the loss.

Miscarriage can begin when your cervix is still closed. You will experience cramping, spotting, or bleeding. Sometimes with bed rest the signs will disappear and nothing more will happen. Your health care practitioner may want to order blood tests to check your hormone levels. If they are declining, then a miscarriage is presumed. Ultrasound (see chapter 19, Pregnancy, p. 462) can confirm it as early as six weeks from your last period (ultrasound can detect the absence of fetal growth and heart movement, but be aware that its long-term effects on your ovaries are unknown). If the process continues, bleeding becomes heavy, cramps increase, and the cervix begins to dilate.

My husband held me and we cried together. The deepest and most obvious feeling was the sense of loss.

Almost as strong was the fear. We did not understand what was happening and why it was happening to us. . . . We were also frightened by the . . . look of what was pouring out of me. . . . It wasn't bad enough that we were losing our baby, but in the midst of all that pain we had to stay strong enough to deal with all that blood. Why hadn't anyone given us any preparation?

You may not believe what is happening. You may feel overwhelmed by helplessness as cramping and bleeding increase. Many women fear that they might bleed to death. You may decide to stay home for comfort, or feel more reassured going to a clinic or hospital.

The process may take just a while, or half a day—it can seem endless. The fetus, amniotic sac, and placenta, along with a lot of blood, may be expelled completely intact. You'll probably know when this is happening; it can be a scary and sad experience. If you are at home and can manage the difficult task of collecting fetus and afterbirth, put them in a clean container and bring them to a hospital-based laboratory for examination. Your efforts may possibly yield information about why you miscarried.

When everything in your uterus has been expelled, you will continue to bleed, but less and less. If you think you are bleeding too much or for too long a time, call your health care practitioner. Sometimes you bleed because fetal tissue remains in your uterus, preventing it from closing up. At that point your practitioner must perform a dilation and curettage (D&C) to clean it out, prevent infection, and enable healing to occur.

Sometimes a fetus dies in the uterus, remaining within for several months. You will know that this is happening because the signs of pregnancy cease. You may feel that something significant is occurring, but not know exactly what. Your breasts decrease in size; your womb does not grow any more. Sometimes there is spotting. Ultrasound and blood hormone level tests will verify your body knowledge. Practitioners will then perform either a D&C or induce labor if it happens later in pregnancy (see chapter 17, Abortion, p. 404). A miscarriage that occurs during the middle or third trimester of pregnancy can be much more traumatic and difficult than an early one.

Clinical terms (some now out-of-date) exist for different stages and kinds of miscarriages: "spontaneous," "threatened," "inevitable," "incomplete," "missed" or "septic" abortion, and for the fetus, "products of conception." Many women feel wounded or insulted when insensitive caregivers use these terms: "When my doctor coolly stated that I'd had an 'incomplete abortion of the products of conception' I wanted to scream, 'That's my *baby* you're talking about!' " Letting your health care practitioner know how you feel allows him or her to respond appropriately and to offer suggestions for further support. Medical caregivers are increasingly aware of the depth and broad spectrum of women's reactions and needs following pregnancy loss. You are entitled to be cared for by someone who has that awareness and sensitivity.

The days, weeks, and months following a miscarriage can be very difficult in all sorts of ways.

We went home from the hospital dazed and tired. I was weak and enormously sad. I don't know that I've ever experienced such deep emotional pain. The loss was so great and so complete in a way that only death is. For the first few days I couldn't talk to anyone, but at the same time it was painful to be alone. I would just cry and cry without stopping. One of the clearest reminders that I was no longer pregnant was all the speedy changes my body went through. Within two days my breasts, which had grown quite swollen, were back to their normal size. My stomach, which had grown hard, was now soft again. My body was no longer preparing for the birth of a child. It was simple and blatant. Tiredness was replaced with weakness. And then there was the bleeding. My body would not let me forget. I knew things would improve once we could make love again and would be even better when we were full of hope. But it seemed so far away.

You may still feel pregnant for a while, your breasts full and tender, your belly enlarged. You may want to get a blood test to determine that the hormones of pregnancy are back to zero. Spotting may continue for several weeks. If your flow increases, or if you have odd or foul-smelling discharge or a fever, contact your health care practitioner. After the bleeding has stopped and your cervix has fully closed again—some practitioners counsel four to six weeks—you can make love that includes penetration with no risk of infection.

Afterward, it can be helpful, although emotionally painful, to try to learn why the miscarriage occurred. Explanations for miscarriage are not easy to come by. Often, testing yields no satisfactory answers. It is your right to learn as much as possible. You may want to have both routine and specialized tests performed, such as cultures for infection and genetic studies of the tissue. Ask for the pathology report. Ask health care practitioners and technicians to fully explain all terminology. If the explanations don't satisfy you, see if further tests can be done. Some of the diagnostic procedures for infertility outlined in the following pages may prove useful. You may prefer not to have any tests; that is fine, too.

Causes

The most common causes of miscarriage are chromosomal abnormalities, infection, undue stress, hormonal imbalances, structural problems of the uterus, or weak cervical muscles. Environmental and industrial toxins can be responsible, as can autoimmune problems, sometimes related to chronic fatigue syndrome. In rare cases a woman will miscarry after certain tests during pregnancy, such as chorionic villi sampling (CVS) or amniocentesis. Blood incompatibility between Rh-negative mother and Rh-positive fetus (which the drug Rhogam prevents, making it a rarity in the Western world) can result in miscarriage.

If tests show that egg and sperm together have failed to divide as they should, this has probably been a random event and the chances of it happening again are small. If the fetal tissue shows genetic abnormalities, you'll work with your health care practitioner on how to proceed from that point. If the fetal tissue is normal, you may find that your hormone levels were insufficient or that your cervix was not strong enough to hold the pregnancy. Both of these conditions can probably be treated.

If you have had two or more miscarriages, you and your partner can get blood tests done to determine whether there is an immunologic cause for your pregnancy losses. These tests check for certain factors that affect blood clotting and for immune system problems.

One miscarriage does not mean that you have a fertility problem. There is a high (55 to 60%) chance that you will have a baby after two or three miscarriages. However, if more than two in a row occur, you may want to begin investigating, with your current health care practitioner, each detail of your next pregnancy. If you are feeling extremely concerned or have experienced more than three miscarriages, and you want help, seek a technically skilled, compassionate infertility specialist. Treatment for multiple miscarriages will vary according to your situation. (For more on specialists and treatment, see "Infertility," p. 531.)

Feelings

Miscarriage evokes myriad emotions. You and your partner may feel buffeted and torn by confusion, relief, shame, anger, sorrow, fear, powerlessness, or despair. Just about everyone feels grief and loss. Thoughtful compassion from family, friends, and health care practitioners is crucial.

Most people didn't know how to give me support and perhaps I didn't really know how to ask for it. People were more comfortable talking about the physical and not the emotional side of miscarriage. I needed to talk about both. It was also difficult for my husband, because people could at least ask how my body was doing. Unfortunately, he would sometimes be completely bypassed when someone called to talk with us, despite the fact that he, too, was in deep emotional pain.

As miscarriage is a physiological event happening to you, you may find that your feelings differ from your partner's in strength and in content, though you both, of course, will experience the loss. Grief may be mixed with guilt; both can cause tension between you. You may wonder if either of you did something "wrong" (too much activity, too much sex, not enough good food, etc.). Acknowledge and talk out your feelings as much as you can. Second- and/or third-trimester miscarriages can be supremely difficult. The effects of a miscarriage can last for months. You may feel a strong resurgence of grief on the date when your baby would have been born, perhaps for years to come.

The first time I got pregnant I miscarried after six weeks. Although I was told that the fetus was only the size of a grain of rice, I deeply grieved the loss. I remember nine months later feeling a deep sadness wash over me and finally I connected it with the fact that if I hadn't miscarried I would have been giving birth that month. My partner hid her grief and began a process of withdrawing from the pregnancy venture. It was just too painful for her to keep participating when the risk for repeated disappointment and loss was so high.

You might want to go through two or three menstrual cycles before you try to become pregnant again. Pregnancy after one or several losses can be terrifying —and also challenging. You will be better able to deal with the anxiety and tension if you have committed support from your partner, friends, and/or support group. If possible, talk with women who have had the same experience to learn how they managed the tension and fear, and then found the courage and optimism to try again.

At first we were stunned, then we were hurt, then we were numb. I have been talking with many women to find that this is a common occurrence that no one speaks of. Women need to be supported and educated about it. I feel like I can go into my next pregnancy with my eyes truly open. Ironically, I thought they already were. Chris and I are healing. He spent the weekend writing a song and I went to an alternative health conference on livestock. Our love for each other is stronger. With great joy, we will begin trying to get pregnant again in a month or so.

ECTOPIC PREGNANCY

Ectopic pregnancy is another form of pregnancy loss, in which the fertilized egg starts developing outside the uterus, usually in the fallopian tube. Between 5 and 10% of women who have had previous tubal surgery may experience ectopic pregnancy, but it can happen to any woman. Ectopic pregnancies are more common in women who have been exposed to DES (see chapter 24, Selected Medical Practices, Problems, and Procedures, p. 637). They are also more common in women who have pelvic inflammatory disease (PID). IUDs can cause scar formation in the tubes, increasing the likelihood of a fertilized egg getting stuck there, or inflammation of the uterine lining, which then "resists" implantation of the fertilized egg. Ectopic pregnancy can be a life-threatening condition that requires immediate treatment. If the tube ruptures, you may experience severe blood loss and go into shock. Because the hormonal changes are similar to those of a normal early pregnancy, you can have all the early signs of pregnancy, such as fatigue, nausea, missed period, and breast tenderness. Abnormal vagi-

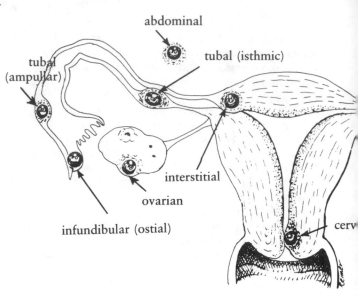

An ectopic pregnancy/Nina Reimer

nal bleeding is a common symptom of ectopic pregnancy. As the pregnancy progresses, causing pressure in the tube, symptoms such as stabbing pain, cramps, or a dull ache may become severe. Neck and/or shoulder pain mean that an ectopic pregnancy has ruptured and there is blood in the abdominal cavity. With good medical care, it is not common for the condition to progress to this point.

Diagnosing an ectopic pregnancy can be tricky. If you suspect something is wrong, ask your practitioner to check your hormonal levels every other day and do a vaginal ultrasound as early as possible to see if there is an embryonic sac in the uterus or tube. Ectopic pregnancy is sometimes misdiagnosed as an early miscarriage. Thus, a blood (pregnancy) test should always be done after a suspected miscarriage to make sure no fetal tissue is present in the tube. It is essential to check any tissue passed from the uterus and to make sure that your hormone levels have returned to zero, to confirm or to rule out ectopic pregnancy.

When the doctor detects an ectopic pregnancy early enough, she or he makes every effort to remove the pregnancy and save the tube. Increasingly often, physicians are using the anticancer drug methotrexate to dissolve embryonic tissue, administering it intravenously or intramuscularly, or injecting it into the tube. Another alternative is a laparascopy, which is generally preferable to major abdominal surgery. Sometimes it becomes necessary to remove the whole tube (in the past, the ovary used to be removed also). Careful surgical technique is important; the less bleeding and consequent adhesions and scar tissue, the better the chance for a normal pregnancy later. Having one tubal pregnancy may increase the chance of another.

It is natural to experience all the feelings that result from a miscarriage, including depression and fright that it could happen again. In addition, you may have had internal bleeding and undergone the trauma of an emergency surgical operation. This experience may change your outlook about future pregnancies. Supportive friends and/or a more structured women's support or pregnancy loss group can help you air and ease your feelings.

STILLBIRTH

Stillbirth means that your baby has died, either *in utero* before labor, or during labor. It is a relatively rare occurrence, which has many causes. But if it happens to you, statistics mean nothing. Your body knows nothing about stillbirth. You are elaborately prepared for the close contact and physical nurturing of your baby. Your breasts are filled with milk, never to be used. (In some cultures, women who lose babies at birth act as wet nurses, nurturing other mothers' babies. They are highly esteemed.) You and your family are ready for the arrival of a new baby, not for a tragic loss.

If you do suffer a stillbirth, the following suggestions can help. If the baby's death takes place before labor and delivery, delivery in the quickest and least hazardous way possible is desirable. You should have the chance to decide whether you want to go into labor spontaneously. Your partner should be present as long as either of you wish. Once the baby has been delivered, birth attendants should handle her or him in a reverent manner and must be especially sensitive if you are planning an autopsy (to find the cause of death). You will decide whether you want to see the baby, either immediately or later on. Many parents hold their babies for as long as they wish, name them if they haven't already done so, and take photos. You and your family must be allowed to grieve in privacy if you need and want to. Hospital personnel should be told that you have lost your baby and offer you a room away from the nursery.

You may need to withdraw at first and not confront a reality that may be too much to bear. You may feel entirely numb. If you ask for help in grieving, we hope those around you will offer it intelligently and humanely, listen empathetically, and comfort you physically if you want that. Platitudes such as "You'll have another baby before you know it" or "Think of your wonderful children at home" have no place in this situation. You are experiencing the death of *this* particular child—no one else will ever replace this baby.

It is important for many families to understand exactly what happened. Most likely, whatever happened was totally beyond your control or the doctor's. (If you do suspect malpractice by your doctor, seek legal counsel and have the facts analyzed.)

A tremendous void and sense of loneliness follow stillbirth, as with all pregnancy loss. Planning a funeral, burial, or memorial service may be an important step in acknowledging your loss. Giving to a favorite charity in your baby's name, or planting a tree, may be something you want to do. During the weeks, months, and even years to come, you may continue to feel very alone in your grief. Your partner and other children in the family will be also dealing with their feelings and with the upset in the household. If you live alone, reach out to others who have experienced and recovered from the loss of a child. They can point out paths to healing. If you do not know anyone to whom this has happened and if no support groups exist in your area, resources are available that may help. Books in which other parents tell the stories of their losses can help you to feel less alone and more sane.

All forms of pregnancy loss shake us to the roots of our beings, thwarting one of our most basic biological instincts: the instinct to protect one's child, born or yet unborn. Today, there is much more understanding of this loss and compassionate guidance for those who experience it. We owe it to ourselves and our loved ones to find the education and support we need to heal.

INFERTILITY

Many people are surprised to learn that *infertility* (the malfunctioning of a man's or woman's reproductive system) is fairly common. It may be a temporary or a permanent condition, depending on the cause and on available treatments. More than 5 million people of child-bearing age in the U.S. experience infertility, including about 8.5% of people in their child-bearing years. In 40% of these cases, male factors are responsible; in 40%, female factors are responsible; in 10%, combined factors are responsible, and 10% are unexplained.

You may *feel* "infertile" when you do not become pregnant after trying for one or two years, or when you have had several miscarriages in a row. (Infertility also takes the form of *repeated miscarriage* or *stillbirths*. In these instances, the problem is not conception but an inability to carry a pregnancy to live birth.)

We can look upon infertility as a *state* or a *condition*. In the early 1990s, both the American College of Obstetricians and Gynecologists (ACOG) and the American Society for Reproductive Medicine classified infertility as a *disease*. Such a classification enables insurance companies to cover certain procedures. Otherwise, out-of-pocket costs can become prohibitively expensive. Physicians define infertility as the inability to conceive after a year or more of well-timed sexual intercourse or insemination. Some women in their late 30s start infertility testing after six months. A woman's fertility begins to drop in her mid- to late 30s and declines even more significantly after the age of 40.

Myths About Infertility

It used to be believed that infertility was "the woman's problem," but that is just not so—man and woman must be diagnosed and treated together. Obviously, if it is the man's problem, treating the woman alone has no value and involves many needless, painful, expensive tests. A man, because of his anatomy, is easier to diagnose: Semen analysis is one of the logical tests to perform first. However, some men refuse to admit that there might be something "wrong" with them.

Another myth is that infertility is not treatable. In fact, 50% of people treated for infertility are able to become pregnant!

Feelings

For most women and their partners, infertility is a major life crisis.

I have always had regular periods. In fact, I used to worry about getting pregnant. I can't believe we have been trying for 10 months to get pregnant and now we can't.

I am 39 years old; finally my life is settled enough to start having a family. Imagine my horror when the doctor did a blood test and told me that even though I had regular menstrual periods my ovarian function was poor, that I was premenopausal, and that my chances of getting pregnant and not miscarrying were low.

I, like every other woman in this society, always believed that I would have children without any problems—as many as I wished and when I decided it was the right time. Unfortunately, after four years of trial and error, tests, operations, et cetera, my husband and I are realizing that life does not always happen the way we plan it. I have found it quite hard dealing not only with our infertility problem but also with the reactions of people around me. I'm sick of people telling me to "relax," "stop thinking it out," "adopt and you'll get pregnant," and all the other wonderful cliches that, although said to be comforting, ring of insensitivity. Friends and family can never possibly know the pain that I feel inside, the anger and resentment I feel every time I see a woman walking down the street with a big belly. How could they understand? How can anyone capable of having children understand?

Initial reactions of shock and denial are common. Sometimes you put your life on hold as you postpone changing jobs, going back to school, and so on because "six months from now you will be pregnant."

I quit teaching five years ago to become pregnant. When that did not happen, everyone wanted to know what I could possibly be doing at home all day if I didn't have kids. Neither a mother nor a career woman, I stayed in limbo because I kept thinking, Maybe it will happen **this** month! *I was drifting, and it is hard to believe so much time has gone by with just this single purpose in mind.*

I always felt in control of my life and body. Now nothing feels in control. I live month to month, period to period. I can't stop medical treatment, because after all this effort how can I walk away empty-handed, defeated?

It may be difficult to spend time with your friends' children. Feelings of envy, jealousy, and "why them and not me?" are common. Because holidays are so child-centered, they can become stressful, lonely, depressing times for you. You may feel isolated from friends and your mate, if you have one. You may each react differently to the infertility crisis.

My husband is disappointed with our failure to conceive, but he could easily accept a child-free life. He says he understands my feelings and sympathizes but doesn't care to hear any more about the subject. His view is "play the cards dealt you"—you go on about your business no matter what. His disappointment is mitigated by involvement in a job he likes and other alternatives. I have not found a satisfactory alternative.

Anger, too, is natural—but where and toward whom to direct it? We want, we need to find reasons. You may feel that something you did in the past caused your present inability to conceive. Could past abortions (even though properly performed), drug or alcohol use, masturbation, or unusual sex practices have caused this form of "punishment"? These experiences do not cause infertility, but we scapegoat ourselves into believing it and then feel terribly guilty. Depression, sadness, and despair are common.

What infertility seemed to do to me was to force a kind of confrontation with lifelessness or death. The fact that there would be no children meant that I was the last line of offense against death. Nobody to carry on who was living. The solution: Disconnect. So I numbed out. I invested back into work, which in the culture has been man's traditional way to combat mortality. If your work lives on, you haven't been wasting your time; there's a purpose to your life.

I grew up surrounded by the idea that if you were willing to work or study hard and always did your best, nothing was beyond your grasp. Generally I have found this to be true. The theory fell apart when I began to deal with my infertility problems. Not only did I become very depressed, but without the help of a friend of mine who shares the same problem, I seriously doubt whether my marriage would have remained intact.

It is only through a great deal of pain and anguish that I have begun to accept the idea that I may never have children. After the initial shock wore off, my husband and I became closer than ever.

Getting Started

You may want to begin learning about infertility, especially from women who have already experienced diagnoses and treatments. They can supplement the information you receive from your physician, and, as important, they know firsthand about feelings and resources, so that you won't flounder or feel abandoned.

Alternative (nonmedical) treatments such as acupuncture, herbal medicine, and relaxation techniques may help you feel and cope better and may also improve your chances of becoming pregnant.

Finding a Physician Who Specializes in Infertility

Your current practitioner, partner, close friends, or an infertility support group can help you find physicians. The most qualified specialists are *reproductive endocrinologists,* obstetrician-gynecologists trained for two additional years in the field of infertility.

It is *crucial* to have a good relationship with your physician, and important for all of your caregivers to be aware of your strong emotions, to respect your mind and body, and to make themselves available when you need them. Clinicians vary greatly in their approach to problems. Ask your physician for her or his track record and expectations. She or he should be willing to assist you in seeking insurance coverage. All of your caregivers should explain words and procedures patiently so that you fully understand them. It may take a while, since you are learning a whole new language and you are under stress. It helps to bring a list of questions to each appointment and to ask your partner or a friend to accompany you for support and clarity. If you don't like your doctor's methods or attitudes, go elsewhere. Confer with a second, even a third, though this may be more difficult in an HMO.

Medical practitioners often use terminology that is hurtful and even blaming in its tone: "hostile cervical mucus," "habitual abortion," "incompetent cervix," and "blighted ovum" do not show any understanding of how difficult infertility or child loss can be.

Causes of Infertility

Fertility is based on several physiological events and their timing. There must be a sufficient quantity of viable sperm and the presence of a mature egg. Sperm must be deposited in your vagina and move upward through cervical mucus to meet the ovum (egg) while it is still in the tube. Timing of intercourse or insemination is important, since an ovum may live as little as 12 or 24 hours, a sperm as little as one or two days. Once the sperm and ovum join and divide to become an embryo, this new organism must implant properly in the uterine lining and proceed to grow. An infertility work-up tests all the links in this chain of events in an orderly way.

CHANGING DIAGNOSES AND TREATMENTS

It is crucial to know that the field of infertility is evolving rapidly. As drug companies, hospitals, and physicians introduce new technologies and drugs into medical practice, the means for determining causes of infertility and the various types of treatments will change. New causes of infertility will be discovered as our environment becomes more toxic. Names and kinds of drugs change rapidly. New techniques and treatments appear regularly; few are studied in a controlled, randomized fashion. Some procedures are tried and true, and others are experimental. Practitioners will agree about the efficacy of some drugs and procedures and differ about others. You have a right to know whether your treatment is new, or part of an experimental study. You also have the right to know about the side effects of each and about the amount of time and money that will be required by diagnosis and treatment. Try to learn about the latest, least invasive, and least taxing treatments. Remember, you can stop whenever you want.

A Man May Experience Infertility Because of

1. *Problems of production and maturation of the sperm.* These can be caused by previous infection, such as mumps after puberty; undescended testicles; chemical and environmental factors; drugs; occupational hazards. Taking hot saunas and baths can cause overly high temperatures in the scrotal sac—affecting sperm production for up to a few months. In addition, a varicocele (a varicose vein in the scrotum) can affect sperm production.

2. *Problems with the movement (motility) of the sperm.* These may be due to chronic prostatitis and abnormally thick seminal fluid. In addition, certain drugs used to treat emotional disorders, stomach ulcers, and hypertension can affect sperm production and motility.

3. *Problems of transport* resulting from scar tissue in the delicate passageways through which the sperm travel; they may be caused by infections or untreated STD. (Intentional blockage is accomplished by vasectomy.)

4. *Inability to deposit the sperm into the cervix,* caused by sexual dysfunction, such as impotence or premature ejaculation, as well as by structural problems in the penis; for example, when the opening is on either the top or the underside of

the penis instead of at the tip. Spinal cord injuries and various neurological diseases can also contribute to this problem.

5. *Other factors* affecting male fertility, such as poor nutrition and poor general health. Marijuana, cigarette smoking, and alcohol if taken in excess can affect sperm quality. Some researchers recommend that men seeking to improve their fertility eat well and take zinc, vitamin C, and vitamin E.

A Woman May Experience Infertility Because of

1. *Mechanical barriers* preventing the union of the sperm and ovum, caused by scarring in the tubes or around the ovaries. Scarring can result from previous PID or pelvic surgery, from infection caused by certain IUDs, or from an abortion that was not properly performed or followed up on. An untreated STD, such as gonorrhea or chlamydia, can also cause scarring and tubal blockage.

2. *Endometriosis* (see chapter 24, Selected Medical Practices, Problems, and Procedures, p. 641) which can cause scarring, tubal blockage, and possible immune responses.

3. *Endocrine problems.* Failure to ovulate regularly or irregular menstrual periods may be caused by a malfunction of the ovaries, pituitary, hypothalamus, thyroid, or adrenal glands. Several specific hormones are secreted at specific times in the normal menstrual cycle. If any one of these is not produced, or is produced in insufficient quantity, the whole cycle can be thrown off. An excess of androgens, including DHEA, may be made by the ovaries and the adrenals. In addition, irregular ovulation decreases the chances of conception, as women cannot count on a consistent cycle with a known fertile time. Women often develop amenorrhea (absence of menstrual periods) following significant weight loss, strenuous exercise, or periods of high stress. The "post-pill syndrome"—seeming to have problems getting pregnant after taking birth control pills—is in question, as an ovulatory problem may have existed even before a woman used the pill. However, women who have irregular periods or who are older when they start their first menstrual periods do seem to be more prone to this (presumed) syndrome. (See chapter 12, Understanding Our Bodies, for more on the hormones of the menstrual cycle.)

4. *Structural problems in the uterus or cervix* due to congenital problems or DES exposure *in utero* is one cause of infertility.

5. *Polycystic ovarian disease,* a complex syndrome usually characterized by lack of regular ovulation, ovaries with multiple cysts, and sometimes extreme overweight. Elevated male hormones may result in increased body hair (hirsutism). You may also have a problem with increased blood sugar levels.

6. *Cervical mucus* that is too thick or too acidic acts as a barrier to the normal movement of the sperm up into the vagina. You can use litmus paper to test the acidity of your midcycle mucus. Some women douche with baking soda 30 minutes before intercourse to change the acidity of cervical mucus. Do not douche if the mucus is alkaline. Infections, such as T-mycoplasma, may cause infertility by changing the quality of cervical mucus and possibly causing early miscarriage.

7. *Immunological response.* You, your partner, or your donor may have sperm antibodies that tend to destroy the sperm's action by immobilizing them or causing them to clump. In some cases, miscarriages are caused by immunological responses. Blood tests can check for this possibility.

8. *Age-related factors.* After age 35, there is a gradual decline in the ability of the ovaries to produce good quality eggs that can be fertilized and become embryos. This decline is more dramatic after age 40.

9. *Other factors,* such as genetic abnormalities, extreme weight loss or weight gain, excessive exercise, poor nutrition, and environmental and industrial toxins, may affect a woman's fertility.

10. *Lack of familiarity with techniques that help to achieve pregnancy.* You may need more information in order to know when you are fertile, how often to make love or inseminate during this time, or what to do to make pregnancy more possible both before and after insemination or making love.

Infertility and planned sex can affect your sexual life. Spontaneity in lovemaking decreases. You have to plan your sex life around your menstrual cycle; it becomes less an act of loving and pleasure and more a medical routine. Recording the time of your sexual relations on a temperature chart may make you feel as if nothing is private or sacred in your life anymore!

I started with the temperature charts. This was quite taxing for me and mentally depressing. I felt very regulated and calculating, both with my own body and in my relationship with my husband. I need not say what it did to our natural sexual impulses. But a child at all cost—this was how we felt.

I was incredibly preoccupied with getting pregnant. Our sperm donor lived 2,000 miles from us and I had an irregular cycle, so there were major logistical hassles to surmount. It became difficult for us to plan

FINDING YOUR FERTILE TIME, AND TECHNIQUES TO HELP ACHIEVE PREGNANCY

If your menstrual cycle is regular, whether it be long or short, you will probably ovulate 14 days (give or take 24 hours either way) before the beginning of your next period. Using fertility awareness techniques (see chapter 13, Birth Control, p. 305), ovulation predictor kits, or basal body thermometer charts, you can determine your most fertile times and have intercourse or inseminations then. You can get a basal body temperature chart from a health care practitioner or from your nearest Planned Parenthood. If you are ovulating normally, from the time of your last period until ovulation you'll have a fluctuating, low temperature (about 98°F or less). About the time of ovulation there's often a dip followed by a rise of 0.6 degrees above baseline, or higher. Some cycles show just a rise but no preceding dip. Once your temperature rises, your fertile time is over. This higher plateau (usually about 98.4°F) is maintained until the day before your next period, when it drops again. You will have to chart your temperature for at least three cycles to find out your ovulation pattern. Or, you can buy a urine test kit from a pharmacy. With the urine test kit you can monitor the amount of luteinizing hormone (LH) in your urine. When the level of LH rises, ovulation usually occurs in the next 24 to 36 hours.

Spacing your lovemaking during this period is important. A man's sperm production decreases if he ejaculates too often, so you should have intercourse or inseminate every 24 hours to keep active sperm in your reproductive tract during your fertile time. It is wise for men to ejaculate two days before this three-day period to stimulate sperm production.

The most effective position for intercourse will be with your partner above and facing you with a folded towel under your hips to raise them. If you are having insemination, also use a folded towel for the same reason. (If your uterus is tilted back, use three or four pillows.) Avoid lubricants, such as jellies, creams, and even saliva. Unless your cervical mucus is too acidic, don't douche immediately before or after intercourse or insemination. If lubrication is necessary, egg white or vegetable oil is the safest choice. Penetration should be as deep as possible, and in intercourse when he reaches orgasm he should stop thrusting and hold quite still, deep in your vagina. Approximately 60 to 70% of the sperm are contained in the first part of the ejaculate.

Since it usually takes only a few minutes for sperm to move through the cervical mucus up to the uterus and fallopian tubes, it is a good idea to stay on your back for about ten minutes.

trips or weekends away, as it seemed like I was always waiting for the stick to turn blue, which would be my signal that it was time to inseminate. She and I stopped kissing good morning in bed because I had a glass basal body thermometer in my mouth. Our morning ritual of breakfast and reading the newspaper changed, as I spent mornings on the phone with the sperm bank or Federal Express because of a sperm shipment. My partner and I became more and more disconnected, and I felt ever more lonely with my quest.

My husband woke me every morning at 6 A.M. so that I could take my temperature. Afterward, he charted it. I needed his involvement.

Diagnosis

During diagnosis (and treatment), keep in mind that you should stay in good health, eat well, and take vitamins containing folic acid (see chapter 19, Pregnancy, p. 444), because it *is* possible that you may become pregnant.

A complete infertility work-up can take six to 12 months. Many tests have to be scheduled at specific times in your cycle and can't be combined. Most tests for women are invasive, painful, often undignified, and emotionally exhausting. Work-ups are expensive, and unfortunately medical insurance coverage is either poor or nonexistent. Some states now have laws mandating insurance coverage for infertility. (See Resolve's "Infertility Insurance Advisor," a booklet offering tips on working with your insurance provider.)

Though the sequence of diagnostic tests may vary with different doctors or clinics, it should include some or all of the following:

1. *A general and medical history of both man and woman.* Your doctor will ask about your menstrual history, including the onset and pattern of your menstrual periods; details about any previous pregnancies, episodes of STD, or abortions; your use of birth control; DES exposure; sexual relations (frequency and position); where you live and whether your job exposes you to any toxins that may affect your reproductive system; lifestyle habits, such as stress, nutrition, smoking, or drinking. Before starting your infertility work-up, have a toxoplasmosis screening, and have tests done for chicken pox (varicella), German measles (rubella), and HIV.

2. *A gynecological examination,* to check your uterus and ovaries, your breasts, and your general development.

3. *Monitoring ovulation.* You will take your basal temperature daily or use a urine test kit to record ovulation patterns.

4. *Hormonal profile.* You will need to have blood tests to check your thyroid levels, as well as levels of follicle stimulating hormone (FSH), luteinizing hormone (LH), estrogen, progesterone, and prolactin. If you have oily skin, acne, or a moderate amount of facial hair, your testosterone level should be checked. Estrogen and FSH blood levels are important to check if you are over 35 years old, to assess ovarian function and the ability of the ovaries to produce eggs of good quality. High FSH levels on day two or three of your cycle may indicate that your chances of pregnancy will not be good.

5. *Semen analysis.* The man will be asked to ejaculate semen into a clean container. It is important that the full ejaculation be collected, usually 1 to 5 cubic centimeters. It must be kept at body temperature and examined microscopically as soon as possible to determine sperm count and motility. A count of over 20 million sperm per cubic centimeter is considered in the normal range; below 10 million per cubic centimeter is considered poor. Yet, men with low sperm counts *can* sometimes impregnate a woman. The sperm must be able to swim in a forward motion and at least 60% should be normal in size and shape. The lab will also look for white blood cells in the sample that could indicate an infection.

If either the motility or the shape of the sperm is abnormal, there are additional tests such as the strict morphology *(Kruger test),* and the *penetration test,* which determines whether the sperm has the capacity to fertilize a specially prepared hamster's egg. Practitioners do not agree about what constitute acceptable percentages of normal forms of sperm.

Because a man's sperm can fluctuate in count and motility for many reasons, he may be asked to repeat the semen analysis at least every six months. If the result is abnormal, your male partner or sperm donor should pursue his own diagnosis before you have further tests done. If you decide to use an anonymous donor, check with the American Society of Reproductive Medicine for a list of reputable sperm banks, and also contact Resolve for its publication "Questions to Ask About Sperm Banks." For more on donor insemination, see chapter 18, Assisted Low-Tech and High-Tech Reproductive Technologies.

You may face a diagnosis of male infertility.

My husband's sperm count was very low; we were both crushed. I don't think my husband believed it was actually happening. In fact, he often talked in the third person, not truly accepting the results. I love him and therefore hurt for him. I didn't know what to say. I couldn't say the typical, "Oh, it's all right," because we both knew it really wasn't all right.

If all male factors are normal, you can choose whether or not to continue with the following tests or procedures, some of which take place in hospitals with radiology facilities; others in physicians' offices or clinics. Remember that you can always say no to a specific test or treatment.

6. *A postcoital test (Sims-Huhner test).* (Some practitioners no longer perform this test, for if the timing is off, it can yield an inaccurate—thus misleading—reading.) Just before you expect to ovulate, you will make love with your partner, inseminate yourself, or be inseminated, and within several hours go to your doctor's office without washing or douching. She or he will take a small amount of mucus from your vagina and cervix to look for live, active sperm. A normal test result shows that sperm have the ability to penetrate cervical mucus and live in this environment. A *sperm antibody test* on both partners' blood, sperm, and cervical mucus may be done if the postcoital test shows immobilized or clumped sperm cells.

7. *A uterotubogram, or hysterosalpingogram.* This test provides visualization of the tubes, establishing a permanent record to use for comparison if future X rays are needed. Doctors perform this procedure before ovulation to prevent possible X-ray exposure of a fertilized egg if conception has occurred (however, whenever you have X rays, you are irradiating all future eggs).

A radio-opaque dye is injected into the vagina and uterus. The dye should pass up through the uterus to the tubes and out into the pelvic cavity, later to be absorbed. A series of X rays is taken during this process. This test can be *very* painful, as the dye produces cramping. The practitioner should give you local cervical anesthesia or an oral medication to help you relax before this test. Taking ibuprofen 30 minutes beforehand can help reduce the pain, as can deep breathing and relaxation techniques. Many clinics give women antibiotics for two to three days before or after the test, to make sure no infection develops. Pregnancy rates are slightly increased in cycles immediately following this test, perhaps because of the dye "cleaning out" any mucus shreds in the fallopian tubes.

8. *An endometrial biopsy.* This test determines whether you are ovulating and whether your uterine lining is thick enough for embryo implantation. It is not done if you might be pregnant, as it could cause a miscarriage. Make sure that it is done after day 21 in your cycle but before you start your period. (Many think that taking such a minute piece of tissue presents no danger to a fetus. Others

avoid possible hazard to a pregnancy by having the woman come in on the day her temperature drops or even at the time her period starts. Some doctors advise using a condom during relations in this cycle so there will be no worry over disturbing a possible pregnancy.)

The doctor inserts a small instrument into your uterus after partially dilating your cervix (this will cause painful cramping), scrapes a tiny piece of tissue from the lining of the uterus (endometrium) and sends it to be examined microscopically. Tissue formed while progesterone is being produced (after ovulation) is different from tissue formed under the influence of estrogen (before ovulation) or in the absence of any hormonal influence.

9. *Laparoscopy.* One of the final infertility tests, laparoscopy allows direct visualization of the tubes, the ovaries, the exterior of the uterus, and the surrounding pelvic cavities. It is the only test that can establish endometriosis. Performed under spinal or general anesthesia, usually on an outpatient basis, it can yield a great deal of information. In laparoscopy, a tiny incision is made near your navel. Carbon dioxide gas is used to inflate the abdomen and allow good visualization of the pelvic organs. Sometimes a dye is flushed through the fallopian tubes to see whether they are open. If endometriosis or scar tissue is found, it can often be removed during the procedure. A *hysteroscopy* may be done at the same time or as a separate office procedure (a small fiberoptic instrument is inserted through the cervix to view inside the uterus). If scar tissue or polyps are present, they can sometimes be removed using the hysteroscope.

In addition to the stress of going for tests and treatments, you may be subject to other pressures at home and at work. Relatives may ask you, "Well, has it happened yet?" Or, worse, they don't say anything, but they look at you and sigh a lot. People you hardly know may comment on your problem. Trying to work and find time to get these tests scheduled is difficult. Many women don't want their bosses to know about their infertility, and that adds yet another pressure: secrecy. When you are going through these tests, once again your sex life comes under scientific scrutiny.

We were supposed to make love at seven o'clock in the morning and then I had to run to my doctor's for the postcoital test. Who feels like making love at seven in the morning during a busy week anyway?

Hopefully, during these hard times, you and your partner can support each other and try to maintain a fulfilling, intimate sex life despite the need to time sex according to your fertile periods. A sense of humor helps.

Treatment

Sometimes, diagnostic procedures result in success, as when, for example, the hysterosalpingogram clears your tubes. In 90% of cases, a reason is found for infertility. At this point, you and your doctor should outline a treatment plan.

Drugs

For women, doctors use a variety of drugs to correct hormonal imbalances, help induce ovulation, and correct problems after ovulation (in the luteal phase). It is important to understand how these drugs work, how they affect you, and how long you should use them. (See chapter 25, The Politics of Women's Health and Medical Care, p. 713, for more information on the informed use of drugs.) The long-term safety of many of these drugs has not been adequately studied, though some good national studies are now under way. Be aware that trade names for these drugs may change.

The drugs used to induce ovulation include clomiphene citrate; human chorionic gonadotropin (hCG, brand name Profasi), a hormone extracted from the human placenta; and human menopausal gonadotropin (hMG, brand names Pergonal and Humegon) extracted from the urine of menopausal women; and a subcutaneous form of pure FSH (brand names Fertinex, Repronex, and Gonal F).

Clomiphene citrate is taken orally, often on the fifth to the ninth day of the cycle. It appears to act directly on the hypothalamus in the brain and causes it to produce more of the hormones FSH and LH, which then stimulate the ovary to ripen and release an egg. About 80% of women will ovulate with the help of this drug, and about 50% of women under 40 will become pregnant, with a 5 to 10% incidence of multiple births. Many women experience mood swings, breast tenderness, hot flashes, headaches, blurred vision, and throbbing feelings in the ovaries at the time of ovulation while they are taking this drug. It can cause the midcycle cervical mucus to dry up, and thins the uterine lining in some women, so request a postcoital test and an endometrial biopsy if you are taking clomiphene for three or more cycles. A potential complication is enlargement of the ovary, which, if undetected, may result in ovarian damage. Ideally, if you are taking this medication, you should have a checkup at the end of each cycle to prevent this complication from developing. Most doctors do not give clomiphene for more than four to six cycles.

hCG, given intramuscularly near the time of expected ovulation, is sometimes combined with clomiphene citrate. It increases LH levels and helps the egg ripen for release.

hMG, a very potent hormone used to induce ovulation, should be prescribed only by an infertility specialist. Treatment with hMG involves frequent deep intramuscular injections and frequent visits to a laboratory for blood tests to check estrogen levels. Most doctors use vaginal ultrasound to check for the number and size of eggs in the ovaries (the long-term effect of ultrasound on ovaries is unknown). A shot of hCG helps release the ripened eggs. Taking these infertility drugs is stressful because your partner will need to give the injections, all of the lab appointments disrupt your work schedule, and the drugs can cost up to $1,500 a cycle! Careful monitoring of the ovarian response reduces the danger of multiple eggs being released from the ovary and consequent multiple births. Ovarian hyperstimulation is also a possible complication of the use of this drug. If it occurs, it happens seven to nine days after the hCG shot.

Gonadotropin-releasing hormone (GnRH, brand names Lupron and Synarel) is often used in combination with one or more of the drugs listed above. GnRH agonists (an agonist being a chemical substance that triggers a particular physiological response) are given to prevent immature eggs from being (prematurely) released. GnRH can be taken via nasal spray or by subcutaneous injection. Some women experience mild to severe hot flashes, vaginal dryness, and mood swings while they are taking the medication, because it causes a temporary menopause-like state. Usually, GnRH agonists are used for five to 14 days.

Bromocriptine (Parlodel) is an oral drug used for women with high levels of the hormone prolactin in the blood. High prolactin levels can affect normal ovulatory patterns and alter the uterine lining. Bromocriptine is taken orally until a positive pregnancy test is confirmed and, in some instances, is continued into a pregnancy.

Problems after ovulation, in the luteal phase of your cycle, may be treated with any or all of the following: clomiphene citrate, hCG, hMG, and natural progesterone. Natural progesterone is available in the form of vaginal suppositories, oral pills, a vaginal gel, or intramuscular injections. It is used until you get your period or until you have a positive pregnancy test. Some doctors suggest continuing progesterone as long as ten to 12 weeks into a pregnancy for women who have had multiple miscarriages, who have conceived via assisted reproductive technologies (ART), or who are over 40 years old. Synthetic forms of progesterone are not used as they may be harmful to fetal development in an unsuspected pregnancy.

Taking fertility drugs is stressful. They are expensive and can cause unpleasant side effects. Some studies show an increase in ovarian cancer for women treated with some infertility drugs; however, researchers are not sure whether it is the drugs themselves or the inherent fact of infertility (especially if a woman never becomes pregnant after treatment) that puts women at a higher risk.

Surgery

Surgical techniques can sometimes correct structural problems of the cervix, uterus, and tubes. *Microsurgery* may repair tubes and remove adhesions. *Balloon-catheter techniques* have also been successful, in outpatient settings, to unblock tubes. *Laser surgery using the carbon dioxide or argon laser,* often in combination with microsurgery, may remove scar tissue or endometrial adhesions. If there is significant tubal damage, *in vitro fertilization (IVF)* may offer more chance of a successful pregnancy than surgical repair of the tubes, but IVF does not have high success rates (see chapter 18, Assisted Low-Tech and High-Tech Reproductive Technologies). Surgery and medications are often used together to treat endometriosis. (See "Endometriosis," chapter 24, Selected Medical Practices, Problems, and Procedures, p. 641.) Unless fibroids are causing blockages, distortion of the uterus, or heavy bleeding, they are not usually removed surgically and do not seem to hinder fertility.

Other Treatments

If you have a cervical mucus problem, you can douche to correct acidity, use estrogen to improve mucus quality, and take a type of cough syrup that thins mucus to treat very thick cervical mucus. Sperm antibody problems are usually treated by intrauterine insemination (IUI) (see p. 539) or with low-dose steroids. However, steroids can mask infections in your body and can cause weakening in your hip-joint bones. Assisted reproductive technologies (see chapter 18) have been used with some success for couples with sperm antibody problems.

Women often have a combination of problems, and treatment may involve combining several medications, many of which are expensive and possibly not covered by insurance.

You can choose to stop the treatments at any time.

By this time I had sunk into a deep depression. Sarah, my partner, who had been ambivalent about having a child, was angry at me for disappearing into this obsession. I had begun to consider more and more invasive procedures. I was both spinning out of control and standing in a dead stillness. I finally realized that I couldn't continue. . . . I began the process of letting go. . . . For the last six months we had been quietly considering international adoption. My partner had worried if she broached this topic I might feel undermined in my efforts to bear a child biologically. . . . I saw that one way or another, a baby would enter our lives.

Some women conceive without any further medical treatment whatever, often after many years of trying, or after adopting a child. How these pregnancies come about is a mystery, and a great joy.

Treatment for Male Infertility

In general, male infertility is more difficult to treat. Various hormones, also used to treat female infertility (clomiphene citrate, hCG, hMG, and pure FSH), are being used. If the tubes that bring the sperm from the testicle are blocked, sperm can be extracted with a needle, joined with your egg in a Petri dish, and replaced in your tube or uterus (see chapter 18, Assisted Low-Tech and High-Tech Reproductive Technologies). A *varicocele* can be corrected surgically or in a nonsurgical procedure using a tiny balloon to block off the vein; a rise in sperm count and motility is usually seen three months after surgery.

If your partner's sperm count is low or has poor motility or morphology, his semen may be inseminated into your cervix or uterus (IUI). This may be combined with ovulation-enhancing drugs such as clomiphene or hMG. If infection is causing a decrease in sperm motility, it can be corrected by treatment with antibiotics.

Intracytoplasmic sperm insertion (ICSI), a micromanipulation technique used during in vitro fertilization (IVF), involves inserting one sperm into the egg. Results have been promising, and fertilization and pregnancies have been achieved. This is an expensive procedure ($2,000 to $4,000) and often not covered by insurance. Some infertility specialists do not consider it experimental.

Different doctors usually treat male and female infertility problems. Men see a urologist and women see a gynecologist, infertility specialist, or reproductive endocrinologist. *Your doctors must communicate with each other.*

Unexplained Infertility

About 10% of women and couples learn, after extensive diagnostic work-ups, that their infertility is unexplained; it has no clear-cut medical cause. Such a diagnosis can give you hope—after all, there is no identifiable problem—or be difficult to cope with. Since new medical treatments are proliferating, it is tempting to hope that the *next* intervention will be the one to work; it can be hard to decide when to stop. You may be told, or you may feel, that the cause of your infertility is "all in your head." But unexplained infertility may be caused by environmental factors. Science has not yet identified all the possible causes of infertility.

Conclusive Infertility—
Grieving Your Loss

In the instance of *conclusive* or *absolute infertility,* you at least have the facts. You must go through the difficult process of adjusting to reality and reexamining your life. You may feel as if "the death of all your babies" has occurred. You may grieve the loss of womanhood, of manhood, of a life dream. All women and men who experience infertility grieve, each in her or his own way, for what has not happened and what cannot ever happen. You can choose to experience this knowledge as consciously as you can or to suppress these very natural but painful emotions. To deny or repress your feelings prolongs the process of their resolution, for somewhere within, you continue to live with the experience. Some people find that the pain never completely goes away, and they accept it as a familiar ache that recurs at unpredictable times throughout life. Some people immediately block their feelings of grief by planning to adopt, but the adoption is more likely to be happy and successful if you can first "work out" your feelings. Grieving can take a long time. Seek the support of friends, family, and other people who have experienced infertility.

After learning of my infertility five years ago, I experienced the usual shock and denial. Unfortunately, I pushed down all other feelings by submerging myself in work. Eventually we adopted a son, and all seemed right with the world. I rarely thought of my infertility. Last fall, for no obvious reason, my infertility again became a prominent concern, and all the feelings I had submerged five years ago resurfaced. I ended up in crippling depression. Only with the help of counseling have I been able to begin to work through the feelings and to address my unresolved grief of never having a pregnancy and a biological child.

It was relieving to meet and talk openly with other couples experiencing infertility. Each of us had our own specific difficulties, but our feelings and reactions were quite similar. After the initial nervousness that accompanied our first two meetings, I began to feel much more accepting and able to deal with the previous two and a half years that had given us two pregnancies and two miscarriages. My almost constant obsession with pregnancy was lifted. I began to feel in touch with myself and somewhat alive again.

ALTERNATIVES

Once it has been determined that you are dealing with infertility, you may want to examine the possibilities and alternatives for the future. You may once again find yourself asking, "Do I really want to be a parent?" Take time to redefine your goals and how you want to live your life. You may want to stop trying to get pregnant and focus on other options, including adoption (see below). Some options, if you want to keep trying, include donor insemination and in vitro fertilization. (See chapter 18, Assisted Low-Tech and High-Tech Reproductive Technologies, for these and other assisted reproductive technologies [ARTs].)

Adoption *

Adoption is one way to create or extend a family. People in many different situations choose adoption. These can include: couples or single women with infertility or with health conditions that might make pregnancy dangerous; lesbians and single heterosexual women who want to have a family and prefer not to pursue donor insemination; and some who value adoption over giving birth out of a concern for children in the world who need families. Adoption is a

---

* See chapter 16, Unplanned Pregnancies, for further discussion.

challenging process, as it involves the complex needs of all people involved: the birth mother, the child, and the adoptive parent(s).* The field of adoption has changed remarkably in the past decade. Adoptions that intend to respect the needs and well-being of all parties are becoming more possible, though they are by no means guaranteed. Adoptions across nationality, race, or culture bring challenges as well as possibilities, as do adoptions of special-needs children and older children.

If you are planning to adopt and if this will be your first child, you have many questions to consider: Do you want to adopt a newborn baby? Do you want a child who "looks like you" as much as possible—that is, of the same race, ethnicity, hair color, etc.? Are you interested in adopting a child from a different race or country or culture? (Please see chapter 16 for more on interracial adoption.) A child with special needs, or an older child? Should you use the services of a private adoption agency or a lawyer representing birth parents? Do you want an open (or semiopen) adoption, in which you and the birth mother (parents) will have some contact, and in which the child you adopt will have easy access to information about the birth parents? Often the adoptive parent has more power than the birth mother and can choose to be more or less responsive. These are questions with practical, ethical, and emotional dimensions. Most of these choices are available to you, and your decisions will shape your experience. Like all parents, you will want to do whatever will be in the best interests of the child. Take care to learn about existing adoption controversies (what should guidelines be? How open should records be? etc.) to guide you in your decisions.

State law governs adoptions in the U.S. Adoption procedures must conform to the regulations of both the state where the adoptive parents reside *and* the state where the child is born. Those procedures, which vary enormously, include determining who should oversee or arrange the adoption (a licensed agency, a lawyer, or a doctor, for example); stating whether a home study is necessary; establishing the length of the postplacement waiting period before legal finalization; and whether reversal is ever possible (e.g., *never* in Texas, even if the birth mother changes her mind the next day).

The adoption process can bring up difficult emotions. Feelings of impatience, anxiety, and vulnerability are common and, for some, of powerlessness and anger. The pain and loss you have experienced if you have constantly hoped for a birth child and undergone invasive medical, and surgical procedures for infertility can make the adoption process seem like taking on additional hoops to jump through. Many women discover that adoption doesn't "fix" infertility—it doesn't

* One professional in the field who has contributed significantly to this understanding of the importance of considering the needs of all three parties—birth parents, adoptive parents, and child—is Joyce Maguire Pavao, Ed.D. Her work has helped to shape the adoption section of this chapter. For more information, see Center for Family Connections, in Resources.

TYPES OF ADOPTION

In *adoptions of children who are kin,* a child is placed with a relative. These are by far the most common. Some are never finalized in court and rest on a sense of responsibility but no legal certainty. *Nonrelative adoptions* consist of adopting a child, unrelated to you, who is born in the U.S. or in another country.

Domestic adoptions (of children born in the U.S.) are usually subject to communication between the birth mother, and sometimes the birth father, and the prospective adoptive parents. Sometimes the birth mother in a private adoption chooses an adoptive home from a book of dossiers of prospective adoptive parents. The prospective parents will sometimes pay some money to the birth mother, typically for living and medical expenses, with state laws governing the purposes and amounts. Birth parents and prospective adoptive parents may also negotiate a plan about future communication between themselves and the child.

It is very important that both birth parents follow state regulations with respect to valid releases, including relinquishment of parental rights.

Lesbian couples in which one partner has or adopts a baby may want to consider having the other partner adopt the baby in those few states where this is possible. (See "Legal Issues" in chapter 10, Relationships with Women.)

International adoptions, (of children born in another country), are subject to each country's requirements and regulations. Usually the adoptive parents adopt their chosen child in the court of the country of her or his birth before they are allowed to leave that country with the child.

Adopting older children (over the age of two). Most older children needing a good home and family have become available for adoption because of some tragedy or trauma in their lives. The adoptive parent(s) rarely, if ever, learn their whole story. Adopting an older child is wonderfully satisfying when it works, but in many instances the child's experience of prior trauma makes it severely difficult to raise them successfully, even with the best professional help and an abundance of love. It is recommended that the adoptive parents have already successfully cared for at least one child whose upbringing has been challenging and, before adopting, make sure to create for themselves a network of other adoptive parents in similar circumstances, as well as connections to potentially helpful professional services.

end the ebb and flow of feelings of loss and longing for children born in our own families. Lesbians who want to adopt must make the often difficult decision about how open to be with the adoption agency or with the birth mother about being lesbian: Many of us feel torn between being openly who we are and the risk of being refused as adoptive parents. (See chapter 10 Resources). The expense of some adoptions can create a strain for adoptive parents. Most private and international adoptions cost a lot of money. To help mitigate expenses, the U.S. Congress has passed a bill giving adoptive families a $5,000 tax credit.

For adoptive parents, the *home study,* which is ideally a series of shared planning sessions with the social worker or agency, can feel like a test of one's potential as a parent. If the home study feels unsympathetic or threatening, you might consider seeking a different social worker or agency. It is important that you feel comfortable with the person doing your home study, and it is also important that the required report does not contain any untruths, which would make the adoption fraudulent.

Given such a mix of feelings and the many decisions to negotiate, it is helpful to talk with other adoptive parents and to join an adoption group (see Resources). Most adoptive families are proud to belong to a growing community. When you decide to adopt, you will feel "pregnant," as a range of emotions from anxiety to joy infuse your daily life until the child is placed in your home. Like all new mothers, you will have a variety of responses as you make the transition from being childless to having a child. And, like any new family, you will all need the support of your family, friends, and community.

Views of adoption in the U.S. have changed remarkably in the last 30 years. Back then, almost everyone considered adoption to be somewhat shameful and surrounded it in secrecy. Over these past few decades, an increasing number of birth mothers have been speaking out about their horrendous experiences in giving over their children for adoption. They have told heartrending stories about how they were misinformed and/or coerced to give up their babies under circumstances they could not control. Many express a passionate desire to know about their children's welfare and to see them if possible. In recent years, more and more teenaged and adult adoptees are demanding access to information about their origins, searching for, and sometimes finding, their birth parents.

Changes in the adoption process resulting in more open adoptions have been slow and hard won, fought for by both adoptees and birth mothers. They have created national organizations that support and assist the searches of adoptees and birth parents for each other. Many believe it is a human right, if not a constitutional right, to know one's biological origins. They are still fighting to change the practices of those adoption agencies that try to keep this knowledge secret. Many adoptive parents also support these organizations.

Today, adoption is not only increasingly common but a matter of pride, public knowledge, and public financial support. Although some women still experience societal and family pressures to give up a child, today it is more likely that adoption becomes a shared planning process. Adoption laws vary from state to state. In an increasing number of states, the law requires that birth parents be counseled fairly and comprehensively in agency adoptions before surrendering children for adoption. If they are not so counseled, the adoption could be reversed, although this is rare.

Searching for a parent or child is not for everyone. Some children and birth mothers never search for each other and never want to. Others do nothing for years until something happens to release in them a desire to know. Loyalty to their adoptive parents often prevents adoptees from expressing a desire to know their birth parents, though they express the dream in many ways, or during counseling. Many adoptive parents fear they will "lose" their children and become childless once again. Birth mothers or fathers fear rejection, not being "good enough" to measure up to their child's expectations, just as they may once have felt "not good enough" to become the parents of their offspring. The experience of a reunion may alleviate these fears. However, no one is ready in exactly the same way or at exactly the same time as anyone else. It is crucial that all family members talk about their fears and wishes. Some families seek therapy for help with this process.

Often, adoptive parents become involved in helping their adopted children search for birth parents. They understand how important this knowledge and these experiences are, especially when the child becomes an adolescent. As adopted children reach their teens, a time of life that often involves a search for identity, they may have very powerful feelings about being adopted that they do not always express. At the time that the adolescent may begin searching for her or his birthparents, the adoptive parents are also preparing for their adopted child's move toward independent adulthood.

Reunions may be brief or temporary, or they may grow into more long-lasting friendships. Sometimes there are painful rejections on one side or another. But most people who have been through it agree that any knowledge is better than no knowledge. For some birth mothers, only a reunion can free them from the pain of having given up their child. For the children, there is healing too. "When I saw how much it meant to her, I wished we had done it sooner," one adoptive mother said. Many adoptees say that the relationship with their adoptive parents improves.

Child-free Living

Many couples and individuals do not wish to incur the risks, expenses, and turmoil of ongoing infertility treatment, or do not choose to adopt a child, and will decide to live without children at home. Too many people still make value judgments about women who don't have children. It is hoped that your family and friends will support your decision. You will have many rich opportunities to love and care for the children who do come into your life.

An extraordinary thing happened to me this Mother's Day. Because I don't have children of my own, I have struggled to honor my own frustrated longings and still sustain my loving connections to other women and their children. Each year in that search has found me in a different place as I extend my capacity to love and care for others. Right now, a lot of my generative energy is going into my work as a teacher, writer, and community health worker. This year, I went to a Mother's Day celebration at the State House recognizing the achievements of Mothers in Recovery and their community supporters. I walked down the many State House steps into a dazzling spring day, and serendipitously joined a group supporting Mothers on Welfare. I said hello to two of the organizers, who teach at the same public university as I do. As I moved out of their circle into the street, an African-American woman walked over and engaged me in an immediately intense, initially suprising conversation. Why did she approach me among so many people moving through their group—because I had stopped to greet my friends in Spanish and English with such delight? Because I was as brightly dressed and bejeweled as she? She told me she was on welfare but, 42 and single with no children of her own, she saw no chance to have them in time. "I'm here," she said, "to show support for family, friends, and neighbors, because it takes more than one or two people to bring up children, and so I help them out." Perhaps recognizing the precious rarity of our multiracial circle of women on the streets of Boston, she added, "We may have come over to this country on different ships, but now we are all in the same boat!"

RESOURCES

For materials on assisted reproductive technology, see Resources for chapter 18.

Infertility—Emotional and Medical Factors

Baran, Annette, and Reuben Pannor. *Lethal Secrets: The Psychology of Donor Insemination, Problems and Solutions.* New York: Amistad Books, 1993.

Becker, Gay. *Healing the Infertile Family: Strengthening Your Relationship in the Search for Parenthood.* Berkeley: University of California Press, 1997.

Carter, Jean, and Michael Carter. *Sweet Grapes: How to Stop Being Infertile and Start Living Again.* Indianapolis: Perspectives Press, 1989. For couples nearing the end of their options.

Cooper, Susan Lewis, and Ellen Sarasohn Glazer. *Choosing Assisted Reproduction: Social, Emotional and Ethical Considerations.* Indianapolis: Perspectives Press, 1998.

Glazer, Ellen, and Susan Cooper, eds. *Without Child: Experiencing and Resolving Infertility.* Lexington, MA: Lexington Books, 1988. Includes the doctor-patient relationship, interaction of religion and infertility, living child-free, and the adoption process.

Leiblum, Sandra, ed. *Infertility: Psychological Issues and Counseling Strategies.* New York: Wiley, 1997.

Marrs, Richard. *Dr. Richard Marrs' Fertility Book.* New York: Delacorte Press, 1997.

Menning, Barbara Eck. *Infertility: A Guide for the Childless Couple.* New York: Prentice Hall, 1988. The first book of its kind. Offers important history.

Resolve, Inc. *Environmental Toxins and Fertility.* Somerville, MA: Resolve, 1995. Available through Resolve: (617) 623-0744.

———. *Infertility Insurance Advisor: An Insurance Counseling Program for Infertile Couples.* Somerville, MA: Resolve, 1994. Available from Resolve: (617) 623-0744.

Salzer, Linda P. *Surviving Infertility: A Compassionate Guide Through the Emotional Crisis of Infertility.* New York: HarperPerennial, 1991.

Sandelowski, Margarete. *With Child in Mind: Studies of the Personal Encounter with Infertility.* Philadelphia: University of Pennsylvania Press, 1993.

Sloan, Gale. *Postponing Parenthood: The Effect of Age on Reproductive Potential.* New York: Insight Books, 1993.

Treiser, Susan, and Robin K. Levinson. *A Woman Doctor's Guide to Infertility: Essential Facts and Up-to-the-Minute Information on the Techniques and Treatments to Achieve Pregnancy.* New York: Hyperion, 1994.

Adoption

See Resources in chapter 16 for a long list of materials on adoption.

Johnston, Patricia Irwin. *Adopting After Infertility.* Indianapolis: Perspectives Press, 1992.

Melina, Lois Ruskai, and Sharon Kaplan-Roszia. *The Open Adoption Experience.* New York: HarperPerennial, 1993. A thorough, practical guide.

Child-free Living

Fleming, Anne Taylor. *Motherhood Deferred.* New York: G. P. Putnam's Sons, 1994. A journalist struggles to become pregnant with new scientific technology, and to balance professional ambitions.

Lisle, Laurie. *Without Child: Challenging the Stigma of Childlessness.* New York: Ballantine Books, 1996.

Pregnancy Loss

Friedman, Rochelle, and Bonnie Gradstein. *Surviving Pregnancy Loss: A Complete Sourcebook for Women and Their Families.* Secaucus, NJ: Carol Publishing Group, 1996. Speaks to couples who have experienced early losses, validating the intensity of their emotional pain.

Panuthos, Claudia, and Catherine Romeo. *Ended Beginnings: Healing Childbearing Losses.* South Hadley, MA: Bergin and Garvey, 1984.

Romeo, Catherine. "Miscarriage: An Ended Beginning." *Boston Parents' Paper* 12, no. 4 (Oct. 1995).

Scher, Jonathan, and Carol Dix. *Preventing Miscarriage: The Good News*. New York: Harper & Row, 1990. Recurrent miscarriage, psychological aspects, and grieving. Lists nationwide self-help support groups.

There Was a Child. 1991. Video by Fred Simon in collaboration with Newton-Wellesley Hospital. Available through Fanlight Productions, 47 Halifax Street, Boston, MA 02130; (800) 937-4113.

Disability

Saxton, Marsha, special ed. "Women, Disability and Reproduction." *Sexuality and Disability* 12, no. 2 (1994).

Organizations

For more adoption organizations, see Resources for chapter 16.

Adoption Support and Networking (AdoptNet)
P.O. Box 50514; Palo Alto, CA 94303-0514; (415) 949-4370

Center For Family Connections, Inc.
P.O. Box 383246; Cambridge, MA 02238-3246; (617) 547-0909; Fax: (617) 497-5952
E-mail: kinnect@aol.com

Center For Family Connections, Inc.
200 Park Avenue South, Suite 916; New York, NY 10003; (212) 777-7270; Fax: (212) 388-1952

Centering Corporation
0531 North Saddle Creek Road; Omaha, NE 68104; (402) 553-1200
E-mail: J1200@aol.com
Nonprofit bereavement publishing company, carrying books and pamphlets, including *Miscarriage* and *Why Mine?*

Childfree Network
6966 Sunrise Boulevard, Suite 111; Citrus Heights, CA 95610; (916) 773-7178

Child Welfare League of America
440 First Street NW, 3rd Floor; Washington, DC 20001; (202) 638-2952; Fax: (202) 638-4004
Web site: http://www.cwla.org

Compassionate Friends
P.O. Box 3696; Oak Brook, IL 60522-3696; (630) 990-0010
Web site: http://www.compassionatefriends.com
Chapters around the country, offers support after pregnancy loss or death of a child.

DES Action
DES-9288
(for address, see chapter 24 Resources)

Endometriosis Association
Information line: (800) 992-ENDO
(for address, see chapter 24 Resources)

National Lupron Victims Network
P.O. Box 193; Collingswood, NJ 08108; (609) 858-2131
Web site: http://www.voicenet.com/~nlvn

Pregnancy and Infant Loss Center
1415 East Wayzata Boulevard, Suite 30; Wayzata, NM 55391; (612) 473-9372
Web site: http://www.babycenter.com/refcap/1422.html

RESOLVE, Inc.
1310 Broadway; Somerville, MA 02144-1731; HelpLine: (617) 623-0744
Web site: http://www.resolve.org
National infertility organization with over 50 chapters in the U.S. Offers medical referrals, newsletters, fact sheets.

Additional Online Resources *

ChildFree Resource Network
http://www.compassnet.com/dmoore/crn

Hygeia: An Online Journal for Pregnancy and Neonatal Loss
http://www.hygeia.org

Infertility Resources
http://www.ihr.com/infertility

Miscarriage Support & Information Resources
http://www.pinelandpress.com/support/miscarriage.html

Sands Support for Parents Who Experience Miscarriage, Stillbirth, or Neonatal Death
http://home.vicnet.net.au/~sands/sands.htm

---

* For more information and listings of online resources, please see Introduction to Online Women's Health Resources, p. 25.

PART FIVE:

Knowledge Is Power

By Paula Doress-Worters (formerly
Paula Brown Doress) with Joan
Ditzion; based on earlier work by Paula
Brown Doress, Norma Meras Swenson,
Diana Laskin Siegal, Robin Cohen,
Mickey Troub Friedman, Lois Harris,
and Kathleen MacPherson

WITH SPECIAL THANKS TO Denise Bergman,
Janine O'Leary Cobb, Linda King, Susan M.
Love, Cindy Pearson of the National Women's
Health Network, Jane Pincus, Lynn
Rosenberg, Wendy Sanford, Stephanie
Studentski, Diana Laskin Siegal,
Mary Yeaton *

Chapter 23

Women Growing Older

I was conversing with a middle-aged friend about a poetry class we both attend. Then the talk turned to personal matters, and she told me about using herbs to manage her hot flashes, while I shared some concerns about my arthritis and needing a cane to get around. We laughed when we realized that though we are past worrying about having periods and getting pregnant, we never really are free of concerns about our bodies.
—A woman in her 70s

* Thanks also to the following for their help with the 1998 version of this chapter: Elena Klein, Judith Lennett, Annekathryn Goodman, Margie Lachman, Jeanne Wei, Frieda Rebelsky, Martha Crozier Wood, Paul Raia of the Alzheimer's Association, Lydia Buki, and Marta Sotomayor of the National Hispanic Coalition on Aging. Over the years since 1984, the following women have contributed to the many versions of this chapter: *Menopause*—Diana Laskin Siegal, Louise Corbett, Tish Anisimov, Lorraine Doherty, Ruth Hubbard, Kathleen MacPherson, Audrey Michaud, Pamela Berger, Irene Davidson, Meg Hickey, Judy Norsigian, and Josephine Polk-Matthews; *Growing Older* —Ruth Hubbard, Edith Fletcher, Barbara Krentzman, Lucile Longview Schuck, Anna Schenke, Anne Smith, and Marian Saunders.

Women of all ages need to know about the challenges that we will face as we age, especially in a society that compounds ageism with sexism, that discriminates against persons with disabilities, that is racist and heterosexist, and that makes life a struggle for people who lack adequate income and assets. All of us can be inspired by the strength, creativity, and contributions of older women. We need to know this so that we can be less ageist to others and less afraid for ourselves. We hope this chapter will help build a movement that can support us through our later years, and a feminism that is strong enough to last a lifetime.

THE CONTEXT IN WHICH WE GROW OLDER

Age and Ageism

Someday each of us will be old if we live long enough. Most of us want to live a long life; yet, our ageist culture values neither aging nor being old and separates people by age and generation. Ageism is

MORE ABOUT WOMEN GROWING OLDER

The New Ourselves, Growing Older: Women Aging with Knowledge and Power by Paula B. Doress-Worters and Diana Laskin Siegal in cooperation with the Boston Women's Health Book Collective (revised, 1994), offers more extensive discussion of many of the topics covered in this chapter.

The original chapter, first included in 1984, was based on discussions held with three groups of women—a midlife group, a menopause collective, and an older women's group—all of whom contributed their wisdom and experiences illustrating different stages of aging. We discovered that women experience so many changes—physical, social, economic, and emotional—during our midlife and older years that we couldn't possibly do them justice in a single chapter. We reached out to many more women and, in 1987, published *Ourselves, Growing Older*, revised in 1994 (see above). This handbook for midlife and older women covers such key topics as aging well, body image, sexuality and aging, menopause, work and retirement, caregiving, dying and death, and many of the health and medical aspects of growing older. A chapter on housing alternatives offers an array of living arrangements that can reduce isolation as well as save money. The money matters chapter offers economic strategies for women in three levels of circumstances: women just making ends meet; women who have some extra to save and invest; and women of wealth seeking ethical investment and donation strategies. Chapters on health care reform and on changing society and ourselves offer ways in which midlife and older women can significantly alter the conditions of our lives.

discrimination because of a person's chronological age. Ageism prevents us from seeing the diversity of older people. Despite common stereotypes of older people, the old are more varied and diverse than younger people. A group of 70- or 80-year-olds will vary more in mental and physical capacity than a group of 20- or 30-year-olds because of variations in the aging process over the years, and because of a lifetime of individuation. Yet, as we age we are more likely to be seen in stereotyped ways and to have our uniqueness and individuality overlooked. Ageism permeates all of our social institutions in subtle and unconscious ways that restrict our lives and affect our thinking. Discrimination against elders appears to be "just the way things are"—until we name and confront it.

Ageism has several sources. Our society overvalues youth and beauty and sets them as a standard for measuring women's value (see chapter 1, Body Image). This is layered on top of a sexist view that women are valuable only for looks and reproductive capacity, so that a woman is regarded as either youthfully beautiful or no longer beautiful. In addition to sexism compounded with ageism, many women also face discrimination based on race, disability status, and sexual orientation. When we are viewed in these stereotyped ways, we must struggle for participation in work and community, as well as to have our contributions taken seriously.

Western industrialized societies tend to isolate old people and others in need of caregiving, to maximize efficiency, and to avoid acknowledging the ultimate interdependence of people on one another. Planning for caregiving of the ill and infirm raises our own fears of infirmity, aging, and possible dependency. Our deep-seated wish to deny this possibility discourages us from planning for our own later years. It makes it less likely that as a society we can plan effectively for the needs of an aging population.

Isolation of elders and dismissal of their skills and wisdom is particularly prevalent in times of rapid social and technological change, when we may forget that we can still learn a lot about living from those who have a greater reservoir of life experience. In a profit-oriented system, ageism often takes the form of devaluing those who are not "productive"—the old, the young, and their caregivers. In today's economy, productivity is being redefined as profitability of a person's work relative to his or her salary. Middle-aged and older workers are increasingly laid off and replaced with younger workers at lower wages. Many are not able to find new employment and must "retire" early. Despite the increasing difficulty of maintaining employment through our 40s, 50s, and 60s, elders are faulted for needing "entitlements" such as Social Security, Medicare, and SSI that most of us contribute to throughout our working years. Because there is no national health care for those under 65, Medicare is criticized as "too expensive"; instead, it should be viewed as a model of a universal single-payer system.

Women face age discrimination at earlier ages than men do, often in our early 40s and sometimes even in our 30s,[1] compared to mid-fifties or later for men. Aging tends to exaggerate or deepen class differences. Wealthy elders are often able to maintain their economic position, while persons with low incomes inevitably grow poorer if they become ill and can't get paid work anymore. Many women find themselves growing older in this situation.

Many studies have confirmed that older workers have excellent skills, a strong work ethic, dependability, and low levels of absence and lateness. Even most employers now know this. But the stereoypes of older workers as inflexible and unwilling to learn new skills overrides these positives for most employers. Therefore, older women seeking employment often must assertively market themselves against this pervasive stereotype.

I did not feel old when I reached the Big Four O, but other people, especially prospective employers, started reacting to the physical appearance of my autumn change. At the employment office, I was advised in a résumé workshop not to list the jobs I had done further than ten years back. I was told not to put my age or date of birth on my résumé. I had gone from being overlooked for not having enough experience to being dismissed for having too much. To make matters worse, the man leading the workshop looked like a lot of my previous employers—he was at least in his late fifties with white hair and pink skin. And here I was African American and over 40. . . . Moreover, here I was pretty used to fighting off racism, as used to it as anybody can be and still hold on to their sanity and I was going to have to add another deficit-inducing category to the list. . . .

But even if I could hide my age on a résumé, how far can that take me? My next step was, as we say in the African-American community, to work out how I was going to keep on pushing. I had to get real comfortable with my age, stop denying the changes people saw on the outside, and deal with what was going on inside. I did have a tremendous fear of using a computer. Yet, I had years of experience in action-research and the writing of reports that would be enhanced in their technical application if I were willing to learn new skills. I decided to take this step and found that there was money available through the Economic Development Corporation of Boston. I also worked with a career counselor to identify how and where to market my new computer skills once I got them. Our planning sessions gave me the confidence to successfully apply for a job in publishing and community action. I am winning!

Even as we ourselves age, we hold ageist attitudes against ourselves and other old people. A woman in her 70s states:

I had always said, "Oh, I want to be with people of all ages, or with young people," but in fact I was avoiding being with people my own age—which would mean admitting I'm an old person—and missing out on a lot because of it! I signed up for a weekend of hiking through the Elderhostel,* and that changed my mind. We're not superwomen by any means, just people interested in vigorous outdoor activity.

Midlife and elder women, on their own and with advocacy organizations, have taken action against stereotyped media images that foster ageism, and they are promoting positive images, diversity, and realism. The Gray Panthers and the Older Women's League (see Resources) at times conduct "media watches."

Every time I see a positive image of an older woman on TV, I write a complimentary letter to the sponsor of the program. And when I see something offensive, I let them know that, too.

There have been successes. For example, the images of midlife and older women depicted in medical journal ads have improved noticeably in the past decade, which may have a small beneficial effect on the attitudes and practices of medical care providers.

Ageism, not age itself, is what limits elders. Every time we speak out, we change attitudes. Affirming ourselves is something that's in the air now. That makes a lot more things possible.

The Feminization of Aging

The single most significant fact about our aging as women is that the population of older persons is overwhelmingly female. Women live, on the average, nearly seven years longer than men. And increasing numbers of women are living a full life span of 80 or more years. The problems that arise with aging—chronic illness, insufficient economic resources, caregiving or needing care, surviving one's relatives and closest friends—are predominantly women's problems. Yet, the researchers and policy makers have mainly been middle-class white men who overlook older women's special concerns, especially those of women of color and of low income. Older persons, on average, are no more likely to be poor than those in other age groups, but those figures apply chiefly to middle-class white men and married couples. Older women living alone, especially women of color, have a high likelihood of living out our years with inadequate income. One-fourth of Latinas over 65 live in poverty. Cuts in federal housing and income support programs are devastating to older women with low incomes.

Large numbers of women outlive their husbands, often by a decade or two, and a significant number even outlive their eldest sons. Older women are more likely to live alone, while older men are twice as likely to be married in their older years; 40% of older women live alone, compared with 16% of older men.[2]

A positive side of our growing numbers is our potentially greater clout as a political constituency. As of January 1, 1996, women over 45 constituted 26% of the adult U.S. population. The government and the press are paying more attention to us. We need to take advantage of this attention to create, demand, and fight for programs that will be responsive to midlife and older women's needs and the needs of an aging population.†

Married or single, women are valuing our friendships with one another more than ever, and learning

---

* Elderhostel (see Resources) is an adult education program for older people. Outdoor activities are only a small part of their offerings. Typically, weeklong courses are given, usually with living arrangements in college dormitories. Many elders are also taking courses for credit and are enrolled in degree programs. Further education is one of the greatest unmet needs of elders.

† The Older Women's League is an important national organization to advocate for midlife and older women's concerns (see Resources for a list of such organizations and information on how to reach them).

that it is women who will most likely sustain us when we are older.

I was brought up to believe that the people in my family were the most important people in my world. I'm still very attached to immediate family members, but I have consciously extended my family to include my "sisters" in the women's community.

My loneliest times were during my marriage. I came out as a lesbian, and my life with women has been a revelation. But so many women I meet don't understand my problems as a single parent and are younger than me. Coming to an older woman's meeting has made me realize that I want to meet more women my own age.

Poverty and Inadequate Income

The authors of this book, along with a growing number of public health professionals, believe that poverty is the primary cause of ill health and diminished well-being. After a lifetime of being unpaid, underpaid, or underemployed, it is no accident that older women are almost twice as likely to live in poverty as are older men.[3]

Many full-time working women do not earn enough to keep themselves out of poverty. As increasing numbers of longtime marriages are ended, growing numbers of formerly middle-class women find themselves at midlife in the situation of women of lower income, raising their children alone and with insufficient resources.

At divorce, few judges include provision for children's higher education or other expenses for children over the age of 18, even those with disabilities. We are often alone with the responsibility at a time in our lives when our wages are shrinking relative to men's. At midlife, our wages increasingly lag behind those of men in our age group: the gap of 82 cents to a man's dollar of our young adult years widens to less than 60 cents to the dollar for the middle-aged group.[4]

Many women participate in work training programs, but some of them are punitive, intended mainly to reduce the welfare rolls and only secondarily to place a woman in a good job. If you are seeking a new outlet for your energies, or simply need to earn money to support yourself, you may want to consider a work training program sponsored by an advocacy organization (see Resources under "Employment and Training for Older Women Workers").

The median income for women over 65 living alone varies by ethnicity: White women, $9,276; Asian-American women, $7,731; African-American women, $5,328; Hispanic women, $5,721.

Consider that in the U.S., the poverty level for a person over the age of 65 is $7,309.[5] (A recent report of the United Nations Development Program sets the U.S. poverty line at $8,122, or half of the 1991 median income. By this standard of older women, only white women are, on average, above the poverty line.)[6]

For women of color, a lifetime of employment problems due to structural racism, and a history of low-wage jobs with low or no benefits, seriously affect retirement income or the ability to plan for retirement. Cuts in Supplemental Security Income (SSI) disproportionately affect women of color, and they specifically target immigrant populations. Many older immigrant women are left widowed, speaking little or no English, to manage on their own. Now that states will have control of funds through block grants, older women with low incomes will be increasingly vulnerable to arbitrary cuts, and immigrant women to total loss of already marginal income.

Health Insurance Coverage

Midlife women face a gap in health insurance coverage when they are too young for Medicare and not quite poor enough for Medicaid.[7] Many women after divorce lose health insurance coverage for themselves and their children. Advocates in Massachusetts are organizing to address this gap in protection for women and children.[8] Compared with white women, African-American women are twice as likely to lack health insurance, and Latinas are three times more likely to be without it; even Asian-American women, who have a slightly higher median income, are 1.5 times less likely than white women to have health insurance.[9]

Women who have been covered under a spouse's employment-related health plan typically lose their coverage when their spouse retires. Since the majority of women are with a partner who is a few years older, many women experience a gap in coverage in their 60s, when paying privately for a nongroup plan can be prohibitively expensive, and when preexisting conditions may make it difficult to get any insurance at all. Coverage is available under COBRA,* but you must be able to pay for it privately.

Unequal Access to Pensions

The majority of women receive no pension other than Social Security payments. Only 20% of women workers receive pensions, compared with 47% of male workers. Women often work in the kinds of marginal jobs and industries that are not unionized and do not provide benefits such as pensions.

Women who work full-time, year-round are less likely than comparably employed men to have an employer-provided pension. Women change jobs more often than men, staying on a job for an average of 4.8 years, compared with 6.6 years for men. Many

* COBRA is federal legislation requiring insurance companies to maintain the option of coverage at group rates for 18 months after termination of employment or eligibility through marriage. The eligible person must pay for the insurance out of pocket.

companies require that an employee put in five to seven years of service to qualify for a pension plan.[10]

The average pension benefit that women receive from a former employer is about $4,330 annually. This is 46% of the average pension that men receive: $9,460 annually. The ratio has actually worsened since 1978, when women's pensions were 51% of men's pensions.[11]

Women in lifelong partnerships with women, or with men to whom they are not married, generally have not benefited from a partner's pension as married women typically do. Recent changes in some progressive workplaces responding to the efforts of gay and lesbian advocates have begun the process of recognizing domestic partners' rights to family benefits.

Widowed or divorced women may find themselves ineligible for their husband's pensions. Many companies offer employees a choice of higher benefits in their lifetime or a reduced rate if spread over both spouses' lifetimes. Thanks to the efforts of the Older Women's League and other advocacy groups, today both spouses must sign off on the decision, giving women more power to protect themselves. Before this change was made, only 5% of widows collected on the deceased spouses' benefits. Many women fail to act in their own long-term interest by going along with a partner's decision to take a larger amount over his lifetime. Women may not want to believe that they will outlive their partner, or they may believe that if they do, their needs will be very minimal. Yet, older women living alone are one of the poorest groups in the U.S.

For those of us who can, it is important to plan for our economic well-being so that we have choices in our later years. Women whose situations are more marginal may want to explore options such as sharing housing or applying for SSI.

In addition to single mothers, another group is often unable to plan for their older years: the growing number of women who take on the care of their grandchildren because of the death, mental or physical disability, addictions, or incarceration of their children, or because they want to help raise an infant born to a teenaged child who may not be ready to manage on her own.

Because we all are growing older, we all have a stake in supporting older women's demands and concerns. We have to work on upgrading women's jobs and salaries as well as learning to plan for ourselves. Many social changes that would help older women to participate more fully in the workplace are similar to those needed by younger women with children: equal pay, caregiving services for children and sick family members, better access to health care, flexibility in jobs, portability of pensions, and universal health care.

Working a nine-to-five job is not the only way of being "productive." We know that we contribute to society whether we are working for pay, raising children or grandchildren, caring for a sick family member, doing creative work, or working in our communities as volunteers. Whatever our differences, we must stand together as we fight for the changes that will recognize and reward our contributions to our families and communities.

THE MIDDLE YEARS

Midlife, the years approximately between 45 and 65, is a major life stage involving emotional, social, and physical changes, of which the biological transition of menopause is just one aspect. It begins for some of us when children leave home or when a parent's health declines.

Exploration and Growth in the Middle Years

The definitions of middle and older years vary from one community to another and may vary by economic class. Women who work at jobs that are physically wearing may experience an earlier onset of chronic conditions associated with aging (see p. 569), and may look forward to slowing down their pace, while women from more privileged backgrounds are more likely to seek new outlets for activity at midlife.

Midlife can announce itself with a surge of new energy—perhaps simply restlessness—or with a growing recognition that we are coming to the end of familiar roles and ways of living.

I loved my work as a nurse. I'd never married or had children. I always denied that I experienced sexism until, when I was 38, a new male nurse was promoted to head of my service. That left me fuming. I used my life savings and then some to go back to college and then medical school. I've never been sorry.

I just want more! More time free of kids to focus on my work; more time to myself, more passion in my marriage, or from somewhere else.

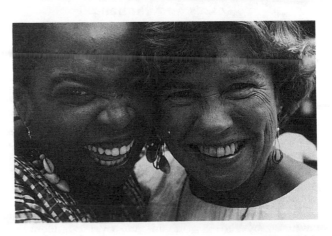

Skip Schiel

I am writing to assure women of middle age or beyond that it is not too late to attend school and begin a career or to switch careers. All my life I had wanted to be a nurse but instead was a secretary. Finally, at age 57, when the youngest of our children graduated from college, I took a year from the workaday world to attend school and become a licensed practical nurse. I made the highest grade in our class on the state board exam. I am not telling this to be boastful but to encourage others who might think they are too old to learn. Seven years later, at age 65, I am happily employed as an LPN [Licensed Practical Nurse]—my lifelong dream.

We may experience a change in our perspective—a heightened awareness of the passage of time and of the value of the time we have left. For today's women over 40, time at home or time devoted to full-time child-rearing without some kind of paid work outside the home is increasingly rare. Both women with low incomes who have always worked, and high-earning women working long hours, may find that only at retirement will they have the freedom to explore other interests or develop new skills, or just relax and enjoy life.

It was a shock when a friend of ours, a middle-aged man, died suddenly. It got me thinking that I don't know how many years Dan and I have left together. . . . Work is still very important to me, but I no longer want it to absorb my whole life. I want to spend time together and have fun.

When I was 50 I was the oldest person in my community and quite conscious of being older. I thought (this seems ridiculous now that I am 76) that I certainly had to plan ahead because I wouldn't have much time left. I wanted to travel a lot, maybe to Africa, in the next five or ten years.

Losses and Challenges During the Middle Years

Statistically, many of the important losses that women face cluster in the 45- to 55-year period. Some losses undermine our image of ourselves as young, healthy, even immortal, as when diseases attack the very wholeness of our bodies. Not as serious as threats to our health, but sometimes causing painful feelings of loss, are the surface signs of aging that challenge us to develop a new body image. As we notice the changes or observe that others respond to us differently, we may keenly feel the loss of our youthful looks, in which we have been taught that much of our value resides. Breast cancer strikes one out of 100 women by age 55 (one in nine over our lifetimes), bringing the threat of surgery or even death. One-third of women are estimated to have had a hysterectomy

by age 60;* the rest of us lose our fertility at menopause at the average age of 51.

Often at about the same time that our fertility ends, our children are going through their adolescent years or leave home. Other important relationships may end or change: our partner or closest friend may die, or we may divorce. Our parents may become ill or die. If we have to care for them or for our partners, we may have to give up or postpone long-awaited changes or adventures. Situations such as these may leave us with less money and/or no health insurance and can cause considerable stress and depression.

Some of our children may encounter stumbling blocks that get in the way of their taking on adult or transitional roles. They may return home soon after leaving, or many years later after an illness, divorce, job loss, or other troubles. They may bring children with them, or move on and leave their children with us.

We may suffer one of the saddest losses—the loss of a child, a more common occurrence since the HIV/AIDS epidemic.† We feel a sense of unfairness, of violation of the natural order of the universe.

The "Dependency Squeeze" of the Middle Years

As our parents live to be older many of us have caregiving responsibilites that may last a long time. When our parents or other close relatives need care at a time when we have demanding jobs, children still at home or returning home, or a partner who is also ill or needs care, we may feel squeezed between conflicting demands. We may feel unable to carry out any of our roles effectively, or that we have no time left for ourselves (see "Caregiving and Needing Care," p. 575).

Caring for grandchildren is an even more unexpected middle- or late-life role, one that is becoming more common.

I was in my late 30s and my other children were all in high school when one of my daughters developed a drug problem, and I had to take her two little ones to raise. I was afraid I couldn't do it. I thought I was done raising kids, and they were babies! But I felt it was my responsibility because they were my blood. I didn't want them to go to foster care. I arranged for day care so I could keep my job.

I raised them both that way, and they still call me Ma. My daughter has been drug-free for several years now, but she has to live away from the temptations of the city. The kids do see her sometimes. They think of

---

* Cancer accounts for only 10.7% of all hysterectomies. Fibroids, the most common diagnosis, account for over one-fourth, yet fibroids will generally shrink after menopause, provided no estrogen is taken. (See "Hysterectomy and Oophorectomy," chapter 24, Selected Medical Practices, Problems, and Procedures, p. 663.)

† See Charlotte Mayerson's *The Death Cycle Machine* (New York: Crown Publishers, 1995), a collection of poems about the death of the author's only child.

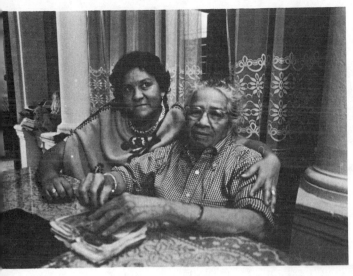

Sarah Putnam

her as an aunt. I am proud that both of my grandkids are doing well now, and that I was able to raise them.

Today approximately 3.4 million children under age 18 are living in households headed by grandparents and other nonparent caregivers.[12] This phenemenon crosses racial/ethnic and socioeconomic lines, though it is more than twice as common in African-American families as in white and Hispanic families.[13] Sometimes, grandparents play a major role in caring for grandchildren for positive reasons, such as providing care when a daughter has to work long hours, or simply to give children more attention than a single parent can provide. When grandparents *raise* grandchildren, it is usually because of a range of personal and social problems of their children: death, divorce, illness, joblessness, drug and alcohol abuse, incarceration, AIDS, or child abuse or neglect. Grandparents are joining support groups and forming coalitions to bring about changes in law to assist in this challenge (see Resources under "Caregiving").

Loss of a Partner

Three out of four women will at some time be widows. Over 11 million widowed women in the United States represent 83% of the widowed population.[14] Many more millions of women have lost "unofficial" partners, male and female. A widowed woman lives, on the average, 18 years after the death of a spouse. The chances of remarriage are low for older women and decrease with age: because three out of four elderly men are married, but only one out of three elderly women is. The majority of men who have lost their wives remarry. Those who remain single have higher rates of death and illness. It is thought that women adjust better to widowhood despite the stresses because of our greater ability to make and keep friends.

The stress of widowhood is enormous. Widows are

particularly vulnerable to disease and often lose or cannot afford health insurance coverage just when it is most needed. Grief is compounded when we:

- have found our main identity in being a wife.
- are isolated and lonely after the initial mourning period.
- find that most of our friends are in couples, and we have to seek new friends as a formerly married person.
- have to seek paid employment for the first time in decades.
- need a crash course in financial planning.

We must negotiate all this while we are still numb with the shock of loss. We need people to call us up, visit, bring food, invite us to do things, shovel the car out, and leave us alone when that's what we want. Yet, some friends may pull back, especially after the initial formalized mourning period, embarrassed or frightened by our grieving or our neediness. Many women have found special support and understanding from other widows (see Resources under "Widowhood"). Ultimately we can build new lives.

Grieving may be complicated when unconventional situations make it hard to be open about our loss and to receive social support from our friends and community.

Years ago, when Trudy discovered that she had cancer, she made sure she wouldn't endure the pain and suffering of the death that was ahead of her. I wish I'd listened more carefully when she held my face in her hand and wept, "I don't want you to suffer with me darling. I don't want you to be burdened with me." Despite my honest remonstrances that I wanted to care for her, to share her pain, she drove to the hills above our home early one Sunday morning and put a bullet through her heart. It pierced my heart too, for it ended our 18 years of life together. Because that life had been lived in such a deep dark closet, Trudy's death caused me to close the door in denial of my lesbian feelings.

It took 11 years for me to begin to creep cautiously from the closet. I emerged by inches, peeking out and withdrawing, discovering at last a new and exciting freedom. I enrolled in a women's studies program at a local univeristy and "bravely" took a class in lesbian literature. Oh wonderful, wonderful coming out.[15]

Sometimes the grieving process brings us through the other side to a new sense of who we are.

My husband died after a seven-year period when his health had been deteriorating and I had been his primary caretaker. My mother died within six weeks of his death. I lost a part of myself, my role as a helping, caring person. I went out to my mother's farm and sat out there for six weeks. I did a lot of different things, but I spent a lot of time writing about what I had left now that I no longer had that identity: Who am I? What I had left was the beginning of a new identity as a feminist and a woman [who] was growing older.

Sometimes in our middle years, losses may occur in quick succession, giving us no breathing time to grieve and recover.

A bad reaction to pseudoephedrine in cold medicine led to a diagnosis of a heart arrhythmia and insertion of a pacemaker. I needed time to assimilate the roller coaster of emotions—the high of being lucky to be alive and with no physical limitations, the loss of my youthful feelings of immortality. I wanted time to integrate all this, and for spiritual reassessment and renewal. But within weeks my wonderful talented son experienced a breakdown, which he believed was a response to my "near death" as he experienced it. He was diagnosed with a major mental illness. I had to put my issues aside, turn off my feelings, and shift into coping mode to make sure he got the help he needed.

Watch out for doctors who want to medicate away legitimate feelings of sadness and rage, or label our normal grieving pathological if it takes "too long." It is a sign of strength to be able to acknowledge feelings of despair, anger, guilt, emptiness, fear, relief, anxiety, and confusion. Particularly in the age of drugs like Prozac, which can be helpful to persons with major depression, the temptation to prescribe medication for the griefs of every life transition and loss can be enormous, as can be the temptation to accept it.

I think now that tranquilizers suppressed or sent underground the pains of that period (divorce, death of mother, betrayal by a lover). These pains still surface with agonizing strength. Maybe if I had fully faced them and "digested" them at the time they happened, this would not be the case.

In the professional literature, there are often unhelpful prescriptive statements about how long grieving should last. Yet, each of us has her own unique rhythm. Talking with women who have "been there" often helps, as does reminiscing, writing, or keeping a journal. It takes enormous energy to rebuild your life. Don't exhaust yourself trying to take care of the emotional needs of others. Take special care of yourself. You will probably need more rest than usual. Go slowly—give yourself time to heal and to regain your trust in the world and in your own capacities.

Our Change of Life: Menopause

The common folk expression "change of life" implies that we have the capacity to change our lives and ourselves. As we pass from our reproductive to our postreproductive years, many women feel more self-confident and self-assertive; some view the change of life as a time of emotional and spiritual transformation. Most middle-aged U.S. women, according to a 1997 national Gallup survey, ". . . welcome menopause as a new and fulfilling life stage." [16]

Menopause (the end of monthly bleeding or periods) is just one aspect of our midlife change. The current debate about hormone use has moved the focus away from the conditions of our lives that often cause us stress to a narrow focus on a transitory biological phenomenon that affects different women in different ways and to different degrees. Many of us in the women's health movement are concerned that menopause is becoming a catchall for all the stresses and losses that women face at midlife. In one large study of midlife women, the cause of depression was less often menopause than multiple sources of worry due to caregiving roles and relationships. [17]

Drug company publicity misuses longevity statistics to imply that we are the first generation of women to live long lives and that our bodies are not made to survive past menopause. Yet, most of the statistical increase in longevity is due to reduced mortality in childhood and in childbirth. Our own experience tells us there have always been long-lived women.

The Medicalization of Menopause

In recent years, pharmaceutical companies have been flooding the popular media and doctors' offices with their literature urging that the majority of women be treated for the "estrogen deficiency disease" of menopause, and to prevent diseases of aging. Paradoxically, this barrage of information may actually reduce our control over our lives by medicalizing our change of life and cutting us off from traditional sources of information. [18] When we rely entirely on medical experts and reject the experiences of older women in our lives, we are left feeling that we have no role models for dealing with normal life transitions like menopause, and we become more vulnerable to manipulative messages from the medical establishment and the media.

As a result of this unrelenting public relations campaign, Premarin (a brand of estrogen) is the number one–selling prescription drug in the U.S. Yet, its use varies by class and by region. For example, middle-class women are frequently pressed to take hormones, while women with low incomes often cannot afford them or the medical visits required to monitor their use, even when they clearly need them, such as after a hysterectomy. [19] Women in Los Angeles, where Hollywood values promote a culture of cosmetic surgery and diets, use hormones at a far higher rate than women in Boston, where the culture does not focus so heavily on maintaining a youthful appearance.

Some overzealous medical providers urge women in their 40s to begin hormone treatments before experiencing the signs of menopause. Some providers encourage women to continue taking birth control pills through their 40s and make the transition directly to hormone treatments—as if the experience of our own body rhythms and patterns would be dangerous.

The myths that frightened our mothers' and grandmothers' generations linked menopause with depression; there were stories of menopause leading to a lifelong mental illness called "involutional melancholia." Myths of women's mental instability had traditionally been used to keep women out of positions of power—raging hormones during our menstrual years and waning hormones at midlife and after. Modern research finds that women at midlife are actually less likely to be depressed than younger women. A recent review of all English-language studies investigating the relationship between natural (nonsurgical) menopause and depression found no evidence of such a link.[20] Although "involutional melancholia" has been dropped from the *Diagnostic and Statistical Manual of Mental Disorders* since the 1960s, some medical care providers are still too quick to prescribe antidepressants and tranquilizers to midlife women rather than listening carefully to their health and medical concerns.

Today, the modern myth of menopause is more body-focused and plays on our fears of losing our youthful looks and sexuality, and of disability and dependency in old age. The biological marker of menopause, which signifies only that our child-bearing years are at an end, has been recast as a transition to incipient fragility and old age—unless, of course, we invest in the medical approach.

In fact, most women take the signs of menopause in stride. A community-based study of over 2,500 midlife women found that the majority were "relieved" or neutral about menopause.[21] Nearly half of the women reported hot flashes, the most common discomfort of menopause, but not all found them bothersome or disruptive.[22]

We in the Boston Women's Health Book Collective view menopause as a normal part of a woman's middle years and favor a self-help approach for most discomforts of menopause, recognizing that some women's discomforts are more severe and that some women may require or prefer medical approaches.

Signs of Menopause

Menopause refers to the ending of menstrual cycles or periods. We cannot know that we have reached menopause until a year without periods has passed. Surgical menopause can be quite different. After hysterectomy, women are more likely to require hormone treatment. Indeed, it has been argued that the high rate of hysterectomy in the U.S. (33% of women have had a hysterectomy by age 60) creates a market for hormone treatment.[23]

The average age of menopause is 51 years, but menopause may occur any time from the mid-40s to the late 50s. The cessation of periods before age 40 is considered *premature menopause*. Smokers tend to go through menopause an average of two years earlier,[24] thereby increasing their risk of bone loss and other effects of an earlier reduction in estrogen level. Women with certain seizure disorders, such as post-traumatic or temporal lobe epilepsy, may also experience early menopause.[25]

We speak of *signs* rather than *symptoms* of menopause, a symptom being a change due to disease while menopause is a natural event. Three signs clearly associated with menopause are cessation of periods, hot flashes, and vaginal changes. Cessation of periods is the only sign experienced by all women. Hot flashes are experienced by most Western women, and vaginal changes by some women during or after menopause. It is also important to differentiate the signs of menopause from signs of aging. Any changes that happen to both women and men as a function of the aging process (wrinkles and graying hair, for example) are not caused by menopause. Body weight and body composition changes may be related to the hormonal changes of menopause.[26]

When physicians view the normal changes of menopause as a deficiency disease requiring medication, they subject women to overtreatment or undertreatment. Some physicians attribute to menopause almost anything reported by women at midlife, overlooking what might be symptoms of gallbladder disease, hypertension, clinical depression, and other serious conditions.[27]

Changes in Menstrual Patterns: The Perimenopause

Confusion about menopause can occur because more of the discomforts and difficulties such as menstrual irregularities, severe PMS, and sometimes even hot flashes occur during the years leading up to menopause, the perimenopausal years. (*Peri* means "around the time of.") By the time we have experienced a year without periods, often the worst of these problems has subsided. All times of hormonal transition, such as puberty, postpartum, and perimenopause, can be chaotic and confusing. Yet, by the time we reach menopause we know we have the resilience to go through these normal life transitions. Some of us have a more difficult time and may need support of one kind or another, but that does not mean that every woman should take medication to prevent distress. Indeed, there is evidence that hormone treatment for menopause simply postpones the transition. It may take about four years, on average, before our menstrual periods stop completely.

During the perimenopausal years, the hormones that control our menstrual cycles slowly change their pattern, the length of periods may change, or the time between periods may become longer or shorter. Occasionally, we may miss a period, sometimes for several months. Some periods may be *ovulatory* (producing an egg) and others may be *anovulatory* (no egg produced), resulting in varying patterns of flow. With reduced estrogen and reduced progesterone, the endometrial lining is thin and our flow may be lighter or last fewer days. When hormonal levels drop further, cycling stops and we no longer have periods. At this time, hot flashes often occur, though they may begin earlier. Some women report hot flashes for years, occasionally even decades, after menopause, though usually not with the same frequency or intensity. It is not known why this occurs.

Heavy Bleeding and Prolonged Periods

Heavy periods (heavy bleeding, flooding, or *menorrhagia*) can be the most annoying and worrisome of perimenopausal patterns. Sometimes periods become so extended and so close together that we seem to be having one continuous period. The flow may clot or gush. We may have a combination of patterns, or fluctuating patterns. Sometimes the flow is so heavy that it washes a tampon out of the vagina and even heavy pads cannot contain it. We may feel faint momentarily. So much blood may be frightening or embarrassing.

The last time I flew in an airplane I perceived that I was flooding (though bolstered by a tampon and two pads) and rushed down the aisle to the bathroom. Blood flowed down my stockings and into my shoes. More dripped onto the carpet. Both bathrooms were occupied, of course. I waited, breathing deeply and resisting the very strong urge to kick in both doors.

Heavy bleeding, particularly common among African-American women, can result from a pattern of prolonged estrogen with reduced progesterone, producing a thick or irregular endometrial lining that may not slough off completely or evenly.

Prolonged bleeding or more than a few brief episodes of bleeding after menopause may be a symptom of cancer. Your health care provider may recommend an endometrial biopsy or dilatation and curettage (D&C), two methods of examining the lining or contents of the uterus. **Do not neglect this step. For most women, heavy or irregular bleeding is a normal part of perimenopause, but for a few it is serious and must be treated.**

Medical Approaches to Heavy Bleeding

To compensate for the body's reduced production of progesterone or prolonged exposure to estrogen, progestins (exogenous progesterone) may be prescribed, usually for the last 10 to 14 days of the cycle. Bleeding usually occurs within 48 hours after the hormone is discontinued, causing the lining of the uterus to slough off more completely than in previous cycles. The next period may then be lighter because the lining has not built up so thickly. Progestins may also be used to interrupt prolonged estrogen production, stimulate a period, and start a new cycle. Some women decide to try small doses of an oral progestin for a very short time or sporadically, depending on the pattern of their periods. There are risks with the long-term use of hormone treatments (see p. 559). It is not a good idea to continue taking oral progestins for more than a few months, or injections that stay in the body for several months. Progestins do not alleviate all bleeding problems.

Some physicians are too quick to propose surgical solutions; they may not have learned to recognize heavy bleeding as a sign of perimenopause. Or they may believe that we no longer "need" our sexual and reproductive organs after menopause. Women whose uteruses or ovaries are removed have higher rates of osteoporosis and heart disease, have a more difficult time during menopause, and are more often given hormone treatment. Some women report a difference in their sexual response after hysterectomy, and may become depressed.

Question any pressure to have surgery unless tests show a malignant (that is, cancerous) condition—not the same as a precancerous condition. Because very heavy or extended bleeding is a frightening, disruptive, and debilitating symptom, we can easily be pressured into taking drastic action. Many women choose hysterectomy simply because of the disruption that flooding causes in their work and social life. We urge women not to agree to a hysterectomy unless a confirmed diagnosis warrants it, including a second opinion from a surgeon, preferably not a colleague of your physician's.

Laser ablation of the uterus, recently approved by the U.S. Food and Drug Administration, provides a less drastic alternative to hysterectomy for the treatment of chronic menorrhagia. A study of the first 65 women to undergo this procedure in the U.S. found that 91% of the women considered it successful.[28]

Many women are learning to cope by talking with other women who have this problem and by discovering new ways to decrease the flow using nonmedical approaches and alternative healing methods, such as acupuncture and herbs (see chapter 12, Understanding Our Bodies, p. 283, and chapter 24, Selected Medical Practices, Problems, and Procedures, p. 657). If you want to consider these techniques, you should know that the most serious heath risk you face, once cancer has been ruled out, is that of becoming anemic. Have your hemoglobin checked regularly, and take iron *only* if yours is low.

Lighter and Fewer Periods

The occasional "missed" period can be worrisome to women who are heterosexually active and fear they might be pregnant. In spite of scanty periods, you can still be fertile, so keep using contraceptives until a year without periods has passed.

It can be reassuring to chart the pattern of your periods and note other body changes, comparing the way they differ from those of pregnancy. For example, if when you miss your period, you are nauseated, or have tender breasts, you may want to have a pregnancy test. If you are experiencing hot flashes or vaginal dryness you are more likely to be menopausal.*

---

* An FSH test can be done to determine menopausal status. An FSH level higher than 40 is menopausal; less than 20 is premenopausal. The test has such a broad indeterminate range that it is rarely useful. It cannot tell you whether you will have another period or whether you can become pregnant. Better to let your body tell you. See chapter 12, Understanding Our Bodies, for more on FSH and other menstrual hormones.

Premenstrual Syndrome (PMS) and Menopause

Some women report more severe premenstrual discomforts (PMS), such as swollen tender breasts, water retention, tension, or anxiety, when periods become irregular. Whether you have had such discomforts for years or begin to have them in the perimenopausal years, you can look forward to relief as periods stop and your hormone cycles level out. This may take several years.

Hot Flashes

In folk wisdom and humor, hot flashes are the sign most commonly associated with menopause. Surveys report that 47 to 85% of women will experience hot flashes, but many women never experience them,[29] and some who have them do not find them bothersome.[30]

It was a freezing December night when I lay in bed, dreading to get up and go down a long cold hall to an even colder bathroom. Then I had a hot flash and, all of a sudden, it was very easy to leave my warm bed! For the rest of the winter I used my nighttime hot flashes this way. My friends laughed when I told them that hot flashes are not all bad!

What is a hot flash? In recent years, physiologists have begun to study hot flashes. Responses that occur during hot flashes include a sudden increase in heart rate, often experienced as palpitations, an increase in peripheral blood flow leading to a rise in skin temperature, and a sudden onset of sweating, particularly on the upper body. When the sweat evaporates, your body cools and you may feel chilled.[31]

Hot flashes can begin when menstrual cycles are still regular or when they are becoming irregular, typically continuing for less than a year after the final menstrual period. For some women they may persist for five, ten, or even more years.[32] In rare instances, hot flashes first begin years after menopause. They vary in frequency, occurring once a month, once an hour, several times an hour, any time of the day or night. We each have our own pattern; it's impossible to know in advance what it will be.

New evidence suggests that women with more intense hot flashes and night sweats tend to have them for more years.[33] If yours feel very intense and self-help or alternative approaches do not help, you may want to consider a short-term (six months) low-dose course of hormone treatment.

Hot flashes can be most disturbing at night when they interrupt our sleep. Drenching sweats may oblige us to change our nightclothes and sheets. The loss of sleep* over many nights can cause fatigue, irritability, and feeling unable to cope—much like depression.

* For help in managing sleep loss, see "Dealing with Insomnia" in chapter 2, Habits Worth Changing in *The New Ourselves, Growing Older* (see Resources).

Removing the ovaries before menopause results in a sudden drop in estrogen levels, causing intense hot flashes, which often begin immediately after surgery. Vaginal dryness may also occur earlier. Most physicians prescribe estrogen treatment at least until a woman has reached the age of a natural menopause. Even when the ovaries are removed after menopause, hot flashes may occur because small amounts of estrogen are still produced by the ovaries postmenopausally. When physicians justify unnecessary surgery by arguing, "You won't need your uterus [or ovaries] any more," or medical texts refer to menopausal changes as "ovarian failure," they demonstrate ageist attitudes and are misleading.

The menopausal ovary is neither failing nor useless. It's simply beginning to shift from its reproductive function to its maintenance function. It's doing in midlife what people do—it's changing careers. (Dr. Susan Love's Hormone Book—see Resources.)

As ovarian estrogen declines, muscle and fat cells produce estrone (a postmenopausal form of estrogen). Generally, the body gradually adjusts to the lower level of estrogen, and for most women, the hot flashes stop or become infrequent. Thinner women have lower levels of estrone than women who are heavier, and thus tend to have more hot flashes.[34]

Self-Help for Hot Flashes

- *Keep track.* Chart your hot flashes in relation to your menstrual periods and other events to identify a pattern.
- *Eat healthfully.* (See "Eating Well," p. 566, and chapter 2, Food) Learn about the nutrient needs of midlife and older women, such as increased calcium to build bone, and about the balance of related nutrients that promote absorption of calcium. To reduce hot flashes, limit caffeine (coffee, tea, cola drinks, chocolate), alcohol, sugar, spicy foods, hot soups, and hot drinks. Very large meals may also trigger hot flashes; try several small meals, with a lighter meal at night. Some women find vitamin B-complex to be helpful.

Each day, eat at least one food rich in phytoestrogens, a weak form of estrogen found primarily in soy products and also in vegetables such as squash, yams, and carrots; in legumes; and in certain fruits, such as papayas.[35] Researchers are investigating the active ingredients in soy. Do not take soy supplements, because they may contain too much of some active ingredients and not enough of others. Rather, eat soy foods, such as soy milk (fortified with calcium and vitamin D), soy yogurt, soy nuts, miso, tofu, and tempeh as part of a healthy diet that includes five servings of fruits and vegetables daily.[36]

Vitamin E, found in vegetable oils (wheat germ, corn, and soybean), brown rice and millet, legumes, corn, and almonds, may minimize or eliminate hot flashes and vaginal dryness. To take a vitamin E supplement, find your appropriate range by starting at 400 IU per day and working up to 800 IU. Do not exceed 1,000 IU, and avoid vitamin E if you are taking digitalis or have diabetes. Though the data on prevention are inconclusive and suggest better results with vitamin E from food sources, some new evidence suggests that women who have breast cancer should not take vitamin E.[37]

- *Keep moving.* Physical activity relieves hot flashes, stress, and depression, and it helps you sleep better. Exercise tones the body and improves cardiovascular, bone, and digestive health.
- *Keep cool.* Dress in layers. Natural-fiber clothing may be more comfortable than synthetics. Fan yourself with whatever is at hand, or collect fans to match your wardrobe as some of our great-grandmothers did. Drink something cool; place something cool where it feels best—on the wrists, temples, forehead. Visualize yourself in a cool place. Lower the thermostat; get an electric fan or an air conditioner. Sleeping in cooler rooms can significantly reduce the frequency and intensity of nighttime hot flashes.
- *Reduce stress.* Hot flashes increase at times of stress. To relax, experiment with a variety of approaches such as meditation, paced breathing, or massage. Changing one's beliefs about hot flashes can make them less distressing.[38]
- *Keep talking.* Break the taboos against menopause. Let people know when you are having a hot flash; reaffirm that it is nothing to be ashamed of. Use positive, not demeaning, humor. A menopause support group or workshop can help you counteract fears and uncertainties with support, information, and humor.

Vaginal Dryness

As we age, the skin and mucous membranes in various parts of our bodies tend to become drier. Thinning vaginal membranes hold less moisture and lubricate more slowly. To help, add moisture to the air in your house and drink eight cups of liquid each day. For a very few women, vaginal dryness is an early sign of menopause; others do not experience it until many years later, and many never do. In a community-based study of women aged 50 to 60, only 20% of 1,109 postmenopausal women reported vaginal dryness, and only 15% of those experienced it as "bothersome."[39]

Vaginal dryness can interfere with sexual spontaneity and pleasure and can be a challenge to deal with. For self-help approaches, see "Sexuality and Aging," p. 563. Tell your health care provider before any pelvic exams so that discomfort can be reduced.

Other Changes Often Incorrectly Attributed to Menopause

Depression and changes in mood, memory, cognition, and the ability to concentrate have been blamed on menopause, but research increasingly shows that women are no more likely to be depressed at midlife than at any other time.[40] Mood swings do occur; they may be more likely at menopause in women who have had PMS and women who have had hysterectomies. Women who quit hormone therapy *abruptly* are also more likely to experience mood swings.[41] When hot flashes and night sweats interrupt sleep, concentration may be affected.

Despite the evidence of a growing number of older women in a variety of professions and creative activities, proponents of hormone treatments emphasize improvements in memory and cognition in an effort to convince women that in order to remain competent in the workplace, they will require medical treatment. A recent study of 800 women from 65 to 95 years of age, half of whom had used estrogen treatment, and one-third of whom were current users, found no effect of estrogen on cognitive function.[42] Some new studies report an effect of estrogen on delaying the effects of Alzheimer's disease, while others show no effect. Many of these studies are flawed, relying on poor research methods, such as participants' recall of whether they took hormones.[43]

Menopause in Other Cultures

Cultural differences influence the experience of menopause. For example, Japanese women report hot flashes at a much lower rate than North American women (indeed, no higher than people of other age groups, 10% of whom report hot flashes). Japanese women tend to use herbal preparations rather than medications and are less likely to use hormones at menopause.[44]

Studies such as this one raise several questions. Is menopause a different, less stressful experience in a culture that values aging and older people, and in which women's roles and choices expand at midlife? On the other hand, do differences in diet reduce the severity of hot flashes? For example, a traditional Asian diet, which includes soy products, rice (a source of vitamin E), and herbs and vegetables (possibly high in naturally estrogenic properties) may explain why hot flashes are infrequently reported by Japanese women. Studies of soy products are under way both in the U.S. and abroad, investigating whether they can lessen the risk of osteoporosis, heart disease, gallstones, and cancer and prevent or reduce hot flashes; the results are still inconclusive.[45]

HORMONE TREATMENT:
MEDICAL MODEL; WOMEN'S CHOICES

Much of the confusion about choosing to take hormones or not stems from the fact that hormones are marketed and prescribed for two purposes: short-term relief from severe menopausal discomforts, and long-term prevention of conditions that can come with aging. Women more often choose hormones for the former, but drug companies are increasingly marketing them for the latter.

The hormone controversy raises an important bio-ethical issue. The standards for using unproven treatments on healthy populations should be more stringent than those for treating persons who are ill and choose to risk something new as a possible cure. We question the ethics of attempting to flood a healthy population with an unneeded medication that may result in new risks. Essentially, women who take hormones over the long term are involved in an experiment.

Whether you take hormones or not, or whether you take them for short-term relief of discomforts or for longer-term prevention of disease, is a decision for you to make. You will want to consider your own history, values, health status, and preferences as well as your understanding of the research studies. If you choose to take hormones for an extended time, continue to reevaluate the risks and benefits by keeping up with new research and discussing it with your health care provider.

Understanding the research results can be confusing because there are different hormone regimens: estrogen alone (estrogen treatment or ET), estrogen with progestins (hormone treatment or HT), and more recently estrogen with testosterone. Research findings about estrogen alone may not apply to estrogen given with another hormone. It can be distressing to read that while hormone treatment has been shown to have several beneficial effects, it also has serious risks, so that sometimes seems that we are being asked to choose from a menu of potential diseases.

Short-Term versus Long-Term Use of Estrogen Treatment or Hormone Treatment

The short-term benefits of estrogen treatment (ET) for the relief of menopausal discomforts, such as hot flashes and vaginal dryness, have been known since 1937 and heavily marketed since the 1960s. After reports in 1975 that women who used estrogen therapy were five to 15 times more likely to to develop endometrial cancer, women became more skeptical of estrogen treatment, and prescriptions for it declined.

To protect against endometrial cancer, a form of hormone treatment combining estrogen with progestin (HT) was developed. **It was hoped that the combined hormone treatment would protect against all forms of cancer; however, the combination of estrogen with progestin protects against cancer of the uterus only, and actually seems to increase the risk of breast cancer.**[46]

Following the decline in their sales, the drug compa-

PROS AND CONS OF HORMONE TREATMENT *

When Hormone Treatment Can Be Helpful

- Ovaries removed before age 45.
- Fractures or high risk of fractures, especially if due to medical risk factors such as surgical removal of the ovaries or steroid use. (If risk is due to lifestyle factors, other approaches work just as well.) Be aware that bone loss can recur after hormones are stopped. One new approach, starting hormones late in life, reduces fractures in old age while not incurring the risk of midlife breast cancer.[47]
- Extreme menopausal discomforts, such as hot flashes and night sweats, which are not manageable with other approaches. Consider low-dose treatment for a short period such as six to nine months, tapering off your dose at the end to minimize the recurrence of hot flashes.
- Vaginal dryness responds to various self-help approaches (see p. 564). Even when it is extreme, estrogen cream in low doses can help. Pills are not necessary.

Do Not Use Hormone Treatment If Any of the Following Conditions Is Present:

- Past or present thromboembolic events (stroke, thrombophlebitis, pulmonary embolus, or heart attack).
- Breast cancer, uterine sarcoma, or any other estrogen-stimulated cancer.
- Severe liver disease or chronic impairment of liver function.
- Unexplained vaginal bleeding.
- Pregnancy or chance of pregnancy (hormone therapy could hurt the fetus).

Consider Avoiding Hormones (Discuss risks and benefits with your health care provider)

- If you have had a hysterectomy for endometrial cancer, consider avoiding hormones. If you decide to use estrogen,† do not use it right away; consult your physician.
- If you have gallbladder disease (taking hormones doubles the risk of gallbladder surgery); nonuterine sarcoma, uterine fibroids, hypertension, migraine headaches, asthma, seizure disorders,‡ heart disease, or

continued on next page

kidney disease associated with fluid retention.

- If you drink more than two drinks of alcohol per day, consider reducing your alcohol consumption or stopping or reducing hormone treatment.

Risks and Drawbacks of Hormone Use

- Increases the risk of breast cancer after long-term use. Combined hormone therapy appears to be riskier than ET.
- Estrogen alone increases risk of endometrial cancer.
- Nausea, weight gain, breast tenderness, uterine bleeding, fluid retention, and/or depression have been reported by some women.
- Depending on dosage and timing, combined hormones can cause monthly bleeding to resume.
- Increased medical visits are required to monitor the effects of hormone treatment.
- One study showed an increased risk of HIV infection in monkeys taking high doses of progesterone, which caused thinning of the vaginal lining.[48] Studies on humans are in progress.

* Information adapted from *Taking Hormones and Women's Health: Choices, Risks and Benefits,* 1995, p. 35. National Women's Health Network, 514 Tenth Street NW, Suite 400, Washington, DC 20004.

† Women who have had a hysterectomy should take estrogen alone because progestins often diminish the beneficial effects of estrogen, may have other unpleasant effects, and bring new risks. Combination hormones protect women who have a uterus against endometrial cancer.

‡ Taking estrogen lowers the seizure threshold, and the risk of seizures increases in women with epilepsy. See Elizabeth M. Sandel, "Sexuality and Reproduction After Traumatic Brain Injury," in J. Lawrence Hall and Nathan D. Zasler, eds., *Medical Rehabilitation of Traumatic Brain Injury* (Philadelphia: Hanley & Belfus, 1996), 557–72.

nies shifted their resources to researching and promoting other benefits of hormone treatment, targeting diseases associated with aging, especially osteoporosis and heart disease, and more recently Alzheimer's disease. Yet, we can often prevent osteoporosis and cardiovascular diseases in simpler and less risky ways (see "Aging and Preventive Health—Special Issues," p. 565) than using hormone treatments that may increase our risk of breast cancer and other cancers.

Testosterone Treatment

Testosterone is one of the class of hormones called androgens, commonly and inaccurately called "male hormones" because they are present in men at higher levels than in women. Androgens contribute to muscle strength, appetite, a sense of well-being, and sex drive. Testosterone levels fall in women after menopause and, more dramatically, after ovariectomy. Yet, it is healthier and less risky to rely on the low levels of testosterone secreted by the ovaries after menopause than to use potentially risky hormone treatments. Testosterone levels in women who have their ovaries have never been demonstrated to correlate with sexual interest or performance.[49]

Testosterone is increasingly prescribed to increase sex drive as well as for other complaints after natural or surgical menopause, but it often brings unwanted side effects and may have serious risks. Some women feel better, but others report rages and anger.[50] The effects can include a permanently lowered voice, facial hair, acne, weight gain, and liver disease (the latter primarily associated with higher doses given to men).

The safety of lower doses given to women has not been adequately investigated. An injectable, as opposed to oral, dose of testosterone has not been associated with liver disease. A 1% testosterone cream applied directly to the clitoris to treat low sex drive reduces systemic absorption and thus limits the side effects.[51]

Testosterone is often prescribed together with estrogen in preparations such as Estratest. In this combination, testosterone counteracts the positive effect of estrogen on lipid levels and can compound the carcinogenic effect of estrogen on the breast and uterus.[52] Women with breast cancer have a higher rate of relapse after surgery when they have higher levels of testosterone in their blood and urine.[53] Though not enough is known about the link between testosterone and breast cancer, certainly it is wise for women with breast cancer to exercise caution.

Making Sense of the New Research on Hormones

In the past, a woman's decision whether or not to use hormones was based on a choice between short-term relief of menopausal discomforts and the possibility of certain risks. Women today are being urged to take hormones earlier, in some cases before experiencing any discomforts, or even signs of menopause, and to take them for longer durations and even indefinitely. Yet, most women are rejecting this approach. The most popular reason for choosing hormone treatment is still short-term symptom relief. (See *Dr. Susan Love's Hormone Book* for a book-length exposition of these issues.)

The ever-growing body of research suggesting that estrogen treatment protects against osteoporosis and heart disease contributes to the trend toward increased and longer-term prescribing of hormones. Yet, more recently, research has been documenting the risks of hormone therapy, especially the risk of breast cancer.[54] Though this research has been neglected and trivialized by the drug companies and many medical care providers, it is finally getting increased public attention.

Hormones and Breast Cancer

The most serious risk of hormones, especially of long-term use, is the increased risk of cancer, especially of breast cancer. Some, but not all, studies suggest that the use of estrogen alone for ten or 15 years may increase the risk of breast cancer by more than 30%. Progestins protect against endometrial cancer, but they do not protect against breast cancer, as they were expected to. Indeed, they may be an additional hazard.[55] Recent data from the Nurses' Health Study shows that combining estrogen with progestins can be even more risky, and the risk increases with age.[56] The use of testosterone with estrogen may compound the carcinogenic effect of estrogen on the breast and uterus (see p. 560).

Smoking and high alcohol consumption increase your risk of osteoporosis and breast cancer. A new study has found that in women who drank alcohol, elevations in circulating estradiol (a type of estrogen) were three times the amount clinically intended.[57] This can increase the risk of breast cancer and may even explain some of the link between breast cancer and hormone treatment. If you are taking hormone treatment and use alcohol, it is important to reduce or eliminate either the alcohol or the hormones.

Hormones and Bones

Osteoporosis, formerly defined as a fracture incurred as a result of brittle or thin bones, has been recast by the drug companies as a disease of thinning bones, turning a risk factor into a disease. Much of this is market-driven as bone density tests and hormone treatment become more common.[58]

Women who are white or Asian,* aged 60 and over, small-boned, short, and slender are most at risk for osteoporosis. Their backgrounds may include insufficient calcium and other important nutrients during the growing years, breast-feeding several children during their teens and early twenties, having had a medically induced menopause (surgical removal of ovaries or chemotherapy or radiation therapy that makes the ovaries nonfunctional). Some long-term steroid medications, such as cortisone for arthritis or asthma, also contribute to osteoporosis, as do several other diseases and treatments (see discussion of iatrogenesis, chapter 25, The Politics of Women's Health and Medical Care, p. 681).

Lifestyle risks that can be modified include smoking,

insufficient exercise, inadequate calcium intake, and excessive use of alcohol. Exercise, especially weight training, is emerging as one of the most effective ways to preserve bone density while building muscle mass and improving balance,[59] all of which prevent falls and fractures. Changing these behaviors—for example, increasing calcium, vitamin D, and other nutrients, and exercising with an emphasis on weight-bearing and muscle-strengthening activity—substantially reduces our risks of osteoporosis and fractures.

Though research shows that estrogen does reduce bone loss, we question the wisdom of treating women beginning at menopause for a condition that occurs typically 20 to 30 years later, and with a medication that carries serious risks. For women at high risk for bone loss, new research suggests that treatment begun in the later years is just as effective. Another new approach is to substantially reduce the dose of estrogen (to 0.3 mg.). One study found that at that dose it was possible to offer estrogen alone without progestins to postmenopausal women without significant risk to the uterus.[60]

Hormones and Heart Disease

Though much has been made of women's increased risk of heart disease after menopause compared with before menopause, women's rates of heart disease have declined by about half since the early 1960s and are lower than those of men at every age.

Hormones reduce heart disease by changing the lipid profile, i.e., slightly decreasing LDL "bad cholesterol" and increasing HDL "good cholesterol."[61] While gynecologists push hormones, cardiologists encourage women and men to exercise, reduce the fat content in their diet, and quit smoking—measures that have successfully decreased the incidence of heart disease.[62]

Estrogen users do appear to have decreased rates of cardiovascular disease (CVD), but hormone users may be healthier to begin with. Women in earlier nonrandomized studies who took estrogen postmenopausally were thinner, were more physically active, and had higher HDL levels, all of which lowered their risk of CVD.[63] In addition, many of the studies excluded women with medical conditions from the hormone trials; thus, the hormone users were at lower risk of CVD to begin with. Though there is an association between taking hormones and better cardiovascular profiles, it has not been proved that taking hormones prevents heart disease.

Only recently have randomized, double-blind trials been conducted to assess the effect of drugs on heart disease for women. The Postmenopausal Estrogen/Progestin Intervention (PEPI) trials investigated the effects of combined estrogen and progestin treatment by comparing estrogen alone, estrogen with Provera, and estrogen with micronized (or "natural") progesterone. The collection of data is now complete, and some results have been reported. For the most part, the positive effect of estrogen on cardiovascular health was

---

* Both white and Asian women have thin bones as they age, but Asian women have a lower fracture rate (see discussion on p. 558 on cultural aspects of diet and menopause).

blunted or cancelled entirely by the addition of progestin. Differences were found depending on the type of progestin and whether it was administered daily or cyclically. The most positive result was found for estrogen taken with micronized progesterone.[64]

While hormone treatment may reduce the risk of cardiovascular disease, women should be aware that no treatment offers absolute protection. An unexpected discovery, in addition, was that all the PEPI treatment regimens raised triglyceride levels—an independent risk factor for coronary heart disease. The use of an estrogen patch is more likely to lower triglceride levels. "If you are unsure of your risk factors for heart disease, the PEPI results suggest that, as part of a regular check-up, [you should ask for] a detailed report including HDL, LDL, triglyceride and fibrinogen levels, as well as total cholesterol."[65]

Hormones and Mortality

New research from the Nurses' Study confirms that women who take hormones live longer, but with some important caveats, including increased risk for some groups. Women who take hormones for longer than ten years incur an increased (43%) risk of breast cancer, so that longevity benefit of taking hormones diminishes with long-term use. Women at high risk for breast cancer increase their risk. Women at high risk for cardiovascular disease benefit most; women at low risk benefit very little. This research suggests that those who take hormones should not take them for too many years and should consider starting later closer to the typical age of onset of the diseases they are trying to prevent.[66]

Deciding About Hormones: Whether, When, How Much, and For How Long?

You may want to take hormones for a short time to relieve discomforts that disrupt daily life and sap energy, weighing the benefits of relief against the risks, including the possibility that the discomforts will recur when you stop. Physicians who criticize women for lack of "compliance" with their hormone regimens may not be providing enough options. Instead, health care and medical providers should provide as much information as possible, respect women's decisions, and help us carry them out.[67]

New research is under way attempting to keep the beneficial aspects of hormone treatments while reducing the negative effects. These "designer hormones" known as selective estrogen receptor modulators (SERMs) are still in the testing stage and little is known about them. Tamoxifen is one SERM that is being tested in women with breast cancer. It seems not to stimulate breast tissue, while still strengthening bone, but it has been found to increase the risk of endometrial cancer (reportedly of a more virulent kind than usually seen). Another SERM called raloxifene strengthens bone while not stimulating either breast or

uterine tissue to become cancerous, however, it does not reduce hot flashes, and may even make them slightly more frequent.[68]

Keep up with new research findings by joining the National Women's Health Network and subscribing to women's health newsletters. Check online resources, such as Medline and Healthgate. (See Introduction to Online Women's Health Resources, p. 25.)

When I read that women menstruate for an average of 37 years, I realized that number came from 50 (average age of menopause) minus 13 (average age of the start of menstruation). Since I started my periods at eleven and stopped at 53, I have already had five more years of estrogen than average. That was one factor in my decision not to take estrogen.

Consider your choices carefully, but remember that the choice to take hormone therapy or not is only one aspect of your change of life, a normal part of a woman's life experience. We can learn from one another ways to manage the typical discomforts that occur. We must not be manipulated into regarding this important turning point in our lives as merely a choice point about medications. At midlife we have the opportunity to expand our lives, to reach out for new and possibly long-delayed experiences, to create lives that reflect our values and desires. We can live our lives more fully and expressively when we refuse to allow ourselves to be defined as a market for drugs, cosmetics, and plastic surgery. Instead, we can assert our pride in the experience and confidence of our years; our considerable and growing numbers give us the potential of becoming a constituency with significant clout.

Support Groups for Menopausal Women

Support groups are an especially important source of strength for midlife women, offering shared experience and "body" information. Best of all, they reduce the sense of isolation as we recognize the social, economic, and political context of our midlife transition.

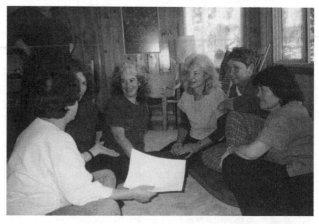

Judy Norsigian

I had never been in any kind of support group before. I thought it would be a discussion group and everyone would be an expert except me, and I'd be embarrassed because I wasn't an expert on anything. But that's not the way this group worked. There's a lot of mutual help; people really listen to each other and laugh a lot. Now I don't worry about menopause or growing older the way I used to.

Validated by the new knowledge that I had the same powerful physical and emotional experiences as all women, I was proud to have gone through menopause and some difficult life changes at the same time. For instance, creating a new life for myself after my divorce. I love my friends and know they have gone through similar changes.

SEXUALITY AND AGING

Sexuality continues throughout our lives. In the middle years, some women first become fully aware of their sexuality.

I was shocked by being so horny after I was divorced, because it's not only sexual. It's aggressive. Certainly not what my mother taught me. It took me a long time to understand that I could lust.

I'm no longer worried about pregnancy; the children are gone; my energy is released. I have a new surge of interest in sex. But at the same time the culture is saying, "You are not attractive as a woman; act your age; be dignified," which means to me, be dead sexually. It's a terrible bind for a middle-aged woman. I say, acknowledge, applaud, enjoy sexuality! Get rid of stereotypes! Change the image of women to include middle-aged beauty and sexuality!

If you are sexually involved with men, remember you can still get pregnant; keep using some form of

PROTECTING YOURSELF

Whether you have sex with men, women, or both, practice safer sex to protect yourself from sexually transmitted diseases and HIV/AIDS. (Review chapters 14 and 15.) Twenty-nine percent of AIDS cases among women reported through June 1997 were diagnosed in women over forty.[69] According to the Centers for Disease Control and Prevention, the number of cases of AIDS among women over 60 has tripled since 1986, and more of them result from heterosexual contact than in the past. Thinning of the vaginal lining and decline of the immune system due to aging make older women more susceptible.[70] Many midlife and older women have less practice in asking a partner to use a condom.

birth control until you haven't had a period for one year. Some midlife women consider the chances of pregnancy to be so low that they rely on abortion as a backup. But if you are certain you do not want a child and would not consider abortion, continue to use birth control for two years after your last period.

Many older women who would like to be sexually active with men lack the opportunity. With each decade of age there are fewer men in their age range, many of whom prefer to date younger women. A divorced woman in her 60s:

I have a great interest in sex, still, and a great desire for it. But what makes it most poignant that I don't have the right partner is that I am capable of giving now to a degree that I never achieved when I was young.

Even married, we may not be as sexually active as we might like if our partners lose interest in sex. Our society admires older men who have relationships with women much younger than themselves, but older women with younger partners become the butt of jokes and derision. Yet, some of us have younger men as partners.

We have to send out signals if a sexual relationship is what we want. I've had a problem if the man is the same age as my son, though after thinking about it I've decided it's okay for me. What really bothers me is my vanity—exposing a middle-aged body to a beautiful younger man.

The joy of making love with a young man who is so full of energy and straightforward is wonderful.

A Duke University study showed that of older men interested in sex, 87% were sexually active, while among interested older women only 60% were sexually active.[71] In fact, the majority of older men are married, while the majority of older women are not. This imbalance is even more pronounced among women of color; the impact of racism on the health and survival of people of color affects the longevity of relationships. As one woman in an older women's discussion group stated:

Some of you say you have husbands at home that won't go anyplace. I have buried three husbands, and I wish I had one to sit home with me now.

Some midlife or older women are considering or having sexual relationships with women for the first time. Others of us have been lesbian for many years, some more or less openly, and others in secret (see chapter 10, Relationships with Women).

Now in my 50s, I am 18 years into what I hope will be a lifelong relationship with a woman. Sex for us is a steady friend. During our busy work week, we cuddle and that's good. On weekends and on vacations, we make time for lovemaking and cherish how it reconnects and refreshes us.

Some older women would rather not have sex at all or prefer to express our sexuality through masturbation and fantasy.

I frankly don't need it, and I don't miss it at all. I had a very, very full sex life—and I was mad about my husband, which is a nice way to be. When he died it was a real shock, but that's 25 years ago now. I've run around with a few men since, but nobody that I really wanted to connect with. You have to have a certain desire toward a person, and I haven't discovered another person that I had that desire for in 25 years now. I'm used to my life the way it is now, and I don't think that my life is incomplete.
                                    —A 73-year-old woman

Many single older women miss not just sex but touching, intimacy, and the excitement of romance.

It's the intimacy that I miss more than the actual sex act. Shared jokes—you know. I'm finding this with a number of women as well as with men, but the whole romantic aspect of my life seems to have gone by. I miss that.
                                    —A woman in her 70s

Physiological Changes

Aging enables us to enjoy sex more. With sexual experience, and after child-bearing, we develop a large, complex venous system in the pelvic area that enhances our capacity for sexual tension and im-

EFFECTS OF DRUGS AND DISEASE ON SEXUALITY

Some drugs, such as Prozac and related antidepressants, depress sexual function or interest. Medication for high blood pressure can prevent erections, as can too much alcohol. (The depressive effect of alcohol becomes more pronounced as people get older.) Fear often interferes with sex after a heart attack or diagnosis of heart disease. Most women find that after an initial recovery period sex is as enjoyable as ever (see table on "Sex and Disability," chapter 11, Sexuality, p. 251, which covers the effects of many physical conditions and treatments). Ask your health care practitioner about the effects on sexual interest, arousal, or functioning of any medications that are prescribed for you or your partner, or check the *Physicians' Desk Reference.*

proves orgasmic intensity, frequency, and pleasure.[72] However, changed estrogen levels or possibly simple aging may produce changes in the vagina. Thinning of the vaginal walls, loss of elasticity, flattening out of ridges, foreshortening or narrowing of the vagina, and dryness or itching may make penetration with penis, finger, or dildo less comfortable or even painful, leading to irritation and increased susceptibility to infection. Doctors, with their gift for nomenclature, call it "senile vaginal atrophy" and describe it in medical texts as occurring five or more years after menstruation ceases. Yet, many women experience vaginal changes earlier in menopause, and others at age 60 or later.

Self-Help Approaches for Vaginal Dryness

Any type of arousing sexual activity with a partner or by ourselves can maintain and improve lubrication. Perineal (Kegel) exercises (see "Anatomy and Physiology," chapter 12, Understanding Our Bodies, p. 274) can help maintain vaginal muscle tone. Or we may find other ways to fulfill our sexual desires (see chapter 11, Sexuality). It is a myth that we must be perpetually sexually active to maintain sexual health.

I had a problem with dryness when I started having sexual intercourse again after a few years [of celibacy]. In a month or two, my vagina began to get wet faster.
                                    —A woman in her 60s

Vaginal dryness at any age may simply mean that you are not ready for penetration. The slower arousal time of older women and men has compensations. A woman in her 40s states:

When Jay used to lose his erection I would think that I had failed as a woman because I couldn't keep him aroused. But now I see that it can mean more time to play around and a chance to start over again so that lovemaking lasts longer.

Water-based lubricants, such as K-Y Jelly or Astroglide, used at the time of lovemaking, can help. Some women have found vitamin E suppositories helpful. If dryness persists, try an over-the-counter moisturizer, such as Replens, which may be used one or more times a week *not* at the time of penetration. If you are still menstruating, remember that these products are not contraceptives, nor do they protect against STDs or HIV/AIDS.

Some prescription and over-the-counter drugs may cause or contribute to dryness. Antihistamines, for example, dry vaginal tissues as well as nasal tissues. Douches, sprays, and colored or perfumed toilet paper and soaps can irritate the tissues of the vulva. If itchiness develops, avoid scratching, which can irritate the delicate tissues and lead to infections and further problems. Itching can be relieved by applying bancha tea or vitamin E oil topically to the pubic and vaginal area.

Aci-gel and other prescription ointments can help itchiness.

Try a variety of lubricants or moisturizers before considering getting a prescription for a low-dose estrogen cream. For vaginal dryness and for "low sex drive," testosterone is increasingly prescribed in cream form. (See above for more on testosterone use.)

Changing Attitudes and Communication

Older women must overcome years of training to initiate sex or consider alternatives to their customary patterns. The physiological changes of aging can invite both men and women, and women with women, to break through old patterns, assumptions, misunderstandings, and miscommunications. Men may misinterpret their slowness to arousal as a sign that their sexual capacities are eroding and, in panic, blame their partner and seek out other (younger) women. Women may fear that their partner's slower arousal is due to changes in their looks, or interpret their own lack of lubrication as loss of attraction to their partner. It is important for both partners in a relationship, whether heterosexual or lesbian, to realize that changes are normal and to talk together to find out what is pleasurable. Such communication may be difficult at first and requires practice. You may want to consider getting some help together. Do what pleases you both, even if it seems unusual or strange at first. A greater capacity for empathy and loving, developed through the years of living, can make sex better.

My immense pleasure and response were for him an incredible high, and that made me feel so marvelous. It was not just the physical part but our delight in each other that was so enormously exciting. It was a circular or spiral effect, because I had not realized that another person could enjoy my passion. Before this, I had experienced my passion and my partner would experience his passion. But this was different. And of course it's very much that way in a lesbian love affair, that delight in the other woman's total experience, the total emotional response. Danny took great pride in that just as a woman does with another woman. He thought it was marvelous that I was multiply orgasmic. After he died, I was in a state of shock for over a year. The mutuality we shared was rare with a man. My subsequent love affairs have all been with women.

I am 74 years old and have been married for 52 years. This is not entirely a matter of luck. We have worked at it. Our good times have been more numerous than our bad times. The medical profession has only recently discovered the healing power of laughter. In our years together we have had a lot of laughs. A sense of humor is as important as food, especially within the confines of marriage. For us, the sharing that comes with having a warm and loving sex life over so many years deepens our joy in one another.

AGING AND PREVENTIVE HEALTH— SPECIAL ISSUES

New research on aging finds that many of the changes of aging, once thought biologically inevitable, are preventable and even reversible. Throughout life we can take active steps to maintain good health and lessen the impact of illnesses or chronic conditions when we get older. Acquiring new habits will serve us well for the rest of our lives: we can stop smoking; exercise more; eat healthfully; and reduce our dependence on caffeine, sugar, alcohol, and tranquilizers to achieve the highest possible quality of life as long as we live.

Activity and Movement in Our Older Years

Activity becomes increasingly important as we age. Without exercise we lose muscle mass, and the ratio of body fat to muscle mass increases as we grow older. Women typically begin to lose bone mass at about the age of 35, often because of physical inactivity and sedentary jobs. Happily, an increasing number of women of every age have rejected this norm and are on the move!

By reading many books and articles on women, mental health, nutrition, and exercise I began to see that my life could and should change. The changes did not come easily. My husband resisted. After all, I was rocking the boat in which we had become quite comfortable. I took up tae kwon do, Eastern self-defense, which appealed to me as a Japanese-American. To my amazement, after a few months of kicking and hitting an imaginary opponent, my chronic insomnia and stiff neck disappeared. Gone also were the painful attacks of gastritis. I began feeling more energetic. . . . I stopped eating white sugar in any form. . . . No more processed food, including white bread, noodles, and spaghetti; in came more fresh vegetables and grains. Out went sleeping pills, aspirin, and other medications; in came vitamins. It was not an overnight sensation. After all, I was trying to undo the damage done over 40-some years. That was more than five years ago. Today, all the ailments that I thought I would have to live with the rest of my life are gone.

—A woman in her 50s

Weight-bearing exercise, such as walking, jogging, and dancing, makes our bones work harder and strengthens the muscles and ligaments supporting the skeleton. Upper body exercise, such as swimming, lifting small weights, and doing push-ups or other arm exercises, is also important. If we continually exercise only one part of our body, we may gain strength in the muscles and bones exercised while accelerating bone loss elsewhere in the body.

Many of the benefits of exercise for older women

are already evident. Exercise can lower blood pressure and reduce atherosclerosis, risks of heart attack and stroke, arthritis, emphysema, and osteoporosis. It is central in finding and keeping a comfortable weight. It helps us sleep, improves bowel functioning, maintains strength and good posture, often relieves depression and hot flashes, and generally makes most people feel better. Women who engaged in moderate or heavy physical activity were found to have increased high-density lipoprotein (HDL) or "good cholesterol" and decreased fibrinogen (a blood-clotting factor) in a sample of 851 middle-aged white women.[73]

After exercise, blood rushes to the skin, bringing with it extra nutrients, raising the skin's temperature, and increasing the collagen content. Skin actually thickens and becomes more elastic and less wrinkled. Delightfully, it is never too late to start exercising.

My grandmother in her early 90s noticed that when she moved around more, her memory improved.

Weight-training programs in nursing homes have increased muscle strength in persons in their 90s.[74] There are forms of exercise that fit almost any kind of physical limitation.

A few tips to help you keep moving even if you don't like "exercise." Fit activity into daily activities by parking a little farther from your destination, or getting off the bus a stop ahead. In bad weather, try walking at a mall, or lift small weights at home. If you do not have an exercise program, start slowly; watch less TV or exercise while you watch. Exercise with a friend for company and support; try walking, yoga, or swimming; take an exercise class to help you overcome sedentary habits. (See chapter 4, Women in Motion, for more.)

Eating Well

Although the same basic principles of healthy eating apply throughout life, nutritional requirements change somewhat with age. You need fewer calories (unless you are working or exercising hard) but the same nutrients and more of certain ones, such as calcium. See chapter 2, Food, for all but the following few items of special interest to older women.

Hints for eating well may become harder to follow in our older years, especially when we can't easily get out to shop or are on a small fixed income and cannot afford to buy fresh foods. As many as 50% of older women over 65 are malnourished because they consume too few calories, proteins, and essential vitamins and minerals.

Changes in our dental health may affect our ability to eat well. If we have teeth and gum or denture problems, it is important to get dental care, but Medicare does not cover dental care. Problems with swallowing should be checked out by a medical care provider. During a temporary period of difficulty in chewing or swallowing, you can puree many nutritious foods or make them into soups. Do not buy the liquid diets often sold in drugstores. They are meant for sick people. They are too expensive for a steady diet, and they lack some of the nutrients found in food.

Calcium, Vitamin D, and Magnesium— A Balance of Nutrients

- *Calcium.* For middle-aged and older women, calcium is an essential nutrient, as it prevents bone loss that can lead to osteoporosis. Since women over 35 absorb calcium less easily, we must make a special effort to exercise more (this is indispensable to helping our bodies absorb calcium), eat a calcium-rich diet, and learn about other nutrients that aid or inhibit calcium absorption so we can get the right balance of such nutrients. If your body can't tolerate milk products (lactose intolerance), see chapter 2, Food, for nondairy sources of calcium. Lactose intolerance may increase with age. Calcium supplements can help us get the recommended 1,500 to 2,000 milligrams. Use the lesser amount if you are taking hormones, the higher if you are not.
- *Vitamin D.* You need 400 to 800 IU a day, for calcium and phosphorus absorption. This is crucial for housebound and/or lactose-intolerant women who do not drink milk. The main sources of vitamin D are sunshine, fatty fish, fortified milk, and fortified cereals. Yogurt and cheese, while good sources of calcium, contain no vitamin D. If you live in a northern climate, you may want to take a vitamin D supplement from November to March and get your vitamin D from sunshine during the rest of the year. Be sure to observe the cautions for preventing skin cancer, such as walking in the early morning, staying out of the midday sun, and using sunscreen.
- *Magnesium.* We need to balance calcium with magnesium in a two-to-one ratio. If your magnesium level drops lower, calcium will be lost. There is some evidence that the older we are, the more magnesium we need, especially when we are under stress. Magnesium can help muscles and nerves relax, and relieve constipation, and it is safer than tranquilizers. Fruits and vegetables contain magnesium.

Other Important Nutrition Information for Older Women

- *Protein.* Because we don't absorb as much protein as we age, try to eat more high-protein foods. However, be sure to balance protein with a sufficient amount of complex carbohydrates. Too much protein relative to other nutrients can interfere with calcium absorption.
- *Water.* Although not a nutrient, water is essential to proper functioning of the kidneys and bowels and therefore to life and health. The basic transport system of the body, it moves all

nutrients, hormones, blood cells, waste products, and oxygen through the body. At menopause, keeping ourselves well hydrated can help counter dryness of the skin, the vagina, and other mucous membranes.

Small changes in diet may be all you can manage, but even cutting down on junk foods helps a lot. If you put off cooking because you are preparing meals only for yourself, try designating one day per week as a cooking day. Fix several dishes, including a main dish and a tasty soup, and then eat them on alternate days, or freeze some in individual portions for later. Exchange meals with a friend or neighbor.

Because we absorb nutrients less well as we age and many of us may not take in enough calories altogether, we may need vitamin supplements. (See discussion of the pros and cons of supplements in chapter 2, Food.) It is always best to try to get as much of the nutrients you need from your food. A recent 12-year study of over 90,000 women found that women who eat a calcium-rich diet reduce their risk of kidney stones, but those who take calcium supplements on an empty stomach increase their risk.[75] If you have a history of kidney stones, make sure you consume lots of fluids to counteract calcium buildup, and check with your physician before taking calcium supplements.[76]

GETTING MEDICAL CARE

Increasingly, medical care has come under the control of managed care, which affects our access to certain tests, treatments, and health care practitioners. (See chapter 25, The Politics of Women's Health and Medical Care.)

Most ob/gyns are not particularly interested in women past menopause, especially when we have already had hysterectomies or refuse estrogen treatment. Internists, family practitioners, physicians' assistants, and well-informed family practitioners and nurse practitioners are often more appropriate health care providers for older women when they have a positive attitude and enough information about aging.

Geriatricians are physicians trained to distinguish disease states from the normal physiological changes of aging. Today, there is a growing consensus that training physicians in geriatrics is necessary to meet the special health needs of an aging population, and efforts are under way to develop the academic teaching and research expertise necessary to carry out that training.[77] There is currently a shortage of primary care physicians who have had *any* specialized training in geriatrics. The U.S. has less than one-third the number of physicians it needs who are geriatricians or who have special training in geriatrics, and less than one-fourth the number of academic geriatricians.[78] A small number of geriatric centers and clinics are mostly located near large medical centers.

Because the health care practitioner or clinic you visit may not have adequate information about the diseases and chronic conditions of aging and about their prevention or the physical changes that affect older women in particular, you may have to educate the practitioners who treat you.

I always try to bring an article with me when I visit a new doctor. The way the doctor reacts tells me whether he or she is someone who will work with me, and respect me as a partner in my health care. If the doctor is dismissive, I don't go back, and I make it known why not. Most of my health care providers have been pleased to have an informed patient who brings new information.

Research on Women and Aging

Until very recently, medical research paid little attention to aging women's health concerns. Even today, it focuses on menopause as the primary midlife health issue, as though reproductive organs were the center of a woman's life, and overlooks occupational health, racial and ethnic differences, and the influence of socioeconomic factors on our health.

Studies, often designed and funded by corporate interests rather than objective researchers, have overfocused on drugs and other interventions for menopause and have been developed with little basic knowledge of the physiology of menopause and hot flashes. In recent years, federal agencies such as the National Institute on Aging (NIA) have invited consumer advocates to meetings and conferences and have paid greater attention to our concerns in developing and funding research projects. As consumers and citizens, we must demand that government and the press investigate the influence and the power of the drug companies in setting the research agenda, which is paid for with taxpayer dollars.

Studies of midlife and menopause rarely address the

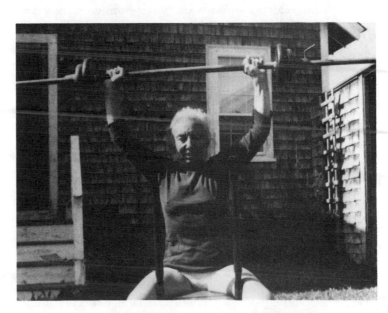

Deborah Wald

needs of women of color, which undermines the ability of health care practitioners to provide appropriate care. Two important studies are under way to remedy this longstanding neglect. The Study of Women's Health Across the Nation (SWAN) is an NIA-sponsored study with seven data collection sites in five states (MA, CA, IL, NJ, PA). At each site, midlife women between the ages of 42 and 52 are to be enrolled for a total study sample of 3,000 women. African-American, Japanese-American, Chinese-American, and Latina women, depending on population concentrations at the sites, will be compared with white women. Another important strength of the study is that it will examine psychological, social, and economic factors as well as more narrowly defined health and medical factors.

The Black Women's Health Study, funded by the National Cancer Institute and conducted by epidemiologists at Howard University and Boston University, aims to enroll 50,000 African-American women, monitoring them every two years through mailed questionnaires. Although the study focuses primarily on younger women's diseases and conditions, it is also looking at some conditions more typical of midlife and older women, such as cardiovascular disease, diabetes, and breast cancer, which affect black women earlier[79] and thus affect their chances of living longer lives. This study has primarily enrolled women who have more formal education on average than the community at large. We and our organizations must continue our advocacy efforts for research approaches that will also reach women with lower incomes and less formal education.

Physicians' Attitudes

Many physicians, like the lay public, are personally ambivalent and frightened by aging and death. Sexism compounds the basic ageism that shapes many physicians' attitudes toward older patients. Physicians and medical personnel view older women's complaints and health problems as neurotic or imaginary far more than they do men's, and at earlier ages. Some have been heard to call aging women "old bags" and other insulting names. Until recently, the medical world seemed to hold the underlying prejudice that after our child-bearing years, we have outlived our usefulness. This is changing somewhat, in part because medical practitioners and institutions have become aware that midlife and older women represent an important market to be courted. New research in gerontology and geriatrics increasingly shows the capacities of older persons for growth and strength, but you must search for a health care provider who is aware of this body of research.

Acute-Care Medicine and Chronic Conditions of Aging

Though demographers have been expecting a surge in needs for long-term care because of the growth in the over-85 population, research has found that higher education and income, along with new techniques of cataract surgery, and hip and knee replacements, have substantially reduced disability levels in the older population.[80] This is an area where medical treatment has made a substantial improvement in quality of life for some elders. Yet, there is a danger that findings such as these may be used to reduce caregiving services and supports for those elders who may have limited access to improved medical care, or who, for whatever reasons, still need caregiving services.

Many of the conditions we may suffer from as we age are not subject to outright "cure"; yet, we have a medical system that is organized primarily around acute care (see chapter 25). Chronic diseases, for the most part, do not respond to daring surgery or high-technology interventions. The ordinariness of diet, canes, physical and occupational therapy, and pain relief medication is boring, and doctors often give us less attention when these are what we need.

Many women also explore alternative approaches to healing to complement conventional medicine, or as an alternative, but these are frequently not covered by health insurance or by Medicare. Better and more appropriate care for older persons requires that nonmedical providers, such as social workers, case managers, and family members, who provide for the care of the chronically ill be recognized and receive compensation. The term "continuum of care" describes a system in which a person receives care appropriate to her condition, provided promptly and efficiently and in the right amount, increasing or decreasing as the person's capabilities change.[81] Health care for elders that fosters autonomy and sociability while limiting unnecessary routinization and medicalization of daily life means increasing funding for supported housing and caregiving. Since conventional care has not met these goals, we wonder whether managed care will meet them, although some managed care organizations do provide case workers for subscribers who need a variety of services. We must keep pressuring policy makers in health institutions and government to fund the health and social services needed by an aging population.

Misdiagnosis and Failure to Treat Reversible Conditions

When we are past 60, and even more when we are over 75, health care practitioners tend to blame all our physical and emotional problems on aging and don't look for treatable disorders. These attitudes and practices are less blatant toward women who have ample financial resources and private physicians. Such women, however, are at greater risk for unnecessary and risky treatments, such as hormone treatment (see p. 554) and cosmetic surgery.

Physicians lacking adequate training in geriatrics may interpret emotional or mental confusion as senility when these may instead indicate poor nutrition, treatable physical malfunctions, grief, or responses to inappropriate medication. Time after time, physicians offer older women tranquilizers, sedatives, antidepressants, and hormones instead of looking for what's really wrong. As one nurse puts it, "When a man complains of dizziness he gets a work-up; an older woman gets Valium."

I was afraid when I broke my wrist that it would take ages if ever to heal, and so I hesitated to do a more "aggressive" type of therapy for it. Now it's much better, and I'm going to begin that therapy. My fear and a stereotype of being old held me back.

Overprescription of Drugs

People over 65 take 30% of the medications prescribed annually in the U.S., though they constitute only 13% of the U.S. population.[82] Many older people take several medications daily for various chronic conditions, often prescribed by different physicians who may not know about the other prescriptions. Health care practitioners frequently neglect the crucial step of finding out what medications a woman is taking, including over-the-counter drugs, before prescribing others. Elders have had so many bad reactions to taking too many medications that this "condition" has been given a name: "polypharmacy." Bring a list of all your medications to your medical appointments. Regularly ask your health care provider to review all your medications. Most physicians don't realize that people over 60 are more sensitive to many drugs and might need lower doses, adjusted to size, age, and nutritional status. (Women at any age may require lower drug dosages than men because of lower body mass and weight.) Some of us prefer other approaches, such as applying heat or massage, or consulting a physical therapist for pain.

As we age become even more sensitive to drugs, metabolizing them more slowly. The kidneys and liver excrete them more slowly, so they stay in the body longer. Also, as we age, muscle mass turns to fat, so drugs that can be stored in fat tissue, such as Valium, stay in the body a longer time, increasing the likelihood of harmful effects or addiction even from low or infrequent doses. A study of older persons admitted to a state mental hospital found that 15% of admissions were tied to drug toxicities rather than to dementia or other mental illness.[83] Some drugs can cause depression (for which we may be offered more drugs) or mental confusion, though symptoms often stop when the medication is stopped.

In nursing homes, many elders are literally "tranquilized" into quiet and compliance. If you believe that you or a relative or friend is being inappropriately or excessively medicated, do all you can to change the situation. Some states have a nursing home residents' advocate called an *ombudsman.*

I went to visit a 94-year-old friend who lives in a nursing home. She was recently diagnosed as having various ailments that require anywhere from three to ten pills a day. She was never told what the pills were or what they were for. When the nurse came to her room to give her the pills, my friend looked her squarely in the eye and said, "The doctor only knows my body and how it works for a short time. I know it for 94 years, and nothing is going in it until I know what it is!"

Physical Impairments and Chronic Conditions Related to Aging

In our 50s and beyond, a lifetime of exposure to occupational health hazards may have caused debilitating disease (see chapter 7, Environmental and Occupational Health). This is even more of a reality for women of color, 40% of whom work in physically demanding or otherwise hazardous occupations, and who are at even higher risk for a number of the chronic diseases and conditions that become more common as we age. African Americans have a one-in-three rate of hypertension, compared with the one-in-four rate in the older population at large. One in ten older white people have type II diabetes, compared with one in five older African Americans and one in three older Hispanics.

Social and economic factors can be more disabling than medical conditions: isolation from family and friends; caregiving for homebound relatives without outside help; and poor medical care due to high cost, lack of insurance coverage, inadequate medical understanding of aging, and maldistribution of doctors. Poverty often causes health and medical problems, and so-called welfare reform has made this worse. Money worries caused by a small, limited income and the fears of cutbacks to Social Security, Medicare, and other government programs add greatly to the unhealthy stresses of daily living. Inadequate income also makes it harder to take care of ourselves in simple but crucial daily ways. It is difficult, for instance, to get enough exercise if sidewalks are not cleared of snow, if we don't feel safe on the streets, or if we have little access to indoor exercise facilities. A worsening economic situation and drastic cuts in social programs make it more difficult each month for thousands of older women to get adequate calories, let alone vitamins and special diets. Some lose their homes or live without adequate heat or air conditioning. Low income severely restricts our access to medical care, especially in a time of reduced government aid. Add to this atmosphere of "benign" neglect the deliberate, punitive withholding of support and services to aged immigrants. Without a major turnaround in social priorities and policies, the health of great numbers of older women will worsen drastically over the next few years, with more emergency hospitalization for anemia, dehydration, and hypothermia (dangerously drastic drop in body temperature), and collapse and deaths from all causes.

Many of the serious health problems affecting midlife and older women are discussed elsewhere in this book because they affect younger women, too (see chapter 24, especially the sections on hypertension, cancer, arthritis, heart disease, diabetes, and arteriosclerosis). *Osteoarthritis* and *hypertension* are the two most common chronic conditions affecting older women. Hypertension, or high blood pressure is a major risk factor for strokes and other cardiovascular conditions; controlling it may be key to preventing many of the most disabling conditions of the older years, including dementia. The troubling but not life-threatening problems and changes that sometimes come with aging—visual impairment, hearing loss, difficulties in walking—along with osteoporosis, which primarily affects women over 60, are discussed below.

Women over 65 are more likely to have two or more chronic conditions and are more likely to have conditions that require help in activities of independent living. This combination of factors increases our risk of nursing home placement.

Each of us ages differently. We should never automatically assume that conditions affecting us are the inevitable result of aging. Be wary of any health care practitioner who dismisses most complaints with "What do you expect at your age?" Many problems are as treatable now as they are at any age. Increasingly, new medical techniques are successfully reducing impairments of mobility and vision that in the past would have limited our independence.

When we do have to give up a degree of independence or a cherished activity because we can't see, hear, or move around as well as before, it may take time to get used to new limits and to find alternative ways to manage. A woman in her 70s, speaking at a meeting of the Older Women's League, introduced her cane as "her new friend."

With my friend, I can still get around. My friend helped me to be here with all of you. I have more than one. I bought wooden ones so I could paint them to accessorize my outfits.

This kind of empowering approach can overcome the stigma many of us attach to canes, hearing aids, and other assistive devices that we fear will make us look "old" but that in fact can keep us active and involved.

Limitations on our ability to drive (during day or night) may force us to give up cherished activities and even social relationships. Invite others to share a cab, or ask for rides, making new friends through sharing transportation. Some councils on aging and some community and religious institutions help elders organize transportation for themselves, or recruit volunteers to provide rides. Many communities provide transportation services for older persons and persons with disabilities, and some offer taxi coupons at reduced rates.

I thought I would have to quit working when my car broke down and I couldn't afford to get it fixed. My knees were hurting me too bad to walk to the bus. But one of my friends who works for the elderly told me about "the Ride." My doctor wrote a letter for me to qualify, and now they pick me up on the days I work. They can't be too specific about the time, so I worked out a flex-time arrangement with my employers.

—A woman in her 60s

Organized around the nuclear family and the individual automobile, society magnifies the isolation of older women, many of whom live alone. To live in more interdependent ways—sharing a house, organizing car pools—might be better for us. We must work for more and improved public transportation and for communities in which it is safe to walk around.

Sensory Loss and Aging

It is common to experience changes in the sharpness of our senses as we grow older. These usually occur so gradually that we adapt without even noticing. Someone else may be the first to point out that we don't seem to be seeing or hearing as well as we used to. We may also lose sensitivity of touch and have difficulty with simple tasks such as fixing a clasp on a necklace, or turning pages or a doorknob. Loss of taste and smell can lead to loss of appetite and even malnutrition for some older people. Declines in vision or hearing more directly affect our interactions with others and may play into ageist stereotypes about the "slowness" or "stodginess" of older persons. Though you may have to work at being up-front about your sensory changes and any adaptations you need, it helps others understand how they can be helpful. Don't hesitate to ask people to speak up and to let them know that your mental abilities are as good as ever.

Changes in Vision

Our eyes have less elasticity by midlife. Far-sighted people may need stronger glasses or perhaps glasses for the first time. Some near-sighted people can give up glasses, except for driving or other distance viewing; others may require bifocals or trifocals. We may have trouble adjusting to them or feel embarrassed about wearing them.

If you experience sudden flashing light or a black area in your field of vision, get medical attention at once. These could be serious symptoms of a detached retina—an emergency. Some women notice black spots in their field of vision, which may become chronic. These should also be checked out, but they do not constitute an emergency. If they become chronic, you can sometimes get rid of them by resting your eyes or by doing eye-rolling exercises.

In our 70s and 80s, or sometimes even decades earlier, cataracts (cloudy lenses) may develop. Although there isn't much evidence yet that these specific conditions can be prevented, some eye care providers recommend vitamin E to their patients. Not much is known about the cause of cataracts, but eye repair is one of the few areas where medicine's heroics really pay off, restoring sight or improving it. A second opinion about eye surgery is a particularly good idea, because some doctors will urge operations when they aren't necessary, or sooner (or later) than is appropriate. If you are having cataract surgery, also investigate postsurgery options in advance. Recent improvements include laser surgery and the possibility of implants placed at the time of surgery, rather than contact lenses or new glasses afterward. Find an ophthalmologist (a medical doctor who specializes in eye diseases) who is experienced in this procedure. Cataract surgery is usually done as an outpatient procedure. Bring someone with you for support, and bring sunglasses. If you are over 65 and "financially disadvantaged," ophthalmologists will provide free medical eye care. For information, call the National Eye Care Project Hot Line at 1-800-222-3937 between 8 A.M. and 4 P.M. Pacific Standard Time.

Glaucoma, a chronic eye disease, usually appears at midlife or later. Excess pressure of fluid inside the eye can damage the optic nerve and cause blindness if untreated. **It is crucial to have an eye exam annually after the age of 45 that includes a test for glaucoma.** Glaucoma affects women more than men and rarely causes early pain or symptoms. Tests done with a tonometer are quick and painless (though some people find them uncomfortable). Optometrists, who measure eye function, can perform tonometry only in certain states. Ophthalmologists have the most accurate diagnostic equipment and skills. If detected early, some mild glaucoma can be treated effectively with drops. More severe glaucoma requires surgical treatment with regular follow-up, since no permanent cures exist.

Coping with Hearing Loss

We take hearing for granted until we suddenly notice that we miss what is being said or must ask people to repeat more often than feels comfortable. Feelings of isolation can be as hard to deal with as the actual hearing loss.

Every once in a while I miss out on parts of a conversation. . . . I discover to my later discomfort that occasionally I act as if I did hear—bright smile, nod of agreement.

Being hard of hearing is an invisible disability. No one knows unless you tell them.

One of the most important things a hard-of-hearing person can do for herself, I have discovered, is to be very assertive. Tell each person you talk with to speak more slowly or more clearly, and force yourself to keep reminding that person if she forgets.

Hearing loss, though common, is not an inevitable accompaniment of aging, though it does seem to run

---

TIPS FOR TALKING WITH A PERSON WITH A HEARING DIFFICULTY *

- Don't talk from another room or from behind her.
- Reduce background noise. Turn off radio or TV if possible.
- See that the light falls on your face, so she can use visual clues.
- Get her attention before speaking.
- Face her directly and on the same level if possible.
- Keep your hands away from your face. Avoid speaking while you are smoking or eating.
- Don't shout. Speak naturally but slowly and distinctly.
- Try to speak at a lower pitch. Many people lose their higher-pitch hearing first. Many women need to lower their pitch to be audible to people with hearing loss.
- She may not hear or understand something you say. If so, try saying it in a different way rather than repeating.
- Recognize that she will hear less well if tired or ill.
- Be patient. Even hints of irritation or impatience hurt.
- Be an attentive listener. Make sure the conversation allows for a balance of speaking and listening for each of you. It's probably easier for her to talk than to listen.

* These tips are adapted from those developed by a community group who present them through skits demonstrating problems and issues.

---

in some families. Hearing loss is the third most common chronic condition among older people. Sixty percent of people over 65, and 90% of those over 75, have some degree of hearing impairment.[84] It tends to be more common and more severe among men than women, but it is a problem for a significant number of women too. The enormous increase in the volume and range of noise accompanying industrialization has contributed significantly to hearing loss in the present generation of people over 65, especially among factory workers and urban dwellers. Baby-boomers face additional risk from years of exposure to loud music. It is crucial to obtain an accurate diagnosis of the cause of hearing loss, because treatment varies depending on whether one has nerve or conduction deafness. Conduction deafness, unlike nerve deafness, can often be corrected with surgery.

I developed a new interest in foreign movies. I was missing a lot at the theater and in American movies, but when I go to a foreign movie, I can read the subtitles so I don't miss a thing—and I'm expanding my horizons!

—A 78-year-old woman

At public events, ask the speaker to speak more loudly. Signing is a way to make cultural events accessible to persons with hearing loss who learn ASL. If you are planning a cultural event, be sure to find someone who will sign.

Hearing aids of many different types exist, but unfortunately there are hucksters who make their money from misleading older people with hearing loss. If you are considering a hearing aid, do some research first. AARP (see Resources) has some helpful material, or ask your health care provider.

Getting Around: Osteoarthritis and Mobility

Osteoarthritis (caused by wear and tear on the joints) is the most common chronic condition among older women, affecting some 25% of us. Osteoarthritis causes pain but is not usually a crippling disease. People who have arthritis and the health care providers who work with them are firm in stating that all arthritis can be helped. Although people with arthritic disorders require more rest than most others, millions of people with arthritis live normal, rich, fruitful lives. Ninety percent of people with arthritis are employable, although some may need help changing to more appropriate jobs. Only 3% of those with arthritis are seriously disabled, and prevention, self-help, early diagnosis, and new methods of treatment are reducing that percentage.[85] Some occupations particularly stress our joints and backs. For example, nurse's aides and LPNs have two and a half times the rate of back disorders as other women workers (see chapter 7, Environmental and Occupational Health).

Managing osteoarthritis involves a balance of exercise and rest, along with pain relief, including drugs. Listen to your body. Exercise gently and slowly, with relaxation between repetitions. Swimming and exercising in water can help. A warm bath or shower on arising can help manage morning joint stiffness and can serve as a nice transition to gentle stretching or limbering exercises. Exercises involving gentle stretching of all involved muscles two or three times a week help reduce pain and maintain mobility.

Don't avoid exercise because of joint pain, but don't do anything that causes or increases pain. If pain occurs, stop. Try another kind of exercise. Try to build up to a half hour each day of moderate activity, for example, 15 minutes of gardening and 15 minutes of walking. Sometimes losing weight can relieve the pain; unlike osteoporosis (see p. 573) which is more common among the very thin, a risk factor for osteoarthritis is excessive weight. Keep warm—people with arthritis are often sensitive to cold, dampness, and changes in barometric pressure, which changes the pressure inside the joints.

It was in that horrible cold, damp January after one close friend died suddenly and another dear friend was terminally ill with breast cancer that I began to have severe back and knee pain on arising. I would roll on my side rather than sit straight up as I had been instructed for my back pain, and on standing, hold on to the bedpost until my knees felt strong enough to hold me. My doctor at my HMO sent me to a physician's assistant in Orthopedics for x-ray and evaluation. The PA felt my back X ray was more alarming than my knee problem and urged me to continue my back exercises at all costs. Happily, I was also referred to a physical therapist to have my back exercises adapted so as not to stress my knees. Exercising every other day allowed my muscles and joints time to recover after each exercise session.

—A woman in her late 50s

If you are considering a move to a warmer, drier climate, try a visit first. Moving can be one of life's most stressful experiences. The loss of friends and an accustomed social environment can be more stressful than weather-related aching joints.

A 78-year old woman began to have pain with some of her accustomed outdoor activity:

[While on a camping trip] I had difficulty climbing stairs at a railroad station. I found I could navigate them by putting both feet on a step before I went to another. I could take some of the easier hikes and avoid the strenuous ones. Professionals and lay friends suggested I continue more or less as I was, testing limits and letting discomfort be the determining factor. If I had pain when I got up after sitting engrossed with a book, I consoled myself with the awareness that this, too, would pass as I limbered up. I accepted these limits to my flexibility and found I could live within them. Then, I found that I didn't have to accept them as completely [as I had]. It all began with borrowing a bicycle and relearning how to ride one. I found out how to take advantage of my strong left hip and soon was braving traffic and riding, once more, with confidence [and] a new sense of my body's resources. Then I learned from a hiking book that all my life I had been walking incorrectly. Soon I began using a more productive method. I began to feel more grounded and, at the same time, freer.

You probably take your feet for granted. If you begin to notice aches and pain, not just when walking but when you rest as well, this may be part of skeletal or bone changes. Foot problems in women are very often caused by the restrictive design of women's shoes or poorly fitted shoes. In one study of female orthopedic patients, 88% of women were found to be wearing shoes that were too small for their feet.[86] High heels distort our walking gait and posture, and they strain other joints, including the back and neck. Well-designed shoes with a firm, supportive arch may prevent fatigue as well as other foot problems, such as bunions. Any existing foot problems may get worse as we age, especially if we have put on weight or are on our feet all day. Women with low incomes and women of color are much more likely to earn their living on their feet, earnings are so low that they often must continue working into old age.

Most managed care plans do not cover routine care by podiatrists, but they will pay for the care of problems and infections caused by neglect of routine foot care. Podiatry visits may be available for homebound elders with low incomes through various elder care programs in your community.

Bone Loss and Osteoporosis

Bone, like skin, blood cells, and other living tissues in our bodies, is constantly replacing itself throughout life. In our teens, if we are physically active and eat a high-calcium diet, we are "putting our money in the bone bank" during the years when it matters most, when we are still growing and building up bone, giving us a lifelong advantage.[87] In our young adult years, bone is replaced at about the same rate that it breaks down, but by our middle 30s, we start to lose bone faster than we replace it, at the rate of about 1% of bone mass every year. Some women lose bone at an accelerated rate at menopause. Another period of increased bone loss occurs in our 70s. Some bone loss in women and men is normal as we age.

Prevention

Throughout life, we can build up bone by eating healthfully, doing weight-bearing exercise, avoiding harmful habits, such as smoking, and avoiding—when possible—medical interventions that contribute to bone loss. It is also never too late to begin.

Health care providers who are up-to-date with the latest recommendations "prescribe" calcium, vitamin C and vitamin D supplements,[88] exercises such as walking and weight-training, special back-exercise regimens, and physical therapy. Exercising in water offers beneficial resistance to movement while placing less stress on joints.

Bone Loss, Osteoporosis, and Fractures

Not all bone loss is osteoporosis, a condition of extreme bone loss leading to fractures. Osteoporosis, when it affects the spine, can be painful and difficult to manage. Relentless publicity campaigns by drug companies give the impression that all women will inevitably suffer fractures unless we take estrogen preventively in our middle years. Only 15% of women who are now 50 who live to be very old will have osteoporosis, and many will never know they "have" it unless they break a bone. Furthermore, bone density declines when treatment is stopped. Most hip fractures

in women occur in our 80s. Therefore, a medical editorial proposes several alternatives, including reserving treatment for women at high risk and starting treatment in our 70s or after fractures occur to prevent recurrent fractures.[89]

In our view, it is more important to prevent fractures than to prevent osteoporosis. In fact, most fractures are preventable with commonsense safety measures (see p. 574) and are not caused by severe osteoporosis. Osteoporosis is more common among light-skinned women; yet, African-American women have the poorest recovery rates from fractures. Asian women have high rates of bone thinning, but they rarely experience fractures. Men who live to be old have as high a risk of fractures as old women. These are among the many seldom-noted facts about osteoporosis and fractures that are obscured by the drug companies' marketing to white women (who are candidates for estrogen treatment and are assumed to have money for their products), while the risks of other groups remain underrecognized.

Diagnosis

During its early stages, osteoporosis produces no symptoms or only mild ones such as backaches or back-muscle spasms. An old woman may be unaware she has osteoporosis until she fractures her spine, hip, or wrist in a simple fall. Postmenopausal women may feel pain in the upper or lower spine lasting for several days and then stopping, which may be caused by disintegrated vertebrae collapsing spontaneously. In a more advanced form, these compression fractures in the upper spine cause a condition commonly called dowager's hump; in rare cases, the resulting shortened chest area may make digesting food more difficult.

Routine X rays cannot clearly show signs of osteoporosis until 30 to 40% of bone is lost, but they may show reduced bone mass caused by other conditions. They do not make a definitive diagnosis of osteoporosis possible. If either you or your health care practitioner suspect *early* osteoporosis, it's best if you can go to a metabolic bone disease service, usually found only in a large urban medical-research center. Bone testing is neither appropriate nor cost-effective as a mass screening technique; it is primarily of use to those at high risk, and even then it is not clear that it improves outcomes.[90]

Early detection is meaningless unless a woman is informed about ways to reduce bone loss and wants to make necessary changes in her eating, exercise, and lifestyle patterns. Since these changes are those that benefit all women, we should be doing them anyway. Thus, the tests are a waste of time and money for most of us.

New Medical Treatments

Several new drugs are now available to treat osteoporosis and fractures. Fosamax (alendronate) is a non-hormonal treatment for osteoporosis. It belongs to a class of drugs called bisphosphonates, which inhibit bone breakdown. The Federal Drug Administration approved Fosamax for treatment, not prevention, after studies over a three-year period showed it to be effective in increasing bone mass (especially of the hip and spine) in older women, and safe for short-term use. Further studies are being conducted to determine its long-term safety. There have been reports of serious complications, such as difficulty swallowing, and over 30 hospitalizations for severe esophageal side reactions.[91] This medication must be used very carefully as directed to avoid side effects. Those who use it most effectively will take a pill first thing in the morning, then exercise for 30 to 45 minutes before eating breakfast.

Another treatment is calcitonin, a hormone produced by the thyroid gland, which regulates blood levels of calcium and thus contributes to building bone. Formerly available only by injection, calcitonin is newly available in a nasal spray, which is less expensive and can be self-administered. Other potential treatments are under study as well, such as etidronate and slow-release sodium fluoride.

For older women with thin, brittle bones, who are at high risk for falls, fractures, or dowager's hump, Fosamax or other new drugs could make a significant difference in quality of life. Our concern is that these new medications be prescribed and used only by those who need them and who are not at risk for complications, and that they not be overpromoted as hormone treatments have been.

Fracture Prevention

Preventive safety measures include reducing overmedication, the main cause of falls in the elderly; eliminating hazards in the home, such as scatter rugs and unsafe bathrooms and staircases; and clearing sidewalks of snow and ice in winter. In one innovative study, nursing home residents wore hip padding, which significantly reduced hip fractures.[92] Thus, after a lifetime of denying ourselves food to meet unrealistic images of thinness, we can don hip pads in our later years to protect ourselves from fractures!

The authors of this book believe that the lowest-risk way to prevent osteoporosis and fractures is to pay attention to prevention throughout life: to eat well, including adequate amounts of calcium; to exercise to build and maintain adequate bone, muscle mass, and balance;[93] and to avoid smoking. Also avoid unnecessary hysterectomies and oophorectomies. In old age, emphasize injury prevention.

Urinary Incontinence and Urinary Tract Infections

With aging, the environment in the vagina and urethra becomes less acid, leading to more urinary tract and bladder infections. This may cause temporary in-

continence, which is easily reversible. If you or someone you are caring for is having this problem, make sure the health care provider checks for an underlying infection (see "Urinary Tract Infections," chapter 24, Selected Medical Practices, Problems, and Procedures, p. 649).

Starting about the time of menopause, you may begin to notice a slight loss of urine as you cough, sneeze, laugh, or exert yourself during strenuous activity. This is called *stress incontinence*. In response to reduced estrogen, the tissues around the urethra begin to thin out just as the vagina does, sometimes making bladder control more difficult. Women who already have a history of this problem may find it getting worse. Perineal (Kegel) exercises (see chapter 12, Understanding Our Bodies, p. 274) to strengthen the muscles of the pelvic floor will help control this problem. If you have never done Kegel exercises, start today, and keep doing them.

Incontinence is more common at older ages, but it is not part of normal aging. Over 30% of women over 65, and over 50% of those in long-term care institutions, have urinary incontinence problems. Sometimes, mobility problems can be a factor when someone can't get to a toilet on her own.

Increasingly, incontinence can be successfully managed, treated, and even cured with both self-help and medical approaches. Getting help when surgery is needed can be challenging, because female reproduction and urology are separate medical specialties. Urologists know little more than the basics about female reproductive organs, while few doctors in either specialty know much about treating middle-aged and older women.* A new medical specialty called urogynecology is developing, consisting of surgeons who specialize in female urinary problems.†

Depression

Being depressed is not typical of aging. Please do not listen to doctors or others who imply that it is. If you lose your appetite, don't feel sexual, can't enjoy anything, sleep too much, or can't sleep, and if such symptoms continue for more than a month and talking to friends doesn't help, you may need professional help (see chapter 6, Our Emotional Well-Being: Psychotherapy in Context). Be aware that low thyroid function, common in older people, can feel or look like depression, but it should be treated as a thyroid problem rather than with antidepressants. Fees for psychotherapy may be prohibitive for many older persons. Coverage for mental health services under Medi-

---

* See *The New Ourselves, Growing Older,* 1994, for a pioneering chapter on urinary incontinence. See also Rebecca Chalker and Kristene E. Whitmore, *Overcoming Bladder Disorders* (New York: Harper & Row, 1990).
† For referral information, send a stamped, self-addressed envelope with your written request to The American Urogynecologic Society, 401 N. Michigan Avenue, Chicago, IL 60611. The society has over 700 members in the U.S. as of 1997.

care for those over 65 years of age and certain people with disabilities is probably as good as under most health insurance plans, but if you join an HMO, you will be limited by its rules.

It is deplorable, yet still true, that many mental health professionals do not care to work with elders.* (They think it's depressing!) You may have to persist to find one who trusts your ability to grow. You may do best with a therapist your own age. Medication can sometimes help depression, but be aware that older people experience more and greater effects from psychoactive drugs, and some drugs may even cause or deepen depressions. Medication should not be a substitute for psychotherapy and should always be carefully monitored.

Memory Loss and Confusion

It can be frightening to realize that simple everyday tasks have become a problem for yourself or a loved one, or to notice a decline in capacity for sound judgment. If you or a friend or family member is increasingly confusing or forgetful, don't assume "That's it! It's all downhill from here." We experience memory lapses throughout our lives, but we worry about them more when we are older.

Memory does not necessarily decline with age. On some tests of memory, elders do as well as college students, such as remembering a span of numbers and knowing word meanings, world knowledge, and the meaning or gist of a passage. Younger persons are better at remembering details. Memory loss is not inevitable or irreversible. Even very ill or frail old people can continue to learn, and declines in intellectual functioning can be reversed by practicing skills like doing math problems and crossword puzzles.[94] We can exercise memory or prevent ordinary memory loss through "mindfulness"—paying attention to everyday tasks—and by making small and large decisions for ourselves.

As one who copes with considerable memory loss at age 68, my major aid is list-making. Knowing that I may well forget an idea or "to-do," I write it down immediately. As a result, I am far better organized than at any earlier time of my life and I accomplish more.

I am still very active socially at the age of 86. When I get up in the morning, I go through my "face exercise." I think about where I am going that day and who I am likely to meet. As their faces come before me, I try to recall as many names as I can.

Severe memory loss and confusion are often diagnosed as dementia (sometimes inaccurately called "se-

nility"). Several reversible causes of memory loss and mental confusion, whose physical signs or symptoms may not be obvious, include drug toxicity (from overmedication or drug interaction), dehydration, hormonal disorders, vitamin deficiency, general malnutrition, chemical or mineral imbalance, hypothermia, anemia or other blood disorders, fever or an acute infection, or endocrine or metabolic disorders. A small stroke, a traumatic event or accident, a series of losses, or an abrupt relocation can also trigger acute confusion and disorientation. Deep feelings of depression and grief can interfere with memory or cause an older person to *appear* disoriented and confused, leading to an inappropriate diagnosis of senility or dementia. If you or a relative experiences these types of symptoms, be sure to get a prompt and thorough assessment from a geriatrician or a specialist in neurological disorders.

Recently, more precise means of diagnosis have identified Alzheimer's disease, alone or in conjunction with a series of small strokes (multi-infarct dementia), as a major cause of severe and permanent memory loss, and confusion. Often abbreviated as SDAT (senile dementia of the Alzheimer type), it affects only 10% of the over-65 population but almost half of those over 85.[95]

The link between Alzheimer's disease and strokes has long puzzled researchers. Some new research suggests that prevention of strokes through quitting or reducing smoking, lowering blood pressure, and controlling diabetes may be the best hope of reducing the risk and severity of SDAT, because strokes are a big contributor to Alzheimer's.[96] Although memory-enhancing drugs may have proved helpful to some, the search for effective treatment of Alzheimer's disease continues.

CAREGIVING AND NEEDING CARE

Life is always changing. The main lesson I have learned over the years . . . is that I have to be flexible. As a widow at age 80 I had been living alone, and it was becoming harder for me to get around. A lot of my friends had died. I knew I needed to make a change. The solution for me was to relocate to a long-term care community close to my daughter. This gave me independence with family support nearby. My move has enabled my daughter and me to renew our relationship. I have a chance to really get to know her as an adult in a more daily way. We have built up a friendship based on a deep understanding of each other. I truly treasure this in my old age.
—An 82-year-old woman

My mother's move to a local long-term care community has worked out beautifully. The place is well-run by an unusually dedicated group of people. I admire my mother's adaptibility at age 82. It's wonderful having her close by. I feel blessed to have this time with her. *—Her 53-year-old daughter*

---

* See Robert Butler, "Emotional Problems and Mental Illness in Old Age" in his groundbreaking classic *Why Survive? Being Old in America* (see Resources for publishing information) for a critique of psychiatry's failure to treat elders.

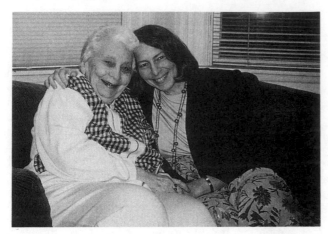

Rob Ditzion

Caregiving—a Gap in Our Delivery of Health, Social, and Medical Services

Women have been caregivers throughout the generations, and even though we have a greater variety of activities and demands today, we are still expected carry out this role. Household members provide 80% of the home care their ailing relatives receive (bathing, dressing, feeding), and women constitute 72% of those family caregivers.[97]

Women are nine or ten times more likely than men to care for an aging parent or spouse's parent. We are also somewhat more likely to care for an aging or ill spouse. Generally, because of the power and privacy of the nuclear family in our society, when a married or partnered person becomes ill, usually a spouse or partner provides care. But when a single, divorced, or widowed person becomes ill, most often a daughter or daughter-in-law steps in to become the principal caregiver. Because of the low birth rate during the Depression, many older women in their 80s and 90s have no surviving children. These women are at higher risk of nursing home placement when they need care, unless they make alternative plans.

When caregiving is work we want to do and is respected by our family and community, it can be rewarding. Too often, however, others simply expect it of us.

We planned for my husband—I was going to be the person who sustained him until his death. We never worked out who would take care of me. It's an unseen social service that women do; if the wife dies first, he finds another woman.

Most often, family care still means women providing care, in isolation, without pay or needed respite or supportive services, and without the security of job retraining, a pension, or even health insurance when the person cared for dies.

We rushed my husband to the hospital with a stroke, and it was a medical miracle. Now I am not so sure it

was a blessing. He is not always rational and cannot be left alone. . . . I had to give up my job. Financially, we are in terrible shape, but disaster will strike when he dies. I am 57 and won't be eligible for anything. I can't see my way out.

A growing number of us are lucky to see our parents live to an old age. Yet, if their health declines, we may also acquire a range of caregiving responsibilities for them. Many of us care for parents and parents-in-law for more years than we spend rearing children. For almost 2 million women in the U.S., elder care responsibilities come while we still have child-rearing responsibilities. Many midlife women today must balance employment with child care and elder care responsibilities.

Family members can be primary care providers but cannot do it all alone. Society must provide and fund policies and programs to support families in their caregiving of the elderly. At the workplace we need flextime, part-time work, job sharing, unpaid leave, and no penalties for those of us who stay home to care for aging parents. In the community we need a continuum of home care services and housing arrangements so that caregiving can be delegated. For example, respite care—even for a weekend—would help relieve a woman carrying a full-time job along with the second job of caregiving. Some agencies that provide home care aides fail to provide adequate training and to carefully check backgrounds of their employees for criminal records, leading to poor care and serious problems such as theft and even in rare cases assault and murder. As the number of home health care aides is increasing nationally, a national registry is needed.[98] Adult day care services can help an employed woman care for an elder living at home by providing support and company during the day. Caregiving can be stressful even in the best of circumstances. Many social service organizations have support groups for caregivers.

Needs of Paid Caregivers

Because of traditional expectations that women provide unpaid labor to care for family members, workers in caregiving occupations, predominantly women, are grossly underpaid. Women of color often occupy the lowest-paid jobs, as in home care and long-term care institutions. These jobs require a lot of standing and lifting, and workers in these jobs are more likely to develop chronic conditions such as leg and back pain. Women who work in such jobs may require care at earlier ages than middle-class white women. Yet, they are less likely to have the means or the insurance coverage to pay for such care.[99] All women concerned with caregiving, whether as family caregivers or caregiving workers, must make common cause to raise the status of caregiving work by affirming its value and demanding that caregivers be paid a decent wage with benefits. Paid caregivers often work in isolation, so it is hard for them to organize. They need support from

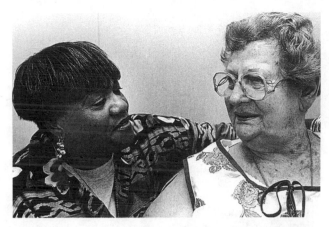

Linda Haas

the people they care for and from their family members.

Interdependence and Accepting Help When We Need It

Women accept and even expect that others will depend on us. Yet, we fear becoming dependent ourselves. Chronic illness or a new disability may be a blow to our pride and our habits of self-sufficiency. It raises the question of who will be there to care for us. On the other hand, some women may feel perfectly entitled to receiving from others what we have given for many decades.

Learning to accept help without resentment or loss of pride is one of the tasks of our later years. It helps when those providing care do so without taking over, or taking away all of an older person's choices. It helps when those needing care can accept offered help graciously.

Making Plans

It's a good idea to talk and plan ahead with family members or friends about the kind of care and living situation we want if we can no longer manage at home. Then, if a crisis occurs, family members or friends will have information (Social Security numbers, insurance policies, doctors, neighbors, financial situation, wills, health care proxy) and if necessary the authority (durable power of attorney) to act on our behalf. It is best to begin this process when we are in good health and to involve the whole family. Family meetings can help family members clarify their expectations of each other about issues of long-term care. If communication is difficult, you can ask an outside person such as a social worker or a member of the clergy to join you. Many families avoid such meetings, dreading the difficult subjects of illness and dependency. We can't predict what will happen in the future, but the more we prepare the more our wishes will be respected (see also the discussion of "advance medical directives," on p. 581).

Living Independently

Despite differences in well-being, living conditions, and income levels, most of us want to be self-sufficient and to live at home as long as possible.

I have a great abhorrence for the ghettos of nursing homes. I would rather struggle with overcoming physical difficulties in my own home than be put in the hands of people that I'm paying and then have to please them so they'll be nice to me.

A variety of services can help us, as individuals or couples, to stay at home even when we need occasional nursing services or help with everyday tasks. Meals on Wheels is a program that delivers hot lunches to elders, usually five days a week. Visiting nurses, physical therapists, occupational therapists, and home health aides are often available to perform needed services in the home.

Home care benefits elders who need help but want to continue to live in their own homes; yet, it is not consistently available in all communities. If you are seeking home care for a relative, it can be challenging to judge quality. If you engage someone through an agency, you may not be able to interview the worker in advance. In recent years, home care services have been touted by policy makers as a means to save money on expensive nursing home services. But even this motivation does not seem to protect home care services from budget cuts. Increasing regulation of hospital and nursing home admissions has left too many elders without any services, and their caregivers without respite. Many are on waiting lists nationwide.

Other available services include transportation, congregate meals, counseling services, senior centers, adult day care, and hospice. Emergency response systems permit older persons with potentially life-threatening conditions to live alone, and some phone companies have special services. Nearly all local area agencies on aging, visiting nurse agencies, and home care organizations will send a trained social worker to evaluate your situation and identify the resources and services that are available to you. Many communities have senior apartments and senior housing subsidized by federal, state, or local agencies.

Alternative Living Arrangements

New patterns of living with others, which can provide companionship and reduce living costs, are emerging for midlife and older women. We may be on our own after the end of a long marriage or relationship, or after children have left home. Many women are becoming roommates or experimenting with alternatives, such as cohousing and communal living. It is important to interview potential roommates or cohousing partners to evaluate their appropriateness for you.

As we grow older, living with others is not only cost-effective but care-effective, because housemates can participate in looking out for one another rather than paying others to do so. Cooperative, intergenerational living with relatives or friends; congregate housing (a managed home with some supportive services where residents have private rooms and share a common space for meals and activities); turning part of a house into an "in-law" apartment; building a separate unit on the same land as a friend or relative; and small group homes are new options. Increasingly, older women have the strength, will, and independence of spirit to make the changes required for new living arrangements.

If you want or will need alternative housing for yourself or a family member, start planning early. Attractive places are hard to find and have long waiting lists. Also, applicants need to be in good health. Waiting until you are sick limits your options.

Assisted Living

These facilities provide elders with a room or apartment as well as a range of services in a communal setting, a middle ground for elders who need daily assistance but not full-time skilled nursing care. Assisted living facilities have a variety of names, such as boarding care facilities, congregate living facilities, or residential care facilities. They are usually not subject to the same regulations as nursing homes, and may refuse "heavy care" elders and others who do not meet their requirements. For some people, their flexibility and lack of medicalization is a plus.

Privately run boarding facilities can be an informal approach to assisted living, especially in states with few regulations. These alternatives may be appropriate when elders do not need nursing care or case management but prefer not to be alone. A geriatric social worker describes such a home in her community:

Two women from Maine triumphed over midlife crises by going into a whole new field of endeavor. After being turned down by eight banks, they finally obtained funds for renovating an enormous old house in a small rural village. They provide room, board, and laundry for a group of 14 elders, most of whom have lived in the area for many years. Using the fruits of a large organic garden and orchard, bartering surplus seedlings for fish and other commodities, they acquired such a good reputation for their food that they were asked to cater weddings and parties. These activities in turn have enabled them to keep their costs— and their rents—fairly low and give the residents the option of participating in the food preparation or festivities.

Life Care or Continuing Care Communities

These communities offer apartment living for people in relatively good health, with medical and social services nearby. Many of these places are so expensive that they serve only the upper and upper middle classes. Some staff and residents may imply that those who are religious or cultural minorities or working class "will not feel comfortable." Only you can decide whether a place is right for you or your family member, and whether the amount of energy you will need to assert your right to be different is worth it, or something you wish to take on at a time of limited energy and need for support. Some communities are run as "co-ops" by the residents, allowing them to avoid federal guidelines prohibiting discrimination against disabled persons and ethnic minorities. Yet, when they work well and are inclusive, the services they provide constitute a model that we as an aging society could adopt to make the older years a time of activity, growth, and safety for all of us.

Many such communities offer a "continuum of care," with assisted living units and a nursing home on the premises. For a sizable entrance fee and monthly charges, residents are guaranteed a permanent place to live and a specified package of medical and nursing benefits to suit the resident's changing needs. Obtain a written agreement specifying the care available, your rights to terminate the contract and receive a refund, the alternative provisions available, and the conditions under which you might be discharged. Find out whether the money you invest goes to the corporation or is returned after your death to your heirs. In communities that emphasize private ownership of units, the latter should be the case. Some communities have closed, causing their residents hardships. Whether nonprofit or for profit, such communities need regulation. Be a prudent consumer: Obtain information in writing, and have the community's financial statement reviewed by your accountant, estate planner, or lawyer.

Nursing Homes

We ourselves, or our relatives, may have to go into nursing homes if we need fairly constant nursing care. On a given day, only 5% of elders live in nursing homes, but 75% of those who do are women. Forty percent of those in nursing homes are 85 years of age and over. One-quarter of all women 85 years and over live in nursing homes. Nursing home care is often poor, with owners putting profits ahead of quality care, paying workers little, and skimping on patients' needs. Almost 40% of all facilities certified by HCFA, the government agency that certifies the 86% of nursing homes that receive Medicare or Medicaid funds, have repeatedly violated federal standards.[100] Protection for nursing home residents is provided by state and federal laws, including the 1987 Nursing Home Reform Act, which set standards for quality of life and quality of care, and provides for unannounced inspections of nursing homes. In addition, residents have many specific rights, including rights to self-determination and to information. Because of the move to transfer Medicaid funds through block grants from the federal to the state governments, the National

Governors Association has been interested in weakening these federal protections. However, advocacy organizations do not foresee such changes from Congress. To find out more about advocating for the rights of nursing home residents, contact the National Citizens' Coalition for Nursing Home Reform (see Resources).

It is important to evaluate nursing homes carefully, as quality of care varies tremendously. Look for signs of group activities, posted calendars of events, and individualized rooms where residents keep some of their own furniture and possessions. Inquire about staff training, staff turnover, the ratio of nurses to residents, and the range of activities. A good source of evaluative information is the ombudsman at your state or area agency on aging. Some are cautious about challenging the nursing home establishment and will give you only the positive recommendations, preferring to say little about the bad ones. Some may give hints, such as "You may prefer to try another one."

The biggest problem in nursing home life is the routinization and medicalization of daily life. Often, in the interest of "efficiency," the routines serve only the sickest residents, depriving healthier residents of a chance to use their full capacities. Some recent innovations include waist-high garden plots for persons in wheelchairs and private rooms for sexual activity, a right won after residents at a rest home instituted a lawsuit to obtain it. A new advocacy organization working with long-term care professionals and family members to enliven nursing home life is called the Eden Alternative. It features a "habitat" approach, involving residents in gardening, caring for pets, and interacting with visiting groups of children, and places the focus more on activity and caring than on treatment.[101] Lacking any meaningful decisions to make, residents of conventional nursing homes become confused and disoriented. Having other people or pets to care for may sustain their attentiveness and memory. Physical and mental abilities deteriorate when we have neither mental stimulation nor chances to exercise and carry out simple tasks on our own.

We are critical of many aspects of conventional nursing home care—the skyrocketing costs, impersonal care, medicalization of everyday life, and lack of privacy and choices for residents. Patients are often discharged as quickly as possible from hospitals, while home care services have been reduced, and the mortality rate is rising sharply as a result (see chapter 25, The Politics of Women's Health and Medical Care). The result is waiting lists for nursing home admission for people who would rather stay at home and could do so if appropriate services existed. Some nursing home residents could return home if they still had homes or home care services. Because nursing home care is essential for some, we must work to improve quality of life and care and innovate ways that give residents more control.

Many nursing homes cannot or will not provide for the needs of women from diverse ethnic cultures who may not feel "at home." Some more progressive nursing homes have tried to compensate for this problem by varying their meals and offering cultural exchange programs:

My mother was much better able to cope with Western food when she could look forward to occasional Eastern meals at the nursing home's new "international nights." Her health and attitude improved, and she began talking to other residents and staff about her native Korean recipes.[102]

Aging and Elder Care in Other Industrialized Countries

The U.S. has not yet made care for the elderly a priority. Some other countries provide innovative support services for elders and their caregivers.

- The Scandinavian countries provide service buses to bring cleaning and laundry, hairdressing supplies, books, and hot food to elders who wish to remain in their homes. Homemakers and personal care attendants are available. An alternative is the service house, where services are available to those who live there. The state pays family caregivers. In Sweden, residences for older people get the most attractive sites with gardens on the balconies.
- New Zealand makes low-interest loans, services, and subsidies available to families who wish to care for elderly relatives at home.
- In England, clusters of about 20 apartments for elders are staffed by a state-employed "helper," who gets people to doctor's appointments and so on. Respite care and short-term placement in nursing homes are available to give caregivers a breather. Caregivers are organized in an advocacy organization.

Many of these services, or equally creative ones, are available or potentially available to elders in this country. However, our programs exist as a patchwork of innovations in a crazy quilt of cutbacks and threatened cutbacks. For instance, chronically scarce funding, often awarded to innovative pilot programs, is not renewed after they succeed and are no longer "new." As a nation, we have not deliberately decided (as have the Scandinavian countries) to make the older years a good time of life, free from financial worry and deprivation. As an ever-greater proportion of the electorate enters the older years, we develop a growing base of support for such a national commitment.

DEATH

At all ages, but more frequently in our middle and older years, we struggle with the reality of death. We lose our parents; as parents we may lose children. People we love die. If we become terminally ill at any age, we have to cope with our imminent deaths. But the impetus to accept the reality of death for ourselves comes for most of us as we grow older.

Here are some excerpts from a discussion group of midlife and older women:

We have the fear that if a person faces death that means she does not participate in life. Actually, it works the other way. The more we acknowledge and recognize death, the more we can live in the present.
—A 52-year-old woman

I am more aware of a mystery and beauty in life since I have accepted death as a personal eventuality for me. Before then, I had thought of death out there; now I know that I am going to die. That has released me for more vivid living. I reach out more. Almost everything reminds me of its connections with other things; my present is many-textured. I do not look to the future with dread. It has to be shorter than my past but it does not have to be less rich.
—A 78-year-old woman

Some of us continue to feel ambivalent and scared about acknowledging death or have difficulty coming to grips with the reality of it for ourselves.

Intellectually I'm very glib about it, but in my gut I can't accept that one day I won't be here.
—A 74-year-old woman

A thought has come to me in the last few years. I doubt that when I die my life will be over—my life with all its loving and caring and striving. Can it be that all my loved ones—mother, sister, other relatives —can all this love be gone? Nothing in nature disappears. Out of our bones, our skeletons, new life comes in some other way.
—An 85-year-old woman

Medical science often distorts our ideas of death. Many doctors view it as an adversary, an evil, a visible defeat. They often use every medical means possible to prolong life for its own sake without considering its quality or whether there is any hope of recovery, ignoring the ill person's wishes. In recent years, increasing recognition of advance directives and living wills has expanded our control over end-of-life issues. Increasingly, physicians and hospital staff receive training to work with patients and family members around these issues. Yet, realization of these goals continues to be problematic. Doctors often delay in responding to or heeding patients' requests for "do not resuscitate" orders or avoidance of heroic measures, such as mechanical ventilation. At the same time, our flawed and inadequate medical care system promotes abuse of the "right to die." Advocates for low-income communities are concerned that if this right is adopted prior to recognition of a "right to care," those without funds or coverage will be pressured to choose the cheaper alternative. A study of over 3,000 patients found a 30% greater likelihood of choosing to reject life-prolonging care among those whose funds were running out.[103]

In response to the excessive medicalization of death, terminally ill people, their friends, and relatives, and concerned professionals created hospices (see Resources), intended as a humane alternative to general hospital or nursing home care. More than a place, a hospice is an idea and a service. The thing we fear most when we are seriously ill is prolonged and unmanageable pain. Hospice workers assist people to manage pain and to die at home or in hospices, which may or may not be attached to a hospital. The patient and family together are the focus of attention. Hospices offer support, understanding, and respite to everyone involved. Bereavement counseling may continue for a substantial length of time beyond the family member's death.

Taking Control of Our Own Death

We know we cannot control whether we die, so we often jump to the conclusion that there is nothing we can do about it. Yet, we do have elements of choice and control. It is possible to choose our place of death —at home or in a hospital or hospice. As long as we are able, we can fight for medical care that allows us to keep our dignity instead of accepting care that is inappropriate for extreme pain and terminal illness. We can authorize a precise disposal of our property, donate vitally needed organs like kidneys and corneas for transplant if we wish, and perform the little details that ensure an easier burden for relatives and friends. Though legal, medical, and theological controversies abound, many of us would like to participate fully in the decision about when and how we will die. The right to control our deaths is part of our basic right to have control over our bodies and our lives.

A woman in her 70s states:

I have been searching for a doctor who would let me participate not just in my health care but in my own death, too.

We want to be able to define for ourselves what we consider a tolerable quality of life, a worthwhile existence.

I've had a lot of things done to my body, and I'm 73. I've made up my mind that enough has been done to me. If something bad happens, something major, I'm not sure I want to be repaired again. No more tampering with my body! I don't want to live to be 100 if I'm all botched up.

You may actively decide to avoid a long, drawn-out period of illness and dependency, or a medicalized death in which life is prolonged by artificial means. Some of us want to choose the occasion and means of our death. According to two distinguished bioethicists, in every state, constitutional and common law support the right of any competent adult to refuse medical treatment in any situation, but this is not the same as the right to commit suicide or to aid someone in ending his or her life.[104] They argue that permitting suicide should not be a way for the medical care system to shirk its responsibility to provide support and comfort care to the dying.

Writing your wishes in an "advance medical directive" can protect your right to refuse unwanted treatments and make your wishes clear to your family members, friends, and medical care providers. A health care institution that will not honor your wishes must, according to federal law, tell you so upon admission so that you can go elsewhere. State laws may vary as to the particulars. Check with your state's attorney general's office for the specifics of your state laws and for copies of forms to use for advance directives and/ or living wills. All 50 states and the District of Columbia authorize some type of advance directive, either a living will or the appointment of a health care agent.[105] Living wills are valid only in cases of terminal illness, not for slow degenerative disease or a very old person with "multiple systems failure." They are also not useful for the person who wants to have every possible treatment tried. For all of these situations, a durable power of attorney for medical affairs is more useful.

To protect loved ones from possible prosecution as accessories, people who might prefer to die supported by family and friends have chosen to go off by themselves when taking a fatal substance. We may even have to forego some of the talking and planning we might want to do in order to protect our loved ones from legal harassment.

I have for years kept a precious bottle somewhere. I talked with my daughter about it and she asked me, "Please, if you are ever ready to do this, tell me first." But I said I couldn't do that because I would be laying too heavy a burden on her; she would certainly feel that it was her job to dissuade me.

—A woman in her 60s

An important way to gain the power to choose our own deaths is working through advocacy organizations to change the laws and social attitudes related to death and dying and challenging legal, medical, and religious control.

Claiming the right to control the ending of our lives in no way minimizes the seriousness or the finality of the decision, nor the pain and grief of those we leave behind. The issues are complex. It is certainly more appropriate for the dying person rather than any outside authority to weigh all the factors involved.

Group Support for a Dying Person

In addition to our individual choices, some of us want to be connected with friends and community when we are very sick and dying.

When Esther, longtime friend and member of our women's group, was dying of breast cancer, she drew upon the love of her three communities, her family, her synagogue, and ourselves, her 25-year-old women's group. With specific people coordinating visits and food arrangements for each group, we took turns doing whatever was wanted or needed. We attended her, sat with her, her husband and sons. We brought cooked food, planted the spring garden she loved, helped her finish the book she was writing. Accepting our offerings, she presided over all activities in a clear firm way, seated in her living-room chair. It was a sad, peaceful rich time; she made it easier for us. She had a gift for giving to each of us in the measure that we gave to her, down to the smallest details, up to the very last moment when she died peacefully with her family around her. It gave us ease to surround her with love.

Now another group member is facing her partner's catastrophic illness, and we along with their other friends are offering similar support. She told us, "We feel buoyed up by our friends' support and caring. We feel surrounded by love."

SURVIVAL SKILLS

In our older years we may feel entitled to do what pleases and satisfies us, to slow down, to let go the strain of former obligations, to express our thoughts and feelings more strongly than ever before.

Getting old can be wonderful if you're not imposed on by other people's rules about how you should be when you're old. I consciously break as many as I can because then I'm breaking through oppression.

—A 65-year-old woman

Old age, because of its time perspective, can be a period of emotional and sensory awareness and enjoyment. I savor life more often. When I draw an iris, I

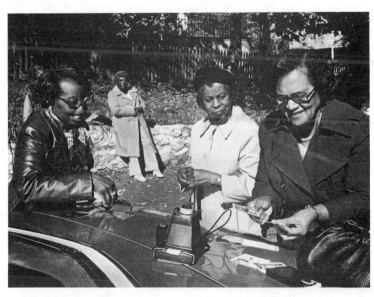

Photography class at Freedom House, Roxbury, MA

see that iris more vividly than I did when my physical sight was better. When I read a book now, I read it more slowly. Several books I have reread.

Elemental things of life have assumed greater importance. I spend more time looking at sunsets. I am more aware of the importance to myself and others of touching (both physical and emotional), of communication, of tenderness. Space and time for quiet reflection is more available for me now. In a strange way, impossible to put into words, I am experiencing a unity beyond space and time.

Sometimes I feel guilty to be happy when there are so many things wrong in the world and I'm not doing something about making joy possible for others. Yet the universe is going to have to get along without me sometime and so I don't have to change everything. Many of my companions are interested in a better, more compassionate world; I don't have to rush to do it all. —A 78-year-old woman

As more of us are living longer, we are learning that our older years can have their own special joys and triumphs. We can enjoy a more leisurely pace, travel, pick up long-delayed projects, and remain as active and involved as possible.

There's a discrepancy between my image of an older person in her 70s and the way I feel. In fact, there's no connection. My concept of a grandmother was of someone who didn't do much. But I became a grandmother at 47. I started a vigorous exercise program at 43 and am still running every day at 76 and love it.

There are so many positive things about being an older black woman—the elasticity of our skin, the strength of our bone structure, our spirituality, the caregiving of our extended families.
—A woman in her 60s

Women most often grow old in the company of other women, frequently surviving our close family members. Though we grieve for the loss of relationships we can never replace, we *can* overcome loneliness and isolation by reweaving and changing family relationships, by nurturing old and new friendships, and especially by reaching out to other women to form connections for support and intimate friendships.

It is important to challenge the stereotypes of elders as rigid, unable to form new relationships or to experience change and growth. Elders often have to be more adaptable than others in order to manage the changes they experience physically, economically, and in their networks of family and friends.

We who wrote this chapter have learned from the many lively, vital, elder women we spoke with that it is possible to live fully for as long as we live.

The 70s have been the best decade of my life. From what I have seen with my friends, it is either the best or the worst. My creative work as an artist is what

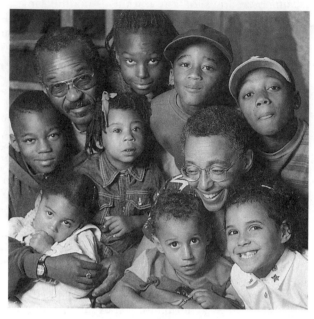

Jenny McKenzie

keeps me alive; my friends keep me happy and contented. If I had to give up people I would never have another happy day, but I would stay alive if I could work. —A 77-year-old woman

Staying in Touch with Our Inner Selves— Spirituality and Emotional Well-Being

Staying in touch with ourselves helps us reach out to others, cope with the hard things in our lives, and keep on growing. There are many ways we can stay in touch with ourselves—writing in a journal, reading a book, exercising, meditating, walking in the woods, taking a long hot shower or bath, camping. For some of us, being connected with a spiritual community helps, too.

Last week, at age 73, I sat in a group of older women discussing religion and spirituality and was reminded of our midweek prayer meetings 60 years ago, except that no woman there was witnessing to the teachings of her childhood church indoctrination but was describing instead her "spirituality." The world's [major] religions have all been founded by men and promote their beliefs, not to mention their reverence of dominance. I don't choose to have men control my moral and spiritual values. In looking within myself for what I value most, I discover I put honesty first, nurturing next, then striving for peace and justice in human relationships and cherishing our earth and universe. I nourish my spirit through music, nature study, and meditation but mostly through relatedness to people I love.

Four years ago, at age 81, I got diabetes. It has impaired my living condition, but it doesn't get me down. In fact, I have always had the feeling that the more we have to fight and overcome, the stronger we are. Obstacles are here to be overcome. That's part of life, and it gives us a good feeling that we are not just little ants, we are fighters. It's not only the physical impairment that has to worry you and the doctor. It is also your state of mind. The healthy mind creates the healthy body, and the healthy body creates the healthy mind. Sometimes a frail body can draw its strength from a courageous mind.

Support Groups and Community Activity for Older Women

Friendship is valuable not only for happiness and mental well-being but for physical health and survival as well. Because aging in this country too often means increasing isolation, the middle and older years are a good time to create a support and friendship network if you don't already have one. Regardless of age, persons with strong social bonds (marriage, friends, group or organizational affiliations) had a mortality rate in one study that was 2.5% lower than those who were relatively isolated. The other important finding was that friendship and support from any of these sources contributed to survival.[106]

It is never too late to reach out for new friends and new activities, or to form a support group. Joining advocacy organizations builds our communities and has the wonderful personal benefit of forging supportive networks of friends and colleagues for ourselves.

I am open to the new adventure of meeting people. Once I was congratulated for having been one of the founders of the Boston Gray Panthers. I had to answer that I didn't deserve any thanks. The Gray Panthers [whose focus is intergenerational activism] deserve thanks from me. Those relationships and that connection mean so much that I am just plain grateful.
—A woman in her 70s

NOTES

1. Paula Rayman et al., "Resiliency Amidst Inequity: Older Women Workers in an Aging United States," in J. Allen and A. Pifer, eds., *Women on the Front Lines: Meeting the Challenge of an Aging America* (Washington, DC: Urban Institute Press, 1993), 134–35.
2. American Association of Retired Persons, *A Profile of Older Americans,* 1996. Informative brochure available free from AARP Fulfillment, 601 E Street NW, Washington, DC 20049.
3. "Poverty Status of Women and Men by Age, Race, and Hispanic Origin, 1993." In C. Costello and B. K. Krimgold,

eds., for the Women's Research and Education Institute, *The American Woman 1996–97: Where We Stand* (New York: Norton, 1996), 314.
4. Institute for Women's Policy Research, "Age Differences in Earnings," *The Wage Gap: Women's and Men's Earnings, 1995,* 4.
5. *1990 Census of Population: Social and Economic Characteristics* (Washington, DC: U.S. Department of Commerce, 1993).
6. "U.S. Poverty Increasing, Study by U.N. Finds," *Boston Globe* (June 12, 1997): A8.
7. Paula B. Doress-Worters, "Choices and Chances: How A Profit-Driven Health Care System Discriminates Against Middle-Aged Women," in M. Brinton Lykes et al., *Myths About the Powerless: Contesting Social Inequalities* (Philadelphia: Temple University Press, 1996), 201–18.
8. Divorce Judgment and Health Insurance Project, c/o Health Care for All, 30 Winter Street, Boston, MA 02108.
9. Young-Yee Yoon, *Women of Color and Access to Health Care* (Washington, DC: Institute for Women's Policy Research, 1994).
10. C. Costello and B. K. Krimgold, op. cit., 148. See "Poverty Status of Women and Men . . ."
11. Ibid., 149.
12. Mary K. Bissell, ed., *The Kinship Care Source Book* (Washington, DC: D.C. Kinship Care Coalition, 1997). Available from the National Committee to Preserve Social Security and Medicare, Washington, DC; (202) 216-0420.
13. Ibid.
14. U.S. Bureau of the Census, *Statistical Abstracts of the United States 1996* (New York: Grosset and Dunlap, 1996): 55.
15. June Patterson, "How to Mend a Broken Heart," in Marcy Adelman, ed., *Lesbian Passages: True Stories Told by Women Over 40* (Los Angeles: Alyson Publications, 1996), 110.
16. Richard A. Knox, "Study Finds Most U.S. Women Welcome Menopause," *Boston Globe* (Sept. 5, 1997): 26A.
17. John B. McKinlay, Sonja M. McKinlay, and Donald Brambilla, "The Relative Contributions of Endocrine Changes and Social Circumstances to Depression in Middle-Aged Women," *Journal of Health and Social Behavior* 28, no. 4 (Dec. 1987): 345–63.
18. Barbara Ehrenreich and Deirdre English, *For Her Own Good: 150 Years of the Experts' Advice to Women* (New York: Anchor, 1989, c. 1978).
19. Paula B. Doress-Worters, op. cit., 1996.
20. Louise Nicol-Smith, "Causality, Menopause and Depression: a Critical Review of the Literature," *British Medical Journal* 16 (Nov. 1996): 1229.
21. Nancy E. Avis and Sonja M. McKinlay, "A Longitudinal Analysis of Women's Attitudes Toward the Menopause: Results from the Massachusetts Women's Health Study," *Maturitas* 13 (1991): 65–79.
22. Sonja M. McKinlay, Donald J. Brambilla, and Jennifer G. Posner, "The Normal Menopause Transition," *American Journal of Human Biology* 4 (1992): 37–46.
23. Susan M. Love with Karen Lindsey, *Dr. Susan Love's Hormone Book: Making Informed Choices About Menopause* (New York: Random House, 1997).
24. McKinlay, Brambilla, and Posner, op. cit.

25. A. Herzog et al. "Reproductive Endocrine Disorders in Women with Partial Seizures of Temporal Lobe Origin," *Archives of Neurology* 43, no. 4 (1986): 341–46.

26. Ann M. Voda, Nancy S. Christy, and Julene M. Morgan, "Body Composition Changes in Menopausal Women," *Women and Therapy* 11, no. 2 (1991): 71–96.

27. Catherine DeLorey, "Differing Perspectives of Menopause: An Attribution Theory Approach," in A. J. Dan and L. L. Lewis, eds., *Menstrual Health in Women's Lives* (Chicago: University of Illinois Press, 1992).

28. Linda Anne Bernhard, "Laser Endometrial Ablation: An Alternative to Hysterectomy," *Health Care for Women International* 15 (1994): 123–33.

29. Fredi Kronenberg, "Hot Flashes: Epidemiology and Physiology," *Annals of the New York Academy of Sciences* 592 (1990): 52–86.

30. New England Research Institute, *Women and their Health in Massachusetts: Final Report* (Watertown, MA: NERI 1991).

31. Fredi Kronenberg, "Giving Hot Flashes the Cold Shoulder—Without Drugs," *Menopause Management* 2, no. 4 (April 1993): 20–25.

32. Kronenberg, op. cit.

33. McKinlay, Brambilla, and Posner, op. cit.

34. Ann M. Voda, *Menopause—Me and You: The Sound of Women Pausing* (New York: Harrington Park Press, 1997).

35. Elaine Moquette-Magee, *Eat Well for a Healthy Menopause: The Low-Fat High-Nutrition Guide* (New York: John Wiley & Sons, 1996). See also Nina Shandler, *Estrogen, The Natural Way* in Resources.

36. Report by Dr. Sadja Greenwood on the Second International Symposium on the Role of Soy in Preventing and Treating Chronic Disease, *Menopause News* 6, no. 6 (Nov./Dec. 1996): 1–2.

37. "Statement on the Use of Vitamin E in Women with Breast Cancer," Dr. Susan M. Love's mailed response to queries from readers of *Dr. Susan Love's Hormone Book* (see Love and Lindsey, *Dr. Susan Love's Hormone Book*).

38. "The Mind and Menopausal Hot Flashes," *Mental Medicine Update: The Mind/Body Medicine Newsletter,* IV, no. 3 (1995).

39. New England Research Institute, *Women and Their Health in Massachusetts,* op. cit.

40. A. Holte, "Influences of Natural Menopause on Health Complaints: A Prospective Study of Healthy Norwegian Women," *Maturitas* 14 (1992): 127–41. P. Kaufert et al., "The Manitoba Project: A Re-examination of the Link between Menopause and Depression," *Maturitas* 14 (1992): 143–55.

41. Love, op. cit., 49.

42. Elizabeth Barrett-O'Connor and Donna Kritz-Silverstein, "Estrogen Replacement Therapy and Cognitive Function in Older Women," *JAMA* 269, no. 20 (May 26, 1993): 2637–641.

43. Jane Sprague Zones and Susan Rennie, "ERT: If It's So Great, Why Aren't We All on It? Part II," *Network News* (see National Women's Health Network in Resources) (Sept./Oct. 1997).

44. Nancy E. Avis et al., "The Evolution of Menopausal Symptoms." *Bailliere's Clinical Endocrinology and Metabolism* 7, no. 1 (Jan. 1993): 17–32.

45. Personal communication, Dr. Margo N. Woods, Tufts University School of Medicine, Boston, MA, Feb. 1997.

46. G. A. Colditz et al., "The Use of Estrogens and Progestins and the Risk of Breast Cancer in Postmenopausal Women," *New England Journal of Medicine* 332, no. 4 (1995): 1589–593.

47. Bruce Ettinger and Deborah Grady, "The Waning Effect of Postmenopausal Estrogen Therapy on Osteoporosis" [Editorial], *New England Journal of Medicine* 329, no. 16 (Oct. 14, 1993): 1192–193.

48. Virginia Mason, "Study Says Progesterone Might Boost HIV Risk," *American Health Consultants' Fax Bulletin* (May 8, 1996).

49. Benjamin C. Campbell and Richard J. Udry, "Implication of Hormonal Influences on Sexual Behavior for Demographic Models of Reproduction," *Annals of the New York Academy of Sciences* 709 (1994): 117–27.

50. Love with Lindsey, op. cit., 273.

51. Sadja Greenwood, *Menopause, Naturally: Preparing for the Second Half of Life* (Volcano, CA: Volcano Press, 1996): 108–9.

52. Love with Lindsey, op. cit., p. 273.

53. S. Greenwood, op. cit., 109.

54. Graham A. Colditz, Kathleen M. Egan, Meir J. Stampfer, "Hormone Replacement Therapy and Risk of Breast Cancer: Results from Epidemiologic Studies," *American Journal of Obstetrics and Gynecology* 168, no. 5 (1993): 1473–480. See also K. K. Steinberg et al., "A Meta-analysis of the Effect of Estrogen Replacement Therapy on the Risk of Breast Cancer," *JAMA* 265, no. 15 (1991): 1985–990.

55. Colditz, Egan, and Stampfer, op. cit., 1473–480.

56. G. A. Colditz et al., op. cit.

57. Elizabeth S. Ginsburg et al., "Effects of Alcohol Ingestion on Estrogens in Postmenopausal Women," *JAMA* 276, no. 21 (1996): 1747–751.

58. Love with Lindsey, op. cit., 79–80.

59. Miriam E. Nelson et al., "Effects of High-Intensity Strength Training on Multiple Risk Factors for Osteoporotic Fractures: A Randomized Controlled Trial," *JAMA* 272, no. 24 (1994): 1909–914.

60. M. Notelovitz et al., "Low-Dose Esterified Estrogens: Prevention of Postmenopausal Bone Loss Without Development of Endometrial Hyperplasia," Abstracts: North American Menopause Society, *Menopause* 3, no. 4 (1996).

61. Azimi A. Nabulsi et al., "Association of Hormone-Replacement Therapy with Various Cardiovascular Risk Factors in Postmenopausal Women," *New England Journal of Medicine* 328, no. 15 (1993): 1069–116.

62. Lynn Rosenberg, "Hormone Replacement Therapy: The Need for Reconsideration," *American Journal of Public Health* 83, no. 12 (1993): 1670–673.

63. Lynn Rosenberg, Julie Palmer, and Samuel Shapiro, "A Case-Control Study of Myocardial Infarction in Relation to Use of Estrogen Supplements," *American Journal of Epidemiology* 137, no. 1 (1993): 54–63.

64. The Writing Group for the PEPI Trial, "Effects of Estrogen or Estrogen/Progestin Regimens on Heart Disease Risk Factors in Postmenopausal Women: the Postmenopausal Estrogen/Progestin Interventions (PEPI) Trial," *JAMA* 273, no. 3 (1995): 199–208.

65. Janine O'Leary Cobb, "Research Results: The PEPI Trial," *A Friend Indeed* 12, no. 1 (April 1995).

66. Louise A. Brinton and Catherine Schairer, "Postmenopausal Hormone-Replacement Therapy—Time for a Reappraisal?" Editorial *New England Journal of Medicine* 336, no. 25 (June 19, 1997): 1821–822. See also Francine Grodstein et al., "Postmenopausal Hormone Therapy," Ibid., 1769–775.

67. "ERT: If It's So Great, Why Aren't We All on It?, or, From Non-Compliance to New Understanding," *The Network News,* National Women's Health Network (Jan./Feb. 1997) (see Resources).

68. "Why Replace Estrogen?" *Menopause News* (July/Aug. 1997): 1–4.

69. Centers for Disease Control and Prevention, "HIV/AIDS Surveillance Report," 9, no. 1, 1997.

70. Robert W. Stock, "When Older Women Get HIV: The Shock and the Isolation," *The New York Times* (July 31, 1997): C1, C7.

71. Jean D. Grambs, ed., *Women Over Forty: Visions and Realities* (New York: Springer, 1989).

72. Mary Jane Sherfey, *The Nature and Evolution of Female Sexuality* (New York: Vintage, 1973), 102.

73. G. A. Greendale et al., "Leisure, Home, and Occupational Physical Activity and Cardiovascular Risk Factors in Postmenopausal Women: The Postmenopausal Estrogens/Progestins Intervention (PEPI) Study," *Archives of Internal Medicine* 156, no. 4 (1996): 418–24.

74. Maria A. Fiatarone et al., "High-Intensity Strength Training in Nonagenarians: Effects on Skeletal Muscle," *JAMA* 263, no. 22 (1990): 3029–34. See also Paula B. Doress-Worters and Diana Siegel, *The New Ourselves, Growing Older* (New York: Simon & Schuster, 1994) chapter 6 "Moving for Health" for more on physical activity and movement for older women and women with physical limitations.

75. Gary Curhan et al., "Comparison of Dietary Calcium with Supplemental Calcium and Other Nutrients as Factors Affecting the Risk for Kidney Stones in Women," *Annals of Internal Medicine* 126, no. 7 (1997): 497–504.

76. Bess Dawson-Hughes et al. "Effect of Vitamin D Supplement on Wintertime and Overall Bone Loss in Healthy Post-menopausal Women," *Annals of Internal Medicine* 115, no. 7 (1991): 505–12.

77. *Will You Still Treat Me When I'm 65?* 1996 Alliance for Aging Research, 2021 K Street NW, Suite 305, Washington, DC 20006, p. 9.

78. Ibid., 9.

79. Lynn Rosenberg et al., "The Black Women's Health Study: A Follow-Up Study for Causes and Prevention of Illness," *Journal of American Medical Women's Association* 50, no. 2 (1995): 56–58.

80. Kenneth G. Manton et al., "Estimates of Change in Chronic Disability and Institutional Incidence and Prevalence Rates in the U.S. Elderly Population from the 1982, 1984, and 1989 National Long-Term Care Survey," *Journal of Gerontology* 48, no. 4 (1993): S153–S166.

81. Institute for Health and Aging, University of California/San Francisco, *Chronic Care in America: A 21st Century Challenge* (Princeton, NJ: The Robert Wood Johnson Foundation, 1996).

82. "The Treatment of Sleep Disorders of Older People," *NIH Consensus Statement* 8, no. 3 (March 26–29, 1990): 2.

83. "Report of the Public Health Service Task Force on Women's Health Issues," *Public Health Reports* 100, no. 1 (Jan./Feb. 1985): 96.

84. American Association of Retired Persons, "Facts About Hearing Loss," *AARP Disability Initiative: Fact Sheet,* 1992.

85. Robin H. Cohen, "Joint and Muscle Pain, Arthritis, and Rheumatic Disorders," in P. B. Doress-Worters and Diana Laskin Siegal, *The New Ourselves, Growing Older.* (See Resources.)

86. Carol Frey et al., "American Orthopaedic Foot and Ankle Society Women's Shoe Survey," *Foot and Ankle* 14, no. 2 (1993): 78–81.

87. Velimir Matkovic, "Calcium Intake and Peak Bone Mass" [Editorial], *New England Journal of Medicine* 327, no. 7 (1992): 120.

88. Robert P. Heaney, "Thinking Straight About Calcium" [Editorial], *New England Journal of Medicine* 328, no. 7 (1993): 503–5.

89. Ettinger and Grady, op. cit.

90. *Agency for Health Care Policy and Research: Research Activities* 194 (June 1996).

91. "Notes on Recent ECRI Reports," *Health Technology Assessment News* (March/April 1996): 7. ECRI is an independent nonprofit health services research agency that provides timely information on health technology assessment. 5200 Butler Pike, Plymouth Meeting, PA 19462; (610) 825-6000.

92. J. B. Lauritzen et al., "Effect of External Hip Protectors on Hip Fractures," *Lancet* 341 (Jan. 2, 1993): 11–13.

93. Nelson et al., op cit. (1994): 1909–914.

94. K. Warner Schaie and Sherry Willis, "Can Decline in Adult Intellectual Functioning Be Reversed?" *Developmental Psychology* 22, no. 2 (1986): 223–32.

95. D. A. Evans et al., "Prevalence of Alzheimer's Disease in a Community Population of Older Persons," *JAMA* 262, no. 18 (1989): 2551–556.

96. David A. Snowdon et al., "Brain Infarction and the Clinical Expression of Alzheimer Disease: The Nun Study," *JAMA* 277, no. 10 (1997): 813–17.

97. Robyn Stone et al., "Caregivers of the Frail Elderly: A National Profile," *The Gerontologist* 27, no. 5 (1987): 616.

98. Alex Pham, "Often Little Is Known About Home Health Aides: With Turnover Rapid, Hiring Carries Risks." *Boston Globe* (Oct. 6, 1997): A1, A6

99. Ronald Angel and Jacqueline L. Angel, *Who Will Care For Us? Aging and Long-Term Care in Multicultural America* (New York: NYU Press, 1997).

100. "Nursing Homes: a Special Investigative Report," *Consumer Reports* 60, no. 8 (Aug. 1995): 518.

101. William H. Thomas, *Life Worth Living: How Someone You Love Can Still Enjoy Life in a Nursing Home* (Acton, MA: VanderWyk & Burnham, 1996).

102. Quoted in "Nursing Homes," in *The New Ourselves, Growing Older,* 252.

103. Kenneth E. Covinsky et al., "Is Economic Hardship on the Families of the Seriously Ill Associated with Patient and Surrogate Care Preferences?" *Archives of Internal Medicine* 156, no. 15 (1996).

104. George J. Annas and Michael A. Grodin, "There's No Right to Assisted Suicide," *The New York Times* (Jan. 8, 1997): A15.

105. Information packet from Choice in Dying (see Resources).

106. Leonard S. Syme and Lisa Berkman. "Social Class Susceptibility and Sickness," in Peter Conrad and Rochelle Kern, eds., *The Sociology of Health and Illness: Critical Perspective* (New York: St. Martin's Press, 1994).

....

RESOURCES

....

Women and Aging

Butler, Robert N. *Why Survive? Being Old in America.* New York: HarperCollins, 1985. The classic work on aging.

Butler, Robert N., and Myrna I. Lewis. *Love and Sex After 60.* New York: Thorndike Press, 1996. Knowledgeable and insightful. Available in large-print edition.

Delany, Sarah Louise, *On My Own at 107: Reflecting on Life Without Bessie.* San Francisco: Harper, 1997.

Doress-Worters, Paula B., and Diana Laskin Siegal in cooperation with the Boston Women's Health Book Collective. *The New Ourselves, Growing Older: Women Aging with Knowledge and Power.* New York: Simon & Schuster, 1994. Contains full chapter coverage of most topics covered in this chapter as well as other topics and resources.

Fogler, Janet, and Lynn Stern. *Improving Your Memory: How to Remember What You're Starting to Forget.* Baltimore, MD: Johns Hopkins University Press, 1994.

Gillick, Muriel R. *Choosing Medical Care in Old Age: What Kind, How Much, When to Stop.* Cambridge: Harvard University Press, 1994.

Griffin, Richard, Frieda Rebelsky, and Radcliffe L. Romeyn. *What's Next? A Guide to Valued Aging and Other High-Wire Adventures.* 1996. Available from Eldercorps, 19 Harrison Avenue, Cambridge, MA 02140. Telephone orders: (800) 585-4909.

Gullette, Margaret Morganroth. *Declining to Decline: Cultural Combat and the Politics of Midlife.* Charlottesville: University of Virginia, 1997.

Jacobs, Ruth Harriet. *Be an Outrageous Older Woman.* New York: HarperPerennial, 1997. Full of humor, empowering suggestions, and success stories.

Kuhn, Maggie, with Christina Long and Laura Quinn. *No Stone Unturned: The Life and Times of Maggie Kuhn.* New York: Ballantine, 1991. Autobiography of a lifelong activist and founder of the Gray Panthers (see under "Organizations").

Macdonald, Barbara, with Cynthia Rich. *Look Me in the Eye: Old Women, Aging, and Ageism.* Minneapolis, MN: Spinsters Ink, 1991.

Nickerson, Betty. *Old and Smart: Women and Aging.* Madeira Park, BC: Harbour Publishing, 1991. Affirming book in large print. Order from your local bookstore, or from Harbor Publishing, P.O. Box 219, Madeira Park, British Columbia, V0N 2H0, Canada.

Pearsall, Marilyn, ed. *The Other Within Us: Feminist Explorations of Women and Aging.* Boulder, CO: Westview Press, 1997. Anthology includes contemporary and classic articles.

Porcino, Jane. *Living Longer, Living Better: Adventures in Community Housing for Those in the Second Half of Life.* New York: Crossroad/Continuum, 1991.

Siegal, Diana Laskin, and Christie Burke. "Midlife and Older Women and HIV/AIDS: My (Grand)mother Wouldn't Do That," in Nancy Goldstein and Jennifer L. Manlow, eds., *The Gender Politics of HIV/AIDS in Women: Perspectives on the Pandemic in the U.S.* New York: New York University Press, 1997.

Weber, Gail. *Celebrating Women, Aging and Cultural Diversity,* 1994. Study with extensive quotes from immigrant women. Available from Regional Women's Health Centre, Women's College Hospital, 790 Bay Street, 8th floor, Toronto, Ontario M5G 1N9, Canada; (416) 586-0211.

Organizations and Sources of Printed Information and Referrals

Alzheimer's Association, Inc.,
National Headquarters; 919 North Michigan Avenue, Suite 1000; Chicago, IL 60611; (800) 272-3900
Web site: http://www.alz.org

American Association of Retired Persons (AARP)
Program Department; 601 E Street NW; Washington, DC 20049; (202) 434-2300
Web site: http://www.aarp.

AARP advocates for the interests of older Americans and has many subdivisions, including Women's Initiative. Publications include *Modern Maturity* and a newsletter, *AARP News.*

American Self-Help Clearinghouse
St. Clare's–Riverside Medical Center; Pocano Road; Denville, NJ 07834; (201) 625-7101; (201) 625-9053 (TDD)

Publications include *The Self-Help Source Book: Finding and Forming Mutual Aid Self-Help Groups,* for $8.

Elderhostel
75 Federal Street; Boston, MA 02110-1941; (617) 426-7788

Short-term, intensive campus-based educational experiences for older adults all over the world. Publishes three seasonal catalogs.

Gray Panthers
2025 Pennsylvania Avenue, NW; Washington DC, 20006; (202) 466-3132

An intergenerational membership organization with a quarterly newsletter, *Network.* Advocates for concerns of elders and other social change issues.

National Hispanic Council on Aging
2713 Ontario Road NW; Washington, DC 20009; (202) 745-2521; (202) 745-2560; Fax: (202) 745-2522
E-mail: nhcoa@mnsinc.com
Web site: http://www.incacorp.com/nhcoa

Advocates for the needs and concerns of older Hispanic Americans.

National Women's Health Network
514 Tenth Street NW, Suite 400; Washington, DC 20044; (202) 347-1140; Fax: (202) 347-1168; National Clearing-house: (202) 628-7814

Educational and advocacy work nationally on midlife women's health issues. Publications include a quarterly newsletter and the pamphlet *Taking Hormones and Women's Health: Choices, Risks, Benefits.*

Older Women's League
666 Eleventh Street NW, Suite 700; Washington, DC 20001-4512; (202) 783-6686; (800) 825-3695

A local and national membership organization that advocates for older women's concerns. Members receive the newspaper *The OWL Observer.* For 24-hour legislative update, call (202) 783-6689.

Special Resources on Selected Issues

Caregiving

Angel, Jacqueline L., and Ronald J. Angel. *Who Will Care for Us? Aging and Long-Term Care in Multicultural America.* New York: New York University Press, 1997.

Caposella, Cappy, and Sheila Warnock. *Share the Care: How to Organize a Group to Care for Someone Who Is Seriously Ill.* New York: Fireside/Simon & Schuster, 1995. The authors began by sharing the care for a friend and went on to organize share the care groups.

Chalfie, Deborah. *Going It Alone—A Closer Look at Grandparents Parenting Grandchildren,* 1994, a publication of American Association of Retired Persons (see Organizations).

Morris, Virginia. *How to Care for Aging Parents.* New York, Workman, 1996. Comprehensive and well researched, with many helpful resource lists.

Sommers, Tish, and Laurie Shields. *Women Take Care: The Consequences of Caregiving in Today's Society.* Gainesville, FL: Triad Publishing Co., 1987. An important book on the politics of women as caregivers by the founders of the Older Women's League.

Employment and Training for Older Women Workers

The Institute for Lifetime Learning, a subdivision of the American Association of Retired Persons (see Organizations), helps older persons pursue educational and/or career changes.

National Caucus and Center on Black Aged
1424 K Street NW, Suite 500; Washington, DC 20005; (202) 637-8400

Runs several work-training programs, including a program to expand the number of African-American administrators in the field of long-term care.

Women Work: The National Network for Women's Employment
1625 K Street NW, Suite 300; Washington, DC 20006; (202) 467-6346; (800) 235-2732

A membership organization rooted in the displaced homemakers movement, dedicated to empowering women from diverse backgrounds and assisting them to achieve economic self-sufficiency through education, training, and employment. Send SASE for referral to a state or local program near you.

Working Today
P.O. Box 681, Times Square Station; New York, NY 10108; (212) 840-6066; Fax: (212) 840-6656
E-mail: working1@tiac.net
Web site: http://www.workingtoday.org

Working Today addresses the problems of a "two-tiered workforce." Its "Good Jobs in the New Economy" campaign promotes the extension of worker protections, such as unemployment benefits, to "second-tier" workers who work less than full time, full year. Newsletter and health insurance coverage plans.

Lesbian and Gay Issues
(see also chapter 10 Resources)

Adelman, Marcy, ed., *Lesbian Passages: True Stories Told by Women Over 40.* Los Angeles: Alyson Publications, 1996. P.O. Box 4371, Los Angeles, CA 90028-4371.

Lynch, Lee and Akia Woods. *Off the Rag: Lesbians Writing on Menopause.* Norwich, VT: New Victorian Press, 1997.

Older Lesbians Organizing for Change (OLOC)
P.O. Box 980422; Houston, TX 77098

National organization for lesbians over 60 and their supporters. Write for its publication "Confronting Ageism: A Facilitator's Handbook."

Senior Action in a Gay Environment (SAGE)
305 7th Avenue; New York, NY 10001; (212) 741–2247

Maintains a list of groups around the country and provides information for starting groups dealing with lesbian and gay aging. Newsletter.

Menopause

Cobb, Janine O'Leary. *Understanding Menopause: Answers and Advice for Women in the Prime of Life.* New York, Plume, 1993. By the author/editor of the newsletter *A Friend Indeed.*

Coney, Sandra. *The Menopause Industry: How the Medical Establishment Exploits Women.* Alameda, CA: Hunter House, 1994. Compelling analysis of the medicalization of menopause and osteoporosis by a leading women's health advocate from New Zealand.

Greenwood, Sadja. *Menopause, Naturally: Preparing for the Second Half of Life.* San Francisco: Volcano Press, 1996. Useful, accessibly written. Covers hormone treatments, including testosterone treatment. Highly recommended.

Love, Susan M., with Karen Lindsey. *Dr. Susan Love's Hormone Book: Making Informed Choices About Menopause.* New York: Random House, 1997. Exhaustive exploration of every aspect of the decision whether to take hormones at menopause. Highly recommended.

McCain, Marian Van Eyck. *Transformation Through Menopause.* Westport, CT: Greenwood, 1991. Exercises and meditations for emotional growth in menopause.

Menopause Handbook. Montreal: Montreal Health Press, 1997. P.O. Box 1000, Station Place du Parc, Montreal QC Canada, H2W 2N1. Single copy is $5.00. Bulk rates available.

Voda, Ann. *Menopause, Me and You: The Sound of Women Pausing.* New York: Harrington Park Press, 1997. Personal experiences of women through the stages of menopause. Scholarly information and tools for monitoring your own changes.

Weed, Susun. *Menopausal Years: The Wise Woman Way.* Woodstock, NY: Ash Tree Publishing, 1992. A thorough and knowledgeable guide to the use of herbal remedies. Covers other alternative remedies as well.

A Friend Indeed: For Women in the Prime of Life
Box 515, Place du Parc Station; Montreal, Quebec H2W 2PI, Canada

An international newsletter for women in menopause and midlife. Reviews of current research and letters from readers. Highly recommended.

Menopause News
2074 Union Street; San Francisco, CA 94123; (415) 567-2368; (800) 241-meno
E-mail: mnews@well.com
Web site: http://www.well.com/~mnews

Meno Times: A Quarterly Journal
The Menopause Center
P.O. Box 6558; San Rafael, CA 94903; (415) 459-5430
E-mail: mtimes@nbn.com

Gives women alternative healing choices in dealing with menopause and osteoporosis.

Aging Well: Nutrition, Movement, and Fitness for Middle-Aged and Older Women

See also chapters 2 and 4 Resources.

Nelson, Miriam. *Strong Women Stay Young.* New York, Bantam, 1997. Explains in lay language the research on preventing bone loss and building muscle. Provides an exercise regimen that will help women who want to keep fit, strengthen their bones, and avoid hormone treatment.

Shandler, Nina. *Estrogen: The Natural Way: Over 250 Easy and Delicious Recipes for Menopause.* New York: Villard, 1997. Cooking with soy, flaxseed, and other ingredients containing vegetable forms of estrogen to minimize the discomforts of menopause without hormone treatment.

Managing Chronic Conditions

Chalker, Rebecca, and Kristene E. Whitmore. *Overcoming Bladder Disorders.* New York: Harper & Row, 1990. Excellent self-help and medical material for women and men; includes incontinence and interstitial cystitis.

Notelovitz, Morris, and Marsha Ware. *Stand Tall! The Informed Woman's Guide to Preventing Osteoporosis.* Gainesville, FL: Triad Publishing Co., 1994.

Cochrane Collaboration Osteoporosis Subgroup
Dr. Peter Tugwell; Dept. of Medicine; University of Ottawa; Ottawa General Hospital; 501 Smyth Road; LM-12 Ottawa, Ontario K1H 8LS, Canada
E-mail: ptugwell@acadvml.uottawa.ca
(See chapter 25, The Politics of Women's Health and Medical Care for more on Cochrane Collaboration.)

National Osteoporosis Foundation
2100 M Street NW, Suite 602; Washington, DC 20037; (202) 223-2226

Send for *Bonewise,* a free information kit for older persons, published with the Administration on Aging. The kit includes *Boning Up on Osteoporosis,* which contains postural tips and exercises.

Nursing Homes

Faces of Care: An Analysis of Paid Caregivers and Their Impact on Quality Long Term Care: 1996 Mother's Day Report. Order from Older Women's League (see "Organizations"). Includes summary of 1987 Nursing Home Reform Act, which governs long-term care institutions.

Matthews, Joseph. *Beat the Nursing Home Trap.* Berkeley, CA: Nolo Press, 1997. Readable and helpful guide that is updated every two years. Also includes information about home care.

American Health Care Association
1201 L Street NW; Washington, DC 20005; (202) 842-4444

Its publication "Thinking About a Nursing Home: A Consumer's Guide for Choosing a Long-Term Care Facility" includes a checklist of questions to ask.

The Eden Alternative
RR1, Box 31B4; Sherburne, NY 13460; (607) 674-5232

Coalition of long-term care professionals and family members of residents advocating for demedicalizing and enlivening nursing home life through a "habitat" approach involving pets and gardening.

National Citizens' Coalition for Nursing Home Reform (NCCNHR)
1424 Sixteenth Street NW, Suite 202; Washington, DC 20036-2211; (202) 332-2275

A coalition of member groups and individuals, including nursing home residents and their families, committed to improving the quality of life and care for long-term care residents.

Death and Dying

Choice in Dying
200 Varick Street; New York, NY 10014-4810; (212) 366-5540
E-mail: cid@choices.org
Web site: http://www.choices.org

Advocates for the recognition and protection of individual rights at the end of life. Newsletter, other publications. Provides copies of state-specific advance directives including living wills and health care proxy forms.

National Hospice Organization
1901 North Moore Street, Suite 901; Arlington, VA 22209; (703) 243-5900
Web site: http://www.nho.org
Publishes a national directory.

Audiovisual Resources

Fanlight Productions
47 Halifax Street; Boston, MA 02130; (800) 937-4113; (617) 524-0980
E-mail: fanlight@tiac.com
Web site: http://www.fanlight.com
Offers excellent videos on women and aging, such as "Tonight's the Night," on intimacy, sexuality, and aging.

Woman on Fire: Menopause Stories. 90-minute video by Kathleen Laughlin. Available from Laughlin & Associates, 709 26th Avenue, Minneapolis, MN 55454-1420. Includes the experiences of women from diverse walks of life.

Additional Online Resources *

The Menopause Mailing List
http://www.howdyneighbor.com/menopaus/index.html

Menopause Online
http://www.menopause-online.com

National Aging Information Center
http://www.aoa.dhhs.gov/naic

National Policy and Resource Center on Women and Aging
http://www.brandeis.edu/hellcr/national/index.html

The Resource Directory for Older People
http://www.nih.gov/nia/related/aoaresrc/resource.htm

SeniorNet
http://www.seniornet.com

Women's Aging Connection
http://www.mainartery.com/woman/womage.html

* For more information and listings of online resources, please see Introduction to Online Women's Health Resources, p. 25.

UPDATERS FOR THE 1998 EDITION ARE LISTED WITH THE SECTIONS BELOW. MUCH OF THIS CHAPTER IS BASED ON EARLIER WORK BY Mary Crowe, Meg Hickey, Judy Norsigian, Norma Meras Swenson, and Terry Thorsos. 1998 EDITION: SPECIAL THANKS TO Mary Costanza, Martha Katz, Mitchell Levine, Cynthia Pearson, and Marcie Richardson for extensive help with different sections of this chapter. CHAPTER COORDINATOR: Judy Norsigian *

Routine Physical Exam and Basic Tests
Diagnostic Tests and Treatments
Surgery
Anemia
Arthritis. Carol Englender
Autoimmune Diseases and Disorders
    Chronic Fatigue Syndrome. Wendy Sanford, with Laurel Berger, Rebecca Rabinowitz, and Pamela Berger
        Fibromyalgia. Beverly Richstone
        Scleroderma. Barbara White
        Sjogren's Syndrome. Barbara Henry
        Systemic Lupus Erythematosus. Barbara Horgan and Kathleen Quinlan

* Thanks also to the following for their help with the 1998 version of this chapter: Linda Andrist, Ann Duerr, Ellen Fineberg-Lombardi, Joseph Hurd, Wanda Jones, Jacqueline Lapidus, Jane Matthews, Noel McIntosh, Allan Rosenfield, Ceil Sinnex, Regina Stolzenberg, Judith Wasserheit, Women's Cancer Resource Center (Berkeley), and the Breast Implant Center (British Columbia Women's Health Center). Over the years, the following have contributed to the many versions of this chapter: Sarah Berndt, Edith Bjornson Sunley, Kris Brown, Edith Butler-Hallstein, Alice Downey, Julia Doyle Sukenik, Susan Keady, Sandra Malasky, and Betty Mitchell (all of the New Hampshire Feminist Health Center), Connie Brooks, Nora Coffey, Craig Henderson, Jeanne Hubbuch, William Kaden, Gail Kansky of the Mass CFIDS Association, Rose Kushner, Lee Liberman, Charlotte Mayerson, Maryann Napoli, David Nathan, Jane Pincus, Gina Prenowitz, and Leslie Walleigh. Original section on Breast Cancer and Breast Problems by the Breast Cancer Study Group (Laurie Ansorge, Cheri DesMarais, Jane Jewell, Elana Klugman, Annette Rosen), Attila Toth, Ruth Tuomala Parker, Jane Hyman Wegscheider, and Nancy Zimmet.

Benign Breast Problems. Susan Troyan, Cathie Ragovin, Judi Hirshfield-Bartek, and Jan Platner
Cancer. Women's Cancer Resource Center; complementary cancer therapies updated by Carmen Tamayo
    Breast Cancer. Susan Troyan, Cathie Ragovin, Judi Hirshfield-Bartek, Jan Platner
    Cervical Cancer. Adele Clarke, Monica Casper
    Ovarian Cancer. Selma Mirsky, Lisa Whiteside
    Uterine Cancer
    Vulvar Cancer. Kath Doyle
Chemical Injury and Multiple Chemical Sensitivity (MCS). Wendy Sanford with Judy Spear
Crabs (Pubic Lice) and Scabies
DES—Diethylstilbestrol. Margaret Lee Braun and Pat Cody, DES Action
Diabetes. Joanne Palmisano, Ruth Thomasian
Endometriosis. Mary Lou Ballweg, Endometriosis Association
Female Circumcision, or Female Genital Mutilation. Nahid Toubia, RAINB♀
Heart Disease, Heart Attack, Hypertension, Stroke, and Other Vascular Disorders. Sheryl Ruzek, with Paula Johnson and JoAnne Manson
Interstitial Cystitis. Vicki Ratner
Toxic Shock Syndrome. Esther Rome
Urinary Tract Infections. Mary Crowe
Uterus and Ovaries. Carol Englender, Mitchell Levine, and others as noted below
    Abnormal Uterine Bleeding
    Cervical Intraepithelial Neoplasia (CIN). Adele Clarke

Hysterectomy and Oophorectomy. Mary Crowe, with Dorothy Reider
 Ovarian Cysts
 Pelvic Inflammatory Disease (PID). Debi Milligan, with special thanks to the Centers for Disease Control
  Pelvic Relaxation and Uterine Prolapse
  Uterine Fibroids

Vagina and Vulva. Carol Englender, Mimi Secor
 Bacterial Vaginosis
 Trichomoniasis
 Vaginal Infections—General Yeast Infections
 Vulvitis
 Vulvodynia. Anne Kahn

This *chapter includes* primarily those health problems that affect large numbers of women or for which it is difficult to get reliable, women-centered information elsewhere. We have also included some alternatives to conventional medical treatments. Please be aware that information is constantly changing, and make use of the resources listed at the end of the chapter, as well as chapter 25, The Politics of Women's Health and Medical Care, for a discussion of the U.S. medical system and suggestions for choosing and using medical care.

ROUTINE PHYSICAL EXAM AND BASIC TESTS

The purpose of a routine physical exam, also called well-woman care or a health maintenance exam, is to provide an opportunity to uncover health problems that may not be readily apparent and to review important preventive health measures. It can also help to establish a more comfortable, ongoing relationship with your health care practitioner.

During any physical exam, a practitioner should take the time to explain exactly what she or he is doing and why. This enables us to learn more about our bodies and ask questions if we are unsure about anything. If your practitioner seems rushed or impatient, try asking her or him to take more time at this visit or at some other time. If your practitioner is not responsive, then consider finding someone else. You might also bring a friend or family member along to act as your advocate. With a practitioner who is respectful, gentle, and informative, you will be able to relax more easily during the exam.

Although health care practitioners can not guarantee the outcome of any exams, tests, or procedures, they have a responsibility to give you all the available information. If you have doubts or feel you need more information, seek another opinion.

As part of a general examination, we should expect these features:

- Questions about our individual and family history regarding medications, medical problems, work, family, and living circumstances.
- A blood pressure and pulse check, along with a height and weight check.
- An examination of the eyes, nose, and throat, skin, and nails.
- Listening to the heart and lungs with the stethoscope.
- An examination of the abdomen, nerves, muscles, and bones.
- A breast examination, with instructions in breast self-exam.
- A pelvic exam, including a rectal exam (especially if you are over 40).
- A Pap test.
- Tests for chlamydial infection and gonorrhea (swabs in the cervix) and possible HIV and syphilis screening (blood tests). See also chapter 14, Sexually Transmitted Diseases.
- A hematocrit (blood test) to check for anemia and a blood lipids test to measure fats such as cholesterol.
- A blood-sugar check if you have a family history of diabetes.
- A urine test, which can detect infection, diabetes, and other problems.
- Referrals for mammography, bone density screening, and colonoscopy may also be appropriate.

Pelvic Examination

This should include an examination of your external genitals (vulva), an internal exam aided by a speculum, a bimanual internal exam, and a rectal examination. If you have been doing regular vaginal self-exams (see p. 593), you will be more familiar with pelvic exams and can tell the practitioner of any changes you

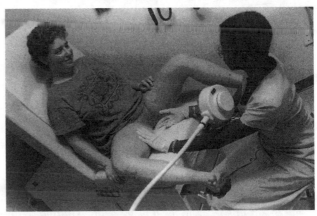

Robin Melavalin

have noticed or simply help her or him understand what is normal for you. If it's your first exam, say so. Ask the practitioner to go slowly and explain what she or he is doing. Be sure to empty your bladder before the exam. Also, your practitioner should "double" glove (put two gloves on the hand that touches your vulva while putting in the speculum), and then remove the top glove after the speculum is in place before doing the internal exam (see below).

When examining the vulva, the practitioner will first check visually for irritations, discoloration, swelling, bumps, skin lesions, size and adhesions of the clitoris, hair distribution, lice, and unusual vaginal discharge. She or he will then check internally with a finger for any Bartholin's gland cysts or pus coming from the Skene's glands. She or he will ask if you ever lose urine when you laugh or cough (urinary incontinence can be a sign of uterine prolapse, rectocele, or cystocele).

Then the practitioner will insert a metal or plastic speculum into the vagina to hold the walls apart. (The speculum should be warmed, if metal, and gently inserted.) She or he will examine your vaginal walls for lesions, inflammation, or unusual discharge; check your cervix (now visible) for unusual discharge, signs of infection, discoloration, damage, or growths; and take a Pap smear for checking abnormal cervical cell growth, and sometimes a smear of vaginal discharge to examine under a microscope or test for chlamydial infection and gonorrhea.

Some women experience pressure in the bladder or rectum with a speculum in place. Relaxing your muscles as much as possible may help. If not, ask the practitioner to readjust the speculum or try a different size.

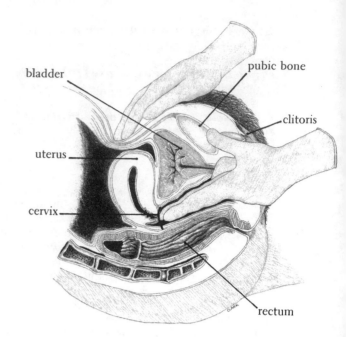

A _bimanual pelvic exam_/Peggy Clark

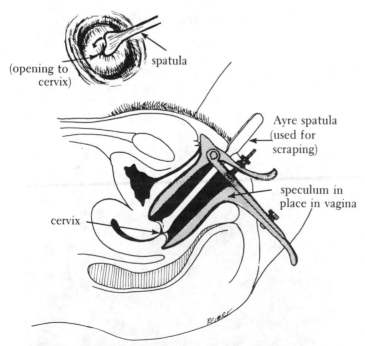

Placement of speculum for a pelvic exam. Spatula scrapes cervix for Pap smear (this is usually painless)/Nina Reimer

Some practitioners keep a hand mirror available. If you wish to watch the exam, ask for help in positioning the mirror and light source. This is an opportunity to learn how and what to look for when examining your cervix in a self-exam.

After removing the speculum the practitioner will insert two fingers of one hand into your vagina, place the other hand on your lower abdomen, and press down on the abdomen, manipulating with the fingers in your vagina in order to locate and determine the size, shape, and consistency of the uterus, ovaries, and tubes. She or he can also locate any unusual growths, tenderness, or pain.

Pressing on the uterus is usually painless, but pressing on the ovaries sometimes causes discomfort. The ovaries are difficult to find, and often the twinge of pain you feel is the only way the practitioner is aware that she or he is touching your ovaries.

The bimanual examination will be more comfortable for you and easier for the practitioner if you are able to relax your neck, abdomen, and back muscles and breathe slowly and deeply, exhaling completely.

To do the rectovaginal exam, the practitioner will insert one finger into the rectum and one into the vagina in order to obtain more information on the tone and alignment of the pelvic organs as well as the ovaries, tubes, and ligaments of the uterus. This exam can also help detect rectal lesions and test the tone of the rectal sphincter muscles. If you are over 35 the practitioner should also check for masses or blood in the rectum (sometimes an early sign of colon cancer). Some women find the rectovaginal exam unpleasant; others don't mind it. You may feel as if you are having a bowel movement as the practitioner withdraws his or her finger from your rectum. Don't worry —you won't.

Some practitioners are much more sensitive and skilled in internal exams than others; some women find it easier to relax than others. You can do Kegel exercises (see chapter 12, Understanding Our Bodies, p. 274) and practice inserting a tampon or speculum before an internal exam to help you practice relaxation.

Self-Examination

Over the past years, an increasing number of women have discovered the benefits of doing vaginal and cervical self-examination. By examining yourself regularly you can learn more about what is "normal" for you: what your discharges look like; the color, size, and shape of your cervix; and the changes in your mucus during the different stages of your menstrual cycles.

Doing self-exam, we see parts of our bodies that we have learned to ignore or fear. By using a speculum ourselves, we use a small part of medical technology to gain back some control over our bodies. Many women have taken self-examination a step further by talking about their experiences and sharing their knowledge with other women in self-help groups.

Self-Examination Tools and Techniques

For cervical self-examination, you will need only a few basic items:

- A light source that can be directed, such as a strong flashlight, and a speculum. Plastic speculums are inexpensive and easier to get than metal; you can get one at a pharmacy that carries medical supplies.
- A lubricant, such as K-Y Jelly or Lubifax, or warm water.
- A mirror with a long handle.
- Antiseptic soap or alcohol.

Find a comfortable setting and get into a relaxed position on the floor or couch. Some women prefer sitting on the floor with a pillow at their back for support.

Familiarize yourself with the speculum and then lie back with your knees bent and your feet placed wide apart. You may want to lubricate the speculum (see above). Hold the speculum in a closed position with the handle pointing upward. Some women prefer to place the speculum into the vagina sideways and then turn it. Experiment until you discover the most comfortable variation for you.

Once you have fully inserted the speculum, grasp the handle and firmly pull its shorter section toward you. This opens the blades of the speculum inside your vagina. Now hold the speculum steady and push down on the outside section until you hear a click; this means that the speculum is locked into place.

For some women, placing the speculum and finding the cervix may take some effort. Breathe deeply and

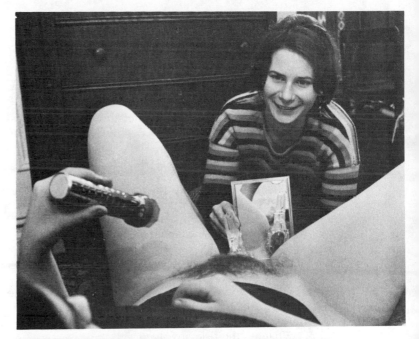

Jeanne Raisler

manipulate the speculum gently while looking into the mirror. Focus the light source on the mirror to help you see better. (A friend can help with this.) With the speculum in the correct position, you will be able to see both the folds in the vaginal walls and your cervix, which looks pink, bulbish, and wet. (If you are pregnant, your cervix will have a bluish tint; if you are menopausal or nursing, it may be quite pale.) Depending on where you are in your menstrual cycle, your secretions may be white and creamy or clear and stretchy. By learning what is "normal" for you, you will more easily be able to identify any changes that may indicate ovulation, an infection, or pregnancy.

Some women prefer to remove the speculum while it is still in its open position, and others close the blades first. Clean it afterward with antiseptic soap or alcohol, and store it for later use.

Pap Smear

The Pap smear is a method for distinguishing normal from abnormal cells of the vagina, uterus, and cervix. It is most accurate in detecting cervical abnormalities. Since the recommended treatments for various kinds of abnormal cells detected by Pap smears remain controversial among practitioners, it will help to understand some basic facts about Pap tests and our treatment options (see p. 656).

To take a Pap smear, a practitioner will, during the speculum exam, use a "cytobrush" or spatula to take one or more samples of cervical tissue from the outside of the cervix and just inside the cervical canal. You may feel a slight scraping sensation. She or he places the gathered cells on a glass slide and "fixes" them to prevent them from deteriorating. A good cell sample is essential for an accurate test. The slide goes to a cytology laboratory for analysis.

DIAGNOSTIC TESTS AND TREATMENTS

Before giving your consent for any of the procedures and/or tests described on the following pages, ask your health care practitioner the following questions (see also "Informed Consent and Informed Decision-Making," chapter 25, The Politics of Women's Health and Medical Care, p. 713):

1. Why does she or he think you need the procedure?

2. What are the benefits of the procedure over others? What are the alternatives?

3. How is it done?

4. What are you likely to feel during and after the procedure?

5. What are the risks involved?

6. What are the negative effects, including effects on future fertility?

7. What may happen if you have no procedure done?

8. How experienced and skilled is the practitioner in doing this procedure? For instance, how many does she or he perform in a year?

Dilation and Curettage (D&C)

A D&C is often used to find the cause of uterine bleeding or to treat it, especially in emergencies. It is also used to diagnose uterine fibroids, endometrial polyps, and uterine cancer. In addition, it may be part of a diagnostic work-up for cervical cancer. It is often performed to prevent infection following an incomplete abortion or after delivery, if part of the placenta is left in the uterus. The diagnostic D&C is rapidly being replaced by vacuum (Vabra) aspiration or endometrial biopsy (see at right).

Many physicians still prefer to do a D&C in a hospital using general anesthesia, but this is not necessary. It can be performed on an outpatient basis using local anesthesia, thereby minimizing the risks and expense, which are both greater with general anesthesia.

D&C involves enlarging (dilating) the opening of the cervix by inserting a series of tapered rods that become progressively wider in diameter. The practitioner then inserts a long, thin metal instrument with a spoon-shaped end (curette) through the cervix into the uterus to scrape out some of the uterine lining. (The doctor sometimes takes a tissue sample from the cervical canal.) The procedure should take five to 15 minutes.

Most women have some bleeding following a D&C and may also pass small clots and/or have cramps for

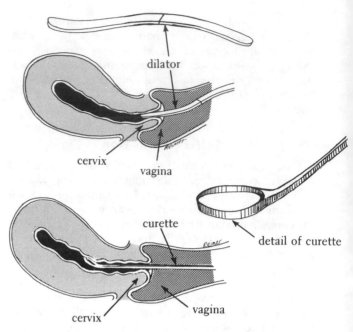

The dilator and curette, instruments for a D&C/Nina Reimer

a couple of days. The risks include infection, hemorrhage, perforation of the uterus or surrounding internal organs, and complications related to the anesthesia used.

Vabra Aspiration

More common now than the D&C for diagnostic purposes is Vabra or endometrial aspiration, which involves inserting a small cannula into the cervix and removing the uterine lining by means of low-pressure suction. This procedure can be done in an office with local anesthesia, thus eliminating the risks of general anesthesia. It usually causes the same mild to moderate cramping as the D&C.

Cervical and Endometrial Biopsy

In a biopsy, a sample of tissue is clipped from the cervix or scraped from the endometrial lining to be examined under a microscope as an aid to diagnosis.

A cervical biopsy is done on abnormal areas of the cervix that appear through visual examination with a colposcope (see "Colposcopy," p. 595). An instrument that looks like a paper punch removes the tissue sample from one or more sites on the cervix.

The biopsy may be done on an outpatient basis, generally without anesthesia. Most women experience some cramping during the biopsy and spotting afterward.

In an endometrial biopsy (which can also be done on an outpatient basis with local anesthesia if necessary), usually a pipelle (a plastic device) is used to obtain a sample of the uterine lining. The procedure may be part of an infertility work-up. It is fairly accu-

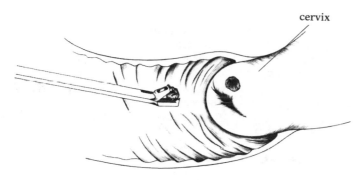

cervix

A cervical biopsy/Christine Bondante

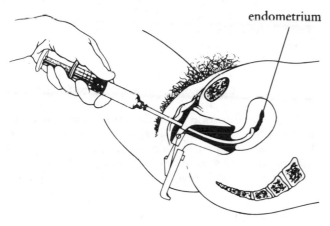

endometrium

An endometrial biopsy/Christine Bondante

rate when used to diagnose cancer of the uterine lining (endometrium).

Colposcopy

This procedure involves the use of a colposcope (a lighted magnifying instrument resembling a small mounted pair of binoculars) to examine the vaginal walls and cervix for abnormalities. It is used with acetic acid wash. A biopsy specimen is usually taken from any abnormal areas for more accurate diagnosis. Colposcopy is useful in the diagnosis of abnormal bleeding. Annual colposcopy is recommended for all DES (diethylstilbestrol) daughters (see p. 636) until any adenosis is healed, usually by the time they are in their late 30s.

A colposcopy is an office procedure that usually involves little or no discomfort. However, it is often combined with a cervical biopsy, which may be painful. Also, it is a prolonged speculum exam, which for some women is physically or psychologically uncomfortable. It is wise to remain lying down for five to ten minutes after a colposcopic exam.

When colposcopic equipment is not available, a less specific test (Schiller's test) is sometimes used. In this procedure, an iodine solution is used to determine areas of the vagina or cervix from which a biopsy specimen should be taken.

Conization or Cone Biopsy

Conization removes a cone-shaped section of the cervix. It is often recommended when a woman has severe dysplasia or cancerous cells confined to the cervix. A diagnostic conization may turn out to be therapeutic if it removes all the abnormal tissue.

A major surgical procedure, conization is done in a hospital with the woman under general anesthesia. Though the edges of the cervical area from which the cone is taken are sutured or cauterized, bleeding and infection are fairly common short-term complications. The removal of too many mucus-secreting glands may affect fertility by causing a decrease in cervical mucus. Sometimes pregnant women suffer a miscarriage after conization because of removal of muscle tissue, though cerclage treatment (which keeps the cervix from opening prematurely) may be possible.

Another option consists of laser treatments of the abnormal area of the cervix. Laser techniques cause few complications and promote faster healing. Laser destroys tissue, however, making it unavailable for laboratory analysis.

After a laser treatment, a Pap smear may show atypical cells for four to six weeks. You should have two followup smears at three-month intervals and two more at six-month intervals before returning to your regular Pap smear schedule.

Cauterization and Cryotherapy

Cautery involves destroying abnormal tissue with a chemical such as silver nitrate or with an electrically heated instrument. It is used by some doctors to treat abnormal cell development (dysplasia), cancer in situ, or cervical erosion (a reddened area that develops around the cervical opening). Sometimes cautery is used to treat chronic cervicitis, vaginal or vulvar warts, or endometriosis involving the cervix or vagina. Cautery can be done in a doctor's office, preferably right

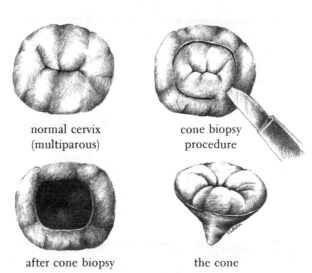

normal cervix (multiparous)

cone biopsy procedure

after cone biopsy

the cone

A cone biopsy/Peggy Clark

after the menstrual period. The practitioner inserts a speculum and applies the cautery tip to the affected area. After treatment a scab forms, allowing healthy new tissue to grow. The scab falls off in a week or so, and complete healing takes seven or eight weeks. Side effects include swelling of the cervix, profuse discharge for two or three weeks, and, rarely, infection or infertility if the cervical glands are damaged.

Cryotherapy, often called cryosurgery and sometimes cold cautery, involves the use of liquid nitrogen to destroy abnormal tissue by freezing. It can be done in an office and takes only a few minutes. It may, however, cause a profuse watery discharge and temporary changes in the cervical mucus. At this time, LEEP (see below) is preferred by many practitioners, because they can obtain tissue for diagnosis at the same time the tissue is removed (cryotherapy, laser treatment, and cautery all destroy tissue).

After either cauterization or cryotherapy, you should not douche, use tampons, or have sexual intercourse for ten to 14 days while your cervix heals. Until healing is complete, Pap smears will be inaccurate and difficult to interpret. *Note:* Cautery and cryotherapy both may cause stenosis (narrowing of the cervical opening), which makes future Pap smears difficult to obtain. As with all procedures for treating cervical dysplasia, there is a very small risk of damaging the cervix and causing infertility problems.

Loop Electrosurgical Excision Procedure (LEEP)

This method has largely replaced conization, cauterization, cryotherapy, and carbon dioxide laser treatment. During a LEEP procedure, a low-voltage, high-frequency radio wave is run through a thin wire loop, which is used to remove abnormal tissue from the cervix. The loop works by scooping out the dysplastic tissue in a matter of seconds. The excised tissue is then examined pathologically for indications of cancer. A major advantage of LEEP and similar techniques is that they combine diagnosis and treatment in the same visit to the medical practitioner. Local anesthesia is used, and the procedure may involve minor discomfort. Cervical healing takes about a month for routine cases.

Laparoscopy

The laparoscope is a lighted tube-like instrument that, when inserted through a small incision made below the navel, allows the physician to see the uterus, tubes, and ovaries.

Laparoscopy is useful in the diagnosis and even treatment of ovarian cysts, ectopic pregnancy, infertility caused by blocked tubes, unexplained pelvic pain or masses, and endometriosis, and in the recovery of an IUD that has perforated the uterus. It is also used in some female sterilization techniques. Much gynecological surgery is now being done laparoscopically, because this approach can make recovery easier and quicker. Laparoscopy is usually done in a hospital after either general or local anesthesia has been given. Before inserting the laparoscope, the practitioner will inflate your abdomen with carbon dioxide to move the intestines out of the way and expose the pelvic organs to better view. With local anesthesia, you may experience an uncomfortable pressure or fullness. You may feel some pain under your ribs for the first few days after a laparoscopy as your body gradually absorbs the excess gas.

Hysteroscopy *

Hysteroscopy involves insertion of a telescope-like instrument inside the uterus, enabling your physician to examine your uterus either directly or on a video screen. Hysteroscopes are available for both office use (often without anesthesia) and operative use (with general or regional anesthesia). The reasons for hysteroscopy include abnormal uterine bleeding, infertility or repeated miscarriage, abnormal growths (fibroids and polyps), and lost IUDs. The risks of hysteroscopy are rare; they include pelvic infection, perforation, allergic reaction to the gas or liquid used to distend the uterus, excessive uterine or cervical bleeding, and adverse reactions to the anesthesia used. There have even been a few deaths from excess fluid absorption.

SURGERY

Surgery may be performed by a physician trained primarily as a surgeon (for example, a gynecologist) or by a physician who has special training in selected surgical procedures. For example, some family practice physicians are trained to do cesarean sections or appendectomies. An important predictor of competency for any given physician is the number of procedures she or he has performed as well as how frequently.

Because a great deal of unnecessary surgery has been performed on women, be careful when deciding on an operation. In some regions, especially where there is an excess of surgeons, unnecessary surgery continues to be a problem.

In contrast to the fast-disappearing "fee-for-service" insurance plans (see chapter 25, The Politics of Women's Health and Medical Care, p. 692), which provided incentives to physicians to do more rather than less surgery, managed care programs generally have reduced the amount of surgery performed (see chapter 25, The Politics of Women's Health and Medical Care, p. 696). The surgical mentality ("When in doubt, cut it out") still prevails in some places, so it is useful to learn as much as you can about when surgery is and isn't necessary.

---

* For an excellent fact sheet on hysteroscopy (stock #CO-016), send a stamped, self-addressed envelope to: Harvard Vanguard Medical Associates, Central Ob-Gyn, One Fenway Plaza, Boston, MA 02215-2523.

Before giving your consent to surgery, you may want to take the following steps:

1. Get a second or even third opinion, preferably from a physician in a different specialty or one who is not one of your doctor's close colleagues. (Many insurance policies and Blue Cross/Blue Shield programs will pay for this second opinion.) Try to find a doctor who is interested in helping you avoid surgery when possible. For example, internists may suggest nonsurgical alternatives not offered by OB-GYNs and general surgeons. Such doctors are sometimes called conservative, meaning that they don't resort to invasive measures unless they believe that it is absolutely necessary to do so. The procedures most frequently found unnecessary after a second opinion are hysterectomy, knee surgery, vein stripping, prostate removal, D&C, cataract extraction, breast surgery, and gallbladder removal.* (See also "Our Rights as Patients," chapter 25, The Politics of Women's Health and Medical Care, p. 713.)

2. Ask your surgeon about studies that show improved outcomes for the procedure in your case. For example, careful studies have shown that much coronary bypass surgery is useless and sometimes even shortens life; yet, the popularity of this procedure is constantly increasing (see the section on heart diseases, p. 644).

3. Ask also about the potential risks and negative effects of the surgical procedure.

4. In a self-help group, or on your own, investigate what alternatives, medical and nonmedical, can be tried before or instead of surgery. Medical researchers themselves now suggest that at least seven common operations may no longer be necessary or may soon be replaced by other, less invasive, treatments: hysterectomy, tonsillectomy, cholecystectomy (gallbladder removal), appendectomy, cardiac revascularization, gastrectomy, and radical mastectomy.

5. Ask whether the surgical procedure has been widely performed, where, and on how many people; check with your insurer to see if it is known and reimbursable. Because there is no regulatory or legal authority anywhere that controls surgery, new experimental procedures are constantly being launched without adequate testing and evaluation.

6. Ask specifically about mortality and morbidity rates in the institution where the procedure will be performed (call your state department of public health). Some hospitals have more careful criteria and much better outcomes than others for certain procedures.

7. Carefully investigate the training and affiliations of the surgeon you are considering. Ask how often she or he performs the proposed procedure.

8. Ask whether you can avoid general anesthesia (one of the major risks of most surgerical procedures) and hospitalization (a major source of postoperative infections) by having the procedure done as an outpatient or office procedure.

9. Talk all this over with your family and trusted friends.

10. Take the time you need to make a careful decision.

Anesthesia

It is just as important to understand the type of anesthesia you will receive as it is to understand the type of surgery you will undergo. Anesthesia can pose a greater risk than the surgical procedure itself. Before surgery, you should be interviewed by the person who will be administering the anesthesia. Be sure to ask the following questions:

1. What type of anesthesia will be administered?

2. Why has she or he chosen this type or combination?

3. How will the anesthesia be given?

4. How may you feel after the surgery?

5. What are the possible risks and benefits of this type of anesthesia, compared with others?†

Be sure to tell the person who will be administering your anesthesia about any allergies to medication, prior anesthesia reactions, current medications you may be taking, and information about your past and current health.

Anesthesia works by blocking pain. There are three types of anesthesia: general, in which you are unconscious; regional or conduction (including spinal and epidural), in which you are awake but numb in a specific region, usually the lower half (or a zone) of your body; and local, in which you are awake and only the area being operated on is numbed. General anesthesia makes you unaware of pain by working on the part of the brain that recognizes pain. Conduction and local anesthesia block the signals sent to the spinal cord and brain from the site that is anesthetized. Another option for certain procedures is *IV conscious sedation,*

---

* This conclusion is the result of second-opinion monitoring programs set up by insurance companies, Medicaid/Medicare, and Blue Cross/Blue Shield.

† Anesthesia capability varies from hospital to hospital as well as from one anesthesiologist or anesthetist to another. Not all facilities offer a choice.

wherein short-acting pain relievers and muscle relaxants are given intravenously (by needle, into a vein).

General anesthesia is administered intravenously, by inhalation, or by a combination of both. When you are given intravenous anesthesia, you will probably first be medicated with sodium pentothal to induce deep sleep.* If you receive inhalation anesthesia, you will inhale it in gaseous form directly into the lungs via a tube inserted down your throat. Most types of anesthesia are administered after you have been given medication to help you relax, which makes the procedure easier for the anesthesiologist and for you. You may experience nausea, confusion, or dizziness for several hours or days after having either type of general anesthesia. Rarely (about once in 10,000 to 20,000 cases) there is a death or paralysis as a direct result of the anesthesia.

Spinal anesthesia is injected into the spinal canal through the membrane that covers the spinal cord. You will feel numb in the legs, in the pelvis, and possibly higher, depending on what anesthesia is needed for your surgery. Spinal anesthesia is most often used for operations within the abdominal cavity.

The anesthetic effects from spinals may last longer than those from general anesthesia. About one woman in 20 will get a postoperative headache that may last for several days, because of small losses of spinal fluid from the injection site. Lying flat on your back for eight to 16 hours after surgery without lifting your head may help relieve your symptoms.

Epidural or caudal anesthesia, frequently used in childbirth, is injected continuously into the space near the base of the spinal column but not into the canal itself. It works by bathing the nerve endings leading to large areas of the body such as the perineum and legs with anesthetic solution. For more on epidural and caudal anesthesia (similar to epidural, sometimes used for rectal and genital surgery), see chapter 20, Childbirth. Always ask whether regional rather than general anesthesia is possible in your case, especially if you have a history of respiratory problems.

In local anesthesia, a solution or jelly that numbs the nerve endings is applied to the mucous membranes, followed by an injection that blocks specific nerves (e.g., an injection of lidocaine given by the dentist).

Before and After Surgery

Because surgery badly depletes the body of nutrients, you will need to eat a diet high in protein, vitamins, and minerals to replenish these losses. You may also want to take supplements of vitamins A, B, C, and D as well as zinc and iron (see also the section on hospitalization, chapter 25, The Politics of Women's Health and Medical Care, p. 706).

* However, you are not truly asleep, and you may hear or even remember conversations of those around you.

ANEMIA

Anemia results from a shortage of red blood cells and/or a low hemoglobin content of these cells, and occurs four times as often among women as among men. (The hemoglobin molecule carries oxygen to every part of the body. When we are anemic, our tissues get less oxygen.) The symptoms, often vague, may include chronic fatigue, irritability, dizziness, memory problems, shortness of breath, headaches, and bone pain. Dark-skinned women may look gray; light-skinned women very pale. Mild anemia may have no noticeable symptoms.

Iron-Deficiency Anemia

Iron-deficiency anemia is by far the most common form in women, often caused by heavy menstrual periods as well as bleeding associated with miscarriage, abortion, childbirth, or surgery for fibroids. Pregnant women are especially prone to anemia because the fetus absorbs much of the iron the mother takes in.

Prevention and Treatments

The best preventive is an iron-rich diet (see the chart in chapter 2, Food, p. 56). Cooking foods in iron pots increases their iron content. If you are still anemic despite eating an iron-rich diet, you may want to take supplements. (Some medical practitioners recommend that pregnant women routinely take iron supplements.) Ferrous gluconate and chelated iron are the most easily absorbed forms of iron. They work best on an empty stomach, but if they cause nausea or cramps, take them with food. Taking vitamin C at the same time will increase absorption of the iron. Even so, some women find through subsequent hematocrit test results that they cannot absorb iron pills. Eating blackstrap molasses has helped some women. Iron pills can cause tarry stools or constipation, which can be remedied by eating more whole grains, bran, and fruit and drinking lots of water. Iron interferes with the absorption of vitamin E. If you are taking vitamin E supplements, be sure to take them at least six hours before the iron. Iron can be given by injection for severe deficiency.

Vitamin-Deficiency Anemias

Pregnant women, women who have had many children, women taking oral contraceptives, and malnourished women can become anemic from a lack of folic acid, an essential B vitamin. You can prevent or treat this deficiency by eating whole grains and dark green vegetables and/or taking folic acid supplements. Vegetarians who eat no animal or dairy products sometimes suffer from pernicious anemia caused by lack of vitamin B_{12} (present in all animal products). Symptoms may include burning or weakness in the legs. Adding brewers' yeast (which often contains vitamin B_{12}), a fortified cereal like Grape-Nuts, spirulina (a microalga), or fermented foods like miso, tempeh, or fermented sprouts to the diet will help. Women who lack a protein called the intrinsic factor, necessary for oral absorption of vitamin B_{12}, will need monthly injections of this vitamin.

Hereditary and Other Types of Anemia

Some forms of anemia can be inherited. Sickle-cell anemia is found in some people of African ancestry, and thalassemia affects people of Mediterranean descent. Also, some African and Mediterranean (especially Italian) women inherit a deficiency in an enzyme called glucose-6-phosphate-dehydrogenase, which causes them to develop hemolytic (red blood cell—destroying) anemia if they take sulfa, aspirin, or antimalarial drugs. This can be a fatal condition.

Finally, anemia can result from chronic illness such as kidney disease, thyroid disease, arthritis, or cancer. Exposure to certain drugs, chemicals, metals, or radiation can occasionally cause anemia.

Testing for Anemia

The hematocrit is a basic screening test for anemia. In this cheap and simple test, blood is taken and the percentage of red blood cells is measured. The normal hematocrit for a woman who is not pregnant is 37 to 47%. If your hematocrit is low, ask for a complete blood count, a lab test done on blood removed from a vein in your arm. In some cases, other specialized expensive tests may be needed. Any new onset of anemia should be thoroughly evaluated, as iron deficiency may not necessarily be the problem.

ARTHRITIS

Although arthritis encompasses over a hundred different joint diseases, women, who get arthritis twice as often as men, most often develop either osteoarthritis or rheumatoid arthritis. The former is a degenerative disease in which the cartilage—usually in the knees, hips, ankles, or spine—gradually wears away. Common symptoms are swelling, redness, and stiffness around the joints. Osteoarthritis, which is most common among older women (affecting about 25%) is not usually a crippling disease.

In rheumatoid arthritis, which affects about 3% of adult women, the body manufactures antibodies that attack the membranes covering the joints. In severe cases, the heart, lungs, and kidneys can be affected. The symptoms include pain, swelling, and redness in the fingers, knees, hips, and back; fatigue; anemia; fever; and weight loss. The symptoms may be mild or severe, spreading to many joints and getting worse over time. In severe cases, the joint supports (cartilage, ligaments, and tendons) become inflamed, and the joints themselves may begin to degenerate. A blood test can distinguish rheumatoid arthritis from other forms of the disease.

Prevention and Self-Help Treatments

Exercise, relaxation, and nutrition can both prevent and treat arthritis, sometimes reducing or eliminating the need for medical treatment. Regular exercise—such as yoga, walking, or swimming—stretches, strengthens, and preserves the joints. Daily rest is especially important when arthritis is severe. Some studies suggest that a diet low in fats can dramatically reduce pain, swelling, and stiffness.[1] Testing can determine what foods trigger an attack—it varies with the individual. Since many foods (such as beef, pork, milk, sugar, chocolate, monosodium glutamate, pepper, alcohol, and artificial preservatives) actually trigger attacks, determining what these foods are and then eliminating them from your diet can be the key to preventing arthritic attacks. Some women find that regular consumption of alfalfa alone (in tea, sprout, or pill form) prevents flare-ups of osteoarthritis, but alfalfa may cause rheumatoid arthritis to worsen. Acupuncture and supplements of vitamin C, B vitamins, and glucosamine (a component of connective tissue) may also be helpful.

Arthritis pain can also be related to stress and depression, making us less motivated to take care of ourselves and thus causing more pain, setting up a cycle that is difficult to break. Meditation, yoga, relaxation exercises, and biofeedback may help us break the stress-depression-pain cycle. The symptoms sometimes abate temporarily during pregnancy. Some menopausal women find that osteoarthritis improves with hormone replacement therapy (HRT).

Medical Treatments

The most common treatment for mild arthritis is aspirin, which relieves both inflammation and pain. Too much aspirin, however, can cause stomach irritation and bleeding. (Taking aspirin with food reduces this irritation.) Ibuprofen and other nonsteroidal anti-inflammatory drugs like naproxen and ketoprofen cause less risk of bleeding and are also available over the counter.

For severe or crippling rheumatoid arthritis, your physician may recommend surgery to repair or replace damaged joints. Other treatments sometimes used for severe rheumatoid arthritis include gold salt taken orally or as injections, antimalarial drugs, immunosuppressant drugs (such as methotrexate) used in cancer therapy, steroids, and other powerful anti-inflammatory agents. These drugs, which can have dangerous side effects, should be recommended only when all other methods have failed.

AUTOIMMUNE DISEASES AND DISORDERS

Chronic Fatigue Immune Dysfunction Syndrome

In November 1988, I came down with a bad flu—or so I thought at the time. My whole body hurt . . . I was so deeply exhausted that a trip to the kitchen for more juice would leave me on my back for hours, without the energy to speak or even keep my eyes open. I called my office and told them I'd be out of work for the week. . . . I never made it back. Three years later, my life is still about the business of getting well.

Chronic fatigue immune dysfunction syndrome (CFIDS), also called chronic fatigue syndrome, is an inappropriate name for a complex illness characterized by a constellation of debilitating symptoms, only one of which is a relentless and immobilizing exhaustion that can make even turning over in bed feel impossible. This exhaustion is not the result of exertion and is not alleviated by rest. Most people suffering from this condition have to reduce their activities considerably.

A puzzling array of other symptoms connected with CFIDS includes low-grade fever, headaches, sleep disorders (insomnia or a tendency to sleep a great deal), tender lymph nodes, muscle and joint pain and weakness, allergies, sore throats, and skin that is slow to heal. There can also be memory loss and an inability to think clearly or to concentrate. It is important for people who have these symptoms for more than three months to undergo a complete medical evaluation. The exam should try to identify any other medical problems that might be masquerading as CFIDS, since other conditions might have specific, effective treatments.

Diagnosis

Though CFIDS has long been difficult to diagnose, recent studies suggest that a diagnostic test may soon be possible. One study indicates that CFIDS may be caused by an unusually small form of an enzyme (Rnase-L), which breaks down RNA, a molecule that is the principle genetic substance of many viruses. People with CFIDS may have a defect in this enzyme, which the body uses to inactivate viruses. When this and other markers common to all or most CFIDS patients have been discovered, it will be easier to make a definite diagnosis of CFIDS. The CFIDS Association tracks and reports on such findings in its quarterly publication (for complete listings, see the Resources section).

For years, most health care providers did not believe CFIDS was an illness because its symptoms tended to be nonspecific. Some medical practitioners speculated that the condition was psychiatric, possibly because they tended to view women's medical complaints as psychological or "emotional." We now know that it is not depression, and recent studies confirm organic sources for the illness.

On top of feeling physically ill, people with CFIDS have had to face the attitudes of those who don't believe we are sick, who think we are lazy hypochondriacs. This makes you defensive, which makes understanding on both ends more difficult.

When people hear that I have chronic fatigue, the response is often "I think I have that," as if it were just normal tiredness. It becomes a kind of joke.

People of all ages, in every imaginable kind of work and living situation, have CFIDS. They need to continue to have tests every few years so that any other conditions they might develop can be ruled out, relieved, or cured.

A growing CFIDS support network has lobbied to get more government funds devoted to this illness. Serious questions about causes, treatment, and transmission are finally receiving public attention. More and more physicians know about CFIDS, and there is printed information for those who want to learn. Over a hundred research projects on various aspects of the illness are under way in Holland, Australia, and Great Britain as well as the U.S.

Meanwhile, many people with CFIDS—often in their most active and fruitful years—have had to stop working and find it hard to carry on with the everyday tasks of their lives. It has been difficult for them to qualify for health insurance or disability payments, because their illness has not had a medically recognized diagnosis. However, a sensitive health care provider can help with managing the symptoms.

Treatments

If you have CFIDS, you may feel not only frequently exhausted and sick but also alone with it. If you have found health care providers who understand CFIDS or are willing to learn, it helps. But family and friends may have pulled away from you in ignorance and confusion about your illness. In our society, women are expected to take care of everyone else, so family members may feel resentful of your need. Or you may have pulled away from them, because even the briefest visit or phone call may be exhausting to you. Also, it can be upsetting to need help, when many of us have prided ourselves on being independent. Whatever the cause, the isolation and loneliness can be painful. Fortunately, a strong, active CFIDS support network offers hot lines, support groups, doctor referrals, a buyer's club for vitamins, and other holistic treatments, as well as publications that can inform you, your health care providers, family members, and friends. One woman writes this word of caution: "Remember that the people selling alternative treatments are in business. People with poorly understood illnesses like CFIDS, especially when we are suffering a lot, can be easy targets for expensive treatments. Pick and choose."

There is no one treatment or approach for CFIDS. The following steps have worked for some women.

1. *Rest.* Arrange to get as much as you need. However, try not to resort to complete bed rest. It is better to move around as much as you can. But when you do feel a little better, don't rush back to normal activity, thinking that if you just try hard

enough your energy will return. This program may involve rearranging your life, but it has helped others to improve. One woman writes:

Regular periods of uninterrupted rest have been essential, particularly in acute phases of the illness. That means periods of time with no phone calls, no doorbells to answer, no unexpected decisions to make, people to deal with, or problems to solve. . . . It was hard for me to arrange, but I do not believe I could have made progress without it.

2. *Help your body heal.* Try to avoid additional stress, and eat a healthy diet. Some people find that certain foods make them feel worse (particularly alcohol, caffeine, sugar, food additives), but no reliable studies have been published supporting the use of any specific diet. One woman tells us: "Eat what is a healthy diet for you. People with CFIDS often need plenty of protein . . . a healthy diet is not the same for everyone. Trust your instincts." Some have tried vitamins, acupuncture, meditation, bodywork, and homeopathic remedies, and have sometimes gotten some relief. But another woman warns: "Massage or acupuncture can stimulate my symptoms and make me worse." Each person has to be treated individually.

3. At times when you do feel better, start a slow, graduated *exercise program* tailored to your needs. It can be as simple as gentle stretching or walking around your apartment. Gradually you will realize that some level of physical conditioning can be achieved.

4. No one medical approach seems to work in all cases. Research trials using low doses of *tricyclic antidepressants* have provided some relief of muscle pain and can improve sleep.

   Issues of safety, benefit, and expense have to be considered on a case-by-case basis.

5. If you apply for *insurance and/or disability benefits,* get assistance from a doctor who understands the illness (see p. 673 in Resources).

6. *Get some support* by calling one of the phone numbers listed in the Resource section for phone counseling or a support group referral. Connect with people who know what you are going through and are familiar with current research and treatments. If you have energy to spare, *join a group* that works to educate the public and to change public policy about CFIDS. Even if you merely sign up, knowing that you are part of such a group may be a boost.

Rest and treatment cost money. This is why changing public policy about medical insurance and disability benefits for persons with CFIDS is crucial. As one woman put it, "This epidemic manages to trigger all the inadequacies and prejudices of America's health care system, particularly in relation to women." For those of us without CFIDS, it should be clear where some of our precious energy needs to go.

Fibromyalgia

Symptoms and Diagnosis

Fibromyalgia is a syndrome of diffuse pain, aching, and stiffness of the muscles, often accompanied by fatigue and sleep disturbance. Fibromyalgia can be distinguished from other chronic pain syndromes by the presence of a well-defined characteristic pattern of tender points, which are unusually painful spots in muscles and in areas where muscles join tendons. The diagnosis is established by applying pressure to each of these sites and observing the person's pain response. A finding of at least 11 out of 18 painful tender points, with a history of widespread pain for at least three months, meets the American College of Rheumatology 1990 classification criteria for fibromyalgia. However, people with fewer tender points may be diagnosed with the syndrome. The results of lab tests and neurological and joint exams are generally found to be normal in the absence of other disease.

While the location of tender points is generally consistent from one person to another, the everyday pain experienced by each person varies considerably in location and intensity and may not always correspond to tender point sites. The quality of pain can also vary from intense aching to widespread burning. Pain often results from exercise intolerance, which causes muscles to remain tired and stiff after exertion, sometimes for several days. However, short periods of inactivity, such as standing or sitting in one position, can also cause pain and stiffness, which may be somewhat relieved or prevented by frequent changes in position. Most people also report morning stiffness upon arising, which may wear off in several hours or last throughout much of the day.

Other symptoms of fibromyalgia can include irritable bladder, headaches, sensations of numbness and tingling, a subjective sense of peripheral swelling without objective signs of swelling, difficulty concentrating, and generalized hypersensitivity to environmental phenomena, such as changes in temperature, humidity, and barometric pressure as well as noise, odors, and so on.

Cause

Although the cause is unclear, more uniform classification criteria for fibromyalgia have enabled researchers to study this problem with greater consistency. Some evidence suggests that decreased responsiveness of the hypothalamic-pituitary-adrenal axis and of the sympathetic nervous system may play a role in fibromyalgia. Greater understanding of the mechanisms of chronic pain, sleep disturbance, and mood is likely to improve our knowledge of this disorder in the near future. Increasingly, physicians are recognizing the physical basis of fibromylagia, so women are less likely to confront automatic assumptions that their problems are psychogenic. Studies have repeatedly shown that the central features of fibromyalgia occur independently of psychological status, although the severity of pain may increase with stress, as in other illnesses.

Treatments

Many people tend to improve if they follow these guidelines:

1. Gentle, daily *aerobic exercise,* starting from as little as three to five minutes and increasing to 20 minutes. It may be difficult to exercise while experiencing fatigue and aching, and it can take more than two weeks before the benefits outweigh the side effects. When they do, you can also try low-impact graded aerobic exercise (swimming, walking), gentle massage, and hot baths. If you also have CFIDS, go very slowly and monitor the effects before continuing.

2. A *consistent bedtime* with adequate amounts of sleep, and one of several *deep-sleep–enhancing medications.* It is often necessary to try different medications in succession and combination before finding the regimen that works best for you. Doctors may prescribe pain-relieving medications that produce serotonins and enhance sleep, such as antidepressants. It is important to note that these doses are often one-tenth of those used to treat depression, which suggests that the benefit is not based on the alleviation of masked depression. If you have brief relapses, a temporary increase in medication may be necessary.

Fibromyalgia is sometimes a chronic, relapsing condition. A long-lasting response to one of these treatment approaches is not always possible, and the condition is not always disabling. With the right combination of medications, exercise, and regular sleep, many women can be helped. Learning as much as you can and becoming actively involved in your own treatment decisions is the best way to achieve as much recovery as possible. Support groups, which have proliferated all over the country, can be extremely helpful in providing up-to-date information, doctor referrals, and encouragement in coping with this chronic and often disabling condition (see Resources).

Another syndrome often confused with fibromyalgia is *myofascial pain syndrome.* Although it has similarities to fibromyalgia, it is distinguished by localized rather than diffuse pain and tenderness. Instead of tender points, it has trigger points that, when palpated, are associated with referred pain at other locations. The referred pain can usually be eliminated by injection at the trigger point with a local anesthetic.

Scleroderma

Scleroderma is an autoimmune disease of unknown cause characterized by activation of the immune system, excessive deposition of connective tissue, and damage to blood vessels. The deposition of excessive connective tissue and the damage of blood vessels cause thickening and scarring (fibrosis) of the skin and malfunction of internal organs, such as the lungs, gut, heart, and kidneys.

Three out of every four people with scleroderma are women, who are typically 30 to 60 years old when the disease begins. Patients with limited cutaneous scleroderma have less skin fibrosis and, early in their disease, usually have problems with Raynaud's phenomenon (sensitivity of the hands and feet to cold), ulcers of the fingers and toes, and heartburn. Patients with diffuse cutaneous scleroderma have more widespread skin involvement, such as on the chest and abdomen, and early in the course of the disease they tend to have more scarring of the lungs, heart damage, and reduced kidney function.

Although some women do quite well despite their disease, scleroderma can devastate the lives of others. Changes in physical appearance and loss of hand function are common problems. The five-year survival rate is 60 to 70%, with severe lung, heart, and kidney involvement the leading causes of death. There is no cure, but effective treatment can be targeted to the organs that are involved. Much more research is needed to better understand this disease and to develop more effective treatments.

For more information, contact the United Scleroderma Foundation or the American College of Rheumatology (see Resources).

Sjogren's Syndrome

An autoimmune disorder, Sjogren's syndrome causes the body's immune system to work against itself, destroying mucus-secreting glands, including salivary and tear-producing tissues. Although Sjogren's is usually not life-threatening, it can be progressive and debilitating and can permanently damage the eyes and mouth if the symptoms are not treated. There are two types: primary and secondary. When Sjogren's occurs alone, it is considered primary. Patients with secondary Sjogren's have an additional connective tissue disease such as rheumatoid arthritis, lupus, polymyositis (inflammation of the muscles), scleroderma (thickening and stiffening of the skin), or polyarteritis nodosa (inflammation of the arteries).

Sjogren's syndrome occurs most commonly among women (90% of patients).

Symptoms

Sjogren's syndrome is often called the "great mimicker" because its symptoms often resemble other diseases, so people are frequently misdiagnosed. Because not all symptoms are always present at the same time, and because Sjogren's can involve several body systems, physicians and dentists often treat each symptom individually and do not view the syndrome as a whole.

Common complaints include dry or parched mouth, burning throat, trouble chewing and swallowing, gritty or sandy eyes, or a sensation of having a film over the eyes. Other symptoms include tooth decay, joint pain, digestive problems, dry nose, dry skin, lung problems, vaginal irritations, muscular weakness, kidney problems, burning tongue, and extreme fatigue.

The tests available to diagnose this disease include measurement of tear and saliva production, blood tests, X-ray exams of major salivary glands, and biopsy of minor salivary glands in the lip.

Causes and Treatments

The cause of Sjogren's syndrome is unknown. Some theories suggest that the causes may include viruses, heredity, and/or hormonal factors.

While there are no known cures for Sjogren's syndrome, treatments can alleviate the discomfort associated with the symptoms. High-quality professional dental care and eye care are extremely important. Artificial tears (preservative-free eyedrops) and salivas, ointments, and anti-inflammatory drugs are among the treatments prescribed, depending on the type and severity of symptoms. The use of a humidifier and protective gear, such as goggles, may also be recommended.

Education and Support

A common thread for many patients is a feeling of isolation, of not knowing anyone else with Sjogren's syndrome, and of not understanding all aspects of the disorder.

Two organizations, the Sjogren's Syndrome Foundation and the National Sjogren's Syndrome Association, provide emotional support to patients and their families, and education and information to both patients and health care professionals. For further information on membership, finding a local support group, or educational materials, see the listing in the Resource section.

Systemic Lupus Erythematosus

Systemic lupus erythematosus (SLE), a connective tissue disease characterized by inflammation, can affect different parts of the body, especially the skin, joints, blood, and kidneys. Its cause is unknown, though certain predisposing traits may be inherited (which may or may not result in the actual development of SLE). Certain drugs (including birth control pills), stress, exposure to sun, infections, and pregnancy can trigger SLE, though the mechanism is unknown. SLE is an autoimmune disorder, which means that the body's immune system becomes defective and produces antibodies against normal parts of the body,

causing tissue injury. A hallmark of this disease is often unusual fatigue, a sign of generalized inflammation. As with arthritis, people with SLE have both flare-ups and remissions (symptom-free periods).

Close to a million women in the U.S. have SLE—ten times more than the number of men affected. Two out of every three of these women are African American, Native American, or Asian American.

Because SLE is so often misdiagnosed and therefore mistreated, it is important for women to learn about the characteristics and symptoms of SLE. Any four of the following could indicate the presence of SLE: (1) facial rash ("butterfly" across the cheeks), (2) other disc-like lesions or rash marks (discoid lupus), (3) whitening of the fingers after exposure to cold (Raynaud's phenomenon), (4) hair loss, (5) mouth or nasal ulcers, (6) arthritis without deformity, (7) inflammation of the lining of the lungs or heart (pleuritis or pericarditis), often indicated by shortness of breath and/or chest pains, (8) light sensitivity, (9) convulsions, (10) anemia or low white blood cell or platelet count, (11) the presence of cells without nuclei (LE cells), (12) repeated false-positive test results for syphilis, (13) excessive protein or cellular casts in the urine. The last few signs can be detected only through lab tests, which you should request if you think you have SLE. Other characteristics include fever, muscle weakness, joint pains and/or redness, and fatigue. While many women with lupus have these symptoms, others simply don't feel well but can't put their finger on a specific problem.

The treatment for SLE will vary from woman to woman. Extra rest, a good diet, and avoiding the sun will help somewhat. The following can provide effective relief from the SLE symptoms, though they sometimes cause other problems: anti-inflammatory drugs such as aspirin, antimalarial drugs (which can cause irreversible retina damage, so regular eye exams are necessary to detect this problem early on), and steroids (which can cause high blood pressure, ulcers, swelling, and other negative effects—use with caution!). Gynecologists tend to know little about SLE, so it is wiser to consult an internist or a rheumatologist: a physician with special knowledge of autoimmune diseases.

SLE is not usually life-threatening, although it can be extremely disabling. Over 90% of women with SLE are alive ten years after diagnosis. Kidney involvement is the most serious complication and can require kidney dialysis as part of the treatment. Pregnancy is potentially problematic, since women with SLE have a higher-than-average rate of miscarriages and often experience flare-ups after the birth.

Because the symptoms are often invisible, vary a lot in severity, and usually come and go (as with many chronic diseases), women with lupus are often accused of being hypochondriacs. Physician ignorance, job discrimination, lack of support from family and friends, and the need to restrict activities are just some of the problems experienced by women with SLE.

Support groups are a key resource for women coping with lupus. If you have lupus, ask your doctor about other women who have this problem, or contact the Lupus Foundation of America (see Resources).

When I first found out I had SLE ten years ago, I was immediately faced with many changes: I had to drop out of school, was hospitalized three times that summer, gave up running five miles a day, and lost 20 pounds by fall. In the years that followed, I learned to cope with my limitations and regain my strength. When my 90-year-old grandmother complains about not being able to do what she used to, I sympathize. For me that happened at 25. Today, after returning to complete a second graduate degree, I work full-time. I control my illness by taking medication daily, but I am still afraid to tell my employer and hate to miss days because of flare-ups. I maintain my health with regular exercise (I swim three-quarters of a mile a day), a good diet, and rest. Acquaintances and even good friends don't always understand when I cancel plans, leave early, or wear long sleeves in summer. But the other lupus patients in a support group I attend understand me; we speak the same language.

BENIGN BREAST CONDITIONS

In adolescence, when our breasts first begin to develop, we usually feel both pleased and awkward. We worry about whether they will be too big or too small, attractive or unattractive. At this age, we sometimes walk hunched over, clutching schoolbooks to our chests in the hope that no one will notice our newly

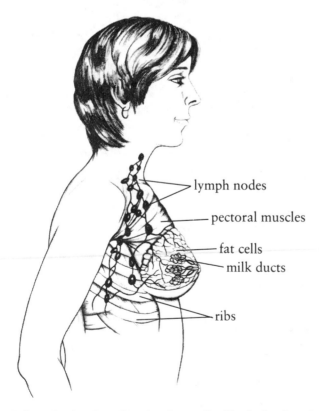

A breast, showing the structure of milk ducts, lymph nodes, and fat cells/Christine Bondante

maturing breasts. At other times, we may stuff tissues into training bras and wear tight sweaters. Our self-images quickly become tied up with our own and others' reactions to our breasts. These reactions can be as confusing and contradictory for grown women as they are for teenagers. Many of us discover that our breasts can be intensely pleasurable to us as well as to those who look at us or with whom we make love. A few women can even experience orgasm from breast stimulation alone. At other times, however, we may be embarrassed or inconvenienced by our breasts. In addition, many of us develop fears concerning our breasts—from the simple fear of sagging to the often overwhelming fear of disease and loss of a breast.

These feelings, both positive and negative, are reinforced by our society's obsessive fixation on breasts. Provocative images of bared breasts are on billboards and magazines everywhere. They are used to sell everything from cars to whiskey. They can also be a factor in getting or keeping jobs. Many men feel free to whistle or stare at our breasts or even to touch them uninvited. Some women may resent or pity us because of our "size." What should be a short-lived adolescent confusion over growing up is prolonged into a lifelong concern with breast size and shape. This sexual context often makes it difficult for us to think about our breasts as functioning parts of our bodies that need health care. It also makes breast problems particularly disturbing.

Wide Range of Normal Breasts

Women have breasts of all sizes and shapes: large, small, firm, saggy, lumpy. One woman's breast may be different in size or shape from her other breast. Nipples may be prominent or inverted. The areola (the area surrounding the nipple) may be large or small, darker or lighter, and it usually has little bumps just under the skin. Sometimes there are long hairs near the edge of the areola.

These individual differences, along with the changes caused by age and menstrual cycles, often produce needless anxiety. Unfortunately, we do not usually have sufficient information about what is normal, either in appearance or in function, to be able to tell when something is abnormal and requires further attention. This lack of information often results in a fear that every change or pain is a symptom of cancer, when in fact most conditions causing change, lumps, or pain are not cancer.

Breast Changes Through the Life Cycle

Our breasts are dynamic organs—they change considerably during our lifetime in response to changes in our body's hormone production. Understanding these changes can help reassure us when we think something is going wrong.

Earliest breast development begins before birth, at the sixth week of fetal development. At that time, the "milk ridge" forms, extending from the axilla (underarm) to the groin (the "milk line"). In humans, this ridge disappears except for the area on the chest that will form a pair of breasts. (In other mammals, the ridge will form multiple pairs of breasts.) Sometimes this ridge does not completely disappear; humans can have small areas of breast tissue in areas along the mammalian milk line. The most common location for this "accessory" breast tissue is in the axilla, although there are reports of its being found all the way down to the vulva. In the fetal period, the breasts continue to develop, regardless of sex, as they respond to placental and maternal hormones. At birth, the breasts are mostly fatty tissue, with a bit of ductal (glandular) tissue underlying sometimes prominent nipples, and they often secrete a "milky" discharge for a few days.

There is then very little change in the breast tissue until puberty. In girls, the ovaries begin production of estrogen a year or two before menstrual periods start. The breasts respond to this estrogen production with growth. At first, this is often most apparent as a firm mass directly behind the nipple—often referred to as the "bud." As most of the breast will develop from this bud, its removal will essentially stop any further breast growth. In the past, before the importance of the bud was understood, this occurred when what was thought to be a suspicious mass in prepubescent girls was surgically removed. Boys may also form small masses and slightly more prominent breast tissue at the time of puberty, which they may find embarrassing, but these usually decrease over time and require no treatment. As puberty progresses, the ductal tissue in the bud grows out into the fatty tissue and branches, forming the ductal tree. Lobules form along the tips of the ducts. The lobules and the ducts make up the glandular portion of the breast. They are surrounded and supported by the stroma, which is the fatty and fibrous tissue that also increases during puberty. One breast may develop more quickly than the other, and it's not uncommon for women to have breasts of different sizes. Most of this growth occurs early in puberty, but some growth continues over the teenage years at a much slower rate.

Following puberty, the stroma and glandular tissue of the breast continue to respond to estrogen and progesterone during the menstrual cycle, with growth and fluid retention at amounts that may be barely noticeable for some but painful for others. In early adulthood, the stroma is dense and fibrous, and the glandular tissue is thickly branching. Most of the lumpiness felt during this time is due to these firm clumps of glandular tissue supported by the dense stroma and surrounded by soft fat. Small cysts (dilation of a lobule or duct with fluid inside) may form, but they are usually very small (less than the size of a BB) because of the dense fibrous stroma surrounding and confining them. Benign (noncancerous) tumors, such as fibroadenomas, may form in the teens and 20s and may grow large enough to be felt as smooth, mostly round rubbery balls, which are mobile—they can be moved easily back and forth in place.

In our 30s, the glandular tissue and dense stroma begins slowly to decrease or disappear. This is called the "involution" of breast tissue. Denser, thicker tissue is replaced by increases in the fatty tissue. As the dense support stroma loosens, small cysts may now fill up further with fluid, ballooning out and, in some women, growing to sizes that can be felt on exam and cause tenderness. This occurs predominantly from the late 30s until menopause, although the timing may vary. As menopause approaches, hormone levels begin to fluctuate, and the cycles to which we were accustomed may become irregular. The breasts may feel the hormone stimulation, so we may notice increased pain and lumpiness. This can be distressing, because it occurs at an age when we are also looking for signs of breast cancer.

The involution of breast tissue continues to occur through menopause and after. Since most benign breast lumps are caused by hormone stimulation, breast lumps that form after menopause are very suggestive of cancer. Cysts no longer form after menopause because the fluid that causes the dilation is no longer produced, once hormone production ends. If a woman is receiving hormone replacement therapy, the involution is slowed and the breasts continue to have symptoms similar to those of the late premenopausal years, because of the continued hormone effects. Some heart, blood pressure, and thyroid medications seem to be linked to benign breast cysts in the postmenopausal years. Benign cysts do not cause cancer, but we may go through a period of stress while awaiting proof that a cyst is not a cancer. Breast pain in the postmenopausal years is usually related not to the breast tissues but to chest wall pain or arthritis of the spine referring pain to the breasts.

Detection: Self-Exam

Almost all lumps (90%) are discovered by women or their partners, either through breast self-exam or incidentally while washing, dressing, making love, and so on.

Breast self-exam is a technique by which you examine your own breasts for suspicious lumps. It is recommended by many health care practitioners and was viewed for many years as an essential component in the detection of breast cancer. However, the most recent scientific evidence indicates that there is insufficient evidence to recommend for or against the teaching of breast self examination.[2]

I just feel so uncomfortable touching myself there. I'm afraid of what I'll find. . . . I can't stand the thought of having my breast removed. I probably won't find it in time, and it will be my fault if I die of it.

American women (60% or more) do not practice breast self-exam regularly, although many have tried it.

BREAST SELF-EXAM

Breast self-exam should be done once a month, right after your period ends, when your breasts are not tender or swollen. If you do not have regular periods, or if you no longer menstruate, examine your breast about the same time every month.

The following steps are based on American Cancer Society guidelines:

1. Begin by looking at your breast in a mirror. Check both breasts for anything unusual, such as discharge from the nipples, puckering, or dimpling.

2. Next, standing in front of a mirror or in the shower, place your right arm behind your head. Soapy hands glide easily over the wet skin, making it easy to check how your breasts feel.

3. Use the finger pads of the three middle fingers of your left hand to feel for lumps or thickening in your right breast. Your finger pads are the top third of each finger.

4. Press firmly enough to know how your breast feels. If you are not sure how hard to press, ask a health care provider. Learn what your breasts feel like most of the time. A firm ridge in the lower curve of each breast is normal.

5. Examine your breasts the same way each time. You can choose to move in a circle, up and down, or from the center out.

6. Now examine your left breast the same way, using your right-hand finger pads.

7. Repeat the exam lying down. Place a pillow under your right shoulder and roll slightly to the left. Put your right arm over your head and examine the outer half of your right breast. Next, examine your left breast by placing the pillow under your left shoulder and rolling slightly to the right, lifting your left arm over your head.

If you find any changes, make an appointment to have your breasts examined by a health care provider.

Source: American Cancer Society

What to Do If You Have a Lump

Words are hardly adequate to describe the panicky anxiety that follows the discovery of a distinct lump that wasn't there before. Cancer is the first thought that flashes into our minds, along with a lot of wild, confused thoughts about "why should this be happening to me." Some women rush immediately to the nearest doctor. Others remain quiet about their lumps, afraid to go to the doctor for fear they have cancer. They can't face the thought of either having the disease or having to undergo a mastectomy, often mistakenly assuming that that is the only possible treatment.

It is important to remember that 80 to 85% of all lumps are not cancer. This is especially true for younger women. If you are premenopausal and the lump is somewhat similar in texture to other areas within your breasts, you may want to monitor the lump for one or two cycles to see if it gets smaller and disappears. Try to check the lump at the same point in your menstrual cycle (about one week after the start of your period). A lump that gets smaller over time is unlikely to be a cancer. A lump that remains the same size or increases in size could possibly be a cancer, so it should be medically evaluated. If less invasive diagnostic approaches (see p. 609) do not provide enough information, a biopsy is always an option.

Lumps that can be felt in our breasts may be cysts,

"FIBROCYSTIC DISEASE"

In the past, physicians used this term to describe general lumpiness of the breast in order to give a diagnosis necessary for insurance forms. The obvious problem is that it describes normal lumpiness, which most women will have at times, as a disease. The diagnosis also meant different things to different physicians. For the physician examining the breasts, "fibrocystic disease" meant lumpy breasts; for mammographers, it meant dense breast tissue; and for pathologists, it was a catchall term to describe 16 to 18 different benign microscopic diagnoses. Over time, it was even said that women with fibrocystic disease were at increased risk of breast cancer. This practice labeled them with a preexisting condition that made it difficult to obtain insurance (not to mention the worry of being "at risk").

This was of concern to a young, then-unknown surgeon named Susan Love, who researched the origin of the term, looking for any evidence of its usefulness in identifying women at risk of breast cancer. In 1982, she published a landmark article in the *New England Journal of Medicine* shooting down this term as a diagnosis, to the benefit of most women. She showed that "fibrocystic disease" described a normal condition of the breast, and that there was no evidence that women with lumpy breasts were at higher risk of breast cancer. It is no longer acceptable to use this term, although some practitioners will use "fibrocystic condition." Pathologists should list the particular microscopic diagnosis.

benign tumors such as fibroadenomas, pseudolumps (clumps of dense glandular tissue and stroma), or cancers. Often it can be very difficult to tell the difference between these on exam alone.

Cysts

Cysts are fluid-filled sacs that develop from dilated lobules or ducts. Cysts can be diagnosed by ultrasound or by removing the fluid and making sure no lump remains. In rare cases, cysts can contain benign (noncancerous) growths called intracystic papillomas. Even more rarely, they may contain an intracystic carcinoma (cancer). These intracystic growths can usually be seen with high-resolution breast ultrasound. Any cyst thought to contain an intracystic growth should be removed by surgical biopsy for microscopic evaluation. Simple cysts (those with no intracystic lesion) require no treatment unless they are causing symptoms of pain or are so big that they prevent you from being able to feel the surrounding breast tissue well on exam. The treatment is to numb the overlying skin, insert a small needle into the cyst, and remove the fluid into a syringe (aspiration). The fluid will often look gray and cloudy, like dirty dishwater, or dark and oily, although it can also be clear yellow. The fluid is not sent for testing because it is a poor indicator of associated cancer. If a lump remains after aspiration or if the fluid has a dark bloody appearance, a biopsy should be done in the area of the cyst. Cysts may refill with fluid after aspiration.

Fibroadenomas

If you are in your teens or 20s and find a lump that does not change, or changes little, with your period, it is most likely a fibroadenoma. Fibroadenomas are thought to form in women in their teens and 20s. Those that appear early may last throughout life. Women may develop one or more fibroadenomas in one or both breasts. Occasionally a fibroadenoma grows large enough to distort the breast's shape. Such fibroadenoma is usually removed surgically. Sometimes the fibroadenoma will grow back, though not necessarily as large as previously. These growths sometimes shrink at menopause, an indication that they may be a normal occurrence. (Cancer rarely, if ever, shrinks.) The main problem is that some less common breast cancers can feel like fibroadenomas. The younger you are, the more likely your doctor will assume that any lump you may have is a fibroadenoma and not a cancer, but there is no way to be certain except by microscopic examination involving a needle or surgical biopsy. Fibroadenomas are rarely associated with cancer.

Pseudolumps

Pseudolumps are areas of dense glandular tissue and stroma, which are normal breast tissue. At times, some areas of the breast may become more stimulated or "turned on" by hormones, and may feel like a large lump. These areas will develop in most women at times during their premenopausal years. In the past, women evaluated for this were often labeled as having "fibrocystic disease" (see box on p. 606). To make sure there is no sign of cancer, these areas should be evaluated medically, usually with good breast imaging and followup exams. At this time, mammography and MRI (see below) are the most common imaging techniques.

Cancer

Breast cancer is quite firm or hard on exam. It usually does not have discrete edges but blends into the surrounding breast tissue. It is usually fixed in place within the breast tissue. However, some types of breast cancer can feel like fibroadenomas, or others like thickening of the tissues. Breast cancers are usually at least half an inch in size before they can be felt and must be even larger to be felt in women with firmer, lumpier breasts. For more information on breast cancer, see p. 623.

Mammograms

A mammogram (an X ray of the breast) can detect, but not prevent, breast cancer. Worldwide evidence now shows that routine mammography screening with or without a clinical exam reduces mortality from breast cancer among women over 50 years by about 30%. Recommendations vary as to how often (every year versus every two years) and at what ages (somewhere between 40 and 50 years) a woman should begin to get regular mammograms. To help you decide

MAMMOGRAPHY QUALITY STANDARDS ACT

Mammography is not perfect (it misses up to 15% of all breast cancers), but it is still the best screening method that currently exists. Until recently, the quality of mammography varied widely across the country, undermining its effectiveness in detecting breast cancer.

The Mammography Quality Standards Act (MQSA) of 1992 requires all mammography equipment and personnel performing mammograms to meet specific, universal standards. In 1997, the Food and Drug Administration (FDA) enacted final regulations to implement this law. Activists also have been calling for regulations requiring that mammography results be communicated directly to all women, and for Congressional appropriation of sufficient funds to implement the MQSA effectively.

what is best for you, discuss this issue with your health care provider.

Before the biopsy of a lump, your doctor may want you to have a mammogram to help determine whether other areas should undergo biopsy.

Advantages and Disadvantages of Mammography

Mammograms do offer important advantages, such as detecting some cancers that aren't yet palpable (easily felt), serving as a map or guide to surgeons, and providing a baseline against which later mammograms can be compared to see whether any unusual changes have taken place in recent years. When mammograms detect cancers that are not yet invasive, the cancers are more likely to be successfully treated. There are also serious drawbacks to the procedure, including misdiagnoses, both through missing cancers that are there and mistakenly identifying benign lumps as cancerous. Technicians may tell you not to wear perfume, powder, or underarm deodorant when you come in for a mammogram because particles on the film may be misread as breast calcifications. The cost of the procedure and the time taken off from work or other activities may be disadvantages as well. With modern mammography equipment, only one case of breast cancer is induced per million women examined per year.

Remember that mammograms only indicate possible cancerous areas. A surgical biopsy of the suspicious area is required to confirm the diagnosis of cancer (see "Which Biopsy Method?" p. 610).

Who Should Have Mammograms?

If you are over 50 years old or if you have already had one or more breast cancers detected, the advantages of mammography for you have clearly been established. Current studies are investigating whether the same benefits hold for younger women.

The breast tissue of premenopausal women is denser and does not show up as well in a mammogram. Overall, mammography has a false-positive rate (indicating cancer where there is none) of about 7%. Estimates of false-negative results (missing a cancer that is present) vary from 4 to 30%. These false-positive and false-negative results are more common among premenopausal women.

There is also evidence that the breasts of younger women may be more susceptible to radiation damage than those of older women. In addition, any woman who starts annual or frequent mammograms at 25 or 35 is clearly increasing the amount of radiation exposure over her lifetime, thus increasing her chances of breast cancer. If a radiation-induced cancer takes 20 years to develop, a 55-year-old woman might develop breast cancer at 75, but a 25- or 35-year-old woman may develop it at 45 or 55.

The decision to have or not to have a mammogram is more complex if you are under 50 and have no suspicious lumps but are considered to be at high risk for breast cancer.* Many doctors argue that high-risk women have the most to gain from mammography—they are more likely to have cancers that mammography can detect. But it may also be that they have the most to lose from it. Perhaps being at high risk means greater vulnerability—less resistance than other people to carcinogens such as radiation. These are questions for which we have no answers. More research is needed.

Most European countries now recommend mammography every two years. In the U.S., most professional groups recommend yearly mammograms for women over 40. The U.S. Preventive Health Services Task Force recommends a mammogram every one to two years. Because the incidence of breast cancer appears to be rising among women in their 30s and 40s, more women are obtaining regular mammograms before the age of 50. They and their physicians hope that earlier detection and earlier treatment of breast cancer will make a positive difference. While mammography is the best screening technique currently available, it has considerable limitations. Researchers should emphasize developing more effective, safe, and economically viable screening methods.

Remember that a mammogram should never substitute for direct examination of a lump, as described earlier in this section.

Medical Evaluation of a Breast Problem

When you seek professional screening, the proper selection of a physician or medical facility is essential. Although your lump or abnormal cells will probably turn out to be benign, on the chance that it is cancer, it is best to go to a breast specialist who has had considerable experience with both cancer and benign conditions, not necessarily a gynecologist. Even though you may have a good relationship with your own doctor, she or he may not keep up with current research on diagnosis and treatment options. A local women's health center or other organizations that are listed in the Resources may help you find a sympathetic and more experienced physician. If you live in a small town, you may want to consider going to the nearest large city with a research or university hospital that keeps up with the current research, uses a "team" approach, and may be more flexible about diagnosis and treatment. Of course, a disadvantage is

* Only a few factors are associated with a high risk of breast cancer: a mother or sister with a confirmed diagnosis of breast cancer before the age of 50, having oneself had breast cancer in the past, or a genetic predisposition coupled with a family history (see p. 612 on genetic testing). Other factors are associated to a much lesser extent with increased breast cancer risk: exposure to radiation; taking menopausal estrogens (30% increased risk with ten or more years of estrogen use); excessive alcohol consumption; lack of regular exercise; not having children at all; not having children over the age of 30; not breast-feeding after the birth of a baby; and being a woman over the age of 50 (the last item being the most significant of these factors).

MAMMOGRAPHY: BREAST X RAYS

1. Recommended as a diagnostic tool in combination with other imaging techniques (ultrasound, MRI, and ductograms) for a variety of breast problems such as solid lumps and cysts, breast pain, abscesses, and nipple discharge.

2. Recommended every six to 12 months for women who have already had breast cancer, regardless of age.

3. Effective as a screening tool for women, reducing breast cancer death rates by 30% for women over 50.

4. Effectiveness for women under 50 remains controversial. Although the American Cancer Society recommends annual mammograms for women in their 40s, the data demonstrate very small benefits in terms of reducing cancer mortality. Furthermore, widespread screening of women in their 40s will inevitably result in unnecessary biopsies as well as missed cancers.

5. Advantages
   Detects *some* cancers before they can be felt, increasing the likelihood that local treatment with breast conservation can be offered.
   Detects some preinvasive cancers, which appear as calcifications within the breast.
   Serves as a map or guide for the surgeon when removing tissue for biopsy.
   Baseline mammograms are useful for comparison with later mammograms, to identify suspicious changes.

6. Disadvantages
   Does not detect all breast cancers—false negatives can be misleading.
   False positives can lead to unnecessary biopsies.

7. If you are about to have a mammogram, ask whether the facility has met quality assurance guidelines as defined in the Federal 1992 Mammography Quality Standards Act. A certificate ensuring that the facility has met these standards should be available for you to examine.

that you may have to travel far from your home (see "Introduction to Cancer," p. 611, and Resources at the end of this chapter).

Try scheduling your appointment after your period.

Your breasts may be lumpy at other times in your cycle, and the doctor may miss a more suggestive lump hidden by the general swelling.

The doctor should inspect your breasts carefully for skin changes as you raise your arms over your head and then lower them to your sides while you are sitting up. Your breasts should also be examined while you are lying down. This procedure is very important, as a lump can sometimes be felt in only one of these positions. The examination may be uncomfortable but is generally not painful. The physician will make a professional, though inevitably somewhat subjective, judgment on whether the lump feels like cancer. Cancers are usually more irregular, harder, and less freely moving than benign growths, but only a biopsy (a procedure to remove part or all of a lump and examine some cells under a microscope for evidence of cancer) can tell for sure, even if a mammogram and/or ultrasound is also done.

Diagnostic Breast Imaging

Diagnostic breast imaging is directed to the area of concern, which may be a lump that can be felt or an abnormality seen on a screening mammogram. The methods currently used are mammography and ultrasound.

Diagnostic mammograms include special angle, spot compression, and magnification views. Special angle views allow the practitioner to see the breast tissue at a different angle or visualize an area of the breast not usually seen in routine screening views. Spot compression views compress only the area of abnormality, spreading out the breast tissue. If the area in question is just overlapping normal breast tissue, it will fade on this view. If the abnormality is being obscured by overlying breast tissue, this view will help make it more clearly visible. Magnification views allow better visualization of microcalcifications (microscopic specks of calcium in the breast, which may or may not be precancerous) to determine their shape, number, and extent. For denser breast tissue, ultrasound may be more useful than a mammogram. Although mammography can show a mass, it can not tell the difference between a solid lump or a cyst.

Diagnostic breast ultrasound has developed tremendously over the past decade as the technology has improved. In the past, ultrasound was used to tell the difference between a solid and a cystic mass. Today, in experienced hands with state-of-the-art technology, ultrasound can look through dense glandular tissue in an area that may have a mass and show the pattern of the underlying breast tissue. This pattern may confirm a separate mass within the dense tissue or show only glandular tissue that has become more prominent (a pseudolump—see p. 607).

Diagnostic breast imaging is an important tool for deciding whether an area should undergo biopsy. It is only a tool and should never be used to provide a definitive answer. If a biopsy is not performed, the area should still be watched over time. The horror stories we see on TV or read about in the papers usually occur when an area thought to be okay was not looked at again.

Which Biopsy Method?

The purpose of a biopsy is to obtain tissue from the abnormal area for evaluation under the microscope. Today, four methods are being used: fine-needle aspiration, core-needle biopsy, incisional biopsy, and excisional biopsy. If the abnormal area cannot be felt, these biopsy methods require mammographic or ultrasound guidance to direct the practitioner performing the biopsy to the correct area.

Fine-needle aspiration is a technique that can be used in the doctor's office. Local anesthetic is used to numb the area. A small (skinny) needle is placed into the area of abnormality, and cells are aspirated into the hub of the syringe. These cells are spread on a microscope slide, stained, and examined under the microscope, as with Pap smears. A cytologist experienced in breast cytology is necessary to make an accurate diagnosis. Even so, this technique is limited, as atypical cells may indicate a range of possible diagnoses ranging from normal cells to atypical hyperplasia (considered benign but a risk factor), carcinoma in situ, or invasive cancer. An atypical diagnosis requires further investigation with a biopsy, which will obtain tissue showing how these cells are situated (the architecture). A normal cytology result is reassuring but should not be considered definitive; that woman should still be followed. A cancer diagnosis could be carcinoma in situ (confined to that spot) or invasive cancer. There have been reports of false-positive results (cytology thought to be cancer but which, on removal, turned out to be benign), so it is important to make sure that the diagnosis from cytology confirms the clinical impression.

Core-needle biopsy (also called true cut biopsy) is a technique that may also be performed in the doctor's office after local anesthesia has been given, or in the mammography suite, using special stereotaxic equipment or with ultrasound guidance. The needle is larger than the one used for fine-needle aspiration. It actually takes a core of tissue, rather than cells, and the specimen is processed like a surgical biopsy specimen, showing the architecture of the tissues. This allows for a more conclusive diagnosis. It is limited by the amount of tissue sampled. The technician must be very accurate to get good samples in the abnormal area and not tissue in front of or behind it. If the diagnosis is cancer, it is very accurate. If the diagnosis is atypical hyperplasia, the area should be removed, as some studies have shown that up to 50% of the time, there is ductal carcinoma in situ in the surrounding tissue. If the core-needle biopsy shows benign tissue without atypical cells, the doctor must make sure the sample came from within the abnormal area.

Incisional biopsies are less commonly performed today. This technique may be performed in the doctor's office or ambulatory surgical suite after local anesthesia has been given. A surgical incision is performed in the skin, and a piece of the abnormal area is removed. This procedure is usually reserved for larger areas of abnormality, where complete removal would cause some deformity in the breast tissue. Core-needle biopsy has largely replaced this technique.

Excisional biopsy is the most common surgical biopsy. It can be performed in the office (depending on the size and location of the area of abnormality), but it is most often performed in the ambulatory surgical suite. It is done using a local anesthetic, with or without some sedation, although some surgeons still use general anesthesia. A surgical incision is made in the skin, and the entire lump or abnormal area is removed and sent for microscopic examination. There is usually some aching in the area for a few days to a week afterward, with some bruising. The cosmetic appearance of the breast afterward depends on the length and location of the scar as well as the amount of tissue removed. Surgeons should try to take out a minimum of tissue around the area (unless the suspicion of cancer is very high) through the smallest incision possible.

This is the most definitive technique for diagnosis, but also the most invasive. If the area to be removed is something that is abnormal on mammogram but not felt on physical exam, the area must be located for the surgeon using a mammography or ultrasound technique called *wire localization* (also known as needle localization). On the day of her biopsy, the woman goes first to the radiology department. With local anesthetic and guidance by the mammogram machine or ultrasound, a needle is inserted into the abnormal area. A long fine flexible wire is then passed through the needle into the area. Then the needle is removed, leaving the wire in place. The tip of the wire becomes bent so that it lodges (hooks) in place within the breast tissue. The excess wire outside the skin is then coiled and carefully taped to the breast. The woman then goes on to the ambulatory surgical suite, where the surgeon removes the tissue around the wire in the area of the abnormality. Usually, the surgeon still cannot feel the abnormality, so it is a somewhat "blind" procedure, requiring accurate placement of the wire and careful dissection to avoid moving or dislodging it. The piece of tissue removed with the wire first undergoes mammography (specimen mammogram) to confirm that the abnormality is within it. It is then sent on to the pathology lab for microscopic inspection. Reported "miss" rates around the country range up to 10%, although institutions experienced in performing these procedures usually miss fewer than 5%. If the abnormality is missed, the procedure should be repeated once the breast has healed well enough to allow compression in the mammogram machine. Accurate placement of the wire by the radiologist not only lowers the risk of missing the area but also decreases the amount of tissue the surgeon must take to assure removal, decreasing the likelihood of any deformity.

The *ABBI* (*Advanced Breast Biopsy Instrumentation*) biopsy technique is a new technique that is gaining in popularity. It is used instead of wire localization and requires specialized, stereotaxic digital mammography equipment. The woman lies on her stomach on a table with a cutout section so that the breast to undergo biopsy hangs through the opening into the area under the table. The surgeon then removes the abnormal area, guided by stereotaxic mammography, through a small surgical incision after giving a local anesthetic. This procedure takes minimal surrounding tissue and rarely misses the abnormal area. It also has the advantage of doing all the steps at the same time so the woman does not have to go from mammography to surgery. Unfortunately, the equipment is expensive, which will probably limit its availability.

Which form of biopsy to use is a decision to be made by the patient, using information provided by her physician (usually surgeon) and tailored to the abnormality in question. The least invasive procedure may not always be the best choice, as additional procedures may still be required for a definitive diagnosis.

Anesthesia

A needle biopsy is almost always done with local anesthesia. A surgical biopsy, which may be excisional or incisional, can be done with either IV sedation and local anesthesia or general anesthesia. Some women consider it too stressful to be awake during the biopsy and thus prefer general anesthesia. Others choose a local because they prefer being awake and/or because they are concerned about the serious health hazards of general anesthesia (see p. 597).

You may meet resistance if you want local anesthesia. Some surgeons recommend general anesthesia out of habit, because they think people are too frightened by the idea of a local, or because they themselves are uncomfortable with a person who is conscious. In most cases, there are no medical reasons why a biopsy can't be done after the patient has been given local anesthesia, with or without sedation.

Before the Biopsy

Decades ago, when a woman had a breast biopsy, if cancer was found a mastectomy would be performed at the same time, with the woman under general anesthesia. This is no longer standard therapy. Today, a diagnosis should first be made, then treatment options discussed with the patient before further surgery is performed. The National Cancer Institute specifically advises against the one-step biopsy (followed immediately by a mastectomy), although many doctors still practice it.

Before the biopsy, you may want to ask the surgeon to cut so as to leave the smallest possible scar, as sometimes doctors are not careful about this. Depending on the size and location of the lump, the incision can sometimes be made along natural wrinkle lines or along the edge of the areola, or under the arm. Any scar, discoloration, or distortion left by the biopsy usually becomes less noticeable over time, though this varies significantly from one woman to another.

Results of the Biopsy

Waiting for the results of a biopsy can be an excruciating experience. Ask when the results will be ready and whether the doctor's office will call you or you should call first. If you haven't heard by the appointed day, call. If the results are *negative,* that means you do not have cancer. *Positive* results mean that cancer was found (see "Breast Cancer," p. 623).

If the Results Are Negative

If you are premenopausal, the doctor may say that the lump is just *fibrocystic,* a word that has unfortunately become a catchall term for noncancerous lumps in younger women (see box on p. 606). You may be so relieved not to have cancer that you don't bother to ask any more questions. However, you should ask the doctor exactly what "fibrocystic" means for your lump. You need to know the names of the conditions detected, whether any tend to recur, and whether any are associated with an increased risk of breast cancer. *Atypical ductal hyperplasia* and *atypical lobular hyperplasia* are linked to a moderately increased risk of breast cancer. If you have one of these types of abnormal cells as well as a first-degree family member (mother, sister, daughter, father, brother, or son) with breast cancer, your risk is even higher.

You have the right to obtain and examine a copy of your medical records. It is a good idea to get a copy of the biopsy test results (pathology report). The information may be helpful in years to come as new data become available about which, if any, types of lumps are associated with cancer. Having your own copy helps when you get second opinions or change doctors.

INTRODUCTION TO CANCER

Most of us (about two-thirds) will never get cancer. Many who do are free of cancer years after their original diagnosis. Why does this illness hold so much terror for us? It is partly due to the constant media attention, treatments that seem almost as bad as the disease, and the uncertainty of cure (60% of those who do get cancer die within five years). For women, there is the added factor that cancer often develops in our sexual or reproductive organs (breasts, ovaries, uterus). Because the conventional treatment—for example, in breast cancer—has been surgical removal, we may fear losing our attractiveness or womanliness in a society that so often locates a woman's identity in her physical attributes. We may also face the loss of certain sexual pleasures. (See the discussion of hysterectomy, p. 663, for example.)

Then there is shame, a "What have I done to deserve this?" feeling that so often sweeps over someone who

GENETIC TESTING AND INHERITED RISK

All breast cancer appears to be associated with alterations in specific genes in one or more breast cells, but research indicates that only 5 to 10% of breast cancer is inherited in the sense that it runs in families. In other words, 90 to 95% of all breast cancer is not inherited. So far, researchers have identified several genes, most notably BRCA1 and BRCA2, which they think are associated with breast cancer. Everyone is born with these genes, receiving a copy of each from her father and mother. If a woman receives an abnormal or mutated copy from either parent, her risk of developing breast cancer may be increased. If she has a BRCA1 or BRCA2 mutation and is from a family with a strong history of breast and/or ovarian cancer (several family members on one side of the family with breast and/or ovarian cancer in several generations, particularly in women under 40; cases of bilateral breast cancer; and/or cases of male breast cancer), her risk of developing breast cancer in her lifetime may be about 70%. At present, there is no accurate estimate of the risk for a woman with one of these mutations who does not have a strong family history of breast or ovarian cancer.

Researchers have developed blood tests that can identify BRCA1 and BRCA2 mutations. Initially, these tests were administered primarily within research protocols; now they are commercially available and are aggressively marketed by the biotech companies that developed them. This is problematic for several reasons. Genetic testing should be considered only in certain limited situations. A positive test result does not mean that the individual will develop breast cancer; it means only that if she has a strong family history *and* a family member with cancer who has had a positive test result for the same mutation, she has a greatly increased *risk* of developing breast cancer. Without this family history, her risk is unknown.* A negative test does not mean a woman will never develop breast cancer; it means that she has the same lifetime risk as most other women in the U.S.

The measures you can take if your test result is positive are quite limited at this time. Some physicians recommend frequent mammography beginning at age 25, or 10 years earlier than the youngest age at which a family member has developed the disease. One problem with this strategy is that mammography is much less effective in younger women because of the density of their breast tissue, and there is no evidence that it will detect breast cancer at an early stage. There are also unanswered questions about the safety of exposing young women who are at high risk of developing breast cancer to repeated X rays.

Another possible strategy is prophylactic—that is, preventive—surgery. This is a drastic step that is reassuring to some women from high-risk families, but its effectiveness is still unproved (see box on p. 613).

Genetic testing can cause great psychological distress and create a variety of problems for individuals and their families. Anyone considering genetic testing needs to get in-depth counseling from a trained genetic counselor. Research centers that conduct tests under a research protocol are more likely to have doctors and other professionals who are experienced in guiding individuals and their families through this complicated process. However, genetic testing is now available through private physicians. Some doctors may suggest it too casually and inappropriately, for example, to assist in a decision about whether or not to prescribe birth control pills or hormone therapy. Far too little is known about the meaning of these genetic tests for physicians to use them as a basis for this type of medical decision. (See also the boxed text on genetic testing in chapter 25, The Politics of Women's Health and Medical Care.)

Undergoing genetic testing may put an individual and her family at risk for discrimination. As of late 1997, only half the states in the U.S. had enacted laws that provided protection against different forms of genetic discrimination. At that time, federal law had only just been introduced in the Congress to protect people from discrimination in insurance, employment, and other areas on the basis of genetic information or the results of genetic tests. Not only the individuals who have been tested but their family members may be denied health or other types of insurance. The results of a genetic test could be used against an individual in a custody dispute, to deny an adoption, to disqualify someone for organ transplant surgery, or in other ways. Current state and federal laws do not adequately protect the confidentiality of individuals who undergo genetic testing; there are numerous ways in which such information could be inadvertently or deliberately disclosed. All genetic testing should be accompanied by complete information, professional counseling, and comprehensive written informed consent.

It is likely that more genes associated with breast cancer and other diseases will be identified. If and when truly effective treatment and prevention methods are developed for women with inherited gene mutations, genetic testing may have more to offer these women. What it has to offer right now is limited and problematic, and the disadvantages far surpass the advantages for most women.

* However, one study of Ashkenazi Jews, who have higher rates of breast cancer than the population at large, showed a 56% estimated risk of breast cancer (*New England Journal of Medicine* 336 [1997]: 1401–408).

PROPHYLACTIC MASTECTOMY

Prophylactic mastectomy is a surgical procedure in which the breasts are removed to avoid the formation of breast cancer. Because there is no known way to prevent breast cancer, and because approximately one out of three women being monitored by medical providers will still develop a breast cancer that will eventually be fatal, some women at high risk turn to this procedure. Although it makes intuitive sense that prophylactic mastectomy would be effective, studies of high-risk populations are inconclusive. Even the best surgeons leave some breast tissue behind under the skin and around the edges. Women may also have additional breast tissue along the mammalian milk line (from the underarm to the groin), which may or may not be noticeable. The remaining breast tissue is still at risk; how much risk is unknown. Animal studies suggest that the risk may still be substantial. These studies of rats and mice in experimental conditions may not relate to what occurs in women. Their results do emphasize the need for caution regarding this operation. Women who choose this surgery should continue to be checked, and studies of such women may provide more information about its risks and benefits. A mastectomy performed for prophylactic purposes should be total, not a subcutaneous mastectomy, which leaves the nipple as well as more tissue under the skin. Breast reconstruction may be performed afterward (see p. 627).

has cancer. And no wonder! All around us, the word cancer is used to describe any particularly immoral or illegal situation. Drugs and juvenile delinquency are "cancers" in our society. Watergate was the "cancer of democracy," not the "heart attack."

This fear and shame means that many of us avoid thinking about cancer even when we ourselves have it. Because of this avoidance, we do not always make the best medical decisions or live as full a life as possible.

What Is Cancer?

Through a process not completely understood, normal cells sometimes become abnormal and begin to grow out of control. These abnormal cells may spread (metastasize) throughout the body, taking over organs and preventing them from functioning. Cancers may be slow-, moderate-, or fast-growing. Each type of cancer has its own particular pattern of growth, spread, and probability of cure or survival time.

Who Gets Cancer?

Although people of all ages can get cancer, it is most often found in older persons, as the disease can take as long as 20 years to reach a detectable state.

Over the past 25 years, the cancer death rate has increased 50% among the black population and only 10% in the white population. The incidence (number of new cases) is also higher among black persons; in some cases (such as cervical cancer), the rate is twice as high for black women as for white women. African Americans continue to be diagnosed later and have lower survival rates for every major type of cancer except stomach cancer. At least part of the reason for these differences may be the discrimination that causes many black people to be exposed more frequently to workplace and environmental carcinogens (cancer-causing substances) than whites, and to have less access to high-quality medical care, nutritious food, and decent living conditions.

Women develop less cancer and die less frequently of it than men do; the gap (except for lung cancer) is widening.* At least part of this difference exists because until recently men consumed much more tobacco and alcohol and were more often exposed to workplace carcinogens. Or there may be something inherent in our immune or metabolic systems that increases our ability to fight cancer. Nonetheless, 265,000 women were expected to die of cancer in 1997.

Terminology

The following terms are frequently misunderstood or misused, even by medical personnel. Ask for careful explanations. It is your right to know exactly what is going on.

Mortality (death) rates tell how many people died of cancer per 100,000 population per year.

Survival rates, generally given for five-, ten-, and 20-year periods, report how long people with specific kinds of cancer usually live. Survival rates are always calculated from the date the cancer was first diagnosed. These rates are most helpful when they are subdivided according to such factors as how far advanced the cancer was at first diagnosis, the type of treatment received, and the age, sex, race, socioeconomic status, and occupation of the people involved.

Cure rates purport to tell how many people are completely cured of their cancers. However, cure rates are generally based on survival rates, resulting in the misleading impression that many people are "cured" who have merely survived for a specified (usually five-year) period. Many people mistakenly believe that a five-year disease-free interval indicates a cure. This is not true.

* From 1950 to 1983, there was a 30% increase in men's cancer death rates and a 6% decrease in women's. However, as women's smoking has increased, our lung cancer rate is also increasing and is now the leading cause of cancer death in women.

Remission is sometimes used loosely to refer to any improvement, at other times in a more technical sense with very strict criteria regarding the amount of change in tumor size and blood test results. Technically, remission means no evidence of disease; it is not a guarantee of no cancer cells in the body. Some cancer therapies will produce technical "remission" of certain symptoms but do not increase the cure or survival rates. Remission rates are usually given as percentages of persons "going into remission" after receiving various types of treatments.*

We should keep in mind that while statistics provide useful information, they can't really predict what will happen to us as individuals.

Causes

Cancer rates increase with exposure to carcinogens (such as radiation, asbestos, some pesticides), smoking, alcohol, or particular dietary habits (see below). Certain genes and viruses have caused cancer in laboratory animals, and similar processes are suspected but not conclusively proved in some human cancers. Yet, it is not clear how these substances cause cancer or why everyone who develops the same kind of cancer does not respond in the same way, either to the disease or to treatments. There are also unexplained cases of spontaneous remission: Approximately 7 to 8% of people with terminal cancer suddenly recover and live out their lives apparently free of the disease. It happens more often with some cancers than with others. These different responses show that our individual immune systems are very important factors.

It seems most likely that cancer is caused by a buildup of one or more factors to the point (different for each person) where the body's immune system can no longer handle the load. For example, smoking will not guarantee that you will get cancer, but it will increase your chances. (Smoking or smoking combined with heavy alcohol consumption accounts for 30% of all cancer deaths. Add smoking to heavy drinking, repeated X rays, constant stress, exposure to pollution,† or excessive overweight, and the risk of cancer goes up.

Both environmental and hereditary elements appear to cause cancer. "Heredity" refers to the traits and tendencies passed on to us by our parents in our genes, whereas "environment" includes all that we eat, breathe, or come into contact with. Most researchers now believe that multiple exposures to carcinogens or other environmental "insults" cause genetic mutations that result in cancer. In some people who already have a genetic predisposition to cancer, it may take fewer exposures to carcinogens to trigger cancer

than in others with no such genetic background. Thus, even though genes may play a role in causing cancer, the environment is a far more significant factor.

Prevention

Although we can do many things to reduce our risk of cancer (such as stopping smoking and limiting X rays), many other factors, such as air pollution and the many environmental carcinogens that bombard us in our daily lives, are not so clearly under our personal control. Diet changes, such as eating more organically grown foods, can be expensive; dietary recommendations are sometimes controversial; and eating is complex behavior that is hard to change.

Thus, cancer prevention means restructuring both our personal lives and the society at large so that a clean environment, safe jobs, healthy food, and less stressful living become top priorities.

Ways to Reduce the Risk of Cancer

Each woman must assess and weigh her individual risk factors when deciding what to do. In the list that follows, factors that seem to be related to breast cancer are marked with an asterisk.

1. Don't smoke, and avoid smoke-filled environments.

2. Avoid frequent X-ray exposure, especially at earlier ages.

*3. Avoid estrogen replacement therapy at menopause, as well as any other medication with estrogen. The relationship between oral contraceptives and breast cancer continues to be very controversial. Some studies have shown that women who begin taking birth control pills at a young age and continue for a long period have a higher risk of breast cancer. Other studies indicate that the Pill lowers women's chances of developing uterine and ovarian cancers. To be on the safe side, women concerned about their risk of breast cancer may want to avoid oral contraceptives.

4. Minimize consumption of smoked, salted, or pickled foods, such as bacon. Avoid additives, preservatives, and refined flour.

*5. Keep fat consumption low—about 15 to 20% of total calories—while ensuring adequate intake of essential fats (see chapter 2, Food, p. 54).

*6. Limit or eliminate alcohol consumption.

*7. Research has shown that people who are overweight (more than 40% above the old "norms") get more cancer and die more frequently of it. In breast cancer, this may be related to estrogen levels. Many studies point to high levels of estrogen

---

* "Long-term remission" refers to a specific number of disease-free years and is preferred to "cure," as people with cancer are often considered to have their disease under control rather than to be entirely cured.

† See chapter 7, Environmental and Occupational Health, for more on environmental and workplace carcinogens.

as a precipitating factor in breast cancer. There is evidence that fat tissue manufactures its own estrogen. Although this process may be helpful during and after menopause as a natural form of ERT, it may also be dangerous to a woman who is very large or who already has elevated estrogen levels.

8. Try to have frequent and regular bowel movements. Increasing exercise and intake of dietary fiber and water may help.

9. Avoid hair dyes made from petroleum bases. According to one study, 20% of non-Hodgkin's lymphoma cases in women are caused by ingredients in hair dyes.

10. Eat a diet high in organic whole grains, vegetables, and fruits rich in bran and fiber.

11. Eat food high in beta-carotene (a vitamin A precursor found in carrots and other yellow and dark leafy vegetables as well as some yellow fruits). Or take supplements of beta-carotene. Be wary of large doses (greater than 10,000 to 15,000 IU daily) of vitamin A, as it can be toxic and is not a substitute for beta-carotene.

12. Eat foods high in selenium (brewers' yeast, eggs, garlic, onions, liver, asparagus, tuna, mushrooms, shrimp, kidney, whole grains, and brown rice). Selenium can be toxic in high doses, so be wary of any megatherapy or supplementation.

Costs

The total costs to the U.S. economy of cancer research and treatments is many billions of dollars per year. Medical treatment for cancer can reach tens of thousands of dollars for an individual, not including hidden costs like transportation, baby-sitters, and loss of income.

Unfortunately, the profit motive affects the way this country tackles cancer. Major research has emphasized high-profit treatments rather than prevention. (Chemotherapy, for instance, can cost up to a thousand dollars per session.) These treatments benefit hospitals, doctors, and the pharmaceutical, insurance, and medical-equipment companies but have not yet brought significant progress in eliminating cancer. Government and industry have done relatively little to clean up the environment, the workplace, or hazardous consumer products. Only recently has the government taken substantial initiative to discourage tobacco use.

What to Do If You Have Cancer

Inform yourself. The first thing to do is learn all you can. Unfortunately, there is no reliable cure for most cancers, and all the once-accepted theories and treatments in the field are now under question. It helps

to be persistent and aggressive in seeking the most up-to-date information and to have someone you trust do it with or for you.

Resist the pressure to rush. Your doctor or your family may pressure you to begin treatment immediately. Yet, most cancers have been developing for two to 20 years before being discovered. Several studies have shown that a short delay of three or four more weeks while you get adjusted to the idea, seek out information, and get second or third opinions should not make any difference in the ultimate outcome of your disease. If you decide then to follow your doctor's original advice, you will feel much better about the decision. If you decide to take another course of action, you may have saved yourself unnecessary treatment or considerable regret at not having made your own choice.

Talk to others with cancer. Try joining (or starting) a group for people with cancer. Being with those who understand and have faced the same problems can provide the kind of practical information and emotional support that is simply not routinely available from those providing conventional medical cancer treatment.

Joining my cancer discussion group is one of the best things that has happened to me since my diagnosis.

In a group founded by those who have cancer, rather than one started by professionals at a hospital or a service organization, you may feel freer to confront all aspects of your situation. These include critical evaluation of both conventional and complementary therapies; the problems surrounding child care, insurance, jobs, and marital relations; and ways of coping with your own fears as well as those of family and friends. If you can't find or create such a group, talk with individuals: people in waiting rooms, people suggested by your doctor, friends, or clergy. Don't hesitate to call persons you haven't met. Many people with cancer are glad to talk about their experiences.

Factors to Consider When Deciding on Conventional Medical Treatment (Surgery, Radiation, and Chemotherapy)

Unfortunately, there has been little progress over the years in effective cancer treatment. Many doctors and hospitals have biased opinions on preferred treatments that they will urge you to accept. Some specialists tend to recommend their own approach; for example, surgeons promote surgery and radiologists radiation. Yet, new research indicates that many factors—age, sex, previous health history, type and stage of cancer—can influence how well a treatment works. The data are changing rapidly, and even those doctors who are familiar with the most recent research often can't agree on how to interpret the information. Ideally, you should have access to a team of specialists to be sure of getting the treatment most appropriate for your cancer and for you.

Because so many variations exist, we cannot give a comprehensive guide to cancer treatments. What we can do is discuss some of the issues and indicate what you need to know in order to make informed decisions. If no one treatment has proved best, it often makes sense to choose the one that will disrupt your body and your life the least.

Although everyone wants the benefits of the most current therapies, it is tragic to give false hope, waste limited finances, or subject already ill persons to painful treatments unless there is good reason to believe that the treatment will pay off with either increased survival time or improved quality of remaining life. We urge anyone considering surgery, chemotherapy, radiation, or any of the alternatives to study carefully what can be reasonably expected from the treatment in her particular case (see also chapter 25, The Politics of Women's Health and Medical Care.)

There are other factors to consider. Choosing anything but the most conventional and locally available treatment often involves traveling quite a distance. This may separate you from loved ones and a familiar environment—important factors in the healing process. Also, most forms of treatment are very expensive, and pursuing a less available treatment may mean even more expense for second-opinion medical visits, travel, noninsured costs. Many women (perhaps having internalized the culture's view of women as secondary) feel guilty about using their own or their family's money on themselves. In making this difficult decision, every woman deserves both the clearest, most current information and the strongest possible support from family and friends. It has clearly become standard practice to obtain at least a second opinion before beginning treatment.

Surgery

Surgery has been the mainstay of cancer therapy for over a century. It helps with local control of the disease and seems to be effective in a few types of cancer (such as nonmelanoma skin cancers and cervical cancer). But surgery is not always the best treatment, and it takes the body a long time to recover from it. It is important to verify that the treatment you are offered is really going to be helpful in eliminating the cancer or at least improving or prolonging your life. See p. 596 for some things to consider before consenting to surgery.

Surgery and Early Detection

Until very recently, most doctors believed that surgery would work if the cancer was removed before it had a chance to spread. For this reason, when possible they would cut a sizable area around the cancer to "be sure to get it·all." They based this approach on the theory that cancer begins in one place (e.g., the lung or breast) and spreads from there.

However, over the past 20 years or more, cancer has been detected earlier and earlier with, in most cases, no corresponding drop in the death rate. This has made many physicians question the entire notion of early detection. Now many doctors are beginning to view some cancers as systemic diseases that tend to show up first in certain areas but are already microscopically present throughout the body. There is evidence to support both theories, and the final answer may lie somewhere in between.

Radiation and Chemotherapy

Radiation (via high-power X rays or internal implants) and chemotherapy (chemicals taken by pill or injection) are supposed to kill cancer throughout the body in places that surgery can't reach. They themselves have carcinogenic (cancer-causing) potential, but theoretically they are more harmful to cancer cells than to normal cells. So far, neither therapy has been very successful in curing or prolonging life in regard to the common cancers such as breast, colon, and lung cancer, although they have reduced some cancer symptoms.

The side effects of chemotherapy are specific to the drug or drug combination. Common side effects include nausea, vomiting, fatigue, hair loss, cessation of menstruation, and suppressed immune function (seriously lowering resistance to infections). The side effects of radiation are specific to the body area being treated (hair loss if hair is in the treatment field, diarrhea if the colon is in the field). Radiation may also cause nausea and vomiting, skin burns, extreme sun sensitivity, and ulcers (body sores that do not heal). Some drugs lessen these symptoms, but they may have their own negative effects. Medication for nausea and vomiting has improved many patients' tolerance of cancer therapy. Marijuana sometimes helps reduce nausea and may be legal in certain situations for people with cancer. Both forms of treatment involve repeated trips to a medical center or hospital.

Chemotherapy and radiation were formerly used only when cancer recurred in the same organ or metastasized elsewhere. Increasingly, doctors recommend radiation and/or chemotherapy immediately after surgery even when there is no evidence of spread (e.g., breast lumpectomy with radiation). In some instances, if the cancer is too advanced for surgery, chemotherapy and radiation are tried without surgery.

Some physicians may overuse chemotherapy and radiation in instances where there's no proven benefit —almost as though they were miracle cures. This is understandable. Most doctors genuinely want to help their cancer patients and are frustrated by the lack of a reliable cure. Most people with cancer feel more reassured when they and the doctor are doing something. Overtreatment is psychologically appealing on both sides; both want to hope that "this time," treatment will make the difference.

Popular articles about cancer often give the impression that chemotherapy is working wonders with all types of cancer. This image makes people more likely to accept treatment under the false notion that it will increase their survival time also. Chemotherapy has shown significant results in a few of the less common types.* In addition, recent evidence shows that chemotherapy offers significant benefits for some women with breast cancer (see "Breast Cancer," p. 623). It is important to determine that chemotherapy has been proved effective for your type of cancer.

It is also important to find out exactly how much increased survival time can be gained. Sometimes the percentages doctors or researchers give are misleading: What is called 50 or 100% increased survival time may mean only two or three months more, or it may mean two or three years more. See the questions that follow.

Many people question whether the possibility of longer survival times is worth the negative effects of these therapies. Others feel that even one more day of life is worth any price. Only you can make this difficult decision with the support of those who love you.

Questions to Ask

An asterisk indicates those questions that doctors frequently do not or cannot give sufficient answers to. Press your doctor to find out and let you know, but also check books, medical journals, and resource centers, and speak to others who have had the same form of cancer as you.

*1. Exactly what form of cancer do I have? Is it slow- or fast-growing?

*2. What therapies are available?

*3. How effective is each therapy? What is the probability of cure? What definition of cure is used?

4. What benefits can I expect? Longer life? Reduced symptoms? Reduced pain? And so on.

*5. Can the therapy prolong life by months? By years?

*6. What percentage of people treated benefit from the therapy: 25%? 50%? 75%? How is that benefit measured?

7. Will I be able to continue my regular activities during and after the therapy? What about sex? Working? Sports?

8. Will the therapy require overnight stays in the hospital, or can it be done on an outpatient basis?

9. What are the potential negative effects? How serious are they? What percentage of people get them? Are they permanent? Are there any drugs that will help alleviate these effects? Do these drugs themselves cause any negative effects? How long does any symptom usually last? How soon after treatment are symptoms likely to begin? (For example, does nausea generally start immediately or within 20 minutes, or several hours later?)

10. How long will the therapy last? Each session? How many sessions?

*11. How many people get recurrences after this treatment, and how soon?

*12. Are there survival, cure, mortality, and remission rates for this therapy for my type of cancer, broken down by such factors as type of cancer, age, sex, race, socioeconomic status, occupation, geographical location, and so on?

13. What are the costs involved? Does insurance usually cover them?

*14. May I speak with some of your other patients? Do you know of any local groups for people with cancer? Any groups for family members and friends?

Alternative (Complementary) Therapies

Complementary, or alternative, cancer therapies have recently gained considerable public attention. Women are seeking these approaches because some conventional medical and surgical therapies have not significantly improved survival rates and are sometimes expensive and painful. In recent years, the medical establishment (including insurers) have started to become more accepting of alternatives to surgery, radiation, and chemotherapy. To date, alternative therapies are most often used along with conventional ones or as a last resort for advanced cancers after conventional treatments have failed. They can also confer an improved sense of well-being even in the absence of a cure (see chapter 5, Holistic Health and Healing).

There are no reliable statistics on survival, recurrence, and mortality for the alternative therapies. However, research into alternative medicine is an evolving science. Centers to conduct such research have existed in European countries and in Russia for several years and are now being set up across the U.S. and Canada, including an Office of Alternative Medicine at the federally funded National Institutes of Health.

Alternative cancer therapies are often reported in what is called anecdotal style: one person who was cured of cancer (or greatly helped) by a certain treat-

* Chemotherapy has produced dramatic increases in five-year survival rates and long-term cures in childhood leukemia, young-adult Hodgkin's disease, and other lymphomas. A child treated for leukemia may gain many precious years of life. However, some children may get another form of cancer later on, caused by the chemotherapy chemicals themselves. It may be inappropriate to call the leukemia treatment a cure in all cases.

ment tells her or his story. Although this makes for inspirational reading, it is hard to confirm individual case histories, and there is no proof that it was the treatment that caused any given instance of a recovery. The key to demonstrating effectiveness is comparing the results of a certain therapy with the results of other therapies. Remember to ask the same questions about these alternative therapies that you would ask about conventional methods.

If you or anyone you know is considering using alternative or complementary cancer therapies, you'll want to know whether they are safe and really work.

You should be aware of these issues:

- Some of these therapies are ineffective, potentially toxic, deceptively promoted, and often expensive.
- Of more than 200 alternative cancer therapies available, fewer than 30% have been tested in large-scale, long-term trials.
- "Natural" or "organic" is not a synonym for safety or effectiveness.

Questions you should ask are these:

- Has the method been evaluated objectively—that is, by researchers other than the proponents of the therapy?
- Has the therapy been tested in large-scale, long-term, controlled trials?
- Has it been evaluated/used in cases similar to my case?
- Is the treatment based on a proven theory?
- Does the potential for benefit exceed the potential for harm?
- Has the Office of Alternative Medicine at the National Institutes of Health gathered any information on the method?

It's a good idea to discuss all the available evidence about a complementary therapy with a receptive health care professional before making any decision regarding its use. If possible, ask your own health care practitioner how the prognosis for your disease would be affected by standard treatments, and whether she or he is familiar with the complementary therapy or therapies you are considering.

In large part because of opposition from the medical world, many alternative health clinics are not well funded or easily accessible. A decision to go to one may mean added and noninsured expenses for treatment, travel, child care, housing, and so on.

Friends and family who disapprove of these therapies may withdraw emotional or financial support. Still, many women have found it worthwhile to push past these obstacles to find complementary sources of healing.

Special Diets and Detoxification Therapies

The most common nutritional alternative cancer therapies, also known as nutritional or integrative approaches, are Gerson therapy, Kelley's nutritional-metabolic therapy, Manner metabolic therapy, the Livingston/Wheeler regimen, the Wigmore treatment, the macrobiotic diet for cancer, the alkaline/acid cleansing diet, Revici therapy for cancer, the Moerman diet, and the grape cure for cancer.

These regimens share several characteristics:

- Usually strict vegan or vegetarian diets, or diets low in animal proteins.
- Diets that are often high in fiber, sugar-free, and low in salt and fat. The result is a diet high in fruits, vegetables, and cereals; high in bulk; and low in calories. This may not meet the needs of many cancer patients, who have high energy requirements because of their high metabolic rate.
- Avoidance of refined and processed products; deep-fried foods; foods containing additives, preservatives, or coloring; caffeine; alcohol; and tobacco.

Diet may be combined with other procedures such as enemas, fasting, and drugs or enzymes that are used to detoxify or "clean" the body of toxins. Sometimes patients undertake these regimens as a last resort, when they are already malnourished and weak. These diets may not produce the desired effect, because they do not provide adequate intakes of protein, iron, calcium, and Vitamin B_{12}. They can be costly to follow because of expensive organically grown goods and vitamin or mineral supplements.

There is evidence that mortality for colon cancer is reduced in strict vegetarians. A vegetarian lifestyle (over 20 years) has also been associated with decreased cancer mortality. Trials of low-fat dietary interventions as adjuncts to breast cancer treatment are currently under way; however, no specific benefits of vegetarian diets for cancer cure have been proved. Health-conscious behavior and a healthy lifestyle including physical activity, control of body weight, and strict adherence to a regimen seem to bring about stronger results than nutrition alone.

The Gerson Diet and Detoxification Therapy

Perhaps the most promising of the nontoxic alternatives is the Gerson diet and detoxification therapy. The diet consists of eating organically grown fresh fruits and vegetables. It forbids salted, processed, or refined foods, and fat. Meat is not allowed in the early stages of treatment. In most cases, the therapy includes tablets and injections of various nutrients, especially potassium and pancreatic enzymes. The Gerson therapy, developed in Austria in the 1920s and 1930s, is one of the few alternatives for which there are records and reports of long-term survival rates. For more information, contact the Gerson Institute of California (see Resources).

Dr. Max Gerson believed that cancer patients have a sodium imbalance in their body in conjunction with a deficiency in the metabolism of fats, proteins, carbohydrates, vitamins, and minerals. The therapy aims to correct these imbalances.

It requires a high level of personal commitment because patients have to eat a raw, vegetarian diet for a year and a half to two years. Patients undertaking this regimen must have access to fresh, organic produce year round and enough time to comply with the treatment. Specifically, patients must prepare fresh vegetable and fruit juices every hour on the hour, take enemas for detoxification, and drink three glasses of fresh, raw calves' liver juice each day.

A modified Gerson therapy (eliminating both hormone supplementation and enemas) has been shown to be effective in improving general conditions in cancer patients. One controlled clinical study showed that there was no difference in survival and quality of life for 78 cancer patients who underwent this regimen compared with conventional treatments. However, the patients receiving conventional treatment experienced more appetite problems and loss of weight than those receiving the Gerson therapy.

Physicians and various health care practitioners have developed other diet therapies. Most of them are similar to the Gerson diet, though there are some discrepancies, especially between raw and cooked foods. Most also include procedures for detoxification (removing wastes from the body through skin, bowels, etc.) and spinal adjustments (see "Chiropractic," chapter 5, Holistic Health and Healing, p. 112). Many people who use the Gerson and other diets experience periods of nausea and headache and occasional pain and fever, which their supporters attribute to the removal of toxins.

Kelley Regimen for Cancer

Donald Kelley believed the historical origins and type of diet to be related to the nervous system. His diet, adopted by Dr. Nicolas Gonzalez, a physician in New York, includes large amounts of carrot juice, a vegetarian diet, coffee enemas, and pancreatic enzymes, along with vitamin and mineral supplements. It is generally tailored to the individual's needs, from purely vegetarian to diets rich in meat.

The Office of Alternative Medicine at the National Institutes of Health is now evaluating this therapy, including claims that there are 50 "successful" cases demonstrating remission of advanced cancer.

Macrobiotics

This vegetarian diet is based on a system originally developed in Japan and reformulated by Michio Kushi in Boston. Macrobiotic theory holds that the incidence and development of cancer is affected by dietary, environmental, social, and personal factors. Its use in cancer treatments is controversial and is based on the belief that cancers are the result of imbalances in the body's yin/yang forces. The diet consists of approximately 50% whole cereal grains; 20 to 30% of organic vegetables; small amounts of soups, beans, sea vegetables, white meat, fish; and limited amounts of fruit. Vitamin supplements are generally not taken.

Evidence suggests that the macrobiotic diet works best with cancers of the breast, cervix, colon, pancreas, liver, bone, and skin. In one clinical study, cancer patients showed no side effects, and there was some degree of tumor regression. In addition, subjective benefits such as reduction of pain were observed.

There is controversy about giving cancer patients a regimen deficient in growth-promoting substances. Its long-term use may lead to deficiencies in vitamins B_{12} and D, and children and critically ill patients may experience severe dietary deficiencies. Macrobiotic philosophy does not encourage patients to combine the diet with conventional cancer therapies.

Meganutrition Therapies

Also known as orthomolecular medicine, a major medical system proposed and developed by two-time Nobel laureate Linus Pauling, meganutrition starts with the principle that cancer patients require larger amounts of vitamins and minerals. Pauling states that large daily doses of vitamin C can aid in both preventing and treating cancer. A study in Scotland supported his claim, but many doctors have vehemently attacked Pauling because similar studies in the U.S. have shown no improvement. Pauling and his associates believe that the American studies had major methodological flaws because they are based on people who had already had chemotherapy (which represses the immune system and may inhibit the vitamin's action). They claim that megadoses of 20 to 600 times the recommended daily allowances of specific nutrients increase immune system activity (T cell number and activity) and restore cell-mediated immunity.

Other researchers have found evidence that megadoses of other nutrients, especially vitamins A and B complex, the provitamin beta-carotene, and trace minerals such as potassium and selenium, can help in the prevention and treatment of cancer. These nutrients are antioxidants: they protect against oxidation, a chemical reaction that can cause profound damage to the cells, thus preventing healthy cells from dying or from proliferating excessively, as occurs in cancer. Despite the protective role of antioxidants in the development of cancer and heart diseases, sound scientific evidence to support a curative role for antioxidants in cancer is lacking.

However, there is increasing clinical evidence that antioxidants may be effective in preventing cancer of the esophagus, mouth, cervix, and lung. In addition, experimental studies on vitamin C have demonstrated that it improves immune system functioning by the production of cytokines (substances that may increase the killing effect of white blood cells) and may resist the formation of metastases (spread of tumors). Beta-carotene and some vitamins, especially A, C, D, and E, are believed to affect the cancer process by strengthening the immune system or as a result of their antioxidant properties. The modulation of immune function by vitamins and trace elements in cancer treatment remains important and affects survival.

Chemotherapy and radiation increase the requirements for antioxidant compounds. However, certain antioxidants may interfere with the therapeutic effect of conventional cancer treatments. High doses of vitamins may reduce the toxicity of conventional chemotherapy and may improve overall well-being.

Care must be taken with any of the megatherapies. Some vitamins, such as A and D, can be toxic themselves at high levels, and for this reason many doctors argue strongly against all megatherapies. Advocates contend that what might be a toxic dose in a healthy person is necessary for someone whose system is responding to cancer.

Herbal Therapies

These therapies often include a combination of different herbs believed to foster anticancer activities. Herbs contain a variety of active ingredients that can have profound effects, both good and bad, on humans. Some herbs are more dangerous than the drugs derived from them. Many herbs have demonstrated anticancer properties in laboratory experiments, although the results are different when the herb is administered to people. Some herbs may be beneficial in controlling the side effects of conventional anticancer treatments. Be aware that herbs can also interact with drugs and that although some herbs are harmless even in large quantities, others should be used cautiously. It is wise to seek the advice of a licensed herbalist.

The most common alternative herbal therapies used for cancer treatment are Hoxsey therapy, Essiac, Taheebo tea (pau d'arco), and green tea.

Hoxsey Therapy

This is a mixture of nine herbs used in conjunction with additional nutrients and hormones. The treatment is offered at the Hoxsey Clinic in Tijuana, Mexico. The cost of Hoxsey treatment is $3,500, which includes a lifetime supply of tonic, visits, medications, and doctor fees. The therapy consists of an external paste(s) or "burning paste" used to "corrode" cancer and an herbal potion (internal formula) that contains potassium iodide, licorice, red clover, burdock, stillingia root, berberis root, poke root, cascara (amarga rather than sagrada), prickly ash bark, and buckthorn bark. The patient consumes a restricted vegetarian diet, and yeast tablets, vitamins, garlic, thymus gland extract, liver, superoxide dismutase, DMSO, BCG (tuberculosis vaccine), bovine cartilage, and hormones are administered. There have been extraordinary claims of cure.

Hoxsey therapy has been evaluated in some clinical series (not controlled clinical studies) on cancer patients, and the results have been positive (increase in survival rates and improvement in quality of life). Seven of the nine herbs have shown some anticancer-related activity in laboratory experiments. Despite intense opposition from conventional medicine, the Hoxsey formula has persisted as a cancer treatment for over 100 years. Mildred Nelson's Hoxsey Clinic is creating a computer database to monitor patients and facilitate research. There has been no reported toxicity from the Hoxsey formula itself; however, toxicity has been reported from some of its components.

Essiac® (or Flor-Essence®)

Essiac is a mixture of at least four different herbs: sheep sorrel (Rumex acetosella), burdock root (Arctium lappa), slippery elm inner bark (Ulmus fulva or Ulmus rubra), and Indian rhubarb (Rheum palmatum). It was said to have been formulated in northern Ontario by an Ojibwa healer "to purify the body and place it back in balance with the great spirit." Nurse Rene Caisse treated thousands of cases in her clinic in Canada and claimed that the tea reduced tumor size and prolonged the lives of people with very advanced cancer. The proponents of Essiac claim that it strengthens the immune system, improves appetite, relieves pain, and improves overall quality of life. The tea can be used in conjunction with conventional treatment and does not require a high degree of involvement.

Essiac therapy was studied in patients who had received it between 1978 and 1982, but researchers were unable to find clear evidence of improved survival. (Other outcomes such as pain control and quality of life were not evaluated.) There are many anecdotal or testimonial reports describing positive outcomes associated with the use of Essiac in individual patients, some of which have been corroborated by physicians. Some of the herbs in Essiac have been shown to have some antitumor activity. Essiac may cause nausea, vomiting, and diarrhea if taken with food or soon after meals. In general, there is weak evidence of effectiveness but little evidence of harm.

Pharmacological and Biological Therapies

These therapies encompass a variety of biological and chemical compounds, some of them derived from "natural" products and some of them synthesized in laboratories. The most common are laetrile, hydrazine sulfate, Iscador and other mistletoe preparations, shark cartilage, and 714X.

Laetrile

A controversial and unconventional therapy, laetrile, produced from apricot pits, releases a cyanide into the system. Like chemotherapy and radiation, it is toxic to the body. Thousands of people have credited laetrile with their recovery from cancer; all these reports are anecdotal.

Despite a blanket condemnation of laetrile by the prestigious Sloan-Kettering research center, some studies at that very institute showed that laetrile delayed metastases of breast cancer in mice. The case for or against the drug is still not resolved. It is illegal in many states.

Hydrazine Sulfate

Hydrazine sulfate is an inexpensive substance proposed specifically to prevent or control cachexia, the wasting process that is the actual cause of death in more than 50% of cancer cases. Its principal proponent is Dr. Joseph Gold, an American oncologist now with the Syracuse (N.Y.) Cancer Research Institute. Dr. Gold reported that cancer patients receiving hydrazine sulfate experienced improved appetite, reduced weight loss, and improved survival. Subsequently, he found specific antitumor effects associated with it and recommended it for patients with breast, colorectal, ovarian, lung, and thyroid cancers; Hodgkin's disease and other lymphomas; melanoma; and neuroblastoma.

Some clinical studies have indicated that there can be adverse interactions if hydrazine sulfate is taken in combination with alcohol, sedatives, or tranquilizers. Gold, along with several Russian researchers, has published subjective and objective evidence of its antitumor effects. Some of these studies reported increased survival rates as well as improvements in appetite and general well-being. Randomized double-blind, placebo-controlled studies in the U.S. showed no benefit from the use of hydrazine sulfate in non–small-cell lung cancer and in advanced colorectal cancer, but these studies contained several flaws. At the proper dosage level, there seem to be few or no adverse effects.

Mistletoe Preparations (Iscador, Helixor, Eurixor)

Rudolf Steiner popularised the use of mistletoe as a cancer therapy in the early 20th century. Dr. Steiner is best known as the founder of anthroposophy, a blend of spiritual and scientific concepts, which he applied to the practice of medicine with a particular focus on the treatment of cancer. Today, mistletoe preparations are principally advocated by and used at anthroposophic medical clinics in Switzerland and Germany, where more than 80,000 patients have been treated since the 1920s. Iscador and Helixor, the most common preparations, can be legally prescribed in European countries. They are not commonly used in North America but can be obtained from European physicians.

Proponents of mistletoe preparations recommend that it be administered as one component of several "holistic" therapies intended to strengthen "higher organizing forces" and enhance natural cancer-fighting abilities. However, mistletoe preparations can be used out of the context of anthroposophic care. The proponents recommend that Iscador be used early in the course of the disease, but it can also be administered in patients whose tumors are advanced and/or inoperable and in conjunction with chemotherapy or radiotherapy. It is claimed that mistletoe preparations stimulate the immune system, cause cancerous cells to revert to more normal forms, improve general well-being, and possibly prolong survival, especially in patients with cancers of the cervix, ovary, breast, stomach, colon, and lung. Mistletoe is said to be less effective for nonsolid tumors such as leukemia.

Local inflammation (redness and swelling) at the injection site and an increase in body temperature, sometimes accompanied by headache and/or chills, are the only side effects reported.

Experimental evidence suggests that mistletoe preparations appear to enhance the resistance of cells to damage caused by mutagenic substances (which cause change in the DNA of chromosomes in the cell) and possibly carcinogenic substances (which cause cancer). Results from the clinical trials have been mixed. However, mistletoe preparations are considered good candidates for further evaluation, and controlled clinical trials are under way.

714X

714X is an unconventional cancer therapy developed in Canada by Gaston Naessens, a French-born Canadian biologist and researcher. 714X is available by prescription under the Special Access Program of Health Canada, but it is not available in the U.S. The Centre d'Orthobiologie Somatidienne de l'Estrie (COSE) in Sherbrooke, Quebec, is the research center responsible for the development, production, and distribution of 714X. In the past six years, the use of 714X to treat breast, lung, colon, prostate, and ovarian cancer has been increasing.

Naessens has studied tiny, motile microorganisms, which he calls "somatids," in the plasma, the life cycle of which can be predictors of the onset of degenerative diseases, including cancer. When the immune system is weakened or disrupted by factors such as chemical pollution, poor nutrition, ionizing radiation, and stress, the somatids go through a longer macrocycle observed in degenerative diseases, including cancer. According to Naessens, 714X prevents the formation of CKF (cocancerogenic factor), a substance responsible for the "passivity" of the immune system of cancer patients. 714X suppresses the secretion of CKF, which in turn results in a "reactivation" of the immune system, halting the progression of the disease.

The use of 714X as an anticancer drug and an enhancer of the body's immune system has yet to be clarified. There are numerous anecdotal reports of improvement in quality of life and stabilization of the disease, especially in breast, lung, and prostate cancer, but no formal clinical trials have been conducted. The theory of disease in which somatids play a central role is not consistent with current thinking about the causes of disease in general or cancer in particular.

This therapy is not toxic, and no severe side effects have been reported.

Shark Cartilage

Shark cartilage is one of the most widely used alternative biological treatments for cancer, although this therapy is not currently reimbursed by insurance. There are many manufacturers of shark cartilage, and the quality of the product is sometimes questionable. Evidence suggests that the anticancer mechanism works by inhibiting angiogenesis (new blood vessel development by tumors). The National Cancer Institute (NCI) suggests that certain proteins block the action of certain metals containing enzymes (metalloproteinases) that help tumor cells invade surrounding tissue. Various animal and in vitro studies identified anti-angiogenesis and immune stimulation factors within shark cartilage. Clinical trials are underway on shark cartilage. Four clinical series and one best-case series have assessed disease response and survival outcomes. Of the 21 patients in the best-case series, 61% reported reduced tumor size, and 87% reported improved quality of life.

Psychological/Spiritual Alternatives

Visualization, meditation, and other psychological and spiritual approaches to cancer are gaining favor with both doctors and the general public. These approaches emphasize people's self-healing capabilities and the ability of the mind to influence the body's recovery (see also chapter 5, Holistic Health and Healing: Navigating Your Way to Better Health).

The therapeutic potential of spirituality and religion has generally been neglected in the teaching and practice of medicine. However, recent research indicates that religious and spiritual well-being is often correlated with increased physical and mental health.

The Simonton Technique

Probably the best known of the psychospiritual approaches to cancer is the Simonton visualization technique, in which the person with cancer learns to picture her or his body's defense system cleansing the body of cancerous cells and replacing them with healthy cells. Some hospitals offer counselors who teach this and other aspects of the Simonton approach. Although too new to have long-term survival statistics, this therapy appears to have been a major factor in the recovery of many people with cancer, including some for whom the conventional treatments had failed.

Prayer and Meditation

Many have found that prayer, meditation, or other spiritual approaches can help transform their experiences with serious illness from a terrifying, hopeless time into a period of personal growth and fuller enjoyment of life. Sometimes this spiritual healing includes "cure," and sometimes it does not. Well-intended prayer from friends or relatives may help overcome the hardships of both illness and treatment. The social support and the relaxation experienced during prayer may provide additional benefits.

Faith Healers and Psychics

If you are considering visiting a psychic or faith healer, research the healer in advance. Making your own decision here is just as important as in any other type of treatment. Do not be rushed into a commitment by well-intentioned friends or deterred by ridicule from nonbelieving friends. Avoid any faith healer or psychic healer who charges exorbitant fees or insists that you must "prove your faith" by refusing all other treatments.

Danger of Blaming the Victim

It is important not to blame the victim for getting cancer ("She brought it on herself, all that repressed anger") or condemning her if she doesn't get well ("She just isn't strong enough; she doesn't really want to get well; she doesn't have enough faith"). Those who have cancer need the support and help, not the judgment, of friends, families, and health practitioners.

Dealing with Pain

Some kinds of cancer are very painful near the end. Often women believe that it is a sign of weakness to take any medicine for the pain, or they are afraid of becoming addicted to medications. Recent studies have shown that pain, including cancer pain, is undertreated by doctors and hospitals. Many medications are available for pain, including morphine. If your pain is not relieved by the strategies you and your medical team are using, ask to consult a pain specialist. If pain is preventing you from living as normally as possible and from enjoying the company of family and friends, you should feel no hesitation in asking for relief.

Remember that metastasis does not inevitably equal death. But if death does seem to be imminent, you can do much to ensure that you live your remaining time as comfortably as possible.

I don't want to die, but since I accepted the fact that I probably will, I am more at peace. It's as if my energy had been used up denying the reality of my own impending death and, when I stopped struggling against the idea, I suddenly felt free. I could begin to think about living again, about what to do with the time I do have. I have my down days, when I ask, "Why me? Why can't I die 20 years from now? Why can't I live to see my children grow up, my grandchildren born?" But these days are fewer and fewer. In a sense, I'm lucky to know about my death in advance. I won't be like those who die unexpectedly with things left unsaid and undone. I've planned what I want to do, who I want to see. I've started working on projects that I had always wanted to do but was too busy for. I can't

*afford to travel or do much special, but then anything
I do now seems special.*

*I am not dying of cancer; I am living with cancer. I
try to deal with the problems caused by my cancer in
my daily life, but my emphasis is on the living, not the
dying.*

BREAST CANCER

If you turned to this section, we hope you will go to
the beginning of the section "Benign Breast Conditions" (p. 604) and read from there. See the section on
breast cancer in chapter 7, Environmental and Occupational Health, too (p. 139). If you ever do have a
breast cancer diagnosis following biopsy, you will be
much better able to cope with it and to decide what to
do next if you have done some reading and thinking
beforehand.

Because breast lumps are so common and most of
them are not cancerous, it is important for us to familiarize ourselves with ways of recognizing and dealing
with them.

If the Biopsy Results Are Positive

No one who has not had the experience can understand the waves of shock, disbelief, fear, and anger
that overcome you after you find out you have cancer.
This emotional trauma comes exactly when you need
to focus all your energy on learning about your treatment options.

The usual first reaction is to do whatever your doctor suggests. This is appealing at a time when you may
need to feel that you are being taken care of, but it has
not always resulted in the best of care. Although most
doctors are well intentioned, they tend to offer only
the treatment they know best. Physicians as a whole
have been slow to accept new therapies, even when
numerous studies have demonstrated that the new approaches have the same or better effectiveness with
fewer negative effects. Many are unwilling or unable
to discuss all the available therapies. Only a few states,
including Massachusetts, California, and Minnesota,
have laws that require patients to be informed of all
the medical options.

At this point, it is advisable to get a second opinion
before committing yourself to a course of treatment.
The National Cancer Institute and the American College of Surgeons can provide lists of appropriate doctors. Using a team approach involving medical
oncologists (cancer specialists), surgical oncologists,
and radiation oncologists may result in the best combination of treatments for your individual situation. Certain centers offer more treatment choices, including
experimental therapies (see "Our Rights as Patients,"
chapter 25, The Politics of Women's Health and Medical Care, p. 713).

Remember, there is no rush. You can take several
weeks to adjust and find out about your options. If
you have had an excisional biopsy, the main cancer is

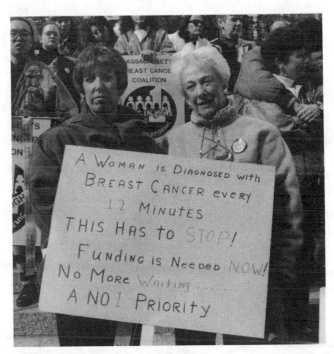

**Rally in support of increased funding for breast cancer
research/**Ellen Shub

already out. In some cases, this could be the end of
surgical treatment within the breast. You can always
decide later to have further treatment such as mastectomy, radiation, or chemotherapy. Some doctors will
try to rush you into a mastectomy by stating that the
biopsy may have "stirred up" the cancer and it is therefore important to proceed immediately. This is an out-
moded theory. If you have had a fine-needle
aspiration (FNA) biopsy and the cancer has not been
removed, surgery within a month of the biopsy is usually recommended.

It is important to get second opinions and learn
about all the available options. No one knows for sure
how long you can safely wait before beginning treatments, and doctors' opinions on this issue may vary
widely. Remember, in order to decide on optimal treatment, you need to know the total size of the tumor,
the status of your lymph nodes, the hormone status of
your tumor, and other tumor characteristics (see the
following pages). Most of this information is available
after the primary surgery and is used to recommend
systemic therapies (hormones or chemotherapy). Evaluating these factors with a team of specialists helps
you to explore your treatment options most effectively.

The entire field of breast cancer medicine is changing rapidly as old, established theories and treatments
are coming under question, while newer techniques
have not been used long enough to be completely
evaluated. While we cannot tell you which therapy
will be best for you, we can point out some directions
to pursue and some pitfalls to avoid.

A good place to begin is the reading list in the Resources. *Dr. Susan Love's Breast Book* by Susan M. Love is especially helpful.

Stages of Breast Cancer

There are several systems for categorizing breast cancer. The most commonly accepted is based on three elements called *TNM:* tumor size or extent, lymph nodes involved with cancer, and whether or not there are distant metastases (breast cancer in other parts of the body). When cancer is first diagnosed, it is "staged" clinically *(clinical stage)* by physical exam and some testing to assess for evidence of metastatic spread. Following the surgical portion of the local therapy the cancer is "staged" pathologically *(pathologic stage)* by microscopic analysis of the breast tissue and lymph nodes removed. The stage of the breast cancer is important because doctors usually base their recommendations for treatment on how well other women with cancer at the same stage and similar history have responded to the treatments. The TNM stage is then grouped into five categories or overall stages.

Stage 0

This refers to noninvasive breast cancer, either ductal carcinoma in situ or lobular carcinoma in situ (see at right).

Stage I

This stage means that there is a small lump (less than or equal to 2 centimeters in diameter), and the lymph nodes or other parts of the body do not appear to be involved.

Stage II

Nodes are palpable and/or tumor size is larger (greater than 2 and up to 5 centimeters). Tumor sizes over 5 centimeters are also included in this category if the lymph nodes are not involved. There is no evidence of distant metastasis.

Stage III

The lump is large (greater than 5 centimeters), and the lymph nodes are involved with cancer. Smaller tumors are included in this category if they involve the skin or chest wall or if the lymph nodes are so involved with cancer they are matted together.

Stage IV

The breast cancer has spread to other parts of the body, as seen on X rays or scans. At this stage, a cancer is not considered curable (although some believe that the newer high-dose chemotherapy may cure some women—see the section on treatments). Mastectomy is not useful unless the breast is infected or ulcerated. The goal of treatment is to control symptoms for as long as possible. Many women with stage IV disease live for years with only occasional symptoms.

In Situ Cancer

Ductal carcinoma in situ (DCIS) and *lobular carcinoma in situ (LCIS)* are two very different entities. Microscopically, in situ cancers are made up of cells that have the appearance of cancer cells but are not behaving like cancer, as they remain within their normal environment—inside the duct or the lobule. In contrast, invasive (also known as infiltrating) breast cancer goes through the walls of the ducts and lobules, invading the surrounding fatty/fibrous portion of the breast tissue where blood vessels and lymphatic vessels lie. Studies have shown that when women with ductal carcinoma in situ are monitored without treatment, 30% develop an invasive tumor within the area of the ductal carcinoma in situ. DCIS is therefore felt to be a preinvasive cancer of the breast. Improvements in mammography have increased this diagnosis from less than 5% of all women diagnosed with breast cancer to over 20% in those undergoing screening mammograms. When patients with lobular carcinoma in situ are followed, 20 to 40% go on to form an invasive cancer (most of which are invasive ductal carcinomas) over 20 years or more. These cancers are not in the area of the LCIS where the biopsy was performed but may occur anywhere within either breast. LCIS is therefore not considered to be preinvasive. Rather, it is a risk factor for the development of breast cancer someday.

Treatment of LCIS

Because lobular carcinoma in situ is not considered to be preinvasive, there is no need to attempt to remove or eliminate it. As a risk factor for breast cancer, it tells us something about the overall biology of the breast cells in general. The 20 to 40% risk of subsequent breast cancer is substantial. Because there is no known method of breast cancer prevention, women currently have two options. One is to be monitored closely with breast exams and yearly mammograms, with the understanding that they will reduce but not eliminate the chance of a fatal breast cancer. With close followup many breast cancers will be detected earlier, with a better prognosis. The other option is to undergo prophylactic (preventive) mastectomies with the understanding that some breast tissue is always left behind and remains at risk. A study is currently investigating the ability of tamoxifen (an antiestrogen drug) to decrease the risk of subsequent breast cancer, and some results should be available by the year 2000.

Treatment of DCIS

Because ductal carcinoma in situ is thought to be preinvasive, treatment options are aimed at eliminating it. How to do this remains controversial. (See the following pages for more on the treatment of invasive breast cancer.) Women who have DCIS may be asked to participate in ongoing studies to find out what treatment is best. In the past, mastectomy was the treatment for breast cancer as a whole, including ductal carcinoma in situ. The risk of recurrence following total mastectomy for DCIS was less than 2%. Since randomized studies of invasive cancer showed breast-conserving therapy to be as effective as mastectomy, many looked to extending these treatments to DCIS. Wide excision with clear margins (similar to lumpectomy as a procedure, but DCIS rarely forms a lump) had local recurrence rates of 10 to 20%, which seemed to continue to increase over time. Half of the recurrences were more DCIS, but the other half were invasive ductal cancers. So, women had a 5 to 10% risk of developing an invasive cancer in the next five to ten years. Having radiation therapy after wide excision decreased the local recurrences by about half. This means the risk of local recurrence is 5 to 10% overall, with a 2.5% to 5% risk of invasive ductal cancer (which is greater than the risk following total mastectomy). Many women find this risk acceptable and choose the lesser procedure. Other women choose mastectomy, knowing that of those women who develop invasive cancer, approximately one out of three will eventually die of the disease. Current studies are evaluating the use of tamoxifen to decrease the risk of local recurrence in women treated for DCIS. These studies should give us more information in the next few years.

Treatments

In making treatment decisions, women frequently feel caught between well-intentioned but competing factions with no way to determine what is best in their particular situation.

After I and the guy I live with had spent almost two hours with the surgeon, we came away convinced that simple mastectomy was the only sensible treatment. I so wanted to be sensible about it all. Then I went to Boston for a second opinion. I went up full of skepticism, feeling that they could never be as convincing as my New York surgeon, but that I must go through the motions to satisfy myself that I had heard the "other side" [in this case, for lumpectomy plus radiation]. It turned out that the "other side" was equally convincing, and I went back to New York feeling really torn. I felt like a statistic that was being wooed by both sides to show how successful their treatments were. "Good instincts," commented an oncologist friend. "That's precisely what it's all about."

This woman, after more research and much agonizing, went back to Boston for a lumpectomy plus radiation.

The decision of what treatment to take is never easy. Sometimes one physician seems more reasonable. Sometimes your intuition will point strongly to a certain option. Sometimes one hospital is more conveniently located. Sometimes a friend's experience is influential. All these factors and more will enter into your final choice, which is often a compromise. In the end, each woman will make the decision in her own way, ideally with the most informed and friendly support possible.

A Brief History and Overview of Breast Cancer Treatments

For many years, the standard practice in the U.S. after a biopsy was to proceed immediately with a mastectomy. Several years of hard work, especially on the part of activist Rose Kushner (who has since died of breast cancer), resulted in a landmark National Cancer Institute (NCI) recommendation in 1979 that breast biopsy be part of a two-step procedure in most cases. A diagnostic biopsy should be performed first, then treatment options discussed with the woman in order for her to make an informed decision.

For the better part of this century, the Halsted radical mastectomy was the usual way to treat breast cancer. In 1960, over 90% of women in the U.S. who had breast cancer surgery underwent this operation, which removes the entire breast plus the underlying muscles and the nearby lymph nodes. Physicians believed that cancer began locally and then metastasized (spread) in a predictable, gradual manner, through the lymphatic vessels to the lymph nodes, filling the lymph nodes before spreading further through the body. They assumed that the more tissue they removed, the more likely that they would "get it all" and thus keep the disease from spreading. Yet, over the years, statistics failed to support this theory. Survival and mortality rates did not improve with these larger operations.

A newer theory began to evolve as researchers discovered more about the biology of breast cancer. Breast cancer in general was found to have a slow growth rate. With current "early" detection methods, most breast cancers have been growing for six to ten years before they are large enough to be seen on mammogram or felt on exam. During this time, cancer cells could be spreading, through blood vessels as well as lymphatic vessels, to other sites within the body. This process of metastasis is not uniform. Not all women will have breast cancer cells that survive outside the breast. The smaller, less aggressive a breast cancer is, the fewer the cancer cells that get into the vessels, and the less likely that any breast cancer cells have metastasized. This is probably why screening mammography is able to reduce the death rate from breast cancer (by 30% in women over 50).

Today, treatment for breast cancer takes the form of *local therapy* (therapy to the breast), and *systemic therapy* (therapy to the whole body). Surgery and radiation are local therapies; chemotherapy and hormone therapy are systemic therapies. Almost all women with breast cancer get some form of local therapy. Systemic therapy is given to those whose cancer is thought to have spread to other areas of the body. Unfortunately, there are currently no tests to tell us whether only a few breast cancer cells have spread, just as there are no tests that show when there are only a few breast cancer cells within the breast. Because doctors think that systemic therapies have a much better chance of eliminating small amounts of cancer spread, they try to look at factors that predict the likelihood of metastasis, rather than wait for larger areas to show up later on X rays or scans. Currently, the strongest predictor remains the axillary lymph nodes on the side of the tumor. Although breast cancer does not have to go through these nodes to "get out," statistically, when breast cancer cells are seen within the lymph nodes, it is more likely there are other breast cancer cells surviving elsewhere in the body. In other words, the lymph nodes are an indicator of the dynamic between the breast cancer cells and the body. As they are only a predictor, even when the nodes are negative (no breast cancer cells seen), some women may still have metastatic cancer, so several minor predictors are also used. For more information on these, refer to the section on systemic therapy (p. 629).

Local Treatment Issues

Breast cancer treatment is still somewhat controversial. There are currently two main issues. First, how much surgery is necessary: Must the surgeon remove just the lump, the lump plus some surrounding tissue, or the entire breast? The second concerns the role of systemic therapies such as chemotherapy and radiation.

According to recent randomized trials (studies) evaluating local therapies for the treatment of early stage (stages I and II) breast cancer, there is no difference in survival rate between the groups who had mastectomies and the groups who had lumpectomies (with or without radiation). Survival is dependent on whether any cancer cells have already spread, and on the effectiveness of the systemic therapy. The only difference local therapy makes is in how likely the cancer is to recur locally within the breast/chest area, requiring more local therapy.

In the larger trial done here in the U.S., the group of women who had lumpectomies without radiation to the rest of the breast had a local recurrence rate of 40%. When radiation was added, the local recurrence rate dropped to 8%. Women with mastectomies had a local recurrence rate of 4%. Again, there was *no* difference in survival among these three groups. However, a 40% local recurrence rate is quite high, so lumpectomy without radiation is not considered an acceptable treatment option. Studies are under way to try to find a group of characteristics identifying a cancer that could be treated without radiation; so far, none have been found.

The two accepted local treatment options are *lumpectomy followed by radiation* (breast-conserving therapy) or *mastectomy.* To be eligible for breast-conserving therapy, the cancer must have microscopically clear margins (no microscopic cancer cells seen at the edge of the tissue removed). The larger the amount of breast tissue removed, the more the shape or size of the breast will be affected. As much as one quarter of the breast can be removed with an acceptable cosmetic result. If more than a quarter needs to be removed, a mastectomy should be performed. Approximately 70 to 75% of women diagnosed with breast cancer are eligible for breast-conserving therapy; yet, many doctors are slow to promote change, and most women in the U.S. still undergo mastectomy. The National Institutes of Health consensus conference concluded in 1990 that breast-conserving therapy is an appropriate treatment for early-stage breast cancer and is preferable to mastectomy, as it is a lesser operation. Women truly have a choice today, as long as the extent of the cancer within the breast allows removal with microscopically clear margins and an acceptable cosmetic result. Radiation may still be recommended after mastectomy if the cancer was larger than 5 centimeters or if more than four lymph nodes contained cancer, to decrease the risk of local recurrence.

Axillary lymph nodes (under the arm) are removed at the time of the surgery to the breast, to aid in decision-making regarding systemic therapy. Years ago, when surgeons thought that removal prevented spread, they tried to strip all the nodal tissue from within the axilla. This disrupted drainage from the arm, and 30 to 70% of women developed permanent arm swelling (lymphedema). Today it is recommended that only level I and II lymph nodes be removed and that care be taken to avoid stripping the lymphatic vessels away from the axillary vein, to decrease the risk of swelling. With this procedure, the risk of lymphedema is down to 2 to 4% but has not been eliminated.

Many surgeons today avoid injury to the intercostal brachial nerve, which goes through the area of the lymph nodes being removed and gives sensation to light touch in the underarm area as well as a patch along the posterior shoulder. All surgeons attempt to avoid injury to nerves that go to muscles.

Procedure Descriptions

Breast-Conserving Therapy

Lumpectomy (also called *tylectomy, wide excision, segmental mastectomy,* or *partial mastectomy*) removes the lump and a varying amount of surrounding tissue with a goal of microscopically clear margins. Adverse effects include scarring and some disfiguring of the breast (although this may be only slightly more than that caused by the biopsy), depending on the size of the lump and the size of the breast.

Quadrantectomy removes the quarter of the breast with the tumor. This surgery is performed mostly in Europe. The problems that occur are similar to those resulting from lumpectomy, but there is more breast disfigurement.

Radiation therapy usually consists of external electron beam treatments to the breast five days a week for five to six and a half weeks. The area surrounding the removed cancerous tissue—the area most likely to contain remaining cancer cells—may receive a higher dose. Adverse effects during treatment include fatigue, muscle pain, swelling of the breast, skin changes (dryness, redness, itchiness), extreme sensitivity to the sun, and possible damage to the heart, when treatment is on the left side. Occasionally (in 5% of women) the radiation causes the ribs to be more brittle and thus more prone to fracture. An inflammation of the lung, not dangerous but painful, can occur in 1 to 2% of women. It responds to anti-inflammatory agents, usually lasts less than a month, and does not recur.

Removal of the Breast

Total mastectomy (also called *simple mastectomy*—as if a mastectomy could ever be simple!) removes the nipple/areola and all of the breast tissue but leaves the underlying muscles and the lymph nodes. Adverse effects include the emotional trauma of losing a breast, numbness of the skin, scarring, and possible posture and balance problems related to the size and weight of the remaining breast if reconstruction is not performed.

Modified radical mastectomy (also known as *total mastectomy with axillary node dissection*) is total mastectomy plus removal of the lower axillary lymph nodes to stage the cancer. Adverse effects are the same as in simple mastectomy, plus occasional arm problems such as fatigue and swelling, and decreased resistance to infection.

Radical mastectomy (also called *Halsted mastectomy*) involves removal of the nipple/areola, all of the breast tissue, the muscles underlying the breast, and a more extensive axillary lymph node removal. This operation is no longer recommended by the NCI and should almost never be performed. Adverse effects include all of the above with the addition of greater deformity. Arm problems are more severe and constant and include weakness. The skin adhered to the rib cage is much more prone to healing problems and future injury.

Reconstruction After Mastectomy

Some women who have had a mastectomy are in situations where they feel comfortable doing nothing to "fill in" the place where a breast is missing. That is, they choose not to get an external prosthesis or a breast implant. Others feel that a visible scar would provoke negative reactions in themselves and others. Some women who have a mastectomy will prefer to use an *external prosthesis,* which will help fill in the area and "match" the other side. Others will choose to have breast reconstruction done by a plastic surgeon, who creates a breast using either one's own tissue or an implant. Nearly all mastectomy patients find that their chest area becomes numb, in some, skin sensations may return, but the area feels different than before the surgery.

With an external prosthesis, you may look as if nothing has changed as long as you wear your bra, which

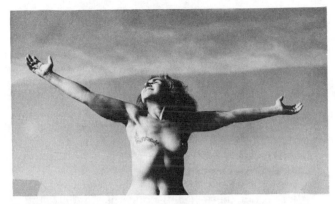

Writer Deena Metzger with a tattoo over her mastectomy scar/Hella Hammid *

holds the prosthesis in place. The prosthesis may shift under your clothes or feel heavy, or hot in warm weather and cold in winter. However, there are always new products coming out as well as improvements in the fit and comfort of prostheses. For example, one company has developed a prosthesis that adheres to the chest wall area by the use of Velcro. While this may seem hard to envision, many women actually like this type of prosthesis and say it helps them feel more secure than the kind placed in a bra. Stores that specialize in prosthesis fitting can custom-make one to fit your anatomy. You can get a temporary prosthesis after surgery; once your scar has healed, you can be fitted for a permanent one. Many health plans cover all or part of the cost of your prosthesis. Medicare will pay for one every year or two if you get a prescription from your doctor. If you have health insurance, ask your insurance company what costs it will cover.

Breast reconstruction can be done at the time of the mastectomy or later. If you feel that you have too many decisions to make all at once—sorting out your cancer therapy as well as what kind of reconstruction to have —don't rush into it. You have plenty of time to decide. Some doctors used to imply that undergoing reconstruction was vain, but over time this attitude has changed; now women are often advised that we will feel better if we have it done. This is a matter of personal choice, and we have the right to learn about surgical options. While nothing can make up for the loss of your breast, reconstruction can help you regain its appearance. Deciding to have breast reconstruction has helped many women both physically and emotionally.

Surgical reconstruction involves either using an implant (see the box on p. 629) under the chest muscle or moving your own tissues, blood vessels, and adjacent tissue from your back, abdomen, or buttocks to your chest area (called a flap reconstruction). Sometimes an implant is used to supplement the tissue transfer operation. Make sure you have a consultation

* This poster is available from Donnelly/Colt: (203) 455-9621.

THE SILICONE CONTROVERSY

Even though silicone gel breast implants were used for more than 30 years, manufacturers never proved their safety or effectiveness. By 1990, women were complaining about symptoms they were experiencing and health problems they were developing, which they attributed to their silicone implants. At Congressional hearings, consumers and scientists testified about these health concerns. In 1992, the Food and Drug Administration (FDA) imposed a moratorium on the sale of silicone gel breast implants, particularly for cosmetic breast enlargement. Exceptions to the ban were made for women who wanted breast reconstruction following cancer surgery, but only if their physicians used approved protocols and participated in a registry.

The moratorium was based on reports of an increased risk of connective tissue diseases and autoimmune disorders, such as lupus and rheumatoid arthritis. Several studies have been done since then, reviewing data from large cohorts of women who have received breast implants. So far, the reports show no indication that implants significantly increase women's risk of these diseases, but women could be suffering from new autoimmune disorders related to silicone gel implant use. We need the results of controlled clinical trials, rather than just a review of medical records, to settle this controversy. The current FDA recommendation is to remove silicone gel implants only if they have ruptured; however, many women choose to have implants that have not ruptured removed in order to avoid a possible rupture or other complications in the future.

Currently, plastic surgeons are using only saline implants because of the controversy surrounding silicone gel. A saline implant still contains silicone, because the saline solution is encased in a silicone envelope or sac. This type of silicone is one of the least reactive substances that can be placed inside the body. It is used in many other medical devices such as indwelling catheters, pacemakers, knee and hip replacements, and implants replacing surgically removed testicles. Most of the controversy over silicone gel implants is about the soft silicone gel that was originally used to fill the sac.

If you have had or are thinking of having implants, ask your doctor for the insert package that comes with the implant. You should also be given an informed consent form that lists the more common possible complications. Some of them, like capsular contracture (hardening of the tissue around the implant), can be quite painful and disfiguring. Ask the doctor about any medical term you don't understand. Make sure you keep a copy of the manufacturer, model, and lot numbers of the implant(s) that come on a sticker attached to your medical records. If there are problems in the future with a particular implant, you will know whether it is the type you have. As with any implant, you should make a point of having regular medical checkups, and be sure to inform your practitioner that you have implants.

with a board-certified plastic surgeon. During the evaluation, she or he will recommend the type of reconstruction that offers the best match to your other breast. Since muscle is taken from one place and moved to where it is no longer functional, you will lose strength at the original site. Ask in what percentage of your surgeon's cases the transferred tissue has died (necrosis). If you smoke or have diabetes, a flap reconstruction may not be appropriate for you, since the blood vessels are narrower or damaged, and healing can be more difficult. If you are active, especially if you enjoy a particular sport, don't forget to ask your surgeon to try to make it possible for you to return to this activity eventually. Once you get a recommendation, ask to speak with other women who have undergone the same procedure with this particular surgeon.

An *implant* is a rubber-like envelope filled with salt water (saline) or silicone (see "The Silicone Controversy," at left). The implant is placed behind the pectoral muscle; then the skin is sewn together, making the area bulge into a breast-like form. Another type of implant, known as an expander, places a hollow sac behind the pectoral muscle, and the overlying skin is sewn together. A valve with a port, which has a tube leading to the hollow sac, is inserted under the skin. Over a three- to six-month period, the doctor injects saline through the port, which expands the sac and stretches the skin out. Once the area has been expanded to a size that matches the other breast, the sac is removed and replaced with a permanent implant.

During the discussion of reconstruction options, it is important to let the surgeon know what size you would like to be. Make sure the surgeon understands what you want; on the basis of previous experience, she or he may have something different in mind.

Whatever type of reconstruction you decide to have, the surgeon can create a nipple and areola using darker, grafted skin or a tattoo technique. This is usually done several months after the reconstruction surgery. Sometimes, with one breast removed, the plastic surgeon will recommend reducing the remaining breast or changing its shape to more closely match the reconstructed breast. You should consider the possible problems that can result, including loss of nipple sensation, before you agree to do this.

BREAST IMPLANTS—ADVANTAGES AND DISADVANTAGES

Advantages of Implants

1. Require a shorter hospital stay, usually one or two days, compared with five days for tissue reconstruction.

2. No evidence that they interfere with mammography or detection of recurrences.

Disadvantages of Implants

1. Contracture is the most common problem. Scar tissue makes the implanted breast firm. For some, firmness is not bothersome; for others, it causes pain and a "wood-like" feeling. Additional surgery may help release scar tissue and correct hardening.

2. Because implants are foreign to our bodies, any infection after surgery may be slower to heal. This is because the implant cuts off the blood supply to the area, thus limiting the circulation of antibiotics in the breast.

3. The implanted breast tends to stay firm, while your other breast will change with aging.

4. Additional surgery may be needed on the other breast to match the implanted breast.

5. Over time, a saline implant can rupture or break. While the body easily absorbs the saline solution, the implanted breast will lose its shape, and the implant will have to be replaced.

Systemic Therapy–Chemotherapy and Hormone Therapy

As mentioned earlier, systemic therapy is given to women whose breast cancer may have spread (metastasized). Decades ago, systemic therapy was given once metastatic disease had been identified (had grown to the point where it would show up on tests such as chest X rays or bone scans). Then studies showed that survival rates improved when systemic therapy was given to women whose lymph nodes tested positive for cancer at the time of their original diagnosis, even though cancer cells could not yet be identified elsewhere. As approximately 25% of node-negative women eventually show signs of metastatic disease, increasing numbers of women in this group are also treated, according to minor predictors such as size of the invasive tumor, presence of vascular invasion, and the differentiation of the tumor. In fact, as many as 75 to 80% of node-negative women are treated with systemic therapy in the hope of catching the 25% who do have microscopic metastatic disease.

Studies have shown that chemotherapy is more effective in premenopausal women than hormone therapy. As women age, hormone therapy increases in its effectiveness, surpassing chemotherapy in the postmenopausal years. In the perimenopausal years, both can be effective and increasingly are used in combination. Chemotherapy reduces the risk of metastatic recurrence by about 30% and hormone therapy by about 25%. What this means is that if a woman has several positive lymph nodes and is therefore thought to have about a 60% risk of metastasis, systemic therapy would reduce that risk to about 45%. If a woman has a small tumor and is node-negative, and her risk of metastatic disease is thought to be about 12%, systemic therapy would reduce the risk of metastatic recurrence to about 9%.

Chemotherapy

Chemotherapy (see p. 616) can cause early menopause, an important consideration for younger women who want to bear children.

Therapy using a combination of drugs, especially the combinations called CMF (cyclophosphamide, methotrexate, and 5-flourouracil) and CAF (cyclophosphamide, adriamycin, and 5-flourouracil) have given better results than the use of single agents (one drug used alone).

The optimal timing of chemotherapy remains unknown. Earlier, it was given after radiation to women who had radiation in addition to surgery. The trend over the past five years has been to give chemotherapy following healing from surgery and either "sandwich" the radiation in the middle (stopping chemotherapy during the radiation) or giving the radiation after the chemo. Giving chemotherapy simultaneously with radiation had been shown to increase the side effects. Some centers are working on protocols to decrease these side effects. Some women may be asked to participate in studies that give both treatments simultaneously.

The optimal choice of drugs, dose, and length of therapy is still being studied as medical oncologists try to find ways to tailor the therapy to particular tumor characteristics. This often involves different recommendations based on the number of cancerous lymph nodes. Studies using tumor markers on the cancer cell are also in progress.

High-dose chemotherapy with *bone marrow transplant* is also an area of active research. Studies suggest that more intensive doses of chemotherapy may be more effective. Unfortunately, higher doses also have the unwanted side effect of killing the bone marrow. To counteract this damage, bone marrow is taken from the woman and "banked" (stored) before chemotherapy. Her own bone marrow is then given back to her after chemotherapy. There is a period of time, between the chemotherapy and return of bone marrow function, when the body remains at high risk of infection because of very low white blood cell counts.

Today, fatal infections occur in only 2% or less of patients in centers experienced in doing the procedure. Women are hospitalized during this stage of treatment to decrease the risk of infectious contact as well as maintain hydration with intravenous fluids.

Stem cell transplant uses a similar technique to restore bone marrow function after high-dose chemotherapy. The bone marrow is not removed, but instead is stimulated to produce a lot of stem cells (immature white blood cells) into the bloodstream, where they can be collected and banked before chemotherapy is given. Afterward, the stem cells are returned to the patient as a transfusion; they will repopulate the bone marrow as well as increase the white blood cell count more quickly. These are still considered experimental therapies. Women undergoing them should participate in research protocols after giving informed consent.

Hormone Therapy

Normal breast cells have estrogen receptors. When estrogen attaches to these receptors, this stimulates growth of the cells. Breast cancer cells may also have these hormone receptors. Hormone therapies are designed to cut off the estrogen supply to such breast cancer cells, inhibit growth of the cancer, and eventually kill it. Both surgery (to remove hormone-producing organs) and medications are used as hormone therapies, although surgery is less common.

Medications

Tamoxifen is the most common therapy. It is a synthetic estrogen that has antiestrogen effects on breast cancer cells. It has estrogen-like effects on the bone and heart and therefore decreases the risk of osteoporosis and heart attack. The current recommendation is to give 10 milligrams twice daily for five years. The side effects include hot flashes in 20% of the women who take it, fatigue, possibly depression in a small percentage of patients, and about a one in 2,000 chance of uterine cancer. *Megace,* a synthetic progesterone, is the second line of therapy. Its side effects include weight gain and hot flashes. Other forms of hormone therapy are being tested in clinical studies, and still more are being developed in the hope of decreasing unwanted side effects while maximizing others, such as osteoporosis prevention.

Surgery

Oophorectomy (removal of the ovaries) may be useful in premenopausal women over 35 but has largely been replaced with chemotherapy and medication. *Adrenalectomy* (removal of the adrenal glands) is another approach to limit estrogen production. (The adrenals make androgens, which can be converted to estrogens in fat cells.)

Special considerations for Stage III

Stage III is considered locally advanced breast cancer. In the past, it was treated with aggressive local therapy. Unfortunately, although better local control was achieved, women still developed metastatic spread and usually died. Today, stage III breast cancer is treated as a systemic disease. Treatment options vary depending on the hospital. Many start with chemotherapy and go on to local therapy, possibly with some systemic therapy to follow. The advantage of this approach is that the tumor within the breast can be monitored to see how effective the chemotherapy is. Sometimes the tumor shrinks enough to allow breast-conserving therapy. In other institutions, high-dose chemotherapy protocols are offered, depending on the number of positive nodes. If chemotherapy is given preoperatively, the number of positive nodes may decrease; the patient would then be ineligible for high-dose therapy. At this time, it is not clear which, if any, of these approaches is more effective, but current research is addressing this issue.

Treatment Options for Metastatic Disease (Stage IV)

Until recently, once metastatic disease could be seen on X rays, it was considered incurable. Treatment was aimed at controlling the disease to prolong life with minimal symptoms. If the cancer was responsive to treatment, women could live five to ten years or more. With higher-dose chemotherapy plus bone marrow or stem cell transplant, some women may be cured. More likely, most patients simply have longer disease-free intervals. Unless your oncologist thinks that cure is possible, or the tumor within the breast is causing bleeding problems or infection, there is no reason for a mastectomy to be performed once metastatic disease has been discovered. Short of high-dose chemotherapy, treatments at this stage are intended to control symptoms, starting with the least toxic therapy.

Future Promise: The Prognosis for Breast Cancer

Approximately one-third of the women who get breast cancer eventually die of it. Some 182,000 new cases are diagnosed every year; about 43,000 women die of breast cancer each year. However, some women may not die for as long as 20 or 30 years or more. Many physicians no longer speak in terms of cure because no one can tell which individuals have been cured. Instead, they refer to long-term remission or survival rates.

Research has found that some groups of women do better than others. Long-term survival is more likely under these conditions:

1. There are no axillary lymph nodes with cancer. This is the most important single predictor found so far (see "Stages of Breast Cancer," p. 624).

2. The cancer is estrogen-receptor (ER) positive. These cancers tend to have fewer or later recur-

rences, no matter what type of treatment is used, although the difference is only 6 to 8%. ER-positive cancer is more common in postmenopausal women.

3. There is tubular carcinoma and no positive axillary nodes. This cancer cell type tends to grow and metastasize very slowly.

4. The tumor cells are well differentiated; that is, they retain more of the characteristics of normal breast cells rather than the embryonic appearance of advanced cancer cells.

Even with these indicators, *it is difficult to make predictions for any specific woman.* Some women with very good prognoses die quickly from the disease, whereas others with more advanced disease live normal life spans. There are still many unknown factors. It may well be that an individual's particular immune system, general health, and possibly mind-body interactions are also involved.

Managed Care and Your Options

It is estimated that by 2000, more than 60% of the U.S. population will be enrolled in managed care. Some health insurance plans attempt to save money by

- refusing to permit you to get a second opinion outside the plan.
- refusing to pay for breast reconstruction.
- insisting that you have mastectomy done as an outpatient.
- refusing to pay for treatment if you enroll in a study.

If any of these happens to you, call your state attorney general's office or consumer protection bureau, and/or the American Cancer Society, for help.

An estimated 1.5 million women or more will face a diagnosis of breast cancer during the next decade. Although all cancers are frightening, breast cancer seems to hold the most terror for us as women. The available information is confusing, and the experts often disagree. This makes it even more important for us to become active participants in all stages of detection, treatment, and decision-making. The information in this section is necessarily brief. You owe it to yourself to take the time to research all the available options and get additional opinions. If you have not read it already, we recommend turning to the general section on cancer next (see p. 611). It has more information on treatments (including alternatives to the accepted trio of surgery, radiation, and chemotherapy). In this section, we have tried to make specific recommendations wherever possible, but so many areas are still unsettled that we can only indicate the issues involved and urge you to find out what new data have become available since the publication of this book.

(see p. 611)

ONGOING STUDIES AND REVIEWS

The Cochrane Collaboration (see chapter 25, The Politics of Women's Health and Medical Care, p. 710) has established a review group on breast cancer. This group prepares summaries of findings from carefully identified and evaluated randomized control trials of the effectiveness of different breast cancer treatments, including an assessment of side effects.

The NCI is conducting several high-priority clinical trials that you may be interested in joining. To find out more about which trials are ongoing, which trials are still open to new participants, and how you might benefit, contact the NCI Cancer Information Service: (800) 4-CANCER.

(see chapter 25, The Politics of Women's Health and Medical Care, p. 710)

Activism and the Changing Epidemic

Since the pioneering efforts of Rose Kushner in the 1970s, the grassroots activism of women with breast cancer and their supporters has been the critical catalyst for increased awareness of and attention to breast cancer issues. The National Breast Cancer Coalition and its over 300 member organizations are responsible for working with Congress to secure hundreds of millions of dollars for breast cancer research. They make it possible for consumers to have a voice in all aspects of breast cancer research and funding decisions through innovative programs such as the Department of Defense Peer Review Breast Cancer Research Program. National groups such as Y-ME and the National Association of Breast Cancer Organizations have provided many thousands of women with much-needed information and support. Grassroots organizations such as 1 in 9 on Long Island, Breast Cancer Action in San Francisco, and the Massachusetts Breast Cancer Coalition have successfully fought to begin research into possible environmental links to the unusually high breast cancer rates in those parts of the country.

While awareness has increased, and screening, detection, and treatment have improved, there is still no true early detection, no prevention, and no cure for breast cancer. Activists must continue to fight for research into the causes of breast cancer, including possible environmental factors; for earlier and more accurate screening and detection methods; for safer and more effective treatments; and for a cure. We must be advocates for ourselves to ensure that we have access to the best possible care and treatment, and can obtain the knowledge we need to make truly informed choices. In addition, as competition for federal research dollars increases, it is crucial that we continue our public advocacy for increased public funding for breast cancer research. It is important not to settle for technological "quick fixes" such as genetic testing, which at present offers little to most women (see p. 612).

Women today are learning that we cannot simply depend on eating well, exercising, and having annual mammograms to protect ourselves. All these things are important, but they will not prevent a woman from getting breast cancer. We need to see beyond the clichés, for while early detection is important, it is *not* your best protection—prevention is the only real protection women can have. As many of us have come to realize over the past decade, the only cure for breast cancer is political action.

CERVICAL CANCER (INVASIVE)

If severely abnormal cells have spread beyond the upper tissue layer (surface epithelium) of your cervix into the underlying connective tissues, you have invasive cervical cancer. A Pap smear (see p. 593) followed by a biopsy can determine this. At first the spread is very shallow and may not involve the lymph or blood systems. In its early stages, cervical cancer is *almost always* curable *(depending on the severity of the lesions and the treatment used)*.

Each year in the U.S. about 17,500 women are diagnosed with cervical cancer. Of the 5,000 women who die annually of cervical cancer, half of them have never had a Pap test.

For more discussion of the causes and prevention of CIN and cervical cancer, see p. 654. Some studies show an elevated risk of cervical cancer in women who are farm workers, cooks, cleaners, maids, and the wives of coal miners.

Most physicians recommend a hysterectomy (removal of the uterus) with close followup in cases of cervical cancer. If the cancer has spread into the lymph or blood systems, physicians usually suggest radiation or hysterectomy/oophorectomy. (Chemotherapy is not as effective as local radiation.) Sometimes a combination of the two is used.

Radiation treatment is given in two ways. If the tumor is large, you will be given external radiation daily over a period of several weeks. During treatment, you will have to make daily trips to the medical center or hospital, which can be exhausting and cause you considerable inconvenience, depending on how far away you live. This is a time to ask family and friends to help with your other commitments and as traveling company and support. Negative effects of the radiation treatment include diarrhea, skin changes, rectal bleeding, and fatigue. Because each person reacts to radiation differently, the amount may have to be increased or decreased depending on your response. The negative effects of the radiation therapy are thought to be short-lived. When the radiation treatment has reduced the size of the growth, internal radioactive materials are placed inside your uterus or in the upper portion of your vagina. You will be hospitalized and given general anesthesia for this procedure. The implants are left inside your body from one to three days while you are in the hospital. This type of treatment directs a greater amount of radiation to a smaller area. Radiation treatment for early invasive cancer has a 60 to 90% survival rate, depending on the size of the tumor and the amount of spread. (See p. 611 for a general discussion of cancer and survival rates.)

Surgical treatment for invasive cancer usually involves a radical hysterectomy.

You should be involved in your treatment and have the final say in all decisions concerning your cancer. If you have any doubts about treatments recommended by your physician, get second and third opinions if you can.

OVARIAN CANCER

Cancer of the ovaries ranks second in the number of new cases and results in more deaths each year than any other cancer of the female reproductive system. More than 26,700 new cases are diagnosed annually in the U.S. alone. Although the incidence of ovarian cancer increases with age (a high percentage of cases is found in postmenopausal women), it may be found in women of any age.[3] Its exact causes are still unknown. Possible risk factors include a family history of ovarian cancer; few or no pregnancies; the use of fertility-stimulating drugs; a history of breast, colorectal, or endometrial cancer; exposure to industrial products, including asbestos, or to high levels of radiation; the use of talcum powder in the genital area; a diet high in fat; and the use of estrogens other than the birth control pill. Oral contraceptive use and multiple pregnancies may decrease a woman's risk for ovarian cancer.*

Diagnosis

Ovarian cancer does not always have clear symptoms. Its warning signs, which may be vague and frequently dismissed as "stress" or "nerves," include indigestion, gas, constipation, diarrhea, irritable bowel syndrome, loss of appetite or weight, a feeling of fullness, lower abdominal discomfort or pain, enlargement or bloating of the abdomen, unexplained weight gain, frequent urination, fatigue, backache, shoulder pain, nausea, vomiting, nonmenstrual vaginal bleeding, pain during intercourse, or an unusual growth or lump.

If you have persistent symptoms or a family history of ovarian cancer, make sure your gynecologist does a thorough evaluation for ovarian cancer. In some cases, you may need to be referred to a gynecological oncologist, who specializes in the diagnosis and treatment of ovarian cancer. There are three tests to ask for that might spot the problem early: a bimanual rectovaginal

---

* Removal of the ovaries has been proposed as an option to protect women against ovarian cancer. Although the benefit of prophylactic oophorectomy has not yet been established, some specialists suggest this surgery for women at high risk.

GENETIC TESTING FOR OVARIAN CANCER RISK

Two known genes, BRCA1 and BRCA2, have been related to an increased risk for ovarian and breast cancers. Evidence of mutation does not mean that a woman will get ovarian or breast cancer. The role of any specific mutation in the development of cancer is still the subject of ongoing research.

About 5 to 7% of ovarian cancer is thought to be associated with an inherited risk factor. Although genetic testing may be helpful to some women with two or more first-degree relatives (mother, sister, daughter) who have ovarian cancer, it has become the subject of great controversy. First, these tests are fast becoming a lucrative business and can be promoted indiscriminately. Second, they may lead to discrimination in insurance and health care (see p. 612). Third, because there is no clear preventive therapy for a woman identified as being at increased risk for ovarian cancer, many people question the whole point of testing. Women who want to be tested need to consider the potential medical, legal, and psychosocial implications of genetic testing. Comprehensive genetic counseling can be useful, especially if the counselors are trained to offer honest and balanced information (see Resources).[4]

pelvic exam,* transvaginal sonography (color flow Doppler ultrasound is available now in some areas), and the blood test CA125-II. Other diagnostic tests may include computerized tomography (CT or CAT scan), pelvic ultrasound, magnetic resonance imaging (MRI), and surgery, the only conclusive diagnostic tool. Ovarian cancer requires exploratory surgery (laparotomy) for diagnosis, staging, and frequently tumor debulking.[5] For more information on staging and different ovarian cancer cell types, including borderline tumors of low malignant potential (LMP), consult the Resource section.

Medical Treatments

Early detection, prompt diagnosis, and accurate staging are necessary for the successful treatment of ovarian cancer. The treatment depends on the stage of the disease at the time of diagnosis, the type of cells that make up the tumor, and how fast the cancer is growing. The current standard medical options for treating ovarian cancer include surgery, chemother-

apy, and/or radiation therapy. Immunotherapies, including interferon, interleukin, bone marrow/stem cell transplants, and monoclonal antibodies, are also available in clinical and/or research settings. Although not necessary for every patient, second-look surgery may be indicated for women at high risk for persistent tumor. (For more about surgical removal of the ovaries, see "Hysterectomy and Oophorectomy," p. 663.)

New cancer therapies become available to patients through clinical trials. Information about some of these investigational treatments is registered with the National Cancer Institute (see Cancer section in Resources). Many women explore supplemental or alternative treatments, alone or in conjunction with mainstream treatments.

Ovarian cancer has a higher cure rate if found early, and a lower cure rate if found in later stages, as is more often the case.[6]

Although scientists are researching new methods like the ROC-Algorithm based on CA125-II,[7] as yet there are no reliable screening measures available for the general population.

Ovarian cancer results in over 14,000 deaths each year. Grassroots women's health activists are beginning to lobby for increased funding for ovarian cancer research and awareness. More efforts are needed to help reduce mortality from this disease and ultimately to prevent it.

UTERINE CANCER

Cancer of the lining of the uterus (endometrial cancer) is the most common pelvic cancer, affecting 14 out of every 10,000 women yearly. Most women with this cancer are past menopause and in their 50s; 10% are still menstruating. If you are very heavy, if you take synthetic estrogen, or if you have diabetes, high blood pressure, or a hormone imbalance that combines high estrogen levels with infrequent ovulation, your risk of uterine cancer is increased. During the early 1970s, there was a sharp rise in the incidence of uterine cancer brought about by to increased use of ERT to relieve menopausal symptoms (see chapter 23, Women Growing Older, p. 559).

Bleeding after menopause is the most common symptom of uterine cancer. For women who are still menstruating, increased menstrual flow and bleeding between periods may be the only symptoms. Unfortunately, the Pap smear is unreliable in detecting the abnormal cells of uterine cancer. Your medical practitioner will probably recommend a procedure for sampling the uterine lining. This could be an aspiration or endometrial biopsy. In some cases, your medical practitioner may suggest a D&C as the first step, because it not only screens for cancer but frequently relieves abnormal bleeding from a variety of less serious causes. Make sure that you have discussed the risks and benefits of all these alternatives before making a decision.

---

* A Pap smear should be part of the pelvic exam, as it may reveal malignant ovarian cells, but it is not a reliable test for ovarian cancer.

Prevention and Self-Help Treatments

Because endometrial cancer appears to be influenced by factors such as obesity, hypertension, and diabetes, controlling these conditions with self-help methods may prevent this type of cancer from developing or spreading.

Medical Treatments

Medical treatment for uterine cancer includes surgery, radiation, and chemotherapy. There is wide disagreement about which is best. Outside the U.S., radiation is used frequently with good results. In this country, hysterectomy is the most common treatment, sometimes with followup radiation after surgery if the tumor was large, if spread to lymph nodes was suspected, or if the cellular changes were more excessive than usual. If you should have a return of the cancer after one of the above treatments, progestin treatments may help slow its spread.

When uterine cancer is found early, the success rate of conventional treatments is very high.

VULVAR CANCER

Women who have had HPV infections (see chapter 14, Sexually Transmitted Diseases, p. 356) seem to be at greater risk for vulvar cancer, although it is relatively rare (5 to 10% of all gynecological cancers). Some experts believe that vulvar cancer rates will rise sharply in the future, largely because of increased rates of HPV infections. Be aware of changes in your vulvar area (especially lesions), and request a biopsy if you find a suspicious lump or lesion. Because vulvar cancer typically grows slowly, early detection can mean the difference between minor surgery and the more emotionally and physically devastating experience of losing one's genitals.

CHEMICAL INJURY AND MULTIPLE CHEMICAL SENSITIVITY (MCS)

As the environments in which we live and work become more polluted, many people, the majority of them women, have developed a multiple chemical sensitivity (MCS) accompanied by debilitating damage to upper airways and/or other organs of the body. Along with acute sensitivity to commonly occurring chemical toxins, they are being diagnosed with various illnesses of the respiratory, neurological, immune, and digestive systems. Some of the chemical triggers of hypersensitivity are pesticides, new carpeting and other building materials, plastics, paints, adhesives, office machinery and supplies (such as correction fluid, felt-tip markers, and printers), auto exhaust, fuels, air "fresheners," tobacco smoke, mothballs, perfumed cosmetics, hairspray, nail polish, and fabrics stabilized with formaldehyde. These toxins are in all our environments and harm all of us; people with MCS are just more susceptible.

As a polysymptomatic condition, MCS varies—sometimes according to the particular toxin and sometimes according to the individual. Symptoms can include irritated eyes, nose, and throat; digestive disturbances and food sensitivities; joint pain; incapacitating exhaustion; drowsiness; disorientation; memory loss; seizures; and a host of other problems. Many persons with MCS have been treated for one allergy or another; but there are indications that MCS is not just an allergic response—it is primarily a neurological disorder, with secondary immune-system impairment. Hormonal instability may well explain why more women than men suffer from MCS. Also, women and children may be more susceptible to toxins because of their lower body weight and their higher ratio of body fat to body mass (toxic chemicals accumulate in fat).

Most of the medical world has not so far recognized MCS, perhaps because the medical model calls for one cause, one set of symptoms, and one cure. Often MCS goes undiagnosed by doctors who are not informed and who send their patients to psychiatrists. Many medical practitioners now realize, however, that MCS is a serious condition that has implications for all of us. Diagnostic tests that have shown abnormalities in hypersensitive patients include BEAM computerized qualitative analysis of EEG studies, MRI, SPECT scans, complete blood count, antibody assays, and various evaluations of organ function (lungs, liver, etc.) and metabolism.

Avoidance is the first line of defense for a chemical-sensitive person. Exercise and detoxification regimens can be helpful, as can nutritional supplements (e.g., antioxidants) to fortify the immune system. Whatever treatment you try, dealing effectively with the symptoms involves a major shift in lifestyle to eliminate the toxins. Besides getting rid of scented personal care and household cleaning products, we need to reduce sources of mold, dust, animal dander, and so on. Strip down your living space gradually, and see how you respond. Some people with MCS have had to move to another house in order to regain stamina. Safe, chemical-free housing is crucial, as are organic foods, to avoid the chemicals used in agribusiness. Many say they feel better on a macrobiotic diet. Air and water filters can also make a difference.

There is a sense among many persons with MCS that in becoming acutely reactive to neurotoxic chemicals, their bodies are showing the cumulative lifetime effects of the same chemical assaults that we all experience. For those who have MCS now, and perhaps for us all, the ultimate "treatment" is cleaning up the environment (see chapter 7, Environmental and Occupational Health).

CRABS (PUBIC LICE) AND SCABIES

Crabs, or Pubic Lice

Phthirus pubis is a roundish, crab-like body louse that lives in pubic hair and occasionally in the hair of the chest, armpits, eyelashes, and eyebrows. You can "catch" crabs by intimate physical contact with someone who has them or from bedding, towels, or clothes that person has used. They are bloodsuckers and can carry such diseases as typhus. The main symptom of crabs is an intolerable itching in the genital or other affected area; they are easily diagnosed because they are visible without a microscope.

Though it may be difficult, try not to scratch. Scratching can transfer lice to uninfected parts of the body. Excessive scratching around the urinary opening can even lead to urinary tract infections.

Medical practitioners usually prescribe a lotion called Kwell,* available by prescription only. This drug should be used with caution: Follow the directions carefully. Vonce, R.I.D., and A-200 pyrinate are safe nonprescription drugs that are almost as effective as Kwell for crabs. Do not use any of these drugs in or around your eyes. If you have crabs in your eyebrows, use an ophthalmic petroleum jelly.

Alternatively, you can try a very hot sauna, a treatment routinely used in Scandinavia (the authors do not know how effective this is). Either way, it's important that all persons with whom you have been in intimate contact, including lovers, family members, and friends, be treated as well.

After treatment, you should use clean clothing, towels and bed linen, because crabs migrate between the body and cloth. Crabs will die within 24 hours after separation from the human body, but the eggs will live for about six days more. Previously used bedclothes, towels, and so on are free of live eggs after a week without use. Anything dry-cleaned or washed in boiling water can be used immediately.

As with scabies, the itch may persist for some time after treatment, especially if your skin is very irritated from scratching. Soothing skin preparations, such as aloe vera and colloidal oatmeal (Aveeno), can ease the symptoms and help your skin heal faster.

The first time I got crabs, I felt embarrassed and humiliated. I'd gone to visit my boyfriend at college, and when I came home I began to itch. I couldn't believe that he would give me something like that—especially since I'd mistakenly associated crabs with people who didn't wash enough. I didn't know what to do, so I just ignored them as long as possible. When the itching became really intolerable, I went to a clinic. Once I learned how crabs are transmitted and that they are both very common and easy to cure, I felt a lot better. The next time I went to visit my boyfriend, I took a bottle of A-200 with me. Turns out he hadn't known what to do either!

Scabies

Scabies are tiny parasitic mites that burrow under the superficial layers of the skin, depositing eggs and

feces and causing intense irritation. Symptoms usually include intense itching (often worse at night) and red, raised bumps or ridges on the skin, which may be found on the hands (especially between the fingers), on or under the breasts, around the waist or wrists, or on the genitals or buttocks. Scratching the area can break the skin, which may then become infected with bacteria.

Scabies is highly contagious. You can get it through close physical contact as well as from infested bed linen, towels, clothing, and occasionally even furniture. If you've never had scabies, it may take a month or more for the skin reaction to develop. During this time, you can pass it to someone else without knowing you have it. Once you've had scabies, however, your skin will react much more quickly, often within a day after reinfestation.

Diagnosing scabies can be tricky because it is easily confused with poison ivy, eczema, allergies, and other skin conditions. If your medical practitioner is unsure of what you have, ask for a scraping to be checked under a microscope. Sometimes physicians will prescribe medication for scabies before they know what you really have, and this might be unnecessary or might cause an allergic reaction. Do not apply the medication until you have a definite diagnosis made from a small scraping of the irritated area.

The most common and effective treatment is Kwell. Apply after a hot bath or shower (avoiding face, eyes, and mucous membranes), leave on for 12 hours, and carefully rinse off. If you need a second treatment, wait two weeks before reapplying.

An alternative to Kwell, often prescribed for pregnant women, is Eurax, whose active ingredient is crotamiton. It should be rubbed into the skin and reapplied after 24 hours.

An old-fashioned treatment using sulfur is making a comeback in popularity among dermatologists. It is especially recommended for treating infants, young children, and pregnant women for scabies. It is considered less irritating than other chemicals that kill scabies, it seems to be less toxic, and it seems to work.

The one disadvantage to the sulfur treatment is cosmetic. It smells like rotten eggs and can stain clothing.

For the adventurous, the recommended mixture is 6% sulfur, 3% balsam of Peru, and the rest petroleum jelly. The mixture is put on the infected areas and left on for 24 hours, with a new application each night for three consecutive nights. Some pharmacists will mix the ingredients for you.

Treatment is important for any friends, lovers, or family members with whom you've had intimate contact. You should also wash any clothing, towels, bedclothes, furniture covers, and so on in very hot water and dry them at the hottest possible temperature.

Even after treatment, you may continue to itch for several days or weeks. This doesn't mean you still have scabies; more likely, your skin is still hypersensitive and needs some time for the irritation to die down. A soothing lotion containing calamine or aloe vera will

---

* This drug should be used very carefully. Its active ingredient, lindane, is a potent pesticide that penetrates the skin and can cause allergic reactions. In addition, lindane has been found to cause tumors in laboratory animals. Pregnant women, infants, and children should not use this drug.

ease the symptoms. If the itching is really intolerable, an antihistamine may help.

DES

A DES daughter with clear-cell cancer:

October will be three years since I was diagnosed with clear-cell adenocarcinoma. At that time I underwent a seven-hour operation to remove my uterus, vagina, fallopian tubes, an ovary, and many lymph nodes. A split-thickness skin graft was used to reconstruct my vagina. As of this date, I'm still trying to understand what clear-cell cancer is, what happened to my body, and how it could have happened to a healthy 25-year-old in the first place. I especially got mad when I found out that there was a reason why this cancer happened and that it never would have happened if DES had been properly tested. It is amazing to me that the people involved in the marketing of DES are so callously indifferent to the fact that it causes cancer.

Overview

DES (diethylstilbestrol) is a powerful synthetic estrogen that was prescribed to an estimated 4.8 million American women between 1938 and 1971, in the mistaken belief that it would prevent miscarriage. In fact, the drug was untested for pregnancy use or safety, and it was aggressively marketed until 1971, when it was found to be linked to a rare form of vaginal cancer in daughters of women who had taken it. DES was manufactured under more than 200 brand names and used throughout the world, most heavily in the U.S., in pills, injections, and suppositories.*

DES crosses the placenta and may damage the reproductive system of the developing fetus. Many reproductive tract injuries are linked to DES exposure. DES may also affect other body systems: endocrine, immune, skeletal, and neurological. For this reason, and to answer questions about whether the children of DES daughters and sons—the "third generation"—will be affected, DES Action and the DES Cancer Network worked to get research funded. The DES Research and Education Amendment passed Congress in 1992, and the largest studies ever done on DES mothers, daughters, and sons are now under way.

Who Is Exposed and How to Find Out

Several million people (mothers, daughters, and sons) have been exposed to DES, most without knowing it. If you were born after 1938, ask your mother whether she had problems with any of her pregnan-

* The use of DES in European countries continued throughout the 1970s (until 1975 in England and the Netherlands, until 1977 in France) and in some countries into the 1980s (until 1981 in Spain and Italy, until 1983 in Hungary). DES was prescribed in every country where U.S. drug companies had markets.

cies or whether she remembers taking anything when she was pregnant with you. (It is generally believed that DES was most widely used between 1947 and 1965, when "wonder drugs" were so popular.)

I didn't remember taking anything besides vitamins during my pregnancy, but when my daughter asked me, we checked, and there it was on the medical record.

If a woman doesn't know whether she took DES, she can check with the doctor she saw at that time. However, many doctors no longer have their medical records, and some refuse to give the information. You may find something in the medical records at the hospital where the birth took place.

Any woman who is not sure whether her mother took DES can get a special exam (see p. 637) from a medical provider knowledgeable about DES exposure. DES Action has referral lists.

Medical Problems and Medical Care

DES Daughters

Clear-cell adenocarcinoma is a rare type of vaginal or cervical cancer linked to *in utero* exposure to DES. Before 1970, clear-cell cancer had occurred only rarely in medical history, and never in women so young. It is estimated that one out of every 1,000 DES daughters will develop clear-cell cancer of the vagina or cervix. The cancer has occurred in girls and women between the ages of seven and 40, with the peak at ages 15 to 22. Although cases of clear-cell cancer have declined in the last ten years (mirroring the decreased use of DES in the 1970s), it was still being diagnosed in the early 1990s, and the upper age limit for developing the cancer is unknown.

Regular DES exams can find clear-cell cancer early so that it can be treated. Clear-cell cancer is fast growing and, in the early stages, sometimes symptomless. The typical treatment for the cancer includes a radical hysterectomy, surgical removal of all or part of the vagina (vaginectomy), and reconstruction of the vagina. Radiation treatment is often used in conjunction with surgery. Eighty percent of the patients survive, but the adjustment to the extreme treatment is difficult.

Structural changes, such as cervical "collars" or "hoods," are also common among DES daughters. They do not need treatment and may disappear after age 30. DES daughters are also more likely than others to have a T-shaped uterus. Some structural changes may contribute to pregnancy problems (see below).

Metaplasia is a normal process whereby tissue changes from one form to another. Although all women have areas of cells undergoing metaplasia around their cervix, this area may be larger in DES daughters with adenosis. Adenosis is the presence of columnar cells where the more usual squamous cells should be. This metaplasia raises two concerns: First, some suspect that this area may be more vulnerable to

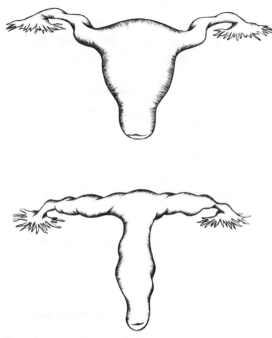

A T-shaped uterus is one of the abnormal changes often found in DES daughters. The uterus may also be smaller than normal. The unusual size and shape may contribute to pregnancy problems for DES daughters, most notably preterm labor/Christine Bondante

precancerous or cancerous changes. Second, pathologists may mistakenly interpret the change as abnormal (dysplasia). Such misdiagnosis can lead to unnecessary treatment with possibly harmful effects.

Dysplasia is more common among DES daughters, and they may want to approach treatment recommendations with caution.[8]

Squamous cell carcinoma, usually of the cervix, is a slow-growing cancer that is sometimes preceded by dysplasia. Research is needed to ascertain whether DES daughters will be at a higher risk for this cancer in later years.

Pregnancy problems are more common in DES daughters, partially because of abnormalities in the uterus and/or cervix. They may have trouble conceiving or carrying a first pregnancy to term because of miscarriage, premature delivery, or tubal pregnancy (pregnancy in the fallopian tube instead of in the uterus). Early in pregnancy, watching for signs of a tubal pregnancy (see chapter 22, Child-bearing Loss, Infertility, and Adoption) may help prevent serious problems. A pregnant DES daughter should always receive high-risk obstetrical care for every pregnancy.

When I got pregnant, I found out that the doctor who was doing my DES exams didn't know anything about pregnancy problems for DES daughters. So I brought him seven articles that DES Action gave me. We both read them, and as a result, he checked my cervix at every prenatal visit. It took 15 seconds and took away tons of anxiety.

Other problems, such as endometriosis, menstrual irregularities, and PID, have been reported by many DES daughters. There is as yet no research on whether these problems are more significant among DES-exposed women.

Contraception for DES daughters poses some special considerations. Birth control pills may be inadvisable because of the possible effects of further estrogen exposure on someone who is already at increased risk of a hormone-related cancer. IUDs for DES daughters are questionable because of the possible cervical and uterine abnormalities. Barrier methods are often the overall safest choice.

The DES Exam

DES-caused changes do not usually show up in regular pelvic examinations or Pap smears. DES daughters should see a medical care provider who is experienced in DES screening. Ask whether the person who examines you is monitoring other DES daughters and if she or he is familiar with the techniques described below.

A DES exam consists of

- careful visual inspection of the vagina and cervix for physical abnormalities.
- gentle palpation of the walls of the vagina.
- separate Pap smears from the cervix and from the surfaces of the upper vagina.
- bimanual exam (feeling the uterus, tubes, and ovaries with the fingers of one hand inside the vagina and the other hand on the abdomen).

The exam may also include iodine staining of the vagina and cervix (normal tissue stains brown; adenosis tissue does not stain) (see Schiller's test, p. 595). Depending on the results of these tests, further procedures may be necessary, such as colposcopy (see p. 595) and biopsy (p. 594).

DES Mothers

DES mothers have an increased incidence of breast cancer. Most studies agree that there is a time lag of ten to 20 years between taking DES and developing a related disease.

If you are a DES mother, get a professional breast exam every year in addition to performing monthly breast self-examination.

DES Sons

Ongoing studies report several areas of concern for DES sons: underdeveloped testes, benign (noncancerous) cysts on the epididymis (the part of the testicle that stores mature sperm), undescended testicles (which may increase the risk of testicular cancer), and sperm and semen abnormalities (which may cause fertility problems). Concerned sons can be examined by a urologist, and DES sons can practice regular self-examination of the testes.

Emotional Issues

For those exposed to DES, all these physical effects often generate emotional effects as well. Living with the necessity of frequent medical examinations, a fear of cancer, knowledge of deformities, and worry about the ability to have a healthy child add to their concerns.

Not surprisingly, some DES mothers feel guilty when they find out that something they took may have harmed their children. Some find it difficult to tell them, though it is essential to do so. Many mothers say they are relieved after telling their children and talking about the health care they need.

I read about the report on DES and its link to cancer back in 1971. I cut the article out of the paper and stuck it in my bureau drawer. Five years later, my daughter was 14 and I knew I had to do something soon. So I found a doctor who knew about DES and how to do the exam, and I finally told my daughter. What a relief!

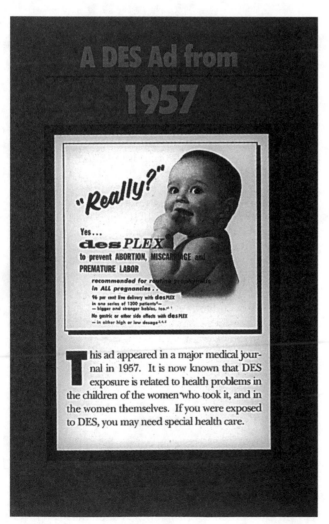

DES Action

It really helped me to talk with other DES daughters. We compared notes, and I went back to my next medical appointment with a list of questions and a friend for moral support. We had a long discussion with the doctor, who was surprised at how much we knew.

DES, which has caused me so much pain, has at least allowed me new and needed understandings. I know to keep myself informed. I would like to work with my doctors. I know that they haven't always read the medical journals. I know that they cannot care about the outcome of my case nearly as much as I do.

Although we know much more about DES than we did ten years ago, daughters, sons, and mothers face unanswered questions about their future health. More research is needed in all areas. Furthermore, some doctors still do not know about the DES exam, special pregnancy problems, and other recent medical findings; their ignorance can result in serious overtreatment or undertreatment. Finally, we need to tell the DES story so that people who have been exposed can receive the medical care they need and so that we can help prevent similar medical mistakes from happening in the future.

DIABETES

Diabetes Mellitus

Classification

Diabetes mellitus is a metabolic disorder characterized by a high fasting blood glucose level. Four major types of diabetes have been defined: insulin-dependent diabetes mellitus (IDDM), non–insulin-dependent diabetes mellitus (NIDDM), gestational diabetes mellitus (GDM), and secondary diabetes that develops in association with disorders or factors such as pancreatic diseases, some genetic syndromes, and the effects of certain drugs, toxins, and chemical agents.

After age 45, about twice as many women as men develop diabetes, and the risk of heart disease and heart-related death is higher for diabetic women than for diabetic men. Diabetes is more common in African-

American and Native American women than among other women.

Ten to 20% of known cases of diabetes in the U.S. are IDDM, also referred to as Type I diabetes. Epidemiological patterns suggest that both genetic and environmental factors contribute to its development. More than 80% of IDDM occurs in children with no known family history of the disease. The presence of a family member with IDDM increases the risk of IDDM in relatives.

IDDM is characterized physiologically by insulin deficiency. Insulin is produced in the beta cell of the pancreas, and in IDDM there is eventual beta cell failure. IDDM has its onset predominantly in youth but can occur at any age. The most common signs include increased thirst, urination, and weight loss in association with a high blood glucose level. Persons with IDDM must take insulin injections to control their blood glucose levels.

Eighty to 90% of all known cases of diabetes in the U.S. are NIDDM, also referred to as Type II diabetes. As with IDDM, both genetic and environmental factors play a role in the development of NIDDM. Persons who develop NIDDM almost always have a family history of NIDDM. The most important risk factor associated with the development of NIDDM is the intake of excessive calories leading to extreme weight gain. The symptoms usually develop slowly and may include fatigue, headache, more frequent urination, leg cramps, blurred vision, and vaginal itching.

Although insulin levels in persons with NIDDM may be normal, mildly depressed, or elevated, almost every person with this disease has insulin resistance (decreased tissue responsiveness to the actions of insulin). This insulin resistance exists both for naturally produced insulin and for insulin taken by injection. For this reason, insulin is not necessarily the treatment of choice in NIDDM. Oral drugs are available that increase insulin sensitivity and lower blood sugar levels.

Many persons with NIDDM do best with a treatment plan that includes a controlled carbohydrate diet designed to reduce weight toward normal, a regular exercise program, and an oral antidiabetic agent. Insulin treatment, either alone or in combination with oral agents, is sometimes necessary with NIDDM. Special circumstances, such as the stress of surgery or an acute illness, may make insulin treatment necessary to control blood glucose in the short-term. It is generally true that once these stresses resolve, insulin can be discontinued.

Gestational diabetes mellitus (GDM) is defined as carbohydrate intolerance of variable severity with onset during late pregnancy. This condition complicates between 1 to 14% of pregnancies in the U.S., with the highest incidence found among African-American, Latina, and Native American women.

An oral glucose tolerance test with a 50-gram glucose load is recommended for screening between the 24th and 28th weeks of gestation. If the fasting blood glucose is above 105 mg/dl or the glucose level is 150 mg/dl or greater one hour after the glucose load, further diagnostic testing is indicated.

High blood glucose levels during pregnancy and abnormalities in the metabolism of other fuels (fatty acids and amino acids) increase the risk of a high-birthweight baby, which, in turn, increases obstetrical risks during delivery. For example, there is a higher risk of cesarean section. Physicians try to help women with GDM use dietary changes to normalize the surge in glucose levels that occurs after meals. Sometimes insulin treatment is necessary as well. *Oral antidiabetic agents are contraindicated for use in pregnancy.* GDM is not associated with a higher risk of birth abnormalities, as is the case with a pregnant woman with preexisting diabetes.

Although most women with GDM return to normal glucose tolerance after birthing, the presence of this disorder during pregnancy indicates a higher risk for the subsequent development of diabetes. If a woman has hyperglycemia during the early trimesters, rather than GDM she may have unrecognized preexisting diabetes, either IDDM or NIDDM, presenting for the first time during pregnancy. Careful postpartum monitoring is important in either case to ensure that maternal diabetes is recognized.

Complications of Diabetes

Persons with diabetes are susceptible to numerous complications. Heart disease, stroke, lower extremity arterial disease, kidney failure, and blindness are all manifestations of an increased incidence of vascular disease in persons with diabetes. To delay the onset and acceleration of these complications, a treatment plan designed to normalize blood glucose, weight, blood pressure, and blood cholesterol is recommended. The use of tobacco is strongly discouraged.

Trends in Diabetes Therapy

Diet and Exercise

Nutritional therapy is fundamental in controlling diabetes. For both IDDM and NIDDM, a major objective is to normalize glucose control and blood cholesterol level, to prevent and treat acute low blood glucose reactions (hypoglycemia), and to prevent chronic complications. For the individual who is taking insulin, an additional goal is to match diet to insulin requirements. For the extremely heavy patient with NIDDM, some long-term weight loss and improved cardiovascular fitness from exercise are primary goals.

The preferred diabetic diet is still a balance of carbohydrates, fat, and protein that emphasizes high fiber, low fat, and restricted sodium intake. Despite the dogma that persons with diabetes cannot eat sweets, studies comparing the effects of refined sweets and complex carbohydrates have shown that there is no significant difference in the post-meal glucose excursion (variation from the normal course) when an equal number of calories is consumed. Diets are best when individualized, and they should be designed by a dietitian knowledgeable about diabetes.

The use of chromium supplementation has gained lay popularity because of studies that show chromium to be helpful in patients with poorly controlled diabetes and chromium deficiency. It is unclear that supplementation is beneficial, since chromium deficiency is unlikely in most individuals who consume a balanced diet. The use of vitamin E supplementation may have a role in preventing microvascular disease, and controlled studies in diabetic patients are in progress.

Oral Medication

In NIDDM, when the first line measures of diet, weight reduction, and exercise fail to restore the blood glucose level to normal, pharmacologic therapy should be considered. Pharmacologic therapy is an adjunct to, not a substitute for, diet and exercise. Three classes of oral agents are now available in the U.S. for use in treating uncontrolled NIDDM: the sulfonylureas (glyburide, glipizide, and glimepiride), the biguanide drug metformin (Glucaphage), and the newly released drug troglitazone (Rezulin). These drugs work through a variety of mechanisms that exert extra-pancreatic as well as pancreatic effects on glucose metabolism. Acarbose (Precose) is a drug that slows carbohydrate absorption and is sometimes used in combination with other hypoglycemic agents in NIDDM.

Insulin Therapy

Insulin is always required in the treatment of IDDM. In 1993, the results of the landmark Diabetes Control and Complications Trial (DCCT) were published. This prospective ten-year study of persons with IDDM was designed to evaluate the influence of tight glucose control on both delaying the onset and slowing the progression of vascular disease in IDDM. Patients were stratified into an intensive treatment group (three or more insulin injections daily or use of an insulin pump) and a conventional treatment group (one or two insulin injections daily). Although patients in the intensive treatment group still maintained blood sugar levels approximately 40% above normal, there was a 40 to 70% reduction in risk of diabetic eye, kidney, and nerve disease compared with patients in the conventional treatment group. This benefit applied to the delay in onset as well as the progression of these complications.

As a direct result of tighter metabolic control, the incidence of hypoglycemia was increased threefold in the intensive treatment group compared with the conventional treatment group. This significant side effect of tighter blood glucose control must be balanced with the benefits of lessening the risk for chronic vascular disease. New technology has made available home blood glucose monitoring devices that can give a nearly exact reading of the blood glucose level using a drop of capillary blood from a finger prick. Self-monitoring of blood glucose levels done frequently during the day can help reduce the unexpected occurrence of hypoglycemia, allowing for prompt detection and treatment, and reduction in the risk for chronic complications.

What to Expect from Your Health Care Provider

If you have diabetes, whether IDDM or NIDDM, expect your health care practitioner to include these practices in monitoring for complications of diabetes:

- A comprehensive physical examination with attention to the cardiovascular system, a neurological examination, and an examination of the circulation and condition of the feet should be performed yearly. Once chronic complications have been detected, quarterly exams are best to closely monitor progression.
- Blood pressure should be normalized, with medication if necessary.
- A full dilated eye examination should be performed at the onset of the diagnosis of NIDDM and within five years of the onset of IDDM. It then should be repeated yearly.
- Albumin is a blood protein that under normal circumstances is barely detectable in the urine. In early diabetic kidney disease, the level of microscopic amounts of albumin is increased and can be measured on a random urine specimen. *ACE inhibitors,* a special classification of blood pressure–lowering medication, have been shown to delay the progression of diabetic kidney disease if given to patients with increased levels of urinary albumin.
- Blood lipids (cholesterol, triglycerides, HDL [*good*] cholesterol and LDL [*bad*] cholesterol) should be normalized, either with diet alone or with diet plus medication.
- Warnings about avoiding tobacco.
- Yearly review of your individualized diet and, if appropriate, weight reduction plan with a knowledgeable dietitian.
- Yearly review of self-management techniques with a certified diabetes educator.
- Periodic review of home blood glucose monitoring results, with attention to changes in insulin regimen or oral antidiabetic drugs, can be guided by the determination of the *glycosylated hemoglobin* (also known as the A1C) *level*. This unique laboratory measurement can give an estimate of the average blood glucose level over the preceding two months. It is recommended that this test be performed at least twice yearly to help guide the appropriateness of therapy.

Since eating is so much a part of our interactions with other people, including family, friends, and co-workers, it is important to communicate your food needs to the people around you if you have diabetes. They need to understand why you are particular about what and when you eat.

Wear an ID bracelet, such as one from Medic Alert, that states you have diabetes and provides a telephone number for use in an emergency. In the event you are not able to speak for yourself, this will identify your medical condition.

If you have IDDM, teach family members and friends how to help you if you show signs of low blood sugar. Always carry juice, glucose tablets, or hard candy with you for emergency situations when your blood glucose level drops below normal. It is also helpful to carry blood-testing strips with you to determine your blood glucose level. These are simple ways to avoid the potentially life-threatening situation of being immobilized by low blood glucose.

ENDOMETRIOSIS

Endometriosis, which can be an extremely painful disease, occurs when tissue similar to the tissue that lines the inside of the uterus (endometrium) grows in other parts of the body. This tissue is sometimes referred to as *growths, nodules, tumors,* or *lesions* and most commonly develops in the pelvic area: on the ovaries, the lining of the pelvic cavity (peritoneum), the ligaments, or the fallopian tubes. Growths may also occur on the bladder, the intestines, or even distant parts of the body—in the arm, lung, or head.

Like the lining of the uterus, endometrial growths usually respond to the hormones of the menstrual cycle. They build up tissue each month, break down, and cause bleeding. Internal bleeding, inflammation, and the formation of cysts and scar tissue results. The immune system appears to be involved in the development of endometriosis and related health problems, and many immune abnormalities have been identified in women with endometriosis.

Endometriosis may cause severe pelvic pain around menstruation, ovulation, and/or sexual activity; excessive menstrual flow; fatigue; painful bowel movements with periods; lower back pain with periods; diarrhea and/or constipation and other intestinal upset with periods; infertility; and other symptoms. It can also cause other severe health problems, including ruptured ovarian cysts, adhesions, a possibly increased risk of ectopic pregnancy and miscarriage, and general debilitation. Some women experience no symptoms.

A 33-year-old woman describes her experience:

I experienced the first symptoms of endometriosis (in my case, very severe pain when having a bowel movement) when I was 19 years old. About five years later I began to have the same kind of pain at midcycle and during my periods. I mentioned this to several doctors, and they seemed unconcerned. A year or two later I began to have premenstrual spotting, which increased in duration as time progressed. I went to at least four different doctors. No one even mentioned endometriosis. . . . At the age of 30 I had new symptoms: chronic, low-level pelvic pain and pain on intercourse, in addition to pain on pelvic examination. At

this time the word "endometriosis" was first mentioned, and a diagnosis by laparoscopy followed a few months later.

A particularly difficult aspect of the disease for many women is that it is chronic. In one survey of 200 women, 60% said that they were unable to carry on normal work and activities, usually for one to three days at a time and sometimes for weeks or even months, not including the time lost because of surgery. One woman calculated that three days lost to pain each month for 20 years added up to a staggering two years of her life. While most people would not make light of two years lost to illness, the recurring nature of this condition—the fact that it comes and goes with the menstrual period and gets better and worse—means that women often don't get recognition and sympathy for the difficulties it causes. A 24-year-old woman states:

The biggest problem is looking very healthy. People don't seem to understand pain and sickness unless they can see physical evidence. This makes you feel absolutely desperate.

Causes and Related Health Problems

Several theories about the cause of endometriosis have been advanced. One theory is the retrograde menstruation theory: that during menstruation, some of the menstrual tissue backs up through the fallopian tubes, becomes implanted in the abdomen, and grows. Research has shown that many women experience some menstrual tissue backup and that an immune system problem and/or hormonal problem allows this tissue to take root and grow in women who develop endometriosis. In addition, many women have endometrial implants but no sign of disease. The definition of endometriosis is changing, since studies such as these imply that immune and endocrine factors in women with endometriosis are more important than simply the presence of endometrial tissue outside the uterus.

A genetic theory about the cause of endometriosis suggests that certain families have predisposing factors. A major international study of families with endometriosis may provide important information in coming years. Tracking families with endometriosis and related health problems has also added greatly to our knowledge of this disease. These related health problems include problems related to *Candida albicans* (both vaginal yeast infections and other signs and symptoms throughout the body), allergies, asthma, eczema, hay fever, food sensitivities, a history of mononucleosis, and a higher than normal incidence of immune system diseases, including chronic fatigue immune dysfunction syndrome, or fibromyalgia, lupus, and thyroid problems. Some of these findings are very new; it will take much more research to determine exactly what is happening.

Another new theory about the cause of endometriosis is based on research spearheaded by the Endometriosis Association, which discovered in 1992 that dioxin, an environmental toxin widely prevalent in the environment from pesticides and herbicides, industrial waste, and incineration, is able to cause severe endometriosis. The more dioxin, the more severe the disease. Additional studies have now been carried out at several research institutions, with the same results. Dioxin and similar chemicals, in research by toxicologists around the world, has been found to disrupt hormones as well as act as an immune toxicant. Additional studies are under way.

Women with endometriosis generally have a history of primary dysmenorrhea; indeed, it is impossible to tell where primary dysmenorrhea ends and endometriosis begins. Given the chronic pain and other difficulties that both primary dysmenorrhea and endometriosis cause, it would be wise to attempt to control primary dysmenorrhea. Some approaches include nonsteroidal anti-inflammatory drugs, nutritional supplements to balance essential fatty acid precursors to prostaglandins, diet and exercise, and avoidance of estrogenic and other endocrine-disrupting chemicals such as dioxin and PCBs. If you or your family have other risk factors, you may also want to control them to improve your health and perhaps decrease your risk for endometriosis. Much more research is needed before we will have definitive answers on the cause, prevention, and cure of endometriosis.

Myths impede both the diagnosis and the treatment of endometriosis. The classical "psychological profile" of the endometriosis sufferer still crops up in both medical literature and the popular media, labeling this "the career woman's disease" and blaming the victim as an upwardly striving, white, educated, egocentric woman in her late 20s or early 30s who has postponed pregnancy in favor of her career. This anachronistic view probably developed because these were the women who tended to have the financial resources, education, sense of entitlement, and private doctors necessary to obtain a correct diagnosis. However, women of color do have the disease, though the medical system has historically overlooked that fact. Also, it is *not* true that the disease typically begins when women are in their late 20s and early 30s. In a very large study from the Association's data registry, 60% of the women experienced their first symptoms of the disease before age 25, and more teenagers are being diagnosed. (The Association has developed a special support program for teens.) Also, contrary to medical myth, early pregnancy—even teenage pregnancy—does not confer immunity to the disease.

Another myth is that menstrual pain is primarily psychological. Many doctors still don't take it seriously, which makes them slow to diagnose endometriosis. Any teenager or woman with severe menstrual cramps or other menstrual problems should seek a very sensitive and knowledgeable physician. The Endometriosis Association offers a special information kit to help you with diagnosis.

Diagnosis

Though physicians can sometimes feel endometrial implants during a pelvic exam, a laparoscopy has been considered necessary for a definitive diagnosis. Endometriosis is sometimes confused with other disorders and diseases (for example, PID, ectopic pregnancy, cysts, cancer, appendicitis, or diverticulitis) that have similar symptoms. Proper treatment cannot occur without proper diagnosis. The Association and others are working on new, nonsurgical diagnostic tests.

Treatments

Choosing a treatment is rarely simple. Several factors may enter into your decision, among them your age, your symptoms, the location of the endometriosis and its severity, your desire for pregnancy, your past experiences with hormones, and your family history.

The aim in treating endometriosis with hormones is to stop the ovary from producing estrogen and also to stop menstruation. Although doctors sometimes recommend pregnancy as a treatment—even stating that it is a cure—it is certainly a dubious one. It is, of course, best to have a child because you want to, not because you have a disease. Pregnancy is not a cure anyway, though it may offer temporary relief. Moreover, dioxin and other pollutants now being linked to endometriosis are passed along to our children when we are pregnant with them and when we breast-feed. Thus, some women with endometriosis are rethinking their child-bearing decisions. No one who has suffered with endometriosis wants to pass it along to their children. And it is not always possible to become pregnant, as women with endometriosis have higher than average infertility. If you have the disease and know you want a child, be aware that delay may make pregnancy less likely if the disease advances.

Hormonal treatments include gonadotropin releasing hormone (GnRH) analogs, danazol, progesterone-like drugs (Provera), and oral contraceptives. The drugs most commonly used by specialists—danazol and the GnRH analogs—are very expensive. All of the hormonal treatments cause problematic side effects for some women. Also, all tend to work to some degree while the woman is taking the drug, but recurrence of the disease within a relatively short time after discontinuing the drug is the rule.

Surgery to treat endometriosis includes a wide range of treatments, from conservative (scraping, cutting, cauterizing, or lasering the growths) to radical (hysterectomy and removal of the ovaries). Radical surgery has been said to be the definitive cure for endometriosis, but research has found the disease can continue or recur even with removal of the ovaries. Surgery through the laparoscope, called *operative laparoscopy,* has rapidly replaced major abdominal surgery in the U.S. and is beginning do so in other countries also.

According to a 28-year-old woman:

THE ENDOMETRIOSIS ASSOCIATION

The Endometriosis Association, founded in 1980, is an international self-help organization with three major goals: supporting and helping women with endometriosis, educating about the disease, and conducting research.

The Association offers lectures and support group meetings, crisis telephone services, networking for special problems (especially for finding sensitive and knowledgeable physicians), and a wide variety of informative, accurate, and highly acclaimed literature on endometriosis and related health problems. The Association's literature includes materials in 14 languages, its popular books *(The Endometriosis Sourcebook),* videotapes, audiocassette tapes of speeches by experts on the disease, a "How Can I Tell If I Have Endometriosis?" kit to help those not yet diagnosed who suspect they have the disease, and other literature.

The Association headquarters is in Milwaukee, Wisconsin; members, chapters, and groups are scattered worldwide. Ending the feeling of being alone, sharing with others who understand what you are going through, counteracting the lack of information and misinformation about endometriosis, and learning from each other are ways those affected by the disease help each other.

Since 1980, the Association has been gathering information from thousands of women who have endometriosis and developed the world's largest data registry on the disease. Part of the Association's research program continues groundbreaking dioxin studies at Dartmouth Medical School, and a variety of other activities are carried out to promote research.

For additional information, call the Association at (800) 992-3636 or fax (414) 355-6065, or write to the Endometriosis Association, International Headquarters, 8585 North 76th Place, Milwaukee, WI 53223, U.S.A.

The hardest part in deciding treatment is picking the lesser of two evils.

In the words of a 33-year-old woman describing 11 years of intensifying symptoms:

Doctors seemed unsympathetic about the fact that by this point I was in almost constant pain. They suggested that I try to get pregnant; I mentioned that intercourse was now quite painful. They shrugged and suggested a few drinks or a few aspirins a day.

Some women, searching for cure and relief from pain (sometimes they have to use prescription pain-

killers for extended periods of time) have turned to alternative forms of healing—visualization, meditation, acupuncture, chiropractic, homeopathy, herbs, and nutritional therapies among them. The Endometriosis Association has found that certain alternative forms of healing can be quite successful for endometriosis. Contact the Association for more information.

In gathering and sharing information, the Association works to build mutual support so that women will not feel isolated. Together we hope to continue our support, education, and research to find better solutions and cures and to recognize endometriosis as the serious health problem that it is.

FEMALE CIRCUMCISION (FEMALE GENITAL MUTILATION)

Female circumcision, also known as female genital mutilation (FGM), is the cutting of parts of a girl's genitals as a ritual of her rite of passage to womanhood in some cultures. The practice is currently known in 28 African countries and among some minorities in Asia. In many African countries and communities, people have never heard of the practice.

There are three basic types of FGM: Type I, or clitoridectomy; Type II, clitoridectomy and removal of the labia minora; and Type III, infibulation, which involves some degree of cutting, as in Types I and II, plus stitching the labia majora to create a hood of skin that covers the urethra and part of the vaginal opening.

FGM has been associated with both immediate and long-term health complications. The immediate complications include excessive bleeding and shock. The long-term health complications of Types I and II are abscess formation, scar neuromas, dermoid cysts, keloids, recurrent urinary tract infections, painful sexual intercourse, and vulval adhesions creating pseudoinfibulation. Additional complications due to the obstruction of the urethra and vagina by scar tissue that may occur in Type III are urine retention and urethral and bladder stones, irregular prolonged menstrual flow, dysmenorrhea, chronic urinary tract infections, and chronic pelvic inflammatory infection, which often leads to scarring of the fallopian tubes and infertility. Since some women who have experienced these complications may not understand the link with their circumcision, health care practitioners need to be prepared to discuss this matter when they observe evidence of FGM.

The U.S. has witnessed a surge of African refugees and immigrants in the last decade because of wars and famine in Africa. The Centers for Disease Control estimate that approximately 168,000 women who have been circumcised or were at risk of being circumcised lived in the U.S. in 1990.* A study by a New York group showed that 28,300 African immigrant women live in New York State. Whatever the exact numbers are, there is little doubt that thousands of women with

* The CDC admits that these estimates are based on very crude calculations and are most likely inaccurate.

FGM are living in the U.S. Many need help to adjust to the sexual norms and pressures on women in this country. Many seek reproductive health care in an environment that at best does not understand them and at worst condemns them by being condescending and alienating.

The media and popular attention to the issue of FGM have focused on the "quick fix" of passing legislation to protect innocent children. While passing laws may be useful, they do not necessarily address the needs of African women. The idea that the state or the majority community can protect children from their own families is unacceptable to many and is probably not even feasible. The best way to prevent circumcision of girls in this country and elsewhere is to empower women to protect their own children. A starting point is to gain the trust of women by providing much-needed health services. Group and individual counseling could help some women come to terms with their fears, denials, and sense of shame about their own circumcision. Women who learn to stay healthy with their circumcisions while rejecting the practice are the best protectors of their own and others' children in the community.

African women who have experienced circumcision need to come together to counsel each other and develop a sense of power from their solidarity. They may also want to talk to women from other cultures who have experienced other forms of violence and abuse to learn from their experience of healing themselves. The important thing is to understand that any of us can be abused by her family or society and that we can help each other heal. Many African women say that the pain they experience from the way they are treated in the U.S. because of the fact they have had FGM is greater than any pain that they experienced because of the operation itself.*

HEART DISEASE, HEART ATTACK, HYPERTENSION, STROKE, AND OTHER VASCULAR DISORDERS

Hypertension, or high blood pressure, and atherosclerosis (sometimes called hardening of the arteries) are diseases that increase women's risk of heart disease and stroke, the leading causes of death in women over age 50. During the past few years, medical scientists have discovered many differences in the way women and men are treated for heart disease. For example, women are often referred for coronary bypass surgery at a later stage of disease than men, and this may be what accounts for their higher death rate from this surgery. Women also receive less complete diagnostic work-ups and are less likely than men to receive coronary bypass surgery. Researchers have found that women who have had heart attacks had many more risk factors and suffered more chest pain

* For more information and resources, contact RAINB♀ (see Resources).

before their heart attack than men but were only about half as likely to have had a cardiac catheterization to assess their heart disease. Dr. Bernadine Healy, a past director of the National Institutes of Health, believes that the new research provides evidence of sex bias in the management of coronary heart disease. What is unclear is whether women are undertreated or men overtreated. Although less attention is focused on the lack of research on hypertension and atherosclerosis in women, these underlying disease conditions are equally ignored by medical researchers.

Many people think of men, not women, as having heart attacks. Most research on the subject has been on men; yet, older men and women (over 60) have similar rates of heart attack. Heart disease is the most frequent cause of death in women over the age of 50. In the Framingham heart study, one of the few longitudinal studies of heart disease in women, 45% of the women with symptomatic heart attacks died within one year, compared with only 10% of the men. Stroke remains the third most common cause of death in the U.S. Black women have a 43% higher death rate from stroke than white women. Stroke is directly related to high blood pressure, which becomes much more common after menopause.

Fortunately, a major research effort funded by the National Institutes of Health—the Women's Health Initiative—will help answer many important questions about heart disease in women. Large-scale, randomized clinical trials are addressing the benefits of hormone therapy, the role of low-fat diets, and other factors affecting heart disease.

What Are These Diseases?

Many forms of heart and circulatory diseases are related to atherosclerosis, a slowly developing disease process in which the passageway through the arteries becomes narrowed and roughened by fatty deposits called plaques. In the most common type of heart disease, called coronary artery disease or ischemic heart disease, the development of plaque blocks one or more of the arteries that supply the heart muscle with blood. When sufficient blood can no longer reach the heart, part of the heart dies from lack of oxygen and other nutrients. This is a "heart attack," or what physicians call a myocardial infarction (MI), coronary thrombosis, or coronary occlusion. When the artery blockage is partial or complete, it may cause chest pain, a condition referred to as angina.

Atherosclerosis can also lead to a narrowing of the blood vessels that supply blood to the brain. Called a stroke, or cerebral hemorrhage, this leads to the death of that part of the brain.

Less common types of circulatory disease are congenital heart disease, phlebitis, valvular heart disease, and cardiomyopathy, including both hypertrophic (thickened heart) and dilated cardiomyopathy. The causes are different for all, and some may lead to congestive heart failure or to arrhythmia (irregular heartbeats).

Who Is at Risk?

The more of the following risk factors you have, the more likely you are to develop atherosclerosis and subsequent heart disease, circulatory problems, or stroke. The first five are the best-established risk factors at present.

- Over age 50 (heart attack is uncommon in women under 50)
- Smoking
- High blood pressure (hypertension)
- Elevated serum (blood) cholesterol (and low HDL cholesterol)
- Diabetes
- Sedentary lifestyle
- Family history of coronary artery disease
- Hysterectomy with removal of both ovaries before age 45 (see p. 664)
- Certain "personality" factors (habitual impatience, hostility, anger, high competitive drive) and stress
- Taking oral contraceptives (particularly if the woman also smokes) (see chapter 13, Birth Control)
- Absence of a social network

Prevention

Considering the seriousness of these diseases, we are disturbed that so few resources are directed toward prevention, compared with emergency care and treatment. We are also concerned that very little is known about how to prevent heart disease and stroke specifically in women. The "experts" have assumed until very recently that what is good for men must be good for women, too. Reducing the risk of heart disease and stroke is very similar to reducing the risk of hypertension. Consider rethinking your current health practices in the following areas:

1. *Smoking.* The more you smoke, the more likely you are to have a heart attack. Women who smoke have at least four times the risk of heart disease as nonsmokers. The risks return to baseline within two to five years of cessation (stopping). Women smokers who take oral contraceptives have a fourfold increase in risk of developing cardiovascular disease. We urge you to give up smoking. For particulars on women and smoking, see chapter 3, Alcohol, Tobacco, and Other Mood-Altering Drugs.

2. *Diet.* Diet is an important factor in preventing heart disease, if it reduces "bad cholesterol," the low-density lipoproteins (LDLs), and increases "good" high-density lipoproteins (HDLs). LDL is associated with coronary heart disease risk, whereas HDLs appear to protect against heart disease in men in whom it has been studied. The relationship between diet and LDLs and HDLs is not yet fully understood, but eating saturated fats tends to raise LDLs, so cutting back on these fats (see chapter 2, Food, p. 48) may help prevent heart disease. However, the food industry has been capitalizing on the low-cholesterol issue by promoting highly processed hydrogenated foodstuffs as beneficial because they are polyunsaturated. On the contrary, when polyunsaturated vegetable oils are hydrogenated (solidified—for example, to form margarine), they are converted to trans fats, which are now strongly linked to a range of health problems, including atherosclerosis. It's wise to avoid such products. Eating fruits and vegetables—at least five servings a day—plays a key role in preventing heart disease.

Current medical advice to avoid foods high in cholesterol and saturated fats may pose problems for women. In an effort to reduce fat intake, some women may eliminate or cut back on dairy products, which may be their main source of calcium. (Inadequate calcium is a factor in the development of osteoporosis and possibly hypertension.)

3. *High blood pressure.* Preventing or treating high blood pressure (see p. 648) will reduce the risk of both heart attack and stroke.

4. *Exercise.* Regular exercise is believed to reduce the risk of heart attack, can definitely lower blood pressure, and in some cases raises beneficial HDL cholesterol levels (see chapter 4, Women in Motion). Women who are sedentary and get little physical activity have three times the risk of heart disease than those who exercise even moderately three days a week.

5. *Weight.* Excess weight may increase cholesterol and blood sugar levels and blood pressure, which increases the risk of heart disease and stroke. A combination of general weight reduction and exercise can be an important strategy for reducing the risk of cardiovascular and circulatory disease in women.

6. *Oral contraceptives.* Women over 40 who use oral contraceptives appear to have an increased risk of heart attack and stroke. If you have other risk factors, including smoking, hypertension, or a family history of cardiovascular disease, carefully consider your decision to use oral contraceptives.

7. *Estrogen "replacement therapy."* Controversy continues over the benefits of ERT for preventing heart disease. There is speculation that women's rate of heart disease rises rapidly after menopause when women lose the protective effect of estrogen. The current thinking is that giving estrogens after menopause decreases the LDL level and increases the HDL level, increasing the body's ability to cleanse itself of cholesterol that could be deposited in arteries. The NIH-sponsored Women's Health Initiative will be providing more infor-

mation on the risks and benefits of hormone therapy.

8. *Stress reduction.* The effects of work-related stress on heart disease in women have not been researched adequately, but it is theorized that multiple role demands on women may increase the risk of heart disease. All stress is implicated in cardiovascular disease. Changing one's life circumstances may not always be possible, but women can often moderate the effects by using stress reduction techniques.

9. For women who already have a history of cardiovascular problems (such as a prior heart attack), *low doses of aspirin* can provide effective secondary prevention.

10. *Regular medical examinations.* Try to get to know your doctor well enough to feel comfortable calling to report possible symptoms of heart disease. In addition to checking blood pressure and cholesterol (the latter at least once every five years), some physicians suggest periodic electrocardiograms to detect "silent" heart attack; over one-third of all heart attacks in women go unreported. Researchers have noted, however, that even when heart disease is detected by noninvasive diagnostic procedures, doctors are less likely to refer women than men for followup diagnostic procedures. Both women and health care providers need to alter their perception of the seriousness of cardiovascular disease symptoms in women.

Heart Attack

Recognizing the Signs of Heart Attack

Unfortunately, the first sign of heart disease can be sudden death from a heart attack. One-fourth of all people who have heart attacks had no previous warning or knowledge of heart disease, and 60% of heart-attack deaths occur before the person reaches the hospital.

Some describe the pain as vise-like or constricting, like a rope being pulled around their chest. Others describe the pain as feeling like a heavy weight crushing their chest. It is useful to know that chest pain can also come from conditions other than heart attack.* Heart pains that occur with exertion but go away with rest indicate angina, a condition that may not be immediately life-threatening but should be evaluated by a physician.

Shooting pains that last a few seconds are common

in young people, and a "catching" sensation at the end of a deep breath usually does not need attention. Chest-wall pain, rarely present at the same time as a heart attack, can often be identified by pressing a finger on the spot, which increases the pain. Hyperventilation (too rapid breathing that changes the carbon dioxide balance in the blood) can cause both dizziness and chest pain.

Getting Help

IF YOU OR ANYONE YOU ARE WITH EXPERIENCES HEART-ATTACK SYMPTOMS, CALL A PHYSICIAN OR AMBULANCE OR GO TO A HOSPITAL IMMEDIATELY. DO NOT WAIT TO SEE WHETHER THE SYMPTOMS GO AWAY! As women, we may be afraid of being seen as "hysterical" or feel that we will be ridiculed for going to the hospital unless we have something "really serious." To ignore heart-attack symptoms is to risk our lives.

Most cities have ambulances staffed by paramedics who are trained to administer cardiopulmonary resuscitation (CPR)† and to monitor the heart rate and rhythm and administer intravenous drugs on the order of physicians with whom they are in contact by radio. It is important to keep calm. Medical personnel often give the person an analgesic drug such as morphine to induce relaxation and relieve chest pain. Oxygen may also be given.

Most urban hospitals have special coronary care units where sudden changes in the rhythm of the heart can be detected immediately and treated, reducing both damage to the heart and the likelihood of death. Every effort should be made to seek emergency medical care from a well-equipped and well-staffed hospital.

Treatments

For women who have had a heart attack or who have been diagnosed as having coronary artery disease or angina, there are two approaches to treatment: medical and surgical. Within the medical and scientific communities, there is considerable controversy over the relative effectiveness of these two approaches.

Coronary bypass surgery, popular in recent years, is done primarily to relieve chest pain. Coronary bypass surgery involves removing a vein from the leg or a mammary artery and attaching it to the coronary artery to "bypass" the obstructed area. Some people experience dramatic relief of pain and can lead physically active lives after surgery. There is no evidence, however, that surgery increases life expectancy, except for those with left main artery disease and severe three-vessel disease. A less invasive and less expensive alter-

---

* Chest pain can also come from muscles in the chest, the lungs, the diaphragm, the spine, the esophagus, or organs in the upper abdomen. Often it is difficult even for medical practitioners to determine the pain's precise origin.

† CPR is an emergency procedure combining mouth-to-mouth resuscitation and closed-chest heart massage. In some U.S. cities, CPR is credited with saving as many as 200 lives a year. To learn CPR, call your local chapter of the American Red Cross or American Heart Association.

native to bypass surgery is angioplasty: a small balloon is inserted and inflated at the site of the obstruction to clear a partially blocked artery. This procedure sometimes needs to be repeated, but it offers the possibility of avoiding more major surgery.

Several excellent studies have shown that more conservative treatment is equal or superior to bypass surgery for most people. This medical approach to treatment focuses on heart conditioning: a program of progressively more strenuous exercise combined with a low-fat diet, relaxation techniques, and drug therapy. Blood pressure is lowered, and participants are urged to stop smoking. (For some participants, any exercise at all is dangerous.)

Before having bypass surgery or angioplasty, even for seemingly intractable pain, a woman may want to consult with a cardiologist who specializes in the medical treatment of heart disease. If your family doctor or a clinic refers you to a heart surgeon who advises surgery, try to get a second opinion from a medically oriented cardiologist who is not part of your surgeon's immediate colleague network. This will ensure that you get a truly different treatment perspective. A final note of caution: The death rates for heart surgery vary enormously from hospital to hospital. Generally, well-known university-affiliated medical centers with specialized coronary surgery teams have the best records. The more frequently the teams operate, the less often their patients die. Never consider undergoing bypass surgery at a hospital where fewer than 200 bypass operations are performed each year (see the section on surgery, p. 596).

Hypertension

Hypertension (high blood pressure) is sometimes called the "silent killer" because it is often symptomless and, when untreated, can lead to heart disease and strokes, the leading cause of death of both men and women in the U.S. Untreated, it can also affect the brain and eyes and cause serious problems during pregnancy.

About 20% of women of all ages in this country develop hypertension at some point in their lives. (Even children may do so.) No one yet knows how hypertension in women 35 and under affects life expectancy—an increasingly important question as larger numbers of women who are or have been taking oral contraceptives move into this age range. (About 25% of all women who use oral contraceptives develop hypertension.) In addition, blood pressure tends to rise naturally with age.

Women of color, especially black women, have a higher incidence of hypertension than white women. This probably is due to a combination of environmental, behavioral, dietary, stress, and genetic factors.

Symptoms

Severe cases of hypertension may be accompanied by warning symptoms such as headache, dizziness, fainting spells, ringing in the ears, and nosebleeds. However, most women have no symptoms of hypertension, so periodic blood pressure readings are important to ensure detection of hypertension in the early stages.

Cause

Approximately 5% of all cases of high blood pressure are caused by glandular or hormonal abnormalities. But in the other 95%, no single obvious cause is found. This is called essential hypertension. Causes other than oral contraceptives and smoking are still being investigated, including diet, properties of the water supply, and the person's size, stress, behavioral patterns, and heredity. Many of these factors may interact to cause hypertension.

Diet, and excess salt intake in particular, is thought to play a key role in causing hypertension. The average American diet contains ten to 15 grams of sodium a day (about five to ten times as much salt as our bodies need). Meat and dairy products contain a fair amount of salt naturally, and canned and processed foods, fast foods, snacks, and soft drinks have large amounts of salt added during processing.

Cadmium, a trace element found in white-flour products and in many water supplies, has been strongly linked to hypertension. Hypertension is much more common in areas where water is soft because of cadmium.

Research shows that those of us who are very overweight are at increased risk for developing hypertension. The stress associated with being fat in a "thin" society may also be an important factor. Although some studies show that losing weight can be effective in controlling hypertension, others indicate that regular exercise is much more important than the amount of weight loss.

Stress is also linked to hypertension. When we are under pressure or tense, blood pressure, breathing rate, and heartbeat all tend to increase. When our lives are continually stressful, we have a greater chance of developing high blood pressure.

Finally, those of us with a family history of hypertension are at somewhat greater risk.

Diagnosis

Blood pressure is described by two numbers (for example, 120/70). The top number is the systolic pressure (the force of the blood in the arteries when the heart is pumping blood out). The bottom number is the diastolic pressure (the force of the blood in the arteries when the heart is at rest between beats). In general, a systolic pressure of above 140 or a diastolic pressure above 90 is considered a sign of hypertension.

Blood pressure varies with the time of day, activity, and stress. Only a consistent elevation of the blood pressure is considered hypertension. At least three elevated blood pressure readings, taken days or weeks apart, should be obtained before hypertension is diagnosed and treated. Some researchers think that a diagnosis of mild or borderline hypertension should be delayed until consistent readings have been obtained over several years, since slightly elevated blood pressures fall by themselves within a few years in a majority of cases. Also, since women normally have higher blood pressure than men, the distinction between normal and borderline hypertension is difficult to interpret. For example, it is normal for blood pressure to rise during pregnancy (temporarily) and after menopause and for it to fluctuate more as part of the aging process.

Because the stress related to a medical exam or procedure may raise blood pressure, make an effort to check your blood pressure when you are not anxious —perhaps at home, at work, or at a neighborhood health center. Large women should be sure to use a cuff big enough to fit around the arm; otherwise, they may get a falsely high reading. Taking blood pressure is an easy skill to learn. Kits with stethoscope and blood pressure cuffs are available in drugstores and many discount and department stores. Increasingly, libraries, senior centers, and shopping centers are also providing this screening service—but don't rely on coin-operated machines, which can give false readings.

Prevention and Self-Help Treatments

You can often prevent hypertension in several simple ways and also lower mildly raised blood pressure —enough, in many cases, to eliminate the need for potentially risky drug treatments.

1. Diet is probably the single most important factor in preventing and treating mild hypertension. Gradually restrict your salt intake by avoiding processed foods and eliminating salt during cooking and at the table. Replace white flour with whole grains whenever possible, and make sure to include enough protein, potassium, and calcium in your diet (see chapter 2, Food). Eating garlic can also help to prevent or reduce slightly elevated blood pressure. Keep your alcohol consumption down to 2 ounces a day or less. Some people also recommend vitamin B and potassium supplements to help the body excrete excess fluids and sodium.

2. Avoid smoking. Studies show that smoking contributes to hypertension.

3. Get together with people in your community to investigate the water supply. If you find that it contains cadmium, try to eat less of this trace mineral in foods (especially white-flour products).

4. Avoid combination oral contraceptives and other estrogens. If you do take the Pill, insist on finding out your blood pressure both before starting and a few months afterward. If your blood pressure is high, don't take the Pill; if it rises, switch to another contraceptive.

5. Regular aerobic exercise (such as fast walking, jogging, or bicycling) often brings elevated blood pressures down to normal.

6. Losing weight if you are very large can prevent or lower high blood pressure. It is most effective in conjunction with exercise. Crash dieting, however, is not recommended.

7. Try to reduce stress in your life. Biofeedback, meditation, and relaxation techniques may help.

Medical Treatments

When the above methods do not work or hypertension becomes severe, you may need drugs. Diuretics, which eliminate water from the tissues, are the most commonly used. Diuretics can have side effects that lead to digestive disorders and exhaustion. They may also affect cholesterol and blood glucose levels. Newer drugs include beta-blockers, angiotensin inhibitors, and calcium channel blockers. These drugs reduce the constriction of the arteries, modify the amount of blood pumped from the heart, or relax the blood vessels. Often a combination of drugs is used. (See chapter 25, The Politics of Women's Health and Medical Care, p. 713, for guidelines in taking drugs.) Hypertension drugs treat only the symptoms of the disease; they do not cure it. You will probably have to take medication for life. Be cautious when physicians recommend drug therapy without attempting less risky methods first. If your hypertension is severe, you will have to evaluate the risk of taking medication against the benefits of preventing a crippling or life-threatening stroke.

Stroke

Because high blood pressure is easily detectable and treatable, stroke is among the most preventable of the causes of death. Yet, true prevention, as described in the previous section, must begin before high blood pressure appears.

Strokes may be very mild—so mild that you or your medical practitioner may not recognize them. They may cause only minor or temporary impairment. These are called transient ischemic attacks (TIAs). When an artery bursts because of high blood pressure, aneurysm, or other causes, either damaging part of the brain or impairing its function because of the pressure of pooled blood, the result is a cerebral hemorrhage. Depending on the type of stroke you have, if you survive, you may experience speech loss, paralysis, or other loss of mental and physical function. Rehabilitation and therapy sometimes achieve remarkable results by helping undamaged parts of the brain to "take over." In only one group of patients—those with obstruction of the left main coronary artery—does surgery improve the chances of survival.

Signs of Stroke or TIA

Any one or more of the symptoms listed in the box call for action, even though they may happen over several hours. Go immediately to a hospital emergency room, or call your regular physician. While less can be done to save a life than in the case of heart attack, prompt treatment may reduce impairment, prevent another stroke, and maximize future functioning.

TOXIC SHOCK SYNDROME

Toxic shock syndrome (TSS) is a rare but serious disease that mainly strikes menstruating women under 30 who are using tampons. Menstrual sponges, contraceptive sponges, and diaphragms used during the menses have also been associated with TSS. Although only a small number of menstruating women have gotten TSS (one to 17 per 100,000 menstruating women), a few of them have died. An increasing number of non–tampon-related cases are showing up in postoperative (male and female) and postpartum patients in hospitals.

TSS is probably caused by a strain of the bacterium *Staphylococcus aureus,* which infects some part of the body, often the vagina, and produces toxins (poisons) that go into the bloodstream, causing a bodily reaction. No one yet knows why some women with *S. aureus* bacteria in their vaginas get TSS and others don't. The following appear to increase the risk of TSS: using higher-absorbency tampons (and leaving tampons in for many hours), postoperative or postpartum infection, and leaving barrier contraceptives (such as the sponge and diaphragm) in the vagina more than 24 hours.

This disease is a syndrome, or group of symptoms. At present, only those people who have all the symp-

---

SYMPTOMS OF STROKE

1. Numbness; tingling; weakness or loss of strength in an arm, leg, or side of the face; or difficulty walking.
2. Blindness in one or both eyes.
3. Speech problems.
4. Intense, mounting headache lasting many hours.
5. Acute, unexplained loss of balance.

---

toms are officially counted as having TSS. However, there are reports of people with a few of the symptoms who may have a milder form of the same disease. The symptoms are as follows:

- A high fever, usually over 102°F.
- Vomiting.
- Diarrhea.
- A sudden drop in blood pressure that may lead to shock.
- A sunburn-like rash that peels after a while. The rashes are easiest to see on a person's trunk and neck, and the peeling is obvious on the palms of the hands or the soles of the feet.

Treatments

If you get any of the aforementioned symptoms during your period and you are using a tampon, remove it immediately. Do not use tampons or any other internal method for catching menstrual blood until you get a culture showing that you have no *S. aureus* in your vagina. TSS can progress extremely rapidly, within hours. It's a good idea to get in touch right away with a medical person, preferably at a medical facility, who can keep track of what is happening to you. For a mild case, the most important thing is to drink lots of fluids and rest if possible.

TSS involving severe dehydration or very low blood pressure may require hospitalization. Although antibiotics do not seem to affect the symptoms once the disease has started, they can still significantly reduce the chance of recurrence. Because this type of *S. aureus* is resistant to penicillin and ampicillin, beta-lactamase–resistant antistaphylococcal antibiotics must be used.

URINARY TRACT INFECTIONS

Urinary tract infections (UTIs) are so common that most of us get at least one at some point in our lives. They are usually caused by bacteria, such as *Escherichia coli,* which travel from the colon to the urethra and bladder (and occasionally to the kidneys). Trichomoniasis and chlamydial infection can also cause UTIs; low resistance, poor diet, stress, and damage to the urethra from childbirth, surgery, catheterization, and so on can predispose you to getting them. Often a sudden increase in sexual activity triggers symptoms ("honeymoon cystitis"). Pregnant women are especially susceptible, as pressure of the growing fetus keeps some urine in the bladder and ureters, allowing bacteria to grow. Postmenopausal women are also susceptible because of hormonal changes. Very occasionally, UTI is caused by an anatomical abnormality or a prolapsed (fallen) urethra or bladder, most common in older women or women who have had many children.

Cystitis (inflammation or infection of the bladder) is by far the most common UTI in women. While the symptoms can be frightening, cystitis in itself is not usually serious. If you suddenly have to urinate every few minutes and it burns like crazy even though almost nothing comes out, you probably have cystitis. There may also be blood in the urine (hematuria) and pus in the urine (pyuria). You may have pain just above your pubic bone, and sometimes there is a peculiar, heavy urine odor when you first urinate in the morning.

It is also possible to get mild temporary symptoms (such as urinary frequency) without actually having an infection, simply because of drinking too much coffee or tea (both are diuretics), premenstrual syndrome, food allergies, vaginitis, anxiety, or irritation to the area from bubble baths, soaps, or douches. Vaginitis can also cause similar symptoms. As long as you are in good health and not pregnant, you can usually treat mild symptoms yourself for 24 hours before consulting a practitioner. Cystitis often disappears without treatment. If it persists more than 48 hours, recurs frequently, or is ever accompanied by chills, fever, vomiting, or pain in the kidneys (near the middle of the back), consult a medical practitioner. These symptoms suggest that infection has spread to the kidneys, resulting in pyelonephritis, a serious problem that requires medical treatment. Some researchers estimate that 30 to 50% of women with cystitis symptoms also have silent kidney infections. Consult your medical practitioner if cystitis symptoms are accompanied by any of the following: blood or pus in the urine, pain on urination during pregnancy, diabetes or chronic illness, or a history of kidney infection or diseases or abnormalities of the urinary tract. Untreated chronic infections can lead to serious complications, such as high blood pressure or premature births (if they occur during pregnancy).

Diagnosis

When cystitis does not respond to self-help treatments within 24 hours or recurs frequently, get a urine test. An ordinary urinalysis is not sufficient to test for cystitis—make sure your medical practitioner takes a clean voided specimen* and does a pelvic exam to

* Wash the area carefully, urinate a little, then collect the rest of your urine in a sterile jar.

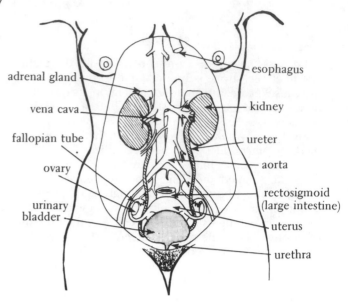

Nina Reimer

rule out other infections. Your urine will be examined for evidence of blood and pus and a culture will be taken. Sometimes, even when you have symptoms, the culture may come back negative (i.e., not show a cause of the infection). False-negative cultures may be due to mishandling or overly dilute urine; you may also get a false negative report if your cystitis is caused by something other than bacterial infection, such as anxiety or stress. On the other hand, a negative culture accompanied by white blood cells in the urine (called acute urethral syndrome) may indicate a chlamydial infection. (See chapter 14, Sexually Transmitted Diseases.) Sometimes women have bacteria in their urine (bacteriuria) without symptoms. If bacteriuria shows up during a routine urine test, you should be treated with antibiotics to prevent kidney infection and other complications.

A sensitivity test, which shows what kind of antibiotics to use, is not always necessary unless there is a large number of bacteria in the urine or you have had many infections or severe symptoms indicating pyelonephritis. Women who have had pyelonephritis repeatedly should be tested for abnormalities of the urinary tract. The usual test is an intravenous pyelogram (IVP) in which a dye injected into the bloodstream collects in the kidneys, showing any blockages or obstructions on an X ray. Ultrasound of the kidneys can identify cysts and tumors.

Treatments

For symptoms that are severe or indicate a kidney infection, medications are usually started immediately. For milder infections, many medical practitioners prefer to wait for culture results before prescribing a drug.

Most UTIs respond rapidly to a variety of antibiotics. Drugs commonly used include antibiotics such as

PREVENTING UTIs, TREATING MILD INFECTIONS AND AVOIDING REINFECTIONS

1. Drink lots of fluid every day. Try to drink a glass of water every two or three hours. (For an active infection, drink enough to enable you to pour out a good stream of urine every hour. It really helps!)

2. Urinate frequently and try to empty your bladder completely each time. Never try to hold your urine once your bladder feels full.

3. Keep the bacteria in your bowels and anus away from your urethra by wiping yourself from front to back after urinating or having a bowel movement. Wash your genitals from front to back with plain water or very mild soap at least once a day.

4. Any sexual activity that irritates the urethra, puts pressure on the bladder, or spreads bacteria from the anus to the vagina or urethra can contribute to cystitis. Make sure that you and your lover have clean hands and genitals before sex, and wash after contact with the anal area before touching the vagina or urethra. To prevent irritation to the urethra, try to avoid prolonged direct clitoral stimulation and pressure on the urethral area during oral-genital sex or masturbation. Make sure your vagina is well lubricated before intercourse. Rear-entry positions and prolonged vigorous intercourse tend to put additional stress on the urethra and bladder. Emptying your bladder before and immediately after sex is a good idea; so is having a glass of water. If you tend to get cystitis after sex despite these precautions, you may want to ask your medical practitioner for preventive tablets (i.e., sulfa, ampicillin, nitrofurantoin); a single dose of a tablet after sex has been shown effective in preventing infections and is usually not associated with the same negative effects as prolonged courses of antibiotics.

5. Some birth control methods can contribute to or aggravate a UTI. Women taking oral contraceptives have a higher rate of cystitis than those not taking the Pill. Some diaphragm users find that the rim pressing against the urethra can contribute to infection. (A different-size diaphragm or one with a different type of rim may solve this problem.) Contraceptive foams or vaginal suppositories may irritate the urethra. Dry condoms may put pressure on the urethra, or the dyes or lubricants may cause irritation.

6. If you use sanitary napkins during your period, the blood on the pad provides a convenient bridge for bacteria from your anus to travel to your urethra. Change pads frequently, and wash your genitals twice a day when you are menstruating. Some women also find that tampons or sponges put pressure on the urethra.

7. Tight jeans, bicycling, or horseback riding may cause trauma to the urethra. When you engage in sports that can provoke cystitis in you, wear loose clothing and try to drink extra water.

8. Caffeine and alcohol irritate the bladder. If you don't want to stop using them, try to drink less of them, and drink enough water to dilute them.

9. Some women find that the routine use of unsweetened cranberry juice, cranberry concentrate supplements, or vitamin C to make their urine more acidic helps to prevent urinary tract problems. The hippuric acid in cranberry juice also helps prevent bacteria from sticking to the bladder lining (mucosa). (If you have an infection, try combining 500 milligrams of vitamin C with cranberry juice four times a day; you can substitute a half cup of fresh cranberries in plain yogurt for the juice.) Whole grains, meats, nuts, and many fruits also help to acidify the urine. Avoid strong spices such as curry, cayenne, chili, and black pepper.

10. Diets high in refined sugars and starches (white flour, white rice, pasta, etc.) may predispose some women to urinary tract infections.

11. Women use a wide variety of herbal remedies to prevent or treat UTIs. Drinking teas made of uva ursi, horsetail or shavegrass, barberry, echinacea, cornsilk, cleavers, lemon balm, or goldenseal may be beneficial to the bladder. You may want to consult an herbalist.

12. Keep up your resistance by eating and resting well and by finding ways to reduce stress in your life as much as possible.

13. Vitamin B_6 and magnesium-calcium supplements help to relieve spasm of the urethra that can predispose to cystitis. This is especially helpful for women who need to have their urethras dilated repeatedly.

ampicillin, nitrofurantoin, tetracycline, sulfonamides (Gantrisin), or Bactrim. (Women who may be glucose-6-phosphate dehydrogenase deficient should not take sulfonamides; see "Hereditary and Other Types of Anemia," p. 599.) The medication may be given in a single large dose or may be spread out over three to ten days. If symptoms persist for more than two days after you start taking drugs, see your medical practitioner again. (You may have organisms resistant to the antibiotics you are using.)

Antibiotics often cause diarrhea and vaginal yeast infections. Eating plain yogurt or taking acidophilus in capsule, liquid, or granule form helps to prevent this diarrhea by replacing the normal bacteria in your intestines killed by the drugs. See p. 668 for information on preventing and relieving vaginal infections.

To alleviate the pain associated with UTIs, you might try acetaminophen. Some practitioners recommend a prescription drug called Pyridium, a local anesthetic that relieves pain but does not treat the infection itself. (Pyridium dyes the urine a bright orange, which will permanently stain clothing. It also can cause nausea, dizziness, and possibly allergic reactions.)

Your practitioner may recommend other surgical procedures, such as stretching the urethral opening and/or making a slit in the urethra to help drainage (internal urethrotomy). Ask for documentation of the effectiveness of these procedures. Surgery is often recommended to correct a prolapsed bladder or urethra, which can be connected with chronic UTIs. Kegel exercises (see chapter 12, Understanding Our Bodies, p. 274) can forestall the need for this surgery and help prevent future infections.

Even with drugs and/or surgery, many women continue to have recurrent urinary tract infections. Sometimes it helps to treat chronic infections with long-term, low-dose medications.

INTERSTITIAL CYSTITIS

Interstitial cystitis (IC) is a painful and debilitating bladder disease that affects approximately 450,000 people in the U.S., 90% of whom are women. Studies indicate that IC, formerly thought to be a postmenopausal condition, occurs in women of all ages. The average age of onset is approximately 40, and 25% of women who have it are under 30.

IC is an inflammatory condition of the bladder wall whose symptoms are similar to those of the common UTI known as cystitis. However, routine urine cultures are negative, and there is usually no response to antibiotics. The symptoms of IC include pelvic pain and pressure, and the urgent need to urinate, sometimes as often as 60 to 80 times a day. There may also be associated vaginal and rectal pain. Pain during sexual intercourse is common. The symptoms may vary from mild to severe.

Because of confusion in defining and understanding IC, many patients have difficulty obtaining the correct diagnosis. IC may be incorrectly diagnosed as urethral syndrome or trigonitis, or patients may be told that there is nothing wrong and that they have a "sensitive bladder." The diagnosis of IC is usually made by a urologist. A complete battery of urologic tests typically produces negative results. Conditions that have symptoms resembling IC include bladder infections, kidney problems, vaginal infections, endometriosis, and STDs. If no infection is present (i.e., urine cultures are negative), and no other disorder is identified, a cystoscopy should be performed, during which a cystoscope, which allows the urologist to look directly inside the bladder, is inserted into the urethra. This must be done with the patient under regional or general anesthesia so that the bladder may be distended enough to enable the pinpoint hemorrhages characteristic of IC to be seen. A biopsy specimen is taken at this time to rule out bladder cancer.

There is no consistently effective treatment or cure for IC. However, treatments are available that may temporarily alleviate the symptoms. The most commonly used treatments include the following:

1. Bladder distention, in which the bladder is stretched by filling it with water while the patient is under regional or general anesthesia.

2. Oral nonsteroidal anti-inflammatory medication, antispasmodics, and antihistamines.

3. Antidepressants, such as amitriptyline (Elavil), which appear to have antipain properties.

4. Elimination of caffeinated beverages, alcohol, artificial sweeteners, spicy foods, citrus fruits, and tomatoes, which may alleviate the symptoms.

5. Dimethyl sulfoxide (DMSO, Rimso 50), a medication instilled directly into the bladder that acts as an antiinflammatory agent.

6. Sodium pentosanpolysulfate (Elmiron), an oral medication believed to coat the bladder wall and protect it from irritants in the urine. It is now available as an "orphan drug" (FDA-approved in 1996).

7. Oxychlorosene sodium (Clorpactin), which appears to decrease symptoms when placed directly into the bladder. Regional or general anesthesia may be necessary for its instillation.

8. Transcutaneous electrical nerve stimulation (TENS unit), a small portable unit worn on the body that is thought to block pain through low electrical nerve stimulation.

9. Surgery (partial or complete removal of the bladder, or very careful removal of certain nerves leading to the bladder). These surgical procedures pose a substantial risk of complications and should be performed only as a last resort when all other conservative treatments fail.

The Interstitial Cystitis Association (ICA) (see Resources), a patient advocacy group, provides information, education, and support to IC patients and their families. The organization is dedicated to raising funds for research and educating the public as well as the medical community about the disease.

UTERUS AND OVARIES

The Cervix

Cervicitis

"Cervicitis" is a term used loosely to describe an inflammation or infection of the cervix. The majority of Pap tests come back with cervicitis noted, but this does not necessarily represent a true disease or disorder. Cervicitis is occasionally a sign that common vaginal infections, sexually transmitted diseases (STDs), or pelvic inflammatory disease (PID) are present. It can also result from a break in the tissue of the cervix caused by an IUD insertion, abortion, or childbirth.

Depending upon the severity and length of infection, you may notice an increased vaginal discharge, pain with intercourse, an aching sensation in the lower abdomen, and/or the need to urinate more frequently. Very severe infections may also bring fever.

Diagnosis
When you touch your cervix, it may feel warmer and larger than usual. Movement of your cervix with your finger may also be uncomfortable. If you examine yourself with a speculum, your cervix will look red and slightly swollen, and you may observe a discharge. If only the cervical canal is affected, your cervix will look normal, but you may see a yellowish discharge coming from within the cervical opening.

If you go to a medical practitioner for an internal exam, be sure to tell him or her whether or not your discharge is normal. (Sometimes scar tissue and normal discharge is mistaken for cervicitis.) A culture and wet mount will determine whether the cause of the infection is bacteria or an STD. In some cases, a Pap smear will also be taken to rule out the possibility of cervical cancer.

Medical Treatments
If tests show that an STD such as gonorrhea, syphilis, or chlamydial infection is responsible, you will get oral or injected antibiotics. For mild cervicitis involving no STDs, medical treatment may be pointless, as the condition is not serious and is likely to return after treatment. For more severe cases, some physicians recommend cryosurgery or electrocautery. Use them only as a last resort, as they can be painful, can lead to fertility problems, and may take about six weeks for healing. Cervicitis unrelated to an STD (see chapter 14, Sexually Transmitted Diseases) need not be treated for the most part.

Self-Help Treatments
When symptoms are mild and not related to PID or serious STDs, the following remedies may help: goldenseal douche (1/4 teaspoon to 1 quart of water two times a day for two to three weeks), vitamin C douche (500 milligrams in 1 quart of water daily for three to four weeks) or vinegar douche. For more information on herbal remedies, see Resources.

To speed healing and strengthen the immune system and for future prevention, you may want to try oral doses of vitamin C (500 to 1,000 milligrams a day), zinc (25 milligrams a day), and vitamin E (400 milligrams a day). You can also apply vitamin E directly to your cervix with your finger. You can use slippery elm as a douche or paste, applied directly to the cervix in a diaphragm or on the end of a tampon.

No matter what treatment you use, try to combine it with extra rest and good nutrition. Avoid using tampons during menstruation.

Cervical Eversion

Cervical eversion (also called ectropion) is a common condition in which the tissue that lines the cervical canal grows on the outer vaginal portion of the cervix, making it red with a bumpy-looking texture smooth to the touch. It has almost a band-like appearance. Eversion requires no treatment unless it is accompanied by infection. Those of us whose mothers took DES during pregnancy are more likely to have a large eversion.

Most women do not have any symptoms; in those who do, the most frequent sign is a slightly increased nonirritating vaginal discharge. For common eversion, no biopsy is necessary, unless there is an abnormal Pap smear. If the discharge is bothersome, use the self-help treatments listed under "Cervicitis."

Cervical Erosion

True cervical erosion is rare and looks like a large or small pinkish-red sore on the cervix beside the cervical opening. It causes little discomfort. Most cases referred to as erosion in the past were really eversion.

Diagnosis
The first step in diagnosis is a Pap smear. If abnormal cells are present, some of the cervical tissue is removed and examined under a microscope (a biopsy) to distinguish cervical erosion, which is benign, from cervical cancer.

Medical Treatments
Ordinarily, no treatment is needed. Some physicians may suggest cauterization or cryotherapy, but this should not be done if your Pap smear is normal.

Cervical Polyps

Cervical polyps appear as bright red tube-like protrusions out of the cervical opening, either alone or in clusters. They consist of excess cervical tissue that "heaps up" within the cervical canal. Polyps, which are very common, are often formed as the body attempts to heal itself after a cervical infection by growing new tissue. Most polyps contain many blood vessels with a fragile outer wall, so that bleeding following intercourse, douching, or self-exam may occur. During pregnancy, polyps may also bleed, when hormonal changes stimulate growth of excess cervical tissue.

Medical Treatments

Polyps do not necessarily require treatment. When they are small and there is little or no contact bleeding, you can usually just keep track of them with regular self-exams. You may want to have them removed if your symptoms change or if the polyp begins to grow. Cervical polyps are rarely cancerous. Occasionally, however, they look like cervical cancer and produce similar symptoms. In that case, you can have a Pap smear, colposcopy, and biopsy to tell for sure.

A polyp can be removed in a doctor's office. The practitioner usually twists the polyp off and cauterizes the base. If your polyp is very large or if you have multiple polyps, you may have to go to the hospital for removal. Sometimes polyps recur after removal.

Cervical Intraepithelial Neoplasia (Cervical Dysplasia)

"Dysplasia" means abnormal cell growth; "cervical dysplasia," "cervical intraepithelial neoplasia (CIN)," and "squamous intraepithelial lesion" (SIL) are terms used to describe abnormal cells on or near the cervix. In most cases there are no symptoms, and the condition is detected by a routine Pap smear.

CIN is not cancer and does not develop into cancer in most cases. CIN occurs along a continuum: At one end the cells are all normal, while at the far-distant other end lies invasive cancer. The several stages or classes of CIN along the continuum can be difficult to distinguish: one stage or class blurs into the next, and different laboratories or physicians may "place" a given cell sample differently. Diagnosis is therefore often difficult, and treatment decisions can be controversial and hard to make. Some women with CIN will develop more severe changes (and at varying speeds), whereas most women's cells will return to normal. There is no adequately reliable way to determine in advance which will happen. Therefore, all cases of diagnosed CIN should be treated and/or watched closely with repeated Pap smears and colposcopy.

Because we can't see CIN and we don't know what is going on, we often feel anxious when we receive this diagnosis. There is no need to panic when a Pap smear comes back abnormal. Most cell changes like those of CIN are very slow. Some physicians may want to rush you into treatment. Because the diagnostic tests are not always accurate, and because medical practitioners vary in their diagnoses and preferred treatments, it is very important to get the opinion of a second medical practitioner and a different laboratory about your condition. Most diagnosed cases of CIN are mild, and the cells return to normal spontaneously. We can monitor any changes by more frequent Pap smears or other diagnostic tests.

The results of Pap smears and other diagnostic tests are classified according to how much of the surface tissue (epithelium) of the cervix is affected and what kind and degree of cell changes exist. Four different classification systems are currently in use, but most physicians use the Bethesda/SIL system now in place (see chart below). Many experts now believe that most CIN is caused by the human papillomavirus (HPV), which is very common and also causes genital warts (see chapter 14, Sexually Transmitted Diseases, p. 356).

COMPARISON OF CERVICAL CANCER CLASSIFICATION SYSTEMS

	Class I	Class II	Class III			Class IV	Class V
The class system	Class I	Class II	Class III			Class IV	Class V
Dysplasia	Benign	Atypia	Mild	DYSPLASIA Moderate	Severe	CIS	Invasive Cancer
Cervical intraepithelial neoplasia (CIN)	Benign	Atypia	CIN I	CIN II	CIN III		Invasive cancer
Bethesda/ squamous intraepithelial lesion (SIL)	Benign	Atypia	Low-grade SIL	High-grade SIL			Squamous cell carcinoma

Prevention

1. It is important to monitor your condition with repeated Pap smears or other tests in addition to employing preventive efforts. Studies show that using a barrier method of contraception (such as the condom or diaphragm) rather than oral contraceptives (the Pill) or an IUD may help to prevent CIN. One study showed that for some women already diagnosed as having CIN, the use of condoms was associated with a return of cervical cells to normal.

2. Some sexually transmitted infections and diseases can contribute to abnormal cervical changes. (See chapter 14, Sexually Transmitted Diseases, for methods of prevention.)

3. Eating foods high in vitamin C and/or taking supplements may help prevent CIN or cervical cancer. After a diagnosis of cervical abnormality, taking folic acid (1 milligram per day) and vitamin C (100 milligrams per day) may help reverse the condition.*

4. We must insist on more research into the connection between occupationally and/or environmentally induced abnormalities and CIN, as well as the role of male partners in CIN and cancer.

*Who Is at Risk of CIN (Dysplasia)
or Cervical Cancer?*
We don't yet know the causes of the cellular abnormalities that we call CIN and cervical cancer. However, certain factors may put you at higher risk for these conditions.

1. If you have an HPV infection (see chapter 14, Sexually Transmitted Diseases, p. 356), you are at a higher risk for CIN. The HPV, which causes condyloma warts, can also cause invisible flat lesions on the cervix. These lesions, which can show up as abnormal cervical cells on a Pap smear or can be seen with a colposcope, are probably more common among women than the visible condyloma warts. Increasingly, evidence suggests that both forms of HPV infection are sometimes contributory factors in the onset of cervical cancer.

2. Recent studies suggest that a protein substance in sperm may cause cellular changes in some women. Women whose partners have cancer of the penis are also at greater risk.

3. Being exposed to synthetic hormones (such as DES or the Pill) may increase your chances of devel-

oping CIN or cancer, because it increases the area of the cervix vulnerable to HPV.

4. Studies have linked cervical cancer with smoking.

5. If you began intercourse at an early age, your risks may be greater. Physical changes in the types of cells that line the vagina occur especially during our teens. As we age, more vulnerable softer cells are gradually replaced by tougher (squamocolumnar) cells. If we begin intercourse before those changes are mostly complete, our cells are more vulnerable to whatever may cause cellular changes.

6. If either you or your partner or both of you have multiple sexual partners, or have had them, your risks of developing abnormal cervical cells may be somewhat greater because of a greater chance of exposure to STDs and other pathogens. Barrier contraceptives (especially condoms) may reduce such risks (see chapter 13, Birth Control). We do not fully understand what causes such changes, but the number of sexual partners of a woman's partner (and not just the number of sexual partners of the woman herself) can affect the level of risk for cervical abnormalities. Some women who have had only one sexual partner have developed cellular changes.

7. If you or your partner works at a job that involves contact with carcinogenic substances (such as those in the mining, textile, metal, or chemical industries), you may be at higher risk for cervical abnormalities.

8. Finally, women with low incomes who do not have access to healthful living and working conditions have a much higher incidence of CIN and cancers, and are more likely to develop such problems at an earlier age than middle-class women. This may also be related to the greater occupational hazards faced by some women and/or their partners as well as their lack of access to good nutrition, and medical care, and Pap screening.

Diagnosis
The first step is the Pap smear. If you have any kind of abnormal result, you should have a second Pap smear to confirm that result. Pap smears can produce false-positive or false-negative readings, and labs can be unreliable. If the smear is abnormal a second time, indicating CIN (not just inflammation), then your physician or nurse-practitioner should perform a colposcopy. In many cases, the colposcopy will show no abnormalities. If an abnormality does appear, your physician or nurse-practitioner may perform a tissue (punch) biopsy. Both Pap smears and colposcopies may be repeated for diagnostic monitoring. With mild dysplasia, there is sometimes a spontaneous return to normal cells.

---

* One hundred milligrams per day should prevent any major deficiency of vitamin C, but many women will want to take more if they are often exposed to conditions that destroy vitamin C in their bodies, such as cigarette smoke.

The FDA recently approved automated reinspection of Pap smears as effective. Insurance companies rarely cover the cost of these tests, which we do not consider necessary for women with no history of abnormal Pap smears. However, if you have ever had dysplasia or CIN and/or have family members who have had cervical abnormalities, or if you are a DES daughter (see box, at right), you may want to invest in this test. Call (800) PAPNET-4 (727–6384) for information and addresses of labs equipped to perform it. (Other new systems for improved Pap testing are under current consideration by the FDA.)

Medical Treatments

Treatments for dysplasia and/or CIN vary from very mild to more serious. What you want is to get appropriate treatment for the condition you have and to avoid unnecessary or inappropriate treatment or surgery. Different practitioners may have varying "preferred" treatments for each diagnosis. This is why second and even third opinions may be important in helping you decide on your treatment. It is important that procedures such as colposcopy, punch biopsy and cone biopsy be done by medical practitioners who have had special training, skills, and experience.

The mildest treatment is the "wait and see" approach with repeat Pap smears and/or colposcopy (see p. 595) and punch biopsy. Regular condom use may also help. The next step up the treatment ladder is destruction of abnormal cells by either cryotherapy, laser, loop electrosurgical excision procedure (LEEP) (see p. 596), or a similar technique called LLETZ (large loop excision in the transformation zone, also called ELECTZ).

When repeated Pap smears or colposcopies confirm severe dysplasia or cancer in situ (CIS, or localized cancer), and if the abnormal area extends into the cervical canal (and therefore cannot be reached for colposcopy or cryotherapy), a cone biopsy (conization or conical) is often recommended. The cone-shaped piece of tissue removed by this procedure is examined to ensure that all borders of the abnormal area were removed. If the abnormal area extends beyond the edge of the removed cone, the physician may recommend a second conization to remove a larger area. Hysterectomy is generally recommended as the appropriate treatment for invasive cancer (see p. 663). It involves major surgery and risks and has other health consequences (see p. 664).

Some of these treatments can be uncomfortable and occasionally somewhat painful. After a cone or punch biopsy, cryotherapy, laser treatment, or LEEP, do not use tampons, douche, or have intercourse for at least three weeks. This minimizes both pain and the risk of infection. Some women experience cramping, tenderness, bleeding, and/or discharges.

A cone biopsy involves some risk of future infertility because it may weaken the cervix. A hysterectomy permanently ends a woman's reproductive capacity. Both surgical procedures can be appropriate and can

----

DES DAUGHTERS AND CIN
by Kris Brown

The type of cancer—squamous cell—that CIN may develop into should not be confused with clear-cell cancer, which is linked to DES exposure (see p. 636). It is not known at this point whether DES daughters are or will be at a higher risk for CIN or squamous cell cancer. Still more research is needed.

DES daughters who have received a diagnosis of dysplasia should be aware of two issues:

1. One study of a small number of DES daughters (born primarily between the years of 1947 and 1965) who had cryosurgery showed cervical stenosis (narrowing of the cervical canal, which can affect menstruation and childbirth) in varying degrees of severity. Non–DES-exposed women in the same study did not experience these side effects from cryosurgery.

2. Metaplasia, a normal process whereby tissue changes from one form to another, may be present in a larger area in DES-exposed than in non–DES-exposed women. Why is this important? Some people believe that the changed tissue may be more vulnerable to precancerous or cancerous change, and pathologists may mistakenly interpret the change as abnormal (dysplasia or CIN). Such misdiagnosis can lead to unnecessary treatment and the possible harmful effects of cervical stenosis.

save women's lives. However, if such a treatment is recommended, it is important to seek a second or even third opinion on whether it is appropriate and what other treatment options may be available, especially for severe CIN or cancer in situ.

Abnormal Uterine Bleeding

"Abnormal uterine bleeding" is a term used to describe a variety of unusual bleeding patterns. You may have unusually light or very heavy periods, bleeding or spotting between periods, or cycles that vary widely in length. Abnormal bleeding is frequently due to hormonal changes and is most common in teenagers just beginning to menstruate or women just entering menopause. Many women in their 30s experience light spotting at the time of ovulation, because of the sudden drop in estrogen. Doctors use a particular term, "dysfunctional uterine bleeding," to describe abnormal bleeding due to a menstrual cycle in which ovulation did not occur—an anovulatory cycle. Periods that are less than 21 days apart and that last for seven days or longer are usually classified as "dysfunctional" bleeding. Women who don't ovulate regularly may have late periods and very heavy bleeding because of a buildup of estrogen. Other possible causes of prolonged, heavy, or irregular bleeding include the IUD, birth control pills, PID, abnormal pregnancy, polyps, fibroids, endometriosis, and cervical or uterine cancer. (See the sections on each of these conditions for information on their treatments.)

Heavy bleeding is a pattern particularly common among black women about the time of menopause. Physicians frequently respond to this problem by recommending hysterectomy, a surgical procedure that is usually inappropriate (see p. 663). As more women seek alternative treatments, it is possible that the exceptionally high rate of hysterectomies among black women[9] will drop.

In postmenopausal women, abnormal bleeding may be caused by estrogen replacement therapy, vaginitis, overgrowth of the endometrial tissues (endometrial hyperplasia), or cancer.

Beware of pressure to have surgery for bleeding unless tests show a malignant (cancerous) condition. This is not the same as a "precancerous condition." Do not agree to a hysterectomy unless you have a confirmed diagnosis that warrants it, including a second opinion. Because very heavy or extended bleeding is such a frightening, disruptive, and debilitating symptom, we can easily be convinced that drastic action, such as unnecessary surgery, is warranted. Try talking with other women who have this problem and learn about alternative approaches (see below and chapter 5, Holistic Health and Healing). The most serious health risk you face, once cancer has been ruled out, is that of becoming anemic. So have your hemoglobin checked regularly, and take iron only if your hemoglobin count is low.

Sometimes, even after extensive testing, no clear-cut reason for abnormal bleeding is found.

Self-Help Treatments

If you are premenopausal, you may be able to stabilize your menstrual flow by reducing stress and changing your diet. Cutting down on animal fat and adding fiber helps to restore normal hormonal balance by lowering cholesterol, which is converted to estrogen in your body. Soy protein, which high in phytoestrogens, can regulate periods. In addition, supplements of vitamins A, E, and C with bioflavonoids, as well as zinc, copper, and iodine, can help regulate heavy bleeding. (Take no more than 10,000 IU of vitamin A twice a day, since larger doses of vitamin A can be toxic. One carrot contains 8,000 IU, and dark green leafy vegetables contain a lot, so you may be able to get increased vitamin A through the food you eat.) Certain herbs (dong quai, wild yam, shepherd's purse) can also help regulate bleeding. Consult a holistic nutritionist, if available, to advise you on dosage. Acupuncture can also help to restore hormonal balance. If you are bleeding heavily, increase your iron intake to prevent anemia (see p. 598).

Medical Treatments

If you are premenopausal and are having light, irregular bleeding, your medical practitioner may suggest waiting a month or two to see whether your system rights itself. (Sometimes stress can contribute to hormonal imbalances.) If abnormal bleeding persists, particularly in women over 40, an endometrial biopsy or D&C should be done to check for endometrial hyperplasia or endometrial cancer. (Such a cancer is very unusual except in women over 50.) If there is no precancerous or cancerous condition, a woman may choose not to have further therapy. If the bleeding is bothersome, hormonal therapy (with progesterone and/or estrogen) may correct the problem. If you want to avoid taking hormones and the bleeding isn't too heavy, you may want to continue self-help measures while observing the amount of bleeding carefully. If you are anovulatory and wish to become pregnant, you may consider taking a fertility drug that stimulates ovulation. Be sure you are informed of the risks associated with such fertility drugs.

Pelvic Inflammatory Disease (PID)

I obtained a copy of my medical records and discovered that I had been complaining of the same problem —pain in my lower right abdomen—for a couple of years. I had severe menstrual irregularities, fevers, bleeding between periods, bleeding after intercourse, pains, and general malaise. Several times I was treated with antibiotics, which brought only some temporary relief. Never was the issue resolved as to what was causing this. Never were my sexual partners or practices mentioned.

Pelvic inflammatory disease (PID) is a general term for an infection that affects the lining of the uterus (endometritis), the fallopian tubes (salpingitis), and/or ovaries (oophoritis). It is primarily caused by sexually transmitted diseases that spread up from the opening of the uterus to these organs (see chapter 14). Annually, nearly one million women in the U.S. are reported to develop PID. In addition, 300,000 women are hospitalized. The cost for treating PID and PID-related problems was about $7 billion in 1996.* These statistics probably greatly underestimate the amount and consequences of PID now occurring. This is primarily because so much PID is undiagnosed.

* The estimated health care costs for the year 2000 are expected to total more than $10 billion (*Women's Health in the U.S.: NIAID Research on Health Issues Affecting Women*, National Institute of Allergy and Infectious Diseases, U.S. Department of Health and Human Services [1997]).

Symptoms

The symptoms of PID vary. They may be so mild that you hardly notice them, but the primary symptom is pain. For instance, you may be aware of tightness or pressure in the reproductive organs or an occasional dull ache in the lower abdomen. On the other hand, the pain may be so strong that you may not even be able to stand. You may feel pain in the middle of your lower abdomen or on one or both sides of the lower abdomen.

You may have some, most, or none of these other symptoms:

- abnormal or foul discharge from the vagina or urethra
- pain or bleeding during or after intercourse
- irregular bleeding or spotting
- increased menstrual cramps
- increased pain during ovulation
- frequent urination, burning, or inability to empty the bladder when urinating
- swollen abdomen
- sudden high fever or low-grade fever that can come and go
- chills
- swollen lymph nodes
- lack of appetite
- nausea or vomiting
- pain around the kidneys or liver
- lower back or leg pain; feelings of weakness, tiredness, depression
- diminished desire to have sex

The intensity and extent of the symptoms depend on which microorganisms are causing the problem, where they are (uterus, tubes, lining of the abdomen, etc.), how long you have had it, what if any antibiotics you have taken for it, and your general health—that is, how much stress you are under and how well you take care of yourself. Doctors characterize PID as acute, chronic, or silent (with symptoms that are not noticed).

Complications

The complications of PID can be very serious. If untreated, PID can turn into peritonitis, a life-threatening condition, or a tubo-ovarian abscess. It can affect the bowels and the liver (perihepatitis syndrome). Months or years after an acute infection, infertility or ectopic pregnancy can result from tubes having been damaged or clogged by scar tissue. PID can also cause chronic pain from adhesions or lingering infection. In the most extreme cases, untreated PID can result in death.

Ninety to 95% of PID is caused by the microorganisms responsible for STDs. These may enter the body during sexual contact with an infected man or

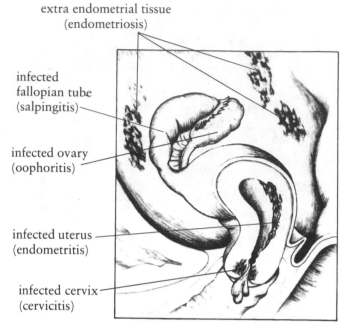

extra endometrial tissue (endometriosis)

infected fallopian tube (salpingitis)

infected ovary (oophoritis)

infected uterus (endometritis)

infected cervix (cervicitis)

PID (full view)/Christine Bondante

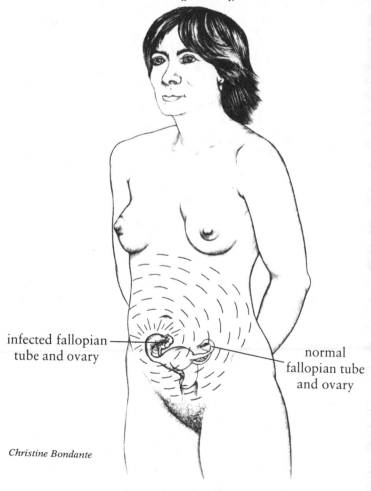

infected fallopian tube and ovary

normal fallopian tube and ovary

Christine Bondante

PID can cause a sharp pain at the most infected site and/or can cause pain throughout all or part of the abdomen/Christine Bondante

woman* and also during an IUD insertion, abortion, miscarriage, childbirth, procedures involving the uterus such as endometrial biopsy, hysterosalpingo-gram (X ray of the reproductive tract), or donor insemination when there has not been careful screening for all STDs. It is not uncommon for male sexual partners of women with PID to have few or no symptoms but to be carrying the organisms that can cause it, so they must be tested and treated as well, and they should use a condom.

My husband had no symptoms at all, although I had been suffering from chronic PID for years. Neither of us could figure out how I got sick. It took us a long time to find a doctor who cultured both of us for organisms. I finally got over it when we both started getting tested and treated according to what organisms were found: chlamydia, mycoplasma, staph, strep.

Doctors may lead women with chronic PID to believe that they are at fault for not responding to antibiotic treatment when in fact it is their sexual partners who need treatment also.

You are at higher risk for developing PID if you are exposed to infected secretions—especially infected semen—during menstruation and ovulation, when your cervix is more open and your mucus is more penetrable. Some researchers hypothesize that certain bacteria can attach themselves to moving sperm and get into the uterus and fallopian tubes. (Birth control pills seem to create dense cervical mucus that prevents sperm from entering the uterus and so reduces the risk of developing PID.) Women using IUDs are also at higher risk during the first four months after insertion. In some parts of the country, gonorrhea still causes most PID. However, in other areas, *Chlamydia, Mycoplasma* and several aerobic and anaerobic microorganisms (those that need oxygen and those that don't) are being found more and more frequently in cervical, endometrial, and tubal cultures taken from women with PID. These organisms may reside in the genital tract for years.

Diagnosis

It would be ideal if, when you got PID, you could know right away exactly which organisms were causing it so you could get the appropriate antibiotics. But such exactness is rarely possible, because pinpointing the organisms often takes some tests that may not be readily available and may be expensive (though it may cost less to get a culture done in the first place than to go to doctor after doctor). Even when you can find a doctor and a lab that culture for organisms such as *Chlamydia* and *Mycoplasma,* you often cannot trust a negative culture result; these organisms are difficult to culture. Sometimes the organisms infecting the uterus and fallopian tubes will not show up in a cervical

* The incidence of PID is very low among lesbians.

culture. Although some doctors rely on blood tests, especially sedimentation rates and white blood cell count, to indicate whether or not you have an infection at all, these are not reliable for diagnosing PID. Sometimes an endometrial biopsy can be useful if hard-to-culture organisms are suspected and not found in a cervical or vaginal culture. However, such a biopsy, if not performed carefully, can further spread organisms from the cervix and vagina to the uterus. In some cases, ultrasound, including vaginal ultrasound, may also be useful. A definitive diagnosis often requires laparoscopy (see p. 596).

If you have PID and a male sexual partner, he must get a test done, too. Frequently, men are diagnosed as having NGU (nongonococcal urethritis). Some of the organisms causing these infections in men (*Chlamydia* and *Ureaplasma,* for example) can cause PID in women. In men, the specimen can be obtained by a urethral swab or by masturbation into a sterile jar, and it must immediately be put into culture media (different for different organisms). The latter method may be important, because men's urethral specimens (like cervical specimens from women) may not contain the organisms living in other parts of the male reproductive or urinary systems.

At the present time, most experts seem to agree that since your health and fertility are at stake, you should not delay getting treatment while waiting for test results.

There is now a growing awareness among gynecologists and urologists about the importance of prompt testing and treatment for PID. Additional research is needed to develop improved, less invasive diagnostic approaches. Some STD clinics and fertility specialists are giving accurate and up-to-date tests and treatments for PID. Call the National STD Hotline, (800) 227-8922, to find out about tests and clinics.

Treatments

PID must be treated just as STDs are; that is, both you and your partner must be treated. If you are treated alone and your partner continues to carry the microorganism(s), you will be reinfected.

When you do start taking antibiotics, you cannot be accurately cultured again until at least a couple of weeks after you stop taking them. Taking the wrong drugs can make organisms more difficult to get rid of. However, it is impractical to suggest that all women with PID wait until cultures are available to take antibiotics. The practical course is to take thorough cultures, begin treatment, and then adjust the treatment according to what is found. Treatment recommendations have recently changed dramatically and include antibiotics such as cefoxitin, doxycycline, and ceftriaxone. The minimum duration of therapy is ten to 14 days because PID is a serious infection. You should receive two different kinds of antibiotics, since more than one organism is often involved. Remember to take all your antibiotic, even if your symptoms are gone, to reduce the possibility of developing antibiotic-resistant strains of organisms. You or your doctor can contact the Centers for Disease Control in Atlanta for the most up-to-date information about effective antibiotics.

Antibiotics can cause yeast overgrowth in the vagina. Treatment may be needed to keep the yeast in check while trying to cure the much more serious PID. Try yogurt or acidophilus for the yeast overgrowth.

I felt like crying today as I filled my prescriptions for antibiotics for PID and suppositories for subsequent yeast. The money is one thing, the visits to the doctor another, but the frustration is the worst. I feel like I'd never have sex again if I knew I'd be cured.

According to the Centers for Disease Control, hospitalization should be strongly considered when (1) the diagnosis is uncertain, (2) surgical emergencies such as appendicitis and ectopic pregnancy must be excluded, (3) a pelvic abscess is suspected, (4) severe illness precludes outpatient management, (5) the woman is pregnant, (6) the woman is unable to follow or tolerate an outpatient regimen, (7) the woman has not responded to outpatient therapy, (8) clinic followup after 48 to 72 hours following the start of antibiotic treatment cannot be arranged, or (9) the woman is an adolescent. Many experts recommend that all women with PID be hospitalized for treatment. Unfortunately, many physicians do not follow these recommendations.

Most women are hospitalized for PID or possible PID when they have acute attacks. In the hospital, you can get intravenous (IV) antibiotics that provide a sufficient concentration of medication in your body to fight the infection. When antibiotic treatment is not successful even then, it is probably because the antibiotics were not the correct ones for the infection and/ or you were reinfected because your sexual partner was not treated successfully. The IV antibiotics may also fail because of problems such as pelvic abscess, septic pelvic thrombophlebitis (an infection of the pelvic veins), or an incorrect diagnosis. You may be told that you have chronic cystitis caused by trauma to the urethra during intercourse, when you really have cystitis accompanying or preceding PID. You may be told that you have infected yourself with organisms from your colon by wiping yourself from back to front, when you really have a sexually transmitted infection. You may be told that you have a spastic colon or that you have an emotional, not a physical, problem, when that is not really true. Try to have your situation thoroughly assessed.

You and your doctor may decide you should have surgery to try to restore fertility by opening closed, scarred tubes (tuboplasty). You may have adhesions: fibrous bands of scar tissue caused by infections. These can bind your internal organs together, causing pain and infertility. In this case, you may decide to have a laparotomy to cut them out. Remember that surgery itself can cause adhesions. Remember, also, that physicians sometimes attribute pain solely to adhesions and fail to recognize the presence of infection.

You may be urged to have a hysterectomy if the doctor thinks that PID has ruined your pelvic organs beyond repair. Also, emergency hysterectomies are done in some cases of acute PID. If the infection is in your urinary tract, which it often is, then hysterectomy does not eliminate it. Some women elect to have hysterectomies in order to get over persistent, debilitating PID, but hysterectomies are rarely necessary for PID.

Personal Issues

Many of us have felt guilt and anger about our own or our partner's sexual experiences that have led to the constant physical problems and pain of PID. We are also angry at a medical system that is not prepared to deal adequately with the growing numbers of women getting STDs, more and more of whom are coming down with PID. Asymptomatic sexual partners may not want to have tests and treatments or may not understand that we need to avoid intercourse with them. They may look for other people to have sex with, which may feel like punishment to us and puts us in further danger of exposure. Unfortunately, instead of expressing our anger outwardly we may just become depressed. It is also enormously frustrating to deal with a doctor who is not willing to pursue a thorough diagnosis. Some doctors do not recognize that we are sexually active, and they disapprove of us for contracting what is so often a sex-related disease, or they doubt the severity and significance of our pelvic symptoms. Finding ourselves untrusted and judged by the medical world can add to the physical and emotional pain we suffer from PID.

It feels like a dirty trick was played on me, doctor after doctor telling me my pain was not in my pelvis but in my head. How many times did I conscientiously and politely ask about getting further tests? I am still mad and sad and bitter. It took months and a lot of pain before I found a doctor who would do what was necessary.

There are many things you can do to help heal yourself while you wait for test results to come back and antibiotics to take hold and work. Very hot baths and heat applied directly to the lower abdomen help relieve pain and bring disease-fighting blood and drugs to your pelvis. A heating pad can be your best friend at this time. Close your eyes and visualize your reproductive organs as healthy, pink, oxygenated, and relaxed. Do not douche or use tampons; to do so may force microorganisms up into your uterus. Do not reuse a douche bag that may be harboring infectious organisms. Have intercourse only when you have felt completely well through an entire monthly cycle and your partners have had negative test results for all

STDs. Sometimes it takes months to feel better after PID. Some women have short bouts of PID months after the initial infection is cleared up, particularly if they abandon their daily health routines or are under too much stress. Acupuncture may help control pain and rebalance energy. You can soak cotton cloth in castor oil, place it on the abdomen, cover it with plastic to prevent greasiness, and then cover it with a heating pad or hot water bottle to bring a maximum amount of heat to the pelvic area. Ginger root compresses and taro root poultices may relieve pain, help eliminate accumulated toxins, keep the area loose and freer from adhesions, and dissolve already formed adhesions. (These are strong medicines and are best used with the guidance of a holistic health practitioner.) Several herbs and teas are useful against infection of the reproductive and urinary tracts. Raspberry leaf tea strengthens the reproductive system. Eliminate sugar and cut down on dairy products (to lessen mucus production); take plenty of vitamins C, A, D, and B complex, as well as zinc. Eat wholesome, fresh foods; avoid stress as much as possible. Eliminate alcohol, tobacco, and other drugs that lower your resistance to disease, and reduce your coffee consumption. You may be unusually tired and run down. Get plenty of sleep. Complete bed rest is recommended but is difficult to achieve. Remember, the most critical element in your healing will be the antibiotic treatment.

To prevent PID, follow these guidelines:

Prevention of PID is like prevention of STDs, because so much PID is caused by sexually transmitted organisms. Birth control foams, creams, and jellies kill some bacteria that can enter the vagina during intercourse. If possible, avoid having intercourse without using a barrier method (condom, diaphragm) of birth control. If you have already had an STD or PID, or if you and/or your male partner have had more than one sexual partner, try to use condoms and avoid using an IUD.

Be aware that PID is an extremely serious problem that needs prompt and skilled attention.

Pelvic Relaxation and Uterine Prolapse

Pelvic relaxation is a condition in which the muscles of the pelvic floor become slack and no longer adequately support the pelvic organs. In severe cases, the ligaments and tissues that hold the uterus in place may also weaken enough to allow the uterus to "fall" or "prolapse" into the vagina. Women sometimes experience pelvic relaxation and/or uterine prolapse after one or more very difficult births, but the tendency can also be inherited. Uterine prolapse is often accompanied by a falling of the bladder (cystocele) and rectum (rectocele) as well.

Often, the first sign of pelvic relaxation is a tendency to leak urine when you cough or sneeze or laugh suddenly. If your uterus has fallen into your vagina, you may have a dull, heavy sensation in your vagina

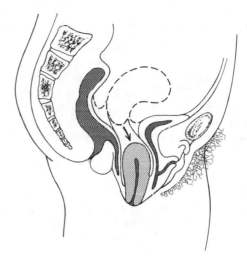

Prolapsed uterus/Christine Bondante

or feel as if something is "falling out." These symptoms are usually worse after you have been standing for a long time.

Prevention and Self-Help Treatments

The best way to prevent pelvic relaxation and uterine prolapse is to do regular Kegel exercises and leg lifts, which strengthen the muscles of the pelvic floor and lower abdomen (see chapter 12, Understanding Our Bodies). One way of determining whether your pelvic muscles are in good shape is to try starting and stopping the flow of urine when you go to the bathroom. If you can't stop the flow, you need to do more Kegels. Some medical practitioners recommend doing the exercise up to a hundred times a day, especially during pregnancy, when the pelvic muscles are under particular stress. You may also strengthen a slightly prolapsed uterus by relaxing in the knee-chest position (kneeling with your chest on the floor and your bottom in the air) several times a day. Some women find that certain yoga positions, such as the shoulderstand and head-stand, relieve the discomfort of a prolapsed uterus.

Medical Treatments

Medical intervention is usually not necessary for pelvic relaxation or even mild uterine prolapse. If the prolapse is severe enough to cause discomfort, you can have a pessary (a rubber device that fits around the cervix and helps to prop up the uterus) inserted. The disadvantages include difficulty in obtaining a proper fit, possible irritation or infection, and the need to remove and clean the pessary frequently. A surgical procedure called a suspension operation can lift and reattach a descended uterus and often a fallen bladder or rectum as well. Many physicians recommend hysterectomy for prolapsed uterus, but it is frequently unnecessary and should be done only as a last resort.

Uterine Fibroids (Leiomyomas, Myomas)

Fibroids are solid benign tumors* that appear on the outside, on the inside, or within the wall of the uterus, often changing the size and shape of it. About 30% of all women will have fibroids by the time they are 35, and they are more likely to affect black women. Although they are of unknown cause, these growths seem to be related to estrogen production: If you are pregnant or are taking oral contraceptives or menopausal estrogens (all of which raise estrogen levels in the body), fibroids may grow more quickly.

Fibroids may be discovered during a routine pelvic exam. Because fibroids keep growing, ask your medical practitioner how many you have and how big they are. If they have grown no further when you have a second exam six months later, a yearly checkup will be sufficient. Ultrasound examination can give more definite information about the number and size of fibroids.

Small fibroids are usually symptom-free. However, very large or numerous fibroids may cause pain, bleeding between periods, or excessive menstrual flow. (Because they usually do not cause abnormal bleeding, if you do have fibroids and abnormal bleeding, be sure to be carefully checked for other causes.) Depending on their size and location, fibroids can also cause abdominal or back pain and urinary problems. Large fibroids rarely make it difficult to conceive or to sustain a full-term pregnancy.

Self-Help Treatments

You may be able to reduce large fibroids by eliminating your intake of synthetic estrogen (found in birth control pills) and stopping estrogen therapy (ERT). Yoga exercises may ease the feelings of heaviness and pressure. If your fibroids cause heavy bleeding, see the self-help treatments in "Abnormal Uterine Bleeding" (p. 656). Visualization techniques may be helpful in dealing with fibroids. Some women try to prevent fibroids by avoiding the hormones usually found in commercial meat, dairy, and egg products and increasing soy in the diet, as well as avoiding processed foods.

Medical Treatments

In many cases, no treatment is necessary, but if you have excessive bleeding, pain, urinary difficulties, or problems with pregnancy, you may want to have the fibroids removed (myomectomy). Sometimes this can be done with laparoscopy or through hysteroscopic resection, wherein the fibroid is shaved off inside the

---

* The word "tumor" is very scary to most of us. It is part of an older language of illness that was used by many of our grandparents, both patients and doctors, to disguise the mention of cancer. Actually, tumors are growths of cells that serve no purpose. Over 90% of all tumors are benign and harmless.

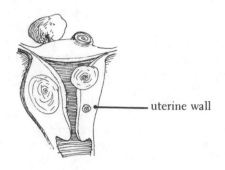

Fibroids (benign growths)/Karen Norberg

uterine cavity; more frequently, myomectomy requires an abdominal incision. In at least 10% of cases, the fibroids will return. (Given enough time and continued hormone stimulation, most women with fibroids are likely to develop new ones.)

Many physicians recommend hysterectomy as a treatment for fibroids in women who are past childbearing age or who do not want more children. This surgery may be unnecessary, particularly for women nearing menopause, when the natural decline in estrogen levels usually shrinks fibroids. Moreover, hysterectomy can have serious consequences for women, including sexual dysfunction and ovarian failure (even when the ovaries are preserved). Myomectomy—done by a surgeon skilled in this procedure—poses no greater risks than hysterectomy and avoids some of the problems associated with hysterectomy. Even large, multiple fibroids can be removed with a myomectomy. Laser surgery to remove fibroids causes less bleeding but is not widely used.

For women near menopause, sometimes the drug Lupron is recommended to help shrink fibroids. Lupron induces an artificial menopause, suppressing the production of estrogen, which promotes fibroid growth. It may be used for several years. Fibroids will grow back after Lupron is discontinued unless the natural onset of menopause continues this lowered estrogen state. A new treatment for women past child-bearing involves injecting a chemical that decreases the blood supply to the fibroids and directly shrinks the tumors.

Ovarian Cysts

Ovarian cysts are relatively common and may result from normal ovulation. Often, they don't cause any symptoms or discomfort. Most ovarian cysts are functional (physiological) and will resolve on their own. A cyst usually develops when a follicle has grown large —as one or more do every month during ovulation— but has failed to rupture and release an egg. Most of these cysts are filled with fluid. Cysts may be accompanied by symptoms such as a disturbance in the normal menstrual cycle, an unfamiliar pain or discomfort in the lower abdomen at any point during the cycle, pain during intercourse, and unexplained abdominal swelling. Found by a routine bimanual pelvic exam, cysts usually disappear by themselves, though some types may have to be removed.

To determine whether a cyst requires treatment, wait a cycle or two for it to disappear. If it persists, a medical practitioner may use ultrasound to augment the pelvic exam. Usually, a pathological cyst, such as a dermoid cyst, a cyst of endometriosis, or cancer will be removed. Such pathological cysts should be removed. Practitioners disagree about the necessity of removing benign cysts, but small functional cysts do not usually cause problems and may be left alone. A large cyst is more of a health risk because it can rupture, causing severe abdominal pain and sometimes bleeding. A large cyst may also twist and damage the blood supply to the ovary. These two uncommon situations require prompt surgery.

If your physician advises removal of the ovary along with the benign cyst, get a second opinion. Removal of the ovary, though a conventional practice, is in many cases unnecessary. Ovaries perform many functions, even after menopause.

Recurrent cysts may indicate a hormonal imbalance or life stresses. Changing your diet, learning how to reduce stress, and using acupuncture may also help to get your system back in balance.

Hysterectomy and Oophorectomy

In 1994, about 556,000 hysterectomies[10] (removal of the uterus) and 458,000 oophorectomies (removal of the ovaries) were performed in the U.S., which has the highest hysterectomy rate in the industrialized world. About one-third of all women have had a hysterectomy by the age of 60. Today, about 90% of hysterectomies are elective—that is, performed by choice and not as an emergency or lifesaving procedure. Various studies have concluded that anywhere from 10 to 90% of these operations were unnecessary. In 1990, the hysterectomy rate had fallen about 20% since the mid-1970s, but many women continue to face recommendations for unnecessary hysterectomies. More physicians are needed who recognize the value of a woman's uterus and ovaries, even when she is in her midlife or beyond.

Both procedures are considered major surgery and risk long-term effects on our health, sexuality, and life expectancy. Certainly, they have saved lives and restored health for many women, but unnecessary operations have exposed women needlessly to risks. Because of the controversy over hysterectomy and oophorectomy rates, many insurance plans now require a second opinion from another physician before agreeing to pay for the procedures.

Because some surgeons recommend these operations inappropriately—for example, as a routine approach to preventing cancer—women need to be informed about when a hysterectomy is truly necessary (see box). The most recent data suggest that African-American women have a somewhat higher

---

WHEN IS HYSTERECTOMY NECESSARY?

Several life-threatening conditions require hysterectomy, including

1. Invasive cancer of the uterus, cervix, vagina, fallopian tubes, and/or ovaries. Only 8 to 12% of hysterectomies are performed to treat cancer.

2. Severe, uncontrollable infection (PID).

3. Rare cases of severe, uncontrollable bleeding.

4. Conditions associated with rare but serious complications during childbirth, including rupture of the uterus.

If you have any of these conditions, hysterectomy may not only save your life but free you from significant pain and discomfort.

Some conditions that are not life-threatening but may justify hysterectomy include

1. Precancerous changes of the endometrium, called hyperplasia. (Remember that most hyperplasia, however, can be reversed with progestational agents.)

2. Severe pelvic infections unresponsive to antibiotics (see the sections on STDs and IUDs in chapter 13, Birth Control).

3. Extensive endometriosis, causing debilitating pain and/or involving other organs. (More conservative surgery and/or medication is usually an effective treatment.)

4. Fibroid tumors that are extensive, large, involve other organs, or cause debilitating bleeding. (However, fibroids can be removed by myomectomy, thereby preserving the uterus.)

5. Pelvic relaxation (uterine prolapse), which is causing severe symptoms. (Uterine suspension, for example, is an alternative treatment in this case.)

Depending on their severity, many of these conditions can be treated without resorting to major surgery. In some cases, observation and explanation is all that is necessary. Fortunately, diagnostic techniques such as sonography, Pap smears, hysteroscopy, and laparoscopy make it possible to avoid or delay many hysterectomies

continued on next page

that might have been done in the past. Unfortunately, most surgeons do not make frequent enough use of such techniques, believing that there is no advantage to saving a uterus, especially if a woman is past her child-bearing years.

Hysterectomies should not be performed for mild dysfunctional uterine bleeding, asymptomatic fibroids, and pelvic congestion (menstrual irregularities and low back pain). These problems can usually be treated with cheaper and safer alternative therapies. If your doctor insists on hysterectomy for one of these conditions, consider changing physicians.

hysterectomy rate than white women, possibly because African-American women are more likely to have fibroids (see p. 662).

For many years, hysterectomy was performed solely for the purpose of sterilization among many poorer women and women of color in the U.S. This abuse led to federal sterilization guidelines in 1979.

OB-GYNs and surgeons sometimes have economic incentives to perform hysterectomies. They are often more profitable than other, less drastic gynecological procedures. Ironically, a myomectomy (see p. 662), which can be more difficult to perform than a hysterectomy, usually gets reimbursed at lower rates. Whenever you have any doubts about the need for hysterectomy and/or oophorectomy, seek one or more other opinions.

Risks and Complications of Hysterectomy and Oophorectomy

Although the death rate from hysterectomy is low (less than 1%), surgical complications from hysterectomy include the following:

1. *Infection.* Most can be treated successfully with antibiotics, but some infections can be severe or even uncontrollable.

2. *Urinary tract complications.* Many women have a kidney or bladder infection following a hysterectomy. Sometimes there is damage to the ureter. In most cases the problem is not serious, but sometimes additional surgery is necessary. In radical hysterectomy (which is performed only in cases of invasive cervical cancer), sensory nerves may be cut, causing loss of the urge to urinate and loss of control over bladder functions. (Injury to the ureters or urinary tract occurs in 2 to 5% of every 1,000 cases.)

3. *Hemorrhage.* About one in ten women require blood transfusions.

Less common surgical complications include the following:

1. *Bowel problems.* These can occur if there is damage to the intestines during surgery. Two percent of all women who have a hysterectomy need further surgery to remove scar tissue from the bowel.

2. *Blood clots.* Clots, which form primarily in the legs, are rare but always dangerous because of the possibility of the clot traveling to the lungs or brain, which can be fatal.

3. *Death or paralysis from anesthesia.*

4. *Postsurgical complications.* These can include abnormal bleeding, improper healing that can cause narrowing of the vagina, and heavy discharge.

Long-Term Risks

Current evidence suggests that for women who are premenopausal, removal of the uterus *with or without* removal of the ovaries approximately doubles the risk of heart attack.[11]

Even if your ovaries are not removed, there is a 20% chance of an earlier menopause. This is usually due to the decreased supply of blood to the ovaries, which causes them to lose their ability to produce hormones, either immediately or over a period of time. Many physicians assure us that we can avoid these risks and symptoms by taking estrogen therapy, but estrogen therapy does not substitute for functioning ovaries and has its own risks (see chapter 23, Women Growing Older, p. 558).

Hormonal responses to hysterectomy vary from one woman to the next, for reasons not yet established. Some women suffer severe hot flashes and lack of lubrication. Others are more fortunate. Some women use hormone therapy for a while, gradually tapering off to nothing.

Other long-term risks include constipation, urinary incontinence (see p. 661), bone and joint pain, fatigue, and depression.

Hysterectomy, Oophorectomy and Sexuality

Many women are concerned about the effect that hysterectomy with or without oophorectomy will have on sexual response. Physicians and popular literature tend to be blandly reassuring and state that any sexual difficulties we may experience are "all in our heads." In fact, there is a physiological basis for these problems, and 33 to 46% of women have difficulty becoming aroused and reaching orgasm after this surgery.[12] Moreover, we now know more about why these changes occur.

First, many women experience orgasm primarily when the penis or a lover's fingers push against the cervix and uterus, causing uterine contractions and increased stimulation of the abdominal lining (peritoneum). Without the uterus or cervix, there may be much less of this kind of sensation.

Second, if the ovaries are removed, ovarian *andro-*

ALTERNATIVES TO HYSTERECTOMY FOR COMMON NONCANCEROUS UTERINE CONDITIONS

CONDITION	CONSERVATIVE SURGERY	PHARMACOLOGIC THERAPIES		OTHER STRATEGIES
		HORMONAL	NONHORMONAL	
Fibroids	Myomectomy Endometrial ablation	GnRH* agonists with add-back therapy Oral contraceptives Androgens RU-486† Gestrinone†	NSAIDs‡	Watchful waiting

Endometriosis	Adhesiolysis
	Excision of endometrial
	  ablation
	Resection of cul-de-sac
	  obliteration
	Nerve blocks
	Uterosacral nerve
	  ablation
		GnRH* agonists with
		  add-back therapy
		Danazol
		Progestins
		Oral contraceptives
		Tamoxifen†
		RU-486†
			NSAIDs‡
			Analgesics
			Anxiolytics
				Watchful waiting
				Biofeedback
				Acupuncture
				Hypnosis
				Lifestyle changes
				  (nutrition, exercise)

Prolapse	Anterior or posterior
	  colporrhaphy
	Laparoscopic or vaginal
	  suspension techniques
		Estrogen		Watchful waiting
				Kegel exercises
				Pessaries
				Electrical stimulation
				Urethral beads
				Periurethral injections
				  of GAX†, collagen,
				  fat, silicon, etc.

Dysfunctional bleeding	Dilation and curettage Endometrial ablation	Progestins Estrogen Oral contraceptives Danazol Prostaglandin inhibitors GnRH* agonists Antifibrinolytic agents Luteinizing hormone agonists		Watchful waiting Antidepressants

Chronic pelvic pain	Adhesiolysis
	Nerve blocks
	Denervation procedure
	Uterosacral nerve
	  ablation
		Danazol
		GnRH* agonists with
		  add-back therapy
		Oral contraceptives
		Medroxyprogesterone
		  acetate
			NSAIDs‡
			Analgesics
			Nerve blocks
			Narcotics
				Watchful waiting
				Counseling
				Biofeedback
				Relaxation techniques
				Trigger point injections
				Acupuncture
				Psychotropics
				Antidepressants
				Physical therapy

* Gonadotropin-releasing hormone.

† Experimental treatment.

‡ Nonsteroidal anti-inflammatory drugs.

From "Treatment of Non-cancerous Uterine Conditions: Issues for Research" (see Resources).

gens, which affect sexuality, may be greatly reduced, thus lowering sexual response. These hormones are not replaced by conventional hormone therapy, but replacement androgens are possible (see below). Even when the ovaries are not removed, hormonal changes may occur if the surgery interferes with the blood supply.

> *I had a hysterectomy two years ago at the age of 45. I went from being fully aroused and fully orgasmic to having a complete loss of libido, sexual enjoyment, and orgasms immediately after the surgery. I went to doctors, all of whom denied ever having seen a woman with this problem before and told me it was psychological. Before surgery, my husband and I were having intercourse approximately three to five times a week, simply because we have an open and loving relationship. Now I find that I have to work at becoming at all interested in intercourse. And I no longer have the orgasm that comes from pressure on the cervix, although I still have a feeble orgasm from clitoral stimulation.*

Third, vaginal lubrication tends to lessen after hysterectomy and oophorectomy.

Fourth, the local effects of surgery may occasionally cause problems. If your vagina has been shortened (see the section on vaginal hysterectomy at right), intercourse may be uncomfortable. Scar tissue in the pelvis or at the top of the vagina from either the vaginal or the abdominal procedure can also cause painful intercourse.

Some of us will find sex unchanged or more enjoyable after hysterectomy. In the words of a woman who had a hysterectomy because of huge fibroids:

> *I had terrible cramps all my life and genuine feelings of utter depression during my periods. My ovaries were not removed, and my libido was not affected. My sexual response, if anything, improved. I also had for the first time no fear of unwanted pregnancy and more general good health.*

Remember, however, that many women do experience genuine loss of sexual desire or response (or both) after hysterectomy, so you must weigh the benefits of surgery against the sexual risk that is *not* "all in the head" and cannot necessarily be predicted in advance. Less drastic approaches than a hysterectomy usually can reduce pain and improve overall well-being.

Androgen replacement therapy is at least partially effective in restoring sexual response. When testosterone (one of the androgens) is administered orally or through injection in a dosage sufficient to restore libido, masculinizing effects may occur, such as lowered voice, acne, and facial hair. However, another way of administering testosterone, with greatly lowered side effects, is through a small slow-release pellet inserted under the skin in the hip region by a simple office procedure every six months. This procedure is quite

HYSTERECTOMY PROCEDURES

These are the common procedures for hysterectomy:

- *Total hysterectomy,* sometimes called *complete hysterectomy.* The surgeon removes the uterus and cervix, leaving the fallopian tubes and ovaries. You may continue to ovulate but will no longer have menstrual periods; instead the egg is absorbed by the body into the pelvic cavity.
- *Total hysterectomy with bilateral salpingo-oophorectomy.* The surgeon removes the uterus, cervix, fallopian tubes *(salpingo)* and both ovaries *(oophor).** "Bilateral" means both sides, though sometimes one ovary may be left if it is not diseased. In rare cases (usually to treat widespread cancer), the surgeon will remove the upper part of the vagina and perhaps the lymph nodes in the pelvic area. This is called *radical hysterectomy.*

Abdominal Versus Vaginal Hysterectomy

Removal of your uterus can be done either through an abdominal incision or through the vagina. Surgeons usually prefer an abdominal approach because it enables them to see the pelvic cavity more completely. The incision is made either horizontally across the top pubic hairline or vertically between the navel and the pubic hairline. Vertical incisions tend to heal more slowly.

Vaginal hysterectomy, useful in cases of prolapsed uterus (bulging of the uterus into the vagina; see p. 661) and for several other conditions, has the advantage of a shorter recovery period and faster healing. In addition, because the incision is made inside the vagina, you will have no visible scar. However, since vaginal hysterectomies are performed less frequently and require greater skill, it is important to find a surgeon who does this procedure regularly. Mistakes during surgery can result in permanent urinary tract difficulties. Other disadvantages include a possible shortening of the vagina, which can result in painful intercourse afterward, and possible temporary severe back pain. Many surgeons now order antibiotics routinely before either abdominal or vaginal hysterectomy.

Oophorectomy: Reasons and Risks

Oophorectomy is removal of the ovary—either one (unilateral) or both (bilateral); the fallopian tube(s) may be removed as well. When both ovaries are removed, a hysterectomy is usually performed at the same time. Common reasons for oophorectomy include ectopic pregnancy, endometriosis, malignant tumors on the ovary, and PID. An enlarged postmenopausal ovary may be cancerous and urgently requires a checkup.

If only one ovary is removed and not your uterus, you will continue to be fertile and have menstrual periods. However, you may experience an earlier menopause. If both ovaries are removed, however, you will experience surgical menopause. Even if one or both ovaries are retained, you may experience symptoms of hormonal loss because of loss of blood supply to the ovaries.

Many surgeons routinely remove the ovaries of women during hysterectomy, whether or not the ovaries are diseased,† if the woman is past 45 or so. For decades, this practice had been one of the most controversial in gynecology. Those in favor of it argue that oophorectomy prevents the possibility of future ovarian cancer, which strikes one in 100 women over 40 and has a cure rate of only 20 to 30%. On the other side, studies show that the actual risk of ovarian cancer following hysterectomy is fairly small (about one in 1,000). Other physicians think the cancer risk is insignificant compared with the risks involved in losing ovarian function: circulatory disease, premature osteoporosis, and sudden menopause, all of which raise the difficult question of hormone therapy (see chapter 23, Women Growing Older).

Oophorectomy affects the hormonal balance of both postmenopausal and premenopausal women, since the ovaries usually continue to produce some hormones after menopause (see "Risks and Complications of Hysterectomy and Oophorectomy," p. 664).

* In Europe and increasingly in the U.S., physicians are leaving in the cervix, hoping that by preserving the cervix, there will be less effect on the function and anatomy of the vagina.
† The terms *diseased* and *healthy* are frequently used carelessly by surgeons when referring to ovaries. Given the rarity of ovarian cancer, ask carefully in advance whether an ovary with a cyst or mild fibrous involvement would be removed as "diseased."

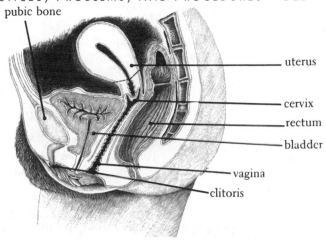

pubic bone
uterus
cervix
rectum
bladder
vagina
clitoris

A *partial* hysterectomy: After surgery the cervix and the stump of the uterus remain, requiring regular Pap tests /Peggy Clark

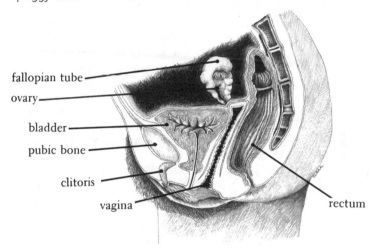

fallopian tube
ovary
bladder
pubic bone
clitoris
vagina
rectum

A *complete* hysterectomy: The uterus is removed, including the cervix (ovaries and tubes are attached to top of vagina)/Peggy Clark

after surgery. This may be due to sudden hormonal changes. Many women are upset. Losing any part of ourselves, especially a part that is so uniquely feminine, is bound to have an impact. You may feel robbed. If you are premenopausal, you may bitterly resent the fact that you cannot have children. Acknowledging feelings of anger and grief after losing a part of yourself or losing some of your sexual responsiveness is an important part of the recovery process.

Thousands of women like me must confront the depression that comes with the loss of their sex lives and the anger they feel when they finally find out that this loss was a side effect of surgery that may have been unnecessary to begin with.

We or our caregivers may or may not recognize posthysterectomy depression promptly. Many gynecologists recommend psychiatric help and prescribe

readily available to British women, but American women have difficulty finding a physician familiar with it.

No long-term studies have been done on the effects of women taking androgen, so skepticism about such therapy is wise.

Even if you were prepared for hysterectomy and did not expect to feel depressed, you may cry frequently and unexpectedly during the first few days or weeks

tranquilizers (or other habit-forming drugs) but almost never encourage treatment of underlying physical or sexual conditions caused by the surgery. Tranquilizers taken together with estrogen therapy may produce negative effects; yet, many physicians routinely prescribe both.

If you are depressed, try to find a women's support group where you can talk about your feelings in a supportive atmosphere. If you can't find a group through a local women's health center, consider starting a postsurgery group of your own. (For information on support groups, see Resources.)

Some women feel only relief following hysterectomy or hysterectomy/oophorectomy, especially when the operation eliminates a serious health problem or chronic, disabling pain.

Self-Help—Recovering from a Hysterectomy or Oophorectomy

After a hysterectomy, you may be in the hospital a few days, depending on the kind of procedure and the amount of anesthesia you had. For the first day or two, you will probably have an IV and a catheter inserted. You will usually be given medication for pain and nausea. Within a day, you will be on your feet and encouraged to do exercises to get your circulation and breathing back to normal. You may also be told to cough frequently to clear your lungs. (Holding a pillow over an abdominal incision or crossing your legs if you had a vaginal incision will help to reduce the pain of coughing.) You may also have gas pains to contend with. Walking, holding on to a pillow and rolling from side to side in bed, and slow deep-breathing exercises will help. You can begin to have light solid foods as well as fluids, when you feel able.

After you go home, you will have light vaginal bleeding or oozing that gradually tapers off. You may also have hot flashes caused by estrogen loss. (Even if your ovaries were not removed, estrogen may be lost because of the possible disruption of blood flow to the ovaries during surgery.) You will probably continue to have some pain that painkillers may not relieve entirely. Consult your medical practitioner if you have excessive pain accompanied by fever or discharge, as this may signal an infection.

Try to arrange for someone to take care of you for the first few days. For at least the first few weeks, ask family and friends for help with household chores and children.

Your practitioner may tell you to avoid tub baths, douches, driving, climbing, or lifting heavy things for several weeks. If you have to drive or have small children at home who need to be carried, ask for suggestions about how to do these tasks safely. Most medical practitioners also recommend waiting six to eight weeks before resuming intercourse and/or active sports. Some women return to these activities much earlier. Start with light exercise, such as walking, and gradually build up to your old routines. Visualizing yourself as healthy and active can speed the recovery process. Full recovery generally takes four to six weeks, but some women feel tired for as long as six months or even a year after surgery.

VAGINA AND VULVA

Vaginal Infections (Vaginitis)—General

All women secrete moisture and mucus from the membranes that line the vagina and cervix. This discharge is clear or slightly milky and may be somewhat slippery or clumpy. When dry, it may be yellowish. When a woman is sexually aroused, under stress, or at midcycle this secretion increases. It normally causes no irritation or inflammation of the vagina or vulva. If you want to examine your own discharge, collect a sample from inside your vagina—with a washed finger, of course—and smear it on clear glass (like a glass slide).

Many bacteria grow in the vagina of a normal, healthy woman. Some of them, especially lactobacilli, help to keep the vagina healthy, maintaining an acid pH and controlling overgrowth of potentially bad bacteria. When infections occur, there may be an abnormal discharge, mild or severe itching and burning of the vulva, chafing of the thighs and occasionally frequent urination.

Some of the reasons for vaginal infections are a general lowered resistance (from stress, lack of sleep, bad diet, other infections in our bodies); too much douching or use of "feminine hygiene sprays"; pregnancy; taking birth control pills, other hormones, or antibiotics; diabetes or a prediabetic condition; cuts, abrasions, and other irritations in the vagina (from childbirth, intercourse without enough lubrication, tampons, or using an instrument in the vagina medically or for masturbation). Postmenopausal women are particularly susceptible. We can also get many of these infections during sex with a partner who has them (see chapter 14, Sexually Transmitted Diseases). Chronic vaginal infections may be a sign of serious medical problems such as HIV infection and diabetes.

Prevention

1. Gently wash your vulva and anus regularly. Pure, unscented mineral oil is a good cleanser and does not dry out the tissues as soap tends to. Pat your vulva dry after bathing, and try to keep it dry. Also, don't use other people's towels or washcloths. Avoid irritating sprays* and soaps (use special nonsoap cleansers for skin very sensitive to plain soap). Avoid talcum powder, as studies have linked it to ovarian cancer.[13]

---

* Feminine hygiene sprays may irritate or cause an allergic reaction in the skin of the vulva. They are at best unnecessary and often harmful. The FDA has suggested, and may soon require, that all feminine hygiene sprays carry a warning on the label.

2. Wear clean, white, all-cotton underpants. Avoid nylon underwear and pantyhose, since they retain moisture and heat, which help harmful bacteria to grow faster. Launder all underwear in hot, soapy water. Be sure to rinse thoroughly.

3. Avoid pants that are tight in the crotch and thighs.

4. Always wipe your genital and anal area from front to back, so that bacteria from the anus won't get into the vagina or urethra.

5. Make sure your sexual partners are clean. It is a good practice for a man to wash his penis daily and especially before making love. Using a condom can provide added protection. If you or your male partner is being treated for a genital infection, make sure he wears a condom during intercourse. Better yet, avoid intercourse until the infection has been cleared up.

6. Use a sterile, water-soluble jelly if lubrication is needed during intercourse (something like K-Y Jelly or Astroglide, for example, not Vaseline). Also, recent studies show that birth control spermicidal gels and creams, which usually contain nonoxynol-9, slow down the growth of trichomonads and possibly monilia. Using these products for lubrication and/or general prevention is a good idea, especially with a new partner you may not know very well. Most lubricants contain propylene glycol, which may cause irritation to a woman.

7. Avoid sexual intercourse that is painful or abrasive to your vagina.

8. Cut down on coffee, alcohol, sugar, and refined carbohydrates. Diets high in sugars can increase sugar in the vagina.

9. Although some women have used unpasteurized, plain yogurt to alleviate mild symptoms of vaginal infections, this practice can prevent proper diagnosis and may even contribute to chronic vaginal complaints.

10. Avoid douching of any kind unless specifically recommended by your practitioner. Although you may "feel cleaner," this practice can destroy the "good bacteria" in your vagina.

11. Take care of yourself. Not eating well or not resting enough makes you more susceptible to infection. Continue most of these beneficial practices —such as proper diet and rest—even after an infection has been treated.

12. Avoid using tampons, especially if you have a history of frequent vaginal infections.

Medical Versus Alternative Treatments

The usual treatment for vaginitis is some form of antibiotic. In the process, however, these drugs disturb the delicate balance of bacteria in the vagina and may actually encourage some infections (such as those caused by yeast) by altering the vagina's normal acid/alkaline balance. Some of these drugs also have unpleasant or even dangerous side effects.

As an alternative to antibiotics for vaginitis, many women are turning to natural and herbal remedies that help to restore the normal vaginal flora and promote healing.[14] For most of them, studies have not shown what the actual effectiveness rates are. For example, you can use herbs to make soothing poultices or sitz baths. You should not rely on these remedies, however, if you have a serious STD (see chapter 14) or an infection that involves your uterus, tubes, or ovaries.

Yeast Infections (Candida, Monilia or Fungus)

Candida albicans, a yeast fungus, grows in the rectum and vagina. In a healthy vagina, the presence of some yeast may not be a problem. When your system is out of balance, yeast-like organisms may grow profusely and cause a thick, white discharge that may look like cottage cheese and smell like baking bread. If a woman has a yeast infection when she gives birth, the baby will get yeast in its throat or digestive tract. This is called thrush and is treated orally with nystatin drops.

Candida grows best in a mildly acidic environment. The pH in the vagina is normally more than mildly acidic (3.5 to 4.5), except when we take birth control pills or some antibiotics, are pregnant, have diabetes, and menstruate (when the pH rises to between 5.8 and 6.8, because blood is alkaline). Obviously, we often find ourselves with a vaginal pH favorable to *Candida,* so preventive measures are especially important.

Microscopic analysis of vaginal secretions (known as a wet mount) is the only way to be sure that the infection is caused by *Candida* and not something else (such as cytolytic vaginosis). Several other conditions (vulvitis, herpes) may respond temporarily to treatment for *Candida* and then recur a short time later, so accurate diagnosis is important.

Once *Candida* infection sets in, treatment usually consists of some form of vaginal suppository or cream. Antifungal external creams such as clotrimazole may reduce or even eliminate the symptoms, sometimes without actually curing the infection. (A vaginal wet mount and yeast culture can determine whether the infection is really gone.) For severe, chronic cases, some of the newer oral antifungal medications may be necessary. Treatment should be based on yeast culture and sensitivity tests. Suppositories and creams have fewer side effects than oral medications, and they can be used during pregnancy.

Another treatment for *Candida* infection involves painting the vagina, cervix and vulva with gentian violet. This is bright purple and it stains, so a sanitary pad must be worn. This procedure really helps, except in occasional cases when there may be a severe reaction to gentian violet.

Self-Help Treatments

Self-diagnosis is inaccurate over half of the time, so it is usually wise to go ahead with self-treatment only after a diagnosis by a clinician. Some of us have had success with the following remedies: inserting yogurt in the vagina, inserting garlic suppositories (peel but don't nick a clove of garlic, then wrap in gauze before inserting in the vagina), and acidifying the system by drinking 8 ounces of unsweetened cranberry juice every day or taking cranberry concentrate supplements. An effective and inexpensive treatment for *Candida* infection is potassium sorbate, commonly used as a preservative in the home brewing of beer. A cotton tampon is dipped into a 3% solution (15 grams of dry potassium sorbate in 1 pint of water) and then inserted into the vagina at night and removed in the morning.

Also try to reduce sugar in your diet, get more rest, don't douche, don't use tampons, and get extra rest if possible.

If you have a male sexual partner, have him apply topical antifungal cream to his penis twice a day for two weeks—especially if he's uncircumcised.

For a long time I felt as though I were on a merry-go-round. I would get a yeast infection, take Mycostatin for three weeks, clear up the infection, and then find two weeks later that the itching and the thick, white discharge were back. Finally, I discovered that reducing my sugar intake and drinking unsweetened cranberry juice would help prevent repeat infections.

Trichomoniasis

Trichomonas vaginalis, or "trich," is a one-celled parasite that can be found in both men and women. Women with trich may have symptoms of vulvar itch and increased discharge, or they may have no symptoms at all. Usually, there is a thin, foamy vaginal discharge that is yellowish green or gray in color and has a foul odor. If another infection is also present, the discharge can vary, sometimes being thicker and whiter. Trich is usually diagnosed by examination of the vaginal discharge under a microscope. It can also cause a urinary infection. It is most often contracted through intercourse (thus, trichomoniasis can be considered an STD), but it can also be passed on by moist objects such as towels, bathing suits, underwear, washcloths, and toilet seats.

The usual treatment for trich is metronidazole (Flagyl)—several pills in one dose. Women with blood diseases, central nervous system disorders, or peptic ulcers should not take this drug. Pregnant and nursing mothers should also avoid metronidazole, as it can pass through the placenta and breast milk to the baby. Many women who take this drug experience unpleasant effects such as nausea, headache, diarrhea, metallic taste, joint pain, and numbness of the arms or legs. In addition, anyone taking metronidazole should avoid alcohol, as the combination can make the effects of both worse.

In some cases, you can treat trich successfully with clotrimazole, which has a 60% cure rate. If you have a stubborn case that has not responded to single-dose treatments and decide to use metronidazole, ask for a single oral dose instead of a three- to seven-day course of pills. This is usually effective and has far fewer negative effects. Because men can also carry and transmit the infection, the Centers for Disease Control recommend that male sexual partners also be treated. Female partners should be examined and treated if trich is diagnosed.

Self-Help Treatments

Although some women have used douches made from vinegar, goldenseal and myrrh, chickweed, and other substances, douching can push organisms farther up into your reproductive system, causing even more serious problems. Douche only with the recommendation and guidance of your medical practitioner.

Garlic suppositories inserted every 12 hours (see at left).

One trichomoniasis specialist advises that taking tub baths, wearing loose clothing (since exposure to air destroys parasites causing infection), and avoiding tampons, douches, and vaginal sprays will help prevent recurrences. Also, use condoms with new male sex partners.

Bacterial Vaginosis (Formerly Called Gardnerella or Hemophilus)

The *Hemophilus* bacterium is one of the most common causes of vaginitis. Like *Candida,* it thrives when the normal pH of the vagina is disturbed. The symptoms are similar to those of trich, though the discharge tends to be creamy white or grayish and is especially foul-smelling (often "fishy") after intercourse. Although the bacterium is fairly easy to recognize on a wet mount, it may be missed or diagnosed incorrectly.

The Centers for Disease Control recommend either metronidazole or clindamycin, taken orally or vaginally for five to seven days, for bacterial vaginosis (BV). Single-dose oral metronidazole may also be effective but less so (40 to 60% cure) than the five- to seven-day treatments. Metronidazole is often used first, because it is lactobacilli sparing and thus carries a lower risk of secondary yeast infections. Vaginal treatment avoids systemic side effects but is more expensive than the five- to seven-day pill regimens. BV may be sexually transmitted, so use a condom during treatment. For chronic BV, male partners may be treated even though research has not found this to be effective. Long-term condom use may be more effective in preventing recurrent BV. Because 5 to 80% of women will have another BV infection within nine months of initial treatment, your clinician may recommend that you return after treatment for a followup vaginal wet mount "test of cure." This is important if you suffer from chronic BV infections. If you have a female sex partner, she should be evaluated and treated if BV is found.

Medicines that are not effective include ampicillin, amoxicillin, erythromycin, doxycycline, tetracycline, Betadine gel or douches, Sultrin cream, Aci-gel, and other over-the-counter douche medications. The vaginal and oral use of yogurt has also not been found to be effective. Alternative treatments may provide temporary relief but not an actual "cure."

Untreated bacterial vaginosis is associated with pregnancy problems and other reproductive problems such as abnormal vaginal bleeding, abnormal Pap smears, UTIs, possibly increased risk of HIV transmission, and PID.

Self-Help Treatments

Self-help treatments include general vaginitis prevention measures (see p. 668) and taking extra vitamins B and C. You can help prevent recurrences by minimizing the use of tampons, avoiding douching, and using condoms (this protects you from the alkaline effect of semen).

Vulvitis

Vulvitis, an inflammation of the vulva, may be caused by external irritants; oral sex; a bacterial or fungal infection; hot tubs; or injury or allergy to common commercial products such as soaps, powders, deodorants, sanitary napkins, synthetic underwear, pantyhose, and topical medications. Vulvitis often accompanies other infections such as vaginitis or herpes. Stress, inadequate diet, and poor hygiene can make you more susceptible to vulvitis. Women with diabetes may develop vulvitis because the sugar content of the cells is higher, increasing susceptibility to infection. Postmenopausal women often develop vulvitis because, as the hormonal levels drop, the vulvar tissues become thinner, drier, and less elastic, making them susceptible to irritation and infection.

The symptoms of vulvitis include itching, redness, and swelling. Sometimes fluid-filled blisters form that break open, ooze and crust over (they may resemble herpes). Scratching can cause further irritation, pus formation, and scaling, as well as secondary infections. Sometimes, as a result of scratching, the skin whitens and thickens. In diabetic vulvitis, the skin may look beefy red; in postmenopausal vulvitis, sores and red, irritated areas often appear.

Women with this problem tend to overclean the vulva, contributing to further irritation. Wash once a day with warm water only.

Prevention

See the section on preventing vaginitis, p. 668.

Medical Treatments

If you have a vaginal infection or herpes, treating these problems will usually clear up the vulvitis as well.

Depending on the cause of vulvitis, your medical practitioner may prescribe antifungal creams. If itching is severe, she or he may prescribe cortisone cream or other soothing lotions. (Low-dose cortisone creams are good for a short time. Fluorinated ones cause thinning and atrophy of the skin if used for a long time.) Postmenopausal women may be given topical estrogen cream or ERT but should not use this for prolonged periods without also adding progesterone to reduce the risk of uterine cancer.

If the vulvitis persists or worsens, you may need a vulvar biopsy to rule out the possibility of cancer. This can be done in an office with the use of local anesthetic.

Self-Help Treatments

Discontinue using any substances that might be a cause of vulvitis (see at left). All commercial preparations may be irritating, including antifungal agents and lubricants containing propylene glycol. Keep your vulva clean, cool, and dry—and remember to wipe from front to back. Hot boric acid compresses and hot sitz baths with comfrey tea are soothing. Use unscented white toilet paper and soft cotton or linen towels and underclothes to prevent chafing. Cold compresses made of plain natural yogurt or cottage cheese also help relieve itching and soothe irritation. Calamine lotion also helps relieve itching. Aveeno colloidal oatmeal bath can be very soothing. Use a sterile, nonirritating lubricant such as K-Y Jelly or Astroglide during intercourse and other genital sex. Finally, try to eat well, get more rest, and find ways of coping with stress.

Vulvodynia

Women with vulvodynia, also known as vulvar vestibulitis, experience excruciating pain, burning, and/or itching in the vulvar area. They may have difficulty sitting, walking, having sex, or doing many of the activities necessary for carrying on a normal life. Vulvodynia has been reported to afflict between 150,000 and 200,000 women in the U.S. alone.

My odyssey took me to 13 medical professionals, including seven gynecologists, two dermatologists, one urologist, and an acupuncturist. I was told that I didn't like sex, that I was imagining the pain, and that my vaginal lips were too fleshy and large. I was tested repeatedly for STDs, but every test came back negative. Some doctors had no idea what was causing the irritation. Others put me through unnecessary and painful procedures, including widening my urethra.

VON WILLEBRAND DISEASE

Do you have: heavy periods, excessive nose-bleeds, easy bruising, bleeding more than one day after dental procedures and surgeries? You may have von Willebrand Disease (vWD), the most common inherited bleeding disorder, which affects up to one in 100 persons worldwide, including one million American girls and women. Yet vWD and other bleeding disorders in women are often unsuspected and undiagnosed.

For a proper diagnosis and treatment plan, contact your local Hemophilia Treatment Center, via the National Hemophilia Foundation at: (800) 42-HANDI.

The cause of vulvodynia is unknown. Theories include bacterial infection, HPV, instability of the pelvic floor, and trauma to the vaginal area as possible causes. Treatments include antihistamines, tricyclic antidepressants such as Elavil, compresses, topical anesthetics, a low-oxalate diet (eliminating most fruits and vegetables), interferon injections, biofeedback, and, as a last resort, surgery. Taking oral calcium citrate before meals, to bind oxalates in the digestive tract and prevent their absorption, may also be helpful.

If you have undiagnosed vulvar pain, monitor your symptoms carefully. If your doctor minimizes your problem or makes you feel insane, try to find one who will take your pain seriously and find a suitable treatment. Above all, remember that help is available. You are not alone, but you'll need to take control of the situation and be persistent in your search for relief.

NOTES

1. See also Dava Sobel and Arthur Klein, *Arthritis: What Works* (New York: St. Martin's Press, 1991).
2. *Guide to Clinical Preventive Services,* 2d edition. Report of the U.S. Preventive Services Task Force, U.S. Department of Health and Human Services (Baltimore, MD: Williams and Wilkins, 1996), p. 73.
3. American Cancer Society, *Cancer Facts and Figures, 1996* (Atlanta: The Society, 1996).
4. William P. McGuire and Faridullah Qazi, "The Treatment of Epithelial Ovarian Cancer," *Ca* 45, no. 2 (1995): 88–101.
5. One study of a small number of DES daughters found that cyrosurgery (a common treatment of freezing the affected tissue) resulted in later problems with maintaining pregnancy.
6. S. Skates, "Statistics, Ethics and Ovarian Cancer," *Ovarian Plus International Gynecologic Cancer Prevention Quarterly* 3, no. 1 (1997): 13.
7. C. Sinnex, "New Ovarian Cancer Detection Test on Horizon," *Ovarian Plus International Gynecologic Cancer Prevention Quarterly* 2, no. 4 (1996): 1–2.
8. Massachusetts Breast Cancer Coalition, January 1997.
9. Toni P. Miles and Kathleen C. Malik, "Menopause and African-American Women: Clinical and Research Issues," *Experimental Gerontology* 29, no. 3–4 (1994): 511. See also by Kristen H. Kjerulff et al., "Hysterectomy and Race," *Obstetrics and Gynecology* 82, no. 5 (1993) 757–64.
10. "1994 Summary: National Hospital Discharge Survey," *Advance Data from Vital and Health Statistics,* no. 278 (1994).
11. Julie R. Palmer, Lynn Rosenberg, and Samuel Shapiro, "Reproductive Factors and Risk of Myocardial Infarction," *American Journal of Epidemiology* 136, no. 4 (1992): 408.
12. L. Zussman et al., "Sexual Response after Hysterectomy-Oophorectomy: Recent Studies and Reconsideration of Psychogenesis," *American Journal of Obstetrics and Gynecology* 40, no. 7 (Aug. 1, 1991): 725–29.
13. B. L. Harlow et al., "Perineal Exposure to Talc and Ovarian Cancer Risk," *Obstetrics and Gynecology* 80, no. 1 (1992): 19–26.
14. For more information on alternative remedies for vaginitis, send for "Home Remedies for Vaginitis," Santa Cruz Women's Health Center, 250 Locust Street, Santa Cruz, CA 95060. Send a stamped, self-addressed envelope and $2.00.

RESOURCES

General

Berger, Sara, and Lawrence Berger. *Native American Women's Health: Directory of Resources.* Albuquerque, NM: Lovelace Research Institutes, 1997. (505) 262-3467.

Federation of Feminist Women's Health Centers and Suzann Gage, illus. *A New View of a Woman's Body.* Los Angeles: Feminist Health Press, 1991.

Fogel, C., and Woods, Nancy. *Women's Health Care: A Comprehensive Handbook.* Thousand Oaks, CA: Sage, 1995.

Fugh-Berman, Adriane. *Alternative Medicine: What Works?* Tucson, AZ: Odonian Press, 1996.

Melpomene Institute for Women's Health Research. *The Bodywise Woman: Reliable Information About Physical Activity and Health.* New York: Prentice Hall, 1990.

National Women's Health Network. *Taking Hormones and Women's Health: Choices, Risks and Benefits.* 1995. $10. Available from the National Women's Health Network, 514 10th Street NW, Washington, DC 20004.

Nissim, Rina. *Natural Healing in Gynecology: A Manual for Women.* San Francisco: HarperCollins, 1996.

Ratcliff, Kathryn Strother, ed. *Healing Technology: Feminist Perspectives.* Ann Arbor: University of Michigan Press, 1989.

Ruzek, Sheryl Burt, Virginia L. Oleson, and Adele E. Clarke. *Women's Health: Complexities and Differences.* Columbus: Ohio State University Press, 1997.

"Special Issue: Women's Health in the 1990s." *American Journal of Preventive Medicine* 12, no. 5, (Sept./Oct. 1996).

Villarosa, Linda, and the National Black Women's Health Project. *Body and Soul.* New York: HarperPerennial, 1994.

White, Evelyn C., ed. *The Black Women's Health Book: Speaking for Ourselves.* Seattle: Seal Press, 1994.

Worcester, Nancy, and Mariamne H. Whatley, eds. *Women's Health: Readings on Social, Economic, and Political Issues.* Dubuque, IA: Kendall/Hunt Publishing, 1994.

Arthritis

Fleming, Linda Frazer. *Releasing Arthritis: The Seven-Year Plan.* Falls Church, VA: LF Publishing, 1990.

Lorig, Kate, and James F. Fries. *The Arthritis Helpbook: A Tested Self-Management Program for Coping with Arthritis and Fibromyalgia.* Reading, MA: Addison-Wesley, 1995.

Sobel, Dava, and Arthur Klein. *Arthritis: What Works.* New York: St. Martin's Press, 1991.

Wallace, Jean. *Arthritis Relief: A Take-Charge Plan of Positive Nutrition, Gentle Exercise, Relaxation, Medical Care and Everyday Coping Tips.* Emmaus, PA: Rodale Press, 1989.

Organizations

The Arthritis Foundation
1330 West Peachtree Street; Atlanta, Georgia 30309; (404) 872-7100
Web site: http://www.arthritis.org

Cochrane Collaboration Osteoarthritis
Contact: Dr. John Kirwan
Cochrane Osteoarthritis Subgroup; Rheumatology Unit; University Department of Medicine; Bristol Royal Infirmary; Bristol, UK BS2 8HW
E-mail: john.kirwan@bristol.ac.uk

National Arthritis, Musculoskeletal and Skin Diseases Information Clearinghouse
1 AMS Circle; Bethesda, MD 20892-3675; (301) 495-4484

Autoimmune Diseases

Chronic Fatigue Immune Dysfunction Syndrome

Bell, David S., *The Doctor's Guide to Chronic Fatigue Syndrome: Understanding, Treating and Living with CFIDS.* Reading, MA: Addison-Wesley, 1994.

Casanova, Kenneth. *How to Apply for Social Security Benefits If You Have CFIDS.* 1998. Available from Massachusetts CFIDS Association, 808 Main Street, Waltham, MA 02154; (781) 893-4415.

Johnson, Hillary. *Osler's Web: Inside the Labyrinth of the Chronic Fatigue Epidemic.* New York: Crown Publishers, 1996.

Massachusetts CFIDS Association. *CFS: A Primer for Physicians and Allied Health Professionals.* 1992. Available from Massachusetts CFIDS Association, 808 Main Street, Waltham, MA 02154; (781) 893-4415.

Organizations

American Association of Chronic Fatigue Syndrome
325 9th Avenue; Box 359780; Seattle, WA 98104; (206) 521-1932
Web site: http://weber.u.washington.edu/~dedra/aacfs1.html

CFIDS Association of America, Inc.
P.O. Box 220398; Charlotte, NC 28222-0398; (704) 362-2343; Information line: (800) 442-3437
Web site: http://www.cfids.org

Fibromyalgia

Ediger, Beth. *Coping with Fibromyalgia.* Edgewood, TX: Fibromyalgia Association of Texas, 1991. Available from Fibromyalgia Association of Texas, Rte. 1, Box 106A, Edgewood, TX 75117; (903) 896-1495.

Starlanyl, Devin, and Mary Ellen Copeland. *Fibromyalgia and Chronic Myofascial Pain Syndrome: A Survival Manual.* Oakland, CA: New Harbinger Publications, 1996.

Journal of Musculoskeletal Pain
Haworth Press; Binghamton, NY 13904; (800) 342-9678

Organizations

The Fibromyalgia Alliance of America
P.O. Box 21990; Columbus, OH 43221; (614) 457-4222

Fibromyalgia Network
P.O. Box 31750; Tucson, AZ 85751-1750; (800) 853-2929

National Fibromyalgia Research Association
P.O. Box 500; Salem, OR 97302
Web site: http://www.teleport.com/~nfra

Scleroderma

American College of Rheumatology
60 Executive Park South, Suite 150; Atlanta, GA 30329; (404) 633-3777
Web site: http://www.rheumatology.org

United Scleroderma Foundation
734 East Lake Avenue, Suite 5; P.O. Box 399; Watsonville, CA 95077; (800) 722-HOPE
Web site: http://www.scleroderma.com

Sjogren's Syndrome

National Sjogren's Syndrome Association
5815 North Black Canyon Hwy, Suite 103; Phoenix, AZ 85015-2200; (602) 433-9844; Information line. (800) 395-6772
Web site: http://www.sjogrens.org

Sjogren's Syndrome Foundation
333 North Broadway, Suite 2000; Jericho, NY 11753; (800) 4-SJOGREN; (800) 475-6473; (516) 933-6365; Fax: (516) 933-6368
E-mail: ssf@idt.net
Web site: http://www.sjorgrens.com

Systemic Lupus Erythematosus (SLE)

National Institute on Arthritis, Musculoskeletal and Skin Diseases. *Systemic Lupus Erythematosus: Handout on Health*. Bethesda, MD: National Arthritis, Musculoskeletal and Skin Diseases Information Clearinghouse, 1997. Available from NAMSIC: (301) 496-8188.

NIAMS Task Force on Lupus in High-Risk Populations. *What Black Women Should Know About Lupus*. Bethesda, MD: National Arthritis, Musculoskeletal and Skin Diseases Information Clearinghouse, 1994. Available from NAMSIC: (301) 496-8188.

Organizations

Lupus Foundation of America
1300 Piccard Drive, Suite 200; Rockville, MD 20850; (301) 670-9292; (800) 558-0121
Web site: http://www.lupus.org/lupus/index.html

Cancer

General

American Cancer Society. *Cancer Facts and Figures 1996*. Atlanta, GA: The Society, 1996.

Boik, John. *Cancer and Natural Medicine: A Textbook of Basic Science and Clinical Research*. Princeton, MN: Oregon Medical Press, 1995

Brady, Judith, ed. *1 in 3: Women with Cancer Confront an Epidemic*. Pittsburgh: Cleis Press, 1991.

Butler, Sandra, and Barbara Rosenblum. *Cancer in Two Voices*. Duluth, MN: Spinsters Ink, 1996.

Dollinger, Malin, Ernest H. Rosenbaum, and Greg Cable. *Everyone's Guide to Cancer Therapy*. Kansas City, MO: Andrews McMeel Pub., 1998.

Information Packages on Unconventional Cancer Therapies, Canadian Breast Cancer Research Initiative. December 1996. Available through the Canadian Cancer Information Service: (905) 387-1153 (in U.S). Also available at http://www.breast.cancer.ca.

Lerner, Michael. *Choices in Healing: Integrating the Best of Conventional and Complementary Approaches to Cancer*. Cambridge, MA: MIT Press, 1994.

National Cancer Institute. *What Are Clinical Trials All About?* Available from the National Cancer Institute, Office of Cancer Communications, 31 Center Drive, MSC 2580, Bethesda, MD 20892-2580; (800) 4-CANCER.

Ramstack, Janet L., and Ernest H. Rosenbaum. *Nutrition for the Chemotherapy Patient*. Palo Alto, CA: Bull Publishing, 1990.

Stocker, Midge, ed. *Cancer as a Women's Issue: Scratching the Surface*. Chicago: Third Side Press, 1991.

Williams, Terry Tempest. *Refuge: An Unnatural History of Family and Place*. New York: Vintage Books, 1992.

Williams, Wendy. *The Power Within: True Stories of Exceptional Patients Who Fought Back with Hope*. New York: Simon & Schuster, 1991.

Workshop on Alternative Medicine. *Alternative Medicine: Expanding Medical Horizons—A Report to the National Institutes of Health on Alternative Medical Systems and Practices in the United States*. Bethesda, MD: NIH, 1995.

Zakarian, Beverly. *The Activist Cancer Patient: How to Take Charge of Your Treatment*. New York: John Wiley, 1996.

Breast Cancer and Breast Implants

Batt, Sharon. *Patient No More: The Politics of Breast Cancer*. Charlottetown, PEI: Gynergy, 1994.

Clorfene-Casten, Liane. *Breast Cancer: Poisons, Profits and Prevention*. Monroe, ME: Common Courage Press, 1996.

ECRI. *High-dose Chemotherapy with Bone Marrow Transplant for Metastatic Breast Cancer*. Patient Reference Guide series, 1996. Order from ECRI, 5200 Butler Pike, Plymouth Meeting, PA 19462-1298; (610) 825-6000.

Gabriel, Sherine E., et al. "Risk of Connective Tissue Diseases and Other Disorders After Breast Implantation." *New England Journal of Medicine* 330, no. 24 (1994): 1697–1702.

Harris, Jay, et al., eds. *Diseases of the Breast*. Philadelphia: Lippincott-Raven, 1996.

Kelly, Patricia T. *Understanding Breast Cancer Risk*. Philadelphia: Temple University Press, 1991.

Kessler, David A., Ruth B. Merkatz, and Rene Schapiro. "A Call for Higher Standard of Breast Implants." *JAMA* 270, no. 21 (1993): 2607–608.

Lorde, Audre. *The Cancer Journals*. San Francisco: Aunt Lute Books, 1997.

Love, Susan M., and Karen Lindsey. *Dr. Susan Love's Breast Book,* 2nd ed. Reading, MA: Addison-Wesley, 1995.

McGinn, Kerry. *The Informed Woman's Guide to Breast Health: Breast Changes That Are Not Cancer*. Palo Alto, CA: Bull Publishing, 1992.

Metzger, Deena. *Tree Essays and Pieces*. Berkeley, CA: North Atlantic Books, 1997. On breast cancer and healing.

Nicholson, Andrew. "Diet and the Prevention and Treatment of Breast Cancer." *Alternative Therapies* 2, no. 6 (1996): 32–37.

U.S. Food and Drug Administration. "Breast Implants: An Information Update." July 1997. Available at Web site: http://www.fda.gov/oca/hotopics.htm

Weed, Susun. *Breast Cancer? Breast Health!: The Wise Woman Way*. Woodstock, NY: Ash Tree, 1996.

Audiovisual Resources

Surviving the Fear. 47 minutes. Available through Great North Enterprises, Suite 012, 11523-100 Avenue, Edmonton, Alberta T5K 0J8; (800) 290-5482.

Tears Are Not Enough. 59 minutes. Available through

Great North Enterprises, Suite 012, 11523-100 Avenue, Edmonton, Alberta T5K 0J8; (800) 290-5482.

Organizations

Coalition of Silicone Survivors
P.O. Box 129; Broomfield, CO 80038-0129; (303) 469-8242

Command Trust Network, National Silicone Implant Information Clearinghouse
11301 West Olympic Boulevard, Box 332; West Los Angeles, CA 90064

Cervical Cancer

Brinton, Louise A., et al. "Occupation and Cervical Cancer." *Journal of Occupational and Environmental Medicine* 37, no. 3, (1995): 357–61.

Coney, Sandra. *The Unfortunate Experiment.* New York: Penguin Books, 1988.

National Cancer Institute. *What You Need to Know About Cancer of the Cervix.* Available from the National Cancer Institute, Office of Cancer Communications, 31 Center Drive, MSC 2580, Bethesda, MD 20892-2580; (800) 4-CANCER.

Posner, Tina, and Martin Vessey. *Prevention of Cervical Cancer.* London: Kings Fund Publishing Office, 1988. Available through the Kings Fund Centre, 126 Albert Street, London NW1 7NF, U.K.

Zahm, Shelia H., and Aaron Blair. "Cancer Among Migrant and Seasonal Farmworkers: An Epidemiologic Review and Research Agenda." *American Journal of Industrial Medicine* 24, no. 6 (1993): 753–60.

Ovarian Cancer

American Cancer Society. "Ovarian Cancer." *CA* 45, no. 2 (1995): Special issue.

Conversations
c/o Cindy H. Melancon; P.O. Box 7948; Amarillo, TX 79114-7949
E-mail: chmelancon@aol.com
Web site: http://www.geocities.com/hotsprings/7938

An excellent newsletter for women who are fighting ovarian cancer. No charge.

American College of Obstetricians and Gynecologists, Committee on Gynecological Practice. *Second Look Laparotomy for Epithelial Ovarian Cancer.* Washington, DC: ACOG, 1995. Available from ACOG: (202) 638-5577.

Greenspan, Ezra M. *What Every Woman and Her Doctor Should Discuss About Ovarian Cancer.* New York: Chemotherapy Foundation, 1997. Available from Chemotherapy Foundation, 183 Madison Avenue, New York, NY 10016; (212) 213-9292.

Heller, Debra S., et al. "The Relationship Between Perineal Cosmetic Talc Usage and Ovarian Talc Particle Burden." *American Journal of Obstetrics and Gynecology* 174, no. 5 (1996): 1507–510.

McGuire, William P., and Faridullah Qazi. "The Treatment of Epithelial Ovarian Cancer." *CA* 45, no. 2 (1995): 88–101.

National Cancer Institute. *Low Malignant Potential Tumor (LMP) PDQ (Physicians Data Query).* Available from the National Cancer Institute, Office of Cancer Communications, 31 Center Drive, MSC 2580, Bethesda, MD 20892-2580; (800) 4-CANCER.

National Cancer Institute. *Ovarian Cancer, PDQ (Physicians Data Query).* Available from the National Cancer Institute, Office of Cancer Communications, 31 Center Drive, MSC 2580, Bethesda, MD 20892-2580; (800) 4-CANCER.

National Institutes of Health. *Ovarian Cancer: Screening, Treatment and Followup—NIH Consensus Statement.* Bethesda, MD: National Institutes of Health, 1994.

Nguyen, Hoa N. "Ovarian Carcinoma: A Review of the Significance of Familial Risk Factors and the Role of Prophylactic Oophorectomy in Cancer Prevention." *Cancer* 74, no. 2 (1994): 544–45.

Park, Robert C. and Michael G. Teneriello. "Early Detection of Ovarian Cancer." *CA* 45, no. 2 (1995): 71–87.

Piver, M. Steven, and Gene Wilder. *Gilda's Disease: Sharing Personal Experiences and a Medical Perspective on Ovarian Cancer.* Amherst, NY: Prometheus Books, 1996.

Rubin, Stephen C., and Gregory P. Sutton, eds. *Ovarian Cancer.* New York: McGraw-Hill, 1993.

Runowicz, Carolyn D. "Advances in the Screening and Treatment of Ovarian Cancer." *CA* 42, no. 6 (1992): 3276–349.

Uterine Cancer

Hummel, Sherilynn, and Lindquist, Marie. *Ovarian and Uterine Cancer: Reducing Your Risk.* New York: Bantam Books, 1992.

National Cancer Institute. *What You Need to Know About Cancer of the Uterus.* Available from the National Cancer Institute, Office of Cancer Communications, 31 Center Drive, MSC 2580, Bethesda, MD 20892-2580; (800) 4-CANCER.

Organizations

American Cancer Society
19 West 56th Street; New York, NY 10019; (212) 586-8700
Web site: http://www.cancer.org

Provides information, booklets, Reach to Recovery (one-on-one counseling by women with histories of breast cancer).

Breast Cancer Action
55 New Montgomery Street, Suite 323; San Francisco, CA 94105; (415) 243-9301
Web site: http://www-med.stanford.edu/bca

Provides education, political advocacy, direct support.

Center for Alternative Medicine Research in Cancer
University of Texas; P.O. Box 20186, #434; Houston, TX 77225
Web site: http://chprd.sph.uth.tmc.edu/utcam

Cochrane Collaboration Breast Cancer Group
Contact: Ms. Davina Ghersi, Coordinator
NHMRC Clinical Trials Centre; University of Sydney; Level 5, 88 Mallett Street, Camperdown 2050, NSW, Australia
E-mail: davina@ctc.trials.su.oz.au

Cochrane Collaboration Gynecological Cancers Group
Contact: Mandy Collingwood, Coordinator
Institute of Health Sciences; P.O. Box 777; Headington, Oxford, UK OX3 7LF
E-mail: cwilliams@canet.org
See also chapter 25, The Politics of Women's Health and Medical Care, p. 710.

Foundation for Advancement in Cancer Therapy (FACT)
P.O. Box 1242; Old Chelsea Station; New York, NY 10113; (212) 741-2790

Gerson Institute of California/Cancer Caring Society
P.O. Box 430; Bonita, CA 91908; (619) 585-7600

Gilda Radner Familial Ovarian Cancer Registry
Department of Gynecologic Oncology; Roswell Park Cancer Institute; Elm and Carlton Streets; Buffalo, NY 14263-0001; (800) OVARIAN
Web site: http://rpci.med.buffalo.edu/clinic/gynonc/grwp.html

Lesbian Community Cancer Project
4753 North Broadway, Suite 199; Chicago, IL 60640; (773) 561-4662

National Breast Cancer Coalition (NBBC)
1707 L Street NW, Suite 1060; Washington, DC 20036; (202) 296-7477
Web site: http://www.natlbcc.org
   Includes the Mautner Project for Lesbians with Cancer. Provides written information and resources; lobbies for legislative concerns.

National Cancer Institute
Office of Cancer Communications
31 Center Drive, MSC 2580; Bethesda, MD 20892-2580; Hot line: (800) 4-CANCER
Web site: http://rex.nci.nih.gov
   Hot line answered at all times except 12:00 midnight to 8:00 A.M.; general cancer and PDQ information available. Also provides names of cancer centers where new research protocols are being conducted. Many publications available in fulltext on the Web site.

National Coalition for Cancer Survivorship
1010 Wayne Avenue, Suite 505; Silver Spring, MD 20910; (301) 650-8868
Web site: http://www.cansearch.org

National Lymphedema Network
2211 Post Street, Suite 404; San Francisco, CA 94115-3427; (800) 541-3259
Web site: http://www.wenet.net/~lymphnet

National Ovarian Cancer Coalition (NOCC)
1451 W. Cypress Creek Road, Suite 207; Fort Lauderdale, FL 33309; (954) 351-9555; (888) OVARIAN
Web site: http://www.ovarian.org

1 in 9/Breast Cancer Group
Nassau County Medical Center; 2201 Hempstead Turnpike; East Meadow, NY 11554; (516) 357-9622

Reach for Recovery
   Contact your local American Cancer Society.

Rosenthal Center for Complementary and Alternative Medicine
Columbia University; 630 W. 168th Street, Box 75; New York, NY 10032; (212) 543-9550
Web site: http://cpmcnet.columbia.edu/dept/rosenthal

SHARE
1501 Broadway, Suite 1720r; New York, NY 10036; (212) 719-0364
Web site: http://www.noah.cuny.edu/providers/share.html
   Self-help support groups for women with breast or ovarian cancer.

United Ostomy Association
19772 MacArthur Boulevard, Suite 205; Irvine, CA 92612-2405; (800) 826-0826
Web site: http://www.uoa.org

Women's Cancer Resource Center
3023 Shattuck Street; Berkeley, CA 94705; (510) 548-9286
Web site: http://www-geography.berkeley.edu/WCRC/2main.htm

Women's Community Cancer Project
c/o Women's Center
46 Pleasant Street; Cambridge, MA 02139; (617) 354-9888

Additional Online Resources

Breast Cancer Information
http://nysernet.org/bcic

OncoLink
http://cancer.med.upenn.edu

Chemical Injury and Multiple Chemical Sensitivity (MCS)

Berthold-Bond, Annie. *Clean and Green: A Complete Guide to Nontoxic and Environmentally Safe Housekeeping.* Woodstock, NY: Ceres Press, 1990.
   Mitchell, Frank, and Patricia Price, eds. *Multiple Chemical Sensitivity: A Scientific Overview.* Princeton, NJ: Princeton Scientific Publishing, 1995.
   Rachel's Environment and Health Weekly. Environmental Research Foundation, Box 5306, Annapolis, MD 21403-7036; (410) 263-1584. E-mail: erf@rachel.clark.net
   Wilson, Cynthia, and Cindy Duehring. *Chemical Expo-*

sure and Human Health. Jefferson, NC: McFarland and Company Publishers, 1993.

Video

Funny, You Don't Look Sick. Video autobiography of a woman with CFIDS and MCS. Order from P.O. Box 851, Watertown, MA 02272.

Organizations

American Academy of Environmental Medicine
10 E. Randolph Street; New Hope, PA 18938; (215) 862-4544
Web site: http://www.healthy.net/pan/pa/NaturalTherapies/aaem/index.html

Chemical Injury Information Network
P.O. Box 301; White Sulphur Springs, MT 59645; (406) 547-2255
Provides members with information and referrals; publishes monthly newsletter, *Our Toxic Times*.

The Environmental Health Network
P.O. Box 1155; Larkspur, CA 94901; (415) 541-5075
Web site: http://users.lanminds.com/~wilworks/ehnindex.htm

MCS Referral and Resources
508 Westgate Road; Baltimore, MD 21229; (410) 362-6400

MC Survivors
Web site: http://www-rohan.sdsu.edu/staff/lhamilto/mcs/index.html

New York Coalition for Alternatives to Pesticides (NYCAP)
353 Hamilton Street; Albany, NY 12210; (518) 426-8246
Offers information packets for people with MCS/environmental illness

DES

Anderson, B., et al. "Development of DES-Associated Clear Cell Carcinoma: The Importance of Regular Screening." *Obstetrics and Gynecology* 53, no. 3 (1979): 293–99.

Apfel, Roberta J., and Susan Fisher. *To Do No Harm: DES and the Dilemmas of Modern Medicine*. New Haven, CT: Yale University Press, 1984.

Dieckmann, W., et al. "Does the Administration of Diethylstilbestrol During Pregnancy Have Therapeutic Value?" *American Journal of Obstetrics and Gynecology* 66, no. 5 (Nov. 1953): 1062–81.

Glendinning, Chellis. *When Technology Wounds: The Human Consequences of Progress*. New York: William Morrow, 1990.

Greenberg, E. R., et al. "Breast Cancer in Mothers Given Diethylstilbestrol in Pregnancy." *New England Journal of Medicine* 311, no. 22 (Nov. 29, 1984): 1393–398.

Herbst, A. L., et al. "Adenocarcinoma of the Vagina: Association of Maternal Stilbestrol Therapy with Tumor

Appearance in Young Women." *New England Journal of Medicine* 284, no. 15 (April 1971): 878–81.

Kaufman, R. H., et al. "Upper Genital Tract Changes and Infertility in Diethylstilbestrol-Exposed Women." *American Journal of Obstetrics and Gynecology* 154, no. 6 (June 1986): 1312–318.

Wingard, Deborah L., and Judith Turiel. "Long-Term Effects of Exposure to Diethylstilbestrol." *Western Journal of Medicine* 149, no. 5 (Nov. 1988): 551–54.

Organizations

DES Action USA
1615 Broadway; Oakland, CA 94612; (800) DES-9288; (510) 465-4011
E-mail: desact@well.com
Web site: http://www.desaction.org
Publishes *DES Action Voice*, a quarterly newsletter with latest research information.

DES Cancer Network
514 10th Street, N.W., Suite 400; Washington, DC 20004-1403; (800) DES-NET4; (202) 628-6330
E-mail: DESNETWRK@aol.com
Offers education, support, and research advocacy.

Video

A Healthy Baby Girl, by Judith Helfand/An ITVS Co-Presentation. Available through Judith Helfand Productions, 2112 Broadway #402A, New York, NY 10023 (212) 875-0456. E-mail: jhp@igc.apc.org. Web site: http://www.itvs.org/babyg. An autobiographical documentary chronicling one woman's experience with cervical cancer caused by DES.

Diabetes

Jovanovic-Peterson, Lois, et al. *The Diabetic Woman*. New York: Putnam, 1996.

Milchovich, Sue K., and Barbara Dunn-Long. *Diabetes Mellitus: A Practical Handbook*. Palo Alto, CA: Bull Publishing Co., 1995

Organizations

American Diabetes Association
1660 Duke Street; Alexandria, VA 22314; (800) 232-3472
Web site: http://www.diabetes.org/default.htm

Cochrane Collaboration Diabetes Group
Contact: Cathy Bennett, Coordinator
Division of Public Health, Nuffield Institute of Health; 71–75 Clarendon Road; Leeds, U.K. LS2 9PL
E-mail: hss6ps@leeds.ac.uk

Disability

Berkeley Planning Associates. *Meeting the Needs of Women with Disabilities: A Blueprint for Change—Bibliography*, Oakland, CA: Berkeley Planning Associates, 1996. Available from Berkeley Planning Associates, (510) 465-7884. Web site: http://www.bpacal.com/publist.html

Ferreyra, Susan, and Katrine Hughes. *Table Manners:*

A Guide to the Pelvic Examination for Disabled Women and Their Health Care Providers. San Francisco: Sex Education for Disabled People, 1982.

Klein, Bonnie. *Slow Dance: A Story of Stroke, Love and Disability.* Toronto: Knopf Canada, 1997.

National Clearinghouse on Women and Girls with Disabilities. *Bridging the Gap: A National Directory of Services for Women and Girls with Disabilities.* New York: Educational Equity Concepts, 1990.

Register, Cheri. *Living with Chronic Illness: Days of Patience and Passion.* New York: The Free Press, 1987.

Resourceful Woman newsletter
Health Resource Center for Women with Disabilities; Rehabilitation Institute of Chicago; 345 East Superior Street, Room 106; Chicago, IL 60611; (312) 908-7997
E-mail: jpsparkle@aol.com

Saxton, Marsha, and Florence Howe, eds. *With Wings: An Anthology of Literature By and About Women with Disabilities.* New York: Feminist Press, 1987.

Webster, Barbara. *All of a Piece: A Life with Multiple Sclerosis.* Baltimore, MD: Johns Hopkins University Press, 1989.

Additional Online Resources

Disabled Peoples' International
http://www.dpi.org

The Invisible Disabilities Page
http://www1.shore.net/~dmoisan/invisible_disability.html

Endometriosis

Ballweg, Mary Lou, and The Endometriosis Association. *Endometriosis Sourcebook.* Chicago: Contemporary Books, 1995.

Carol, Ruth ed. *Alternatives for Women with Endometriosis: A Guide by Women for Women.* Chicago: Third Side Press, 1994.

Kennedy, Stephen H., et al. "A Comparison of Nafarelin Acetate and Danazol in the Treatment of Endometriosis," *Fertility and Sterility* 53, no. 6 (June 1990): 998–1003.

Weinstein, Kate. *Living with Endometriosis: How to Cope with the Physical and Emotional Challenges.* Reading, MA: Addison-Wesley, 1987.

Organization

The Endometriosis Association
8585 North 76th Place; Milwaukee, WI 53223; (800) 992-3636 (in the U.S.); (800) 426-2363 (in Canada)
Web site: http://www.endometriosisassn.org

Female Circumcision (Female Genital Mutilation)

Carr, Dara. *Female Genital Cutting: Findings from the Demographic and Health Surveys Program.* Calverton, MD: Macro International, 1997.

Toubia, Nahid. *Female Genital Mutilation: A Call for Global Action.* New York: RAINB♀, 1995.

Organization

RAINB♀ (Research, Action and Information Network for the Bodily Integrity of Women)
915 Broadway, Suite 1109; New York, NY 10010-7108; (212) 477-3318

Heart Disease, Heart Attack, Hypertension, and Stroke

Ayanian, John Z., and Arnold M. Epstein. "Differences in the Use of Procedures Between Women and Men Hospitalized for Coronary Heart Disease." *New England Journal of Medicine* 325, no. 4 (1989): 221–25.

Douglas, Pamela S., ed. *Cardiovascular Health and Disease in Women.* Philadelphia: W. B. Saunders, 1993.

Eaker, E. D., et al. "Epidemiology and Risk Factors for Coronary Heart Disease in Women." *Cardiovascular Clinics* 19, no. 3 (1989): 129–45.

Hardman, A. E., et al. "Brisk Walking and Plasma High Density Lipoprotein Cholesterol Concentration in Previously Sedentary Women." *British Medical Journal* 299, no. 6709 (1989): 1204–210.

Khan, Steven S., et al. "Increased Mortality of Women in Coronary Artery Bypass Surgery: Evidence for Referral Bias." *Annals of Internal Medicine* 112, no. 8 (1990): 561–69.

Legato, Mariane J., and Carol Colman. *The Female Heart: The Truth About Women and Coronary Artery Disease.* New York: Simon & Schuster, 1991.

Matthews, Karen A., et al. "Menopause and Risk Factors for Coronary Heart Disease." *New England Journal of Medicine* 321, no. 10 (1989): 641–46.

Steingart, Richard M., et al. "Sex Differences in the Management of Coronary Artery Disease." *New England Journal of Medicine* 325, no. 4 (1991): 226–30.

Wenger, Nanette K. "Coronary Heart Disease in Women 1996." *Seminars in Reproductive Endocrinology* 14, no. 1 (1996): 5.

Organization

American Heart Association
(800) 242-8721
Web site: http://www.amhrt.org
Many local chapters.

Cochrane Collaboration Hypertension Group
Contact: Mr. Michael Brand, Coordinator
Cochrane Hypertension Group; Audie L. Murphy Memorial Veterans Hospital; VA ACOS/AC (1106); 7400 Merton Minter Boulevard; San Antonio, TX 78284
E-mail: htncrg@merece.uthscsa.edu

Hysterectomy and Oophorectomy

Carlson, Karen J., et al. "Indications for Hysterectomy." *New England Journal of Medicine* 328, no. 12 (1993): 856–60; and Letters to the Editor, *New England Journal of Medicine* 329, no. 4 (1993): 275–76.

Harber, Becca, "Alternative Healing for Fibroids and Cysts." *WomenWise* 13, no. 4 (1990/91): 5.

"Incidence and Prevalence of Hysterectomy." *Activities of the U.S. Public Health Service,* 1995.

Kritz-Silverstein, Donna, et. al. "Hysterectomy, Oophorectomy, and Heart Disease Risk Factors in Older Women." *American Journal of Public Health* 87, no. 4 (April 1997): 676–80.

Oldenhave, Anna, et al. "Hysterectomized Women with Ovarian Conservation Report More Severe Climacteric Complaints Than Do Normal Climacteric Women of Similar Age." *American Journal of Obstetrics and Gynecology* 168, no. 3 (1993): 765–71.

Payer, Lynn. *How to Avoid a Hysterectomy: An Indispensable Guide to Exploring All Your Options Before You Consent to a Hysterectomy.* New York: Pantheon Books, 1987.

———. "The Operation Every Woman Should Question." *McCall's* (June 1995): 54–56.

Strausz, Ivan K. *You Don't Need a Hysterectomy: New and Effective Ways of Avoiding Major Surgery.* Reading, MA: Addison-Wesley, 1993.

U.S. Senate Subcommittee on Aging. *Unnecessary Hysterectomies: The Second Most Common Major Surgery in the United States: A Hearing Before the Subcommittee on Aging of the Committee on Labor and Human Resources, United States Senate, 103rd Congress, 1st Session, May 5, 1993.* Washington, DC: U.S. GPO, 1993.

Organization

Hysterectomy Educational Resources and Services (HERS)
422 Bryn Mawr Avenue; Bala Cynwyd, PA 19004; (610) 667-7757

Video

Costa, Barbara, and Denisce Dilanni. *Sudden Changes: Post-Hysterectomy Syndrome.* 1985. Excellent 29-minute color video. Examines the reasons for the high number of hysterectomies performed on women every year, the alternatives available, the side effects, and the aftereffects. Includes interviews with doctors, other professionals, and women who have undergone the operation. Available from The Cinema Guild, 1697 Broadway, Suite 506, New York, NY 10019 (212) 246-5522.

Urinary Tract Infections/Disorders and Interstitial Cystitis

Brody, Jane. "Interstitial Cystitis: Help for a Puzzling and Extraordinarily Painful Illness of the Bladder." *The New York Times* (January 25, 1995): B7.

Burgio, Kathryn, et al. *Staying Dry: A Practical Guide to Bladder Control.* Baltimore, MD: Johns Hopkins University Press, 1989.

Chalker, Rebecca, and Kristene E. Whitmore. *Overcoming Bladder Disorders: Compassionate, Authoritative Medical and Self-help Solutions for Incontinence, Cystitis, Interstitial Cystitis, Prostate Problems and Bladder Cancer.* New York: Harper and Row, 1990.

Gartley, Cheryle, ed. *Managing Incontinence.* Ottawa, IL: Jameson Books, 1985.

Hanno, Philip. "Interstitial Cystitis." *Urologic Clinics of North America* 21, no. 1 (1994): 1–176.

Kilmartin, Angela. *Cystitis: The Complete Self-Help Guide.* New York: Warner Books, 1980.

Sant, Grannum R. "Interstitial Cystitis." *Monographs in Urology* 12, no. 3 (1991): 37–63.

Wein, Alan, and Phil Hanno, eds. *Urology* 49, no. 5A (Supplement May 1997). Entire issue devoted to interstitial cystitis.

Organization

Interstitial Cystitis Association (ICA)
P.O. Box 1553, Madison Square Station; New York, NY 10159-1553; (212) 979-6057
Web site: http://www.ichelp.com

Uterus, Cervix, and Ovaries; PID

Malesky, Gale, and Charles B. Inlander. *Take This Book to the Gynecologist with You: A Consumer's Guide to Women's Health.* Reading, MA: Addison-Wesley, 1991.

U.S. Department of Health and Human Services. *Treatment of Non-cancerous Uterine Conditions: Issues for Research—Conference Summary.* Washington DC: USDHHS, 1994.

Wasserheit, Judith N. "Pelvic Inflammatory Disease and Infertility." *Maryland Medical Journal* 36, no. 1 (Jan. 1987): 58–63.

Vagina/Vulva

National Vulvodynia Association
P.O. Box 4491; Silver Spring, MD 20914-4491; (301) 299-0775
Web site: http://www.sojourn.com/~nva

Resources for Topics Not Covered in This Chapter

"Chronic Hepatitis C." *Education Initiatives in Gastroenterology* (Aug. 25, 1997). Special issue.

Harriton, Monique B. *The Whiplash Handbook.* Springfield, IL: CC Thomas, 1989.

Solden, Sari. *Women with Attention Deficit Disorder: Embracing Disorganization at Home and in the Workplace.* Grass Valley, CA: Underwood Books, 1995.

National Headache Foundation
428 West St. James Place; Chicago, IL 60614; (773) 388-6399; (800) 843-2256

By Norma Meras Swenson with Wendy
Sanford and Judy Norsigian;
"Our Rights as Patients"
by George Annas
"Evidence-Based Medicine"
by Carol Sakala

BASED ON EARLIER WORK BY Hilary Salk,
Norma Swenson, Judith Dickson Luce, and
Wendy Sanford

WITH SPECIAL THANKS TO Nancy Krieger,
Anne Kasper, Ellen Shaffer, Steffi
Woolhandler, Karen Kahn, Jacqueline
Lapidus, Arnold Relman, Philip R. Lee, Roz
Feldberg, Julie Friesen, Anne-Emmanuelle
Birn, Nancy Worcester, and Mariamne
Whatley * †

Chapter 25

The Politics of Women's Health and Medical Care

* Thanks also to the following for their help with the 1998 version
of this chapter: Denise Berg, Lucy Candib, Joanna Gomes, and
Gayle Martin. Over the years since 1969, the following people have
contributed to the many versions of this chapter: Amy Alpern,
David Banta, Gene Bishop, Robin Blatt, Lucy Candib, David Clarke,
Mary Fillmore, Mary Howell, Sherry Leibowitz, Judy Norsigian,
Barbara Perkins, Joan Rachlin, Sheryl Ruzek, Kathy Simmonds,
Mary Stern, Nancy Todd, Karen Wolf, and Nancy Worcester.
† We are basing the analysis in this chapter both on thousands of
personal accounts and on the work of a wide range of people and
groups: feminist writers and other investigative journalists; feminist,
radical, and progressive physicians and nurses; medical educators;
health workers and practitioners of all kinds; public health
researchers; lawyers and health law experts; medical historians and
medical sociologists; ethicists; public-interest groups; and
government specialists; as well as social and feminist critics of
many different persuasions.

We are living in a time of great change in the U.S. health, medical, and social support systems. Unfortunately, the changes we are experiencing today, a result of shifts in the global economy as well as the "welfare reform" act of 1996,[1] are eliminating the social safety net constructed during earlier periods as minimal protection for the elderly and those with low incomes. Many people have depended on this net for access to health care. These new social policies have already resulted in increasing rates of poverty and, therefore, ill health. If citizens don't work to change these policies, there are likely to be greater levels of illness than there have been since the early 20th century.

At the same time that our country's social welfare system is being dismantled, our health and medical care system is undergoing rapid change. Over the last 30 years, this system has been transformed from a system that was moderately profitable for some to an exorbitantly profitable industry that values financial gain over the social good of maintaining a healthy population.

This chapter addresses the impact of these changes in social and economic policy on the lives of women, and shows how they make women's experiences of earning a living, caring for our families, and obtaining satisfactory health and medical care services much more difficult than at any point in the recent past. The chapter also provides some of the information women

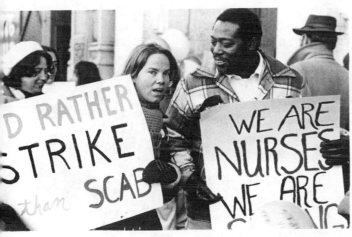

Sarah Putnam

need to survive the health and medical care systems. As we face these vast changes and new social policies, we will need even greater knowledge and commitment to negotiate the system in order to get the care we need as well as to organize for change.

WHY FOCUS ON WOMEN AND HEALTH?

I think you would have been proud of the way I handled the situation with the surgeon. Despite a fair amount of crying on my part, I was able to demand a second opinion for my diverticulosis treatment and the most conservative treatment possible. My surgeon was appalled when I balked at surgery Monday without what I felt was adequate time to discuss the situation or get another opinion. I really think that if it wasn't for my experience with the Women's Health Collective and the support of my friends and family, I would have a temporary colostomy right now.

I, extremely well informed, well connected, verbally aggressive, have had to summon all my resources to get what I wanted in my treatment for breast cancer: medical care that was consistent with the findings of the latest literature and that took into account my needs as a woman.

As a young woman interested in one day having a family, I was never told that cimetidine [medication for ulcers] should not be used in pregnant patients or women of child-bearing potential unless, in the judgment of the physician, the anticipated benefits outweigh the potential risks. I should have been informed of this and given the opportunity to make the decision myself in consultation with the doctor. My family raised me to trust doctors, but I no longer can do that.

As a visiting nurse I learned to listen to patients, to speak their language, to let them set their own priorities for care, to teach them when they were ready. I also learned to evaluate the health care system through their eyes. Each day I confronted an irrele-

vant, noncaring, inadequate health care system that refused to consider the personal, social, cultural, and economic needs of the patient.

This isn't a health care system; it's a crapshoot!
—From a feminist doctor

These are just a few of the thousands of women who are speaking out about their dissatisfaction with the medical care system and with physicians and other medical personnel who have

- not listened to us or believed what we said.
- lied to us.
- treated us without our consent.
- not warned us of risks and negative effects of treatments.
- overcharged.
- experimented on us or used us as "teaching material."
- treated us poorly because of race, class, sexual identity, age, or disability.
- offered us tranquilizers or moral advice instead of medical care or useful help from community resources (self-help groups, battered women's services, etc.).
- administered treatments or performed operations that were unnecessary, sometimes mutilating and too extreme for our problem, some of which resulted in permanent disability or even death (iatrogenesis).*
- prescribed drugs that hooked us, sickened us, changed our entire lives.
- abused us sexually.
- withheld knowledge or necessary treatment.
- refused to prescribe or even discuss high-cost treatment options that might be uniquely beneficial.

Clearly, men experience some of these problems as well. But in general, men are treated with more respect and use the medical care system less often than women. In fact, women use the health and medical care system twice as often as men, not just for our own care but because we are so often responsible for children, partners, aging parents, and other relatives as well. In addition, women are about 75% of all health care workers in hospitals and about 85% in the system as a whole. We carry out most doctors' orders—treatment regimens like special diets, medications, daily

---

* Iatrogenesis occurs when illness, impairment, or death results from medical treatment. Some examples are cancers caused by diethylstilbestrol (DES), pelvic inflammatory disease (PID) or hysterectomy caused by an IUD or untreated STD, death or disability due to anesthesia accident (particularly when the surgery may not have been necessary), electrocution or burns from hospital equipment, medication errors, infection from respirators, crippling or fatal strokes due to the birth control pill, addiction to tranquilizers, and illness or death resulting from infant formula feeding in hospitals.

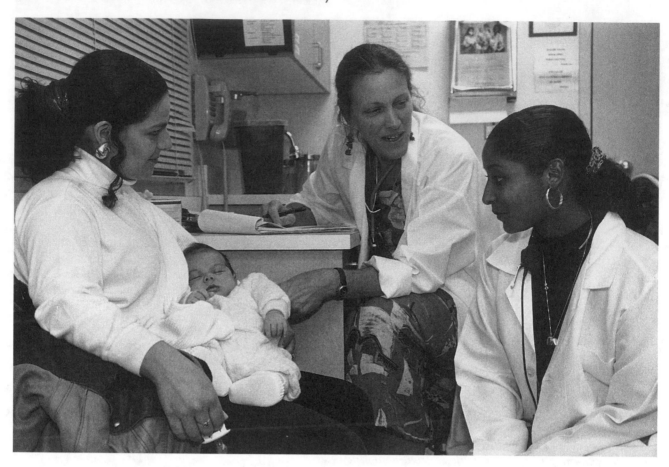

Ann Dowie/The Picture Cube

activity supervision, and so on—either as paid workers in some part of the system or, increasingly, as unpaid workers at home. Most "patient communication" for and about family members' health and illness flows through women: we report signs, changes, symptoms, and responses to treatments and medications. We are most of the teachers about health both in the home and in the system, informing people about how to take care of themselves and what to do when problems arise. At home, we are usually the first to be told when someone doesn't feel well, and we help decide what to do next, usually going with the unwell person to seek care. If care is unavailable or unaffordable, we are usually left to manage on our own.

As women many of us provide as much of our unpaid caregiving labor to assist family members or people in our communities who are disabled, elderly, or chronically ill as we do to raise young children. Frequently, we sacrifice earning potential and future Social Security or retirement benefits in order to do so. We may be put in the position of taking on serious, life-and-death caregiving responsibilities without adequate support or resources. Moreover, in our communities, we are the majority who give thousands of hours of volunteer labor to local organizations, staffing blood-pressure clinics and managing blood drives, and keeping AIDS support networks and hospice op-

tions available. We are also most of the lowest-paid workers in nonprofit and community service organizations, acting as citizens in the public interest, advocating for better health for everyone.

Paradoxically, power in the current health care system does not reflect the massive volunteer labor of the overwhelming numbers of women who keep the system going at all levels. Women have the largest portion of the responsibility but not the requisite authority we deserve in return. Despite increases in the percentage of female doctors in recent decades—and women's overwhelming presence throughout the system—the health and medical care field overall persists in being among the most male-dominated, sexist, racist, and resistant to change of any of society's major institutions in the U.S. Possible reasons for this resistance include

- the exceptional prestige, social power, earnings, and professional autonomy bestowed on physicians by society (even in the age of managed care).
- relatively few women or people of color in leadership positions.
- the enormous profitability of all the industries associated with health and medical care, which now make up one-fifth of the U.S. economy.

As the health care industry becomes increasingly profit-oriented, the pressure of this male-dominant culture on women is likely to increase. It is essential that we understand the economic and social forces that shape the health care industry if, as women, we want to participate in creating a system that meets our needs.

THE POLITICAL CONTEXT

Assumptions About Women by the System

The medical care system has traditionally made certain assumptions about women as patients, workers, and caregivers:

- Our labor is available free or at low cost, especially as caregivers of ailing partners, parents, or in-laws.
- We should be dependent on spouses/partners or employers for access to insurance and care.
- Because women use the system more often, we should pay higher insurance premiums.
- "Poor" women and women of color are liabilities, while insured women are "markets" and "billable" resources.

Women will have to take the lead in making sure that these assumptions are not built into any proposals for changing the way health, medical, and social services are financed and delivered.

Factors That Affect Women's Health

Poverty and Racism

Poverty, which disproportionately affects women and children and all people of color, is the most basic cause of ill health and early death in our society. People with low incomes have more illnesses and die in greater numbers and earlier than people with more income and education.[2] Many health problems result from malnutrition, workplace dangers, inadequate sanitation and housing, joblessness, environmental pollution, excessive stress, malnutrition, or violence. The violence of racism contributes significantly to the poorer health status and outcomes of people of color. (Recent research has begun to identify specific disease effects of racism.)[3] Much medical thinking, however, blames people who suffer the effects of poverty; for instance, doctors accuse "poor" women of not taking proper care of ourselves or our children, or they see drug use and depression in "poor" families as individual, preventable failures of character rather than as markers of economically and socially depressed community development.[4]

The 1996 "welfare reform act" is likely to have a major impact on the health of women with low incomes. Medicaid programs, which offered at least minimal access to medical care, will be cut drastically as federal welfare "block grants"—finite sums—are left to the states to spend and distribute as they see fit.[5] We are seeing a loss of the very programs that reduce people's need for costly medical care: job training, food-assistance programs, reproductive health services, and health education in the community. These cuts in the federal budget will accelerate rates of illness and death. Most city and county health systems are experiencing increasing patient loads, rising costs, deteriorating facilities, and decreasing budgets, with no relief in sight. Many immigrants are losing access to medical care under "welfare reform."

Racism may create more barriers to obtaining needed care, and to survival, than social class. For example, even allowing for social class, black babies continue to die at higher rates than white babies living in the same geographic area. This is primarily due to low birthweight among black babies, which is almost entirely preventable. Medicine's usual response to the infant death gap between the races—costly neonatal intensive care centers—has been unsuccessful. That is because what is needed is not more expensive machines but more investment in the community to counter the effects of racism and poverty on the health of expectant mothers.[6]

Those of us who are women of color need medical care more often than white women do, but we frequently get less. For example, we are less likely to get preventive screening or the most modern treatment or followup care for cancer and, as a result, do not survive as long after diagnosis. This is especially true of breast cancer. Similarly, even though hypertension is 82% higher among women of color, we receive no more treatment than white women.[7]

In addition to lack of care, many women with low incomes and women of color have received more abusive and damaging care than other women. Women who do not speak English fluently are often treated by medical providers as if we are stupid. "Poor" women are more likely to be used as "teaching material" in hospitals, so that physicians in training can practice the craft they will use later on wealthy private patients.[8] Because of stereotyping, some practitioners offer different diagnoses and different treatment to women of color and lower-income women, even when they have the same symptoms as white, middle-class women. Paradoxically, when women decide not to return for care, our absence gives rise to medical providers' accusations of "noncompliance." Again, women are blamed.

Overwork

The combination of paid work outside our homes and unpaid work within our homes affects our overall health. Alone, with children, or even with a partner, we may find juggling the combination of work and home responsibilities overwhelming. We may have little personal time. But we all need time to be alone, to exercise, to learn a new skill, to laugh out loud because we are relaxed and having a good time—not just once or twice a year, but often. Sometimes even sex seems like just one more thing we have to do, not the fun or pleasure it's supposed to be.

Pleasure is a strange word. It is so long since I have had a really good time that I can't even remember—maybe since before my last child was born. Right now I think it would be like pleasure if I could just stop, just sit and do nothing, because it feels like there is never enough time to do everything no matter where I am, and everybody is counting on me and waiting for me to come and do what needs to be done. . . . Pleasure, I think maybe if I had nothing else to do I would read a book for a while, if I could keep from feeling guilty.

This is not to say that men never "help out" in the home, but most studies show that fewer than 10% of men living with women and children share truly equally in tasks of child-rearing or household work.[9] Most men maintain an expectation that after eight or more hours of working, they are entitled to rest, relaxation, recreation, and pleasure at home or elsewhere.[10] Even in Sweden, where men and women are in the workforce nearly equally, recent studies have shown that as the working day draws to a close, stress hormone levels in the blood begin to rise for women as they start to anticipate the "second shift" of their day, while for men they begin to go down in anticipation of going home, where they will relax and do little or no work.[11] It isn't that women never enjoy tasks performed routinely for our households or families. But as pressures increase, it is clear we need support of all kinds, or risk becoming ill from overwork.

The primary source of women's overwork is the current world economy and social structure (see "Poverty and Racism," p. 683), as well as society's presumption that women's unpaid labor will continue to take up the slack created by changes in the health system and in wider society. We work harder and harder to do it all, like Superwoman, to survive in an economy that profits, literally, from our sacrifices.[12]

Lack of sleep, lack of support, and limited opportunities for genuine pleasure, relaxation, or exercise not only build up stress and hidden resentments but are serious risks to good health. This condition is called overwork, or stress, which is not simply psychological but has physical effects ranging from moderate strain on the heart, for example, to occasional heart attacks or strokes. When we realize that all over the world most women are working approximately twice as many hours as men, and girl children usually work harder than boys, we must look at the overwork in women's lives as a socially created health problem—a situation we must change. Stress is not simply some kind of special women's "mental health" issue. Women may live longer than men, but we suffer more from all chronic diseases. Rest, pleasure, and support for ourselves are not selfish desires but essential to our health and well-being as well as the well-being of all our communities.

Overwork must become a women's issue and a women's health issue. The many resources needed to keep ourselves and our communities healthy include

- more widely available high-quality day care for young children.
- more diverse and stable elder care services, including adult day care, in-home services, long-term care, and respite coverage.
- better after-school programs.
- improved community and public services, including safe and equal exercise and recreation opportunities for women and girls.
- good shelters for homeless and battered women with permanent funding support.
- health coverage de-linked from employment.
- more support for nonprofit, public interest organizations working on community health issues.
- tax or Social Security credits for unpaid family caregiving.
- tax credits for child-rearing costs, like day care.
- equal pay for equal work.
- paid family and medical leave.
- a shorter work week.
- time off to work in and for the community.

We must demand that all workplaces, including tax-exempt institutions like religious institutions, schools, and government, openly acknowledge women's double workload and risk of overwork, and reinforce the principle of family supports and equal sharing of household labor. This is a matter of women's health, and community health, now and in the future.[13]

Medicalization* and Social Control of Women's Lives

It is good practice for medical professionals to be aware of the many factors that may be part of a woman's health picture. However, many have carried this to an extreme and actually claim expertise in matters that society has never before considered medical: adolescence, overactivity in children, sex, diet, child abuse, exercise, criminality, and aging, to name a few. This phenomenon, called medicalization, allows medical people to become the "experts" on how normal experiences of life, or social problems, should be defined and "managed."[14] The most striking example of this process is the medicalization of women's lives in all areas of reproductive health, sexuality, and aging. For example, consider how often women are expected to go to physicians for normal life events, like having a baby or entering menopause. Because physicians are trained to look for problems and to respond with

* For a thorough discussion of medicalization, see Irving Kenneth Zola, "Medicine as an Institution of Social Control" in *Socio-medical Inquiries* (see endnote 14); for an historical discussion of medicalization and iatrogenesis, see Ivan Illich, *Medical Nemesis* (Pantheon, 1976).

interventions like drugs, surgery, and medical devices, we are often led to see our normal life events as full of potential problems and to accept interventions when they aren't necessary. For instance, studies show that having a baby at home or with a midwife can be an equally safe and often more satisfying option for low-risk child-bearing women than hospitalization (see chapters 19, Pregnancy, and 20, Childbirth). Yet, most physicians tell women that hospital birth is always the safest approach. The drug industry reinforces medicalization by supporting and promoting the research that transforms women's major life transitions into fearful problems requiring technical, pharmacological solutions available only through medical professionals.

Medical "care" often extends to value judgments about our behavior and life choices as well.

When I told my doctor (foolishly) that I'm a lesbian, the whole visit turned into a moral lecture and he never really paid attention to my problem. I walked out when he recommended a psychiatrist.

These moral judgments carry a weighty power, though they are no more "scientific" than the judgments of a priest or rabbi.[15] When we "deviate" by not conforming to norms of womanhood, or "fail to comply" with medical advice, we discover how powerful medicine can be. For example, in the past many women were sterilized without their knowledge or consent because physicians thought they had "too many babies" (see "Sterilization," chapter 13, Birth Control, p. 331). Some physicians have sought court-ordered cesarean sections, declaring women "unfit mothers" when we refused this surgery; some women have had their children taken from them by the courts because a physician judged them "potential child abusers" for refusing medical treatments during pregnancy.

We may not question the role physicians have taken in our lives because our dependence began very early, when our mothers took us regularly to "the doctor." It is crucial, however, that we look more closely at the doctor/patient relationship and secure independent sources of information and support to help guide our decisions.

The Doctor-Patient Relationship

In part, medicine has achieved social control over women's lives through the special sanctity of the private physician/patient relationship. The relationship between a woman and her doctor is often one of profound inequality on every level, an exaggeration of the power imbalances inherent in many client-professional relationships in our society. This is more likely to be true in a male physician/female patient relationship, but it can be true of female doctor/female patient encounters as well, often aggravated by racial or social class distances. As in any relationship in which we are less powerful, we tend to evaluate what happens in a medical encounter in terms of our own behavior rather than the doctor's. For example, if we

don't understand something, we may feel inadequate or intimidated and find it hard to muster the courage to admit this and ask for an explanation we understand. Often we believe that a doctor's superior education, training, experience, and (sometimes) age automatically produce infallible judgment.

There may always be something about the "laying on of hands" that calls up the child in us and makes us feel dependent, especially when pain and fear are present. Some physicians deliberately work to increase this natural phenomenon into a special kind of dependency in which the patient turns to the physician in a child-like way for guidance. When a woman raises real, matter-of-fact questions, a doctor may say, "What's the matter, don't you trust me?" or "I can't take care of you if you don't believe in my advice." Many doctors believe that if a woman becomes overly dependent it is because she "needs" or wants to be.

Work by many feminist sociologists and even some women physicians shows the importance of changing this imbalance and improving communication.[16] Our stories are crucial for correct diagnoses as well as for choice of treatment options, and we need to insist that our providers listen to them and act upon them. Sociologist Ann Oakley has shown in the most extensive work on this subject that some physicians seek to contradict and replace a woman's own knowledge and sense of herself and her problem with the doctor's own convictions about what is "really" going on, medically speaking.[17] Increasingly, in rushed encounters, doctors no longer engage openly in that exercise of persuasion but rather quietly wait, apparently listening, murmuring "Uh-huh," from time to time until the moment of prescription arrives. Without further information, we may not know enough to challenge whether a prescription is even appropriate.

I explained everything as clearly as I could, and went over my general healthy condition, which showed my cholesterol is fine and my blood pressure is high only when I come in to her office. I was due for an annual checkup, but she's so busy it can't be done until May! She never once looked me in the eye, busy writing, and all of a sudden she gave me this prescription for hormones, which I never have taken, and said, "You should be taking estrogen." I was so annoyed and surprised I didn't have the nerve to ask her why, without a checkup and in the absence of any real reasons, I should now go on this drug.

So many doctors only know how to prescribe and they feel that they haven't helped if they haven't prescribed. As someone who has seen doctors a lot in my life for asthma, I can tell you that they always prescribe. I've reached the point where I just rip up the prescription or monitor the doses because I know my body.

Today, the problem of communication in the doctor/patient relationship has much more serious consequences than ever before. As more of us receive medical care through managed care (MC) plans (see "The Language of the Medical Care System" p. 692), we will be seeing doctors who are in charge of both our medical care and the decisions about how to pay for it. Under MC, most "primary care" visits are limited to 15 minutes—insufficient time to raise, let alone resolve the most pressing issues women want to raise. MC also encourages doctors to save costs, not necessarily to provide the best care (see p. 696). This is not only a conflict of interest but a dangerous situation.

It is crucial that we make whatever efforts we can to improve doctor visits (see p. 685). Even when we are well-informed and sure of our ground, it can be difficult to speak up and to bring up doubts and misgivings with a doctor or other practitioner. Immersed in the propaganda about women's "need" for dependency, and comfortable with their authoritarian role as many still are, doctors may react with surprise and even hostility at our "aggressiveness" when we insist on being partners in our health and medical care decisions. We must not let their reactions prevent us from persisting. If necessary, we must remind them that the advice to "take charge of your own health care" and "get informed," which we proposed in this book 25 years ago, is now coming from many well-known critics and writers in this country.[18] **Whenever possible, bring someone whom you trust with you.**

MC may make it more difficult, but over time, you may find you can build a satisfactory relationship with a committed and ethical doctor.

Friends now marvel at my close relationship with my current doctor and my ability to talk back, question, and disagree with him and his colleagues. He respects me and trusts me to tell him what is going on, and I in turn trust him to listen, make suggestions, and consult with me before any action is taken. When I don't want a procedure done or feel the psychological burden of making yet another trip to the lab or to his office is just too much for me on an occasion, I will tell him and he understands me most of the time. I have finally after many, many years found someone willing to take into account my whole medical history and apply it to my current situation.

Sexual Abuse

One of the consequences of the imbalance in the doctor/patient relationship is that some doctors abuse their power. Not only have women reported increasing numbers of cases of rape by their doctors over the past ten years, but between 5 and 10% of doctors have admitted in surveys and interviews to having had sexual relations with their patients.[19] To explain their behavior, these doctors say that they believed such relations were either harmless or actually beneficial or "therapeutic" to the women involved. It is not uncommon for women who are sexually abused by a doctor to be persuaded that he has fallen in love with them and to agree to "consensual" sex. This is not a sign of naïveté or psychopathology on our part. The physicians involved have abused a trust that every woman has learned to place in them.

Because of the broken trust involved, sexual abuse by health care practitioners may produce the kind of severe damage found in father-daughter incest. Yet when the woman turns to or is referred to a psychiatrist, she may be blamed for having "caused" the abuse. Worse still, a few psychiatrists seduce the woman once again.[20] It takes enormous courage for women to come forward and speak out about sexual abuse by doctors. Frequently, no one believes us, and in one case, nurses reporting their eyewitness experiences of patient abuse for three years were ignored by hospital administrators until another physician caught his anesthesiologist colleague in the act. One dentist abused dozens of patients, including young girls, before one woman spoke out and he was exposed.

In spite of the fact that the Hippocratic oath and the ethics codes of all medical and mental health societies specifically forbid sexual relations with patients, the medical profession has made minimal effort to discipline those who breach the code. The few cases of sexual abuse that reach state boards of registration in medicine frequently drag on for months and are then resolved with inadequate controls on future abuse. Some women physicians have taken a stronger stand on sexual abuse. For the most part, the medical profession appears primarily concerned with covering up for a colleague who commits what are often tactfully called "indiscretions."

In the words of a woman psychiatrist:

I reported a psychiatrist who had had sex with two of his patients to the medical society. I called back two months later to find out what had been done. They told me the doctor denied everything, and it was his word against the patients', so they were dropping the matter. When I persisted, the chairman of the ethics committee told me, "You know, my dear, we are not a consumer organization."[21]

Recent legislation requires that a physician's loss of hospital privileges (and certain other disciplinary actions) be reported to a central registry. Hospitals hiring or granting privileges to a new doctor, for example, are required to check this registry first.

If you notice any sexually inappropriate, peculiar, or irresponsible behavior on the part of any health care practitioner, you may feel more empowered by discussing the experience with others. A local women's group or rape crisis center may be able to help you. One woman we know wrote her story in detail, naming her abuser, and circulated it in the hospital where the doctor had privileges. Many other women then came forward. It took years, but eventually his license was suspended.[22] **To support your case, it is important to make and keep a written or taped record of what happens.** Also, consider discussing your experience with a reliable lawyer or women's law group. They may know aspects of the law on rape or sexual harassment of which you are unaware (see chapter 8, Violence Against Women).

The Women's Health Movement(s)

Almost 30 years ago, women of all ages and backgrounds joined together in local communities and nationwide to fight for better health care for women, and for everyone, by maintaining a critical perspective and by challenging the medical establishment, the profit motive, the professions, industry, and government. This effort, known as the Women's Health Movement, has significantly changed the way many women and providers think about women's health and medical care. Activists have formed local and national organizations and have fought in legislatures, hospitals, and courts for improvements in research, care, and products used by women—often successfully (see chapter 27, Organizing for Change: U.S.A.).[23] Many became doctors and other health care providers. Over the years women of color from a broad range of ethnicities and communities, lesbians, women with chronic illnesses and disabilities, and older women have created many women's health movements, writing new agendas for better health in our communities.

The successes of the Women's Health Movement include substantial federal funding of research into women's diseases at the National Institutes of Health (NIH), women's health legislation introduced regularly at the state and federal levels, and increases in the numbers of women physicians and scientists. The subject of women's health now has a visible place in the media. Nonetheless, the health of women and children

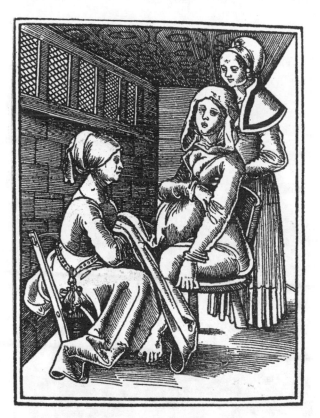

A midwife attending a child-bearing woman (sixteenth-century illustration)/Corbis-Bettmann

is not improving. As the health insurance and delivery systems increasingly come under corporate control, many of the advances for women achieved by health activists are being reversed.[24] Many of the government-sponsored research efforts are tied firmly to the *biomedical model* of women's health, focusing mainly on chronic diseases and little, if at all, on the social and economic factors that affect our health. (A focus on race, ethnicity, and social class in several government-sponsored meetings during 1996 and 1997 indicates that this may be changing.)

Currently, only a handful of underfunded women's groups are able to sustain an active presence and critical, public-interest voice in advocating for women's health. These groups often depend on volunteer labor —increasingly harder to come by as women retreat from the public sphere because of the burdens of work and family responsibilities.

There is much work to be done. It is not enough to provide or improve medical care for everyone, to have more women physicians, to stop abuses of patients' rights, or to increase access to existing health and medical care for the poor and uninsured—goals that are essential and laudable. Women need a role not only as researchers and policy-makers but also as citizens and community members in the actual governance of health care programs. We need to broaden our focus from the clinical and biomedical to the politi-

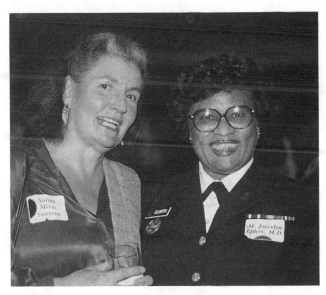

Dr. Joycelyn Elders (right), during her tenure as Surgeon General in the Clinton administration, and Norma Meras Swenson of the BWHBC, receiving awards from Educational Equity Concepts in New York, 1993/Sarah Swenson

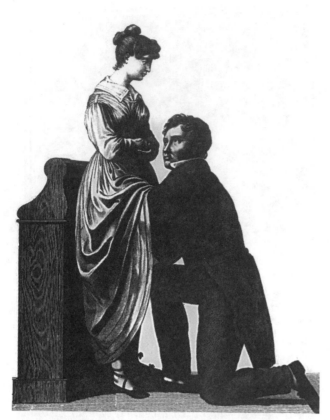

A gynecological exam (nineteenth-century illustration)/
Corbis-Bettmann

cal and economic issues of women's power and control over systems that have so much power over us. Women also need to reclaim the domain of self-help knowledge. Preventive and nonmedical healing methods should be available to all who want them. We need to expose the way the medical establishment suppresses these alternatives (home birth and midwifery, for example) and to assert that such alternatives are human rights.[25] (See chapter 20, Childbirth.)

At the Boston Women's Health Book Collective, we continue to believe in the healing powers within all of us, in our ability to help one another by listening, talking, caring, and touching—and in the power of small groups as sources of information sharing, strength, support, and healing. We still believe that we, as women, are the best experts on ourselves. The more we understand how vulnerable we become—both to disease and to dependency on experts—when isolated from one another, the more we see supportive group experience and community action as essential resources for health, for everyone. These groups may range from small consciousness-raising or self-help and support programs to large numbers of women and communities organized for political action.[26]

THE HEALTH CARE INDUSTRY

The health care industry in the U.S. is roughly a three-armed structure, sometimes called the "medical-industrial complex."* There are medicine and the medical establishment,† the pharmaceutical/hospital supply industries, and the insurance/"managed care" industries. Although the U.S. has always had a private, profit-making system, it has always been balanced by some government funding and regulation. Today, the balance has shifted toward greater control by large corporations and less power in the hands of doctors, patients, and the government. In this section, we look at each of these elements and how they have participated in driving up the costs of U.S. medicine.

Almighty Medicine

Despite increasingly poor press, most people still have a deep belief in U.S. medicine, whose institution and ideology have penetrated so totally into the fabric of our lives over the past 50 years that many of us may be unaware of its influence on our thinking and beliefs. Similarly, many have stopped questioning corporate power and profits in a culture where the fear of joblessness or lack of health insurance makes us grateful just to be employed.

Myths and Facts About Medicine

The power of medicine in our society rests on several widely held myths, which have in good part been created by aggressive and highly successful public relations campaigns of the wealthy American Medical Association (AMA) and the giant health "charities" (American Cancer Society, American Heart Association, etc.). TV programs glorifying doctors and heroic medical care (often sponsored by medical groups) reinforce these myths. Brought up as most of us are to "believe" in medicine, it is hard at first to realize how we are influenced (even at times manipulated) by this propaganda.

Myth: *U.S. medical care is the best in the world.*

Fact: The U.S. spends more money on medical care, uses more medical technology per capita than any country on earth, and has one of the highest ratios of

---

* For a critique, read Arnold S. Relman, "The New Medical-Industrial Complex" (special article), *New England Journal of Medicine* 303, no. 17 (Oct. 23, 1980): 963–70.

† We use "medicine" to mean both the tangible personnel and institutions of the medical system like physicians and hospitals, and the discipline, field, or profession of medicine. We also mean the intangible arrangements of beliefs, ideology, and assumptions that influence or control our daily habits in ways most of us are not aware of (as do "the family" and "religion"). By "medical establishment," we mean the cluster of organized physician, hospital, drug, and insurance groups like the American Medical Association (AMA), the American College of Obstetricians and Gynecologists (ACOG), the American Hospital Association (AHA), and the Health Care Corporation of America (HCA—a huge managed care corporation), which pay enormous sums to influence public opinion, legislation, and policy on health and medical matters.

doctors and hospitals to people. Wealthy potentates and world leaders come here from all over the world to be treated by medical specialists. Yet, as a country caring for its own people, the U.S. lags behind all other industrialized countries in life expectancy and ranks 22nd in infant mortality rates: two crucial basic indicators of health in the general population.[27] Recent policy studies confirm that our system is, in fact, one of the worst in the industrialized world by these and other measures like comparative costs, scale of U.S. gross domestic product investment, physicians' earnings, and the ratio of uninsured people relative to health outcomes.[28] We would be better off spending more money on general social improvements, especially in nutrition, fertility control, education, housing, and access to community services, which contribute most to improvements in mortality rates and the general health of populations.

Myth: *Medical care has been responsible for the major improvements in the U.S. and in the world's health.*

Fact: The best scientific epidemiology shows that many dreaded infectious diseases (typhoid, smallpox, scarlet fever, measles, whooping cough, diphtheria, influenza, tuberculosis, pneumonia) were believed "conquered" in the past century, but this was almost certainly because of improved nutrition, sanitation, and housing as well as rising levels of education and income, not medical care. The incidence rates of these diseases were already falling when medical treatments and vaccines were introduced. With the exception of smallpox and probably polio, vaccines helped speed the decline of these diseases only minimally.[29] The disappearance of infectious diseases is a major source of our greater life expectancy in this century, leaving the chronic diseases, for which medicine has as yet provided no cures. Difficult as it is to believe, mortality from most of the chronic diseases, which are our leading causes of death today, has remained virtually unchanged throughout the century.[30] Through neglect, however, some infectious diseases, like tuberculosis, are beginning to return.

Myth: *Medical treatments in current use have been proved safe and effective.*

Fact: Most accepted treatments, therapies, and medical technologies in use today have never been evaluated *scientifically* in terms of benefit. Fetal heart monitors and radical mastectomies are only two examples of technologies coming into widespread use and over a long time before being evaluated fully. The highest standard of scientific evaluation—randomized or controlled clinical trials (RCTs, CCTs)—is difficult to achieve because it is time- and labor-consuming and expensive. As a result, only 10 to 20% of all procedures used in medical practice have been scientifically shown to be of benefit (see "Evidence-Based Practice and the Cochrane Collaboration" box on p. 710).

Most doctors, even those recently trained, still have limited ability to evaluate studies, medical treatments and technology, and they often base their recommendations simply on what colleagues do, or on what they think may work. As we were told by an assistant professor of medicine at Harvard Medical School:

Too frequently, practicing physicians indulge in cookbook medicine: they open the latest medical journal and inflict the latest recipe on patients, assuring their patients that, on the one hand, they are receiving "the latest thing" and, on the other hand, that they are "not guinea pigs."... In fact, the practicing physician is often extending some scientist's last experiment into the community setting—and without obtaining the patient's informed consent! At the same time, the scientist who performed the original experiment five years ago and who wrote the paper two or three years ago has long abandoned that approach in favor of something with more promise for a real cure.

Fact: Until recently, most nonreproductive medical research has been done only on men, and the results have been applied, inappropriately, to women. Such a process is far from scientific. In 1990, the National Institutes of Health (NIH) issued new guidelines to ensure that women would be adequately represented in all NIH-funded research of potential relevance to women. Thus, this situation should improve over time, but it is important to remain critical of many therapies applied to women.

Myth: *Medical care keeps us healthy.*

Fact: Although deep down many of us may believe that medicine has created and sustained our health through skill and technological advances in the past 50 years, public health studies show that our health is primarily the result of social, economic, and environmental conditions: the food we eat, the water we drink, the air we breathe, the environment we live in, the work we do, and the habits we form. These factors in turn result primarily from the education we have, the money we are able to earn, and the other resources we are able to command in taking care of ourselves. Still other factors may contribute to good health and long life: control over one's personal life, influence over the larger forces that affect all our lives, loving friendships, and a supportive community. Some researchers feel that strong religious beliefs also contribute to good health and long life.

Drugs, surgery, and medical technology (kidney dialysis machines or blood transfusions, for example) are invaluable tools, which can prevent death and prolong life, and many people would not be alive today without them. While few of us would want to live without these skills and emergency resources available to us and our families, they are not at base what keeps us healthy. Even what we do alone isn't the key. We may pursue good health by ourselves or within families, seeking personal medical care when we become ill. However, only group or community action can prevent the massive threats to our health that come from the environment.

Every one of these myths encourages us to trust medical professionals, to lean on their reassurances, and to follow their orders. Especially when we are sick, it is difficult to be anything but trusting and compliant; being sick is frightening, and we need to feel comforted. Because medical professionals offer false reassurances more often than we'd like to think, we must be as critical as we can, get all the information possible, and ask friends and family to help us. (See "Our Rights as Patients," p. 713.)

The Medical Monopoly

Modern "scientific" medicine's virtual monopoly of the U.S. health care system is slowly being challenged, but it remains a major force in determining the types and quality of care available to us, because in the past large sums were spent, often illegally, to crush competition from other healing systems and practitioners. Doctors have used and continue to use their power, for example, to eliminate midwives as competitors. Today, a majority of the insured pay out-of-pocket for access to holistic healing approaches (see chapter 5, Holistic Health and Healing).[31] (Health plans in some states now offer coverage for a range of alternative healing practices—an indication that the insurance industry, in its drive for profit, is breaking the medical monopoly.[32])

Physicians who practice conventional medicine (also called either the biomedical model of medical care or allopathic medicine) created a virtual monopoly in the early 20th century through control over state licensing laws that defined what the practice of medicine should be and who could be called a doctor. These laws provided state-sanctioned penalties for those who were not "properly" trained and licensed. At the same time, the medical profession also gained absolute control over its education process, thus becoming a "legally enforced monopoly of practice."[33]

Medicine was allowed to expand without limits, with tax dollars supporting medical education, research, and hospital operations, but with virtually no mechanisms of accountability to society. (Other public services paid for by tax dollars—for example, public utilities and public education—are expected to be accountable to users.*) As a result, we ended up with medical care that costs more than anywhere else in the world and a preponderance of specialists. Many rural

areas and most inner cities go without any primary care doctors in their communities.

Medicine's monopoly was further consolidated in the 1940s when the government made federal funds available for hospital construction (Hill-Burton law), and the "Blues" (Blue Cross/Blue Shield) were created to reimburse doctors and in-hospital care—the beginning of the "fee-for-service" system. Backed up by the private insurance industry, hospitals became the base of medical care in this country after World War II and supported the exclusion of nonphysician health care practitioners. Substantial federal funding for Medicare, Medicaid, and medical research in 1965 dramatically increased the volume of federal money flowing into medicine (see "The Insurance Industry," p. 693).

The power of medicine began to shift with the arrival of nonprofit, prepaid health maintenance organizations (HMOs) in the 1970s. Though organized medicine attempted by fair means or foul to halt the trend to prepaid care, younger, more progressive physicians saw HMOs, like group practices, as saner and just as financially rewarding as private practice. Though HMOs put physicians on salaries, the doctors continued to control medical decision-making. The medical monopoly thus made a divided and uneasy alliance with "managed care" until recently. Now that profit-making managed care companies are taking medical decision-making out of the hands of doctors, and profits go to stockholders, more progressive forces in the medical community have begun to revolt.

The Drug Industry

Unlike most Western democracies, the U.S. does not regulate the price of prescription and over-the-counter drugs charged by the drug industry, so that we pay on average about three times what citizens in other countries pay for their medicines.[34] Unlike the United Kingdom or Australia, the U.S. government's unwillingness to limit the scale of profit enjoyed by this industry at public expense is a result not only of heavy lobbying by pharmaceutical companies, but a strong pro-business bias in both Congress and the Executive Branch. Sales of prescription drugs in 1996 were estimated at about $85 billion, averaging 20 prescriptions per family in the U.S. Pharmaceutical companies regularly show a return on investment of over 26%, routinely outperforming almost all other parts of the industrial sector. The advertising budget for this sales volume is about $12.5 billion. More is spent on marketing than on research, and most of it for prescription drug promotion targeted to physicians.[35] Now, the industry has begun advertising directly to potential patients, for example, the TV ads that urge women to "Ask your doctor about Fosamax."

Despite legislative efforts to curb industry gifts to medical students, drug companies continue successfully to woo practicing physicians, medical school faculty and development offices, specialty societies, and medical residents by offering "research" opportunities

---

* Accountability in the case of the medical profession would mean a requirement to be responsive to our perceived needs and wishes in recognition of the fact that as taxpayers we have supported medical education, research, hospital construction, and much of the medical care given in hospitals, nursing homes, and clinics. From managed care corporations we need another kind of accountability.

and luxurious travel symposia as well as by sponsoring educational programs in hospitals and schools. There is evidence that the information distributed through these symposia favors the sponsor's products. Medical schools and training programs have become increasingly dependent on funding from drug companies. Because medical school training in pharmacology is largely inadequate, doctors become permanently dependent on drug companies for information (or misinformation). (See Sidney Wolfe's article listings in Resources.) As a result, physicians often cannot or do not protect us from ineffective or dangerous drugs. Often they simply don't know the possibly serious negative effects, or they continue to prescribe the drugs anyway, based on personal observation or the belief that any negative findings (always challenged by the drug companies) have been inaccurate. (For instance, some physicians continued to prescribe diethylstilbestrol [DES] for a variety of fertility-related purposes after they knew about its effects on fetuses during pregnancy. See also fen-phen, p. 63.) The "off-label" (not approved by FDA) use of prescription drugs is a growing problem. Doctors often prescribe the advertised brand-name drugs, which are more profitable to the drug companies, rather than using generic drugs, which are cheaper for the consumer and equally effective. They also often encourage us to believe that a visit to the doctor is not complete without a prescription to "solve" the problem.

Although some drugs save lives and enhance many people's quality of life, research reveals increasing numbers of both new and older drugs to be dangerous or useless.* The General Accounting Office (GAO) reports that Medicare/Medicaid pays $40 million a year for drugs shown to have no effectiveness. Each year, at least 1.5 million people go into the hospital because they have adverse reactions to drugs, or get sick because they are taking too many (*polypharmacy*). Women receive about two-thirds of all prescription drugs, and the most profitable drugs made by the industry worldwide continue to be oral contraceptives, injectable contraceptives (like Depo-Provera), and prescription mood-altering drugs—all risky in some ways and all targeted mainly to women. The larger societal question—whether the prevalence of drugs, and drug or pill solutions to life's problems, models drug-dependency for the younger generation—is still being debated.[36]

The Food and Drug Administration (FDA) was created to protect the public from the dangers of adulterated food and harmful or useless drugs (see chapter 2, Food, for more on the FDA). Over many years, the efforts of some conscientious FDA staff, prompted and

HEALTH AND MEDICAL CARE TECHNOLOGY

The proliferation of new, expensive, and invasive technologies continues to escalate, driving up costs and increasing profits. Some experts claim that as much as 70% of health care costs go toward paying for advanced technologies. However, the systems to evaluate the safety and usefulness of these technologies are weak and are often destroyed by Congress. The FDA has some authority over devices used inside the human body, but little over those on or outside it. Even when there is clear evidence of harmfulness, or uselessness, we as a society lack effective measures to stop the use of high-tech procedures. (See "Our Rights as Patients," p. 713, for information on reporting problems to the FDA.)

Much medical technology is used in women's health, specifically birth control, infertility, childbearing, and menopause. The majority of routine obstetrical interventions are of limited effectiveness. Some birth control methods go on the market even when important questions about long-term safety and relatively rare adverse effects are still unanswered.

Women's health activists are sometimes divided on this issue. Some women's advocacy groups seek to educate the public and pass laws requiring that certain technologies be covered by health insurance benefits. Without such coverage, few women would be able to take advantage of expensive high-tech procedures such as in vitro fertilization (IVF), producing great inequities in women's care. Other women's health advocacy groups argue that mandated insurance coverage is premature in the absence of better evidence of a technology's safety and effectiveness, and drives up costs for everyone.

encouraged by the pressure of consumer groups, activists, investigative reporters, and members of Congress, have sometimes led to effective, though limited, protection as well as to increased consumer participation in the regulatory process. The FDA now offers the *FDA Consumer* newsletter and has a program of consumer participation in most of its scientific advisory committees. It now has a women's health unit. Its work on tobacco during the Clinton administration, under the leadership of David Kessler, will remain one of its finest accomplishments.

Yet, old ways change slowly: the drug companies still often have the dominant influence over FDA decisions—sometimes even after an FDA committee has denied approval or raised safety questions. The FDA's budget has never been adequate to compete

---

* Work by Ralph Nader's Health Research Group shows consistently that even in industry-sponsored studies of all drugs approved between 1938 and 1962, for example, only 12% are effective for their prescribed use, and at least 15% have no effectiveness whatsoever. Yet, most of these drugs are still on the market.

THE LANGUAGE OF THE MEDICAL CARE SYSTEM

Everyday talk in the media creates confusion between health (our well-being, which for the most part we take care of ourselves) and medicine (institutionalized care from licensed medical practitioners). Many of us say "health care" when often we mean "medical care." We say "health system" when referring to the "medical system": the entire patchwork of public and private, profit and nonprofit medical services. Increasingly, we hear about the "health care industry," an indication of the increasing share of our economy that medical care has come to occupy.

To understand current debates about health care and the options available, we need to understand the terminology of health care financing and delivery, include the following terms:

Capitation. This refers to the practice in a managed care (MC) company in which providers are allotted a fixed sum for each *person* they care for in the (usually profit-making) plan, during a month or year, rather than being reimbursed one fee for each service provided, as in traditional FFS practice. In order to increase earnings and keep his or her job, the physician must care for these patients for some figure less than what the capitation provides. This creates a conflict of interest for the physician, who has a permanent, built-in incentive to undertreat and sometimes gets bonuses for saving money for the company.

Fee for Service (FFS). An insurance system by which medical care providers bill third-party payers for each medical visit, treatment, or service provided as a separate job—a fee for a service. FFS is based on the indemnity insurance principle: if you get sick and need services, the insurance company will cover those services. The premiums of people who don't get sick partly subsidize the payments for those who do. FFS gives the maximum incentive for medical care providers to do more and charge more, especially in hospitals. Because FFS offers the maximum choice of doctors, it remains popular among consumers.

Health Insurance. Any system, private or public, that provides payment for health and medical care to those enrolled or eligible to receive it. This health insurance coverage is in exchange for premiums or sums received, and varies according to specific terms or agreements, such as "fee-for-service," "prepaid" plans, etc. (see below). Originally, Blue Cross/Blue Shield began the insurance system, mainly to cover hospitalization. In general, insurance covers mostly medical care and could rightly be called medical insurance. However, this is changing, and increasingly some plans cover preventive care or other "health" services.

Health Maintenance Organization (HMO). An HMO is organized to deliver office-based medical care, tests, and necessary hospitalization for subscribers who pay one prepaid annual or monthly fee (packages vary). HMOs may be nonprofit or for-profit and can be set up by government, insurance companies, unions, or other groups. Nonprofit HMOs traditionally have been managed by doctors and employ their own staff, including primary-care doctors, specialists, and nurses as well as pharmacists. Plan coverage varies, but expensive procedures, drugs, and hospitalization are restrained. Nonprofit HMOs are the oldest type of managed care and have the best performance record so far. As the for-profit trend in HMOs grows, pressure on doctors in nonprofit HMOs to undertreat will increase.

Independent Practice Association (IPA). An IPA is an organization that contracts with doctors who are in private practice to care for patients enrolled in different HMOs and other MC health plans. IPAs "sell" physician services wholesale to insurers, for much less cost than the physician's regular private fee in a FFS system. Thus, plan patients receive care for less cost to the plan than the fee physicians charge their regular patients.

Insurer, Third-Party Payer. The insurer is the corporation or association that "sells" the plan(s) to the individual or business, receives the premiums or fees from the employers or individuals, contracts with the provider(s) to perform the health and medical care services, and actually pays those providers. Increasingly, the for-profit corporate insurer is also deciding which treatments and services recommended by a provider will be "allowed" or paid for in the plan; insurers may also hold their providers accountable for making a profit for the insurer.

Managed Care (MC). Managed care is any system of health care financing and delivery that relies on financial incentives and the monitoring of provider decisions to control medical costs and limit the use of services. These plans generally claim to cover most "medically necessary" services, ambulatory medical visits, partial or full costs of medications, and hospitalization. Historically, MC organizations such as nonprofit, physician-managed HMOs were set up on the prepaid insurance premium principle: employers, unions, or individual subscribers made a set monthly or annual payment for all services covered by their plan. Enrollees saw only those salaried providers who belonged to the plan, and out-of-pocket expenses were limited to co-payments at visits and some pharmacy costs. This kind of MC is still available in some places, but the newer MC forms are now more dominant (see IPAs, above, and PPOs, below). Many of these are for-profit arrangements that put providers in the untenable position of making decisions about care in terms of the impact on their salaries and employment as well as on company profit. Another drawback for some is the more limited choice of providers. (See "Managed Care, Mangled Care, or Management Care?," p. 696). MC often focuses on routine disease detection and preventive services and may reduce hospitalization and unnecessary or risky treatments, but all plans may cancel policies or deny needed care in the face of serious illnesses.

Medicaid, for the poor of any age, and ***Medicare***, for the elderly on Social Security, poor or not, are frequently confused. Both programs are federally legislated and funded health insurance. Both are currently moving recipients out of fee-for-service into managed care plans to reduce costs. Medicaid benefits vary widely by state, and under the new "welfare" law, funding will be through finite federal "block grants" that states will spend on people they define as poor. Medicare is entirely federal, designates approved providers, and has the most effective standards and regulations to protect recipients. Recent efforts by conservatives may succeed in deregulating Medicare. In other proposals, wealthy Medicare beneficiaries may be asked to pay much more. Presently, all recipients pay the same.

Preferred Provider Organization (PPO).

In a PPO, one of several MC approaches, doctors and hospitals may form corporations to give volume discounts to insurance companies to help lower copayments for subscribers who choose from a large list of providers in private practice. The insurer pays the providers on a FFS basis, but the cost of each service is significantly less than if paid by a private individual. PPOs are rarely nonprofit, but out-of-pocket costs for subscribers who use network providers are relatively limited.

Single Payer.

This is a principle similar to public utilities in which one national, centralized nonprofit utility, or a government agency like the Social Security Administration, would be responsible for both collecting and disbursing the money needed to pay medical care bills, thus eliminating the private insurance industry. Health care providers could remain in the private sector. Canada works on a similar principle and covers everyone in the country for much less than the U.S. now spends, while still allowing consumers to choose their own providers. With agreed-upon fee schedules for providers, and systemwide access for consumers, Canada's system produces fewer very sick people. A single payer would replace the approximately 1,000 (profit-making) U.S. insurance companies now handling medical claims, of which a few are now giant corporations with assets in the billions. Two independent federal agencies and many independent analysts agree that a single-payer system would save the most money and provide the most equitable care, largely because it would eliminate the 20 to 25% of premiums now wasted on administration, marketing, and the excessive profits earned by today's MC companies.

Utilization Review.

As a part of managed care, managers—often nurses, but increasingly midlevel managers with little or no health training—review in advance all of a doctor's requests to provide services (tests, treatments, hospitalizations, etc.) and either approve or deny those requests. Most of the tragedies and scandals reported in the media about managed care have come from this practice, when needed care was denied and patients were severely injured or died as a consequence.

against the huge financial resources the drug industry musters for PAC contributions, lobbying, court cases, and the production of new products. For example, the FDA cannot successfully monitor all drug advertising. As a result, the achievements of public-interest groups, such as the National Women's Health Network, are always threatened. Today, the antiregulatory climate of a conservative Congress and the possible use of SLAPPs (Strategic Lawsuits Against Public Participation) by industry make lobbying in the public interest particularly difficult.

At the very least, as the health care industry continues to undergo restructuring, the drug industry should be required to submit to certain basic reforms and the payment of much more severe penalties for misconduct. Consumer and public-interest groups and the media have to become better-than-ever watchdogs of the FDA and also must press for better regulatory systems at the state and local levels.

The Insurance Industry

The insurance principle has become the dominant approach in shaping U.S. medical care systems, with insurance coverage generally tied to employers. Until recently, all "third-party" reimbursement systems—private, profit-making insurance systems, Blue Cross/Blue Shield (the "Blues," now moving from nonprofit to for-profit), and public programs (Medicare, Medicaid)—have rewarded doctors and hospitals by reimbursing them on a "fee-for-service" (FFS) or indemnity basis, similar to automobile collision insurance. Dominated by physicians' interests, the FFS insurance system has always been problematic. There is great incentive to overtreat those who can afford to pay, especially insured women. For employers, the cost of providing health benefits has become astronomical and virtually uncontrollable, making their companies less competitive. In addition, this method of providing health care siphons off public monies, Medicare and Medicaid, into a profit-making system that greatly benefits the hospital and drug industries, insurance companies, and medical providers and leaves fewer resources for education, housing, job training, and other essential public health services.

The principle of relying on health insurance for access to health care has never benefited women. Women are the majority of the 80 million uninsured or underinsured adults as well as most of those dependent on government programs for health and medical care.[37] We are seen as "overusers" of the system because of our reproductive health and other "normal" but medicalized needs, and thus we either pay more or have a difficult time getting health insurance coverage for these needs. Abortion coverage, for example, is totally random, depending on which state, which insurance company, and which employer is involved. In general, women subscribers pay more out-of-pocket than men do for health insurance, and the poorer we are the higher the proportion of our income we pay. We are also more likely than men to care for dependent family members and thus are often unable to work outside our homes. Many of us who do work outside are now "locked in" to jobs we might rather leave, or take jobs we might not like, in order to keep or obtain employer-covered health insurance for ourselves or our children.

For many women, insurance coverage has become like a revolving door because of lost employment, lost coverage, changes in employer policy about coverage, moving to part-time work, and many other factors. Recent changes in federal law have helped to some extent, and states are mobilizing on an issue-by-issue basis, but these piecemeal efforts will likely be inadequate to improve this situation. Under the Kennedy-Kassenbaum bill, which took effect in July 1997, women and children can at least obtain insurance despite a preexisting health condition and can transfer their coverage if they change jobs or health plans, but the law still has serious shortcomings.[38] Federal legislation has also made provisions for divorced or widowed women, who may stay on their ex-partner's group plan through special federal legislation (COBRA). Only a few, however, can afford the premiums.

These laws do not alter the discrimination against women by the insurance industry, nor the discrimination that is built into the structure of women's employment in the U.S. As the insurance and managed care giants swiftly take over delivery of the bulk of women's health and medical care services, our needs for change and accountability from the system will only intensify.

HEALTH SYSTEM TRANSFORMATION IN THE 1990s

Corporate Power and the Free Market Economy

Certain shifts in the U.S. economy help to explain the dramatic changes in the health care system in the late 20th century. Beginning in the 1980s, conservative political policies in the U.S. increasingly shifted power to the states and to corporations. We are told that a free market economy, in which corporations are successfully creating profits and thus wealth, benefits the society as a whole by "trickling down" the wealth to poorer people. Yet, in recent years, we have seen corporations "downsize," laying off thousands of employees. Worker benefits, especially health care, have shrunk. Salaries for most workers have remained stagnant while the salary and benefit packages of CEOs have exploded. This is especially true within the "health industry," where the nonprofit principle itself is under systematic attack (see below).

Unrestrained profits, low taxes, and low government investment in human development inevitably produce a small percentage of people who control the lion's share of a country's wealth.* [39] Some members of the shrinking middle class are becoming more racist and prejudiced against immigrants and the "poor," as evidenced in their support of "welfare reform" and the anti-immigrant legislation of the late 1990s. With almost one-fifth of our population living below the poverty line,[40] and more than 40 million people without health insurance, the overall health of the country is already suffering. Costs will eventually rise again as more people enter the system in emergency, requiring expensive crisis care.

Health Care and Profits

When health care is turned over to private enterprise, the driving motive in providing care is profit, just as in any other industry. The need to reduce costs, and even to optimize profits, competes with a commitment to optimum health care, despite industry rhetoric and the many conscientious medical practitioners who care about their patients. For this reason, most wom-

---

* In 1996, the richest 1% of people in the U.S. owned 40% of the nation's wealth, more than the entire combined wealth of the bottom 92% of the population. (Statistics provided by United for a Fair Economy, 37 Temple Place, 5th floor, Boston, MA 02111. [617] 423-2148. Web site: http://www.stw.org)

WHERE DOES THE MONEY GO?

- About 15% of the U.S. gross domestic product (GDP) now goes for health and medical care. Though its rise has slowed somewhat recently, this is about 50% more than Sweden or Canada, two-thirds more than Japan, and twice that spent in Great Britain—all countries with better health outcomes.
- Per capita spending on hospital and physician services for the insured is 25 to 50% greater than for the uninsured.
- Nursing home costs have been increasing more than 10% annually, inching toward $75 billion.
- Unnecessary services and administrative and advertising costs amount to at least $600 billion annually. Administrative costs, largely because of the many health insurers (close to 1,000) and their thousands of employees, the many different billing systems used, and the range of variations in plan packages, account for more than 40% of total health and medical care expenditures—more than in any other nation.
- Physicians' earnings and hospital costs continue to rise well ahead of inflation; for many, profits are increasing sharply. In the U.S., doctors are paid more than twice as much as they are paid in any other industrialized or Western country.
- Technological innovations, many of unproven value, may account for 70% of health and medical care costs.
- Our tax dollars now support more than half the medical enterprise in all its forms, including medical education; yet, U.S. taxpayers have fewer government controls or accountability mechanisms for how that money is spent than those in any other country.[41]

en's health activists have long opposed the profit motive in health and medical care systems.

Like many mainstream citizens, most women's health activists believe in the principle of the public good and the public interest. Many services are provided by governments that benefit the community as a whole: police, firefighting, land conservation, education, roads, and bridges, to name a few. Similarly, we believe health is a public good, not a commodity to be sold in the marketplace like a car. There are many social needs that a free market cannot possibly fulfill effectively, and health and medical care is one of them.

Corporate Takeover of Health Care

Though voters had been consistently in favor of a single-payer system, in which the government would pay directly for health care and universal coverage would be achieved, the Clinton administration's plan in 1993 capitulated to the power of the medical establishment and the insurance industry. The administration proposed a plan that was unwieldy and failed to gain support in the business community, the health care industry, or Congress, primarily because key leaders of affected industries had organized to prevent legislation long before Clinton's election.[42] Special interest groups and political action committees (PACs) spent more than at any time in their history to aid this defeat.

The failure of Clinton's legislation was followed by an immediate corporate takeover of the system that has already had grave consequences for the health of consumers and for health care workers. Some major corporate trends of the mid- to late 1990s have been these:

1. *The growth of managed care:* Within the next few years it is likely that almost all U.S. residents will be receiving their care through one of several kinds of managed care systems (see box on p. 692).

2. *Mergers and acquisitions:* Large health care corporations are acquiring a larger share of the health care market, leading to greater control over the workers and the facilities. Community-based hospitals that once provided low-cost or free care may not continue to do so as they are bought out by profit-making corporations.

3. *Downsizing:* Some hospitals are closing; others are reducing their staff. The loss of small community hospitals is likely to make health care increasingly inaccessible outside of major urban areas; fewer and fewer options are available for the uninsured and for those who no longer qualify for Medicaid; nonprofit teaching hospitals, expected to take up the slack, are increasingly overwhelmed.

4. *De-skilling:* Hospitals, nursing homes, and other community-based centers are hiring less and less skilled personnel; for example, skilled nurses are being replaced by aides and others with very little training (see "What Every Patient Should Know About Nursing Care" box on p. 708).

Women and children are facing an unprecedented health care crisis as nonprofit clinics close and free care pools dry up. Recent estimates claim that one in four people are unable to obtain care.[43] These are not people on welfare but those who have low-paying jobs that do not provide health insurance coverage. Though several proposals have been made to insure the children of these families,[44] few of the proposals recognize the fundamental truth that the best way to help children is to help their mothers and fathers.

Loss of Consumer Power

The power of "users," "consumers," "clients," "subscribers," or "citizens" to influence the health and medical system is more limited now than at any time since the 1950s. Business executives and policymakers, mostly but by no means all male, have designed a health care system primarily for the convenience and financial gain of the "health" and insurance corporations, the physicians, the investor-owned hospitals, and the medical industries. The "consumer" in this scenario is not the patient and policyholder, but the employers who "provide" health benefits to employees! Employers negotiate with these corporations to offer a variety of plans, with different costs and benefits—or none at all. As the new "consumers," employers decide how cheaply they can purchase "packages" of benefits for different employee groups. While in some companies the unions may play a role in this process, union weakness often forces a choice between health and other benefits. Roughly half of all companies that offer health benefits offer only two plans, which they select.[45] Increasingly, this coverage excludes dependent partners and children. Many companies do not offer health benefits to incoming employees at all.

After 40 years of recognized, established legitimacy in both progressive and mainstream circles—on boards, in community advisory groups, at public hearings, and in organizations—the women's health and consumer or community activists who represent patients trying to obtain decent care now barely have a voice. As "subscribers" to plans we never devised, we come up against the corporation that employs the doctor caring for us. In most states, we cannot sue managed care corporations because of existing ERISA* legislation, although recent state challenges hope to remove this barrier.[46]

Nonetheless, some consumers and consumer groups have influenced legislation to curb some of the worst problems, for example, securing two-day hospital stays for maternity care (for women who want it), and forbidding outpatient mastectomies. Often it is the more powerful actors, such as medical groups and larger nonprofit corporations, that actually wield the winning influence. Creative alliances among consumer organizations and practitioner groups will likely be essential in any successful challenge to the powerful managed care industry, which is trying to close any remaining nonprofit loopholes.

We will have to unite to defend the basic principles that health and medical care are not commodities, and that consumers should be able to speak for ourselves and make the system accountable to us directly.[47]

---

* ERISA: Employment Retirement Income Security Act, originally designed to protect pensions and other employee benefits.

MANAGED CARE, MANGLED CARE, OR MANAGEMENT CARE?

We need to know how to evaluate the strengths and weaknesses of different health plans so that we can make good "choices" when choice is available, get what we need from the plans in which we are enrolled, protect ourselves from problems, and be able to work to change the system in ways that will benefit everyone.

Nonprofit Managed Care: A Long Tradition

HMOs have a tradition more than 25 years old. The fundamental principles of MC—prepaid premiums, combining outpatient and hospital care, and controlling costs through reducing expensive tests, unnecessary treatments, and hospitalization—have brought benefits to many women and their families, mostly through nonprofit HMOs: prepaid systems with a "closed panel" of salaried doctors (see "The Language of the Medical Care System," p. 692). However, only a few such physician-directed, nonprofit HMOs still exist today.

Some of the benefits from nonprofit HMOs have included

- a focus on primary and preventive care and a reasonable commitment to providing optimum care.
- providers collaborating across their disciplines to determine diagnoses and the best, most cost-effective treatments.
- reasonable, round-the-clock access to emergency care.
- the return of some portion of any surplus income to the system, where it is used to improve care or is returned to subscribers in the form of a refund.
- the benefit to consumers when state and federal laws have required that a certain ratio of the HMO's governing board include actual users of the system and that grievance procedures be open and accessible to subscribers.

If we are given an opportunity to look at MC plans directly, or through our employers, or as part of organizing state legislation designed to correct MC problems, these are some basic features to fight for, along with the nonprofit principle itself.

Though women consumers have had mixed experiences with nonprofit HMOs, research has shown health outcomes to be quite good. The financial incentives to physician-managers to skimp on care have mostly been balanced by nonprofit HMOs' commitment to reducing costs by keeping people healthy.

For-Profit Managed Care

Because of the success of nonprofit HMOs in reducing costs while providing high-quality care, employers, who wanted to reduce rising insurance premiums but opposed government-based reform, threw their support behind MC as the "only solution" to the health care crisis. In addition, the federal government has been hesitant to criticize MC because it seems the best solution for reducing the rising costs of Medicaid and Medicare.[48] As a result, we saw a major swing in the marketplace from FFS toward MC during the 1990s.

Today, however, nonprofit HMOs are no longer the dominant form of managed care; for-profit corporations are rapidly taking over the health care market. Because the primary goal of the corporation is profit rather than the provision of good health services, for-profit managed care has many drawbacks. There is continuous pressure to offer lower quality and fewer services to make larger profits, without creating a "product" so completely unsatisfactory that employer/consumers refuse to buy. Complaints are ignored whenever feasible, and "damage control" of the corporate image takes precedence over investigation and responsiveness to complaints. Reports of lack of coverage, denial of coverage, or inadequate coverage for many important services, especially specialist care, mental health treatment, and care for those with chronic illnesses and disabilities, are becoming routine. Not surprisingly, critics have dubbed these new for-profit managed care systems "mangled care." Another name could be "management care" for a system that provides top management and the doctor-managers of health care corporations with optimum care and compensation, largely at the expense of women.

Medicare and Medicaid Managed Care

As Medicare and Medicaid recipients are moved gradually from FFS to MC systems, it is unclear how women—those most dependent on both government programs—will fare. Some analysts consider FFS care under Medicare a kind of crown jewel, a model of what a good federal program should be—even though there have been some problems. Although Medicare has a better image than Medicaid, which serves poorer and sicker populations, neither system is wracked by fraud and abuse, as right-wing rumors suggest. Government involvement in the new MC programs, so long as Medicaid and Medicare exist as federal programs, provides patients certain essential guarantees and protections—oversight, complaint, and redress mechanisms—whatever their other limitations. The federal agency decides whether a facility or individual may be a Medicaid provider, and the federal agencies involved will monitor and evaluate these providers.

Whether the MC approach will really save the government money or whether patients will receive good-

THE TITANIC OF MANAGED CARE

The profit motive in health, even when controlled somewhat by minimal state legislation, is guaranteed to produce more uninsured and more poor people. Here's how it works. As sicker people—people with preexisting conditions, now permitted access to insurance by federal law; people with low incomes on Medicaid; and elderly people on Medicare—are permitted to enter the pool of those in managed care systems, the cost of providing care will go up. The premiums charged for everyone will then no longer be enough to guarantee the level of profit needed to show growth and pay stockholders. Premiums will then have to go up again; new limitations will have to be developed to strip down the terms of some policies, so that people pay more, receive less service, or find their policies canceled altogether. Once this happens, another whole group of employers or individual subscribers can no longer afford the premiums, and another batch of uninsured people is added to the existing numbers. Many estimate that at this rate, more than half of all U.S. children will be uninsured just after the turn of the century.[49] If the trend continues, the pool of uninsured and underinsured could reach 100 million.

quality care remains to be seen. For-profit managed care corporations have done well financially because they have been able to attract young, healthy subscribers.[50] For older and sicker people who require more expensive and time-consuming care, managed care has not yet been proved to be as effective as FFS care.[51] MC corporations are attracted to hefty amounts of Medicare and Medicaid dollars, but it is hard to see how money could be "made" on sicker and older people.

Evaluating For-Profit Managed Care

Many conscientious experts are already at work trying to evaluate this new, profit-making managed care system in terms of cost, access, and quality. However, private corporations own almost all of the information they generate and, unless compelled to by law, will not make that information available for outcome studies, complaints, cost-effectiveness studies, or comparisons with other systems. Thus, figures to prove or disprove cost savings and improvements in for-profit systems of managed care may be very difficult to obtain. Also, differences in results between types of plans may depend on which kinds of people are enrolled in them: If some plans are able to enroll only younger, healthier, employed people and keep out those who need the most care, they may show greater savings than those systems that must enroll a mix of people, some of whom are sicker.[52] In addition, good results one year may not necessarily mean good results the next year. For example, a big merger of two corporations may suddenly create a lot of competition for a third corporation. Budgets for advertising, marketing, and promotion may shoot up suddenly for that third company, leaving fewer resources for patient care. If the goal is to maintain the same profit levels, patients will suffer.

In the meantime, as women who use the system do evaluative work of our own, it is important to emphasize that cost, access, and quality are not the only issues. These systems should be evaluated on the basis of accountability and gender/race justice, taking into account the impact of these systems on women and people of color, who have different bodies and different needs than white men. In evaluating for-profit managed care systems, we can ask ourselves: Who decides? Who benefits? Who pays the most? Who profits, how much, and at whose expense? Are these arrangements fair and reasonable, given the costs and the impact on us? What kind of information, from what sources, is available in helping us to make critical decisions? When the answers to our questions are not satisfactory, women have been organizing speakouts and meeting to publicize the ways in which for-profit MC is not meeting our needs.

Limiting Corporate Power

As MC has become more widespread, aggressive and profitable, and as abuses and medically unsound denials of care increase, more government action is inevitable. President Clinton created a special bipartisan commission to study the impact of for-profit managed care. Coalitions have formed in several states to support legislation that would create special managed-care offices to protect consumers. These state-level offices would help consumers in choosing plans, monitor managed care practices, and review grievances. They would attempt to set minimum standards for plans to be offered in their states and to introduce legislation to limit insurance companies.[53] Otherwise, MC will become a "race to the bottom." States with the weakest and poorest consumers, unable to organize in their own interests, will be forced to accept the poorest and most inadequate care.[54]

The big question is whether any government or citizen power can challenge successfully the large insurance and managed care companies in this country. MC executives claim that the defeat of the Clinton plan was a message sent by voters to the corporations to take over the system. It is essential that women, in particular, send a message back to those corporations that today's MC programs are not what we asked for or wanted, that there has to be a better way, and that we will insist upon it.

Some progressive medical people who care about quality and the institution of medicine are beginning to talk of mobilizing against the new system because it is not what they had in mind, either, especially since doctors are losing both control and money. Dr. Arnold Relman, health reform activist and former editor of the *New England Journal of Medicine,* believes that the only acceptable future for medical practice in the context of managed care is to be functioning in physician-directed, physician-salaried, nonprofit, HMO entities.[55] Other medical leaders believe that large employers will gradually bypass profit-making managed care corporations and the insurance industry altogether. Even some Medicaid programs are proposing direct contracting with providers, bypassing insurance programs.

In fact, these kinds of challenges to the power of corporate health care are already beginning. Some trends are very important: (1) Very large groups of doctors are forming their own corporations in order to compete with the insurance and managed care corporations; thus far, only one or two have been even moderately successful, but others will be watching them to see if they can survive in the long term. (2) Coalitions of very large employers in some major cities, or major industries (such as the Big Three automakers) are already negotiating directly with providers for coverage in order to avoid paying high profits to a third party. (3) Small cities and communities are attempting to "self-insure" rather than pay huge premiums for indifferent care.

All these efforts have much to recommend them and may help to improve care, reduce costs, and limit profits. In the long run, all of them would have to grow significantly to actually change and challenge the profit-making system. None directly address women's needs or the de-linking of health coverage from employment.

Choosing a Managed Care Plan

Though often we have little choice of health plans, in some states employers are required to offer their employees different options. If you have a choice, you may want to consult some of the surveys of MC HMOs carried out in recent years. One is by Consumers' Union, publisher of *Consumer Reports* and one of the most respected consumer organizations in the country. Others have been done by *U.S. News and World Report* and *Newsweek* magazines. All worked with teams of policy experts and providers. Their criteria and results are too long to list here, but we urge you to look for them at your local library (see Resources). You can also get involved with state-level consumer action groups, many of which are establishing criteria for what good MC plans must be and incorporating these criteria into model legislation. Also investigate the work of ECRI focused on technology assessment, evidence-based medicine, and many other consumer concerns (see Resources).

REFORMS NEEDED TO MEET WOMEN'S NEEDS

Women's health activists believe that health plans should have the following features in order to meet our needs as women:

- benefit packages and insurance systems that are not linked to welfare, employment, income, or health status.
- comprehensive benefits: reproductive/ gynecological/child-bearing, occupational/ environmental, mental, dental, long-term care.
- an emphasis on genuine primary care for women—readily accessible, coordinated care that emphasizes prevention and is based on ongoing relationships with providers over time.
- access to midlevel practitioners (midwives, nurses) and other health practitioners of our choice—not just doctors.
- access to trained doctors and nurses in times of crisis, and especially during hospitalization.
- full coverage of illness care, without penalties or cancellations.
- full coverage of home dialysis, home birth, hospice care, and the special treatment needs of HIV-positive and substance-abusing pregnant women.
- long-term care, rehabilitation and disability services.
- coverage of all necessary drugs.
- confidentiality of medical records and protection from genetic discrimination (see p. 717).
- specific mechanisms of accountability and evaluation that are clear to all parties and are binding on the caregiving system, so that users have a basis and right of redress when providers fail to meet obligations.
- just compensation or redress when the system fails or damages us.
- community-based services near home.
- choice of providers.
- global budgeting* for hospitals and other institutions to control costs fairly.
- an independent advocate (ombudsprogram) to guarantee fair adjudication of complaints and claims.

Many women are also calling for broader reforms in the U.S. health and social service systems, such as

- recognition of women's unpaid labor as health workers in community, family, and home (via income-tax credits or Social Security credits, and respite services that give time off for full-time caregivers in the home).
- more training, upgrading, and pay equity for nonphysician women health workers.
- better-quality, unbiased women's health information.
- consumer- and community-based research on appropriate elements of primary care for women.
- recognition of patients', consumers', and the community's rights and roles, especially women's, in system planning and policy decision-making and governance.
- elimination of all existing insurance discrimination against women.
- a single-payer system that would provide universal access and equity by eliminating profits and administrative waste through public control (see p. 693).
- rigorous elimination of waste and fraud, and limits on excess administrative activity such as advertising and marketing.
- the training and retraining of health professionals in the economic/cultural/ psychological and race/gender/age determinants of health and effective caregiving.
- better technology assessment and evaluation research, with results publicly available. (See box, "Evidence-Based Practice and the Cochrane Collaboration," p. 710.)
- mechanisms for national health planning (such as existed in the 1970s).
- clinical practice standards, with input and review by consumers/patients.
- controls on the drug industry to reduce exorbitant prices and focus research on new treatments instead of profitable copies of existing drugs.
- improved investment in and recognition of public health programs.
- better monitoring of the health status, needs of and services for vulnerable populations (young, elderly, those with disabilities, AIDS, etc.) in managed care programs.
- public policies that establish an individual's right of ownership over her or his genetic material as well as control over who has access to her or his genetic information.

* Global budgeting is any annual, government-established target or spending limit for health expenditures. In other countries, it has been used to control wasteful expansion of already half-empty facilities and duplication of high-tech services such as CAT scanners by hospitals competing for doctors and patients. In its most extreme form, annual limits that are too stringent would be set for health care expenditures, as several states are now preparing to do in response to welfare reform.

WHY OTHER INDUSTRIALIZED COUNTRIES DO BETTER

Other industrialized countries, especially the European countries and Japan, spend consistently about half as much as the U.S. does on health care, and they get much better results. (For instance, Canada, the United Kingdom, and the Netherlands provide universal care for less than 10% of their GDP.)[56] They do this through many different mechanisms, but most include

- national planning and multisector investment (balancing investments in education, jobs, housing, and public health, etc., resulting in less need to overspend on medical care).
- taxing the very wealthy fairly and appropriately (now at much higher rates than in the U.S.).
- global budgeting for hospitals and other institutions, and caps on charges by individual providers.
- universal coverage and comprehensive benefits.
- price controls on the drug industry, and some limits on profit generally.
- technology assessment and uniform practice guidelines.
- controlling supplies of expensive equipment.
- emphasizing primary care and limiting the use of specialists.

A focus on public health is key. In 1991, Canada, Germany, and Japan spent 72% of their total health expenditures on public health. These countries have better overall health statistics (lower infant mortality rates and higher life expectancy) than the U.S., which spent more per capita on health but spent only 44% of total health expenditures on public health.

To be fair, some countries exploit female labor in the health and medical care system, and many of them have also devised employer-dependent systems that are in trouble when the economy contracts and that don't work as well for women. Also, corporate-model health systems are making inroads overseas as part of the greater globalization of this industry (see Navarro in Resources). But none of these countries has a health care system with costs as far out of control as ours, and, for the most part, their people are much healthier. While some critics suggest that these are primarily white, homogeneous populations that ought not be compared with the U.S. "melting pot" and immigrant groups, the reality is that many of these countries also now have diverse populations. They simply do not intend to have an undereducated, underskilled, unhealthy workforce.

With the political will, the U.S., too, could have a national health system that is cost-effective and serves everyone's needs. Belief in the market system runs deep, however, in this country. Until the present system fails or dissatisfies enough people, government intervention will continue piecemeal, resulting in doz-

ens of foolish and expensive efforts that will address the worst abuses but not the underlying system.[57]

WOMEN AS HEALERS

Our History

The history of women as healers in all cultures is a crucial dimension of our history as women and puts us in touch with a power that has rightfully belonged to women throughout the ages. Women's research worldwide is still uncovering the missing pieces of this story (see Resources). Midwives and "wise women" healers have been primarily poor and working-class nonelites in most cultures around the world. As such, they have often been revered and loved in their communities but have not been recognized by historians (most of whom have been white, privileged, and male) as significant matter for history. In the West, first the church and then medical men have suppressed women healers, burning them at the stake in the European Middle Ages and colonial America, and refusing hospital privileges to midwives in the 20th century. Many women in the dominant Eurocentric culture have internalized these views, looking with contempt or fear at women who work in "marginal" communities beyond medicine's watchful eye. Though women still practice healing arts in many non-Western cultures, Western medical dominance pervades ministries of health throughout the world, creating competing or parallel belief systems and practices, and driving pride and faith in indigenous women healers further underground. Yet, many women everywhere will, if pressed, admit that we still carry some remnants of beliefs and practices we learned from mothers or aunts, and may call upon them in times of crisis, even in the face of the very best modern medical advice. What has happened in the evolution and suppression of women as healers is critical to our understanding of the relationship between medicine and women today. It can help us to see the vast and fundamental difference between women's healing practices and the contemporary enterprise of modern, commercialized medicine. For women thinking of becoming health workers, healers, or activists, one essential step is to clarify and confront the profound differences in philosophy, beliefs, and practices between modern Western medicine and the many other healing approaches.

Women Physicians

Today, about 18% of all physicians in the U.S. are women, as are about 42% of medical students. By the year 2010, women are expected to be about 30% of the physician workforce.[58] These gains are often hailed as a triumph for women, though a closer look shows that—as in most other fields—mostly elite white women have benefited. Moreover, women tend to cluster in the primary care disciplines and mostly in institutional settings with regular hours; in other words, women doctors are concentrated in the lower-status, lower-paying specialties and positions.[59]

Women who seek health or medical care all over the world have admitted their desire to be cared for by a competent woman, rather than a man, though there are always exceptions. Women express over and over again the belief that female physicians and health care workers will be different from their male colleagues, that they will listen and understand and be sensitive and caring. How realistic is this hope?[60]

Unfortunately, many women emerge from the stressful and dehumanizing medical training process (see "Medical Training and Its Impact on Women" in previous editions of this book) expecting prestige, money, and position just as male physicians do. What's more, many are eager to prove that they can be as good as any male physician according to the male-centered criteria of the profession: clinical competence; emotional detachment; dependence on the very latest tests, drugs, technologies, and procedures; and financial success. Because they have not usually chosen to question the underlying medical ideology, they are often virtually indistinguishable from their male counterparts. These women physicians can be a great disappointment for some women patients.

At the medical plan I belong to, I chose one of the two women doctors because I believed a woman would *be less likely to push drugs and surgery, and would look with me first for the less invasive nonmedical alternatives. In the first visit, she suggested not only thyroid medication but also a "routine" X ray; she talked crisply, rapidly, coolly, with many complicated medical terms. I felt as if I were sitting across from a medical school curriculum.*

It is a mistake, therefore, to assume that women physicians are the answer to the inadequacies of the medical system. Unfortunately, the public and even the medical community have quickly elevated women doctors to the status of "experts" on the feelings, experiences, and health needs of all women. In health books, talk shows, conferences, and magazines, female physicians are replacing the voices of women speaking our own truths. Women physicians sometimes study and write about us, the "patients," in exactly the objective way women's health activists once criticized male doctors for doing.

Recent studies do indicate that women physicians have a slight edge in communication skills over their male counterparts, and that many patients appreciate this.[61] There are also women doctors who have survived the training, kept alive their warmth and compassion, and remember what it's like to be a woman patient. Though they are not common, they can make a great difference.

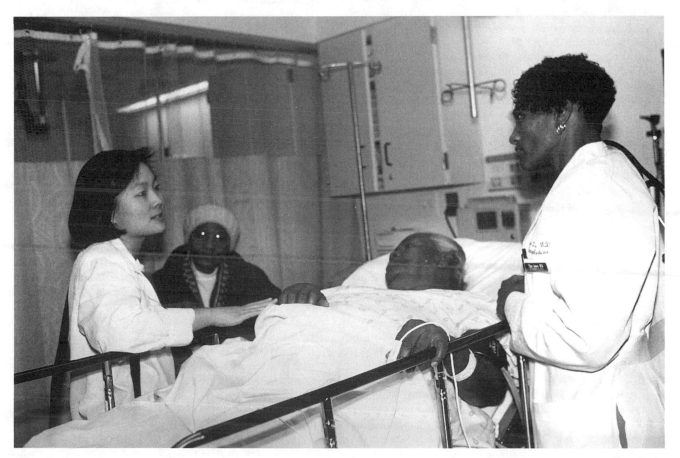

Ellen Shub

For the first time, I left a doctor's office feeling absolutely wonderful. I felt that she was genuinely concerned for my well-being as a person. I knew that if I had any further complications, I could call and discuss them with her without feeling as if I were "eccentric."

Rate a woman physician as you would any doctor—for skill, honesty, quality of communication, flexibility, intellectual curiosity, ability to really listen, and respect for you as a person.

Nonphysician Health Workers in the Medical Care System

The medical system in the U.S. is like a pyramid, with highly paid male doctors and administrators at the top and underpaid and undervalued women forming the vast base. While about 82% of doctors are still men, about 70% of all medical care workers are women: doctors, nurses, physical therapists, medical technicians, secretaries and other clerical workers, service and maintenance staff, and more. People of color, usually hired for the most menial jobs and paid rock-bottom wages, are concentrated at the very bottom of this system.

When we go for care, particularly to a hospital or an HMO, we encounter mainly women. These nonphysician women health care workers are part of the same medical system that has been so strongly criticized throughout this book; like many physicians, some of these workers overly medicalize our health problems, focus too much on technology, and are too busy to offer empathic care. Many women hospital and HMO workers, however, truly want to offer supportive care, but like most other women workers, they work within a structure over which they have little or no control. They are often overworked and tremendously frustrated in their jobs. It is important to support all of these women as they fight for more control over their work so that they are able to deliver more humane, person-oriented care under good working conditions.

Nurses

Following the male physicians' takeover of health and medical care shortly after the turn of the century, becoming a woman physician was rare. Nursing was one of the few options open to women who wanted constructive and useful health-related work.

Most nurses still come from the middle or working classes, where people of color are concentrated; most physicians still come from the mostly white, middle or upper classes. The entry of more women into medical practice is changing this mix somewhat and sometimes creates unfamiliar tensions between women doctors and women nurses, often as a result of class and lifestyle differences. Of about one million nurses—registered nurses (RNs) and licensed practical nurses (LPNs)—about 95% are women. Nursing has histori-cally been a relatively low-status occupation, like other women's jobs, though graduate nurses and "advance practice" nurses, such as nurse-practitioners and nurse-midwives, now command quite good salaries. Nurse-practitioners (about 1% of nurses) became popular a decade ago because they saved private physicians and health maintenance organizations (HMOs) time and money. The current health care crisis has made their services, and those of other nonphysician primary care providers, more marketable. Certified midwives, nurse-anesthetists, and nurse-practitioners have developed extra skills and a strong professional identity.

This professionalization, however, is controversial among some nurses because it emphasizes more education and credentials as well as a doctor-like relationship to patients and keeps nurses divided from other health care workers. Nurses also express the concern that extra responsibilities and functions do not always bring additional recognition or compensation. Professionalization doesn't guarantee control over working conditions, job security, or access to clients. When specially trained nurses threaten to compete with physicians, their existence becomes more precarious. Their freedom to work is still in the hands of physicians, administrators, legislators, and, increasingly, managed care executives. Ironically, some health care plans that once sought out specially trained advance practice nurses to replace doctors as primary care providers are today switching gears and bringing in relatively low-paid primary care doctors whom they think will be more successful in attracting healthy middle-income enrollees.

Regular RNs now also perform many delegated medical functions: doing physical examinations, conducting tests, drawing blood, starting IVs, doing EKGs, and so on. Many nurses have become skilled in using diagnostic and treatment machines, and they see this as expertise that should help them professionally. But physicians and managers retain full control over who uses the technology, when it is used, and what diagnoses are made.

Nurses have always seen nursing as quite distinct from medicine. In the "caring versus curing" split that always fragments medical care, nurses traditionally do the caring—the day-to-day, hands-on work with patients and their families, and the listening, explaining, and teaching, with a special emphasis on prevention. As Lucy Candib, Mary Howell, Michelle Harrison, and other feminist physicians have pointed out, medicine undervalues caring because of sexism (women's work is less valuable), because of medicine's continual fascination with ever more complex technology, and because hospitals are increasingly becoming big businesses. Caring work doesn't use medical supplies, drugs, or expensive machines, nor does it generate profits.

Working conditions for nurses have never been the best. In hospitals, which still employ the majority of nurses, most nurses face dangerous understaffing, occupational hazards, insufficient job mobility, and, de-

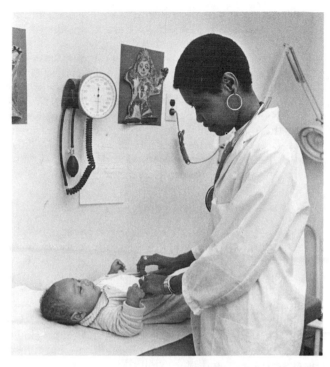

Spencer Grant/Stock, Boston

spite nurses' huge responsibility, a lack of overall administrative power (e.g., control over budgets or nursing rules and regulations).

Today, the corporate reorganization of health care is having a devastating impact on the nursing profession as hospitals rapidly convert from nonprofit to for-profit institutions. MC and hospital conversions have led to wholesale layoffs of skilled nursing personnel, without regard for the impact on patient safety or quality of care. Nurses, once the chief coordinators, administrators, and monitors of the patients' experience, are instead being hired to represent corporate interests in reducing skilled care and in limiting benefits and services. Nurses who are managers of care increasingly oversee not nurses but people who have been hired as "aides" but have little or no experience in caregiving: security guards, housekeepers, transport workers, and janitors. *As a result, the quality of care for hospital patients is plummeting, but the RNs who must manage an unqualified staff are put in the position of being held* legally *responsible if anything goes wrong!*[62] (See box, "What Every Patient Should Know About Nursing Care," p. 708.)

The glut of nurses produced by massive layoffs is creating an employers' market and much more difficult working conditions. Many nurses are now looking for work, and nursing schools are closing down. Nurses' frustration with the nursing role is at an all-time high, partly because the women's movement has affirmed women's capabilities and worth and has inspired women to express their entitlement to better conditions. This has led to several developments.

There is a resurgence of nurses organizing in health care unions and other associations. The struggle for

better working conditions has erupted into nursing strikes, which, unfortunately, are not usually supported by the public. Striking nurses are often seen as abandoning patients and deserting their posts, reinforcing every stereotype of "female selfishness" that lurks not far below the surface in U.S. society. Occasionally, though, in cases where quality of care has been successfully linked to working conditions for nurses and other health care workers, striking nurses have received substantial community support—for example, the Kaiser strikes in California during the 1980s.

Some nurses are beginning to explore seriously how to develop strategies that provide meaningful opportunities for lesser-skilled workers as well as for themselves, and to create alliances with their local communities based on a mutual interest in quality care. Nurses active in working for change emphasize that they want to be able to care directly for patients and to be valued and paid well for this work. They believe the effectiveness of medical care would improve dramatically with this shift, because caring plays much more of a role in actual "curing" than medicine has been willing to admit.

Several nursing organizations are lobbying with increased activity at state and national levels, and groups like NursesNOW (a part of the National Organization for Women) seek change through political and legislative strategies. One successful campaign ended all barriers to third-party reimbursement by insurance companies and by Medicaid for nursing care, which made a big difference in the autonomy and job satisfaction of many nurses with specialized training, even though this perpetuated the FFS system. In general, though, nurses have far fewer financial resources for lobbying and for political action than does the medical establishment; legislative change will, at best, be slow, and it needs the combined efforts of both consumers and other supportive professionals. For example, we may improve access to nurse-practitioners and nurse-midwives by getting involved in trying to change state legislation and regulation that may be opposed by local medical societies.

The growing mix of frustration and assertiveness among nurses comes through vividly in the words of one nurse:

We have put up with so much. Our contributions are barely mentioned; the labor of our backs is never recognized. We have come to the point where we actively discourage others from becoming nurses. We are beginning to question whether we want to continue to be the mainstay of the "health industry" and all its concomitant pollutants.

We nurses must begin to believe in ourselves. We must look at our numbers and consider the sum total of our shared experiences. We must rejoice that our hands can soothe, that our arms can lift those that cannot move, that our eyes can show what is in our hearts. . . . They have made us handmaidens—we will not be machines! The dictatorship of the dollar must end. It is time that we nurses . . . define the structure of our work. We can be creative. We know we are strong. And we know we are right.

Public Health Workers

Public health workers have several important roles in keeping populations healthy. First, they work to try to prevent outbreaks of disease and epidemics. Second, they are responsible for keeping our food and water safe and clean, so that disease is not spread through these sources. And third, through research, public health experts find out why illnesses and conditions that cause disease and death are widespread among certain populations, so that these illnesses can be treated and, eventually, prevented through education, health promotion, and/or immunization programs. Public health analysts may also look at the social, economic, and environmental causes of disease, including race, class, and gender. In addition, they organize and manage health and medical care services that are paid for by state and local government, including hospitals, clinics, and many other services.

Most public health workers are employed by the government. While those doctors who practice clinical medicine treat individuals, public health researchers study whole populations or subpopulations to discover and help halt the rise of diseases such as polio, TB, cancer, and HIV/AIDS. Public health research has taken the lead in identifying smoking-related diseases and their costs as well as in planning public information campaigns that help people quit smoking.

Most public health workers, until recently, have been doctors; today, public health schools accept both men and women students from many backgrounds. While women presently constitute half or more of most student bodies in public health, women faculty in leadership positions remain sparse, and most of them are physicians. People of color are often drawn to public health, intending to work with communities of color. But women and men of color, especially non-physicians, find it increasingly difficult to get financial support for this training, since government funding is shrinking. Graduates are gravitating toward the private sector, where MC is starting to take over the care of low-income and elderly people.

Pharmacists

More women are becoming pharmacists than ever before, and because pharmacists are such a valuable community resource, this is encouraging. While we used to think of them as druggists who just filled the doctors' prescriptions, in fact, they are much better trained than the average physician to communicate and explain about medicines. They know more about drug interactions, over-the-counter medications, and what food and drink should and should not be taken in combination with medications. It can be very helpful to discuss your medications with your pharmacist.

Pharmacists, too, are suffering from the corporatization of health care, especially the expansion of national drugstore chains such as Walgreens and Osco. These chains have driven many independent druggists out of business. Cities and towns have fought back, sometimes successfully, but it takes organizing and commitment. In addition, many community pharmacies are being squeezed out by MC corporations, which want the profits which result from bulk purchases in pharmacies they run themselves. Some states have successfully challenged restrictions HMOs want to place on where a prescription can be filled.

Allied Health Workers

Physical and occupational therapists, social workers, nutritionists, and other allied health workers, most of whom are women, can help us make the daily changes essential to a swift recovery or to preventing illness. Their techniques speed healing, help us live with physical limitations, and ease the helplessness, loneliness, and fear that often come with sickness. Yet, they can rarely fully use their knowledge and skills. The system is set up so that patients do not have easy access to them and often don't know that these services exist for them unless a doctor tells them so. Each profession is separate from medicine, setting its own standards and training its own workers in distinct and vital skills. Ask to see one of these workers if you think they might be at all helpful to you.

SURVIVING THE SYSTEM: CHOOSING AND USING MEDICAL CARE

Choice

When we need medical care, we want as much choice as possible. As in most aspects of our lives, economic status, sex, and race limit our choices. Because there is a severe maldistribution of doctors, where we live may also be a limiting factor. Prepaid medical plans and other MC organizations, although sometimes convenient, increasingly limit choices even for those who can pay. For those who can't afford to pay, there may soon be no choices—and no care. For example, more and more hospitals are turning away women in labor if they cannot prove they can pay, even though it is against federal law. In most settings, elderly poor women are forced to pay for many of their drugs and for increasing amounts of their care, often when they can least afford it. Women with low incomes, women of color, working-class women, lesbians, older women, and disabled women seeking medical care face language or culture barriers, physical-access barriers, prejudice, and abuse that further limit "choice." As our choices evaporate, it becomes more necessary to improve our skill at evaluating care and to create fair and equitable complaint and grievance systems wherever medical care is given.

Choosing a Primary Care Practitioner

What Is Primary Care?

Primary care (PC) refers to a basic, general form of caregiving that emphasizes prevention, continuity, and coordination of care. Ideally, we should seek care first from primary care practitioners who will then refer us to specialists as necessary. A good primary care practitioner is trained to give well-person care and checkups. She or he monitors mild, uncomplicated conditions and recommends appropriate treatments, recognizes more serious complications that require more specialized evaluation and treatment, coordinates specialists' care and institutional treatments, helps act as an advocate in decisions about medical treatment, provides continuity when many different people are involved, and may help us evaluate our experiences afterward. Primary care practitioners do not necessarily have to be physicians; nurse-practitioners and physician's assistants also make very good providers. Today, almost all managed care plans assign patients to a primary care physician, who makes decisions with you about your care and who writes the orders that allow you to get drugs or to be referred to other doctors or health workers.

Primary care physicians have been looked down upon by other specialists. Specialty areas such as surgery, radiology, anesthesiology, and psychiatry have always been regarded as more dramatic and prestigious than primary care (and more lucrative). Today, however, MC companies are limiting referrals to these specialists and are searching for more primary care physicians. This is a change that may benefit consumers, as primary care physicians are better trained to deal with patients as whole persons and to oversee care on all levels.

Nurse-Practitioners or Certified Nurse-Midwives

A skilled nurse-practitioner (NP) or nurse-midwife (CNM) may well be more satisfying and appropriate and less expensive in giving primary care than a physician. Both handle routine exams and problems. Although both NPs and CNMs always work in consultation with MDs, some have agreements that permit relatively autonomous practices, and they refer to their backup doctors only rarely; others work within doctors' offices, MC plans, hospitals, or clinics and are in daily consultation with them. Depending on the situation, a specially trained nurse may be able to make referrals, write prescriptions, and give out health and medical care information relatively independently of doctors, and some health centers now give them this job. Some have better performance records than doctors. One drawback is that in some plans and group practices, NPs act as gatekeepers and may prevent you from having a face-to-face conversation with your doctor when that is what you want. MC plans vary enormously in their use of what some "medical experts" call, condescendingly, "physician extenders."

Physician's Assistants

Physician's assistants (PA) are trained to carry out certain routine physical patient care tasks normally performed only by physicians or surgeons and not, in general, by nurses, whose tasks are sharply limited and regulated. Virtually all PAs are trained by doctors as apprentices, and have special licenses. They usually work with a particular physician or in a practice with one or more physicians, and often they are good primary care providers. This consultative model frequently offers more time for counseling and questions. In many states, PAs can make referrals and write prescriptions. In some states they perform early abortions.

Family Practice Physicians

These practitioners are specialists, different from old-time general practitioners (GPs) in that they have gone through a residency in family medicine and most have taken a specialty board examination in family practice as well. Family practitioners treat families and individuals of all ages, and some include delivering babies, frequently with fewer interventions than their OB-GYN counterparts. Some family practice physicians set up group practices and have admitting privileges at a hospital; today most have also been drawn into MC plans as primary care doctors except in very remote rural areas or in urban centers, where they are major providers for people with low incomes and for specific ethnic communities.[63] Recently, the family practice specialty decided that all residents in family medicine must learn to do obstetrics, and it is also introducing teaching about women's health.

Primary Care Internists

A reasonable choice for primary care is often an internist: a specialist with residency training in internal medicine. However, until recently most internists actually subspecialized (circulatory, heart, digestive problems, etc.), and only a few have had special training in primary care. Traditionally, some internists had an unspoken "gentleman's agreement" to refer most women to OB-GYNs for routine care, whereas they themselves preferred to care for male patients and their systemic problems. However, women have serious nonreproductive medical problems that the internist, not the OB-GYN, is specifically trained to treat —for instance, heart conditions, cancers, and other chronic illnesses; difficulties with basic bodily functions such as metabolism, elimination, breathing, and so on; or problems created by contraceptive or tranquilizer use.

Obstetrician/Gynecologists

For more than a decade, women have been 40% or more of those newly trained in OB-GYN, and many men feel that they are being driven out of the field. The truth is that many women prefer to see female

OB-GYNs and are pleased that more women are entering the field. Many women have used OB-GYNs not only for reproductive care but as their primary care physicians. This is changing, however, as many managed care plans insist that women have nonspecialist primary care practitioners who then may refer them to OB-GYNs or nurse-midwives as needed. OB-GYNs are not trained for primary care, even if some health plans hire them for this work with women.

Still, today the majority of OB-GYNs are seeing healthy women who turn to them for routine well-woman care, and they attend at least 90% of all births, more than 80% of which are normal and uncomplicated. Since OB-GYN training is neither necessary nor appropriate for these services, the trend toward women having other primary care providers is a positive change. OB-GYNs are surgical specialists, trained especially to diagnose and treat diseases of the reproductive organs, manage childbirth complications (about 5 to 15%, maximum, of all births), and perform gynecological surgery. With this kind of training, and a tendency to suspect a psychological origin for the physical pain many women report, OB-GYNs may miss important nonreproductive illnesses. They may overprescribe tranquilizers and refer to psychiatrists inappropriately. They are also likely to offer treatment solutions more drastic, invasive, and permanent than is necessary—hysterectomy, for example, is still done too often—and they may offer few alternatives, medical or nonmedical, for common problems. Some know little about women past menopause and may not appreciate the nonhormonal aspects of the midlife transition or of aging; they are also often insensitive to women's emotional needs during childbirth, and to the health concerns of lesbians. Their surgical talents, however, are extremely important, when needed, and many women prefer their care.

Largely because women return to them so often for expensive, routine office visits, for delivering babies and for surgery, OB-GYNs have had among the highest incomes of any physicians in office-based community practice. As a result, the American College of Obstetricians and Gynecologists (ACOG) is one of the most effective medical specialty societies, with the financial resources to maintain multiple lobbyists in Washington, DC, and many state or regional offices around the country, which often influence legislation. Their work is funded lavishly by the pharmaceutical industry.

Surviving the Hospitalization Experience

Hospitalization involves risks, isolation, and sometimes fear. It's often difficult to make contact with physicians or nurses who know your case and to get clear information from them when you do. Being in the hospital may involve costs and, especially for women, worries about those at home. Because most of us will continue to use hospitals, we have to be aware of how to use them as well as possible in today's corporate climate.

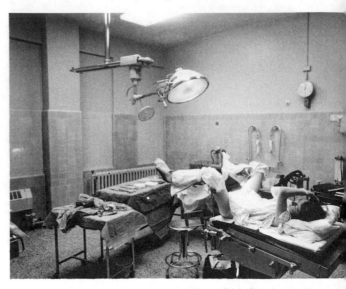

James Holland/Stock, Boston

First of all, make sure you need to be hospitalized. Consider all your outpatient medical and nonmedical alternatives. If the procedure is elective (postponable, nonemergency), get a second or even a third opinion. A few insurance and Medicaid programs will pay for this. Investigate outpatient surgical possibilities, which may be less invasive, may use local anesthesia, may be cheaper, and will allow you to go home sooner (maybe too soon, but because you've received fewer drugs, you may recover sooner).

Once hospitalization seems necessary, find out as much as you can. Ask health care practitioners, friends, and neighbors about their recent experiences, and look into the policies of the hospitals you may be obliged to use. For example, one mother was upset to discover that the hospital would not allow her to stay with her seriously ill child; another woman learned that her partner could not be with her during her cesarean section; still another woman discovered that her lesbian lover was excluded from the intensive care unit because she was neither "family" nor spouse and therefore had no "legitimate" claim.

If possible, bring someone with you when you are being hospitalized who can act as your advocate and help you make decisions (see "Our Rights as Patients," p. 713) throughout your stay. In most cases today, hospitalization periods are relatively short, as health plans don't want to pay for lengthy stays. As a result, you are usually sicker while you are there, and you need more care when you return home. Once you are hospitalized, the following information may be helpful:

- Whenever you are in a hospital, you have a right to know the name of the one doctor in charge of your case.
- Find out who is caring for you. Not all of the people caring for patients in the hospital are nurses.

- Try to forge an alliance with the nursing staff, once you know who they are. Nurses are still the true coordinators of your total care and keep their own records that are often separate from the doctors'; nurses' judgments can influence the whole course of your care. Remember that they work under constraints that may severely limit their ability to advocate for you.

- Whenever tests or X rays are proposed, be sure to ask why, and ask to see the results, as well as receiving verbal reports. The rapid expansion of technology in hospitals vastly increases overall hospital cost and further depersonalizes care; such technology is often applied inappropriately if there is money to be made, creating iatrogenic illnesses and problems. At other times you may need a test and find you will have to fight to get it.

- There are nearly continuous outbreaks of infection in most hospitals that are increasingly resistant to antibiotic treatments. Called *nosocomial* infections, they are produced within the hospital environment and carried largely by doctors and nurses and other personnel, some of whose antiseptic techniques are careless. Such infections complicate surgery, delay recovery, and may cause secondary illness or even death if undiagnosed or untreated (as in the case of some newborns). If you are hospitalized, try to go home as soon as is reasonable, but don't be afraid to insist on the care you need. Once home, be alert for signs of secondary illness caused by hospitalization—infection, swelling, redness, fever.

- In a wide range of operations, local anesthesia can be used instead of general anesthesia. Local anesthesia enables you to recover more quickly and doesn't carry the same risk of death.

- Because rates of error in administering medications remain high, find out as soon as you can what medicines have been prescribed for you, by whom, for what purpose, and how often you must take them. Ask nurses which medications they are giving you, try to keep a record of them, and cross-check with your doctor(s). Resist routine tranquilizers and sleeping pills if at all possible.

- Because hospital food is frequently not nutritious, ask friends to bring you good food daily. Hospital water at the bedside has repeatedly been shown to be contaminated by bacteria, such as *Salmonella,* so bottled spring water is also a good idea. Also consider taking vitamins, especially vitamin C, unless your doctor has objections on the grounds that they would interfere with medications or other treatment.

- Wearing your own sleepwear, robes, and so on, may make you feel more like yourself.

- As you leave the hospital, ask for a copy of your records to be sent to your home (lab or X-ray results may be available as part of your hospital record, depending on your state's laws). These records may be useful in the future, and some hospitals destroy records after a short period of time (state laws vary).

- If the hospital wants to discharge you before you feel able to go home, insist on staying, especially if there will be no one to care for you at home. The hospital may also prefer to transfer you to an extended care facility (a temporary stay in a nursing home) before you go home. Sometimes this will be what you need; however, because there may be a financial incentive for this transfer (as when the managed care plan or hospital owns the nursing home), you might want to seek a second opinion. (See "Our Rights as Patients," p. 713.)

Emergency Rooms

Accidents and emergencies, alcoholism, heart attacks, drug abuse, and mental illness bring many people to emergency rooms, sometimes on a regular basis. If they are part of hospitals, emergency rooms (ERs) are required by law to take all comers. As a result, people without regular medical providers or the ability to pay for health care use ERs as a way to access regular care as well as in emergencies. Since it is so expensive, MC plans tend to limit these visits. And since even nonprofit hospitals are under pressure to limit "free" care, they, too, are trying to eliminate this service. As a consequence, some cities have few places where emergency care is available. On the other hand, we have heard of many instances in which MC subscribers were discouraged from going to the ER, but went anyway because they knew they were in a crisis that demanded immediate attention. Don't be intimidated if you feel sure there's something wrong. For a list of symptoms and conditions requiring emergency care see "Our Rights as Patients," p. 713.

Where to Find (and Not to Find) the Information We Need

To have some control over our lives and to be informed participants in our health and medical care, we need a lot of information about our bodies and about the health system. We need to know what options are available. We need to know which forms of care have not been adequately studied—and are therefore "experimental"—and which forms of care have been adequately studied and have been shown to be either effective or ineffective or even harmful. We need to know the risks that are involved with each choice. Knowledge gives us the ability to make choices.

Today, much more independent health and medical information is available than there was even ten years ago. Some of it is trustworthy; some of it is not. It is crucial for our health that we get information from sources that are both accurate and independent—that is, sources able to evaluate the material from technical, public interest, user, and feminist perspectives. The

WHAT EVERY PATIENT SHOULD KNOW ABOUT NURSING CARE

Today, more and more patients have learned to ask important questions when their doctor tells them they need a particular treatment, operation, or medication. Patients need to learn to ask similar questions about nursing care. They also need to ask about the availability of nurse practitioners in health plans, physician practices, hospitals, and other facilities.

Here are some questions patients can ask:

In the Hospital

- Will a registered nurse be assigned to care for me?
- Does your hospital have primary nursing?
- What is the nurse-to-patient ratio on the floor or unit where I will be in the hospital?
- Will a nurse be available to check on me at least once an hour?
- What other health care workers will be working with my nurse?
- Have these health care workers received special training to do this work? What are their duties?
- Does your hospital use a lot of agency or temporary nurses [the nursing equivalent of temps]?
- Does your hospital use a lot of float nurses [the nursing equivalent of assigning a pediatrician to take care of an adult oncology patient]?
- Are nurse-practitioners or clinical nurse specialists used by the facility to provide clinical care or education for staff?
- Will nurses prepare me for my discharge and make sure nursing care is available to me at home if I need it?
- What are my options for managing pain and other problems at home?
- Will nurses educate my family members about the care I will need after the hospital?

Subacute (and Nursing Home) Facilities

Many patients today are discharged from the hospital while they are still acutely ill to so-called subacute facilities and nursing homes; many women will seek nursing home care for a family member. In these cases it is important to ask the following questions:

- How many deficiencies—and of what type—did you receive on your last federal/state survey (70% of all nursing homes are out of compliance with federal requirements).

- Will a registered nurse be responsible for my care? (Although the name "nursing home" suggests that there are a great many registered nurses providing care, in fact, very few registered nurses are employed in most nursing homes.)
- Are your nurses educated in and able to deliver sophisticated and effective pain and symptom management?
- What is the education and training of your nurses?
- What is the ratio of RNs and other types of nursing personnel to the residents—particularly on different shifts?
- What was the nursing and nursing aide turnover rate during the past year?
- Are nurse-practitioners or nursing specialists used by the facility to provide clinical care or education for staff?

(See also chapter 23, Women Growing Older, p. 578.)

Home Care

- Is your home care agency state licensed and Medicare certified? (Fewer than 50% of home care agencies are Medicare certified.)
- Can you provide all the care I might need in the home?
- Are services available 24 hours a day, seven days a week?
- Will I have a consistent registered nurse care manager?
- Will this case manager also deliver my hands-on care?
- Will the nurse caring for me have expertise with my particular medical problem or in pain and symptom management?
- What are the requirements your agency has for hiring registered nurses? Do you hire mainly new graduates, or do you have a mix of new graduates and nurses with five years or more of experience?
- How many visits per day do you expect your nurses to make?
- What resources (educational seminars, professional development courses, time off to attend conferences) do you provide to educate nurses to make sure they are up to date clinically?
- Are nurse-practitioners available to provide my home care?

How to Complain

If in any setting you find it difficult to get good nursing care, you should be prepared to complain to managers, administrators, physicians, or politicians. Keep in mind that many deficiencies in nursing care today may have little to do with the willingness of individual nurses to provide that care. Problems often stem from lack of staff or lack of time allotted to deal with patients' needs. Complaints should therefore not scapegoat individuals but rather question overall organizational policies. (See "Our Rights as Patients," p. 713, for more on complaint mechanisms.)

best information describes "evidence-based practice": practices that are supported by research that uses rigorous scientific methods to evaluate medical care and that is free of commercial or professional biases. (See "Evidence-Based Practice and the Cochrane Collaboration" box on p. 710.)

Ourselves

We know a lot about our bodies; we must listen to and trust what our bodies are telling us. Our awareness of change in ourselves or those we care for is often the first and most important indicator of sickness. Most of what doctors learn about us, we tell them. We learn much from the women in our lives: our mothers, sisters, aunts, grandmothers, and friends. Convincing medical personnel that our knowledge is valuable may be quite difficult.

Reading

Reading is important, but we must make sure that our sources are as accurate as possible. Magazines and newspapers, a common resource, have their problems (see box, "The Media and Women's Health"). Look for progressive and feminist magazines and journals. Consumers can also buy the *Physicians' Desk Reference (PDR)* or ask for it in local libraries to find out what the drug industry says about the drugs it manufactures. *The Medical Letter* is a public-interest drug evaluation guide. Be sure to see other consumer guides to drugs as well (see Resources). Beware of booklets and brochures in your doctor's office, as they are usually from the drug industry. They tend to downgrade nonmedical or nonpharmacological approaches and are slow to present innovative alternatives or prevention orientations.

Databases and the Internet

The two leading medical databases are MEDLINE (medical articles) from the National Library of Medicine, and CINAHL (references to nursing and allied health literature). These and other databases may be available through your local public library. Sometimes a trained librarian will search or show you how to

THE MEDIA AND WOMEN'S HEALTH

Many of us depend on mainstream media like television, magazines, and daily newspapers for our understanding of women's health issues and key points of the ongoing health system debate. Many conscientious reporters and editors in a few key organizations, like PBS and NPR, work hard to provide documented facts and thorough analyses that distinguish between the public interest and special interests; some producers and editors try to offer discussions that illuminate all sides of a debate. Nonetheless, the mainstream media are heavily influenced by the health industries' special interest groups. Many publications have a pro-medicine and "gender-neutral" bias, rejecting woman-centered or feminist perspectives. The few consumer rights stories that appear rarely make it clear how women specifically are treated or mistreated by both the health insurance and medical care delivery systems. The overwhelming majority of health care reporting is heavily biased in favor of the financial needs of business, the health industries and professions, and the federal budget. Though "horror stories" of individual patients who suffer under MC plans may appear with regularity, these stories rarely invite the viewer to understand what citizens and activists need to do in order to change the system. Even the best news and editorial contributions in the mainstream media are now swamped by the massive campaigns and commercials of the managed care industry.

Among the most pervasive biases of the media have been their generally unquestioning acceptance of the profit motive in health and medical care. The mainstream media have failed to emphasize the health industries' spectacular rise in PAC donations to key members of Congress and the influence of this money on the political process in health reforms. The biggest story of all—that consumers favor overwhelmingly a universal, comprehensive health care system ("single payer," see p. 693)—has been practically eliminated from news and editorial consideration in the mainstream media.[64]

The mainstream media have missed the importance of consumer involvement in decision-making and oversight. Stories of the few malpractice suits that result in huge damage awards distort the reality that thousands of consumers suffer from damaging care and never receive redress. Finally, the media have virtually ignored women's central and unique place in the entire health care and medical care system—as

continued on next page

workers, caregivers, and decision-makers. Women's health activists' long history of watchdogging Congress, the drug industry, the medical professions, and the FDA—in the public interest as well as women's interests—usually remains invisible, even in the best media presentations.

Though many try to be even handed, reporters work on tight deadlines and are inclined to use well-packaged, well-placed materials from the special interest groups, which are always available for immediate use. They are also sometimes careless about identifying whether invited spokespeople and "experts" interviewed represent special health industry interests or political interests, rather than the public interest. Similarly, they may quote study outcomes or results of polls without explaining how these were conducted or who paid for them. Often, they are not skilled enough to understand the scientific meaning of words used by researchers like "significant," "prove," or "cure," or to realize that a study of six women is not enough to make the result a scientific breakthrough. As media consumers we need to be aware of these biases and deficiencies and to find ways to make the media more accountable to women's, and everyone's, health concerns and problems with the current system.

search the database (sometimes for a fee). Increasingly, the databases are available on CD-ROM, and library patrons can search them for free. MEDLINE is now free on the Internet. For ease of use, try the service offered by the National Library of Medicine at http://www.nlm.nih.gov. (For more informaton on Internet resources, see Introduction to Online Women's Health Resources, p. 25.)

Self-Help Groups

These are one of the most important sources of courage and information. Different from medically run or hospital-run self-care or self-help groups, these small informal groups of women meet throughout this country to help each other learn about birth control, fertility awareness, menopause, breast cancer, DES, hysterectomy, cervical self-exam, lupus and other autoimmune diseases, and many other topics. When groups focus on one specific issue, they are often better able than many physicians to keep abreast of the most current research.

Such groups are organized in ways that reflect the values of the women's health movement. They are nonhierarchical; every member plays an equal part. Information is free. Implicit in these groups is the belief that women can understand medical information, that it "belongs" rightfully to us, and that we need to feel empowered by it. Group members' experiences are an important source of information about health, illness, and treatment. By comparing notes and trading

EVIDENCE-BASED PRACTICE AND THE COCHRANE COLLABORATION
by Carol Sakala

Randomized controlled trials (RCTs) provide especially high-quality information about the effects, if any, of specific forms of care. They provide an excellent basis for determining "evidence-based practice," or practice supported by sound research. In RCTs, each person enrolled in a study is assigned randomly to a study group. If the studies are done well, the researchers can conclude that the groups were comparable, with the exception of the "variable of interest"—the care given or withheld. Compared to other types of studies, differences in outcome in RCTs are more reassuringly related to the care being studied.

In general, we can get the soundest information about the effectiveness of health and medical practices by combining results of well-conducted RCTs that address similar questions. This pooling of results is known as a "systematic review" or a "meta-analysis." Researchers have used this approach to confirm that specific medical practices do indeed "work" and offer specific benefits. Meta-analysis also shows that many other common practices are ineffective or even harmful, while many others involve trade-offs between benefits and risks. The effectiveness of many health and medical practices has not been carefully studied using RCTs and meta-analysis.

One of the most valuable resources in researching evidence-based practice is the Cochrane Collaboration (CC) (see "Resources for Evidence-Based Practice" below). CC is a rapidly growing international network of researchers, clinicians, and others who create and publish systematic reviews of RCTs and update the reviews as new trials become available. The reviews are available by subscription, and abstracts of all completed reviews are available on the Internet at no charge. Currently, over 30 Collaborative Review Groups are preparing reviews on such topics as breast cancer, depression/anxiety/neurosis, menstrual disorders, pregnancy and childbirth, subfertility, osteoporosis, osteoarthritis, and tobacco addiction. New groups are forming around topics such as fertility regulation, gynecological cancer, HIV/AIDS, pain/palliative care/supportive care, and drug addiction.

A valuable and unprecedented undertaking, the Cochrane Collaboration still has important limitations. Since CC is based on controlled trial studies that have been funded and reported, it necessarily represents the values, interests, and biases of those who carry out and fund clinical trials, including medical industries, medical practitioners, and medical settings. Funded trials, for example, tend to reflect biases toward intervention and more invasive treatment; preventive approaches are much less adequately studied. Commercially valuable forms of care tend to be more widely used and better studied than care that has little or no commercial value. Trials tend to focus on expected benefits and short-term effects, with much less exploration of potential risk and longer-term effects. Many outcomes that are of interest to care recipients have not been well studied. In other words, the topical databases that are being created do not yet reflect a proactive vision of services that would best meet people's needs.

There is great need for "consumer" voices in the Cochrane Collaboration to provide the perspectives of those who participate in trials and receive care. Consumers are in an excellent position, for example, to question assumptions that many professionals take for granted and to raise questions about the inevitable limitations of this project. The experience of HIV/AIDS activists and breast cancer activists suggests that consumers can use the information available through Cochrane resources to help shape research agendas. By policy, CC encourages broad participation in all areas of its work. Collaborative Review Groups are required to be multinational and to include at least one "consumer" member. A Consumer Network (see below), which welcomes any interested participants, has been established to help ensure that users of health and medical services have a voice throughout the organization. A "Comments/Criticism" procedure enables anyone who identifies concerns about specific reviews to provide feedback and help shape regular updates. Every Cochrane group has an administrator, and some have World Wide Web sites, Internet discussion groups, and/or a newsletter. These channels offer opportunities for women's and other health advocates to become involved in this important undertaking.

Resources for Evidence-Based Practice

British Medical Journal. Contains a ten-part series for nonexperts on finding and assessing medical information, beginning with the July 19, 1997, issue. Web site: http://www.bmj.com

Centre for Evidence-Based Medicine, Research and Development, National Health Service, England. *Searching for the Best Evidence in Clinical Journals.* Web site: http://cebm.jr2.ox.ac.uk/docs/searching.html

Centre for Reviews and Dissemination, National Health Service, England. *Search Strategy to Identify Reviews and Meta-analyses in Medline and CINAHL.* Web site: http://www.york.ac.uk/inst/crd/search.htm

Centre for Reviews and Dissemination, National Health Service, England. *Systematic Reviews, Health Technology Assessment and Evidence Based Healthcare.* Web site: http://www.york.ac.uk/inst/crd/sites

Cochrane Collaboration. The best place for centralized information of interest to consumers is on the Internet at http://som.flinders.edu.au/fusa/Cochrane. For information on the Cochrane Consumer Network, visit their Web site or contact Hilda Bastian, Coordinator, Cochrane Consumer Network, Australasian Cochrane Centre, Flinders Medical Centre, Bedford Park, SA, Australia 5042.

The Cochrane Library is a subscription-based resource that includes full text of all completed systematic reviews within the Cochrane Collaboration. It consists of four major databases, updated and reissued quarterly, available in CD-ROM. U.S. distributor: Update Software, Inc., 936 La Rueda, Vista, CA 92084; (760) 727-6792.

Entwistle, Vikki A., Ian S. Watt, and James E. Herring. *Information About Health Care Effectiveness: An Introduction for Consumer Health Information Providers.* London: King's Fund Publishing, 1996. (Promoting Patient Choice series.)

Hope, Tony. *Evidence-Based Patient Choice.* London: King's Fund Publishing, 1996. (Promoting Patient Choice series.)

Lerner, Jeffrey C. "The National Patient Library: Evidence-based Information for Consumers," *International Journal of Technology Assessment in Health Care* 14, no. 1 (1998).

Research and Development Directorate, National Health Service Executive. *Cochrane Electronic Library: Updated Self Training Guide and Notes.* Web site: http://libsun1.jr2.ox.ac.uk/nhserdd/aordd/evidence/clibtrng.htm

School of Health and Related Research, University of Sheffield, England. *Netting the Evidence: A SCHARR Introduction to Evidence Based Practice on the Internet.* Web site: http://www.shef.ac.uk/uni/academic/R-Z/scharr/ir/netting.html

stories with other women, we learn how to use the information we get from both medical and nonmedical sources. Independent of medical care institutions and professionals, these groups are not hampered in exploring nonmedical therapies and practitioners or in questioning, challenging, and evaluating accepted ones.

Some groups already exist (see chapters 24, Selected Medical Practices, Problems, and Procedures, and 27, Organizing for Change). We have to initiate others as the need arises. When you find one or two other women who want to get together, that is a good beginning. You can also try an ad in the local paper to start a group.

Health Information Centers

There are a few good (and fairly stable) independent health information centers women can turn to. Examples are the BWHBC's Women's Health Information Center in Somerville, Massachusetts; the Center for Medical Consumers and Health Care Information in New York City; and Planetree Health Resource Center in San Francisco. The Clearinghouse of the National Women's Health Network (NWHN) is another national resource. In these centers—a cross between a library and a hot line—anyone can come to read, learn, and sometimes talk about health and medical care: what the controversies are, what home remedies women have tried, the risks and possibilities of various medical and nonmedical treatments. Workers at these centers may also be willing to help you select a health care practitioner and/or put you in touch with women who have gone through experiences similar to yours. Many women's health centers and community groups, such as the Emma Goldman Clinic in Iowa and the Feminist Health Centers in Concord and Portsmouth, NH, offer similar services on a more limited basis.

As community funds dry up and hospitals take on a larger corporate existence, more and more health information centers will not be community run but hospital-run or health plan–run, with all the limits outlined below. The authors of this book strongly believe that health information centers should be part of each neighborhood and/or region, located in public libraries or other community settings, and free of commercial bias. They should be community controlled, with a definite consumer and public interest perspective, and with plentiful information on where to go for additional resources. Consumers will have to fight for them and convince others they are worthwhile and worth paying for.

Sources of Information Within the Medical Establishment

Doctors

Although most of us learned while growing up to turn to doctors for health and medical information, our experience reveals that there are many limits to what they can or will tell us. Some doctors are happy to give over-the-phone commonsense information that can be extremely helpful. Others send complete reports in writing after a checkup. But the information we get from doctors is increasingly limited by

- the sexism, racism, homophobia, and class bias of much of their training.
- how little time they budget to teach patients.
- their frequent mistrust of our ability to understand or make good use of complex information.

- their tendency not to keep up with the latest research or their inability to evaluate it.
- their lack of knowledge about prevention, self-care, and less invasive procedures.
- pressures from drug company representatives to push certain medications.
- the desire to appear "sure" and "dependable," which creates an unwillingness to admit to uncertainty or controversy.
- their unfamiliarity with and distrust of nonmedical alternatives and holistic healing traditions.

And, most seriously:

- financial incentives not to recommend the best care if it costs the MC plan more money.
- the inability to spend adequate time with patients for appropriate diagnosis. It can be frustrating, even humiliating, to try to get information over the phone or in person from doctors who don't want or are unable to give it. We may try to get test results and find that the doctors will not give them to us. We may leave an office or clinic with many questions. We must remember in these situations not to blame ourselves. We have a right to be treated with respect and to get the information we need. (See "Our Rights as Patients," p. 713.)

Even when our doctors provide information, it may not be "the best." Commonly, our providers make clinical decisions on the basis of what other colleagues in the area are doing, what local "opinion leaders" recommend, what seems to work in their own clinical experience, what they learned during their professional education, or what they may have read in one or two professional journal articles.

This is not evidence-based practice. For these reasons, we urge you to consult doctors for their advice and information as you always have, but not to rely solely upon what they say. Take someone with you who can observe the interview. Write down your questions, ask them all, and record the answers. Check an independent source, like *Practice Guidelines** or a health information center, to be sure the course recommended is really the best for you in this case.

Classes or Groups Sponsored by Hospitals, Physicians or HMOs (Often Called Self-Care Groups)

Some of the more practical physicians and medical centers, in part because of pressure from women's and consumer health activists, offer groups or classes in everything from childbirth to smoking cessation to weight management or posthysterectomy or mastectomy adjustments. These groups help up to a point, mainly because they give you a chance to talk with

* Available from Agency for Health Care Policy Research (see Resources).

OUR RIGHTS AS PATIENTS

by George J. Annas,

Edward R. Utley Professor and Chair, Health Law
Department, Boston University
School of Public Health

Each of us has specific legal rights that protect us in our daily lives, including a number of particular rights as consumers of medical care services. In any medical setting, your most important right is the right to control what happens to your body, to decide about your treatment. You have the right to information about all reasonable treatment alternatives and the right to decide among these, although you may have to go outside your health plan if you choose certain ones. All competent adults have the right to refuse any treatment, even if such a refusal means you will likely get sicker or even die.

Informed Consent and Informed Decision-Making

The doctrine of informed consent is founded on two fundamental propositions:

1. It's your body and you should be able to decide what is done with it.

2. You are likely to make a better decision about what is done with your body if you are provided with information on which to base a rational decision.

No one can treat or even touch you until you make an informed decision to accept or reject treatment. When physicians and patients take informed consent seriously, their relationship can be a true partnership, with shared authority, decision-making, and responsibility. Physicians must provide you with at least the following information:

1. a description of the recommended treatment or procedure.

2. a description of the risks and benefits of the recommended treatment or procedure, with a special emphasis on the risk of death or serious disability.

3. a description of alternative treatments and procedures, together with the risks and benefits of each.

4. the likely results if you refuse any treatment.

5. the probability of success, and what the physician means by success.

6. the major problems anticipated in recuperation, including how long it will be until you can resume your normal activities.

7. any other information patients in your situation generally receive, such as cost and how much of the cost your health plan will cover.

You have a right to know if a drug is being used for a purpose not approved by the FDA. (Check the *Physicians' Desk Reference* or package insert for the approved purposes.) This situation is extremely common among women, because most routinely used obstetric drugs, many hormonal preparations, and some psychiatric drugs are given for purposes not specifically approved by the FDA.

For consent to be informed, you must also understand all that is being explained. It is not enough for a physician or other practitioner to simply catalogue the risks and benefits in a quick or complicated manner, to do it when you are under the effects of medication, or to tell you in English if it's not your first language. You should ask as many questions as you have, and wait until they are answered to your satisfaction before proceeding. You can ask for a written statement of the treatment plan in order to monitor your care or in case you choose to seek a second opinion later. Where no medical emergency exists, take as much time as you need to think about your decision. You can make a decision and later change your mind, because informed consent includes the right to refuse during as well as before any treatment. And you must agree voluntarily, without coercion or pressure applied by the physician or others.

Despite the fact that it is the physician's legal duty to ensure informed consent, some doctors and hospitals do not do so. Insist on an unpressured discussion with your physician. It is not uncommon for patients to be told little or nothing about the risks of treatments and medications being proposed for them. Physicians and hospitals may also try to take advantage of the few legal exceptions to the informed consent requirements.

It is essential to read any consent form very carefully and to inquire about any vague or technical terms before signing, because your signature suggests—often incorrectly—that you were informed. The form can be used as evidence of consent. Some hospitals ask patients to write out their understanding of the proposed procedure in their own words. You may cross out, reword, or otherwise amend a prepared form before signing it. Insist on getting a second opinion if

continued on next page

you have any unanswered questions about proposed treatment or surgery. You have a right to a copy of any form you sign. If you are in a health maintenance organization (HMO) or other managed care setting, you also have a right to know how your physician is being paid and whether he or she can make extra money by not treating you, or by not recommending expensive care.

Research

Under certain conditions, medical personnel are obligated, legally and ethically, to give you specific detailed information before you consent to treatment, as when:

1. the provider uses an unproven (experimental) medical, surgical or psychiatric treatment, and the chance of success is therefore unknown.

2. a randomized clinical trial or study is being carried out that may involve giving certain people no treatment or a treatment that may be inferior, in order to compare results with a newer treatment.

Because so much research goes on in teaching hospitals, it is important to determine whether or not you are being treated with standard or experimental therapies. Also, the line between treatment and experimentation is often unclear, and because physician-researchers may not adequately protect us, we must continually ask questions about recommended treatments. Experimental situations require that researchers keep a record of our statements, that we understand and agree to the experiment, and that we realize that the probability of a good outcome is uncertain. If the research is taking place in an institution that derives part of its support from public funds, federal regulations require the creation of a special committee called an institutional review board (IRB), which includes both medical personnel and nonmedical community representatives. This board must first grant approval to the project and then review the consent form. In this instance, the researcher is obligated to give you a copy of any informed consent form you sign, as well as the identity of a person who can provide you with more information about the research.

What Other Rights Do We Have?

The law does not yet recognize all the rights we should have, although women's and consumer health activists are working to expand these rights through lawsuits and legislation. In 1997, President Clinton suggested that Congress pass a National Patient Bill of Rights. We can still ask that physicians and institutions recognize even those rights not legally required. Certain rights are guaranteed by the Constitution, federal and state laws and regulations, and case law. Several decisions made by hospitals or other private groups may also affect our rights as consumers.

Reproductive Rights

The U.S. Constitution implicitly guarantees each one of us a right to privacy, and the U.S. Supreme Court has ruled that this right protects a woman's ability to make personal decisions concerning abortion, sterilization, contraception, and other reproductive matters. As recently as 1992, the Court confirmed a woman's right to liberty in seeking an abortion. The Supreme Court did, however, rule that states may restrict this right in ways that do not "unduly burden" women before the time after which the fetus might live outside the womb. For example, states may constitutionally require a 24-hour waiting period before an abortion is performed (see chapter 17, Abortion).

The Right to Refuse Treatment

You have a legal right to refuse any medical treatment at any time, even if you have consented to it previously. This right applies to all competent adults and all mature minors (i.e., those who can understand and appreciate the information necessary to give informed consent). Simply disagreeing with your physician's recommendation does not mean that you are incompetent. In life-or-death matters involving decisions for "incompetent" patients, however, physicians and hospitals may try to resist your choice to refuse treatment on behalf of someone else. All states have passed laws that, through the use of a living will or health care proxy, allow competent people to authorize the withholding or withdrawal of medical treatment, even though such an order may lead to their death after they become incompetent. Of course, you must sign a health care proxy to authorize another person to make medical decisions for you before you become incompetent. Remember, too, that accepting one part of the treatment plan does not mean that you must accept it all, and you always have the right to leave the hospital if your wishes are not respected (with the exception, in some cases, of a psychiatric facility; see chapter 6, Our Emotional Well-Being: Psychotherapy in Context.) Enlisting the support of a family member or other advocate may be particularly helpful in such situations.

The Right to Receive Care in Emergencies

You have a legal right to treatment if you are experiencing a medical emergency and get to a hospital emergency room. Moreover, if either transfer or discharge from an emergency department will threaten or adversely affect a patient's condition, then treatment must be rendered, regardless of your ability to pay. The physician's role is central. First, the physician has a duty to determine whether an emergency exists. If one does, law and medical ethics require the physician to treat you or to find someone who can. Conditions that require immediate attention include heavy bleeding, heart stoppage, breathing stoppage, profound shock from any cause, ingestion of or exposure to a rapidly acting poison, pregnancy with active labor, severe head injuries; sudden and complete changes in personality, and anaphylactic reaction (severe allergic response). Emergencies can be less serious, however; they could include broken bones, fevers, and cuts that require stitches.

Other than emergency care, there is no legal "right to health care." When combined with the high costs of medical care, this means that many people receive either inadequate care or no care at all. There are a few entitlement programs for pregnant women and low-income, elderly, or physically challenged persons, although many of them are being cut back—for example, Medicare and Medicaid payments (which are constantly being cut and the eligibility requirements made more stringent) and monthly Social Security payments for those who are temporarily disabled, regardless of age. Contact your local legal services office for a full list of the various programs and their eligibility requirements.

Rights Regarding Medical Records

You have a legal right to see, obtain, or have access to your hospital and medical records. But in reality, many patients are never informed of this right and find it difficult and costly to obtain their records. In addition, many facilities keep medical records only for the limited period of time specified by state law. There are also variations from state to state about medical versus psychiatric records, hospitals' versus doctors' or nurses' records, and minors' versus adults' records. It is advisable to have copies of all medical encounters for future reference and to make sure they are accurate.

Physicians' records are also confidential, but state laws and regulations usually require physicians to make them available to patients. Most physicians will give you copies of your records and test results if you ask. Otherwise, your only recourse may be to hire a lawyer who will demand the records through either a letter or, in rare circumstances, a lawsuit. When selecting a physician, ask how the physician feels about making records available.

Contract Rights and Health Plan Rights

The patient has a right to a copy of the entire health care insurance or health care plan contract, and to competent counseling in selecting a health plan. The patient has a right, regardless of source of payment, to examine and receive an itemized and detailed explanation of all services rendered. The patient has a right to timely prior notice of termination of eligibility for payment for services, or denial of a health care benefit, and an opportunity to contest such denial in a timely and fair manner.

No health plan may interfere with or limit communication between the patient and physician or the patient and primary care provider. Health plans must disclose to members any and all financial arrangements that might encourage physicians to limit or restrict care, specialty referrals, or advocacy for noncovered alternatives. Many states require health plans to pay for emergency services based on what a prudent layperson would see as an emergency. Health plans must provide timely access to an independent appeals mechanism for benefit denials or terminations.

How Can We Enforce Our Rights?

Our rights as patients mean little if we are unable to enforce them effectively. The method of enforcement will depend on state laws and the right involved. Listed on the following pages are some of the most common ways to exercise and enforce our rights. Further information and possible assistance can often be obtained by contacting local women's health groups, consumer groups, or legal services organizations (see chapter 27 Resources).

Patient Advocacy

Probably the best way to safeguard your rights is to bring someone as an advocate to all medical encounters. Your advocate may be a friend, relative, or women's health care worker—anyone you trust enough to share confidential health information with and who will help you assert your rights. Before your medical visit, discuss

continued on next page

with your advocate what you expect—and what you want—to happen. Make sure you both understand what kinds of diagnostic tests, treatments, or surgical procedures are being proposed. Ask your advocate to keep a record of events that occur while you are unable to be aware of them. Try to anticipate those situations that in the past have made you feel powerless or inadequately informed. Make a list of the questions you want to ask. If more than one physician is involved in your case, your advocate can help coordinate your care. If the medical staff raises questions about your emotional or psychiatric stability (and thereafter dismisses your concerns and complaints), an advocate can speak up for you.

Although few private physicians mind the presence of a relative or friend during office visits or examinations, hospitals may be more restrictive. Be as firm as you can about wanting your advocate with you, and if your provider refuses unreasonably, you may want to make a change if you can.

Large hospitals and health plans may employ patient advocates or patient representatives who can be helpful in cutting through red tape. Yet, because they represent the hospital, these advocates may not be free to represent your interests when they conflict with the interests of the hospital or doctor. Despite this, some patient representatives do an excellent job on behalf of patients. Ask the nurse how to get in touch with the patient advocate or patient representative, or call the hospital switchboard.

Complaint Mechanisms

If you are unhappy with the results of a medical encounter, do not be afraid to complain. Make a written record of the events as soon as they occur, and draft a letter that clearly states what happened and when. If friends or family members have firsthand knowledge of the events, ask them to record their thoughts and observations right away. If your complaint is against a licensed health professional, send it to the appropriate licensing board, and send a copy to the relevant county and state professional societies. You can also contact a local women's health group for assistance and encouragement. When complaining about a facility (hospital, nursing home, clinic, etc.) that is licensed by the state, contact the appropriate licensing agency as well as the consumer protection division of the attorney general's office. If you have reason to think you have received an experimental drug, or if you experience a strong drug reaction, report this to your local FDA (see p. 717).

Consider sending a letter of complaint to the following people or organizations: the doctor involved; the doctor who referred you; the administrator or director of the clinic, hospital, or managed care organization; the local medical society; the organization that will pay for your visit or treatment if different from the organization that provided the care (e.g., your union, insurance plan, or Medicare); the local health department; the neighborhood health council or community boards; community agencies; local women's groups, women's centers, magazines, and newspapers.

It is sometimes useful to discuss your intentions with the health care provider before actually lodging any complaints, since this may provide the incentive necessary to improve the situation. Make certain, though, that all your medical records and supporting materials are in order before you discuss the matter with your provider, since once they are put on notice about your discontent, they may become more defensive and limit or manipulate the information included in your record.

Contrary to the protestations of the medical profession and the insurance companies, patients are not responsible for the cost of malpractice insurance, which in turn drives up the cost of medical care. Doctors who practice bad or careless medicine are responsible, and malpractice suits are one way we as patients can be compensated for the harm those doctors cause. Litigation, though, is an expensive, time-consuming, and often frustrating means of recourse. Unless you have suffered serious injury, lost some earnings (past or future), incurred large medical bills, or experienced serious emotional harm, litigation will probably not be worth the effort.

In order to recover in a lawsuit against a health care provider or drug/device manufacturer, the plaintiff must prove by a preponderance of the evidence, that

1. the physician, nurse, hospital, or health plan had a responsibility to you, the patient (which generally exists as a matter of law).

2. duty was breached (usually because conduct fell below the "standard of care").

3. you were harmed.

4. the harm was a direct result of the breach, or of negligent behavior.

If you feel you have been injured, you will probably want to seek a lawyer. Make sure that your lawyer has had extensive experience with malpractice cases. Both NOW and the American Civil Liberties Union usually maintain reliable attorney referral lists. Attorneys take malpractice cases on a "contingency fee" basis and don't charge clients for their time in pursuing the matter unless they win (in which case they claim a percentage of the recovery, usually 30 to 40%); some, however, charge for out-of-pocket expenses regardless of outcome. You should interview at least three lawyers about your case before picking one.

Reporting Problems to the FDA

Tongue depressors, Band-Aids, tampons, diaphragms, IUDs, and cervical caps, as well as more obvious things like kidney dialysis machines, are classified by the FDA as medical devices. If you have any problems, even minor ones, with a medical device or prescription, or over-the-counter drugs, report them to the FDA, which records complaints in publicly available databases. (Your name will not appear in the public report.) Reporting a problem to your physician alone does not guarantee that the FDA will learn about it. Reports to the FDA are the only way to make public the problems women are having and to assess their frequency. Manufacturers are supposed to pass on reports of problems to the FDA, but often they do not. The FDA acts only in response to complaints. It will not initiate investigations. Write to the FDA, 5600 Fishers Lane, Rockville, MD 20857. Keep a copy of your complaint for future reference. You might also want to look for a women's group to find out what health activists are doing on the issue, if anything, or to access a support group of women with a similar problem, or even a plan for legal action, as happened with tampons and toxic shock, the Dalkon shield, breast implants, Depo-Provera, and Norplant.

other people in your situation, trade ideas, feel less alone, and perhaps learn a few skills. Such groups often emphasize "self-care"—that is, those activities the providers have decided you can carry out for yourself. Be aware that these classes and groups have a major limitation: Their main goal is a smoothly functioning medical system with compliant patients. They rarely offer nonmedical alternatives or a chance to criticize accepted practices or practitioners.

Living with Uncertainty

In giving up our unquestioning trust of the information we get from doctors and other medical personnel, we also give up the (often false) comfort that comes from their frequent reassurances that we are getting "the best treatment possible." Often we and our health practitioners have to make decisions without complete information, because not even the "experts" know

GENETICS, WOMEN'S HEALTH, AND HUMAN RIGHTS

Genetics used to be considered a subspecialty of medicine. Now some individuals in the medical and biotechnology fields view medicine as a subspecialty of genetics. Because this dominance is a growing trend in medicine and medical research, the media report daily on the role of our genes in everything from disease susceptibility, to sexual orientation, to criminal behavior, and even to such things as our lifelong tendency to be optimistic or pessimistic. The centuries-old "heredity vs. environment" debate has now swung sharply to heredity.

The Boston Women's Health Book Collective has joined others in criticizing this tendency toward the "geneticization" of our health and lives, also called "genism" and "gene mania." We question the overzealousness on the part of some researchers and others to find genetic explanations for complex medical and social conditions. In fact, inherited genetic conditions are responsible for only a small fraction of illness and disease.

An overemphasis on genes opens the door to "blaming the victim": if people become ill, the responsibility does not reside with the industries that poison our environment or the employers unwilling to invest in eliminating occupational health hazards. Rather, the locus of responsibility is shifted to the people who get sick because they have "bad genes." Increasingly, research indicates that many, if not most, mutations to our genes result from environmental influences.

Because women continue to carry most of the burden of medical care decision-making as well as most of the caregiving responsibilities in their families, we believe women deserve high-quality unbiased information about all genetic issues. Moreover, most of the controversial genetic testing issues thus far are concerned with conditions having the greatest impact on women: prenatal testing, breast cancer, and Alzheimer's disease.

We believe that much of the planned research and marketing of genetic tests and gene therapies should not proceed in advance of a wider public discourse on issues such as the following:

- What public policies will best ensure that we will control access to our own genetic material and information?
- How can we better preserve the confidentiality of general medical records so that genetic information is released only with the consent of the individual?

continued on next page

- How can we prevent genetic tests from being marketed and widely used before their usefulness and the ethics of their use have been established?
- How does the pursuit of genetic tests, therapies, and "enhancements" affect our attitudes toward disability and our tolerance for difference among us all? How can we prevent genetic research from being used to further stigmatize particular racial and ethnic groups?
- How can we best ensure that genetic counseling is nondirective and that no genetic testing is done without informed consent as well as thorough pre- and post-test counseling?
- What public policies will best prevent the misuse of genetic information and any resultant genetic discrimination in insurance, housing, employment, custody, medical care and adoption?
- What are the most ethical ways to obtain genetic samples (e.g., from blood and tissue) and make them available for research? Can informed participation and informed consent be assured and, if so, how?*

These matters are human rights issues and debate about them must involve *all* of us, not only scientists and medical specialists but also policy makers, religious groups, disability rights activists, social scientists, health consumers, public health workers, and both women and men. We are, after all, much more than the sum of our genes.

* Contact the NIH Office of Research on Women's Health for the report from a June 2, 1997, meeting sponsored by the National Institutes of Health, the National Action Plan on Breast Cancer Working Group on Tissue Banking, and other organizations.

enough about certain problems to suggest that one approach is necessarily better than another. Yet, physicians often believe that they have to act sure even when they are not. Especially when we are scared, it can be deeply reassuring to believe them. Learning about the controversies and alternatives rather than blindly trusting what our doctors tell us, therefore, may mean living without the particular kind of certainty or hope that they offer. Often what we need most is courage in the face of uncertainty.[65]

NOTES

1. Barbara Ehrenreich, "Spinning the Poor into Gold: How Corporations Seek to Profit from Welfare Reform," *Harper's Magazine* 295, no. 1767 (Aug., 1997): 44–52.
2. Oliver Fein, "The Influence of Social Class on Health Status: American and British Research on Health Inequities," *Journal of General Internal Medicine* 10, no. 10 (Oct. 1995): 577–86; and S. Leonard Syme and Lisa F. Berkman, "Social Class, Susceptibility and Sickness," in Peter Conrad and Rochelle Kern, eds., *The Sociology of Health and Illness: Critical Perspectives* (New York: St. Martin's Press, 1994), 29–34.
3. Nancy Kreiger and Stephen Sidney, "Racial Discrimination and Blood Pressure: The CARDIA Study of Young Black and White Adults," *American Journal of Public Health* 86, no. 19 (Oct. 1996): 1370–378; and Wornie L. Reed. "Suffer the Children: Some Effects of Racism on the Health of Black Infants," in Peter Conrad and Rochelle Kern, eds., *The Sociology of Health and Illness,* 314–27.
4. Sally Satel, "The Politicization of Public Health," *The Wall Street Journal* (Dec. 12, 1996).
5. Peter Edelman, "The Worst Thing Bill Clinton Has Done," *Atlantic Monthly* (March 1997): 43–58.
6. Marie McCormick, "The Canary in the Coal Mine," *Harvard Public Health Review* (fall 1994): 76; and Reed, op. cit.
7. Steffi Woolhandler et al., "Medical Care and Mortality: Racial Differences in Preventable Deaths," in Phil Brown, ed., *Perspectives in Medical Sociology* (Belmont, CA: Wadsworth, 1989): 71–81; and The Commonwealth Fund Commission on Women's Health, *Prevention and Women's Health: A Shared Responsibility* (New York: Commonwealth Fund, 1996).
8. Diana Scully, *Men Who Control Women's Health: The Miseducation of Obstetrician-Gynecologists* (New York: Teachers College Press, 1994).
9. Arlie Hochschild, *The Second Shift* (New York: Avon, 1990).
10. ———, *The Time Bind: When Work Becomes Home and Home Becomes Work* (New York: Metropolitan Books, 1997).
11. Piroska Ostlin, "Gender, Social Class and Equity," in Eeva Ollila et al., eds., *Equity in Health through Public Policy: Report on the Expert Meeting in Kellokoski, Finland, November, 1996* (Helsinki: STAKES, 1997): 99–106.
12. Women's Research and Education Institute, *Women's Health Insurance Costs and Experiences* (Washington, DC: WREI, 1994): Young-Hee Yoon, *Women's Access to Health Insurance* (Washington, DC: Institute for Women's Policy Research).
13. Rhona Rapoport and Lotte Bailyn, *Relinking Life and Work: Toward a Better Future* (New York: Ford Foundation, 1996). A report to the Ford Foundation.
14. Irving Kenneth Zola, "Medicine as an Institution of Social Control," in *Socio-medical Inquiries* (Philadelphia: Temple University Press, 1983): 247–68.
15. Janice Raymond, "Medicine as Patriarchal Religion," *The Journal of Medicine and Philosophy* 7 (1982): 197–216.

16. Sue Fisher. *In the Patient's Best Interest: Women and the Politics of Medical Decisions* (New Brunswick, NJ: Rutgers University Press, 1986); Alexandra Todd, *Intimate Adversaries: Cultural Conflict Between Doctors and Women Patients* (Philadelphia: University of Pennsylvania Press, 1989); and Lucy Candib, *Medicine and the Family: A Feminist Perspective* (New York: Basic Books, 1995).

17. Ann Oakley, *The Captured Womb: A History of the Medical Care of Pregnant Women* (New York: Blackwell, 1984).

18. C. Everett Koop, on *The Health Beat Project,* WCVB Channel 5, Boston, 1997.

19. Ann W. Burgess and Carol R. Hartman, eds., *Sexual Exploitation of Patients by Health Professionals* (New York: Praeger, 1986).

20. Anita Diamant, "Bedside Manners: Of Doctors, Patient Abuse, and Regulation, Again," *Boston Phoenix* (Nov. 10, 1981).

21. Personal communication, Women's Medical Association members investigating physician sexual misconduct, 1985.

22. Personal communication with hospital patient initiating action. See also Sidney Wolfe et al., *Questionable Doctors* (Washington, DC: Public Citizen Health Research Group, 1996).

23. Judy Norsigian, "The Women's Health Movement," in Kary Moss, *Man-Made Medicine: Women's Health, Public Policy and Reform* (Durham, NC: Duke University Press, 1996); and Norma Swenson, "The Women's Health Movement," in Gloria Steinem et al., eds., *Reader's Companion to U.S. Women's History* (Boston: Houghton-Mifflin, 1997).

24. Commonwealth Fund Commission on Women's Health, op. cit.

25. Marsden Wagner, "The Global Witch-Hunt," *Lancet* 346 (Oct. 1995): 1020–22.

26. Norsigian, op. cit., and Swenson, op. cit.

27. Derek Bok, "Health Care," in *The State of the Nation: Government and the Quest for a Better Society* (Cambridge: Harvard University Press, 1997): 243.

28. Bok, op. cit.

29. John McKinlay and Sonja McKinlay, "Medical Measures and the Decline of Mortality," in *Sociology of Health and Illness* (1994), op. cit., 10–23.

30. Ibid.

31. David M. Eisenberg et al., "Unconventional Medicine in the United States: Prevalence, Costs, and Patterns of Use," *New England Journal of Medicine* 328, no. 4 (1993): 246–52.

32. Oxford Health Plans, telephone interview, 11/24/97.

33. Zola, op. cit.

34. Personal communication, pharmaceutical company executive; Jeanne Kassler, "The Pharmaceutical Industry," in *Bitter Medicine: Greed and Chaos in American Health Care* (New York: Carol Publishing Group, 1994); and U.S. Senate Committee on Aging, *Staff Report of the Select Committee on Aging, U.S. Senate, 102nd Congress, 1st Session* (Washington, DC: U.S. Government Printing Office, 1991).

35. Bok, op. cit.

36. Dr. Philip R. Lee, U.S. Department of Health and Human Services, *The Nightline Show with Ted Koppel,* ABC (March 19, 1997).

37. Paula Doress-Worters and Diana Siegel, *New Ourselves, Growing Older* (New York: Simon & Schuster, 1994): 221–48.

38. Women's Legal Defense Fund, *What the New Health Insurance Reform Means for Women and Their Families* (Washington, DC: WLDF, 1997); also Robert Kuttner, "The Kassebaum-Kennedy Bill: The Limits of Incrementalism," *New England Journal of Medicine* 337, no. 1 (1997): 64–67.

39. Robert Kuttner, op. cit. See also United Nations Development Program, *Human Development Report 1997* (New York: UNDP, 1997). Also see John Cassidy, "Who Killed The Middle Class? The Mystery That Our National Self Image Hangs On," *The New Yorker* 71, no. 32 (March 1996): 113–25.

40. John M. Goshko, "U.S. Poverty Increasing, Study by UN Finds," *Boston Globe* (June 12, 1997): A8.

41. Bok, op. cit.

42. Kuttner, Robert. *Everything for Sale: The Virtues and Limits of Markets* (New York: Alfred A. Knopf, 1997); and Haynes Johnson and David S. Broder, *The System: The American Way of Politics at the Breaking Point* (Boston: Little Brown, 1996). Also see Jacob S. Hacker, *The Road to Nowhere: The Genesis of President Clinton's Plan for Health Security* (Princeton, NJ: Princeton University Press, 1997).

43. Bok, op. cit.; see also Richard Knox, "1 in 4 Find Health Care Unavailable," *Boston Globe* (Oct. 23, 1996); citing Karen Donelan et al., "Whatever Happened to the Health Insurance Crisis in the United States," *JAMA* 276, no. 16 (1996): 1346–350.

44. "Implementing Health Insurance for Children," *The News Hour with Jim Lehrer,* PBS (Aug. 25, 1997).

45. Marcia Angell and J. Kassirer, "Quality and the Medical Marketplace: Following Elephants," *New England Journal of Medicine* 335, no. 12 (1996): 883–84.

46. "Closing the ERISA Loophole," *American Medical News* (March 17, 1997): 19. See also Kuttner, "The Kassebaum-Kennedy Bill," op. cit.

47. Marc A. Rodwin, "The Neglected Remedy: Strengthening Consumer Voice in Managed Care," *American Prospect* 16, no. 34 (1997): 45–50.

48. *Physicians for a National Health Program Newsletter* (Nov. 1996).

49. Louise Lief, "Kids at Risk: Uninsured Children Increasingly Come from the Middle Class," *U.S. News & World Report* 122, no. 6 (April 28, 1997): 66.

50. Angell et al., op cit.

51. *Boston Globe* (March 13, 1997).

52. Howard Larkin, "Not All Health Plans Live Up to Potential," *American Medical News* 40, no. 39 (Oct. 1997).

53. Health Care for All, Legislative Report, Boston, spring 1997.

54. Helen Halpin Schauffler and John Wilkerson, "National Health Care Reform and the 103rd Congress: The Activities and Influence of Public Health Advocates," *American Journal of Public Health* 87, no. 7 (July 1997): 1107–112.

55. Telephone interview, March 20, 1997.

56. Bok, op. cit.

57. Kuttner, "The Kassebaum-Kennedy Bill," op. cit.

58. Margaret Hynes, *Who Cares for Poor People? Physicians, Medicaid, and Marginality* (New York: Garland Publishing, [publication forthcoming]).

59. President, American Medical Women's Association, address at American Medical Student's Association conference, Galveston, Texas, Feb. 3, 1996.

60. Michelle Harrison, *A Woman in Residence* (New York: Fawcett Book Group, 1993).

61. Lucy Candib, "The Gender of the Doctor: What Is the Difference in Practice?" Cabot Series Primary Care Lecture, Harvard Medical School, Dec. 12, 1996.

62. Suzanne Gordon, "What Nurses Stand For," *Atlantic Monthly* 279, no. 2 (Feb. 1997): 80–88; and J. Duncan Moore, "Nurses' Patient-Care Outlook Grim," *Modern Healthcare* (June 17, 1996): 22.

63. Hynes, op. cit.

64. Vicente Navarro, *Why the United States Does Not Have a National Health Program* (Amityville, NY: Baywood, 1992); see also *Physicians for a National Health Plan Newsletter* (spring 1994).

65. Harold J. Bursztajn, Robert M. Hamm, and Archie Brodsky, *Medical Choices, Medical Chances: How Patients, Families and Physicians Can Cope with Uncertainty* (New York: Routledge, 1990).

RESOURCES

Books and Reports

Adams, Diane L., ed. *Health Issues for Women of Color: A Cultural Diversity Perspective*. Thousand Oaks CA: Sage Publications, 1995.

Alvarez, Luz. *Homenaje a Nuestras Curanderas: Honoring Our Healers*. Oakland, CA: Latina Press, 1997.

Andrews, Charles. *Profit Fever: The Drive to Corporatize Health Care and How to Stop It*. Monroe, ME: Common Courage Press, 1995.

Bayne-Smith, Marcia. *Race, Gender, and Health*. Thousand Oaks, CA: Sage Publications, 1996.

Bodenheimer, Thomas S., and Kevin Grumback. *Understanding Health Policy: A Clinical Approach*. Norwalk, CT: Appleton & Lange, 1995.

Bok, Derek. *The State of the Nation: Government and the Quest for a Better Society*. Cambridge: Harvard University Press, 1996.

Brown, Richard E., et al. *Women's Health-Related Behaviors and Use of Clinical Preventive Services: A Report to the Commonwealth Fund*. Los Angeles: UCLA Center for Health Policy Research, 1995.

Conrad, Peter, and Rochelle Kern. *The Sociology of Health and Illness: Critical Perspectives*. New York: St. Martin's Press, 1994.

Families USA. *Doing Without: The Sacrifices Families Make to Provide Home Care*. Washington, DC: Families USA, 1994.

———. *Hurting Real People: The Human Impact of Medicaid Cuts*. Washington, DC: Families USA, 1995.

Fee, Elizabeth, and Nancy Krieger, eds. *Women's Health, Politics, and Power: Essays on Sex/Gender, Medicine, and Public Health*. Amityville, NY: Baywood Publishing, 1994.

Focus on Women's Health. *Women's Health Research and Policy: A National Directory*. Philadelphia: University of Pennsylvania Publications, 1996.

Fogel, Catherine Ingram, and Nancy Fugate Woods, eds. *Women's Health Care: A Comprehensive Handbook*. Thousand Oaks, CA: Sage Publications, 1995.

Hubbard, Ruth, and Elijah Wald. *Exploding the Gene Myth*. Boston: Beacon Press, 1993.

Kaufman, Sharon R. *The Healer's Tale: Transforming Medicine and Culture*. Madison, WI: University of Wisconsin Press, 1993.

Macklin, Ruth. *Enemies of Patients*. New York: Oxford University Press, 1993.

Miller, Marc S., ed. *Health Care Choices for Today's Consumer: Families USA Guide to Quality and Cost*. Washington, DC: Living Planet Press, 1995.

Moss, Kary L. *Man-Made Medicine: Women's Health, Public Policy, and Reform*. Durham, NC: Duke University Press, 1996.

National Latina Health Organization. *National Welfare Reform: An Analysis of Its Impact on Latinas*. Oakland, CA: National Latina Health Organization, 1995.

Office of Research on Women's Health. *Women's Health in the Medical School Curriculum: Report of a Survey and Recommendations*. Washington, DC: National Institutes of Health, 1997.

Payne Epps, Rosalyn, and Susan Cobb Stewart, eds. *The Women's Complete Healthbook*. New York: Delacorte, 1995.

Perkins, Jane, and Lourdes Rivera. *Medicaid Managed Care: 20 Questions to Ask Your State*. Los Angeles: National Health Law Program, 1995. Available from the National Health Law Program: (310) 204-6010.

Reverby, Susan. *Ordered to Care: The Dilemma of American Nursing, 1850–1945*. New York: Cambridge University Press, 1987.

Rosser, Sue V. *Women's Health: Missing from U.S. Medicine*. Bloomington: Indiana University Press, 1994.

Rowland, Diane, et al. *Medicaid and Managed Care: Lessons from the Literature*. Menlo Park, CA: Kaiser Family Foundation, 1995.

Ruzek, Sheryl Burt, et al., eds. *Women's Health: Complexities and Differences*. Columbus: Ohio State University Press, 1997.

Sidel, Ruth. *Keeping Women and Children Last: America's War on the Poor*. New York: Penguin Books, 1996.

Starr, Paul. *The Social Transformation of American Medicine*. New York: Basic Books, 1982.

Teitelman, Robert. *Profits of Science: The American Marriage of Business and Technology*. New York: Basic Books, 1994.

U.S. Department of Health and Human Services. *Health United States: 1995*. Hyattsville, MD: USDHHS, 1996. Annual.

· U.S. General Accounting Office. *Continued Vigilance Critical to Protecting Human Subjects.* Washington, DC: GAO, 1996.

Wear, Delese. *Women in Medical Education: An Anthology of Experience.* New York: State University of New York Press, 1996.

Women's Research and Education Institute. *Women's Health Insurance Costs and Experiences.* Washington, DC: WREI, 1994.

Worcester, Nancy, and Mariamne H. Whatley, eds. *Women's Health: Readings on Social, Economic, and Political Issues.* Dubuque, IA: Kendall/Hunt Publishing, 1994.

Articles

Albelda, Randy, "Farewell to Welfare But Not to Poverty," *Dollars and Sense* 208 (Nov./Dec. 1996): 16–19.

Bennett, Trude, "Reproductive Health and Welfare Reform," presented at the American Public Health Association Meeting, San Diego, CA, 1995.

Brownlee, Shannon, and Matthew Miller, "The Lies Parents Tell About Why They Work," *U.S. News and World Report* (May 12, 1997): 58.

Dresser, Rebecca, "What Bioethics Can Learn from the Women's Health Movement," unpublished manuscript (contact author at Case Western Reserve University School of Law).

"Foundations That Fund/Have Funded Anti-Immigration Organizations," *Hampshire College Population and Development Program,* 1996.

Fugh-Berman, Adriane, "Training Doctors to Care for Women," *Technology Review* (Feb./March 1994): 35–40.

Health Care for All, "What You Should Know About Columbia/HCA," *Health Care for All's Legal Network* (1996).

"How Good is Your Health Plan," *Consumer Reports* 61, no. 8 (Aug. 1996): 28–42.

Jacobs Institute of Women's Health, "Women's Primary Care in Managed Care: Clinical and Provider Issues," *Insights* 1 (Jan. 1997): 1–9.

Korn, Peter, "America's 10 Best Hospitals When You're Having Your Baby," *Self* magazine (Dec. 1996): 141–57.

Krieger, Nancy, et al., "Racism, Sexism, and Social Class: Implications for Studies of Health, Disease, and Well-Being," *American Journal of Preventive Medicine* 9 Supp. (Dec. 1993): 82–122.

Krieger, Nancy, and Sally Zierler, "Accounting for Health of Women," *Current Issues in Public Health* 1, no. 6 (1995): 251–56.

Leigh, Wilhelmina A., "The Health of Women: Minority/Diversity Perspective, An American Perspective," presented at the Canada/USA Women's Health Forum, Aug. 1996.

Mann, Charles, "Women's Health Research Blossoms," *Science* 269 (Aug. 1995): 766–69.

Parsons, Donna, "Insurance Companies Sock It to Battered Women," *On the Issues* (summer 1996): 14–15.

Phillips, B. J., "Charity Begins in CEO's Pay," *Philadelphia Inquirer* (Jan. 19, 1997).

Relman, Arnold S., "The Future of Medical Practice," *Physician Executive* 22 (Jan. 1996): 23–25.

———, "Physicians and Business Managers: A Clash of Cultures," *Health Management Quarterly* 16, no. 3 (1994): 11–14.

Russell, Mary, "Converting to For-Profit Health Care: What Advocates Should Know," *States of Health* 5, no. 8 (Nov. 1995) (Families USA).

Saxton, Marsha, "Disabled Women and the Medical System," unpublished manuscript (on file at the Boston Women's Health Book Collective).

Shaffer, Ellen R., "Power, Money, Feelings and Women's Health: How to Take Control in the New Health Care Environment," Presentation to American Psychological Association, 1996. Work in progress (E-mail author: eshaffer@jhu.edu).

Spragins, Ellyn, "Does Your HMO Stack Up?" *Newsweek* 127, no. 26 (June 24, 1996): 56–63.

Taylor, Humphrey, " 'Public Health': Two Words Few People Understand Even Though Almost Everyone Thinks Public Health Functions Are Important," *The Harris Poll* 1 (Jan. 6, 1997).

Turshen, Meredeth, "Unhealthy Paradox: A Nation of Immigrants Debates Harsh Immigration Controls," *Current Issues in Public Health* 2, no. 2 (1996): 61–67.

Uhlman, Marian, "Hospital Bosses Are Growing Richer," *Philadelphia Inquirer* (Jan. 19, 1997): A1.

Weisman, Carol S., Barbara Curbow, and Amal J. Khoury, "The National Survey of Women's Health Centers: Current Models of Women-Centered Care," *WHI* 5, no. 3 (1995): 103–17 (Jacobs Institute of Women's Health).

Withorn, Ann, "Let's Pretend: The Dilemmas of Workfare," *Otherwise* 1, no. 2 (April 18–May 1, 1996): 16–17.

Wolfe, Sidney. "Why Do American Drug Companies Spend More Than $12 Billion a Year Pushing Drugs? Is It Education or Promotion? Characteristics of Materials Distributed by Drug Companies: Four Points of View," *Journal of General Internal Medicine* 11, no. 10 (1996): 637–39.

Audiovisual

The Harvard Guide to Women's Health (CD-ROM) by Carlson, Karen J., Stephanie A. Eisenstat, Terra Ziporyn.

Periodicals

Consumer's Guide to New York's Managed Care Bill of Rights
Citizen Action of New York; 94 Central Avenue; Albany, NY 12206; (800) 636-BILL
E-mail: canyalb@aol.com

Health Letter and *Worst Pills, Best Pills News*
Public Citizen Health Research Group (see "Organizations" below for address and phone)

Journal Watch Women's Health
1440 Main Street; Waltham, MA 02154; (617) 893-4610
Published by the Massachusetts Medical Society

Public Citizen News
1600 20th Street, NW; Washington, DC 20009; (202) 588-1000
E-mail: public_citizen@citizen.com
Web site: http://www.citizen.org
 Best gender-neutral critique of loopholes in federal systems, many women's health examples.

States of Health
Families USA Foundation; 1334 G St. NW; Washington, DC 20005; (202) 628-3030
E-mail: info@familiesusa.org
Web site: http://www.familiesusa.org

Organizations

The Agency for Health Care Policy and Research Executive Office Center
2101 East Jefferson Street, Suite 600; Rockville, MD 20852; (800) 358-9295
Web site: http://www.ahcpr.gov

American College of Surgeons
55 East Erie Street; Chicago, IL 60611-2797; (312) 664-4050
E-mail: postmaster@facs.org
Web site: http://www.facs.org

American Friends Service Committee
National Women's Program; 1501 Cherry Street; Philadelphia, PA 19102; (215) 241-7000
E-mail: afscinfo@afsc.org
Web site: http://www.afsc.org

Center for Research on Women and Gender
University of Illinois at Chicago; 1640 West Roosevelt Road; Chicago IL 60608-6902; (312) 413-1924

Council for Responsible Genetics
5 Upland Road, Suite 3; Cambridge, MA 02140; (617) 868-0870
E-mail: crg@essential.org
 Publishes position papers on genetics issues and the newsletter, *Genewatch*.

ECRI
5200 Butler Pike; Plymouth Meeting, PA 19462-1298; (215) 825-6000
 Conducts technology assessment research and publishes periodic news releases.

Health and Medicine Policy Research Group
332 South Michigan Avenue, Suite 500; Chicago, IL 60604; (312) 922-8057
 Produces a series of reports and conference proceedings on urban women's health.

National Association of Women's Health Professionals
175 West Jackson Boulevard, Suite 1-1711; Chicago, IL 60604; (312) 786-1468; Fax: (312) 786-0376
Web site: http://www.nawhp.org

National Women's Health Information Center
(800) 994-WOMA
Web site: http://www.4woman.org

New England Research Institute
9 Galen Street, Suite 117; Watertown, MA 02174; (617) 923-7747

Office of Research on Women's Health
National Institutes of Health; Building 1, Room 201; Bethesda, MD 20892
Web site: http://ohrm.od.nih.gov/orwh
 The goal of this important government office is to strengthen and develop research in women's health issues, to ensure that women are included in research studies, and to increase the number of women in biomedical careers.

Physicians for a National Health Program
332 South Michigan, Suite 500; Chicago, IL 60604; (312) 554-0382
 Focus on single-payer issues; produces *PNHP Newsletter* and other publications and audiovisual material.

Public Citizen Health Research Group
1600 20th Street NW; Washington, DC 20009; (202) 588-1000
Web site: http://www.citizen.org/HRG
 Ralph Nader's group that watchdogs drugs, doctors, and federal agencies.

Women's Health Advocate Newsletter: An Independent Voice on Women's Wellness
10310 Main Street, #301; Fairfax, VA 22030
E-mail: jeanshaw@hevanet.com

Women's Health: Research on Gender, Behavior, and Policy
The Graduate School & University Center; City University of New York; 33 W. 42nd Street; New York, NY 10036-8099
 Journal with women's studies, social science perspective.

For more online resources, please see Introduction to Online Women's Health Resources, p. 25.

By Nalini Visvanathan, based on earlier
work by Vilunya Diskin

WITH SPECIAL THANKS TO Gabriela Canepa,
Marilen Danguilan, Betsy Hartmann, and
Jennifer Yanco*

Chapter 26

....

The Global Politics of Women and Health

The health of women in the U.S. and the health of
women around the world are connected in significant ways. This chapter invites readers to be aware
of these connections and to become part of a growing international women's health movement.

As we enter the 21st century, women everywhere
are confronting a global market of powerful political,
financial, and commercial interests that promote consumer societies. In their pursuit of profits in the global
economy, the players often exploit economically depressed countries and their people. By fostering uniform patterns of production and consumption, the
global market economy threatens the economic and
ecological systems of local and indigenous peoples.
Moreover, the globalization process changes the priorities of national governments by undermining their
ability to provide for the impoverished, the sick, and
the infirm. This situation is detrimental to women's
health and well-being worldwide.

The contemporary international women's health
movement, made up of women's groups and nongovernmental organizations (NGOs), has its roots in various indigenous uprisings and feminist organizing
activities, spanning more than a century of European
colonial empire-building and liberation struggles.[1]
Grounded in a history of subjugation and impoverishment, women in the global South† see health in the
broad context of political, social, and economic rights
—a view generally shared by Northern women committed to progressive social politics. However, responding to the continuing assault on abortion and
other reproductive freedoms, many North American
women health activists have emphasized reproductive
health over other critical social and economic rights,
thus failing to address adequately the needs of women
who face multiple social, economic, and health prob-

* Thanks also to the following for their help with the 1998 version
of this chapter: Mayra Canetti, Shobha H. Gurung, Jeanne
Koopman, Veronica Nielsen-Vilar, Laura Tandara, and April Taylor.
Over the years since 1969, the following women have contributed
to the many versions of this chapter: Anita Anand, Asoka
Bandarage, Elizabeth Coit, Jane Cottingham, Betsy Hartmann,
H. Patricia Hynes, Marilee Karl, Una MacLean, Judy Norsigian,
Annie Street, and Norma Swenson.

† "The South" and "Southern" are used interchangeably with
"Third World," denoting a political entity composed of nations
once colonized by European rulers.

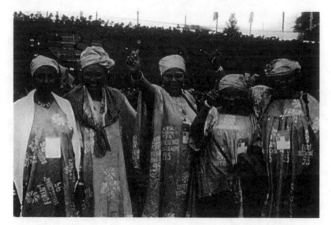

Kenyan delegates to the N.G.O. Forum, Huairoo, China (Beijing Conference, 1995)/Robin Melavalin

lems. The resulting tension has divided the movement worldwide along the lines of race, class, religion, and ethnicity, bringing into question the vision expressed by the feminist slogan "Sisterhood is Global." At the same time, many women who were silenced in the past have become active and are speaking out. The 1995 Beijing Fourth World Women's Conference, which brought together the largest gathering of women the world had seen to date, generated a progressive agenda for women's rights and forged new solidarity for the work that still needs to be done.

WOMEN, GENDER, AND DEVELOPMENT

Southern women, emerging from colonial rule in the post–World War II world, faced new challenges in the form of Western concepts of "development." The success of the Marshall Plan in rebuilding Europe after the war prompted Western nations to launch a similar enterprise for bringing the colonized nations of Africa,

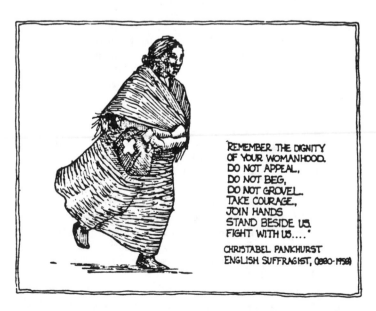

REMEMBER THE DIGNITY OF YOUR WOMANHOOD. DO NOT APPEAL, DO NOT BEG, DO NOT GROVEL. TAKE COURAGE, JOIN HANDS STAND BESIDE US, FIGHT WITH US...."

CHRISTABEL PANKHURST ENGLISH SUFFRAGIST, (1880-1958)

Karen Norberg

The international women's health movement has become a major force in United Nations policy-making conferences and other gatherings. Here are examples of what women have been doing to link themselves internationally.

1975

The successful U.N. *First World Women's Conference,* Mexico City, led the U.N. General Assembly to declare 1976–1985 as the U.N. Decade for Women, underscoring the conference theme, "Equality, Development, Peace."

1976 to 1985

United Nations *International Women's Decade.* For the first time, a vast body of information and statistics was collected, reviewed, and desegregated by gender to map the social, demographic, and economic situation of women. Women's contributions were made visible in arenas where they had been ignored or overlooked, especially in agricultural labor and food production. Once largely excluded from the political process on every continent, women began to be recognized as the subjects of development rather than as targets of programs and patronage.

1979

The Convention on the Elimination of All Forms of Discrimination against Women (CEDAW) was adopted by the U.N.

1980

Progress on the World Plan of Action, adopted in Mexico City, was reviewed in mid-decade at the *Second World Women's Conference* in Copenhagen.

1985

Women's NGO Forum, Nairobi, Kenya, End-of-Decade U.N. Conference on Women. The final document, titled "Forward-looking Strategies for the Advancement of Women," which was unanimously adopted at this conference, articulates ambitious objectives for women, including the elimination of illiteracy by the year 2000, the elimination of all forms of discrimination, a life expectancy of at least 65 years, and the opportunity for employment.

1987

Fifth International Women and Health Meeting, San Jose, Costa Rica. For the first time, this international feminist meeting was held outside Europe and was attended by large numbers of participants from Latin America and the Caribbean. It highlighted issues of concern to women in the region.

1990

Sixth International Women and Health Meeting, Manila, the Philippines. Over 400 women from 60 countries participated. Strong representation from Asian countries brought concerns of women from that region to the fore.

1991

World Women's Congress for a Healthy Planet, Miami, Florida. In this breakthrough event for the global women's movement, feminist environmental groups, notably the Women, Environment and Development Organization (WEDO), brought together women from around the world to create "Women's Action Agenda 21," an action guide for incorporating women's issues and rights into local, national, and international environment and development decision making.

1992

U.N. Conference on Environment and Development, Rio, Brazil. The women's agenda set in Miami the previous year was accepted by the participating nations.

1993

U.N. Human Rights Conference. Recognizing women's rights as human rights, this conference placed women's issues—violence, sexual abuses, and reproductive abuses—within the framework of the U.N. human rights declaration.

1993

Seventh International Women and Health Meeting, Kampala, Uganda. An opportunity for African women to participate on a large scale.

1994

U.N. International Conference on Population and Development (ICPD), Cairo, Egypt. The concept of reproductive health replaced a focus on population control and its language of "fertility reduction targets," which dehumanizes women and facilitates abusive practices.

1995

Social Summit, Copenhagen, Denmark. Women were an integral part of this first United Nations conference to focus on issues of social justice. The Copenhagen Hearing on Economic Justice and Women's Human Rights featured personal testimonies of women from across the globe.

1995

U.N. Fourth World Women's Conference, Beijing, People's Republic of China, reiterated the importance of gender justice and equality in the home and the workplace in matters of production (waged work) and reproduction (unwaged household tasks and responsibilities).

1996

U.N. Habitat Conference, Istanbul, Turkey, emphasized housing rights for all and partnership between women's grassroots and community-based groups, and local authorities and the private and public sectors.

1997

Eighth International Women and Health Meeting, Rio de Janeiro, Brazil, assessed the real gains for women's health from previous conferences against the larger picture of women's everyday realities. It called for a transformation of the state through public discussion and legislation, and for greater accountability of the private sector. It acknowledged the need for building new forms of solidarity, and noted that abortion and HIV/AIDS were not issues just of health but of gender and social justice.

Asia, Latin America, and the Caribbean to the path of industrialization for economic development. Development planning emphasizes the Western development model of capital infusion, industrialization, and technology transfer in the belief that the benefits of economic growth "trickle down" to the poorest sectors of the population. Economists who favored this approach to development were supported by other social scientists who saw development as a "modern-

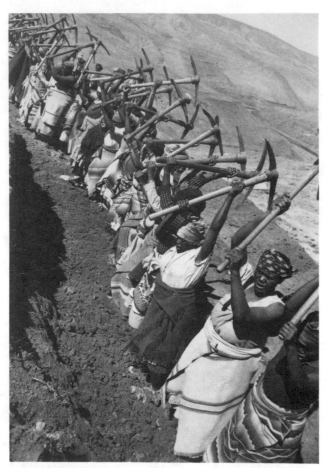

Women building a cross-country road in Lesotho/United Nations/D.P.I.

ization" project. This liberal and Eurocentric vision attributes the "underdevelopment" of Southern countries to their traditional societies and authoritarian political structures.

The late 1960s saw wide acknowledgment of the failure of "trickle-down" theory to eradicate poverty, especially for poor rural southern women, compelling Third World leaders and intellectuals to call for alternative forms of development. A notable response was the "Basic Needs" approach of the International Labor Organization (ILO), which addressed growing poverty by increasing employment and income-generation opportunities for poor women to ensure that their needs for food, shelter, and clothing were met.[2]

In 1970, the publication of Ester Boserup's *Women's Role in Economic Development*[3] galvanized a group of liberal feminists in Washington, DC, to create a field that would address women and development issues. Many of these women joined in an effort that became known as Women in Development (WID). By building on research that documented women's work and economic productivity, and through advocacy for integrating women into development programs, WID feminists aimed to give women skills in generating income and to bring them into the workplace. Accepting the basic "trickle-down" assumptions of the

development paradigm that guided agencies funded by the U.S. government, the objective of WID has been to bring women within the fold of these development programs rather than to question the basic assumptions of the model.[4] When modernization-oriented development policy failed, WID stressed equity for women as the solution. The advocacy work of WID led to the passage of the Percy Amendment in the U.S. Congress that stipulated the inclusion of women as beneficiaries for development programs funded by USAID (United States Agency for International Development).

During the 1970s and 1980s, international funding agencies supported programs that targeted maternal and child welfare, often incorporating the concept of family planning.[5] Although family planning can play an important role in women's health, the expanding allocations for family planning often have eroded health care budgets and significantly reduced their scope (for example, in India[6]).

In the 1980s, the "efficiency" approach—Structural Adjustment Programs (SAPs)—became the underlying theme of the "development" establishment, guided by the International Monetary Fund (IMF) and the World Bank[7] (see box on p. 727).

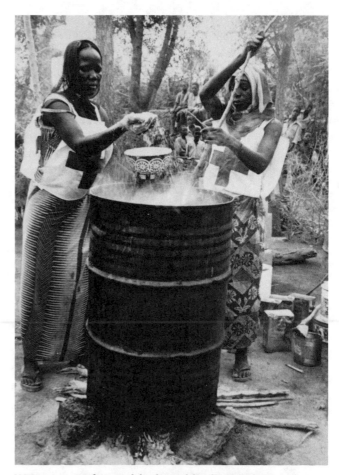

Women preparing enriched porridge in Chad/International Federation of Red Cross and Red Crescent Societies/Liliane de Toledo

INTERNATIONAL LOAN POLICIES AND WOMEN'S LIVES: STRUCTURAL ADJUSTMENT PROGRAMS (SAPs)

The origins of the SAPs imposed on several African and Latin American countries (and later some Asian countries) can be found in the fluctuations in world trade during the 1970s after oil prices rose sharply. At the same time, prices of primary products (Africa's principal exports) plummeted. Seeking to invest the oil revenues, Northern banks made loans to already heavily indebted nations. These loans supported Western development schemes that were often based on faulty assumptions.* When the debtor nations in Latin America and Africa were unable to continue paying interest on the debts, the IMF intervened by floating the loans, which were conditional on governments instituting severe measures to bring their economies "back on track." These "conditions" took the form of Structural Adjustment Programs (SAPs), whose stated objective was to maximize production and economic growth and to integrate the country into the free market.

These SAP packages reduced government spending on public sector services and programs, devalued the currency to make exports cheaper and imports more expensive, and deregulated industries to make them more attractive for foreign investors (thus replacing public sector enterprises with private firms). Because SAPs often prescribed wage cuts and massive cutbacks in social services such as health education, alongside privatization, they set in motion a sequence of unemployment, high interest rates, and soaring food prices. Studying the impact of these "efficiency" approaches, feminist scholars have documented the increased domestic burden on women, who have assumed care of the elderly and the sick, processed and prepared foods once cheaply purchased in the market, and taken up formal and informal employment to make ends meet.[8] Many women have been laid off by government offices after having gained admission in large numbers to clerical, secretarial, and supervisory positions.[9] Others have been pushed into the informal sector to sell household products for additional income. In sub-Saharan Africa and elsewhere, young girls are losing the gains they had made in access to education, as free state education systems are slashed. Faced with these conditions, women are resorting to desperate means of survival, and prostitution has significantly increased in many urban areas of the Third World.[10] Health care systems gutted by SAPs are even less prepared for the increased prevalence of STDs and HIV. According to an informed observer, "In India health-care cuts in the early 1990s intensified epidemics of malaria, diarrhea, and encephalitis. . . . In Tanzania female life expectancy declined by six years during the adjustment process imposed by the World Bank and IMF in the 1980s; in Zimbabwe maternal mortality rates doubled in the first three years of adjustment in the early 1990s."[11]

* In the early 1980s, a program was initiated in Kenya to automate agriculture by providing loans for the purchase of tractors, combines, and other farm equipment. However, no plan was made to train persons for their maintenance, nor were spare parts provided for servicing. As a result, when machinery broke down, it was often abandoned in the fields. Within a year of the inception of this "development" plan, Kenya's landscape was littered with rusting tractors, and the Kenyan government was left to repay the loans—with interest.

In 1987, a Third World women's network of researchers and practitioners called Development Alternatives with Women for a New Era (DAWN) published a manifesto calling for a radically different vision of development, wherein women would be at the center of the process, empowered through grassroots mobilization and organization that would bring fundamental changes in power relations.[12]

In the U.S., other feminist approaches to development besides WID have emerged, with different political underpinnings. In the late 1970s, Marxist feminists began to challenge the liberal assumptions of the WID model. These scholars, whose approach has been titled Women and Development (WAD), have studied women in exploitative work settings, particularly the export processing zones. Socialist feminists of the Gender and Development (GAD) school argue that gender relations and domestic issues, not women and employment alone, should be the focus of research and program development, with priority given to issues of domestic violence, child care, and household work.[13] These three major feminist schools of thought—WID, WAD, and GAD—continue to evolve and to exercise varying levels of influence on social and economic policy.[14]

WOMEN, WORK, AND THE WORLD ECONOMY

Across the globe, women are represented in greater numbers in the light industries that manufacture food products, garments, textiles, and electrical and electronics products. Even in areas where women do not provide the actual labor for industry, their work is instrumental. In sub-Saharan Africa, for example, where the mines, plantations, and seaports that fuel Western economies are built using highly exploitative systems of male migrant labor, women are left behind

LENDING ON A HUMAN SCALE: MICROCREDIT AND MICROENTERPRISES

The success of two lending programs in South Asia has generated a range of lending programs worldwide for individual women to finance microbusiness initiatives and for groups collectively to guarantee loans for individual members. The Grameen Bank of Bangladesh initiated loans for rural women who were ranked among the poorest with little or no resources. The extraordinarily high repayment rate of these loans enabled their reinvestment in an ever-widening circle of poor women unable to gain credit through formal banking channels.[15]

As a trade union, India's Self-Employed Women's Association (SEWA) is a membership organization that mobilizes women in the informal sector to bargain collectively for fair prices for goods they produce, such as milk, joss sticks (scented votary candles), and ladies' garments. SEWA runs a bank to encourage savings, and it provides credit for business and personal purposes on attractive terms. Unlike Grameen, SEWA does not use peer pressure to enforce payment. Nevertheless, repayment levels are very high, since the bank is part of a larger support system that promotes solidarity and motivates individual responsibility.[16]

Inspired by the success of these two credit programs in the nongovernmental sector, the World Bank has launched multimillion-dollar microcredit programs. Small amounts of money (approximately $100) are lent to thousands of women to foster or initiate a source of income-generation such as a milk cow or a vegetable vending business. In February 1997, a microcredit summit in Washington, DC, brought together several heads of state to pledge their support to this approach to economic development for poor women. We must note here, from the perspective of progressive feminist development advocates, that in today's global economy where the states have retreated from their responsibilities, the emphasis on innovative approaches to credit for women is a palliative—not a panacea—for social development.

—often for years at a stretch—to tend livestock, grow food, raise families, and build their communities. These contributions of women's labor are rarely acknowledged, nor is the huge burden placed on women's emotional and physical resources by this system.

Third World women's labor is integral to the international economy in three principal areas: (1) they are employed in export-processing industries by domestic firms and transnationals operating offshore in Asia, Latin America, and the Caribbean; (2) they are recruited as cheap migrant labor for the oil-rich countries of the Middle East and the metropolitan centers of Southeast Asia and Europe; and (3) they are maneuvered into sex work by state promotion of tourism and a lucrative trade and traffic in sex that target children as well. In the U.S., they take up domestic work with wealthy families or join sweat factories. While domestic labor accounts for a large proportion of international migration by women, professionally skilled women increasingly contribute their services to the output of the global economy. Hospitals and clinics in Europe, the U.S., and Canada are staffed by immigrant women doctors and nurses, who are filling critical shortfalls in health care services.

Global Factories/TNCs

The restructuring of the global economy has enabled transnational corporations (TNCs) to move production from Northern sites to Third World countries while retaining concentration of capital and authority in the industrialized world, including some wealthy Southeast Asian nations. Some scholars argue that assembly-line work in the export-processing zones, often women's only source of paid employment, offers women an escape from the pressures of conforming to traditions that restrict their mobility and limit their earning potential.[17] Such liberation, however, is often purchased at a high cost to their health. Substandard work environments and heavy work demands reduce women's fitness for work within a few years, at which point they are replaced by lower-paid younger women in a repetitive cycle that works to the advantage of employers.

Women are resisting these exploitative conditions through responses ranging from union formation, demonstrations, and marches to acts of retaliation and subversion. Malaysian workers reacted to an increase in the work pace by using the local cultural phenomenon of spirit possession to bring work to a halt. In other Asian countries, women workers are organizing to challenge foreign corporations' unfair practices, and they are winning decisively. Recently, U.S. TV talk show host Kathie Lee Gifford attracted public criticism when an investigative report showed that her brandname jeans were being manufactured in New York sweatshops by underpaid women working in substandard conditions. Goaded by public outrage, the U.S. government has recently instituted labor laws to regulate sweatshops. However, when women begin to organize for better wages and working conditions, industries often pick up and move to another country or community.

Health hazards abound in TNC workplaces. In the electronics industry, one of the safest and cleanest of the exporting industries, toxic chemicals and solvents sit in open containers and fill the air with powerful fumes. The stress of peering through a microscope for 7 to 9 hours at a time, straining to meet quotas at a pay rate of $2 per day, has a major health impact. Electronics assembly workers often lose the 20/20 vision required for the job through chronic conjunctivitis, nearsightedness, and astigmatism. In Penang, Malaysia, women wear gloves and boots to dip circuits into open vats of acid, but when the vats leak, burns are common, and the workers sometimes lose fingers in painful accidents.[18] Textile and garment industry conditions rival those of any 19th- or 20th-century Western sweatshop. Workers are packed into poorly lit rooms where summer temperatures rise above 100°F; textile dust, which can cause permanent lung damage, fills the air. Stress is probably the most invidious health hazard. Visits to the bathroom are a privilege; in some cases, workers must raise their hands for permission and wait up to half an hour.

In Nicaragua, in 1993, more than 850 women led the first big strike against Fortex, a Taiwanese textile company, protesting inhuman working conditions and physical and emotional violence. Many of these women reported that they were constantly subjected to sexual harassment as well as to other forms of humiliation, including having to eat on the floor, being restricted from using the restrooms, and being under constant surveillance. This surveillance included requiring that they totally undress at the end of every shift, with the excuse of making sure they were not stealing company property.[19]

Women working in the agricultural sector are often part of a migrant labor force whose working conditions include long hours of backbreaking labor, overexposure to the elements, direct contact with dangerous pesticides, and inadequate health facilities.[20]

The transnational corporations have deliberately targeted women for exploitation. If feminism is going to mean anything to women all over the world, it's going to have to find new ways to resist corporate power internationally.[21]

Migrant Domestic Workers

I was recruited to work as a domestic helper in the Kingdom of Saudi Arabia. I had to pay US$140 in placement fees plus 100 Saudi Riyals (US$28) to be deducted from my monthly salary each month for the next six months. My contract stipulated a monthly salary of US$200.

On May 1, 1994, I departed for Saudi Arabia and worked there for nine months. My work as a domestic helper included cleaning the entire two-story house and taking care of my employer's five children. I woke up at around four or five o'clock in the morning and started working without having any breakfast. We only had one main meal a day served at around three o'clock in the afternoon. All the food for all members of the household was placed on the table in a big plate. The first to eat were the male members of the family, followed by the female members, and only then could the servants and employees of the family eat whatever

was left. I always felt hungry because I had to work very hard in the day.

My employers did not pay me on a monthly basis. I only received the equivalent of US$100 in January 1995, and not US$200 each month as stipulated in my contract. I wanted to go home because I felt physically weak from lack of food, lack of sleep, and too much work. But my employer would not allow me to go. Because I could not finish my work on time, my employer would constantly beat me and slap me. I got weaker every day, and eventually I was brought to the doctor and given some medicines. By then everything was hazy.

Finally, on January 28, 1995, my employer brought me to the airport. I was entrusted to an Arab man. He told me that he would only give me my passport and air ticket if I would have sex with him—I refused. He took hold of my arm and forced me to drink something. I cannot remember what happened after that but I am sure that I was raped. I also do not know how I managed to return to the Philippines. My passport indicated that I arrived on January 31, 1995. Apparently, some Filipinos who were on the same plane that I took to Manila brought me to the mental institution as I was not in my right mind anymore. They also contacted my family in Mindanao, who immediately came to Manila to see me. On February 7, 1995, I was discharged from the hospital and brought to the Kanlungan Center for Migrant Workers for temporary shelter. Kanlungan is a nongovernmental organization that provides support services to Filipino migrant workers. I stayed there for two weeks with my husband. During this time, Kanlungan assisted me in retrieving my passport and air ticket, which were with the Filipinos who brought me to the hospital.

—Susan Paciano[22]

Asian women from countries with low economic growth and high trade deficits (the Philippines, India, Thailand, Sri Lanka, and Bangladesh) are the principal sources of cheap labor for the oil-exporting Middle East countries and the newly industrialized countries of Southeast Asia. Lured by salaries that are high compared with those in their own country, women leave the security of their homes and take up jobs as domestic workers that are exploitative, demeaning, and underpaid and that expose them to sexual harassment by the males in the family.[23] It is estimated that migrant women working as "maids" provide child care for almost two million children in Asia.[24] Caribbean women provide similar and even affluent homes in the U.S. Poor rural women and even educated urban women migrate, responding to family pressures and their strong sense of filial duty to aging or impoverished parents. Not only do migrant domestic workers support their national economies by acquiring foreign currency, but their work in the home releases educated middle-class women of the receiving countries to contribute their skills and services to their countries' economic growth.

The abuse of domestic workers and their legal prosecution for alleged violations of local law have raised international protests. Domestic workers are organizing and have demanded their rights in different continents and at several international women's conferences. They are demanding fair wages, humane treatment, and permits for permanent residence and family reunification. With help from local activists, many migrant domestic workers have successfully sued abusive employers and won their civil rights.

Sex Trade

Many global factories not only force young women and girls to work long hours under unhealthy conditions, but serve as conduits for the sex trade. In Nepal, for example, carpet factories may lure young women on false pretenses to work in the brothels of Bombay or Calcutta. Last year, around 200 Nepali women were found working in the brothels in India and sent back home, many of them having become infected with HIV. The Nepali government refused to let the plane land. It was only with intense pressure from local NGOs that the government backed down. These women, no longer welcome in their families, were taken into rehabilitation centers to equip them with skills to earn their livelihood. Yet, no amount of rehabilitation can return them to their health or their rightful place in society.[25]

There is a clear link between international trading in a free market dominated by capitalist nations and firms—be they Japanese, North American, or European—and the emergence of a powerful, ubiquitous sex industry trafficking in women and children. A multibillion-dollar industry, sex trafficking contributes to the revenues of governments in Third World countries as well as of local and transnational businesses. The formation of the international Network of Organizations in Support of a New Convention Against All Forms of Sexual Exploitation was a recognition of the international character of the sex industry. (For information, contact Coalition Against Trafficking in Women, in Resources.)

Tourism has become an important source of national income in the Third World, in some cases the third or fourth largest source of foreign currency. A strong incentive for tourism is the availability of women in these countries—either explicitly as prostitutes, or disguised as hospitality girls, massage and bath attendants, performers in sex shows, or hostesses and waitresses in clubs. Sex tour operators in Europe, the U.S., and Japan objectify and commodify young women and children in Southeast Asia, packaging together the erotic and the exotic. Even though prostitution is illegal in nearly all of the U.S., some travel agencies in New York, California, and Florida have entered the sex tour business. Equality Now, a group based in New York City, recently called on 2,500 women's groups to petition the U.S. State Department and the Queens, New York, District Attorney to investigate sex tour operators.[26]

Women enter this type of employment out of eco-nomic necessity and because there are often no alternatives for them. In Thailand, for instance, the gap in incomes and opportunities between the city and the countryside is enormous. For women from poor rural backgrounds, migration to urban centers provides an earning power that is astounding compared with normal rural budgets. Many families—indeed, entire villages—have raised their standard of living through the bodies of their daughters.[27]

Prostitution and the Military

The close relationship between the military and prostitution has been exposed and denounced by women's groups in the Philippines, the United Kingdom, and elsewhere.[28] The closing of American naval bases in the Philippines in 1991 was a triumph for local women's groups and activists who had battled the establishment for many years. Within a few years, however, the American naval fleet was back in the Philippines, making "rest and recuperation" stops for U.S. soldiers. President Clinton's Acquisition and Cross-Servicing Agreement (ACSA), a U.S./Philippine military pact that legitimizes the naval visits, encourages the use of Asian women to service the sexual needs of American soldiers and sailors, thus raising questions about the U.S. commitment to women's reproductive health, which it vigorously promoted in the 1994 Cairo conference[29] (see box on p. 733).

Military occupation, in times of war or peace, institutionalizes violence against the citizenry in many forms. Former Korean "comfort" women, who were enslaved by the Japanese military during World War II, have demanded a public apology as well as reparations from the Japanese government. While fewer than 200 of these women are still living, they have organized to make their demands heard and have publicly testified at the Asian Human Rights Tribunal in Beijing.[30] The recent case of three American servicemen based in Okinawa who were convicted for the rape of a young Japanese schoolgirl reignited demands by Japanese citizens of Okinawa to close U.S. bases. These citizens cite the continual sexual assault on women and children, traffic accidents, and environmental destruction from 50 years of occupation by the U.S. military.

Differing Perspectives on Prostitution

Some women's groups label prostitution as commercial sex work, and prostitutes as commercial sex workers who must mobilize to make their work environment safer. A leading voice for this viewpoint is San Francisco–based COYOTE (Cast Off Your Old Tired Ethics), headed by Margo St. James, which works for the rights of prostitutes as workers.* Others see prostitution as a violation of human rights. For example, the U.S.–based Coalition Against Trafficking in Women has stated the following:

---

* See also Gail Pheterson, *The Prostitution Prism* (Amsterdam: University of Amsterdam Press, 1996).

Those who want prostitution recognized as "commercial sex work" argue that when prostitution is destigmatized and regulated, the more "professional" the prostitute will become and the more "dignity" will be given to her and her "work." Professionalizing prostitution neither dignifies nor upgrades the women in prostitution. It merely dignifies and professionalizes the sex industry and the men who buy the bodies of women and children in prostitution. It gives them more dignity and professional credibility than they have ever had, or could get anyplace else—and, this time, in the name of women's rights!

Prostitution is a practice that violates the human dignity and integrity guaranteed to all persons in the Universal Declaration of Human Rights. This Declaration proclaims that all human beings are born free and equal in dignity and rights. Any form of sexual exploitation, including prostitution, abrogates this human dignity.[31]

VIOLENCE AGAINST WOMEN

In addition to the sex trade, other forms of violence continue to be a major threat to women's health. Violence was a priority issue in the agenda of the 1995 Beijing Fourth World Women's Conference. Researchers report that "at a global level the health burden from gender-based victimization among women aged 15 to 44 is comparable to that posed by other risk factors and diseases already high on the world agenda, including HIV, TB, sepsis during childbirth, cancer and cardiovascular disease."[32] Violence in society can be traced to the increasing poverty and degradation in the lives of millions of people, and women bear the heaviest toll. Violence against women continues to be a tool used in armed conflict. The conflict between the Serbs and the Croats reminded the world that sexual violence such as rape and forced pregnancy continue to serve as weapons of wars in which women's bodies have become the battlefield (see chapter 8, Violence Against Women).

Another form of violence against women is female circumcision, or female genital mutilation (FGM), which affects two million girls and women worldwide every year (see chapter 24, Selected Medical Practices, Problems, and Procedures). Although the practice is concentrated in parts of the African continent, global migration patterns have made it a significant health issue in other parts of the world as well. The enormous media exposure given to this issue in recent years has led to more open discussions in countries where it is taking place. Dr. Nahid Toubia, founder of RAINB♀, a U.S.–based organization working against this practice (see chapter 24 Resources) says this:

The real obstacle to progress is the lack of political commitment from African governments who condemn the practice in international forums and then censor their own grassroots organizations working on this and other women's rights issues.[33]

VIOLENCE AGAINST WOMEN: A GLOBAL TREND

The following examples indicate the extent of domestic violence and its impact on women.[34]

- Worldwide, studies indicate that 20% to over 50% of women have been beaten by an intimate male partner.
- In South America, one study found that 70% of all crimes reported to the police involved women being beaten by their husbands.
- In the U.S., up to one-third of women patients in hospital emergency rooms are there because of injuries sustained in domestic violence.
- In Papua New Guinea, a survey found that over half of married women in cities had been battered, and almost one in five of these women had gone to a hospital after being beaten.
- A study in Alexandria, Egypt, showed domestic violence as the leading cause of injury to women, accounting for 25% of all visits by women to trauma units.
- In a survey in the Kisii District of Kenya, 42% of women reported being "beaten regularly" by their partners.
- In Jamaica, a study among girls aged 11 to 15 years found that 40% reported their first sexual intercourse as "forced."
- In a nationally representative sample of Canadian women, 20% of those who had ever been married reported being physically assaulted by their current or former partners.

REPRODUCTIVE RIGHTS AND HEALTH

Women all over the world increasingly see reproductive-rights issues as central to self-determination. A healthy attitude toward our bodies adds to our self-respect, and such self-awareness is the first step toward playing an active role in our communities.

An Argentinean woman:

When we were children we were not allowed to explore our bodies; there were no names for the different organs that compose our genitalia. Our entire genital area, from the clitoris to the anus, was referred to by words such as "bottom," "down there," etc. As Catholic women we are not given a realistic way of being accepted by God: the model that we are given is that of the Virgin Mary, virgin and mother; a model impossible to follow for any woman, one that will always present us as being at fault, which, at the same time, makes us feel that we don't have the right to our own sexuality. We are only allowed to view sex as a way to

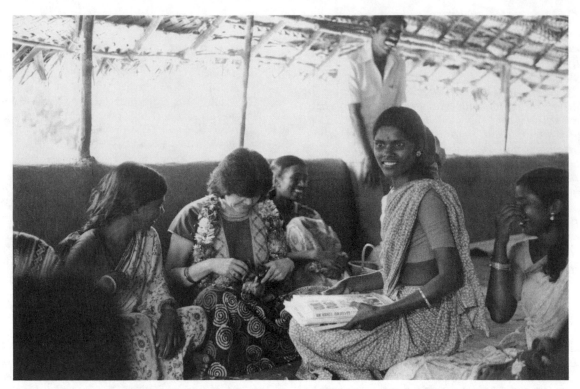

Women in India discussing *Our Bodies, Ourselves/Unitarian Universalist Service Committee*

have a family and not as something pleasurable—sex for pleasure is a sin.[35]

The overall reproductive health of Third World women has received less attention than the regulation of their fertility. Declining mortality has led to a growing population in the global South and a growing urgency among planners and international donors to funnel resources into family planning programs rather than the expansion of primary health care. At the NGO forum in Cairo, a woman from East Africa spoke of the conditions in local heath clinics: "Plenty of contraceptives, but not a single aspirin." (Some important exceptions to this approach have been in Costa Rica, Sri Lanka, and the socialist countries of China, Cuba, and Sandinista Nicaragua, which developed model health care systems and improved the general health status of the population.) The long-standing neglect of Third World women's health—general and reproductive— has had disastrous results, as is evidenced by high rates of maternal mortality, HIV, and cervical cancer.

STDs are increasing in incidence, and HIV is raising the death toll for women in the countries of sub-Saharan Africa and in Thailand. The AIDS pandemic has had grave consequences for women, who are increasingly being infected at younger ages than men. Their greater vulnerability to HIV and STDs has made them the target for discrimination. Although women are more likely to contract HIV from men than men are from women, HIV transmission is often blamed on women. As in the case of fertility control, men's

responsibility in the transmission process is downplayed. And in countries where women have few legal rights, widows are deprived of their inheritance when the husband dies of AIDS; ironically, it is these same women who provide care for the sick and dying in their homes and in the community and who bear the burden of maintaining households.

Maternal mortality, with highest levels in South Asia and sub-Saharan Africa, is the third leading cause of death among women in Latin America and the Caribbean. Between 30 and 50% of these deaths are due to complications from clandestine abortions. In Colombia, studies have demonstrated that approximately 94% of the deaths attributed to maternal morbidity could have been avoided if the women had had access to better health care.[36] In South Asia, which has some of the highest maternal mortality rates in the world, women's low status is a major contributory factor. Socioeconomic and cultural factors, distance, and delayed treatment all contribute to mortality rates.[37]

A reproductive health problem that disproportionately affects poor Southern women is cervical cancer, a leading cause of female mortality in the Third World. African-American women, socially and economically disadvantaged, also have a higher incidence of cervical cancer compared with white women. "There is a clear socioeconomic gradient in the incidence, linking it to poverty.[38] . . . An estimated 75% of all cases occur in the developing countries where only 5% of the global resources for cancer control are available."[39]

Cervical cancer is one of the more "curable" cancers

CAIRO CONSENSUS STIRS NEW HOPES, OLD CONCERNS

by Betsy Hartmann, Director of the Population and Development Program at Hampshire College in Amherst, Massachusetts, and co-coordinator of the Committee on Women, Population, and the Environment [40]

The 1994 International Conference on Population and Development (ICPD) held in Cairo, Egypt, has been widely heralded for reaching a remarkable new consensus on population policy. The new consensus embraces several positive changes. It endorses a broader reproductive health strategy, in which women have access not only to contraceptives but to sexuality education, pregnancy care, and treatment of sexually transmitted diseases. The plan also highlights the need for male responsibility in birth control. These provisions have spurred some long overdue reforms in population programs.

Embedded in the new population consensus, however, are several contradictions that carry negative consequences for women, health, and human rights.

Unsustainable Development

The Cairo conference tended to reinforce the economic status quo. Specifically, the Cairo plan of action calls for more efficient government, higher levels of foreign investment, and greater reliance on the private sector and nongovernment organizations, rather than any substantive measures to redistribute wealth in an effort to eradicate poverty. It frequently calls for "sustained economic growth within the context of sustainable development." Whatever this vague formulation means exactly, population stabilization is at the heart of it. Ever since the time of Malthus, elites have advocated reducing population growth as a panacea for poverty; in the new consensus, it's also the key to environmental sustainability, receiving far more attention than efforts to change harmful patterns of production and consumption.

Currently, the industrialized nations with only 25% of the world's population consume 75% of the world's energy and 85% of its forest products while generating 75% of pollutants and wastes. Furthermore, military activities cause up to 20% of all global environmental degradation. The Cairo consensus puts the lid securely on this Pandora's box, keeping such issues scaled from public scrutiny.

Empowering Women?

Despite its essentially conservative analysis of development and the environment, the consensus appears to be based on progressive principles because it endorses the empowerment of women. However, its plan of action pays scant attention to the empowerment of poor men. In addition, it glosses over the differences between women in terms of race, class, and nationality—all are lost in the broad category of "women."

The focus on women's empowerment was not purely an opportunistic calculation, however. In the new consensus, empowering women equals reducing population growth. The trouble with this approach is that it narrows the definition of empowerment to those factors—namely, education for girls and reproductive health services for women—that appear to have the most immediate impact on fertility but the least impact on transforming social and economic relations. Educating girls, while certainly a worthy goal, nevertheless is politically safer than other forms of empowerment, like unionizing women workers or reforming legal and land-tenure systems, which would give women greater control over resources.

Undermining Health

Another empowerment strategy favored by the new population consensus involves increasing women's access to "reproductive health services." Although this may offer potential for reforming population programs, it cannot compensate for the continuing deterioration of public health.

Ever since the 1970s, when population control became a major strategy of Western governments and multilateral lending agencies, family planning has not only been divorced from basic health care in many Third World countries but has been funded at its expense. In Bangladesh and India, spending on population control absorbs one-quarter to one-third of the annual health care budget, and in Indonesia, almost twice as many family planning clinics as primary health care centers have been built. These skewed priorities contribute to unacceptably high death rates among the poor from preventable and treatable illnesses and conditions. Ironically, the lack of basic health care in countries such as Bangladesh slows the decline of fertility. High infant and child mortality rates are often linked to high birth rates because families must have many children just to ensure that a few will survive.

continued on next page

In terms of funding strategies, the Cairo plan of action still favored family planning over reproductive health by a margin of two to one. Moreover, much of the proposed funding for reproductive health programs has not materialized.

Politics of Choice

Population officials generally favor long-acting, provider-dependent methods of contraception (female sterilization, the IUD, injectable hormones, and implants) over barrier methods such as the condom and the diaphragm. These high-technology methods, which are considered more effective, give women little control over contraception. Presently, barrier methods account for less than 5% of contraceptive use in the Third World; in more developed countries, such methods account for nearly 25% of contraceptive use.

Barrier methods have many advantages: their use entails fewer side effects, helps protect both women and men against sexually transmitted diseases, and does not interfere with lactation. Because of the rapid spread of HIV/AIDS in many Third World countries and because of pressure from women's health activists, population agencies finally are recognizing the importance of barrier methods and have, at long last, increased research on improving them. However, long-acting, provider-dependent methods continue to dominate the contraceptive agenda.

Last but not least, the Cairo commitment to reproductive health founders on its failure to endorse women's right to safe, legal, and accessible abortion. An estimated 50 million abortions occur worldwide every year, and almost half of all abortion procedures are illegal. Illegal abortion, in turn, is responsible for an estimated 20 to 25% of maternal mortality. In Latin America, complications of illegal abortion are regarded as the main cause of death of women in their reproductive years. Safe abortion thus poses one of the most important reproductive health interventions that any nation can take.

The Cairo plan of action states that in countries where abortion is legal, it should be provided safely, and that in all countries women should have access to high-quality services if they suffer abortion complications. Yet, the plan also states that "in no case should abortion be promoted as a method of family planning." It leaves the legality issue up to the whims of "the national legislative process." The battle to make abortion safe, legal, and accessible is far from over.

In fact, at home and abroad, the fundamental paradox of the new population consensus is that while it endorses women's empowerment, it accepts the economic and political status quo, which condemns so many women to a life of poverty.

with early diagnosis and treatment. Yet, in the Third World, the absence of screening facilities, essential equipment, and diagnostic services reduce the chances of cure. The data show that age is a factor in the onset of this cancer and that the majority of cases are among women 35 and older.[41]

It is clear that family planning services alone cannot alleviate these serious problems. Yet, family planning has for decades been the focus of the major aid efforts aimed at women in the Third World, often at the expense of other important health services. In addition, critics of current population policies and programs highlight the link between reproductive health problems and social and economic development—for example, the link between women's increasing susceptibility to HIV infection and the oppressive socioeconomic structures that perpetuate poverty.[42] Despite some modest progress in the population policies of affluent nations, these important public health and feminist perspectives are often missing (see box on p. 733).

The Pharmaceutical Industry

Among the most powerful and profitable TNCs in the world, the pharmaceutical industry continues to exploit Third World health systems. SAPs have undermined regulatory barriers in many countries, allowing drug companies to promote their products with impunity, often without advising women of the side effects. The high-dose birth control pill was first tested on women in Puerto Rico and later in El Salvador, with severe consequences to their health. Drug companies have long dumped banned and unmarketable drugs on Southern countries. Recently, some U.S.–based groups and individuals have promoted quinacrine for chemical sterilization in Asian and Latin American countries. Claiming that they are reducing maternal mortality among poor Third World women, they are openly defying a World Health Organization statement that quinacrine should not be used for nonsurgical sterilization.[43]

A tragic result of the export of Western medicine and pharmaceuticals all over the world under the guise of sharing "expertise" has been the devaluation and persecution of indigenous health systems. In many places, however, women are organizing to revitalize traditional healing systems. One such example is the Shodhini Network in India (see box on p. 735).

Everywhere, women have become a strong force to be reckoned with. At the local, national, regional, and international levels, we are challenging economic and political systems based on the exploitation of our labor and our bodies—systems grounded in racism and sexism and driven by the pursuit of profit. Everywhere, women are organizing to transform communities and to build a world where power and resources are distributed in ways that promote human well-being for all instead of profit for a few. There is much to be done. The Resource section lists some of the many women's organizations around the world that are

SHODHINI—WOMEN, HEALING, AND HERBS

Shodhini is a network of women health activists who have gathered information about common gynecological problems and traditional plant remedies collected from women healers from various parts of India. These remedies have been in use for hundreds of years but are rapidly disappearing from people's knowledge.

Their book *Touch-me, Touch-me-not* is an outcome of action research and attempts to rediscover the efficacy of common herbal remedies in healing a wide range of disorders, particularly gynecological ones. Among the book's offerings:

- Symptoms, diagnosis, and treatment of menstrual problems, vaginal infections, urinary infections, uterine problems, backache, etc.
- Exhaustive, simple-to-use indices by symptoms, plants, and ailments.
- Tested herbal recipes for gynecological problems.
- Women's perceptions, beliefs, and experiences about their health.
- Experiences of the self-help process.

(See Resources for Shodhini's address and book ordering information.)

working to realize this vision. Look around; you will find a group in your own community. Acting together we *can* change the world.

NOTES

1. Saskia Wieringa, ed., *Subversive Women: Historical Experiences of Gender and Resistance* (London: ZED Books, 1995). See also Amrita Basu, *The Challenge of Local Feminisms: Women's Movements in Global Perspective* (Boulder, CO: Westview Press, 1995) and Leda Maria Vieira Machado, "We Learned to Think Politically," in Sarah A. Radcliffe and Sallie Westwood, eds., *"Viva": Women and Popular Protest in Latin America* (New York: Routledge, 1993).
2. Rosi Braidotti et al., *Women, the Environment and Sustainable Development: Towards a Theoretical Synthesis* (Atlantic Highlands, NJ: Zed Books, 1994).
3. Ester Boserup. *Women's Role in Economic Development* (New York: St. Martin's Press, 1970).
4. Eva M. Rathgeber, "WID, WAD, GAD: Trends in Research and Practice," *The Journal of Developing Areas* 24 no. 4 (1990): 489–502.
5. Caroline O. Moser, *Gender Planning and Development Theory, Practice and Training* (New York: Routledge, 1993).
6. Imrana Qader, "Primary Health Care: A Paradise Lost," *IASSI Quarterly* (Indian Association of Social Science Institutions, New Delhi) 14, nos. 1–2 (1995): 1–20.
7. Moser, op. cit.
8. Diane Elson, "From Survival Strategies to Transformation Strategies: Women's Needs and Structural Adjustment," in Lourdes Beneria and Shelley Feldman, eds., *Unequal Burden: Economic Crises, Persistent Poverty and Women's Work* (Boulder, CO: Westview Press, 1992).
9. Takyiwaa Manuh, "Ghana: Women in the Public and Informal Sectors under the Economic Recovery Programme," in Pamela Sparr, ed., *Mortgaging Women's Lives* (Atlantic Highlands, NJ: Zed Books, 1994), 61–76.
10. Adetoun Ilumoka, "Nigeria," in Nalini Visvanathan, "Beyond Commitments: Policies and Practices," *Political Environments* 4 (summer–fall 1996): 44–47.
11. Betsy Hartmann, "Cairo Consensus Stirs New Hopes, Old Concerns," *Forum for Applied Research and Public Policy* 12, no. 2 (summer 1997): 33–40.
12. Gita Sen and Caren Grown, *Development, Crises, and Alternative Visions: Third World Women's Perspectives* (New York: Monthly Review Press, 1987).
13. Kate Young, "Gender and Development," in Sara Hlupekile Longue, ed., *Gender and Development Readings* (Ottawa: Canadian Council for International Cooperation, 1992).
14. Nalini Visvanathan et al., eds., *Women, Gender and Developmental Reader* (Atlantic Highlands, NJ: Zed Books, 1997).
15. Andreas Fuglesang and Dale Chandler, *Participation as Process—Process as Growth: What We Can Learn from Grameen Bank, Bangladesh* (Dhaka: Grameen Trust, 1993).
16. Kalima Rose, *Where Women Are Leaders. The SEWA Movement in India* (London: Zed Books, 1992).
17. Linda Y.C. Lim, "Capitalism, Imperialism and Patriarchy: The Dilemma of Third World Women Workers in Multinational Factories," in June Nash and Maria Patricia Fernandez-Kelly, eds., *Women, Men and the International Division of Labor* (Albany: State University of New York Press, 1983), 70–91.
18. Barbara Ehrenreich and Annette Fuentes, "Life on the Global Assembly Line," *Ms.* (Jan. 1981): 56.
19. Boston Women's Health Book Collective, *Nuestros Cuerpos, Nuestras Vidas* (publishing is forthcoming).
20. See Sonia Jasso and Maria Mazorra, "Following the Harvest: The Health Hazards of Migrant and Seasonal Farmworking Women," in Wendy Chavkin, ed., *Double Exposure: Women's Health Hazards on the Job and at Home* (New York: Monthly Review Press, 1984), 86–89.
21. Saralee Hamilton (an American Friends Service Committee staff person working on the issue of women and global corporations) in Ehrenreich and Fuentes, op. cit., 60. See also the newsletter of the Pacific Studies Center for the Global Electronics Information Project, 222B View Street, Mountain View, CA 94101; (650) 961-8918.

22. Gina M. Alunan and Teresita Cuizon, "Human Rights Violations Against Migrant Workers: The Stories of Susan Paciano and Teresita Cuizon," in Niamh Reilly, ed., *Without Reservation: The Beijing Tribunal on Accountability for Women's Human Rights* (New Brunswick, NJ: Center for Women's Global Leadership, 1996), 77–78.

23. Noleen Heyzer et al., eds. *The Trade in Domestic Workers: Causes, Mechanisms and Consequences of International Migration* (Atlantic Highlands, NJ: Zed Books, 1994).

24. Ibid.

25. Shobha H. Gurung, personal communication.

26. "Sex Tours Abroad Find U.S. Market," *Boston Sunday Globe* (June 15, 1997).

27. Pasuk Phongpaichit, "Bangkok Masseuses: Holding Up the Family Sky," in "Tourism: Selling Southeast Asia," *Southeast Asia Chronicle* 78 (April 1981): 23.

28. Cynthia Enloe, *Bananas, Beaches and Bases: Making Feminist Sense of International Politics* (Berkeley: University of California Press, 1990).

29. Marilen Danguilan, "Philippines," in Nalini Visvanathan, "Beyond Commitment: Policies and Practices," *Political Environments* 4 (summer–fall 1996): 44–46.

30. Heisoo Shin, "The Situation of the Comfort Women: An Update," in Niamh Reilly, op cit., 43–44.

31. Janice G. Raymond, *Report to the Special Rapporteur on Violence Against Women, The United Nations, Geneva, Switzerland* (Amherst, MA: Coalition Against Trafficking in Women, 1995), 11.

32. Lori Heise et al., *Violence Against Women. The Hidden Health Burden* (Washington, DC: World Bank, 1994); 17.

33. Dr. Nahid Toubia, personal communication.

34. Lori Heise et al., op cit.

35. *Nuestros Cuerpos, Nuestras Vidas,* op cit.

36. Ibid.

37. Sereen Thaddeus and Deborah Maine, "Too Far to Walk: Maternal Mortality in Context," *Social Science and Medicine* 38, no. 8 (1994): 1091–110.

38. World Health Organization, *Women's Health: WHO Position Paper. Fourth World Conference on Women, Beijing, China. 4–15 September 1995* (Geneva: WHO, 1995): 14.

39. Ibid., 27.

40. Betsy Hartmann, op cit.

41. Jacqueline D. Sherris et al., *Cervical Cancer in Developing Countries. A Situation Analysis* (Washington, DC: World Bank, 1993).

42. See Paul Farmer et al., eds., *Women, Poverty and AIDS* (Monroe, ME: Common Courage Press, 1996).

43. *Reproductive Health Matters* 6 (Nov. 1996): 142–46.

....

Resources

....

Books

Abzug, Bella, and Devaki Jain. *Women's Leadership and the Ethics of Development.* New York: United Nations Development Programme, 1996.

Asian and Pacific Women's Resource Collection Network. *Health.* Kuala Lumpur: Asian Pacific Development Center, 1990.

Bajpai, Smita, and Mira Sadgopal. *Her Healing Heritage: Local Beliefs and Practices Concerning the Health of Women and Children.* Gujarat, India: Centre for Health Education, Training and Nutrition Awareness, 1996.

Banderage, Asoka. *Women, Population, and Global Crisis.* London: Zed Books, 1997.

Barry Kathleen. *Female Sexual Slavery.* New York: Avon Books, 1979.

Boston Women's Health Book Collective. *Our Bodies, Ourselves: List of Over Fourteen Foreign-Language Editions.* Available from BWHBC, P.O. Box 192, West Somerville, MA 02144.

Center for Reproductive Law and Policy. *Women of the World: Formal Laws and Policies Affecting Their Reproductive Lives.* New York: Center for Reproductive Law and Policy, 1995.

Chant, Sylvia. *Gender, Urban Development and Housing.* New York: United Nations Development Programme, 1996.

Doyal, Lesley, *What Makes Women Sick: Gender and the Political Economy of Health.* New Brunswick, NJ: Rutgers University Press, 1995.

Farmer, Paul, et al., eds. *Women, Poverty and AIDS: Sex, Drugs and Structural Violence.* Monroe, ME: Common Courage Press, 1996.

Fenton, Thomas P., and Mary J. Heffron. *Women in the Third World: A Directory of Resources.* Maryknoll, NY: Orbis Books, 1987.

Gomez, Elsa, ed. *Gender, Women and Health in the Americas.* Washington, DC: PAHO, 1993. Also published in Spanish.

Hardon, Anita, et al. *The Provision and Use of Drugs in Developing Countries.* Amsterdam: Het Sphinhuis Publications, 1991.

Hartmann, Betsy. *Reproductive Rights and Wrongs: The Global Politics of Population Control.* Boston: South End Press, 1995.

Hosken, Fran P. *The Childbirth Picture Book.* Lexington, MA: WIN News, 1982. Available in Hindi, Gujarati, Tegulu, and Bengali.

———. *The Universal Childbirth Picture Book.* Lexington, MA: WIN News, 1982. Available in Arabic, English, French, and Spanish.

Heyzer, Noeleen, et al., eds. *A Commitment to the World's Women: Perspectives on Development for Beijing and Beyond.* New York: United Nations Development Fund for Women (UNIFEM), 1995.

Isis International. *Violence Against Women in Latin America and the Caribbean: A Bibliographic Catalogue.* Santiago, Chile: Isis International, 1990.

Koblinsky, Marge, et al., eds. *The Health of Women: A Global Perspective.* Boulder, CO: Westview Press, 1992.

Latin American and Caribbean Women's Health Network. *The Right to Live Without Violence: Women's Proposals and Actions.* Santiago: Isis International, 1996.

McClain, Carol, ed. *Women as Healers: Cross-Cultural Perspectives.* New Brunswick, NJ: Rutgers University Press, 1989.

Panos Institute. *Triple Jeopardy: Women and AIDS.* London: Panos Institute, 1990.

Parikh, Rita. *In the Name of Development: Exploring Population, Poverty and Development.* Ottawa: Inter Pares, 1995.

Parker, Richard. *Bodies, Pleasures and Passions: Sexual Culture in Contemporary Brazil.* Boston: Beacon Press, 1991.

Pietila, Hilkka, and Jeanne Vickers. *Making Women Matter: The Role of the United Nations.* London: Zed Books, 1994.

Sai, F., et al. "The Role of the World Bank in Shaping Third World Population Policy," in Godfrey Roberts, ed. *Population Policy: Contemporary Issues.* New York: Praeger, 1990.

Schuler, Margaret, ed. *Freedom from Violence: Women's Strategies from Around the World.* New York: UNIFEM, 1992.

Sen, Gita, and Rachel Snow, eds. *Power and Decision: The Social Control of Reproduction.* Cambridge, MA: Harvard University Press, 1994.

Sen, Gita, Adrienne Germain, and Lincoln Chen, eds. *Population Policies Reconsidered.* Cambridge, MA: Harvard University Press, 1994.

Shodhini. *Touch-me, Touch-me-not: Women, Plants, and Healing.* New Delhi: Kali for Women. (To order, send $10.00 international money order to Kali for Women, B¹/₈ Hanz Khas, New Delhi 100016 India.)

Smyke, Patricia. *Women and Health.* London: Zed Books, 1991.

Taylor, Jill, and Sheelagh Stewart. *Sexual and Domestic Violence: Help, Recovery and Action in Zimbabwe.* Harare, Zimbabwe: Women and Law in Southern Africa, 1991.

Toubia, Nahid, ed. *Women of the Arab World: The Coming Challenge.* London: Zed Books, 1988.

Turshen, Meredeth. *The Politics of Public Health.* New Brunswick, NJ: Rutgers University Press, 1989.

United Nations Development Programme. *Human Development Report 1997.* New York: Oxford University Press, 1997. An annual statistical report.

Werner, David. *Where There Is No Doctor: A Village Health Care Handbook.* Palo Alto, CA: Hesperian Foundation, 1992. Available in Spanish, English, Portuguese, Swahili, and Hindi.

Werner, David, and B. Bower. *Helping Health Workers Learn: A Book of Methods, Aids and Ideas for Instructors at the Village Level.* Palo Alto, CA: Hesperian Foundation, 1982.

Women Living Under Muslim Laws. *WLUML Dossier for NGO Forum, International Conference on Population and Development, Cairo 1994: Women's Reproductive Rights in Muslim Communities and Countries—Issues and Resources.* Lahore, Pakistan: WLUML, 1994.

Women's Global Network on Reproductive Rights Uganda Chapter. *Report on First African Regional Meeting of Women and Health, 23–27 October, 1989.* Kampala: WGNRR, 1990.

Women's Health Interaction. *Uncommon Knowledge: A Critical Guide to Contraception and Reproductive Technologies.* Ottawa: Inter Pares, 1995.

World Health Organization. *Women's Health: Across Age and Frontier.* Geneva: WHO, 1992. Prepared for the 1992 World Health Assembly on Women's Health.

Articles

Berer, Marge. "The Quinacrine Controversy Continues." *Reproductive Health Matters* 6 (Nov. 1995).
———. "The Quinacrine Controversy One Year On." *Reproductive Health Matters* 4 (Nov. 1994): 99–106.

Fletcher, Suzanne W., et al. "Report of the International Workshop on Screening for Breast Cancer." *Journal of the National Cancer Institute* 85, no. 20 (1993): 1644–656.

Grundfest-Schoepf, Brooke. "AIDS Action-Research with Women in Kinshasa, Zaire," *Social Science and Medicine* 37, no. 11 (1993): 1401–413.

Henshaw, Stanley K. "Abortion Law and Practice Worldwide." Presented at Abortion Matters, an international conference, Amsterdam, 1996.

Ireland, Kevin. "Sexual Exploitation of Children and International Travel and Tourism," *Child Abuse Review* 2 (1993): 263–70.

Jaising, Indira, and C. Sathyamala: "Legal Rights . . . and Wrongs: Internationalising Bhopal," in *Women, Ecology and Health, Development Dialogue* (1992): 1–2.

Lurie, Peter, and Wolfe, Sidney M. "Unethical Trials of Interventions to Reduce Perinatal Transmission of the Human Immunodeficiency Virus in Developing Countries." *Lancet* 337, no. 12 (Sept. 18, 1997): 853–55.

Paxman, John M., et al. "The Clandestine Epidemic: The Practice of Unsafe Abortion in Latin America." *Studies in Family Planning* 24, no. 4 (July/Aug. 1993): 205–26.

Pheterson, Gail. "The Whore Stigma: Crimes of Unchastity." *Women's Global Network for Reproductive Rights Newsletter* 58, no. 2 (1997): 8–12.

Richter, Judith. " 'Vaccination' Against Pregnancy: The Politics of Contraceptive Research," *The Ecologist* 26, no. 2 (1996): 53–60.

Sadasivam, Bharati. "The Impact of Structural Adjustment on Women: A Governance and Human Rights Agenda." *Human Rights Quarterly* 19, no. 3 (1997): 630.

Toubia, Nahid. "Female Circumcision as a Public Health Issue." *New England Journal of Medicine and Surgery* 331, no. 11 (Sept. 15, 1994): 712–16.

Audiovisual Materials

Abortion Stories from North and South, a 55-minute video by the National Film Board of Canada. Documentary examines abortion cross-culturally in Ireland, Japan, Thailand, Peru, Colombia, and Canada. Available from the Cinema Guild, 1697 Broadway, Suite 802, New York, NY 10019.

The Double Day (Doble Jornado), a 56-minute 1975 film. The efforts of Latin American working women to achieve equality in the home and workplace—a "double day." Classic. Available from the Cinema Guild, 1697 Broadway, Suite 802, New York, NY 10019.

Global Assembly Line, a 60-minute, 16-mm film. Produced by Lorraine Gray, Anne Bohlen, and Patricia Fernandez. A documentary about the impact of factory work on women and their families in the U.S. and free trade zones of developing countries. Available from New Day Films, 22D Hollywood Avenue, Hohokus, NJ 07432; (201) 652-6590.

Legacy of Malthus, a 1-hour video documentary revealing the impoverishment of Indian peasants who are targeted for government population policies. Directed by Deepa Dhanraj, 1994. Available from Women Make Movies, 462 Broadway, Suite 500E, New York, NY 10013; (212) 925-0606.

La Operación, a 40-minute 16-mm film. A powerful documentary about female sterilization abuse and economic development in Puerto Rico. In English and Spanish with subtitles. Available from the Cinema Guild, 1697 Broadway, Suite 802, New York, NY 10019.

Something Like a War, a 1-hour video documentary exposing India's national family planning campaign with its emphasis on female sterilization. Directed by Deepa Dhanraj, 1991. Available from Women Make Movies (see *Legacy of Malthus* for address).

Still Killing Us Softly: Advertising's Image of Women, a 30-minute, 16-mm, 1987 film. An examination of the advertising industry's manipulation of sex roles to sell products. Available from Cambridge Documentary Films, Inc., Box 385, Cambridge, MA 02139.

The Ultimate Test Animal, a 40-minute video available in all formats. This documentary examines the history and controversy around the use of the birth control injection Depo-Provera, primarily in the U.S. Available from the Cinema Guild (see *La Operación* for address).

Periodicals

Manushi
C/1202 Lajpat Nagar 1; New Delhi 110024, India

A feminist magazine (*manushi* means "woman") that encourages women to write in and tell their stories as well as analyze their situations and move toward a shared understanding. Lively, interesting, it reflects the Indian woman's often harsh reality. Published in English and Hindi, it deserves wider circulation.

Radical America
38 Union Square; Somerville, MA 02143

An excellent monthy socialist journal covering a variety of topics not exclusive to women but with a feminist perspective when women are discussed.

WIN News (Women's International Network News)
187 Grant Street; Lexington, MA 02173

A quarterly covering a wide range of topics of concern, including statistical data and reports on conferences.

Organizations

(Many publish periodicals and other materials.)

Asian-Pacific Resource and Research Centre for Women (ARROW)
2nd floor, Block F; Anjung Felda, Jalan Maktab; 54000 Kuala Lumpur, Malaysia; (60-3) 292-9913
E-mail: arrow@po.my.jaring
Web site: http://www.asiaconnect.com.my/arrow

Association for Women in Development (AWID)
1511 K Street NW, Suite 825; Washington, DC 20005; (202) 628-0440
E-mail: awid@igc.org

Boston Women's Health Book Collective
P.O. Box 192; West Somerville, MA 02144

The Women's Health Information Center includes many foreign-language books, periodicals, and documents as well as English-language materials on women's international issues. Send for literature lists.

Center for Women's Global Leadership
Rutgers University; 61 Clifton Avenue; Douglas College; New Brunswick, NJ 08901-8535; (732) 932-8782

Many publications on women's human rights, including testimonies from several U.N. women's conferences.

CHETNA (Centre for Health Education, Training and Nutrition Awareness)
Lilavatiben Lalbhai's Bungalow; Civil Camp Road, Shahibaug; Ahmedabad 380 004, Gujarat, India; (91-079) 866-695; 866-856; Fax: (91-079) 866-513

CIDHAL
Apdo, Postal 579; Calle des Flores No. 12; Col. Acapantzingo; Cuernavaca, Morelos, Mexico

A documentation center for Latin American women, CIDHAL holds classes, produces pamphlets on women's health and education, organizes meetings and study groups. It also offers clinical services and holistic approaches.

Coalition Against Trafficking in Women
P.O. Box 9338; North Amherst, MA 01059; Fax: (413) 367-9262

Has consultative status with the United Nations Economic and Social Council (UNESCO).

Committee on Women, Population and the Environment
c/o Population and Development Program, Hampshire College; P.O. Box 5001; Amherst, MA 01002; (413) 582-5506
E-mail: cwpe@igc.org

Produces *Political Environments.*

DAWN (Development Alternatives for Women for a New Era)

Women and Development Unit; UWI Pinelands; St. Michaels, Barbados; (809) 426-9288

Feministische Frauengesundheits Zentrum (FFGZ Feminist Women's Health Center)
Bambergerstrasse 51; 10777 Berlin 30, Germany

Health Action Information Network (HAIN)
9 Cabantuan Road; Philam Homes; Quezon City 1104, Philippines; (63-2) 929-8805
E-mail: hain@mnl.sequel.net

Health Action International (HAI)
Jacob van Lennepkade 334T; 1053 NJ Amsterdam, The
Netherlands; (31 20) 683-3684
E-Mail: Barbara@hai.antenna.wl

An international network of consumer and professional groups whose main concern is to resist ill treatment of consumers by multinational drug companies.

Inter-African Committee on Traditional Health Practices
Affecting Women
c/o ECA/ATRCW; P.O. Box 3001; Addis Ababa, Ethiopia;
(25-11) 515793; or, Inter-African Committee; 147 rue de
Lausanne; CH-1202 Geneva, Switzerland; (41-22) 732-
0821

International Women's Health Coalition
24 East 21st Street, 5th floor; New York, NY 10010; (212)
979-8500

Produces in-depth analyses of women's reproductive
health issues. Works with selected groups in particular
Southern countries.

International Women's Rights Action Watch
Women, Public Policy and Development Project; Humphrey Institute of Public Affairs; University of Minnesota;
301 19th Avenue South; Minneapolis, MN 55455; (612)
625-5093

Produces a regular newsletter, *The Women's Watch.*

International Women's Tribune Center
777 UN Plaza, 3rd floor; New York, NY 10017; (212) 687-
8633
E-mail: iwtc@igc.org

Clearinghouse for information on women's issues and
organizations worldwide. Produces *The Tribune Newsletter.*

Inter Pares
58 rue Arthur; Ottawa, Ontario K1R 7B9; Canada; (613)
563-4801

Educational programs on development issues; funds
overseas groups that address underdevelopment and
poverty.

ISIS Internaciónal
Esmerelda 636, 2o piso; Casilla 2067, Cor. Central; Santiago, Chile; (56-2) 638-2219
E-mail: isis@reuna.cl
and, ISIS International; P.O. Box 1837; Quezon City Main;
Quezon City 1100, Philippines; (63-2) 435-3408; 436-0312
E-mail: isis@phil.gn.ape.org

ISIS is an international women's information and communication service with a resource and documentation
center. It provides original and in-depth feminist analyses
of a wide variety of topics.

ISIS WICCE
P.O. Box 4934; Kampala, Uganda; (256 41) 266007;
266008
E-mail: isis@starcom.co.ug

Latin American and Caribbean Women's Health Network
Casilla 50610; Santiago 1; Santiago, Chile; (56-2) 634-9827
E-mail: rsmlac@mail.bellsouth.cl

Produces the *Women's Health Journal.*

Saheli
Unit Above Shop; 105–108 Shopping Center; Defense
Colony Bridge (South Side); New Delhi 110024, India;
(91-11) 461-6485

A group of feminists working to build awareness of
women's issues and rights in India. It began by organizing against dowry burnings and tortures and now covers
a broad range of women's issues, including health and
reproduction.

Shodhini
J-1881 Chittaranjan Park; New Delhi 110019, India.
See text for information on Shodhini.

Sos Corpo
Rua do Hospicio; 859-4o Andar, Boa Vista, Apt. 14;
Recife, PE 50050 Brazil

A women's health activist organization.

Taller Salud
Apartado 2172; Hato Rey, PR 00919; (809) 767-6908

A self-help, advocacy, and activist collective that produces publications and carries out community-based
health education projects.

Women's Action Group
P.O. Box 135; Ivory House, 5th floor; 95 Robert Mugabe
Road; Harare, Zimbabwe; (263) 4702986

Women's Environment and Development Organization
355 Lexington Avenue, 3rd floor; New York, NY 10017-
6603; (212) 973-0325
E-mail: wedo@igc.org
Web site: http://www.wedo.org

Women's Global Network for Reproductive Rights
(WGNRR)
NZ Voorburgwal 32; 1012 RZ Amsterdam, The Netherlands; (31-20) 620-9672
E-mail: office@wgnrr.nl

The organization's newsletter and annual maternal
mortality campaign and reports are indispensable women's health activist resources.

Women's Global Network for Reproductive Rights
Uganda Chapter; Plot I 2/4, City-House; William Street;
Kampala, Uganda

Women's Health Action Foundation (formerly Women
and Pharmaceuticals Project)
PB 94263; 1009 AG Amsterdam, The Netherlands

Produces excellent materials on fertility regulation
technologies and attempts to improve women's health
services and to increase the role of women in developing
health policies and programs.

Women's Health Project
P.O. Box 1038; Johannesburg 2000; South Africa; (27-11) 489-9917
E-mail: womenhp@sn.apc.org
   Produces *Women's Health News*.

Women's Living Under Muslim Law
Shirkat Gah Women's Resource Centre; 208 Scotch Corner, Upper Mall; Lahore, Pakistan; (92) 42 666 1874
E-mail: brain!sgah!info@uunet
   Produces *Women Living Under Muslim Law Newsheet*.

A longer version of this chapter and bibliography is available from the author, who can be reached c/o the BWHBC, 240A Elm Street, Somerville, MA 02144.

By Eugenia Acuña, with Judy Norsigian
and Jane Pincus

WITH SPECIAL THANKS TO Caty Laignel,
Meizhu Lui, Suzanne Nam, and the thousands
of women organizing around the country for
social justice in health care *

Chapter 27

Organizing for Change: U.S.A.

GETTING TOGETHER

Women may begin to work together to change the conditions of our lives for many reasons. We may start to organize ourselves when we're angry or when we become fed up with a particular situation. We may see a common health need, or want to learn something about ourselves; maybe we start out to support a friend or relative.

Working together with other women can be a powerful experience. The strength of collective action can not only change a situation but propel us in numerous other ways. We can receive much-needed support from our peers and model it for other women; we can break our isolation through sharing experiences and working against the forces that divide us, like sexism, racism, homophobia, and classism.

You can meet other women working on health is-

sues through friends and neighbors, at your workplace, at a public meeting, or by placing an ad in a newspaper, a notice on a bulletin board, or, if you have access, through the Internet. If you already belong to an organization, you may want to become part of a subgroup within it, like the Women's Caucus of the American Public Health Association or the reproductive rights committee of a local NOW chapter. You can work from within the system as health workers or from the outside as a "consumer" pressure group seeking institutional change (e.g., a local childbirth group).

Once a group starts to meet, the need for information and for taking effective action generates its own energy and fuels enthusiasm. At first, women may drift in and out, but usually the group settles down to a steady number of people. Many questions come up about how to proceed. Here's a sampling:

The Issue(s)

- What will be the scope of our work? What is the background of the issue?
- How many women are affected?

* Thanks also to the following for their help with the 1998 version of this chapter: Hannah Doress, Cynthia Pearson, Julia Scott, Susan Evans, Laura Whitehorn, and Susan Rosenberg. Over the years since 1976, the following women have contributed to the many versions of this chapter: Norma Meras Swenson, Judy Norsigian, Jane Pincus, and Rachel Lanzerotti.

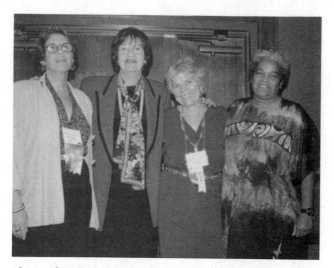

Photo of Gail Gordon, Ruth Sidel, Helen Rodriguez-Trias, and Linda Rae Murray/Donya Arias, courtesy of the American Public Health Association

- What research has been done already? By whom?
- Are the women most affected centrally involved in efforts to create solutions?
- Who and what is the opposition? What do we want to accomplish?
- What approaches to the problem are we considering? What is the possibility of success with these approaches?
- Are other organizations or individuals already working on the problem? If they are, how can we work together?
- Will our work give women a sense of power? Will our work help inform members of the public and motivate them to work for more improvements in women's health? Will it tangibly improve the quality of life and accessibility of good health and medical care for women?

The Group

- Should we close it to new members or keep membership open? (The former increases stability and minimizes the need to keep orienting new people, whereas the latter allows for valuable new resources and energies.)
- How should we make decisions? By consensus? By majority vote?
- How do we ensure that mothers can participate (pay for or provide child care, make meetings at accessible times)?
- Do we want our group to have diversity in terms of race, class, age, and physical ability? Or do we want our group to be only of our ethnicity, race, age, or sexual orientation in order to empower ourselves and our community?
- If we want a diverse group, how do we make our group accessible? (Some locations may prevent women with certain disabilities from attending;

POSSIBILITIES FOR GROUP ACTION

- Focus on a specific topic such as infertility, pelvic inflammatory disease (PID), endometriosis, fibroids, access to services, being teenagers, herbal remedies.
- Organize a "Know Your Body" course.
- Start an information hot line for birth control and abortion information, postpartum support, help for women who are raped or beaten, or any other issue. Publish listings of the better community resources where women can go for basic well-woman care, breast cancer treatment, abortion services, infertility help, midwifery care, and so on. Start a childbirth education group to provide information about both hospital and out-of-hospital birthing options.
- Work to change a local health care facility, for example, by adding services such as translation or expanded hours.
- Discuss ways you might address racism, classism, and other forms of oppression in your community.
- Get child care/day care into clinics and hospitals.
- Mobilize with other parents around issues concerning children's health: immunizations, cost of medications, street safety, violence on TV and in films, and so on.

new immigrants may not know their way around; people may need help with transportation costs, etc.)
- How much money do we need? How can we get it? What resources other than money do we need? How much can we achieve without money?
- How will we handle conflict among ourselves? Will we be able to stop discussing business to deal with strong, unresolved, maybe even unvoiced feelings or personality clashes?
- How mainstream do we want to be? An activist addresses this issue:

As Asian women activists, we challenge the model minority myth, which is used by U.S. mainstream society to win the consent of the elite in our communities. At the same time, we run the danger of succumbing to this myth and co-opting ourselves if we go about trying to establish the most successful and professionalized nonprofit operations, forgetting the desire for a fundamentally different society which led us to walk down this path in the first place.[1] —Anannya Bhattacharjee*

* Of Workers' Awaaz, founding member of Sakhi (an organization of South Asian women in New York, working on domestic violence issues).

the interviewer's question. Doing all this is a great way to break through shyness and stage fright.

Working with the media can have serious drawbacks. Inevitably, distortions occur, even when you are careful about what you say. You may be quoted out of context or misquoted so badly that you seem to be saying the opposite of what you intended. If this happens frequently, you may need to pull back for a while. But try again. Over time it becomes clear which reporters are most reliable, sympathetic, and trustworthy.*

2. *Allies inside government agencies and health institutions* can be useful sources of information (e.g., about upcoming meetings, proposals for new technologies, studies) and can help develop strategies for achieving specific goals. Sometimes these contacts can offer invaluable advice about how best to approach a key official. By offering assistance from the "inside," these women and men who support the women's health movement can make significant contributions.

3. *Writing letters* to legislators and key officials about specific legislation, institutional policies, and regulatory proposals is an effective way to influence policy-makers. Write clearly and concisely, as a group or as private individuals, and point out why your position is in the best interests of women and possibly other constituents of the official addressed. It is important to thank officials for their efforts on your behalf. There will always be a next time!

4. *Forming coalitions,* so that more groups and individuals will support the same cause, can increase political influence as well as establish stronger bonds for future collaboration. Coalitions can provide an excellent means of exchanging new information and ideas, comparing different strategies for change, and even organizing into a larger organization or movement.

When I heard that local authorities near Syracuse were harassing a midwife who had attended a home birth that had complications, I got on a plane to find out how our group could lend its support. The only way we can establish and/or preserve the option of home birth is to challenge repeatedly the unscientific and outrageous assertions made by certain physicians and policy-makers. They want to "stamp out" home birth and even freestyle birth centers by persecuting midwives who make these options possible. We cannot let this happen.

* An excellent media resource is *Promoting Issues and Ideas: A Guide to Public Relations for Non-Profit Organizations*, $24.95. Available from The Foundation Center, 79 Fifth Avenue, New York, NY 10003-3050.

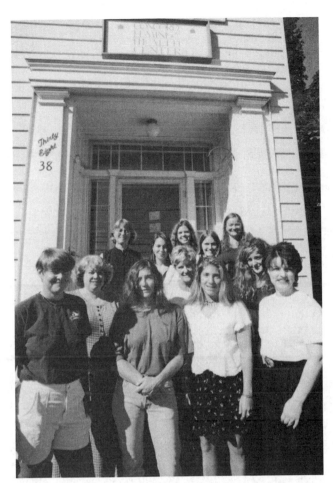

The Concord Feminist Health Center Staff, August 1997/ Steve McColloughy

Some Resources and Tactics

1. *Using the media effectively*—knowing when and how to get publicity when we need it—is essential to all our efforts to bring about change, since most people get almost all their information from TV, movies, newspapers, radio, and magazines. To get the best media coverage possible, it is essential to develop your *speaking skills* for press conferences and interviews with media people both "on" and "off" stage, *writing skills* for press releases and newspaper articles, and *graphic skills* for flyers, posters, and brochures. Sometimes you can find people to donate their graphics and layout services. It is useful to identify journalists sympathetic to your issue and to develop good relationships with them.

In our group, very few women had experience speaking publicly to or before the media. So we set aside some meetings to role-play, to practice speaking before a group, and to learn how to say the most important things in the least amount of time. We also practiced saying the things we wanted people to hear even if it was not related to

5. *Using new technology.* For some of us, cyberspace is quickly becoming part of our everyday lives. New ways of communicating through the Internet, E-mail, and the World Wide Web can be effective and at times inexpensive ways to communicate with women who are doing similar work across the country and around the world. The World Wide Web also has a tremendous amount of information about women's health (see Introduction to Online Women's Health Resources, p. 25). Most low-income and working-class communities lack access to electronic media, but this is rapidly changing. Many public libraries are providing community access, as are some larger community-based organizations. Some colleges and universities also provide access to community members organized around issues of mutual interest. A 30-year-old lesbian and former campus activist tells of her experience in community-building on the Internet:

E-mail has been a powerful tool for community-building in Boston. I have a list geared toward queer women which reaches about 300 people. We send information about queer and progressive political actions, benefit parties, and cultural events. We also provide space for roommate, job, and creative classifieds. My goal is to create linkages between political, artistic, and social communities and to assist them with outreach.

I am on other mailing lists, some for events listings and some for political action. I also use the World Wide Web pages where organizations provide letters you can edit and send to legislators and policy-makers. Being able to personalize a letter drafted by an organization I support and to send it instantly allows me to do more in less time, and avoid retyping, which would aggravate my repetitive strain injuries. The use of the Internet saves valuable resources like trees and funds for envelopes and postage but has some of the same pitfalls as regular mail, in that your messages may be discarded or lost, and you may not get forwarding addresses.

The biggest problem with the Internet is that most people don't have access to it, usually for financial reasons. . . . My advice to organizers is to have a clearly defined mission and to make participation as easy as possible (and requiring as few keystrokes as possible).

Developing a Strong Group

Building Leadership

Key to building an organization or organizing a project is building and sustaining leadership. Many of us have been taught that we should do everything ourselves. This approach may seem more effective than having to train someone else, and it may increase our sense of self-confidence in the short run. In the long run, however, it will exhaust us and prevent new leaders from emerging. A healthy organization supports new leadership by delegating tasks and training less experienced women.

In addition, leaders need to be nurtured and supported. This means supporting them in their roles, volunteering to take on some of their tasks, and forgiving mistakes. Leaders need to hear positive comments as well as thoughtful feedback on errors or hurtful ways of leading.

If you see yourself as a follower rather than a leader, think about taking the leap. Give voice to your ideas and thoughts; take action. Expect that you will make mistakes; the important thing is to take risks and learn from your mistakes, so you won't have to repeat the same ones again.

Developing and Sustaining a Base

The people from your community who are not in your group are invaluable. They are your most important resource, your advocacy base. They can be mobilized to write letters and to attend meetings and demonstrations. They may, at some point, join your group.

If your group represents many communities, it's important to support the members in maintaining and developing ties with their constituents.

I have been working with families of various backgrounds, providing direct services, counseling, advocacy, interpretation, translation, and so on. I work eight hours a day, plus sometimes at nighttime and during the weekend, trying to do my best to help people. I go to people's houses, talk to them, give them information about health care, take pregnant women to the health center and to the WIC office, bring people to ESL classes, go with them to the welfare office, to doctors' appointments, take them to Boston City Hospital to get free care if they are uninsured. I cannot say no to people. When people come to you, that means they really need you, that's what I'm thinking. My boss once told me he has to teach me how to say no sometime.
—A Vietnamese outreach worker

Dealing with Conflict

Even when we initially see ourselves as a homogeneous group, there may be differences among us. As Latinas, for example, we may be indigenous, or of African or European descent, or all of the above. We may be Native American women from the reservation or from the city, with a doctorate or with little or no formal schooling. As African Americans we may have wide differences in income; we may come from urban, rural, or suburban areas. As Asians we may span many countries, languages, or cultures. As white women we may be students or on welfare. Depending on how long we have been in the U.S., our language skills will differ, as will our traditions.

As women we usually have more in common than

WOMEN OF COLOR
ORGANIZING FOR CHANGE

- Opened in 1988, the Native American Women's Health Education Resource Center (NAWHERC) offers community-based activities—support and self-help groups, youth tutoring services, and advocacy/outreach—as well as health education information. In September 1991, the NAWHERC helped open the Women's Lodge/Shelter, a shelter for abused women and/or children. Working through the resource center, the Native Women's Reproductive Rights Coalition, a coalition of women from over 11 Northern Plains nations, came together in 1990 to create an agenda and statement of reproductive rights for Native American women.
- The National Latina Health Organization was formed to raise Latina health consciousness. The NLHO promotes self-help methods and self-empowerment processes as a vehicle for Latinas taking greater control of health practices and lifestyles. They are committed to working toward the goal of bilingual access to high-quality health care and the self-empowerment of Latinas through educational programs, outreach, and research. All programs are bilingual.
- The National Asian Women's Health Organization began in 1993 and works to improve the health status of Asian women and girls.
- The National Black Women's Health Project, a self-help and health advocacy organization, promotes the health and wellness of African-American women, girls, and their families (see p. 747).

See Resources for addresses.

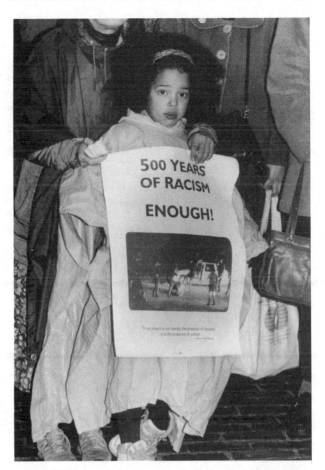

Skip Schiel

we have differences. Yet, inevitably, conflict will occur. In part, our socialization sets up the situation for conflict but also for reconciliation. We have been taught to be competitive (for men, for beauty) and to avoid competition. We've been told to keep quiet and that women can't be leaders.

Sometimes competition for leadership or recognition can be hurtful. Built-up resentment may suddenly burst forth. There may be overt or subtle racism; resources may not be shared fairly.

It is important to sort out and try to resolve these issues without allowing them to consume all of the group's time and energy or to divert the original purpose of the group. At the same time, a group needs to be flexible and to be able to refocus as issues change.

THE SANTA CRUZ
WOMEN'S HEALTH CENTER

The beginning of 1982 marked a turning point in the Santa Cruz Women's Health Collective/Center (SCWHC), when the Bilingual Outreach Program was launched. A mobile health unit (a van equipped with medical and educational supplies) began providing health information, counseling, and referrals directly to three Latino neighborhoods in North Santa Cruz County. The mobile health unit and staff served as a link between Latinas and the bilingual health services offered at the clinic operated by the SCWHC.

A multiracial group of women designed and developed this project for the SCWHC. The dream was to create a bilingual outreach program that would serve the needs of Latinas in our community. The goal of the program was to bring basic information about women's health care to the Latina/o and low income community

continued on next page

santa cruz women's health center

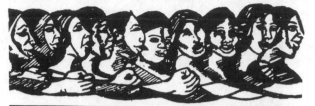

250 locust street
santa cruz, ca 95060
(408) 427-3500

and to give women the information they needed to take more control over their lives and the lives of their children and families. Our process was based on the exchange of information, knowledge, and experience. We learned an enormous amount from the women we served.

The mobile health unit contained a minilab and a library, and it served as a resource center with health information and community referrals. Its staff provided health education classes and counseling, covering such topics as nutrition, high blood pressure, anemia, pregnancy, prenatal care, birth control, and abortion.

The mobile health unit ultimately provided a catalyst for the historic and present-day ethnic and cultural diversification of the staff, clients, and board of directors of the Santa Cruz Women's Health Center. The mobile unit was discontinued but eventually culminated in the formation of Familia Center, a community center run by and for Latinas/os in the barrio of Santa Cruz. Once a project of the SCWHC, Familia Center is now a successful independent Latina/o nonprofit organization. The SCWHC has survived the corporatization of health care, Medicaid managed care, and the demise of many other feminist and neighborhood health centers. Today, the SCWHC provides full primary care services for a diverse clientele of over 3,000 women and children.

For current publications of the SCWHC, see Resources.

NATIONAL WOMEN'S HEALTH NETWORK

The National Women's Health Network, this country's only national membership organization devoted exclusively to the health of all women, influences health policy at the local and national level. Founded in 1975, its membership has grown to over 11,000, and it includes several hundred organizations that represent a constituency of half a million people. Today, its annual budget is $550,000, and it has five staff members at its national headquarters in Washington, DC, and dozens of interns and volunteers. Its committees work on a wide range of women's issues, including reproductive health, access to health care, women and HIV/AIDS, cancer, menopause, and hormone treatments. The Network also maintains a Women's Health Information Clearinghouse.

Among other accomplishments over the past two decades, the NWHN has

- testified at numerous U.S. Senate and House hearings on unsafe birth control pills and devices, drug reform laws, contraceptive research priorities, nurse-midwifery practice, treatment for DES daughters, and unsafe hospital childbirth practices.
- won, with other groups, a precedent-setting lawsuit requiring drug companies to publish patient package information on the risks of menopausal estrogen drugs.
- testified at U.S. Department of Health, Education and Welfare hearings on sterilization abuse and recommended safeguards to ensure informed consent and bilingual patient information.
- organized the first major rural women's health conference in Appalachia in June 1981.
- successfully pressured the federal government to spend $1.5 million to study the effectiveness of the cervical cap and make it available to women nationwide.
- filed a worldwide class-action lawsuit against the A. H. Robins company on behalf of all women damaged or potentially damaged by the Dalkon Shield IUD.
- persuaded the FDA to streamline its approval process for women's condoms and other barrier contraceptives.
- produced the first educational brochure about AIDS prevention that highlighted the risks facing women.

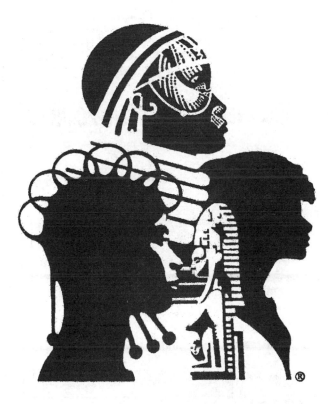

National Black Women's Health Project
Empowerment Through Wellness

The National Black Women's Health Project Logo

- mounted a multiyear campaign to persuade the government to undertake large, long-term studies of the health of older women and possible prevention of breast cancer, which finally resulted in the Women's Health Initiative and WomenCARE.

To contact the NWHN, see Resources.

THE NATIONAL BLACK WOMEN'S HEALTH PROJECT: OUR STORY

The National Black Women's Health Project (NBWHP), founded in 1981, is an internationally known grassroots health advocacy organization. Run by black women for black women, NBWHP rises daily to the challenge of qualitatively enhancing the lives of our sisters.

The mission of the NBWHP is to improve the health of black women through wellness education and services, self-help group development,

and health information and advocacy. NBWHP works

- at the primary prevention level, with individuals and groups.
- at the community action level, where groups influence local health policies that affect them.
- at the national policy level, where the perspectives of African-American women influence policy-makers and the public.
- at the international level, where self-help tools are offered to women in developing nations.

Through a broadened concept of health and an active program, NBWHP enables black women to live, love, and work in new and more authentic ways.

Programs

NBWHP is organized around a core program of services that are provided to our members, our constituents, and the general public.

Self-help group development is the primary focus of NBWHP. Our self-help program is the outreach vehicle through which most of our organizing, leadership development, and advocacy is conducted. The self-help process, used to unearth vital health information, allows each participant to analyze her life and understand her own decision-making abilities. The process of empowerment encourages personal responsibility and commitment to change.

NBWHP works in partnership with seven historically black colleges and universities to establish drug abuse prevention self-help groups.

Walking for wellness, the fitness component of self-help groups, involves sisters walking in groups for 20-minute periods three times a week.

The Public Policy and Education Program researches, analyzes, and promotes public policies that will improve the health status of black women. Consequently, we address a range of health access and equity issues as well as health conditions specific to black women.

SisteReach, an international project, provides self-help group development and technical assistance to women outside the U.S.

Vital Signs, NBWHP's newsmagazine, is distributed to our members, health care providers, and community groups.

To contact the NBWHP, see Resources.

WE ARE TOMORROW'S ABORTION PROVIDERS: MEDICAL STUDENTS FOR CHOICE

In the spring of 1993, tens of thousands of medical students across the country opened their mailboxes at home to find a crudely drawn "joke book" that rewrote old racist, sexist, and other vicious brands of "jokes" and directed them at abortion providers. Coming as it did, virtually on the heals of the murder of Dr. David Gunn, an abortion provider in Florida, it became suddenly obvious to many of us that we, as future physicians, were targets of antichoice extremists.

We then noticed that abortion was excluded from most medical school curricula and residency training programs. This meant that not only were we ill prepared to counsel women about their reproductive health options, but we were even less prepared to provide abortion services if our patients chose that option. Finally, we learned that the vast majority of U.S. counties lack even one abortion provider, and that the absence of trained providers was becoming the largest barrier to choice for women.

Medical students across the country began to come to the same conclusion: If we wanted to learn about abortion in school, be trained in abortion in residency, and find support as future abortion providers, we were going to have to take matters into our own hands.

Today, we are a national nonprofit organization called Medical Students for Choice. We are over 100 schools strong and represent more than 3,100 students nationwide. Our goals include

- reforming the curricula in medical school and residency programs to include abortion.
- expanding opportunities for students to gain clinical experience in reproductive health care through our internship program.
- increasing awareness of the issue among policy-makers.
- supporting grassroots efforts by students around the country.

We are committed, as future physicians, to ensuring that all women have access to a full range of reproductive health services.

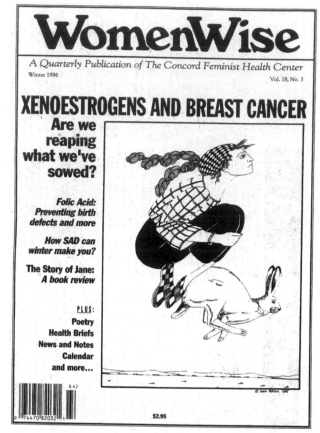

Womenwise (cover of newsletter from the Concord Feminist Health Center)/Sudie Rakusin

THE NORTHWEST COALITION FOR ALTERNATIVES TO PESTICIDES

Founded in 1977, NCAP is a five-state, grassroots membership organization that works to stop the use of pesticides as a preferred method of pest control in the Northwest and elsewhere. NCAP influences public policy on pesticides, educates the public, and works to involve citizens in pest management decisions. NCAP promotes sustainable resource management, prevention of pest problems, the use of alternatives to pesticides, and protection of the individual's right to be free from pesticide exposure.

NCAP plays many roles in the pesticide reform community. Our members serve as educators, policy-makers, critics, and community organizers. We respond to information requests from around the world and participate in ongoing dialogue and strategy-sharing with other activists. Our direct policy initiatives and community organizing efforts focus largely in the Northwest, but via our information services and sharing of model policies, we have influenced policy in many localities in other states and countries. NCAP recognizes that society's dependence on pesticides will be broken only when viable alternatives are available and used. Consequently, our emphasis is not primarily on stricter regulation of pesticides but on the development and implementation of alternative pest control practices and ecologically sound policies.

Over the last 20 years, NCAP has successfully guided the development of comprehensive model pest management policies for forests, schools, roadsides, ground water protection, and state agencies. Real-life examples of citizens successfully replacing conventional pesticides with viable alternatives serve to encourage more individuals and communities to try a different approach.

To contact NCAP, see Resources.

THE PROJECT ON WOMEN AND DISABILITY

The Project on Women and Disability (PWD), which began in 1988 as a project of the Boston Women's Health Book Collective, is a nonprofit organization that serves women whose lives are affected by disability. This includes women with disabilities, mothers, partners, and friends of disabled people, and women working in disability services.

The mission of PWD is to eliminate sex and disability bias in our society, to promote women with disabilities as equal and active members of the workforce and the community, and to enlist men and women as our allies. Among our primary goals are high-quality health care and reproductive rights for disabled women. PWD provides training, discussion and support groups, information, referral, and a quarterly journal on women and disability issues called *WILDA* (Women in Leadership/Disability Issues).

Where do you go for help if you're a divorced mother of two and you're disabled and can't find housing? I've called all the women's hot lines and centers, and none of them could comprehend my disability. It seems that women's services don't understand disability, and disability agencies don't understand the needs of disabled women. In this group, it was such a relief to talk to each other about what it really means to be a female with a disability.

To contact PWD, see Resources.

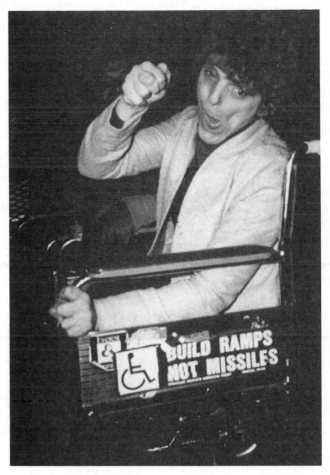

Ellen Shub

WOMEN ORGANIZING IN PRISONS

Almost every woman in prison has led a life defined by racism, poverty, and violence—all risk factors for HIV.

—Laura Whitehorn

Women in prisons face added challenges to organizing that women on the outside do not have to contend with. Along with the lack of freedom, incarcerated women exist in an atmosphere designed to quell expression, unity, and organization—an atmosphere of isolation and degradation. HIV-positive women in prisons also face serious challenges, including limited access to high-quality health care and little or no HIV awareness information.

The percent of women prisoners is on the rise, and a disproportionate number of incarcerated women are black, Latina, or Native American.

continued on next page

The needs of female prisoners, especially those with HIV, have not been met by prison officials. In response, women in prisons have been organizing.

PLACE (Pleasanton AIDS Counseling and Education) was formed in 1991 by women inmates (many of them political prisoners) at FCI-Pleasanton in California (now called FCI-Dublin). Run and organized entirely by incarcerated women, the purpose of PLACE is to provide HIV education and counseling to female inmates. PLACE provides a peer-taught eight-week class on the social and medical aspects of HIV with the assistance of prison staff and makes regular presentations on AIDS/HIV and hepatitis C at orientation sessions for new inmates and pre-release seminars for women who are due to be released. PLACE also provides other ongoing programs, including inviting outside speakers and holding AIDS video showings. In 1993, PLACE organized a showing of the Names Project Quilt at FCI-Dublin. Women at the federal prison in Danbury, Connecticut, made a panel for the Names Quilt with more than 100 names on it.

ACE Against the Odds, a film about a prison-based AIDS counseling and education (ACE) program, describes the advantages of a peer counseling approach and includes role-playing sessions that vividly, sometimes humorously, depict the reality of women's lives (see Resources).

NOTE

1. Linda Wong, "Dragon Ladies," *Sojourner: The Women's Forum* (Nov. 1997): 34.

RESOURCES

Books

Acuña, Eugenia. *Empowerment Workshops on Women's Health.* New York: Hunter College Community Empowerment Training Project, 1995. Available in English and Spanish through Hunter College Community Empowerment Training Project, Box 613, 425 East 25th Street, New York, NY 10025.

Annas, George. *The Rights of Patients: The Basic ACLU Guide to Patient Rights,* 2nd ed. Totowa, NJ: Humana Press, 1992.

Bair, B., and S. E. Cayleff, eds. *Wings of Gauze: Women of Color and the Experience of Health and Illness.* Detroit: Wayne State University Press, 1993.

Children in Hospitals, Inc. *Children in Hospitals. Consumer Directory of Massachusetts Hospitals, 1996–1997.*

Needham, MA: Children in Hospitals, Inc. Available from Children in Hospitals, Inc., 31 Wilshire Park, Needham, MA 02192; (617) 482–2915. Updated every two years.

Dan, Alice J., ed. *Reframing Women's Health.* California: Sage Publications, 1994.

Hope, Anne and Sally Timmel. *Training for Transformation: A Handbook for Community Workers.* Vols. 1–3. Gweru, Zimbabwe: Mambo Press (P.O. Box 779, Gweru Zimbabwe), 1989.

Hubbard, Ruth. *The Politics of Women's Biology.* New Brunswick, NJ: Rutgers University Press, 1990.

Kahn, Si. *How People Get Power.* Washington, DC: NASW Press, 1994.

———. *Organizing: A Guide for Grassroots Leaders.* Washington, DC: NASW Press, 1991.

Lykes, M. Brinton, et al., eds. *Myths about the Powerless: Contesting Social Inequalities.* Philadelphia: Temple University Press, 1996.

Molina, Carlos W., and M. Aguirre-Molina, eds. *Latino Health in the U.S.: A Growing Challenge.* Washington, DC: American Public Health Association, 1994.

National Clearinghouse on Women and Girls with Disabilities. *Bridging the Gap: A National Directory of Services for Women and Girls with Disabilities.* New York: Educational Equity Concepts, 1990.

National Congress of Neighborhood Women. *The Neighborhood Women's Training Sourcebook.* Brooklyn, NY: National Congress of Neighborhood Women, 1993. Available through NCNW: (718) 388-0285.

ProChoice Resource Center. *Strategies for Action: A Grassroots Organizing Manual.* Mamaroneck, NY: ProChoice Resource Center, 1997. Available from ProChoice Resource Center: (914) 381-3792; (800) 733-1973.

Richie, Beth. *Compelled to Crime: The Gender Entrapment of Battered Black Women.* New York: Routledge, 1996.

———. *The Empowerment Program: A Curriculum for Health Education Groups for Women at Rikers Island.* New York: Hunter College Center on AIDS, Drugs and Community Health, 1990.

Ruzek, Sheryl. *The Women's Health Movement: Feminist Alternatives to Medical Control.* New York: Praeger, 1978. A classic.

Shah, Sonia, ed. *Dragon Ladies: Asian American Feminists Breathe Fire.* Boston: South End Press, 1997.

Walters, Shirley, and Linzi Manicom. *Adult Education: Understanding Feminist Mythologies.* London: ZED Books, 1996.

White, Evelyn C., ed. *The Black Women's Health Book: Speaking for Ourselves.* Seattle: Seal Press, 1994.

Articles

Bell, Susan. "Political Gynecology: Gynecological Imperialism and the Politics of Self-Help," *Science for the People* (Sept./Oct. 1979): 8–14. A classic.

The National Black Women's Health Project. *Self-Help Developers' Manual,* rev. ed. 1990. Available from the Project at 175 Trinity Avenue SW, 2nd Floor, Atlanta, GA 30303.

Periodicals

The Fight for Reproductive Freedom
Civil Liberties and Public Policy Program (CLPP)
Hampshire College; Amherst, MA 01002-5001; (413) 582-5645
E-mail: clpp@hampshire.edu
Web site: http://hampshire.edu/~clpp
A newsletter dedicated to issues concerning women students.

Health Facts
Center for Medical Consumers; 237 Thompson Street; New York, NY 10012-1090
Regular, clear, in-depth, referenced discussion of key issues for consumers.

Instantes
A bilingual newsletter of the National Latina Institute for Reproductive Health (see "Organizations").

Off Our Backs
2423 18th Street NW, 2nd Floor; Washington, DC 20009; (202) 234-8092
A feminist newspaper with excellent regular coverage of women's health issues.

Reproductive Freedom News
The Center for Reproductive Law and Policy
120 Wall Street, 18th Floor; New York, NY 10005; (212) 514-5534
A newsletter covering legal aspects of reproductive issues.

Audiovisual Materials

ACE Against the Odds, 30-minute video about a prison-based AIDS peer counseling program. Available from the Women's Prison Association, 110 2nd Avenue, New York, NY 10003; (212) 674-1163. E-mail: rubyrae@aol.com.

Healthcaring from Our End of the Speculum, 35-minutes. A good introductory film covering many different women's health concerns. Available from Women Make Movies, 462 Broadway, Room 500, New York, NY 10013; (212) 925-0606. E-mail: rnso@wmm.com.

La Operacion, a 40-minute 16-mm film. A powerful documentary about sterilization abuse, particularly among Puerto Rican women. Available from The Cinema Guild, 1697 Broadway, Suite 802, New York, NY 10019; (212) 246-5522. E-mail: cinemag@aol.com.

Taking Our Bodies Back: The Women's Health Movement, a 33-minute 1973 film. A classic general film on women's health. To be updated in the early 1990s. Available from Cambridge Documentary Films, Box 390385, Cambridge, MA 02139; (617) 484-3993; E-mail: cdf@shore.net. Web site: http://www.shore.net/~cdf

We Are Not Who You Think We Are. About women in prison. Video/Action Fund, 1000 Potomac Street, NW, Washington, DC 20007; (202) 338-1094.

Women of Substance. About women who use drugs. Video/Action Fund, 1000 Potomac Street, NW, Washington, DC 20007; (202) 338-1094.

Organizations

American Academy of Physician Assistants
950 N. Washington Street; Alexandria, VA 22314-1552; (703) 836-2272
Web site: http://www.apa.org

American Medical Women's Association (AMWA)
801 North Fairfax, Suite 400; Alexandria, VA 22314; (703) 549-3864; Fax: (703) 838-0500
Web site: http://www.amwa_doc.org/index.html
National organization of 12,000 women physicians and medical students dedicated to promoting the personal and professional well-being of women physicians and improved health care for all women. AMWA is active on such issues as reproductive rights, domestic violence, breast cancer, and osteoporosis.

Asian Health Project
T.H.E. Clinic for Women, Inc.
3860 West Martin Luther King Boulevard; Los Angeles, CA 90008; (213) 295-6571
Provides multilingual health information and a wide range of health services to Asian and Pacific communities in Los Angeles County. Multilingual publications on sexual and reproductive health and hygiene for both women and men.

Asian Women's Center
(212) 732-5230; (888) 888-7702
Free confidential services for battered women in the N.Y. area, including a 24-hour hot line, emergency shelter, counseling, advocacy, support groups, and legal assistance.

Association of Physician Assistants in Obstetrics and Gynecology
P.O. Box 1109; Madison, WI 53701

Boston Reproductive Rights Network (R2N2)
P.O. Box 686, Jamaica Plain, MA 02130
A grassroots feminist reproductive rights organization. Organizes demonstrations, picket lines, coalitions, leafleting, clinic defense, conferences, and media campaigns. Publishes *Reproductive Rights Newsletter.*

Center for Science in the Public Interest
1875 Connecticut Avenue, NW, Suite 300; Washington, DC 20009-5728
E-mail: cspi@cspinet.org
Web site: http://www.cspinet.org
Excellent resources, including posters on food and nutrition. Publishes *Nutrition Action.*

Choice in Dying
200 Varick Street; New York, NY 10014-4810; (212) 366-5540
Web site: http://www.choices.org
Works through educational, judicial, and legislative action for recognition of the right to die with dignity. Provides information and advice for consumers and professionals concerned with dying and the development of a living will.

Concord Feminist Health Center
38 South Main Street; Concord, NH 03301; (603) 225-2739
Publishes an excellent quarterly, *WomenWise,* which covers a wide variety of topics on women and health.

The Federation of Feminist Women's Health Centers (FFWHC)
633 E. 11th Avenue; Eugene, OR 97401; (541) 344-0966; Fax: (541) 344-1993
An association of women's health projects, working to secure reproductive rights for women and men, to educate women about the healthy functioning of our bodies and to improve the quality of women's health care.

The Foundation Center
79 Fifth Avenue; New York, NY 10003-3050; (212) 620-4230
Web site: http://fdncenter.org
Publishes *Promoting Issues and Ideas;* provides extensive information on funding sources.

Gray Panthers
1424 16th Street NW, Suite 602; Washington, DC 20036; (202) 387-3111
Nonprofit advocacy organization working on national health and medical care reform.

Health Research Group
c/o Public Citizen
1600 20th Street NW; Washington, DC 20009; (202) 588-1000
Web site: http://www.citizen.org
Ralph Nader–affiliated research and advocacy group. Consumer-oriented publications on drugs, medical devices, occupational and environmental health, health insurance and benefits programs, and related topics.

Latina Rights Initiative (LRI)
Puerto Rican Legal Defense and Education Fund
99 Hudson Street, 14th Floor; New York, NY 10013; (212) 219-3360
Works to establish legislation and legal precedent to enable Latinas to assert their civil rights and to position Latinas' interests into the national and international civil rights agenda.

Latina Roundtable on Health and Reproductive Rights
116 East 16th Street, 7th Floor; New York, NY 10003; (212) 533-9055; Fax: (212) 982-3321
E-mail: latinarights@mindspring.com

Lyon-Martin Women's Health Center
1748 Market Street, Suite 201; San Francisco, CA 94102; (415) 565-7674
A model community clinic staffed and run by women. Committed to providing high-quality, affordable, accessible, nonjudgmental, comprehensive health care to all women, focusing on lesbians, with special outreach to women of color, low-income women, older women, and differently abled women.

Medical Students for Choice
1436 U Street NW, Suite 104; Washington, DC 20009; (202) 667-5881
Web site: http://www.ms4c.org
Organized to ensure an adequate number of abortion providers and to address violence against them.

Montreal Health Press
Box 1000, Station G; Montreal, PQ H2W 2N1, Canada; (514) 282-1171
E-mail: mhpmontreal@msn.com
Web site: http://www.worldsfinest.com/mhp/eng/indexe.html
Publishes *A Book About Birth Control, A Book About Menopause, A Book About Sexually Transmitted Diseases, A Book About Sexual Assault,* and poster kits on female and male reproduction, birth control methods, and abortion. English and French.

Mujeres Project
418 Villita, Building 246; HemisFair Plaza; San Antonio, TX 78205; (210) 222-9417
Advocacy group and resource center that provides information on reproductive health and rights, particularly for Latinas.

National Asian Women's Health Organization (see p. 745)
250 Montgomery Street, #410; San Francisco, CA 94104-3401; (415) 989-9747

National Black Women's Health Project (NBWHP) (see p. 747)
1211 Connecticut Avenue NW, Suite 310; Washington DC 20005; (800) 444-6472; Fax: (202) 833-8798

National Clearinghouse on Women and Girls with Disabilities
Educational Equity Concepts, Inc.
114 East 32nd Street; New York, NY 10016; (212) 725-1803
Web site: http://www.onisland.com/eec
Actively promotes equal opportunities through educational programs and materials that address the intersections of race, disability, and low income. Special concerns: teenage pregnancy and parenting and sex role stereotyping; the special educational needs of women and girls with disabilities.

National Health Law Program
2639 South La Cienega Boulevard; Los Angeles, CA 90034; (310) 204-6010
E-mail: nhelp@healthlaw.org
Web site: http://www.healthlaw.org/index.html
   Publishes the *Health Advocate* newsletter and other materials. Covers many issues of concern to women.

National Latina Health Organization (NLHO)/Organizacion Nacional de la Salud de la Mujer Latina (see p. 745)
P.O. Box 7567; Oakland, CA 94601; (510) 534-1362; (800) 971-5358
Web site: http://clnet.ucr.edu/women/nlho
   Offers bilingual classes and workshops on health issues, training for self-help, and publications.

National Latina Institute for Reproductive Health (NLIRH)
1200 New York Avenue, Suite 300; Washington, DC 20005; (202) 326-8970; Fax: (202) 371-8112
   A pro-choice organization working to enhance the quality of life for Latinas nationwide, especially their reproductive health, through advocacy, networking, information, and education and by impacting public policy. They are committed to promote and defend access to appropriate, comprehensive health information and services for Latinas.

National Women's Health Network (see p. 746)
514 Tenth Street NW, Suite 400; Washington, DC 20004; (202) 347-1140 (Voice); Clearinghouse: (202) 628-7814
   A national consumer/provider membership organization; monitors and works to influence government and industry policies. Publishes *Network News.*

National Women's Studies Association
7100 Baltimore Boulevard, Suite 501; University of Maryland; College Park, MD 20740; (301) 403-0525
E-mail: nwsa@umail.umd.edu
Web site: http://www.feminist.com/nwsa.htm
   Large membership organization promoting feminist and women's studies in all educational institutions as well as the larger community.

Native American Women's Health Education Resource Center (NAWHERC) (see p. 745)
P.O. Box 572; Lake Andes, SD 57356-0572; (605) 487-7072
E-mail: nativewoman@igc.apc.org

New Day Films
22-D Hollywood Avenue; Hohokus, NJ 07432; (201) 652-6590
Web site: http://www.newday.com
   A cooperative distribution organization of independent media producers who make films and videotapes about social, political, and cultural issues, including women's experience and health.

Northwest Coalition for Alternatives to Pesticides (NCAP) (see p. 748)
P.O. Box 1393; Eugene, OR 97440; (541) 344-5044
E-mail: info@pesticide.org
Web site: http://www.efn.org/~ncap

Nurses for National Health Care
P.O. Box 441021; Somerville, MA 02144
   Nurses working together with consumers and other health care workers to support the creation of a national health care program in the U.S. that promotes the health of every person.

The Project on Women and Disability (see p. 749)
c/o Janna Jacobs
43 Waban Hill North; Newton, MA 02167; (617) 969-4974

Research Action and Information Network for Bodily Integrity of Women (RAINB♀)
915 Broadway, Suite 1109; New York, NY 10010; (212) 477-3318; Fax: (212) 477-4154
E-mail: nt61@columbia.edu
Web site: http://www.rainbo.org
   Focuses on female genital mutilation (FGM)

Santa Cruz Women's Health Center (see p. 745)
250 Locust Street; Santa Cruz, CA 95060; (408) 427-3500

Sakhi for South Asian Women
P.O. Box 20208, Greeley Square Station; New York, NY 10001; (212) 695-5447
E-mail: sakhiny@aol.com
Web site: http://www.sakhi.com
   Community-based organization committed to ending exploitation and violence against South Asian women. Outreach, advocacy, leadership development, and organizing.

South Asian Women for Action (SAWA)
2 Wheeler Road; Bolton, MA 01740;
Web site: http://www.sawa.way.net
   A collective of women of South Asian descent formed for mutual support, creative expression, and political activism against discrimination.

Taller Salud
Apartado Postal 192172; San Juan, Puerto Rico 00919-2172
   Puerto Rican women's educational and advocacy organization that offers materials in Spanish on topics such as breast cancer, AIDS, and sexuality.

Vancouver Women's Health Collective/Le Collectif de la Sante des Femmes de Vancouver
1720 Grant Street, Suite 302; Vancouver, BC V5L 2Y7, Canada; (604) 255-8285
   A resource center promoting a self-help approach to health care, with files, books, and journals on all aspects of women's health. The collective also offers a practitioner referral directory, phone line for questions or referrals, and workshops on health topics.

Women Make Movies
462 Broadway, Room 500; New York, NY 10013; (212) 925-0606
E-mail: rnso@wmm.com
A leading distributor of films by and about women in the U.S. Has an excellent collection of films about women's health and reproductive rights.

Women Organizing and Diversity
Women Organizer's Project of ECCO (Education Center for Community Organizing)
c/o Hunter College School of Social Work; 129 East 79th Street; New York, NY 10021; (212) 452-7132

Women's Health Action Mobilization (WHAM)
P.O. Box 733; New York, NY 10009; (212) 560-7177
Web site: http://www.echonyc.com/~wham/wham.html
WHAM is a direct-action group demanding, securing, and defending reproductive freedom and high-quality health care for all women. Its actions range from escorting women into clinics to dropping banners off the Statue of Liberty. Contact the New York group for affiliates in other cities.

Women's Health Empowerment and Training
Proyecto Mujer, Salud y Poder
Box 613, Hunter College; 425 East 25th Street; New York, NY 10010; (212) 481-5141
E-mail: eacuna@shiva.hunter.cuny.edu
Workshops, support groups, curriculum, and facilitator trainings on Latina reproductive health and empowerment.

Women's Legal Defense Fund (WLDF)
1875 Connecticut Avenue NW, Suite 710; Washington, DC 20009; (202) 986-2600
E-mail: info@wldf.org
Web site: http://www.afjorg/wldf.html
Through legislative channels, policy-making, and advocacy, works to shape a society that offers equal opportunity to every person, that responds to women's basic economic and health needs, and that embraces policies that enable women and men to live with dignity and participate fully in every aspect of family and community life.

Additional Online Resources *

Alliance For Justice
http://www.afj.org

Feminist Activist Resources on the Net
http://www.igc.apc.org/women/feminist.html

Feminism and Women's Resources Page
http://www.ibd.nrc.ca/~mansfield/feminism

Public Interests Groups' Hub
http://www.essential.org

WebActive Directory
http://www.webactive.com/webactive/cgi-bin/wniadirsearch?Women

Women Leaders Online, E-mail discussion: wlo@wlo.org

* For more information and listings of online resources, please see Introduction to Online Women's Health Resources, p. 25.

Index

salt, 444, 445; hypertension and, 647, 648; reducing, 48–49

Santa Cruz Women's Health Collective/Center (SCWHC), 745–746

Santeria, 117

Satter, Ellyn, 53

saturated fats, 48, 49

scabies, 342, 634–35

Schiller's test, 595

school meals, 56–57; government programs for, 59

scleroderma, 602

scopolamine, 491

Seaman, Barbara, 309

search engines, 28

Searle Corporation, 68

sebaceous glands, 275

Seconal, 80

secondhand smoke, 84

second opinions, 597, 623, 663, 707

second-parent adoption, 218, 223

sedative-hypnotics, 80

sedatives, 78

segmental mastectomy, 626

selective estrogen receptor modulator (SERMs), 562

selenium, 615

self-care groups, 712, 717

self-defense, 173

Self-Employed Women's Association (SEWA), 728

self-examination: breast, 275, 605, 606; vaginal, 269–74, 593

self-help groups, see support and self-help groups

Self-Help Resources, 28

self-injury, 171

semen analysis, 536

Semicid spermicide, 305

senile dementia of the Alzheimer type (SDAT), 575

sensory loss, 570–72

sensuality, 243

septic abortion, 325, 328, 329

seroconversion, 362

serotonin, 125

714X, 621

sex industry, 172–73, 362; international, 730–31

sex information, obstacles to, 289

sexism, 106, 122, 702; ageism and, 568; HIV/AIDS and, 360, 361; in insurance industry, 694; in sexual relationships with men, 230–31; violence and, 159

sex organs, see reproductive system

sex preselection, 427, 429–30

sex-role stereotypes, see gender roles, traditional

sex toys, 367

sexual abuse, 170–72; by doctors, 686–87; eating disorders and, 61, 63; pregnancy and history of, 458

sexual assault, see rape

sexual harassment, 147–48, 160–62, 233

sexual health care, 255

sexuality, 229–62; aging and, 563–565; breast-feeding and, 507; celibacy and, 236–37; changes in, of rape survivors, 167; during childhood and adolescence, 234–535; communicating about, 247–248; disability and, 248–53; hysterectomy and oophorectomy and, 664, 666; of l/b/t women, 209–11; models of response, 237–238; oral contraceptives and, 315; postpartum, 511; problems with, 256–57; social influences on, 230–234; substance abuse and, 76; testosterone and, 255–56; see also lovemaking

sexually transmitted diseases (STDs), 188, 263, 324, 341–58, 447, 563; birth control methods and, 288, 289, 292, 298–300, 323, 326–30, 343, 345; cervical disorders and, 653, 655; home testing for, 346; infertility from, 533, 534; legal issues of, 348; PID and, 657–59, 661; prevention of, 344–46, 406; rape and exposure to, 168; social problems of, 345–46; in Third World, 727, 732; treatment of,

346–47; see also HIV/AIDS and other specific diseases

sexual orientation, 179–83

shared power, 188–89

shark cartilage, 622

shiatsu, 111

shift work, 147

Shimizu, Jenny, 201

Shodhini, 735

shoulder injuries, work-related, 146

sickle-cell anemia, 313, 443, 463, 599

silicone gel breast implants, 628

Simonton technique, 622

Sims-Hubner test, 536

single mothers, 520–21

single-payer system, 693, 695

single women, 187; l/b/t, 212–13; safety of, 188

Sjogren's syndrome, 602–3

Sjogren's Syndrome Foundation, 603

skin, effect of exercise on, 566

skin cancer, 314

skin disorders: environmental causes of, 136–37; oral contraceptives and, 315

sleep: fibromyalgia and, 602; menstruation and, 281

Sloan-Kettering research center, 621

SMART Recovery, 82

Smith, Margaret Charles, 452–53

smoking, 75, 83–85, 691; alcohol use and, 77–78; cancer and, 64, 561, 613, 614, 655; diabetes and, 639, 640; environmental hazards interacting with, 137; heart disease and, 645, 647; HIV and, 371; hypertension and, 648; infertility and, 534; Norplant and, 320; nutritional needs and, 53; oral contraceptives and, 312–13, 316; osteoporosis and, 561, 573; during pregnancy, 446; public health programs on, 704; quitting, 84–85; stress and, 31; withdrawal from, 76

snack foods, 47; advertising of, 68

social control of women's lives, 684–685

☆☆☆☆☆ **Puzzle 27**☆

My number is a square
number.

☆☆☆☆☆ **Puzzle 27**☆

My number is a factor
of 10,000.

☆☆☆☆☆ **Puzzle 27**☆

My number is even.

☆☆☆☆☆ **Puzzle 27**☆

My number has two digits.

☆☆☆☆☆ **Puzzle 28**☆

My number is a factor of 1000.

☆☆☆☆☆ **Puzzle 28**☆

My number is not a factor
of 10,000.

☆☆☆☆☆ **Puzzle 28**☆

My number is a multiple of 50.

☆☆☆☆☆ **Puzzle 28**☆

My number is a multiple of 8.

Introduction
Landmarks in the Number System

Mathematical Thinking at Grade 5

Grade 5

Also appropriate for Grade 6

Marlene Kliman
Cornelia Tierney
Susan Jo Russell
Megan Murray
Joan Akers

Developed at TERC, Cambridge, Massachusetts

Dale Seymour Publications®
Menlo Park, California

The *Investigations* curriculum was developed at TERC (formerly Technical Education Research Centers) in collaboration with Kent State University and the State University of New York at Buffalo. The work was supported in part by National Science Foundation Grant No. ESI-9050210. TERC is a nonprofit company working to improve mathematics and science education. TERC is located at 2067 Massachusetts Avenue, Cambridge, MA 02140.

This project was supported, in part,
by the
National Science Foundation
Opinions expressed are those of the authors
and not necessarily those of the Foundation

Managing Editor: Catherine Anderson
Series Editor: Beverly Cory
Revision Team: Laura Marshall Alavosus, Ellen Harding, Patty Green Holubar, Suzanne Knott, Beverly Hersh Lozoff
ESL Consultant: Nancy Sokol Green
Production/Manufacturing Director: Janet Yearian
Production/Manufacturing Manager: Karen Edmonds
Production/Manufacturing Coordinator: Joe Conte
Design Manager: Jeff Kelly
Design: Don Taka
Illustrations: DJ Simison, Carl Yoshihara
Cover: Bay Graphics
Composition: Archetype Book Composition

This book is published by Dale Seymour Publications®, an imprint of Addison Wesley Longman, Inc.

Dale Seymour Publications
2725 Sand Hill Road
Menlo Park, CA 94025
Customer Service: 800-872-1100

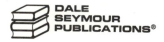
DALE
SEYMOUR
PUBLICATIONS®

Order number DS47043
ISBN 1-57232-796-0
1 2 3 4 5 6 7 8 9 10-ML-01 00 99 98 97

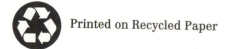
Printed on Recycled Paper

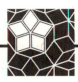

T E R C

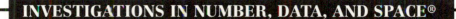

Principal Investigator   Susan Jo Russell

Co-Principal Investigator   Cornelia C. Tierney

Director of Research and Evaluation   Jan Mokros

Curriculum Development

Joan Akers
Michael T. Battista
Mary Berle-Carman
Douglas H. Clements
Karen Economopoulos
Claryce Evans
Marlene Kliman
Cliff Konold
Jan Mokros
Megan Murray
Ricardo Nemirovsky
Tracy Noble
Andee Rubin
Susan Jo Russell
Margie Singer
Cornelia C. Tierney

Evaluation and Assessment

Mary Berle-Carman
Jan Mokros
Andee Rubin
Tracey Wright

Teacher Support

Kabba Colley
Karen Economopoulos
Anne Goodrow
Nancy Ishihara
Liana Laughlin
Jerrie Moffett
Megan Murray
Margie Singer
Dewi Win
Virginia Woolley
Tracey Wright
Lisa Yaffee

Administration and Production

Irene Baker
Amy Catlin
Amy Taber

Cooperating Classrooms for This Unit

Betsy Hale
Arlington Public Schools
Arlington, MA
Judy Hanlon
Winter Hill Community School
Somerville, MA
Jo-Ann Pepicelli
Curtis Guild School
Boston, MA

Technology Development

Douglas H. Clements
Julie Sarama

Video Production

David A. Smith
Judy Storeygard

Consultants and Advisors

Deborah Lowenberg Ball
Marilyn Burns
Mary Johnson
James J. Kaput
Mary M. Lindquist
Leslie P. Steffe
Grayson Wheatley

Graduate Assistants

Kent State University
Richard Aistrope
Kathryn Battista
Caroline Borrow
William Hunt

State University of New York at Buffalo
Jeffrey Barrett
Julie Sarama
Sudha Swaminathan
Elaine Vukelic

Harvard Graduate School of Education
Dan Gillette
Irene Hall

Revisions and Home Materials

Cathy Miles Grant
Marlene Kliman
Margaret McGaffigan
Megan Murray
Kim O'Neil
Andee Rubin
Susan Jo Russell
Lisa Seyferth
Myriam Steinback
Judy Storeygard
Anna Suarez
Cornelia Tierney
Carol Walker
Tracey Wright

CONTENTS

TEACHER NOTES

WHERE TO START

The first-time user of *Mathematical Thinking at Grade 5* should read the following:

When you next teach this same unit, you can begin to read more of the background. Each time you present the unit, you will learn more about how your students understand the mathematical ideas.

Investigations in Number, Data, and Space® is a K–5 mathematics curriculum with four major goals:

- to offer students meaningful mathematical problems
- to emphasize depth in mathematical thinking rather than superficial exposure to a series of fragmented topics
- to communicate mathematics content and pedagogy to teachers
- to substantially expand the pool of mathematically literate students

The *Investigations* curriculum embodies a new approach based on years of research about how children learn mathematics. Each grade level consists of a set of separate units, each offering 2–8 weeks of work. These units of study are presented through investigations that involve students in the exploration of major mathematical ideas.

Approaching the mathematics content through investigations helps students develop flexibility and confidence in approaching problems, fluency in using mathematical skills and tools to solve problems, and proficiency in evaluating their solutions. Students also build a repertoire of ways to communicate about their mathematical thinking, while their enjoyment and appreciation of mathematics grows.

The investigations are carefully designed to invite all students into mathematics—girls and boys, members of diverse cultural, ethnic, and language groups, and students with different strengths and interests. Problem contexts often call on students to share experiences from their family, culture, or community. The curriculum eliminates barriers—such as work in isolation from peers, or emphasis on speed and memorization—that exclude some students from participating successfully in mathematics. The following aspects of the curriculum ensure that all students are included in significant mathematics learning:

- Students spend time exploring problems in depth.
- They find more than one solution to many of the problems they work on.

- They invent their own strategies and approaches, rather than relying on memorized procedures.
- They choose from a variety of concrete materials and appropriate technology, including calculators, as a natural part of their everyday mathematical work.
- They express their mathematical thinking through drawing, writing, and talking.
- They work in a variety of groupings—as a whole class, individually, in pairs, and in small groups.
- They move around the classroom as they explore the mathematics in their environment and talk with their peers.

While reading and other language activities are typically given a great deal of time and emphasis in elementary classrooms, mathematics often does not get the time it needs. If students are to experience mathematics in depth, they must have enough time to become engaged in real mathematical problems. We believe that a minimum of five hours of mathematics classroom time a week—about an hour a day—is critical at the elementary level. The plan and pacing of the *Investigations* curriculum is based on that belief.

We explain more about the pedagogy and principles that underlie these investigations in Teacher Notes throughout the units. For correlations of the curriculum to the NCTM Standards and further help in using this research-based program for teaching mathematics, see the following books:

- *Implementing the* Investigations in Number, Data, and Space® *Curriculum*
- *Beyond Arithmetic: Changing Mathematics in the Elementary Classroom* by Jan Mokros, Susan Jo Russell, and Karen Economopoulos

This book is one of the curriculum units for *Investigations in Number, Data, and Space.* In addition to providing part of a complete mathematics curriculum for your students, this unit offers information to support your own professional development. You, the teacher, are the person who will make this curriculum come alive in the classroom; the book for each unit is your main support system.

Although the curriculum does not include student textbooks, reproducible sheets for student work are provided in the unit and are also available as Student Activity Booklets. Students work actively with objects and experiences in their own environment and with a variety of manipulative materials and technology, rather than with a book of instruction and problems. We strongly recommend use of the overhead projector as a way to present problems, to focus group discussion, and to help students share ideas and strategies.

Ultimately, every teacher will use these investigations in ways that make sense for his or her

particular style, the particular group of students, and the constraints and supports of a particular school environment. Each unit offers information and guidance for a wide variety of situations, drawn from our collaborations with many teachers and students over many years. Our goal in this book is to help you, a professional educator, implement this curriculum in a way that will give all your students access to mathematical power.

Investigation Format

The opening two pages of each investigation help you get ready for the work that follows.

What Happens This gives a synopsis of each session or block of sessions.

Mathematical Emphasis This lists the most important ideas and processes students will encounter in this investigation.

What to Plan Ahead of Time These lists alert you to materials to gather, sheets to duplicate, transparencies to make, and anything else you need to do before starting.

INVESTIGATION 2

Multiples and Factors up to 1000

What Happens

Session 1: Skip Counting and Other Ways to Multiply Students count around the class by factors of 100 and their multiples. They use what they know about counting by 25 to make predictions about counting by 50 and 100. Partners then brainstorm strategies for remembering difficult factor pairs.

Sessions 2, 3, and 4: Factor Pairs from 100 to 1000 Students first find all the factor pairs of 100, and they write about how they know they found them all. They use their knowledge of factor pairs of 100 to find factor pairs of multiples of 100, such as 200 and 300. Working in pairs, they make two different rectangles containing 1000 squares. Groups then brainstorm a list of all the factor pairs of 1000.

Session 5: Exploring Rectangles of 1000 Squares After learning a system for numbering the individual squares that make up their 20 × 50 and 25 × 40 rectangles, students find the squares that correspond to certain numbers. They compare strategies for finding the squares on the two different rectangles (20 × 50 and 25 × 40). Finally, they make a class display of 10,000 squares.

Mathematical Emphasis

- Using knowledge of landmarks up to 100 (including factors of 100 and multiples of those factors) to explore landmarks up to 1000
- Becoming familiar with factors and factor pairs of 1000
- Developing a variety of strategies for exploring number composition, such as repeated addition, skip counting, finding factors, finding factor pairs, and using a calculator to check divisibility
- Reading, writing, and ordering numbers to 1000
- Developing a sense of the magnitude of 1000
- Becoming familiar with skip-counting patterns (sequences of multiples such as 25, 50, 75, . . .) leading to 1000

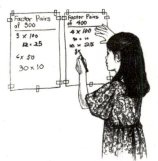

INVESTIGATION 2

What to Plan Ahead of Time

Materials

- Square tiles: have available for use as needed (Sessions 1–4)
- Scissors: 1 per pair (Sessions 2–4)
- Tape: at least 1 roll for every 4 students (Sessions 2–4)
- Overhead projector (Sessions 1–4, optional)
- Calculators: available (Sessions 2–4)
- Chart paper (Sessions 2–4, optional)
- Notebook paper: 1 sheet per student (Session 5)

Other Preparation

- Make a 20 × 50 or 25 × 40 rectangle of graph paper for each pair of students. (Session 5)
- Make a 50 × 20 grid for class display. The grid should be large enough for everyone in the class to see. You might use square-inch graph paper, either a roll or smaller sheets taped together. Or you could draw a 50 (across) by 20 (down) grid of squares, 1 inch or larger, on the board. If you have a very small class, you could use centimeter paper. (Session 5)
- Duplicate student sheets and teaching resources, located at the end of this unit, in the following quantities. If you have Student Activity Booklets, copy only the transparency and extra materials marked with an asterisk.

For all sessions

A supply of 300 charts (p. 158): 3–5 per student, available for use as needed

For Session 1

Student Sheet 8, Find the Counting Numbers (p. 119): 1 per student (homework)

For Sessions 2–4

15 × 20 grid (p. 122): 10 per pair, plus approximately 20 extras.* Note: Make all copies of this grid directly from the master on p. 122 or from the same copy of the master to ensure that all grid squares are the same size.

One-centimeter graph paper (p. 157): 5–7 per student, available for use as needed, and 1 transparency*

Student Sheet 9, More Factor Pairs (p. 120): 1 per student (homework)

Student Sheet 10, Counting Backward (p. 121): 1 per student (homework)

Sessions Within an investigation, the activities are organized by class session, a session being at least a one-hour math class. Sessions are numbered consecutively through an investigation. Often several sessions are grouped together, presenting a block of activities with a single major focus.

When you find a block of sessions presented together—for example, Sessions 1, 2, and 3—read through the entire block first to understand the overall flow and sequence of the activities. Make some preliminary decisions about how you will divide the activities into three sessions for your class, based on what you know about your students. You may need to modify your initial plans as you progress through the activities, and you may want to make notes in the margins of the pages as reminders for the next time you use the unit.

Be sure to read the Session Follow-Up section at the end of the session block to see what homework assignments and extensions are suggested as you make your initial plans.

While you may be used to a curriculum that tells you exactly what each class session should cover, we have found that the teacher is in a better position to make these decisions. Each unit is flexible and may be handled somewhat differently by every teacher. While we provide guidance for how many sessions a particular group of activities is likely to need, we want you to be active in determining an appropriate pace and the best transition points for your class. It is not unusual for a teacher to spend more or less time than is proposed for the activities.

Ten-Minute Math At the beginning of some sessions, you will find Ten-Minute Math activities. These are designed to be used in tandem with the investigations, but not during the math hour. Rather, we hope you will do them whenever you have a spare 10 minutes—maybe before lunch or recess, or at the end of the day.

Ten-Minute Math offers practice in key concepts, but not always those being covered in the unit. For example, in a unit on using data, Ten-Minute Math might revisit geometric activities done earlier in the year. Complete directions for the suggested activities are included at the end of each unit.

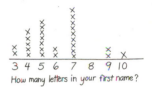

For full directions and variations, see p. 96.

Activities The activities include pair and small-group work, individual tasks, and whole-class discussions. In any case, students are seated together, talking and sharing ideas during all work times. Students most often work cooperatively, although each student may record work individually.

Choice Time In some units, some sessions are structured with activity choices. In these cases, students may work simultaneously on different activities focused on the same mathematical ideas. Students choose which activities they want to do, and they cycle through them.

You will need to decide how to set up and introduce these activities and how to let students make their choices. Some teachers present them as station activities, in different parts of the room. Some list the choices on the board as reminders or have students keep their own lists.

Extensions Sometimes in Session Follow-Up, you will find suggested extension activities. These are opportunities for some or all students to explore a topic in greater depth or in a different context.

They are not designed for "fast" students; mathematics is a multifaceted discipline, and different students will want to go further in different investigations. Look for and encourage the sparks of interest and enthusiasm you see in your students, and use the extensions to help them pursue these interests.

Excursions Some of the *Investigations* units include excursions—blocks of activities that could be omitted without harming the integrity of the unit. This is one way of dealing with the great depth and variety of elementary mathematics—much more than a class has time to explore in any one year. Excursions give you the flexibility to make different choices from year to year, doing the excursion in one unit this time, and next year trying another excursion.

Tips for the Linguistically Diverse Classroom At strategic points in each unit, you will find concrete suggestions for simple modifications of the teaching strategies to encourage the participation of all students. Many of these tips offer alternative ways to elicit critical thinking from students at varying levels of English proficiency, as well as from other students who find it difficult to verbalize their thinking.

The tips are supported by suggestions for specific vocabulary work to help ensure that all students can participate fully in the investigations. The Preview for the Linguistically Diverse Classroom (p. I-21) lists important words that are assumed as part of the working vocabulary of the unit. Second-language learners will need to become familiar with these words in order to understand the problems and activities they will be doing. These terms can be incorporated into students' second-language work before or during the unit. Activities that can be used to present the words are found in the appendix, Vocabulary Support for Second-Language Learners (p. 100). In addition, ideas for making connections to students' language and cultures, included on the Preview page, help the class explore the unit's concepts from a multicultural perspective.

Materials

A complete list of the materials needed for teaching this unit is found on p. I-17. Some of these materials are available in kits for the *Investigations* curriculum. Individual items can also be purchased from school supply dealers.

Classroom Materials In an active mathematics classroom, certain basic materials should be available at all times: interlocking cubes, pencils, unlined paper, graph paper, calculators, things to count with, and measuring tools. Some activities in this curriculum require scissors and glue sticks or tape. Stick-on notes and large paper are also useful materials throughout.

So that students can independently get what they need at any time, they should know where these materials are kept, how they are stored, and how they are to be returned to the storage area. For example, interlocking cubes are best stored in towers of ten; then, whatever the activity, they should be returned to storage in groups of ten at the end of the hour. You'll find that establishing such routines at the beginning of the year is well worth the time and effort.

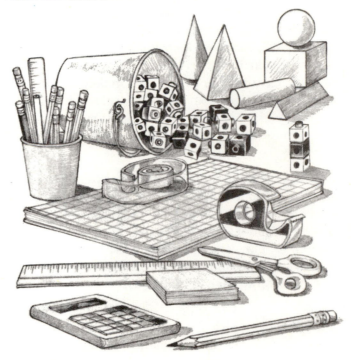

Technology Calculators are used throughout *Investigations*. Many of the units recommend that you have at least one calculator for each pair. You will find calculator activities, plus Teacher Notes discussing this important mathematical tool, in an early unit at each grade level. It is assumed that calculators will be readily available for student use.

Computer activities at grade 5 use two software programs that were developed especially for the *Investigations* curriculum. The program *Geo-Logo*™ is used for activities in the 2-D Geometry unit, *Picturing Polygons,* where students investigate the properties of geometric figures while drawing them on the computer. *Trips* software, which helps students use tables and graphs to explore how things change over time, is used with the unit *Patterns of Change.*

How you use the computer activities depends on the number of computers you have available. Suggestions are offered in the geometry units for how to organize different types of computer environments.

Children's Literature Each unit offers a list of suggested children's literature (p. I-17) that can be used to support the mathematical ideas in the unit. Sometimes an activity is based on a specific children's book, with suggestions for substitutions where practical. While such activities can be adapted and taught without the book, the literature offers a rich introduction and should be used whenever possible.

Student Sheets and Teaching Resources Student recording sheets and other teaching tools needed for both class and homework are provided as reproducible blackline masters at the end of each unit. They are also available as Student Activity Booklets. These booklets contain all the sheets each student will need for individual work, freeing you from extensive copying (although you may need or want to copy the occasional teaching resource on transparency film or card stock, or make extra copies of a student sheet).

We think it's important that students find their own ways of organizing and recording their work. They need to learn how to explain their thinking with both drawings and written words, and how

---

---

to organize their results so someone else can understand them. For this reason, we deliberately do not provide student sheets for every activity. Regardless of the form in which students do their work, we recommend that they keep a mathematics notebook or folder so that their work is always available for reference.

Homework In *Investigations,* homework is an extension of classroom work. Sometimes it offers review and practice of work done in class, sometimes preparation for upcoming activities, and sometimes numerical practice that revisits work in earlier units. Homework plays a role both in supporting students' learning and in helping inform families about the ways in which students in this curriculum work with mathematical ideas.

Depending on your school's homework policies and your own judgment, you may want to assign more homework than is suggested in the units. For this purpose you might use the practice pages, included as blackline masters at the end of this unit, to give students additional work with numbers.

For some homework assignments, you will want to adapt the activity to meet the needs of a variety of students in your class: those with special needs, those ready for more challenge, and second-language learners. You might change the numbers in a problem, make the activity more or less complex, or go through a sample activity with those who need extra help. You can modify any student sheet for either homework or class use. In particular, making numbers in a problem smaller or larger can make the same basic activity appropriate for a wider range of students.

Another issue to consider is how to handle the homework that students bring back to class—how to recognize the work they have done at home without spending too much time on it. Some teachers hold a short group discussion of different approaches to the assignment; others ask students to share and discuss their work with a neighbor, or post the homework around the room and give students time to tour it briefly. If you want to keep track of homework students bring in, be sure it ends up in a designated place.

Investigations at Home It is a good idea to make your policy on homework explicit to both students and their families when you begin teaching with *Investigations*. How frequently will you be assigning homework? When do you expect homework to be completed and brought back to school? What are your goals in assigning homework? How independent should families expect their children to be? What should the parent's or guardian's role be? The more explicit you can be about your expectations, the better the homework experience will be for everyone.

Investigations at Home (a booklet available separately for each unit, to send home with students) gives you a way to communicate with families about the work students are doing in class. This booklet includes a brief description of every session, a list of the mathematics content emphasized in each investigation, and a discussion of each homework assignment to help families more effectively support their children. Whether or not you are using the *Investigations* at Home booklets, we expect you to make your own choices about home-

work assignments. Feel free to omit any and to add extra ones you think are appropriate.

Family Letter A letter that you can send home to students' families is included with the blackline masters for each unit. Families need to be informed about the mathematics work in your classroom; they should be encouraged to participate in and support their children's work. A reminder to send home the letter for each unit appears in one of the early investigations. These letters are also available separately in Spanish, Vietnamese, Cantonese, Hmong, and Cambodian.

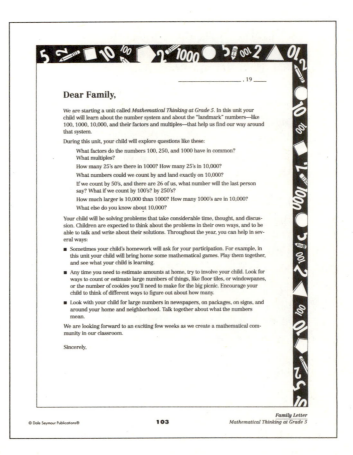

Help for You, the Teacher

Because we believe strongly that a new curriculum must help teachers think in new ways about mathematics and about their students' mathematical thinking processes, we have included a great deal of material to help you learn more about both.

About the Mathematics in This Unit This introductory section (p. I-18) summarizes the critical information about the mathematics you will be teaching. It describes the unit's central mathematical ideas and how students will encounter them through the unit's activities.

Teacher Notes These reference notes provide practical information about the mathematics you are teaching and about our experience with how students learn. Many of the notes were written in response to actual questions from teachers, or to discuss important things we saw happening in the field-test classrooms. Some teachers like to read them all before starting the unit, then review them as they come up in particular investigations.

Dialogue Boxes Sample dialogues demonstrate how students typically express their mathematical ideas, what issues and confusions arise in their thinking, and how some teachers have guided class discussions.

These dialogues are based on the extensive classroom testing of this curriculum; many are word-for-word transcriptions of recorded class discussions. They are not always easy reading; sometimes it may take some effort to unravel what the students are trying to say. But this is the value of these dialogues; they offer good clues to how your students may develop and express their approaches and strategies, helping you prepare for your own class discussions.

Where to Start You may not have time to read everything the first time you use this unit. As a first-time user, you will likely focus on understanding the activities and working them out with your students. Read completely through each investigation before starting to present it. Also read those sections listed in the Contents under the heading Where to Start (p. vi).

Teacher Note ▶ **Powers of 10: How Much Larger, and How Many Times as Large?**

Understanding relationships among powers of ten is an essential part of understanding the structure of our number system. When students first begin exploring powers of ten, they are often surprised at just how much larger each power of ten is than the one before. Even students who have memorized the place headings, and the fact that each is ten times more than the previous one, may not have a sense of the size of these numbers.

For example, some students may at first assume that it is just as far from 1 to 1000 as it is from 1000 to 1,000,000. They may be likely to respond "1 million" to questions such as: "What's 1 thousand more than 1 thousand?" or "What number is 10 times as large as 1 thousand?" In order to grasp relationships among powers of ten, students need a chance to develop their intuition about the magnitude of large numbers, and time to explore just how much larger each successive power of ten is.

Most upper elementary students are familiar with number patterns that grow according to an additive rule: You *add* 10 in order to go from one multiple of 10 to the next; you *add* 2 in order to go from one even number to the next. Each multiple of 10 is always 10 larger than the previous one; each even number is always 2 more than the one before.

Fewer students are familiar with number patterns that grow according to a multiplicative rule (or exponentially): you *multiply by 10* in order to go from one power of ten to the next; you *multiply by 2* in order to go from one power of two to the next. While each power of ten is 10 times as large as the previous one, each successive power of ten is increasingly larger than the one before.

Many of the activities in this unit are designed to help students develop their understanding of relationships among large numbers. You can provide additional ways for students to explore the distance between large numbers. For example:

- Use counting sequences to emphasize distance between large numbers.

  I listed the numbers we said when we counted around the class by 500's up to 10,000. How many people counted to get to 1000? How many counted to get to 13,000? If each person said only one number, how many people would we need to get to 100,000? How do you know?

- Provide opportunities for visualizing the distance between numbers. Some students will find it easiest to think about the distance between numbers visually. The 20 × 50 and 25 × 40 rectangles of 1000 squares and the Many Squares Poster in Investigation 4 can help them. For example, you might draw two or three horizontal lines across a Many Squares Poster to divide it into horizontal strips. The strips do not need to be equally spaced. Post the poster at the front of the room, and ask students to make a few quick estimates of which strip different numbers would be in.

  Which strip would 10 be in? Why do you think so? What about 100? 1000? 5000? 7500?

- Encourage students to make additive and multiplicative comparisons. When students are working with numbers of different sizes, they might compare *how much larger* and *how many times as large* one is than the other.

  We found that 100 is one of the factors of 10,000. How much larger is 10,000 than 100? How many times as large?

Multiples of 10	How much larger than previous multiple of 10?
10	—
20	10
30	10
40	10
50	10
60	10
70	10

Powers of 10	How many times as large as previous power of 10?	How much larger than previous power of 10?
1	—	—
10	10	9
100	10	90
1000	10	900
10,000	10	9000
100,000	10	90,000
1,000,000	10	900,000

D I A L O G U E ☐ B O X

Ways to Solve 46 × 25

This class has been working on Student Sheet 12, Multiplication Clusters. Now, in a follow-up discussion (p. 57), they are sharing their strategies for thinking about one of the problems in the fifth cluster, 46 × 25.

4 × 25	10 × 25
40 × 25	50 × 25
6 × 25	46 × 25

Rachel: I didn't finish getting the answer yet, but I made a plan for how to find it. If you do the answer of 50 × 25, and you take away the answer of 4 × 25, you get 46 × 25. You can get 50 × 25 if you add 40 × 25 and 10 × 25. So you do that, and then you minus 4 × 25.

Maricel: I did it her way. I knew that 4 × 25 is 100. Then you think of 40 × 25 as ten times that. It's like ten 100's, so it's 1000. Then, ten 25's is 250. You go 10 × 25 plus 40 × 25 to get 50 × 25. 1000 plus 250 is 1250. Then you have to take away the 4 × 25 . . . 1250 minus 100 is 1150.

Antonio: I started with 40 × 25, because I knew that from the rectangles we made. Then you need another 6 × 25. It's like three 50's, because 25 is two 50's—so it's 50, 100, 150. So you put it together and the answer is 1150.

Cara: I got 50 × 25 the way Maricel did. I knew it would be 100 less than 1250, so 1250 take away 100 is 1150.

Robby: I noticed that 50 × 25 is the same as 5 × 10 × 25. So I started with 10 × 25—that's 250. You need five of those. I knew that's 1250 because 5 × 25 is 125, so 5 × 250 must be 1250. Then you just need to take away 4 × 25, or 100.

Marcus: I put together 40 × 25 and 4 × 25 and half of 4 × 25 to get 46 × 25. You put the 40 and the 4 together, that's 44, and then half again of the 4 to get 46 × 25. So it's 1000 plus 100 plus 50.

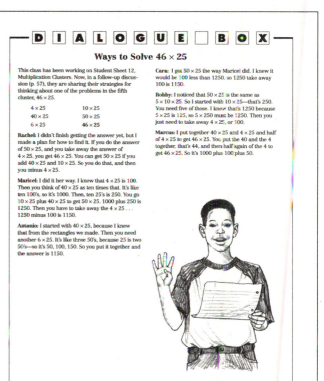

The *Investigations* curriculum incorporates the use of two forms of technology in the classroom: calculators and computers. Calculators are assumed to be standard classroom materials, available for student use in any unit. Computers are explicitly linked to one or more units at each grade level; they are used with the unit on 2-D geometry at each grade, as well as with some of the units on measuring, data, and changes.

Using Calculators

In this curriculum, calculators are considered tools for doing mathematics, similar to pattern blocks or interlocking cubes. Just as with other tools, students must learn both *how* to use calculators correctly and *when* they are appropriate to use. This knowledge is crucial for daily life, as calculators are now a standard way of handling numerical operations, both at work and at home.

Using a calculator correctly is not a simple task; it depends on a good knowledge of the four operations and of the number system, so that students can select suitable calculations and also determine what a reasonable result would be. These skills are the basis of any work with numbers, whether or not a calculator is involved.

Unfortunately, calculators are often seen as tools to check computations with, as if other methods are somehow more fallible. Students need to understand that any computational method can be used to check any other; it's just as easy to make a mistake on the calculator as it is to make a mistake on paper or with mental arithmetic. Throughout this curriculum, we encourage students to solve computation problems in more than one way in order to double-check their accuracy. We present mental arithmetic, paper-and-pencil computation, and calculators as three possible approaches.

In this curriculum we also recognize that, despite their importance, calculators are not always appropriate in mathematics instruction. Like any tools, calculators are useful for some tasks, but not for others. You will need to make decisions about when to allow students access to calculators and when to ask that they solve problems without them, so that they can concentrate on other tools and skills. At times when calculators are or are not appropriate for a particular activity, we make specific recommendations. Help your students develop their own sense of which problems they can tackle with their own reasoning and which ones might be better solved with a combination of their own reasoning and the calculator.

Managing calculators in your classroom so that they are a tool, and not a distraction, requires some planning. When calculators are first introduced, students often want to use them for everything, even problems that can be solved quite simply by other methods. However, once the novelty wears off, students are just as interested in developing their own strategies, especially when these strategies are emphasized and valued in the classroom. Over time, students will come to recognize the ease and value of solving problems mentally, with paper and pencil, or with manipulatives, while also understanding the power of the calculator to facilitate work with larger numbers.

Experience shows that if calculators are available only occasionally, students become excited and distracted when they are permitted to use them. They focus on the tool rather than on the mathematics. In order to learn when calculators are appropriate and when they are not, students must have easy access to them and use them routinely in their work.

If you have a calculator for each student, and if you think your students can accept the responsibility, you might allow them to keep their calculators with the rest of their individual materials, at least for the first few weeks of school. Alternatively, you might store them in boxes on a shelf, number each calculator, and assign a corresponding number to each student. This system can give students a sense of ownership while also helping you keep track of the calculators.

Using Computers

Students can use computers to approach and visualize mathematical situations in new ways. The computer allows students to construct and manipulate geometric shapes, see objects move according to rules they specify, and turn, flip, and repeat a pattern.

This curriculum calls for computers in units where they are a particularly effective tool for learning mathematics content. One unit on 2-D geometry at each of the grades 3–5 includes a core of activities that rely on access to computers, either in the classroom or in a lab. Other units on geometry, measurement, data, and changes include computer activities, but can be taught without them. In these units, however, students' experience is greatly enhanced by computer use.

The following list outlines the recommended use of computers in this curriculum:

Grade 1

Unit: *Survey Questions and Secret Rules* (Collecting and Sorting Data)
Software: Tabletop, Jr.
Source: Broderbund

Unit: *Quilt Squares and Block Towns* (2-D and 3-D Geometry)
Software: *Shapes*
Source: provided with the unit

Grade 2

Unit: *Mathematical Thinking at Grade 2* (Introduction)
Software: *Shapes*
Source: provided with the unit

Unit: *Shapes, Halves, and Symmetry* (Geometry and Fractions)
Software: *Shapes*
Source: provided with the unit

Unit: *How Long? How Far?* (Measuring)
Software: *Geo-Logo*
Source: provided with the unit

Grade 3

Unit: *Flips, Turns, and Area* (2-D Geometry)
Software: *Tumbling Tetrominoes*
Source: provided with the unit

Unit: *Turtle Paths* (2-D Geometry)
Software: *Geo-Logo*
Source: provided with the unit

Grade 4

Unit: *Sunken Ships and Grid Patterns* (2-D Geometry)
Software: *Geo-Logo*
Source: provided with the unit

Grade 5

Unit: *Picturing Polygons* (2-D Geometry)
Software: *Geo-Logo*
Source: provided with the unit

Unit: *Patterns of Change* (Tables and Graphs)
Software: *Trips*
Source: provided with the unit

Unit: *Data: Kids, Cats, and Ads* (Statistics)
Software: Tabletop, Sr.
Source: Broderbund

The software provided with the *Investigations* units uses the power of the computer to help students explore mathematical ideas and relationships that cannot be explored in the same way with physical materials. With the *Shapes* (grades 1–2) and *Tumbling Tetrominoes* (grade 3) software, students explore symmetry, pattern, rotation and reflection, area, and characteristics of 2-D shapes. With the *Geo-Logo* software (grades 3–5), students investigate rotations and reflections, coordinate geometry, the properties of 2-D shapes, and angles. The *Trips* software (grade 5) is a mathematical exploration of motion in which students run experiments and interpret data presented in graphs and tables.

We suggest that students work in pairs on the computer; this not only maximizes computer resources but also encourages students to consult, monitor, and teach one another. Generally, more than two students at one computer find it difficult to share. Managing access to computers is an issue for every classroom. The curriculum gives you explicit support for setting up a system. The units are structured on the assumption that you have enough computers for half your students to work on the machines in pairs at one time. If you do not have access to that many computers, suggestions are made for structuring class time to use the unit with five to eight computers, or even with fewer than five.

Assessment plays a critical role in teaching and learning, and it is an integral part of the *Investigations* curriculum. For a teacher using these units, assessment is an ongoing process. You observe students' discussions and explanations of their strategies on a daily basis and examine their work as it evolves. While students are busy recording and representing their work, working on projects, sharing with partners, and playing mathematical games, you have many opportunities to observe their mathematical thinking. What you learn through observation guides your decisions about how to proceed. In any of the units, you will repeatedly consider questions like these:

■ Do students come up with their own strategies for solving problems, or do they expect others to tell them what to do? What do their strategies reveal about their mathematical understanding?

■ Do students understand that there are different strategies for solving problems? Do they articulate their strategies and try to understand other students' strategies?

■ How effectively do students use materials as tools to help with their mathematical work?

■ Do students have effective ideas for keeping track of and recording their work? Does keeping track of and recording their work seem difficult for them?

You will need to develop a comfortable and efficient system for recording and keeping track of your observations. Some teachers keep a clipboard handy and jot notes on a class list or on adhesive labels that are later transferred to student files. Others keep loose-leaf notebooks with a page for each student and make weekly notes about what they have observed in class.

Assessment Tools in the Unit

With the activities in each unit, you will find questions to guide your thinking while observing the students at work. You will also find two built-in assessment tools: Teacher Checkpoints and embedded Assessment activities.

Teacher Checkpoints The designated Teacher Checkpoints in each unit offer a time to "check in" with individual students, watch them at work, and ask questions that illuminate how they are thinking.

At first it may be hard to know what to look for, hard to know what kinds of questions to ask. Students may be reluctant to talk; they may not be accustomed to having the teacher ask them about their work, or they may not know how to explain their thinking. Two important ingredients of this process are asking students open-ended questions about their work and showing genuine interest in how they are approaching the task. When students see that you are interested in their thinking and are counting on them to come up with their own ways of solving problems, they may surprise you with the depth of their understanding.

Teacher Checkpoints also give you the chance to pause in the teaching sequence and reflect on how your class is doing overall. Think about whether you need to adjust your pacing: Are most students fluent with strategies for solving a particular kind of problem? Are they just starting to formulate good strategies? Or are they still struggling with how to start? Depending on what you see as the students work, you may want to spend more time on similar problems, change some of the problems to use smaller numbers, move quickly to more challenging material, modify subsequent activities for some students, work on particular ideas with a small group, or pair students who have good strategies with those who are having more difficulty.

Embedded Assessment Activities Assessment activities embedded in each unit will help you examine specific pieces of student work, figure out what it means, and provide feedback. From the students' point of view, these assessment activities are no different from any others. Each is a learning experience in and of itself, as well as an opportunity for you to gather evidence about students' mathematical understanding.

The embedded assessment activities sometimes involve writing and reflecting; at other times, a discussion or brief interaction between student and teacher; and in still other instances, the creation and explanation of a product. In most cases, the assessments require that students *show* what they did, *write* or *talk* about it, or do both. Having to explain how they worked through a problem helps students be more focused and clear in their mathematical thinking. It also helps them realize that doing mathematics is a process that may involve tentative starts, revising one's approach, taking different paths, and working through ideas.

Teachers often find the hardest part of assessment to be interpreting their students' work. We provide guidelines to help with that interpretation. If you have used a process approach to teaching writing, the assessment in *Investigations* will seem familiar. For many of the assessment activities, a Teacher Note provides examples of student work and a commentary on what it indicates about student thinking.

Documentation of Student Growth

To form an overall picture of mathematical progress, it is important to document each student's work in journals, notebooks, or portfolios. The choice is largely a matter of personal preference; some teachers have students keep a notebook or folder for each unit, while others prefer one mathematics notebook, or a portfolio of selected work for the entire year. The final activity in each *Investigations* unit, called Choosing Student Work to Save, helps you and the students select representative samples for a record of their work.

This kind of regular documentation helps you synthesize information about each student as a mathematical learner. From different pieces of evidence, you can put together the big picture. This synthesis will be invaluable in thinking about where to go next with a particular child, deciding where more work is needed, or explaining to parents (or other teachers) how a child is doing.

If you use portfolios, you need to collect a good balance of work, yet avoid being swamped with an overwhelming amount of paper. Following are some tips for effective portfolios:

- Collect a representative sample of work, including some pieces that students themselves select for inclusion in the portfolio. There should be just a few pieces for each unit, showing different kinds of work—some assignments that involve writing, as well as some that do not.

- If students do not date their work, do so yourself so that you can reconstruct the order in which pieces were done.

- Include your reflections on the work. When you are looking back over the whole year, such comments are reminders of what seemed especially interesting about a particular piece; they can also be helpful to other teachers and to parents. Older students should be encouraged to write their own reflections about their work.

Assessment Overview

There are two places to turn for a preview of the assessment opportunities in each *Investigations* unit. The Assessment Resources column in the unit Overview Chart (pp. I-13–I-16) identifies the Teacher Checkpoints and Assessment activities embedded in each investigation, guidelines for observing the students that appear within classroom activities, and any Teacher Notes and Dialogue Boxes that explain what to look for and what types of student responses you might expect to see in your classroom. Additionally, the section About the Assessment in This Unit (p. I-19) gives you a detailed list of questions for each investigation, keyed to the mathematical emphases, to help you observe student growth.

Depending on your situation, you may want to provide additional assessment opportunities. Most of the investigations lend themselves to more frequent assessment, simply by having students do more writing and recording while they are working.

Mathematical Thinking at Grade 5

Content of This Unit   Students explore factors and multiples of 100, 1000, and 10,000—important landmarks in our number system. They solve problems and puzzles that involve building numbers in different ways, such as skip counting (25 + 25 + 25 + 25 = 100) and multiplying factor pairs (10 × 10 = 100). They use their knowledge of factor pairs of 100 to help them find factor pairs of multiples of 100 up to 1000, and factor pairs of 10,000. They also use their knowledge of relationships among landmark numbers up to 10,000 to develop strategies for solving computation problems. This unit will help students become acclimated to a mathematics class in which the emphasis is on developing strategies, solving problems for which there is no single procedure, and constructing conjectures about mathematical ideas based on evidence that they gather themselves.

Connections with Other Units   If you are doing the full-year *Investigations* curriculum in the suggested sequence for grade 5, this is the first of nine units. It has connections with nearly every other unit in the fifth grade sequence, both in its content and in its emphasis on ways of thinking and doing mathematics. The number work in this unit is specifically continued and extended in the Computation and Estimation Strategies unit, *Building on Numbers You Know.*

Many of the activities in this unit assume some exposure to the array model of multiplication with factor pairs up to 10 × 10. This topic is addressed in two *Investigations* grade 4 units, *Arrays and Shares* and *Packages and Groups*. Investigation 2 in *Arrays and Shares* may be particularly helpful if your students need additional background.

This unit can be used successfully at either grade 5 or grade 6 at any time of the year, depending on the previous experience and needs of your students. It offers a way to help students focus on thinking, working, and talking mathematically, and helps you assess student understanding of some key mathematical content.

Investigations Curriculum ■ Suggested Grade 5 Sequence

▶ *Mathematical Thinking at Grade 5* (Introduction and Landmarks in the Number System)

Picturing Polygons (2-D Geometry)

Name That Portion (Fractions, Percents, and Decimals)

Between Never and Always (Probability)

Building on Numbers You Know (Computation and Estimation Strategies)

Measurement Benchmarks (Estimating and Measuring)

Patterns of Change (Tables and Graphs)

Containers and Cubes (3-D Geometry: Volume)

Data: Kids, Cats, and Ads (Statistics)

Investigation 1 ■ Exploring Numbers and Number Relationships

Class Sessions	Activities	Pacing
Sessions 1, 2, and 3 (p. 4) RECTANGLES AND FACTOR PAIRS	Introducing the Mathematical Environment Building Number Rectangles Special Math Words Number Shapes Discussion: Names for Numbers Homework: Factor Pairs from 1 to 25 Homework: Skip Counting Extension: Factor Pair Rectangles Extension: Number Boxes Extension: Primes Under 100	minimum 3 hr
Sessions 4, 5, and 6 (p. 16) NUMBER PUZZLES	Homework Review: The Rectangles We Made Using Puzzle Clues Teacher Checkpoint: Solving Number Puzzles Make Your Own Number Puzzle Homework: What's the Number? Homework: Make an Impossible Puzzle	minimum 3 hr

◐ Ten-Minute Math ■ Exploring Data

Mathematical Emphasis

- Describing numbers and number relationships with the terms *factor, multiple, prime,* and *square*

- Reasoning about number characteristics such as multiple, factor, even, odd, prime, and square

- Representing factor pairs as dimensions of a rectangular array

- Developing, discussing, and comparing strategies for solving problems about number relationships

- Understanding that problems may have one solution, more than one solution, or no solution

- Communicating about mathematical thinking through written and spoken language

Assessment Resources

Collaborating with the Authors (Teacher Note, p. 13)

Using Mathematical Vocabulary (Teacher Note, p. 14)

Talking About Calculators (Dialogue Box, p. 15)

Teacher Checkpoint: Solving Number Puzzles (p. 20)

Solving a Number Puzzle (Dialogue Box, p. 24)

Materials

Overhead projector
Square tiles
Letter-size envelopes
Calculators
Centimeter rulers
Student Sheets 1–7
Teaching resource sheets
Family letter

Investigation 2 ■ Multiples and Factors up to 1000

Class Sessions	Activities	Pacing
Session 1 (p. 28) SKIP COUNTING AND OTHER WAYS TO MULTIPLY	Counting Around the Class Strategies for Remembering Factor Pairs Homework: Find the Counting Numbers Extension: Counting by Larger Numbers Extension: Help with Difficult Factor Pairs	minimum 1 hr
Sessions 2, 3, and 4 (p. 35) FACTOR PAIRS FROM 100 TO 1000	Teacher Checkpoint: Factor Pairs of 100 Factor Pairs of Multiples of 100 Building Rectangles with 1000 Squares What Rectangles Did We Make? Homework: More Factor Pairs Homework: Counting Backward	minimum 3 hr
Session 5 (p. 44) EXPLORING RECTANGLES OF 1000 SQUARES	Numbering Squares in Our Rectangles Displaying 10,000 Squares Extension: 1000 Square Rectangles Extension: How Big Is 10,000?	minimum 1 hr

◔ **Ten-Minute Math** ■ **Exploring Data**

Mathematical Emphasis

- Using knowledge of landmarks up to 100 (including factors of 100 and multiples of those factors) to explore landmarks up to 1000

- Becoming familiar with factors and factor pairs of 1000

- Developing a variety of strategies for exploring number composition, such as repeated addition, skip counting, finding factors, finding factor pairs, and using a calculator to check divisibility

- Reading, writing, and ordering numbers to 1000

- Developing a sense of the magnitude of 1000

- Becoming familiar with skip-counting patterns (sequences of multiples such as 25, 50, 75 . . .) leading to 1000

Assessment Resources

Two Important Ways of Building Numbers (Teacher Note, p. 33)

Counting Around the Class (Dialogue Box, p. 34)

Teacher Checkpoint: Factor Pairs of 100 (p. 35)

Observing the Students (p. 37)

Finding Factor Pairs of Multiples of 100 (Dialogue Box, p. 42)

Relationships Among Factor Pairs of 1000 (Dialogue Box, p. 43)

Materials

Square tiles

Scissors

Tape

Overhead projector

Calculators

Chart paper

Notebook paper

Student Sheets 8–10

Teaching resource sheets

Investigation 3 ■ Multiples and Factors up to 10,000

Class Sessions	Activities	Pacing
Session 1 (p. 50) COMPARING FACTORS OF 100, 1000, AND 10,000	Counting to 100, 1000, and 10,000 Homework: What Could You Count By? Extension: What Could We *Not* Count By?	minimum 1 hr
Sessions 2, 3, and 4 (p. 55) MULTIPLICATION AND DIVISION CLUSTERS	Solving Multiplication Clusters Teacher Checkpoint: Multiplication Clusters Sharing Our Cluster Strategies Making Our Own Problem Clusters Solving Division Clusters Division Cluster Strategies Homework: Writing About Multiplication Clusters Homework: Make Your Own Cluster	minimum 3 hr
Session 5 (p. 66) FACTOR PAIRS OF 1100	Assessment: Finding Factor Pairs of 1100 Homework: Factor Pairs of 950	minimum 1 hr

◐ Ten-Minute Math ■ Quick Images

Mathematical Emphasis

- Using knowledge of landmarks up to 1000 (including factors of 1000 and multiples of those factors) to explore landmarks up to 10,000

- Developing multiplication and division strategies that rely on landmarks up to 10,000

- Becoming familiar with skip-counting patterns (sequences of multiples such as 250, 500, 750 . . .) leading to 10,000

- Becoming familiar with some factor pairs of 10,000

Assessment Resources

Powers of 10: How Much Larger, and How Many Times as Large? (Teacher Note, p. 54)

Teacher Checkpoint: Multiplication Clusters (p. 56)

About Cluster Problems (Teacher Note, p. 62)

The Relationship Between Division and Multiplication (Teacher Note, p. 63)

What About Notation? (Teacher Note, p. 64)

Ways to Solve 46×25 (Dialogue Box, p. 65)

Assessment: Finding Factor Pairs of 1100 (p. 66)

Assessment: Finding Factor Pairs of 1100 (Teacher Note, p. 68)

Materials

Chart paper

Calculators

Class lists of Factor Pairs of 100 and 1000

Overhead projector

Student Sheets 11–20

Teaching resource sheets

Investigation 4 ■ Reasoning About Landmarks up to 10,000

Class Sessions	Activities	Pacing
Session 1 (p. 74) CLOSE TO 1000 AND CLOSE TO 0	Close to 1000 Close to 0 Homework: Close to 1000 and Close to 0 Extension: Close to 1000: Using Negative and Positive Integers	minimum 1 hr
Sessions 2, 3, and 4 (p. 81) USING LANDMARKS UP TO 10,000	Choice Time: Numbers to 10,000 Homework: Problems from Close to 1000 Homework: Problems from Close to 0 Extension: Different Paths to 1000 Extension: Further Exploration of the Many Squares Poster	minimum 3 hr
Sessions 5 and 6 (p. 89) REASONING ABOUT 1000 AND 10,000	What Can You Say About 10,000? Assessment: Add a Clue Factor Pairs of 10,000 Choosing Student Work to Save Homework: Another Add a Clue	minimum 2 hr

◐ **Ten-Minute Math** ■ **Quick Images**

Mathematical Emphasis

- Using knowledge of landmarks up to 10,000 (including factors of 1000 and multiples of those factors) to solve a variety of puzzles and problems

- Developing mental and written strategies for finding sums and differences of three- and four-digit numbers

- Reading, writing, and ordering numbers to 10,000

- Developing a sense of the magnitude of 10,000

Assessment Resources

Playing Close to 1000 and Close to 0 (Teacher Note, p. 79)

Observing the Students (p. 85)

About Choice Time (Teacher Note, p. 87)

Assessment: Add a Clue (p. 91)

Observing the Students (p. 92)

Choosing Student Work to Save (p. 93)

Assessment: Add a Clue (Teacher Note, p. 94)

Materials

Numeral Cards

Many Squares Posters

Letter-size envelopes

Students' Number Puzzle Recording Sheets from Investigation 1

Square tiles

Class lists of Factor Pairs of 100 and 1000

Overhead projector

Calculators

Student Sheets 21–30

Teaching resource sheets

Following are the basic materials needed for the activities in this unit. Many of the items can be purchased from the publisher, either individually or in the Teacher Resource Package and the Student Materials Kit for grade 5. Detailed information is available on the *Investigations* order form. To obtain this form, call toll-free 1-800-872-1100 and ask for a Dale Seymour customer service representative.

Square tiles: about 70 per student pair

Numeral Cards: 1 deck per pair, 2 decks for class (manufactured; or use blackline masters to make your own)

Many Squares posters: 2 per class (packaged with this book)

Calculators

Large 50 × 20 grid for class demonstration

Letter-size envelopes (32–56, to hold puzzle clues)

Overhead projector

Chart paper

Notebook paper

Scissors

Tape

Centimeter rulers (optional)

The following materials are provided at the end of this unit as blackline masters. A Student Activity Booklet containing all student sheets and teaching resources needed for individual work is available.

Family Letter (p. 103)

Student Sheets 1–30 (p. 104)

Teaching Resources:

    Sample Puzzle Clues (p. 111)

    Number Puzzles 1–28 (pp. 112–118 and 150–156)

    15 × 20 Grid (p. 122)

    Numeral Cards (p. 147)

    One-Centimeter Graph Paper (p. 157)

    300 Chart (p. 158)

    Quick Image Dot Patterns (p. 159)

    Quick Image Geometric Designs (p. 160)

Practice Pages (p. 161)

Related Children's Literature

Dee, Ruby. *Two Ways to Count to Ten*. New York: Henry Holt, 1972.

Lord, John. *The Giant Jam Sandwich*. Boston: Houghton-Mifflin, 1972.

Pittman, Helena Clare. *A Grain of Rice*. New York: Hastings House, 1986.

Seuss, Dr. *The 500 Hats of Bartholomew Cubbins*. New York: The Vanguard Press.

Working with numbers 1000 and greater can be challenging even for adults, as few of us have had opportunities to develop our intuitions about the magnitude of such numbers. Even those of us who routinely perform calculations with large numbers may have little sense of what these numbers actually mean and how they relate to smaller, more familiar numbers.

The activities in this unit are designed to help students develop a sense of the size of numbers up to 10,000. The focus is on 1000 and 10,000 and their factors and multiples—termed *landmark* numbers because they are important landing places in our number system. Familiarity with these landmark numbers is a cornerstone of good number sense.

Throughout the unit, students explore relationships among these numbers. They find ways to draw upon their knowledge of landmarks as they develop strategies for solving computation problems. For example, consider how using landmarks could help us solve a problem like 83×25. Rather than using an algorithm to multiply, we might solve the problem *mentally,* using reasoning such as this:

> I know there are four 25's in 100, so forty 25's (or ten times as many) would be 1000. Eighty 25's would be 2000, and three more 25's makes 2075.

This unit also introduces a particular way of approaching mathematics:

- As students solve games and puzzles in groups, they learn to work cooperatively, to explain their thinking and reasoning to others, and to listen to and learn from their classmates.

- As students build and investigate models of numbers with graph paper and square tiles, they see that visual and concrete models can help them gain important insights into mathematical ideas.

- As students solve problems in ways that make sense to them, they come to value their own unique problem-solving approaches and computational strategies.

- As students use calculators to explore number relationships, they find that the calculator can be more than just a quick way to do computation—it can also be a valuable tool for mathematical investigation.

- As students pose their own problems and puzzles and exchange them with classmates, they learn that they can use mathematics creatively.

- And, as they explain and write about their solution processes, sharing their ideas with each other, they come to appreciate that there are many valid ways of approaching a mathematical problem.

Many of these approaches may be familiar and comfortable for your students; others may be new and might seem difficult. Writing about one's thinking and reasoning, for example, can be challenging for people at all levels of expertise. Use this unit as an opportunity to focus on approaches that are new or difficult for your students. As you take the time to show students what you value in a community of mathematics learners, students will begin to adopt new ways of thinking about and doing mathematics themselves.

Mathematical Emphasis At the beginning of each investigation, the Mathematical Emphasis section tells you what is most important for students to learn about during that investigation. Many of these understandings and processes are difficult and complex. Students gradually learn more and more about each idea over many years of schooling. Individual students will begin and end the unit with different levels of knowledge and skill, but all will gain greater knowledge of the relationships among numbers up to 10,000 as they develop strategies for solving puzzles and problems involving large numbers.

Throughout the *Investigations* curriculum, there are many opportunities for ongoing daily assessment as you observe, listen to, and interact with students at work. In this unit, you will find three Teacher Checkpoints:

Investigation 1, Sessions 4–6:
Solving Number Puzzles (p. 20)

Investigation 2, Sessions 2–4:
Factor Pairs of 100 (p. 35)

Investigation 3, Sessions 2–4:
Multiplication Clusters (p. 56)

This unit also has two embedded assessment activities:

Investigation 3, Session 5:
Finding Factor Pairs of 1100 (p. 66)

Investigation 4, Sessions 5–6:
Add a Clue (p. 91)

In addition, you can use almost any activity in this unit to assess your students' needs and strengths. Listed below are questions to help you focus your observation in each investigation. You may want to keep track of your observations for each student to help you plan your curriculum and monitor students' growth. Suggestions for documenting student growth can be found in the section About Assessment (p. I–10).

Investigation 1: Exploring Numbers and Number Relationships

■ How do students describe numbers and number relationships? Do they understand terms such as *factor, multiple, prime,* and *square?* How (accurately) do they use them?

■ How familiar and comfortable are students with number characteristics such as multiple, factor, even, odd, prime and square? Can they use knowledge about such characteristics to solve problems? For example, do they know that 92 is an even number? That 20 is a multiple of 4? That 4 is a factor of 20?

■ How do students represent the factor pairs as the dimensions of rectangular arrays? How do they make rectangles to find factor pairs? Do they use knowledge of familiar factor pairs? Do they transform one rectangle to make another? Do they have an organized way to find all the possible rectangles for a given number?

■ What strategies do students use to solve problems involving number relationships, such as the number puzzles? Are they developing efficient strategies? How do they discuss and compare them? Are they refining their strategies over time?

■ How comfortable are students solving problems which may have one solution, more than one solution, or no solution?

■ How do students communicate their ideas and strategies? How clearly and confidently do they articulate these ideas and strategies, both orally and in writing?

Investigation 2: Multiples and Factors up to 1000

■ What strategies do students use to explore landmarks up to 1000? For example, do they use their knowledge of landmarks up to 100, such as factors of 100 and multiples of those factors?

■ How familiar are students with factors and factor pairs of 1000? Do they use what they know about factor pairs of 100 to find factor pairs of 200, 300, and other multiples such as 1000?

■ What strategies do students use to explore number composition? Are they comfortable using a variety of strategies, such as repeated addition, skip counting, finding factors, finding factor pairs, and using a calculator to check divisibility?

■ How do students read, write, and order numbers to 1000 in a variety of situations? How comfortable are they in doing so?

■ What evidence do you have that students are developing an understanding of the magnitude of 1000? For example, do they have a sense of how much larger 1000 is than 100? than 10?

■ How familiar and fluent are students with skip-counting patterns leading to 1000? Can they see a relationship between counting by a number and multiplying by that number?

Investigation 3: Multiples and Factors up to 10,000

■ What knowledge of landmarks up to 1000 do students use to explore landmarks up to 10,000?

■ What multiplication and division strategies have students developed that rely on landmarks up to 10,000? For example, can they find an answer to a multiplication problem by doubling one of the factors in a known pair? Can they use known factor pairs to help them solve division problems?

■ How familiar and fluent are students with skip-counting patterns leading to 10,000? Can they see a relationship between counting by a number and multiplying by that number?

■ In what ways have students shown that they are developing familiarity with some factor pairs of 10,000? What factor pairs do they know by heart? What strategies do they use to find other pairs?

Investigation 4: Reasoning About Landmarks up to 10,000

■ What knowledge of landmarks up to 10,000 do students use to solve a variety of puzzles, and problems?

■ What strategies do students use to add and subtract three-and-four-digit numbers?

■ How do students read, write, and order numbers to 10,000? How comfortable are they in doing so?

■ What evidence do you have that students are developing a sense of the magnitude of 10,000? Do they have a sense of how much larger it is than 1000, than 100, than 10?

Thinking and Working in Mathematics

Mathematical Thinking at Grade 5 provides the chance for you to observe students' work habits and communication skills. Think about these questions as you decide which routines, processes, and materials will require the most ongoing support, guidance, and opportunities for practice.

■ Are students comfortable and focused working together in pairs? in small groups?

■ Do students expect to devise their own strategies for solving problems, or do they expect you or another student to tell them exactly what to do? Do they understand that different people may solve problems in different ways?

■ Are students familiar with the basic mathematics materials used in this Investigation? Do they know how to use them? Do they have strategies to use these materials as tools when solving problems?

■ Can students work well when materials are available? Do they take them out and put them away efficiently?

■ Can students express their ideas orally? Who participates in discussions? Do the same students always speak up? Who never speaks?

■ Do students have ideas about how to record their work, or does writing and drawing about mathematics seem new to them?

■ Can students give reasons for their ideas? Do they use examples to help explain their ideas? Do they make generalizations from seeing patterns and relationships?

■ Can students choose an activity from among several that are offered, then move smoothly to a second activity when finished with the first?

■ Can students use a calculator to do basic arithmetic? Can they determine if an answer obtained with the calculator is reasonable, and if necessary, check it? Do they notice the decimal point on the calculator screen? Do they have some idea of what it means? Do they know the meaning of 0.5?

In the *Investigations* curriculum, mathematical vocabulary is introduced naturally during the activities. We don't ask students to learn definitions of new terms; rather, they come to understand such words as *factor* or *area* or *symmetry* by hearing them used frequently in discussion as they investigate new concepts. This approach is compatible with current theories of second-language acquisition, which emphasize the use of new vocabulary in meaningful contexts while students are actively involved with objects, pictures, and physical movement.

Listed below are some key words used in this unit that will not be new to most English speakers at this age level, but may be unfamiliar to students with limited English proficiency. You will want to spend additional time working on these words with your students who are learning English. If your students are working with a second-language teacher, you might enlist your colleague's aid in familiarizing students with these words, before and during this unit. In the classroom, look for opportunities for students to hear and use these words. Activities you can use to present the words are given in the appendix, Vocabulary Support for Second-Language Learners (p. 100).

possible, impossible   While solving number puzzles that give several clues to identify a number, students find that some puzzles have several *possible* answers, and others are *impossible* to solve.

even, odd   Even and odd are among the number characteristics that students identify as they solve number puzzles and find factors of large numbers.

row   Grids of 1000 and 10,000 numbered squares help clarify patterns in the number system, and one way that students track patterns is by *rows* of squares.

Investigations

Exploring Numbers and Number Relationships

What Happens

Sessions 1, 2, and 3: Rectangles and Factor Pairs   Students make as many different rectangles as they can from a set of square tiles. They draw the rectangles on graph paper, record the dimensions of their rectangles, and list the factors that the dimensions represent. They then solve tile puzzles that develop both geometric and numeric meaning for the terms *factor, multiple, prime,* and *square*.

Sessions 4, 5, and 6: Number Puzzles   In small groups, students solve number puzzles by sharing four clues and working together to find one or more numbers that fit all the clues. Students also write sets of clues to make their own puzzles.

Mathematical Emphasis

- Describing numbers and number relationships with the terms *factor, multiple, prime,* and *square*
- Reasoning about number characteristics such as multiple, factor, even, odd, prime, and square
- Representing factor pairs as dimensions of a rectangular array
- Developing, discussing, and comparing strategies for solving problems about number relationships
- Understanding that problems may have one solution, more than one solution, or no solution
- Communicating about mathematical thinking through written and spoken language

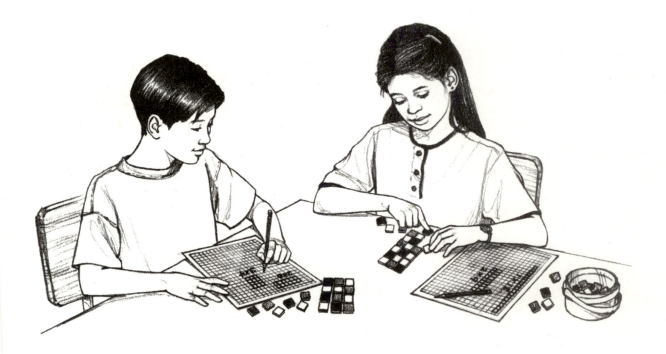

What to Plan Ahead of Time

Materials

- Overhead projector (Sessions 1–3)
- Square tiles: 70 per pair (Sessions 1–6) (Use any squares of uniform size—cubes, game tiles, cardboard squares.)
- Letter-size envelopes (to hold number puzzles): 16 per class and 14 more for the optional challenge puzzles (Sessions 4–6)
- Calculators
- Centimeter rulers (optional)

Other Preparation

- Plan how students will work together in pairs and groups of four. Some teachers find it helpful to arrange desks in clusters of four.
- Duplicate student sheets and teaching resources, located at the end of this unit, in the following quantities. If you have Student Activity Booklets, copy only the items marked with an asterisk, including any transparencies needed.

For Sessions 1–3

Family letter* (p. 103): 1 per student. Remember to sign and date it before duplicating.

Student Sheet 1, Number Shape Clues (p. 104): 1 per student

Student Sheet 2, Factor Pairs from 1 to 25 (p. 105): 1 per student (homework)

Student Sheet 3, Skip Counting (p. 106): 1 per student (homework)

One-centimeter graph paper (p. 157): 5–7 sheets per student, and 1 transparency*

For Sessions 4–6

300 chart (p. 158): 5–8 per student, and 1 transparency.* Alternatively, prepare for each student one laminated 300 chart or one chart copied onto transparency film, making reusable charts.

Sample Puzzle Clues* (p. 111): enough copies to provide one set of clues per group of 4 students

Number Puzzles 1–8* (pp. 112–115): 2 of each for the class, cut apart and placed in prepared envelopes (see below). Note that the starred challenge Number Puzzles 9–14* (pp. 116–118) are optional.

Student Sheet 4, Number Puzzle Recording Sheet (p. 107): 1 per student

Student Sheet 5, Make Your Own Puzzle (p. 108): 1 per student

Student Sheet 6, What's the Number? (p. 109): 1 per student (homework)

Student Sheet 7, Make an Impossible Puzzle (p. 110): 1 per student (homework)

- Prepare envelopes to hold the puzzle clues. Clearly label each envelope with the puzzle number, using a star to identify any challenge puzzles. Make two identical sets of clues for the class to share.

- If your students have not previously worked with the *array* model of multiplication (presented in *Investigations* grade 4), allow extra time for practice with making tile rectangles and representing those rectangles and their dimensions (factor pairs) on graph paper.

Rectangles and Factor Pairs

What Happens

Students make as many different rectangles as they can from a set of square tiles. They draw the rectangles on graph paper, record the dimensions of their rectangles, and list the factors that the dimensions represent. They then solve tile puzzles that develop both geometric and numeric meaning for the terms *factor, multiple, prime,* and *square.* Student work focuses on:

■ describing numbers and number relationships with mathematical terms such as *factor, multiple, prime,* and *square*

■ representing factor pairs as dimensions of a rectangular array

Materials

■ Overhead projector

■ Square tiles (70 per pair)

■ 300 chart

■ One-centimeter graph paper (5–7 sheets per student, and 1 transparency)

■ Family letter

■ Student Sheet 1 (1 per student)

■ Student Sheet 2 (1 per student, homework)

■ Student sheet 3 (1 per student, homework)

■ Centimeter rulers (optional)

■ Calculators

Activity

Introducing the Mathematical Environment

Begin this session with a brief discussion about the kind of work students will be doing in this unit. Have available a calculator, square tiles, a 300 chart, and one-centimeter graph paper to display.

intro.

In mathematics for the next few weeks, you'll be solving problems, playing math games, and learning about very large numbers, like 10,000. You won't have a math textbook, but you'll work with pencil and paper, and with certain mathematical tools—calculators, square tiles, 300 charts, and graph paper.

As you show these tools, ask students if they are familiar with any of these materials, and how they have used them in the past. You might show students where you store the materials you will be using in math class and discuss your procedures for handling and storing these materials. The **Teacher Note,** Caring for and Storing Materials (p. 12), offers some ideas for workable routines.

Mathematicians use tools just like these when they solve problems. They also work hard to communicate about their work. They talk about it, write about it, draw pictures, and build models so they can their share their ideas with other people. Just like mathematicians, you'll be doing all these things.

When you are working on a math problem, I will often ask you to use words and pictures, in addition to numbers, to explain how you solved it. Lots of times I will ask you to talk about how you solved a problem—either with your

partner, a small group, or the whole class. This is how you'll share your ideas and strategies for thinking about the math problems you are working on.

Like adult mathematicians, many of you will invent ways of solving problems on your own. I look forward to hearing all your ideas.

Invite students to speculate briefly about the kinds of mathematical thinking they might be doing in the coming weeks.

If you plan to use math journals or math folders, this is an appropriate time to introduce them. Explain that they are a way to collect the writing and drawing students will be doing during math class.

Building Number Rectangles

Students work in pairs for this activity. Distribute 70 square tiles and 2–3 pieces of graph paper to each pair.

This year in math class, we'll sometimes use materials like these tiles to help us understand more about mathematics. Today we'll be using them to learn more about numbers.

Review the procedures you established for using and caring for materials like the tiles. Explain that students may use calculators as needed. If you have a calculator for each student, you might let students keep one in their math folder. Allow some time for students to explore the calculators as necessary. The **Dialogue Box,** Talking About Calculators (p. 15), gives some examples of short activities to use as needed.

If students are unfamiliar with calculators, you may need to schedule additional time with individuals or small groups. You might also ask students who know how to use the calculator to work with those who don't.

Then give the following instructions for building number rectangles. You may want to put reminders on the board:

- **With your partner, pick a number between 10 and 30.**
- Count out that many tiles. Use all the tiles you counted out to make a rectangle. For example, if you picked the number 21, you would count out 21 tiles and then make a rectangle with those 21 tiles.
- Write down what size rectangle you made—how many tiles across it is, and how many tiles down. Use the graph paper to record each rectangle.
- See if you can make a rectangle of a different shape using the same number of tiles. Keep going until you've made all the rectangles you can.

Students may use calculators to help them determine what rectangles they can build. If pairs do not have enough tiles to keep each rectangle they build, they may take the first ones apart to make others. You may provide centimeter rulers as tools for recording.

Some students may ask if two rectangles with length and width reversed (such as a 3 × 4 rectangle and 4 × 3 rectangle) are the same. Acknowledge that it might sometimes be important to list both, but for this work with tiles, these rectangles are "the same."

Some students who select 16 or 25 may not build a square because they think that a square is not a rectangle. If you notice this happening, explain that mathematicians think of squares as special rectangles. Rectangles have at least two equal sides; squares have all four sides equal. Similarly, for students who chose numbers like 11, 13, 17, 19, 23, or 29, you may need to explain that a "line" of tiles 1 square wide is a rectangle.

As students work, circulate to observe how they generate and record their rectangles, and whether they understand that the dimensions of the rectangles are factors of the numbers. Notice which students have an organized way to find all the rectangles for a number, such as trying to make a rectangle 1 wide, 2 wide, and so on, until they began repeating themselves; finding one rectangle that works and transforming it (for example, by halving the length and doubling the width) to make another rectangle; and using knowledge of factors and factor pairs.

If you think some students would benefit from seeing their classmates' strategies, call the class together and ask one or two students to show how they are finding all the rectangles for a number.

Students who finish early can choose a different number and continue to build all the rectangles they can with the new number of tiles. As pairs are finishing, call the class together for a brief discussion of their results.

What number did you work with? What rectangles did you make? How do you know you found all the rectangles?

Record students' responses by outlining the rectangles on the overhead transparency of graph paper and labeling their dimensions as shown below. Or, draw and label the appropriate rectangles—including the "inside" squares—on the board.

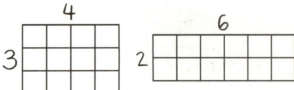

For Further Practice   Students who have not had previous work with the array model of multiplication may benefit from more practice making rectangles with tiles and drawing each rectangle on graph paper. Write a few numbers less than 50 on the board, such as 18, 13, 40, and 42. Students use their tiles to make all the rectangles they can for each number. After they make a rectangle, they outline it on graph paper and label its length and width. This visual model is the foundation for work students will be doing in Investigation 2.

Choose one of the numbers students used and discussed in the previous activity.

When you were building tile rectangles, some of you found the dimensions of all rectangles with (18) tiles. [*Throughout this discussion, substitute for the number 18 whatever number you have chosen as an example.*] **We give the dimensions of rectangles in pairs—for example, 3 × 6, 2 × 9. These pairs for rectangles with (18) tiles are called** *the factor pairs of (18).*

What are all the factor pairs of (18)? How do you know?

Write "Factor pairs of (18)" on the board, and list the factor pairs as students name them. When students suggest a factor pair that duplicates one listed, but with the factors reversed (such as 3 × 6 and 6 × 3), list the two pairs next to each other. Explain that since they describe the same rectangle, we will count them as the same factor pair. If students suggest pairs that include decimals, such as 1.8 and 10, you might encourage them to find more such pairs (as good practice with decimals), but explain that mathematicians think of *factors* and *factor pairs* as including whole numbers only.

If these are factor pairs of (18), what are the *factors* **of (18)? How do you know?**

Write the title "Factors of (18)" on the board, and list the factors as students name them. See the **Teacher Note**, Using Mathematical Vocabulary (p. 14), for additional ideas on introducing and using mathematical vocabulary.

Factor pairs of 18	Factors of 18	Multiples of 18
3 × 6	3, 6, 2,	36
2 × 9	9, 1, 18	54
1 × 18		72

We've just listed the factors of (18). What are some *multiples* **of (18)?**

As you list students' responses, emphasize the difference between factors and *multiples.*

Many people get the words *factor* **and** *multiple* **mixed up. They are not the same, and it's important to learn the difference. What could you say to help someone remember which is which?**

As students offer their ideas, start a class Math Words chart to help students remember the meanings of these and other terms they will encounter during this unit. One class came up with this chart:

<table>
<tr><td>

Multiples

- Multiples of a number are what you say when you count by that number.

- Multiples of 18:
  18, 36, 54, 72 . . .

- Multiples are times a number, and you keep going up.

</td><td>

Factors

- When you times the factors of a number, they equal that number.

- Factors of a number are the sides of rectangles with that number of tiles.

- Factors of 18:
  1, 2, 3, 6, 9, 18

- You find factors on the calculator by doing divide by.

- A factor is a number that fits into another number evenly.

</td></tr>
</table>

❖ **Tip for the Linguistically Diverse Classroom** Make your Math Words chart comprehensible to students with limited English proficiency by adding visual representations and examples for each defining rule that students suggest. For example:

When you times the factors of a number, they equal that number.

$$6 \times 4 = 24 \qquad 3 \times 8 = 24 \qquad 2 \times 12 = 24 \qquad 1 \times 24 = 24$$

You find factors on the calculator by doing divide by.

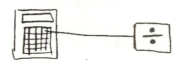

Number Shapes

For this activity, students work independently but share approximately 70 square tiles with another student. Each individual needs a copy of Student Sheet 1, Number Shape Clues, and a piece of plain paper or graph paper for recording rectangles.

P-104

Students read each given clue, find and record a number that fits the clue, draw rectangles to demonstrate that their number fits, and record the factor pairs for their rectangles. As students work, circulate to observe whether they under-stand the terms *wide, rectangle,* and *square* as used in the clues. If necessary, briefly review the meaning of these terms.

❖ **Tip for the Linguistically Diverse Classroom**   As visual cues, suggest that students make simple drawings of a tile, a rectangle, and a square over those words where they appear on the student sheet.

For More Challenge   Students who finish quickly might be encouraged to find more numbers that satisfy each clue. They can also compare answers with another pair, and if the answers differ, check that both satisfy the clue. See the **Teacher Note**, Collaborating with the Authors (p. 13), for more about your role and your students' roles in finding the right level of challenge for everyone in the class.

Discussion: Names for Numbers

Gather students' answers for the first problem on Student Sheet 1, Number Shape Clues, and record them on the board.

What do you notice about all the rectangles you found that are 2 tiles wide?

Students may describe these as *even numbers, multiples of 2,* or *numbers that have 2 as a factor.*

What other numbers could we write on this list?

Students may recognize that any even number—even large numbers such as 100 and 1000—could go on the list.

Let's look at problem 3—numbers that could be made into only one rect-angle. What are some numbers you found? Do the rectangles you made all have 1 as a dimension? Does anyone know what these numbers are called?

Explain that these are called *prime numbers*. This is the mathematical name for numbers with only two factors—1 and the number itself. (Mathematicians do not consider 1 itself to be a prime number.) Add *prime number* to the class Math Words chart, asking students to suggest ways that they can remember what this term means. Students may be interested to know that numbers that are not prime are called *composite numbers;* add this term to the chart if you like.

What about the numbers that can be made into squares? What is different about them?

Explain that numbers that can be made into squares are called *square numbers.* These numbers are the product of a single factor multiplied by itself. They can be written as $3^2 = 9$, $4^2 = 16$, and so on. Add *square number* to your Math Words chart. If students seem interested, you might add that the number that is multiplied by itself is called the *square root* of the number. Thus, 5 is the square root of 25; 6 is the square root of 36. You might illustrate this with a diagram:

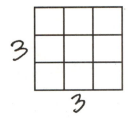

$3^2 = 9$

3 is the square root of 9.

Continue the whole-class discussion of Student Sheet 1, Number Shape Clues.

Sessions 1, 2, and 3 Follow-Up

(handwritten: ← P. 108 103)

🏠 **Homework**

Factor Pairs from 1 to 25   After Session 1, send home the family letter or *Investigations* at Home booklet and a copy of Student Sheet 2, Factor Pairs from 1 to 25. Give each student 3–5 pieces of one-centimeter graph paper. Explain that they are to draw rectangles on the graph paper to show the factor pairs for each number from 1 to 25. They label the dimensions of each rectangle, and they list the factor pair that each rectangle shows. Allow two nights for this assignment.

When students have finished, they record at least one thing they have discovered about the rectangles and factors for these numbers. For example, they might note which numbers have the most factors, which numbers have the fewest factors, or how many numbers have 2 as a factor.

❖ **Tip for the Linguistically Diverse Classroom** Offer students a visual way to record their discoveries. For example, they might *circle* the numbers that have the fewest factors, and draw a *box* around the numbers that have the most factors.

(handwritten in left margin: EXPLAIN SQUARE + SQUARE ROOT)

Skip Counting   After Session 3, send home Student Sheet 3, Skip Counting. Students record the first 20 numbers they would say if they counted by a large one-digit number, such as 7 or 9, or a small two-digit number, such as 11 or 12. They might use a 300 chart to help them.

Factor Pair Rectangles   After completing the Session 1 homework, students use graph paper and colored pencils to make a colorful and permanent display of the rectangles showing the factor pairs for the numbers 1 to 25. They can develop their own ways to arrange or color-code their rectangles; for example, they might decide to color the *primes* red and the *squares* blue.

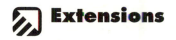

Number Boxes   Students choose some numbers that have many factors (such as 24, 30, 36, and 48) and find all the three-dimensional rectangular blocks they can make with each number of square tiles. For example, with 36 tiles, they can build a block that is $2 \times 9 \times 2$, one that is $6 \times 3 \times 2$, and so on.

Primes Under 100   Students find all the prime numbers less than 100 (or 50). They can use a 300 chart and calculators.

Teacher Note ▷ *Caring for and Storing Materials*

Before introducing concrete materials (such as tiles, calculators, or interlocking cubes), think about how you want students to use and care for them, and how they will be stored in your classroom.

Introducing a New Material Students will need time to explore any new material before using it in a structured activity. By freely exploring a material, students will discover many of its important characteristics. Once having had the chance to make their own decisions about how they would like to use a material, they will be more ready to use it as a tool in a specific activity. Although some free exploration should be done during regular math time, many teachers make materials available to students during free time or before or after school.

Establishing Routines for Using Materials
Establish clear expectations regarding the use and care of materials. Students generally find math manipulatives very engaging, and are eager to use them. Consider having students suggest rules for how materials should and should not be used. Students will often be more aware of rules and policies that they have helped create.

Plan how materials will be distributed and cleaned up at the beginning and end of each class. Some teachers assign one or two students each week to be responsible for passing out and collecting materials. Most teachers find that stopping 5 minutes before the end of class gives students time to clean up materials, put their work in their folders, and double-check the floor for any stray materials or pencils.

Caring for and Storing Materials Store materials where they are easily accessible to students. Many teachers use plastic tubs or shoe boxes arranged on a bookshelf or along a windowsill. Students should view materials as useful tools for solving problems or illustrating their thinking— the more available they are and the more frequently they are used, the more likely students are to use them. Model this by using materials yourself when you are solving a problem, and encourage all students to use them.

If materials are used only when someone is having difficulty, students can get the mistaken idea that using materials is a less sophisticated way to solve a problem. Mathematicians frequently use concrete materials and build models to solve problems and explain their thinking. Encourage your students to think and work like mathematicians.

Collaborating with the Authors

Teacher Note

Every unit in this curriculum is a guide, not a prescription or recipe. We tested these activities in many different classrooms, representing a range of students and teachers, and we revised our ideas constantly as we learned from students and teachers. Each time we tried a unit in a classroom, no matter how many times it had been tried and revised before, we always discovered new ideas we wanted to add and changes we wanted to make. This process could be endless, but at some point we had to decide that the curriculum worked well enough with a wide range of students.

We cannot anticipate the needs and strengths of your particular students this particular year. We believe that the only way for good curriculum to be used well is for teachers to participate in continually modifying it. Your role is to observe and listen carefully to your students, to try to understand how they are thinking, and to make decisions, based on your observations, about what they need next. Modifications to the curriculum that you will need to consider throughout the year include:

- changing the numbers in a problem to make the problem more accessible or more challenging for particular students

- repeating activities with which students need more experience

- engaging students in extensions and further questions

- rearranging pairs or small groups so that students learn from a variety of their peers

Your students can help you set the right pace and level of challenge. We have found that, when given choices of activities and problems, students often do choose the right level of difficulty for themselves. You can encourage students to do this by urging them to find problems that are "not too easy, not too hard, but just right." Help students understand that doing mathematics does *not* mean knowing the answer right away. Tell students often, "A good problem for you is a problem that makes you think hard and work hard. You might have to try more than one way of doing it before you figure it out."

The *Investigations* curriculum provides more than enough material for any student. Suggestions are included for extending activities, and some curriculum units contain optional sessions (called Excursions) to provide more opportunities to explore the big mathematical ideas of that unit. Many teachers also have favorite activities that they integrate into this curriculum. We encourage you to be an active partner with us in creating the way this curriculum can work best for your students.

Students learn mathematical words the same way they learn other vocabulary—by hearing it used correctly, frequently, and in context. Young children learn words by hearing their families use language appropriately. When they make mistakes—"Look at the big doggy," says a young child pointing at a horse—family members use the correct word and the child gradually learns the distinctions among all the four-footed animals that at first look like "doggies."

We don't ask young children to memorize definitions; rather, we try to find lots of opportunities for them to hear words being used in meaningful ways. Learning mathematical vocabulary is no different.

When you speak to students, try to use mathematical vocabulary as often as you can. Connect mathematical terms with more familiar words that students may know, and use these terms in contexts that make sense to students. For example:

> Antonio and Kevin made a rectangle from 24 tiles. The rectangle is 8 tiles across and 3 tiles down. Its *dimensions* are 8 by 3.

> While we counted around the class by 25's, Toshi listed the numbers we said on the board. Look at what she wrote. Do we have the *multiples* of 25 on the board?

Throughout the *Investigations* curriculum, we will point out mathematical terms that are important for you to use in context. Don't insist that students use these terms. It is important that students express their ideas and describe their strategies clearly and accurately, using whatever words are comfortable for them. However, as you use mathematical terms frequently, students will become used to hearing them and will begin to use them naturally. Even young children can learn to use mathematical vocabulary accurately when they hear it used correctly in the context of meaningful activities.

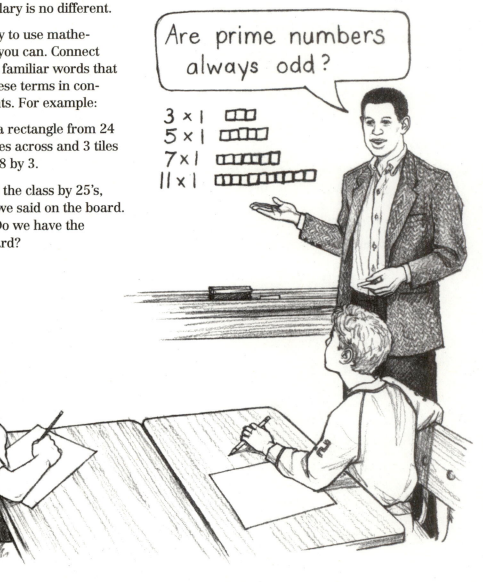

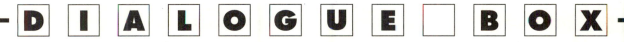

Talking About Calculators

The following vignettes illustrate how Mrs. Jackson introduces the calculators her class will be using.

[*First, she discusses their proper handling.*] **Before we start, should I throw it to you? Here, catch!**

Various students: No! Don't throw it!

What about this? [*She punches several numbers at once, roughly.*]

Rachel: Mrs. Jackson, you're going to ruin it!

Exactly! These are electronic devices. Please respect them.

[*The teacher then helps students locate familiar symbols on the keypad.*] **What do the buttons on the right side do?**

Heather: Take away, plus, multiply, divide.

What about down next to the equals sign?

Antonio: A dot.

Christine: The decimal point.

Oh, the decimal point. OK. And what about over on this other side [*the +/– key*]**?**

Antonio: Plus and take away.

What do you think that might mean?

Zach: It's minus . . .

Jeff: Like on Jeopardy, when they answer a question wrong they get minus.

Zach: It changes the number. Minus is under zero and plus is over zero.

What button clears the display?

Greg: C.

Lindsay: You can also turn it off, then on again.

[*To model sensible calculator use, the teacher gives students the chance to do some computations and to determine whether the answer is reasonable.*] **If I said to you, multiply 653 times 680 . . . don't do it yet! What if your answer came out to be 1200?**

Various students: No way! Way off!

What do you think this person did with those two numbers to get 1200 something?

Katrina: Maybe they didn't hit one of the keys and they thought they did.

Alani: Or maybe they hit the wrong number.

Marcus: I think maybe they plussed them instead of times-ing them.

[*It's also useful to talk about decimals on the calculator display.*] **Corey just made up a division problem and got 5.2631578. What does that mean?**

Yu-Wei: That's about 5.

Greg: It's a little more than 5.

Heather: More than 5 and less than 6. It's even less than 5 and a half.

Mei-Ling: It's close to 5.25—about five and a quarter.

[*The calculator is good for exploring patterns.*] **Try this. Press clear. Press the plus sign, then 2, then the equals. Keep pressing the equals, slowly. What's it doing?**

Corey: Going up by 2's. . . . Even numbers!

Marcus: Multiples of 2.

Does it only work with 2? Prove it to me.

Marcus: I made it go by 5's. You do plus 5 and it's like 5 times 1, then you do it again, and it's like 5 times 2 is 10. . . .

Greg: I did it by 4's.

Lindsay: The calculator did our tables for us!

Try this. Pick a number to count by, but don't tell your partner. Push + , then your number, then = a few times. See if your partner can guess your number by pressing only the equals sign.

Then work together to figure out how many times you'd have to hit the equals sign to get as close to 100 as you can.

Number Puzzles

Materials

- Square tiles (70 per group)
- 300 charts (5–8 sheets or 1 reusable copy per student)
- Sample puzzle clues (1 set per small group)
- Number Puzzles 1–8 (2 duplicate sets, in labeled envelopes)
- Number Puzzles 9☆–14☆ (2 duplicate sets, in labeled envelopes, optional)
- Student Sheet 4 (1 per student)
- Student Sheet 5 (1 per student)
- Student Sheet 6 (1 per student, homework)
- Student Sheet 7 (1 per student, homework)
- Calculators

What Happens

In small groups, students solve number puzzles by sharing four clues and working together to find one or more numbers that fit all the clues. Students also write sets of clues to make their own puzzles. Their work focuses on:

- reasoning about number characteristics such as *multiple, factor, even, odd, prime,* and *square*
- developing, discussing, and comparing different strategies for solving problems
- understanding that problems may have one, many, or no solutions
- writing about mathematical reasoning

 Ten-Minute Math: Exploring Data   For ongoing practice in recording and analyzing data, which will be the focus of other units in the grade 5 curriculum, try the Ten-Minute Math activity Exploring Data. Remember that Ten-Minute Math activities are designed for use in any 10 minutes outside of math class, perhaps before lunch or at the end of the day. Plan to repeat the activity three or four times over the period you spend working in Investigations 1 and 2.

To start the activity, you or the students choose a question about themselves. In order to keep this a short activity, the data they collect must be something they immediately know or can observe easily in the class. For example:

In what country were you born?

How many pockets are you wearing today?

How did you get to school?

What kind of pet do you or someone in your family have, if any?

As students supply their individual pieces of data, quickly graph the data using a line plot, list, table, or bar graph. Ask students to describe what they see in the data, generate new questions, and, if appropriate, make predictions about how the data might be different if they were to ask the same question another time.

For full instructions and variations, see p. 96.

Homework Review: The Rectangles We Made

Open the session with a brief homework review. Working with a partner, students compare the rectangles they made for homework. They check to make sure that they both found all the rectangles for the numbers 1 to 25. They also share what they observed about the rectangles. Then, a few volunteers share their observations with the class.

What are some things you noticed about your rectangles for 1 through 25?

❖ **Tip for the Linguistically Diverse Classroom** Encourage students to hold up their paper and point to specific rectangles and numbers as they share their observations with the rest of the class.

Possible observations include the following:

> Every other number has a factor of 2.
>
> 24 has the most factors.
>
> Some of the rectangles are squares.
>
> 1 is the only number that has a single factor.
>
> Some numbers have only 2 factors.

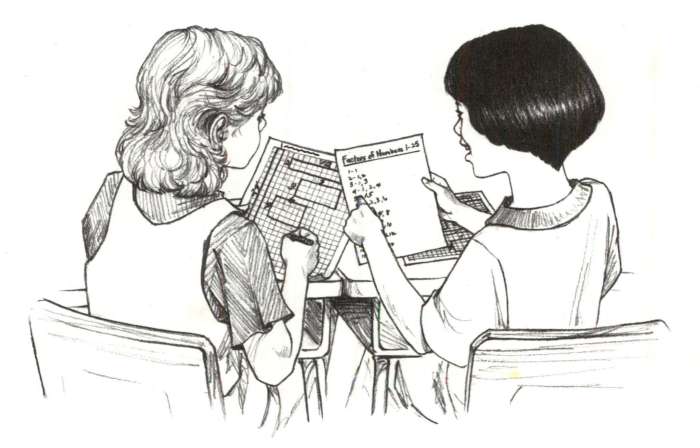

Using Puzzle Clues

Form small groups for this introduction to the number puzzles that the class will be doing for the next three sessions, and again in Investigation 4. Four per group is ideal, since that gives each student exactly one clue. If some groups of three are needed, each student gets a clue, and the extra clue goes to a different student with each new puzzle.

Each group should have a set of the four clues for the sample puzzle (p. 111). Make 300 charts and calculators available.

❖ **Tip for the Linguistically Diverse Classroom** Place second-language learners in groups with English-proficient students. For visual aids in later discussion, the students should save everything they record in the process of solving their puzzle (for example, listing multiples of 15 or marking them on the 300 chart, then crossing out those that are even numbers).

Your set of clues contains one clue for each person in the group. Pass out one clue to everyone in your group. Share your clues by reading them to each other. Your goal is to find a number that fits all four clues.

If you have a question, check with everyone in your group before asking me. If everyone in the group has the same question, raise your hands and I'll come to help you.

Put extra copies of the 300 chart in a convenient place and explain that students can get more if they need them.

If students are unfamiliar with the 300 chart, explain that some people may find these useful in solving number puzzles. Without explaining their use further, give students the chance to find their own ways to use the charts. While groups are working, observe whether anyone uses the 300 chart. During the follow-up discussion, ask any students who have used the charts to explain what they did. If no one uses the charts, you might model using them yourself. The **Dialogue Box**, Solving a Number Puzzle (p. 24), describes several different ways to solve this sample puzzle, including strategies that involve 300 charts.

As students work on the puzzle, circulate to make sure that everyone is participating, that students are listening to one another, that no one is dominating or hoarding all the clues, and that students are discussing any questions group members have.

When all groups have finished, call students together to discuss how they solved the puzzle.

See p. 24

How did your group go about finding the answer? How did you decide that your answer was correct?

One student representative from each group explains how the group used the clues to solve the puzzle. After each explanation, ask if the other group members have anything to add. Encourage students to explain the thinking and reasoning they used to arrive at their answers. Focus on the idea that different students or groups solved the puzzle in different ways.

❖ **Tip for the Linguistically Diverse Classroom** As students explain their strategies, ask them to use visual aids, pointing to relevant parts of their written records as they explain how their group solved the puzzle.

Did you need everyone's clue to solve the puzzle? Why or why not?

Give students a chance to discuss whether they think the answer to the puzzle would change if only three of the clues were used. (There would be more than one solution, because it is impossible to narrow the answer down to just one number with only three of these clues.)

Be sure to collect the sample puzzle clues from each group before you distribute the clues for the next activity.

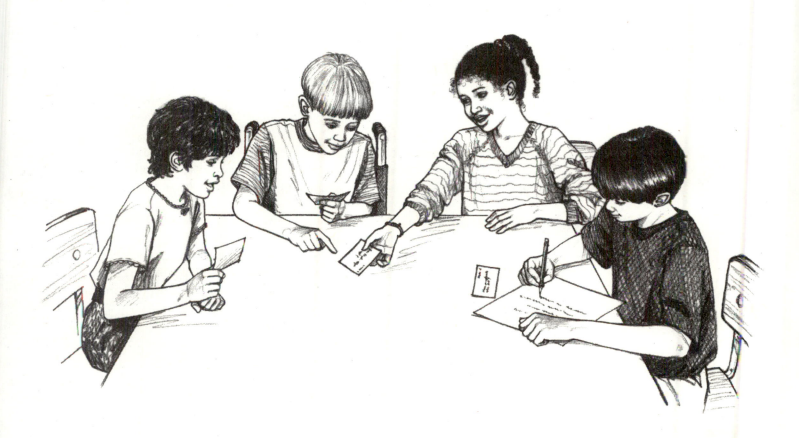

Teacher Checkpoint

Solving Number Puzzles

Teacher Checkpoints are places for you to stop and observe student work (for more information, see About Assessment, p. I-10). However, keep in mind that this entire unit is designed to help you assess your students' understanding of mathematical ideas.

Before You Begin The eight basic number puzzles for this activity (Puzzles 1–8) contain clues about numbers and number relationships. As in the preceding activity, students work together in groups of four to find numbers that fit all the clues. Puzzles 1–4 include clues about the use of square tiles ("My number of tiles will make a square"). Puzzles 5–8 are at the same level of difficulty, but their clues use mathematical terms such as *factor, multiple, prime,* and *square,* ("My number is a square number"), rather than descriptions of what can be made with square tiles.

Decide how many puzzles you want students to try, depending on the time available and the level of your students. You might set a goal for each group of solving three or four different puzzles or even all eight puzzles. Many groups will be able to solve six to eight puzzles in about an hour.

Some teachers designate a certain amount of time (perhaps a single session or an hour split between two sessions) for number puzzle work. Groups then do as many puzzles as they can in that time period, perhaps beginning with one or two puzzles that everyone in the class solves, and then choosing others to work on.

Set up a "puzzle pool" where groups can trade in their envelopes as they finish each puzzle. Also have available extra copies of the 300 chart, if each student does not have a reusable copy.

Introducing the Activity Each group needs at least 70 square tiles and a set of clues for one puzzle. Each student should also have a copy of Student Sheet 4, Number Puzzle Recording Sheet, for writing down their group's answers.

In the envelope that I have given each group, there are four clues for the number puzzle your group will solve first. Some puzzles have more than one answer. Try to find *all* the answers. When you have finished a puzzle, check it off on your recording sheet and write all the answers you found. Then put the clues back in the envelope, return the puzzle to our puzzle pool, and get another one. Be sure to take a different puzzle each time.

Show students where they can return the puzzles and pick up new ones. Remind students that they can take extra copies of the 300 chart if they need them. Encourage students to work without calculators (although calculators may be used if students feel they really need them).

Observing the Students   As students work, circulate to observe whether they are using terms such as *factor, multiple, prime,* and *square* when they talk to one another. Observe whether group members are participating in finding answers, listening to one another, and explaining their reasoning. You may need to remind some students that the clues on puzzles 1–4 are about a number, not about a rectangle. Try to observe each group at least once with the following questions in mind:

- What strategies do students use as they consider each clue (skip-counting orally, skip-counting on the hundred chart, knowledge of multiples?)
- Are they using the terms *multiple, factor, prime, square, odd* and *even* as they talk to one another?
- Do they use these terms correctly in context?
- Are students explaining their reasoning to each other?
- Can students explain what numbers each clue helped them eliminate?
- Can students say how they found all of the solutions (if there is more than one)?

Challenge Number Puzzles   The use of number puzzles 9☆–14☆ is optional. These challenging puzzles require more sophisticated reasoning about numbers and number relationships, and one of the puzzles is impossible. None of them involve the use of square tiles. Put the starred puzzles in a separate location, as a "challenge puzzle pool," for students who finish early. Students who finish the challenge puzzles could try making up their own, then work in groups to try solving each others' puzzles.

 # 11

Sharing Solution Strategies   At the end of the allotted puzzle time, bring the class together to share their answers and the strategies they used to find them. You might organize class sharing in one of the following ways:

- Choose one or two of the puzzles that everyone in the class solved. A member of each group explains how that group approached the puzzle and what answer they arrived at.
- Post a large sheet divided into a section for each of the puzzles. Groups record their answers to each of the puzzles they solved. Students compare the answers their own groups arrived at with those of other groups. Then, as a class, students discuss any discrepancies. For example:

  Some groups thought this puzzle was impossible, and some found an answer. Which do you think is correct? Why? Why do you think someone might have thought this puzzle was impossible?

- If different groups solved different puzzles, pair up students who worked on different puzzles. These students take turns explaining their solution process to their partner who did not do the puzzle. As they work, circulate to listen to their explanations. Can they explain what numbers each clue helped them eliminate? Can they say how they are sure they found all the answers? Can they say how they know the puzzle is impossible? Can the students learning about new puzzles put their partners' explanations in their own words?

Note: Remind students to keep their Number Puzzle Recording Sheet in their math folder, as they will continue working on these and other puzzles during Choice Time in Investigation 4. If they have reusable 300 charts, these should also be saved for use during that same Choice Time.

Following are the answers for number puzzles 1–8 and 9☆–14☆. However, we urge you to try the problems yourself first, to better understand the mathematical thinking students are doing. Use these answers for confirmation of your solutions.

Puzzle 1—16

Puzzle 2—24

Puzzle 3—20, 40

Puzzle 4—1, 3

Puzzle 5—150

Puzzle 6—120, 240

Puzzle 7—36

Puzzle 8—2, 7

Puzzle 9☆—12

Puzzle 10☆—6, 14

Puzzle 11☆—impossible

Puzzle 12☆—350

Puzzle 13☆—99

Puzzle 14☆—154

Activity

Make Your Own Number Puzzle

Distribute a copy of Student Sheet 5, Make Your Own Puzzle, to each student. This sheet gives three clues for a number puzzle and asks students to write a fourth clue that will give the puzzle just one answer.

❖ **Tip for the Linguistically Diverse Classroom** Pair second-language learners with English-proficient students to complete this student sheet.

When students finish their puzzle, they join with another student and trade clues. Partners check each other's new clue to see that it really does give the puzzle only one answer.

When students have finished sharing in pairs, bring the class together. To help students recognize the wide variety of clues that can be added, record all their clues on chart paper to display. You might group them by the resulting answer.

The three given clues yield the following possible numbers: 27, 45, 63, 81, and 99. Below is a list of clues students in one class wrote to narrow the possibilities down to one answer:

It is a rectangle 3 × 9. (27)

It's a multiple of 5. (45)

It's between 50 and 75. (63)

It's a multiple of 7. (63)

It can make a square. (81)

It's a multiple of 11. (99)

It's 1 away from a 3-digit number. (99)

The sum of the digits is 18. (99)

It's over 90. (99)

You say it if you count by 11. (99)

Sessions 4, 5, and 6 Follow-Up

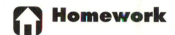 **Homework**

What's the Number?   Students complete Student Sheet 6, What's the Number? They might use a 300 chart to help them. Be sure students understand that three of the four puzzles have more than one answer, and one of the puzzles is impossible—there is no number that fits the clues.

....

❖ **Tip for the Linguistically Diverse Classroom**   Before sending the sheet home, pair second-language learners with students who are fluent in English to read aloud each problem as needed.

....

Student Sheet 6 answers:

1. possible numbers: 2, 5, and 10.

2. impossible

3. possible numbers: 41, 43, and 47

4. possible numbers: 4, 16, and 36

Do Sheet 5

Make an Impossible Puzzle   After students have done Student Sheet 5, Make Your Own Puzzle, in class, send home Student Sheet 7, Make an Impossible Puzzle, and a 300 chart. Consider sharing their added clues in class the following day.

The three given clues yield the following possible numbers: 21, 42, 63, and 84. Following are some sample clues that students in one class wrote to make the puzzle impossible:

It's under 18.	It's a multiple of 5.
It isn't even or odd.	It has 9 as a digit.
It's more than 100.	The sum of the digits is more than 13.
It's a square number.	The sum of the digits is 7.
It's between 45 and 60.	

....

❖ **Tip for the Linguistically Diverse Classroom**   Encourage students to use visual recording techniques—such as listing multiples of 7 and crossing out those that don't fit the remaining clues—as their answer for question 2. Students may use their primary language to write their fourth clue and their explanation of why that clue makes the puzzle impossible.

....

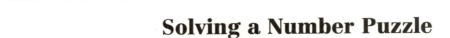
Solving a Number Puzzle

Working in groups on the activity Using Puzzle Clues (p. 18), these students have solved the sample four-clue puzzle. Now a representative from each group comes to the overhead projector and, with a blank transparency or a transparency of the 300 chart, demonstrates how his or her group solved the puzzle. As the students describe their strategies, the teacher records their steps on the board in brief notes, as shown at the end of this dialogue.

Let's review the clues for this sample puzzle. [*The teacher writes the clues on the board.*] **The number is a multiple of 15. It's odd. It's greater than 50, and it's less than 100. OK, let's hear how all the groups solved the puzzle.**

Matt [*from group A*]: We used the 300 chart. We circled the multiples of 15 that are less than 100 and greater than 50. [*He circles 60, 75, and 90 on a transparency of the chart.*] Then it tells you to only use the odd ones, so we went back and crossed out 60 and 90. [*He crosses these out.*] So it's 75.

1	2	3	4	5	6	7	8	9	10
11	12	13	14	15	16	17	18	19	20
21	22	23	24	25	26	27	28	29	30
31	32	33	34	35	36	37	38	39	40
41	42	43	44	45	46	47	48	49	50
51	52	53	54	55	56	57	58	59	60̶
61	62	63	64	65	66	67	68	69	70
71	72	73	74	(75)	76	77	78	79	80
81	82	83	84	85	86	87	88	89	90̶
91	92	93	94	95	96	97	98	99	100
101	102	103	104	105	106	107	108	109	110
111	112	113	114	115	116	117	118	119	120
121	122	123	124	125	126	127	128	129	130
131	132	133	134	135	136	137	138	139	140
141	142	143	144	145	146	147	148	149	150
	153	154	155	156	157	158	159	160
		166	167	168	169	170
					179	180

Amir [*from group B*]: We used the chart, too, but we crossed out the numbers under 50 and over 100. [*He crosses them out on a transparency of the chart.*] Then we crossed out all the even numbers. [*He crosses these out.*] We were left with the multiples of 15 clue. Between 50 and 100, there's 60, 75, and 90. The only one of those that wasn't crossed out was 75. [*He draws a box around 75.*]

1	2	3	4	5	6	7	8	9	10
11	12	13	14	15	16	17	18	19	20
21	22	23	24	25	26	27	28	29	30
31	32	33	34	35	36	37	38	39	40
41	42	43	44	45	46	47	48	49	50
51	52	53	54	55	56	57	58	59	60
61	62	63	64	65	66	67	68	69	70
71	72	73	74	[75]	76	77	78	79	80
81	82	83	84	85	86	87	88	89	90
91	92	93	94	95	96	97	98	99	100
101	102	103	104	105	106	107	108	109	110
111	112	113	114	115	116	117	118	119	120
121	122	123	124	125	126	127	128	129	130
131	132	133	134	135	136	137	138	139	140
141	142	143	144	145	146	147	148	149	150
151	152	153	154	155	156	157	158	159	160
161	162	163	164	165	166	167	168	169	170
	173	174	175	176	177	178	179	180
		186	187	188	189	190
					199	200

Christine [*from group C*]: We wrote down the multiples of 15 less than 100. That's 15, [*she writes as she says them*] 30, 45, 60, 75, 90, and, that's all we can go. Then it said more than 50 [*she crosses out the numbers less than 50*], and it can't be 60 or 90 because that's even. [*She crosses out 60 and 90.*]

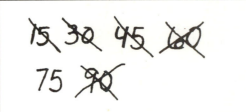

Continued on next page

Desiree [*from group D*]: We wrote down the multiples of 15 under 100. Then we crossed out the even numbers. [*She writes 15, 30, 45, 60, 75, and 90, then crosses out the 30, 60, and 90.*] Then, our paper was a mess, so we rewrote the numbers that were left. [*She writes 15, 45, and 75 underneath.*] That was 15, 45, and 75. We crossed out the ones under 50 [*she crosses out 15 and 45*], so we had 75.

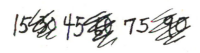

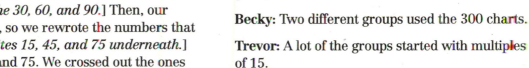

Toshi [*from group E*]: We also wrote down the multiples of 15 under 100. But we crossed out the ones under 50 first [*crosses out 15, 30, and 45*]. Then we crossed out the even ones [*crosses out 60 and 90*], so we got 75 left.

What a lot of different ways to solve the same problem! What do you notice about how different groups found the answer?

Becky: Two different groups used the 300 charts.

Trevor: A lot of the groups started with multiples of 15.

Natalie: One of the groups listed the numbers they found partway through.

Manuel: Some of the groups did sort of the same thing in different orders.

Did you need everyone's clue to solve the puzzle? Do you think you would have all come up with 75 for your answer if you only had three of the clues?

As the class continues, students explore what their answers would be if they had used only three of their clues. They find that if they used only three clues, they would be left with several numbers.

Group A	Group B	Group C	Group D	Group E
• 300 chart	• 300 chart	• list mult of 15 < 100	• list mult of 15 < 100	• list mult of 15 < 100
• circle mult of 15 < 100 and > 50	• cross out > 100	• cross out < 50	• cross out evens	• cross out < 50
• Cross out odds	• cross out < 50	• cross out evens	• wrote odds	• cross out evens
	• cross out evens		• cross out < 50	
	• circle mult of 15			

Multiples and Factors up to 1000

What Happens

Session 1: Skip Counting and Other Ways to Multiply Students count around the class by factors of 100 and their multiples. They use what they know about counting by 25 to make predictions about counting by 50 and 100. Partners then brainstorm strategies for remembering difficult factor pairs.

Sessions 2, 3, and 4: Factor Pairs from 100 to 1000 Students first find all the factor pairs of 100, and they write about how they know they found them all. They use their knowledge of factor pairs of 100 to find factor pairs of multiples of 100, such as 200 and 300. Working in pairs, they make two different rectangles containing 1000 squares. Groups then brainstorm a list of all the factor pairs of 1000.

Session 5: Exploring Rectangles of 1000 Squares
After learning a system for numbering the individual squares that make up their 20 × 50 and 25 × 40 rectangles, students find the squares that correspond to certain numbers. They compare strategies for finding the squares on the two different rectangles (20 × 50 and 25 × 40). Finally, they make a class display of 10,000 squares.

Mathematical Emphasis

- Using knowledge of landmarks up to 100 (including factors of 100 and multiples of those factors) to explore landmarks up to 1000

- Becoming familiar with factors and factor pairs of 1000

- Developing a variety of strategies for exploring number composition, such as repeated addition, skip counting, finding factors, finding factor pairs, and using a calculator to check divisibility

- Reading, writing, and ordering numbers to 1000

- Developing a sense of the magnitude of 1000

- Becoming familiar with skip-counting patterns (sequences of multiples such as 25, 50, 75, . . .) leading to 1000

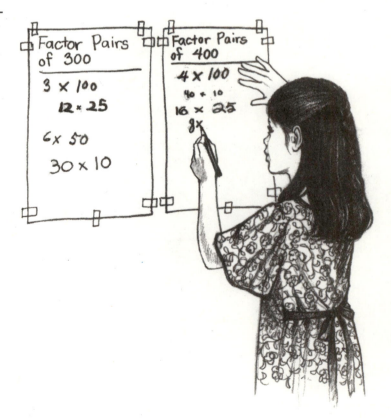

What to Plan Ahead of Time

Materials

- Square tiles: have available for use as needed (Sessions 1–4)
- Scissors: 1 per pair (Sessions 2–4)
- Tape: at least 1 roll for every 4 students (Sessions 2–4)
- Overhead projector (Sessions 1–4, optional)
- Calculators: available (Sessions 2–4)
- Chart paper (Sessions 2–4, optional)
- Notebook paper: 1 sheet per student (Session 5)

Other Preparation

- Make a 20 × 50 or 25 × 40 rectangle of graph paper for each pair of students. (Session 5)

- Make a 50 × 20 grid for class display. The grid should be large enough for everyone in the class to see. You might use square-inch graph paper, either a roll or smaller sheets taped together. Or you could draw a 50 (across) by 20 (down) grid of squares, 1 inch or larger, on the board. If you have a very small class, you could use centimeter paper. (Session 5)

- Duplicate student sheets and teaching resources, located at the end of this unit, in the following quantities. If you have Student Activity Booklets, copy only the transparency and extra materials marked with an asterisk.

For all sessions

A supply of 300 charts (p. 158): 3–5 per student, available for use as needed

For Session 1

Student Sheet 8, Find the Counting Numbers (p. 119): 1 per student (homework)

For Sessions 2–4

15 × 20 grid (p. 122): 10 per pair, plus approximately 20 extras.* **Note:** Make all copies of this grid directly from the master on p. 122 or from the same copy of the master to ensure that all grid squares are the same size.

One-centimeter graph paper (p. 157): 5–7 per student, available for use as needed, and 1 transparency*

Student Sheet 9, More Factor Pairs (p. 120): 1 per student (homework)

Student Sheet 10, Counting Backward (p. 121): 1 per student (homework)

Skip Counting and Other Ways to Multiply

What Happens

Students count around the class by factors of 100 and their multiples. They use what they know about counting by 25 to make predictions about counting by 50 and 100. Partners then brainstorm strategies for remembering difficult factor pairs. Their work focuses on:

- skip counting by factors of 100 and their multiples
- developing strategies for using known factor pairs to find other factor pairs

Materials

- Square tiles, available for use as needed
- 300 charts, available for use as needed
- Student Sheet 8 (1 per student, home-work)
- Overhead projector (optional)

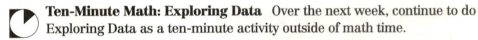 **Ten-Minute Math: Exploring Data** Over the next week, continue to do Exploring Data as a ten-minute activity outside of math time.

You or the students decide on something to record about themselves. For example:

How many letters are in your name?
What color are your shoes today?

As students supply their own pieces of data, quickly note them in a line plot, list, table, or bar graph. Students describe what they can see in the data, generate new questions, and, if appropriate, make predictions about how the data might be different if they were to ask the same question another time.

For full directions and variations, see p. 96.

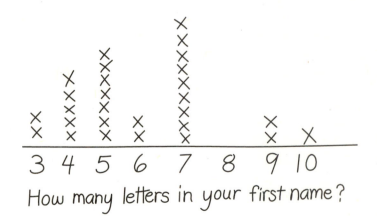

How many letters in your first name?

Counting Around the Class

You all know how easy it is to count by 2's and by 5's and by 10's. Today we're going to try counting by some larger numbers. We'll do it by counting around the class, taking turns saying the number that comes next.

We're going to start out counting by 25's. The first person will say "25," the second will say "50," the third will say "75," and so on.

Count around the class, asking for volunteers who haven't yet said a number to say the next number in the count. Stop at about 225 to look back.

We're up to 225 counting by 25's. How many students have counted so far? How do you know?

Encourage students to figure this out without actually counting heads.

If we keep counting by 25's, and everyone in the class says one number in the count, what number will we end with?

Again, encourage students to explain how they could find the answer without actually doing the counting. Record students' predictions on the board. Then ask the class to count by 25's again, specifying the order so that each student understands when his or her turn will be. As students count, put the numbers they say on the board. Seeing the sequence of numbers that have been counted so far will help some students know what comes next.

How do your predictions compare to the number we actually ended with? Were all your predictions in the 25's table?

Let's count again by 25's, but this time we'll start in another part of the room, with Trevor.

Count around the class by 25's again, starting with a different person. Then try counting around by 50's. Ask students to predict the ending number, without counting, and to explain their predictions. Record their predictions on the board.

As students count around the class by 50's, you may want to stop them one or more times to look back on how many students have counted so far. When students have finished the count, ask them to compare their predictions to the number they really ended with.

During this activity, observe what strategies students use for determining how many of them have counted so far and for predicting the ending number. The **Dialogue Box**, Counting Around the Class (p. 34), illustrates some strategies that students sometimes use in making predictions.

Different Ways of Naming Thousands As students do this activity, notice how they say number names. When counting by 100's, some will say: "9 hundred, 10 hundred, 11 hundred, 12 hundred . . ." Other students will say the same numbers this way: "9 hundred, 1 thousand, 1 thousand 1 hundred, 1 thousand 2 hundred . . ."

Of course, both ways are correct. If there seems to be any confusion, encourage students to find different ways of saying the same number and explain their reasoning. Seeing the numbers on the board as they count by 100's may increase their understanding. That is, when counting out loud, they may find it natural to continue saying "hundreds," but when they see the written number, they may recognize that it can also be expressed as a number of thousands and number of hundreds.

Counting by Hundreds Ask students where they would end up if they counted around the class by 100's. Students make their predictions and explain their reasoning. If there is much disagreement in the predictions, you may want to count around by 100's to check.

Now I'm looking for another number to count around the class by, and I want to be sure that somewhere in the count, someone will say 100. What are some numbers we could use?

As students give their answers and explain how they know someone would say 100, record their responses on the board. Then count up to 100 by a few of the numbers they suggest.

What if we wanted to be sure that somewhere in the count, someone would say 200? 400? 1000? What numbers would work?

Students talk with a partner about how to figure this out without actually doing the counting. For example, one strategy is to count by multiples of numbers that work for 100. If someone in the class will say 100 when you count by 4's, then someone will say 200 when you count by 4's.

What are some other large numbers that are easy to count by? What makes them easy to count by?

Some students find it easy to count by numbers that are 10, 100, or 1000 times a familiar counting number, such as 2 or 5. Plan for another class time (or time outside of class) for students to count around the class with some of the large numbers they think will be easy.

Note: In this activity, students worked with a powerful way of building numbers, *repeated addition,* as they counted around the class. In Investigation 1, students explored building numbers with *factor pairs*—that is, they found a pair of numbers that can be multiplied together to form a given product. Students will continue to work with these two ways of building numbers in many different activities throughout the unit. See the **Teacher Note,** Two Important Ways of Building Numbers (p. 33), for more on the relationships between these two ideas.

Strategies for Remembering Factor Pairs

When we counted around the class, we used the answer to one problem to help find the answer to another problem. That is, we knew that counting around by 25 would get us to _____ [*whatever ending number applies to your class*], and we used that to predict what number we'd end with if we counted by 50 and 100.

Now we're going to think about factor pairs, and see how we can use easy factor pairs to remember harder ones.

Write on the board or overhead:

$6 \times 8 =$

Suppose a fifth grade friend of yours had trouble remembering the answer to 6×8. What are some ways your friend might remember it?

If students have difficulty getting started, encourage them to think about how *they* remember 6×8. You might also suggest thinking about how they could use the answer to one problem to find another:

Suppose your friend knows that $3 \times 8 = 24$. How could she use that knowledge to find the answer to 6×8? How else could she find the answer to 6×8?

As students suggest possible strategies, record their suggestions on the board. Possible strategies include the following:

- Doubling either 3×8 or 6×4. "6×4 is 24. 6×8 is twice that, so it's 24 and 24—that's 48."
- Combining two known factor pairs. "The 5's are easy to remember, so you can start at 6×5, and then add on 6×3. That's 30 and 18."
- Counting up or down from a known factor pair. "If you know 5×8 is 40, you can just add 8 more to get 6×8, so that's 48."
- Counting by 8 to find six 8's. "8, 16, 24, 32, 40, 48."

Now write $9 \times 7 =$ on the board or overhead. Ask students to take a few minutes to talk with a neighbor about ways they might help someone remember the answer to 9×7. Record their ideas.

Strategies for Remembering Factor Pairs   Write these multiplication pairs on the board:

$8 \times 7 =$ $7 \times 6 =$

$9 \times 6 =$ $8 \times 9 =$

Some students find these factor pairs hard to remember. Can you think of others that are hard to remember?

As students suggest other factor pairs that they find difficult, add these to the list on the board. For now, restrict the pairs to one-digit numbers.

For the remainder of the session, students work with a partner. They take turns choosing a factor pair that they find difficult—either one of the pairs on the board or one of their choice. With their partners, they brainstorm and record a list of strategies for remembering that particular pair.

Circulate to observe the strategies students are listing. Encourage students to list all the strategies they can think of. Using square tiles or 300 charts might help some students find relationships among factor pairs.

Session 1 Follow-Up

Homework

Find the Counting Numbers   Students complete Student Sheet 8, Find the Counting Numbers. They may use 300 charts to help them find all the numbers that fit each clue.

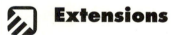

❖ **Tip for the Linguistically Diverse Classroom**   Before sending the sheet home, pair second-language learners with students who are fluent in English to read aloud each problem as needed.

Student Sheet 8 answers:
1.   4, 20, 25, 50, 100
2.   25, 50, 100, 200
3.   2, 4, 6, 10, 12, 20, 30, 50, 60, 100, 150, 300

Extensions

Counting by Larger Numbers   Students choose a multiple of 5 between 25 and 50. With a group of three to five people, they then count several times around by that number, writing down the numbers that are said during the count.

Help with Difficult Factor Pairs   Each student lists the factor pairs he or she personally finds difficult to remember. Students work alone or with a partner to list strategies for remembering each of those factor pairs. They return to their lists of difficult factor pairs and strategies periodically throughout the unit, cross off the pairs that no longer seem difficult, and, with a partner, brainstorm and list additional strategies for the pairs they still find difficult.

Two Important Ways of Building Numbers

In this unit, students work with two important ways of building numbers: repeated addition, and factor pairs (or multiplication). Some activities in the unit, such as Counting Around the Class (p. 29), focus on repeated addition; others, such as Building Number Rectangles (p. 5), focus on factor pairs; and some are designed to invite a variety of approaches. Each approach offers a different view of number composition.

Repeated Addition   With repeated addition, we build up a number step by step as we add the same quantity over and over again. The "in-between" numbers we make when we build a number in this way form a pattern: They are the multiples of the number we are repeatedly adding. We get the same pattern of multiples in reverse by repeatedly subtracting the same number over and over again.

$0 + 50 = 50$ $50 + 50 = 100$ $100 + 50 = 150$
$150 + 50 = 200$ $. . . 950 + 50 = 1000$

$1000 - 50 = 950$ $950 - 50 = 900$
$900 - 50 = 850 . . .$ $100 - 50 = 50$ $50 - 50 = 0$

Factor Pairs   With factor pairs, we work with only three numbers: the two factors we multiply together and their product. Each factor divides the product evenly. Building numbers with factor pairs is conceptually more complex than building numbers with repeated addition, since there are no "in-between" numbers.

$$50 \times 20 = 1000$$
$$1000 \div 20 = 50$$
$$1000 \div 50 = 20$$

The Relationship Between Repeated Addition and Factor Pairs   The two approaches are rather closely related. Consider the two numbers in a factor pair. When we multiply them together, we get a product: $50 \times 20 = 1000$. We get the same number if we add one number in the factor pair the other number of times. That is, if we add 50 twenty times, we get 1000. And if we add 20 fifty times, we also get 1000.

Some students will begin to recognize these relationships between repeated addition and factor pairs. For example, they may be able to explain how knowing factor pairs of 1000 can help them find numbers they can count by to get to 1000. Other students may be fluent with both ways of building numbers, but not yet be ready to articulate the relationship between the two. Still others will not recognize the similarity between skip counting (50, 100, 150, . . .), adding the same number on paper $(50 + 50 + 50 + . . .)$, and finding a series of multiples ($50 \times 1 = 50$, $50 \times 2 = 100$, $50 \times 3 = 150$, . . .).

It's important that all students develop a flexible repertoire of number composition strategies, whether or not they are able to explain relationships among them. Building numbers in different ways can provide a strong foundation for many kinds of mathematical thinking, such as reasoning about number, inventing mental arithmetic strategies, and analyzing relationships among the four basic operations.

DIALOGUE BOX

Counting Around the Class

In the activity Counting Around the Class (p. 29), students have just gone around the entire class counting by 25's. The teacher explains that next they will be counting around the class by 50's. As students make their predictions for an ending number, some begin to recognize that what they know about counting around the class by 25's can help them make predictions about counting by 50's.

Before we count by 50's, let's predict what number we'll end with. How can you make your predictions without counting?

Tai: Count the people in the room and times by 50. That's 23 [the number in the class] times 50.

Christine: Or you can take 50 and add it 23 times.

Jeff: 50 times 23 is like 25 times 23 and another 25 times 23, or 25 forty-six times.

Sofia: When we counted by 25's, we got 575. This is another 25 for each person. So it's 575 plus 25 times 23.

Amy Lynn: We already know that 25 times 23 is 575. So it's 575 and 575. You can take the two 500's and add them together. That's 1000. Then 75 and 75 is 150. So it's 1150.

Maricel: It's just double it! 50 is double 25, so you double what we got when we counted by 25.

Heather: 50 times 23 is like 100 times 11 and a half, because you double the 50 to get 100 and you take half of 23. That's easier—you just go 11 and a half times ten is 115, and that times another ten is 1150.

Noah: I've got a different way to do it. You also could do it by number of people at each table. Every table of 4 is 200. There's [*he counts the tables*] 1, 2, 3, 4, 5, 6 tables. So it's six 200's.

Kevin: That won't work. There's a table of 3.

Robby: You can still do it by 4's and then take away the one that's not there. So there are 6 tables and let's make believe they are all 4's. So, 200, 400, 600, 800, 1000, 1200. And then take away 50 for this table of 3 . . . 1200 take away 50 is like, 200 take away 50 and then the 1000—1150.

Duc: A group of 4 is 200 and a group of 3 is 150.

Julie: There's five tables of 4. That's 200, 400, 600, 800, 1000. Then there's one group of 150. You add them up. 1000 plus 150 is 1150.

Leon: It's simple. It's like money. When we did the 25's, it was like 25, 50, 75, and a dollar for a table of 4. Five tables of 4 is five dollars. This [the 50's] is like two dollars for a table of 4, so it's ten dollars. Then 25, 50, 75 for a table of 3, so it's now a dollar fifty for a table of 3. It's ten dollars and a dollar fifty. Eleven dollars and fifty cents.

Duc: It's a pattern. A dollar for a table of 4 if you count by 25, two dollars if you count by 50. Everything is twice as much because 25 times 2 is 50.

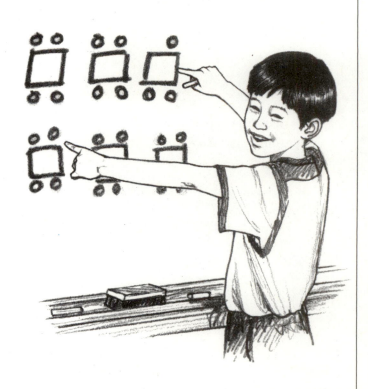

34 ■ *Investigation 2: Multiples and Factors up to 1000*

Factor Pairs from 100 to 1000

What Happens

Students first find all the factor pairs of 100, and they write about how they know they found them all. They use their knowledge of factor pairs of 100 to find factor pairs of multiples of 100, such as 200 and 300. Working in pairs, they make two different rectangles containing 1000 squares. Groups then brainstorm a list of all the factor pairs of 1000. Their work focuses on:

- developing a sense of the magnitude of 1000
- becoming familiar with factor pairs of 1000
- finding relationships among factor pairs of different multiples of 100

Materials

- One-centimeter graph paper (5–7 sheets per student, and 1 transparency)
- 300 charts remain available
- Square tiles and calculators remain available
- Chart paper (optional)
- 15 × 20 grid (10 per pair, plus extras)
- Scissors (1 per pair)
- Tape (1 roll per 2–4 students)
- Overhead projector (optional)
- Student Sheet 9 (1 per student, homework)
- Student Sheet 10 (1 per student, homework)

Let's start by thinking about some of the things we've done so far in this math unit. Who can tell us how we used calculators to find "paths to 100"? What were some ways we got to 100 when we counted around the class? Who remembers what we did with our square tiles and our graph paper? How can we use 300 charts to identify factors of a number?

....

❖ **Tip for the Linguistically Diverse Classroom** Have examples of graph paper, 300 charts, square tiles, and calculators to display as you refer to them. Model a quick example of skip counting as a reminder of this approach. Write the numbers on the board as you count.

....

After a brief review of the tools and techniques the class has been using, introduce today's activity.

Today you're going to work with a partner to find all the factor pairs of 100. You may use any of the tools and approaches we have used in class—graph paper, 300 charts, square tiles, calculators, skip counting.

Activity

Teacher Checkpoint

Factor Pairs of 100

Students work in pairs, with each student recording all the factor pairs of 100 on his or her own paper. They record each factor pair only once; thus, if they record 1 × 100, they do not also record 100 × 1. When they think they have found them all, students explain in writing how they know this is all the factor pairs of 100.

Observing the Students   While students are working, try to observe each pair at least once. What are students' strategies? How well-developed is their ability to explain their strategies? As you circulate, keep the following questions in mind:

■ How do they go about finding factor pairs of 100? Do they find and record factor pairs in a systematic way? What numbers do they try before they decide they have found all the factors?

■ What tools do they use to find the answer—calculators? mental arithmetic? skip counting? graph paper? 300 charts? knowledge about divisibility?

■ Do students have strategies for using one answer to find others? For example: "I know that 10 × 10 = 100, so 20 × 5 also works, because you can double the 10 to get 20 and then take half the other 10 to get 5."

■ Do pairs work cooperatively, or does one member tend to dominate?

■ Are students able to write clearly about how they know they found all the factor pairs?

If students have difficulty with the final writing, ask them to tell you orally what they think. If they can tell you clearly, ask them to write down just what they told you. If they cannot, ask a few questions to help them to express their thinking.

You wrote down that 2 × 50 is a factor pair of 100. How did you find that factor pair? I noticed you didn't write down a factor pair with 3 in it. How did you decide that there wasn't a factor pair with 3? Did you try 5 to see if it worked? 50? 99?

If students have difficulty finding factor pairs of 100, suggest that they use graph paper to make all the rectangles that have exactly 100 squares. For additional activities that focus on factor pairs of 100 and multiples of 100, review the *Investigations* grade 4 unit, *Landmarks in the Thousands*.

Sharing the Factor Pairs of 100   On a part of the board you will not need for a while, or on several pieces of chart paper, create lists that can remain posted throughout this unit. You will need ten lists, headed as follows: Factor Pairs of 100, Factor Pairs of 200, Factor Pairs of 300, . . . up to Factor Pairs of 1000. Introduce these lists after everyone has finished the checkpoint activity.

Invite students to share the factor pairs of 100 they found and their strategies for finding them. On the first list, write the factor pairs in order. Explain that over the next few days, students will be finding factor pairs for other multiples of 100 and adding them to these lists.

Factor Pairs of 100
1 × 100
2 × 50
4 × 25
5 × 20
10 × 10

Note: Some students may suggest pairs of numbers that include decimals, such as 12.5 and 8, that have 100 as a product. Encourage them to find more such pairs of numbers and record them on the lists, but explain that mathematicians think of factors as whole numbers only.

Factor Pairs of Multiples of 100

Now you're going to work on the lists of factor pairs for 200 and 300. Do you think you could use what you know about factor pairs of 100 to find factor pairs of 200 and 300?

Students work in pairs on this activity for 5–10 minutes. They may use calculators, 300 charts, square tiles, and graph paper as needed.

Observing the Students Circulate to observe how students are approaching the task. Some will have no difficulty using what they know about factor pairs of 100 to find other factor pairs. For example, to find factor pairs of 200, they might double one factor in a factor pair of 100, or they might use a calculator to divide factors of 100 into 200. Other students may need to find some factor pairs of 200 another way before they begin seeing relationships between factor pairs of 100 and 200.

Students who finish early can try to find *all* the factor pairs of 200 and 300, or they can find a few factor pairs for other multiples of 100, such as 400 or 800.

When you observe students who need more practice, suggest that they circle skip-counting patterns that lead to 100 on a 300 chart, and then extend these patterns to reach 200. As necessary, point out that the number they are counting by is one member of the factor pair, and the number of times it is counted (circled) is the other member of the factor pair.

Sharing Our Discoveries   After most students have found several factors for 200 and 300, bring the class together to share the factor pairs they found and their strategies for finding them. The **Dialogue Box**, Finding Factor Pairs of Multiples of 100 (p. 42), illustrates some student strategies you may hear in your class.

Record on the class lists the factor pairs students found. Encourage students to continue adding to these lists in their free time (this is also suggested as home-work for these sessions). Remind them to record each factor pair only once— that is, if they record 25 × 8, they do not also record 8 × 25.

Note: Keep the Factor Pair lists on display, as you will be referring to them later in this Investigation and also in Investigations 3 and 4.

Activity

Building Rectangles with 1000 Squares

What's the largest number we created a Factor Pair list for? (1000) How much larger is 1000 than 100?

Some students may explain that 1000 is 900 more than 100; others will say that it is 10 times as large.

Hold up one of the 15 × 20 grids you have duplicated for student use.

How many squares do you think there are on this grid? How could we find out?

Most students will recognize that they could find out by multiplying the number of squares across by the number of squares down. A few may suggest adding the number in each row or column.

Would a rectangle with 1000 of these squares fit on your desk? Would it fit on the bulletin board? Would a long, narrow strip of 1000 of these squares fit along the length of the classroom?

Gather a few quick estimates from students, and record students' ideas about how big 1000 squares would be. Explain that students are now going to make rectangles with 1000 squares, so they will be able to check to see if their estimates were close.

Model the following instructions for making the rectangles as you present them to the class. Jot examples and key phrases on the board to remind students what to do. Include simple drawings wherever possible.

(handwritten note) SAVE ALL 20×50 OR 40×25 GRIDS FOR NEXT ACTIVITIES

(handwritten)
1 × 1000
2 × 500
4 × 250
5 × 200
10 × 100
8 × 125

20 × 50
25 × 40

- I'm going to give ten of these grids to each pair. You are to make two *different* rectangles from your grids. Each rectangle should have 1000 squares. You should not be able to turn one of your rectangles around to make the other one.

- It's hard to count lots of squares accurately, so make sure you double-check before you cut.

- Record the dimensions of each rectangle on the back.

- If you need to make any marks on your rectangles, use pencil so that it's easy to erase if you make a mistake.

Student pairs will find it easier to use a work surface larger than a student desk. Depending on the layout of the classroom, students may either work on a table, at two desks pushed together, or on the floor.

Distribute scissors and ten grids to each pair. Leave additional grids in a convenient place so that students can take more if they need them. Distribute a roll of tape to each pair, or for two pairs to share.

When students have completed their rectangles, each student chooses one. On a separate piece of paper, the students write about how they know their rectangles have 1000 squares.

Pairs who finish early can make a third rectangle (of different dimensions) with 1000 squares, or they can continue to find factor pairs of other multiples of 100 for the class lists.

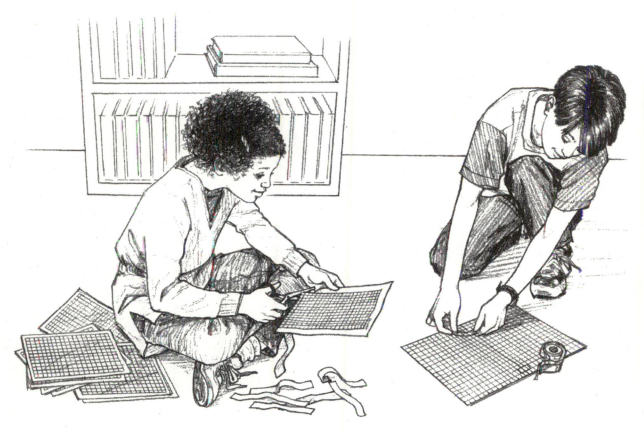

What Rectangles Did We Make?

As pairs complete their rectangles, group each pair with another pair to compare their work. Pairs show each other their rectangles, and they explain how they made them and how they know each one has 1000 squares. Together, the four students brainstorm a list of all the rectangles that would have 1000 squares.

Class Discussion When the small groups seem to have found all the rectangles they can, bring the class together.

What's one rectangle you made? How did you find those dimensions? Did anyone make a different rectangle?

Students hold up their rectangles for others to see. Remind students that the dimensions of the rectangles with 1000 squares are the factor pairs of 1000. Write the dimensions of each different rectangle on the class list of Factor Pairs of 1000. Record each dimension pair only once. As students explain how they found the different rectangles, you may hear strategies like these:

■ Beginning with a known size rectangle, such as 1 × 1000, then halving one side and doubling the other to create a different rectangle.

■ Using a calculator or skip counting to find factor pairs of 1000.

■ Building on their knowledge of factor pairs of 100 (or multiples of 100).

Ask if the class has found all the factor pairs of 1000, and how they can know for sure. Some students may suggest a systematic strategy for checking, such as ordering the factor pairs and checking numbers that are not in the factor pair list to see if they divide 1000 evenly, or starting at 1 and checking successive numbers to see if they are factors of 1000.

Post each one of the different rectangles of 1000 squares on a bulletin board, on the wall, or on a section of the classroom floor. Gather students around the display.

How do we know that each of these rectangles has 1000 squares?

The **Dialogue Box**, Relationships Among Factor Pairs of 1000 (p. 43), illustrates how trying to "prove" that the different rectangles all have 1000 squares can lead students to a deeper understanding of factor pairs and the array model of multiplication.

You may want to engage the class in testing some of the predictions they made earlier about the size of 1000 squares. For example, to test a prediction that a strip of 1000 squares would fit along the length of the classroom, someone could try laying a 1000 × 1 rectangle across the floor or along the wall.

For Session 5 of this Investigation, each pair will need either a 20 × 50 or a 25 × 40 rectangle. Some pairs will have already made one or both rectangles. Pairs that have both can give one to a pair that has not made either. Some students may need additional time during the school day to make their rectangles. If necessary, students can make a suitable rectangle for homework using additional 15 × 20 grids.

Sessions 2, 3, and 4 Follow-Up

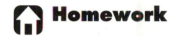

Homework

More Factor Pairs   After you have started the class lists of Factor Pairs (100 to 1000), students choose a multiple of 100 and work at home to find and record several factor pairs of that number on Student Sheet 9, More Factor Pairs. When they come to class, they can add their factor pairs to the appropriate list if they are not already listed. Encourage students to check that they agree with what their classmates have added to the lists. They should watch for factor pairs that are recorded more than once—such as 25 × 8 and 8 × 25—and remove one of the duplicate pairs.

Counting Backward   Students start at a multiple of 100 and count *backward* by one of the factors on the class factor pair lists. Because backward counting sequences are less familiar, this process requires students to think more carefully about number sequences and number patterns. Students record their counts on Student Sheet 10, Counting Backward. Students choosing a number less than 300 might use a 300 chart to help them.

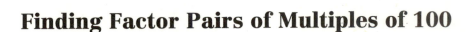
Finding Factor Pairs of Multiples of 100

While working on the activity Factor Pairs of Multiples of 100 (p. 37), student pairs have just spent several minutes finding a few factor pairs of 200 and 300. The teacher then brings the class together to share their discoveries and to extend their findings to larger multiples of 100. Notice that the students have used a variety of strategies, including finding multiples of one of the numbers in a factor pair, using repeated addition, drawing upon knowledge of familiar multiplication facts, and reasoning about divisibility.

What did you discover for factor pairs of 200 and 300? Did you find a way to use what you know about factor pairs of 100?

Danny: For 200, all you have to do is double it, and for 300 you triple them.

Marcus: But just one of them. I can't say it! It's like, we moved it up the 100's tables. We doubled one side for the 200's and tripled one side for the 300's.

Let's use 50 × 2 as an example. What would you do to turn it into a factor pair of 200?

Mei-Ling: Add 50, so that's 100 × 2.

Greg: You could also change the 2 into a 4 to get 50 × 4.

What about making 50 × 2 a factor pair of 300?

Greg: 50 × 6.

Mei-Ling: 50 plus 50 plus 50 . . . 150, times 2.

OK, now take 50 × 2 and tell me how you can make it a factor pair of 700.

Trevor: 350 × 2 . . . 50 × 7 is 350, times 2.

Cara: It's easier to do 7 × 2 is 14, so I'd make 14 × 50.

Let's look at another factor pair of 100—what about 25 × 4? Can you get to 200 starting with 25 × 4?

Jeff: 27 × 4, because it's twice as much so you go up by 2.

Amir: No, you added. You need to double. It would work for 50 × 4.

Mei-Ling: It wouldn't work because 27 is not a factor of 100.

Cara: Sometimes that doesn't matter. You also need to check other numbers like 3, 4, 6, 7, 8, 9 . . . Like, 8 works for 200, but it doesn't work for 100.

How could we find a factor pair for 400 starting with 25 × 4?

Danny: 25 × 16, because 25 times 4 is 100, and all you had to do is keep going with the 4's tables and keep going up by 4's.

Alani: You go 4, 8, 12, 16. The first 4 is 100, 8 is 200, 12 is 300, and 16 is 400.

Can you make 25 × 4 into a factor of pair 900?

Cara: 36, because you go 4 × 9—so 36 × 25.

Relationships Among Factor Pairs of 1000

During the whole-class discussion, What Rectangles Did We Make? (p. 40), students posted on the board six different rectangles they made with 1000 squares: 8 × 125, 25 × 40, 20 × 50, 5 × 200, 10 × 100, and 4 × 250. In discussing whether they had done all the factor pairs of 1000, the class discovered that there were two rectangles no one had made—the 1 × 1000 and the 2 × 500. Four students offered to make these so their collection would be complete. The two new ones were too long to post with the others, so the class laid them out as best they could on the floor.

In the following discussion, as the students explain how eight rectangles that look so different can all have 1000 squares, they extend their understanding of the array model of multiplication to large numbers, and they use mathematics to develop their ideas about size and shape.

How can this one [the 1 × 1000 rectangle] have the same number of squares as that one [the 20 × 50 rectangle]? This one's real long and really skinny, and the other one's real short and fat.

Natalie: Because of length and width.

Corey: Because if you cut that one [1 × 1000] into shorter strips and put them together, you can make the other one [the 20 × 50].

Lindsay: If you cut that one [2 × 500] down the middle, it'd be the same [as the 1 × 1000].

Yu-Wei: You could count by 10's, and cut them all up in strips of 10. You'd get the same number of strips for each one.

Jasmine: Or 100's. The same number of 100 strips.

Other students: Or 50's. Or 200's.

Desiree: You could cut them all into strips and put them into one line and it would always equal 1000.

Jasmine: Break 'em all up into little squares, and you'd have 1000 little squares for each one.

How do you know they have 1000?

Matt: You don't need to cut. You can just do 1000 in half to get 500, and double the 1 to get 2. You can keep going and do it on every one. To make all of the rectangles we did.

What about 5 × 200? How do you get that with Matt's way?

Matt: If you start with 5 × 200, you can do it. Double the 5 and half the 200 is 10 × 100.

Natalie: They're all related because they're always from 1000. The rectangles all have 1000.

Corey: They're all factor pairs of 1000.

Leon: Count both sides and multiply on a calculator, and you'd get 1000 for each one.

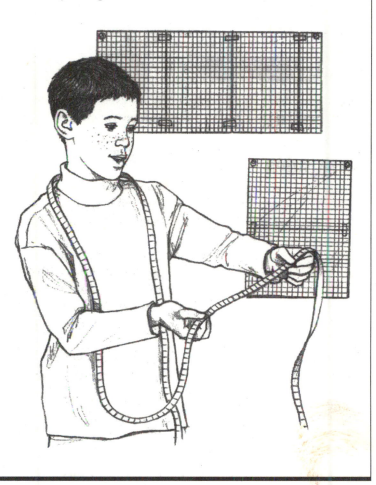

Session 5

Exploring Rectangles of 1000 Squares

Materials

- 20 × 50 or 25 × 40 rectangles of graph paper, made previously (1 per pair)
- Large 50 × 20 grid for class demonstration
- Notebook paper (1 sheet per student)

What Happens

After learning a system for numbering the individual squares that make up their 20 × 50 and 25 × 40 rectangles, students find the squares that correspond to certain numbers. They compare strategies for finding the squares on the two different rectangles (20 × 50 or 25 × 40). Finally they make a class display of 10,000 squares. Their work focuses on:

- reading, writing, and ordering numbers to 1000
- becoming familiar with skip-counting patterns (sequences of multiples such as 25, 50, 75, . . .) leading to 1000
- becoming familiar with important landmarks up to 1000, including the factors of 1000 and multiples of those factors
- developing a sense of the magnitude of 10,000

Activity

Numbering Squares in Our Rectangles

Have students make these first. use 15×20 grid paper & tape together

READ TO CLASS

Continue to bottom of P. 45

collect work when done.

Before You Begin For this activity, each pair needs either a 20 × 50 or a 25 × 40 rectangle. Pairs should double-check that their rectangle is the correct size. If necessary, allow time for students to change or redo their rectangles.

The Numbering System Use the large 50 × 20 grid to demonstrate how everyone will number the squares on their rectangles. The sequence of numbers begins in the upper left corner and proceeds from left to right across each row.

This rectangle is 50 squares wide and 20 squares long. If we started numbering the squares with 1 in the upper left corner and went across the row, what would this next square be? three more squares across? the last square in the row? the first square of the second row? the last square of the second row? the square in the lower right corner? How do you know?

As students explain how they are determining the numbers for the squares, demonstrate their strategies on the large rectangle. For example, if a student explains that you can find the 200 square by counting by 50's down the rightmost square in each row, you might write in the numbers down the last column (50, 100, 150, 200) to demonstrate.

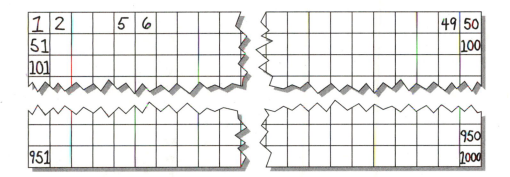

Continue asking students to find the numbers for squares on your large rectangle until you are satisfied they understand the numbering system and that they are developing ways of finding particular squares *without counting by 1's.*

Finding Six Particular Squares Direct students' attention to their own rectangles. Explain that with their partners, they will be finding some numbers on their grid, the same way they did on the big one. In addition to their rectangle, each student needs a sheet of notebook paper.

First decide how you and your partner will position your rectangle—with the long way across, or the long way down. Either way is OK. On your paper, write the dimensions of your rectangle, like this:

_____ squares across and _____ squares down

These are the numbers [*write them on the board*] you will be finding on your rectangle:

250   375   461   500   640   750

While you are doing this activity, you can fill in a few other numbers to help keep track of where you are—but don't write in *every* number. Use only pencil, so you can erase easily.

When you have found all six squares, I want each of you to write about this on your paper [*write on the board*]:

Describe how you found 640 on your rectangle.

Before students begin work, you might do a trial run to make sure students can apply the numbering system to their rectangles.

Let's do one number together first. Find the square that would be numbered 100 on your rectangle. In pencil, write 100 in the correct square. Then explain how you found it to another pair of students.

Circulate to make sure students are applying the numbering system that you demonstrated, and that they are not counting or numbering every square on their rectangles.

❖ **Tip for the Linguistically Diverse Classroom** Pair students so that one who writes comfortably in English can describe how they found 640, while the other partner supports the description with numerical records. For example:

> We counted by 100's, down every two rows (50 + 50), until we got to 600. We knew 640 would be 10 less than another whole row of 50 so we went another whole row and then counted back 10 squares.

$$50+50 + 50+50 + 50+50 + 50+50 + 50+50 + 50+50 + 50 - 10$$
$$\quad \smile \qquad \smile \qquad \smile \qquad \smile \qquad \smile \qquad \smile \qquad \smile \quad \smile$$
$$\quad 100 \qquad 200 \qquad 300 \qquad 400 \qquad 500 \qquad 600 \quad 650 \quad 640$$

Each pair now proceeds, finding the six numbers and writing their descriptions of how they found the square for 640. When they finish, they meet with a pair that used a different rectangle (or that used the same rectangle in a different orientation), and they share their strategies for finding 640 and a few of the other numbers.

Observe students to see how they are finding the numbers. Encourage them to use skip-counting patterns, multiples, or other strategies. If it is not clear how some students are finding numbers, ask them individually to locate a few more numbers and to tell you how they are doing it. Possible student strategies include the following: (1) filling in the number of the rightmost square in every row (or every other row); (2) marking multiples of a number such as 25 or 50; (3) filling in the multiples of a small number, such as 5, across a row in the middle of the rectangle, and then counting up or down by the width of a row to find other squares.

Students who finish early might repeat the activity, using a rectangle with different dimensions.

Activity

Displaying 10,000 Squares

With our rectangles, we've been working with one thousand squares [write 1000 on the board]. **Does anyone know how to write the number ten thousand?**

As you hear the correct response, write 10,000 on the board.

How many of your rectangles with 1000 squares would you need in order to have 10,000 squares?

Students briefly discuss this question with a partner; then a few share their answer and how they got it. Possible strategies include keeping track of the number of times you need to add 1000 until you reach 10,000; knowing that 10,000 means 10 one thousands; or dividing 10,000 by 1000 on a calculator.

Ask for ten volunteers to each donate one rectangle for a class display of 10,000 squares. Post the rectangles, with edges touching, on the board or on a section of the wall.

Session 5 Follow-Up

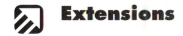 **Extensions**

1000 Square Rectangles   Ask the class to count the total number of rectangles of 1000 squares in the classroom. These might include all the 1000 square rectangles made in the previous sessions, or just those used in Session 5. Students determine how many squares there are in all these rectangles put together, and they write about how they found their answers.

❖ **Tip for the Linguistically Diverse Classroom**   Students who are not writing comfortably in English may use numbers and pictures to show how they found their answers.

The next day, you might find a place to post all the rectangles—perhaps in the hallway—to get a sense of the magnitude of the number they found that represents all those squares.

How Big Is 10,000?   Pose the following questions to students:

> A school orders 10,000 pencils. When they are delivered, they will be stored until next year. How much storage space is needed?

> Would they fit in a student desk? in the drawers of a teacher desk? in a closet? Would you need a whole classroom?

> What if the order were for 100,000 pencils? for 1,000,000 pencils?

Multiples and Factors up to 10,000

What Happens

Session 1: Comparing Factors of 100, 1000, and 10,000 In small groups, students find numbers they can count by to land exactly on 100, 1000, and 10,000. They discuss how knowing factor pairs of 100 and 1000 can help them find factor pairs of 10,000.

Sessions 2, 3, and 4: Multiplication and Division Clusters Students work with clusters of multiplication and division problems that focus students on using their knowledge of factor pairs for 100 and 1000 and their multiples to solve problems.

Session 5: Factor Pairs of 1100 As an assessment activity, students find factor pairs of 1100 and write about how they found them.

Mathematical Emphasis

- Using knowledge of landmarks up to 1000 (including factors of 1000 and multiples of those factors) to explore landmarks up to 10,000

- Developing multiplication and division strategies that rely on landmarks up to 10,000

- Becoming familiar with skip-counting patterns (sequences of multiples such as 250, 500, 750, . . .) leading to 10,000

- Becoming familiar with some factor pairs of 10,000

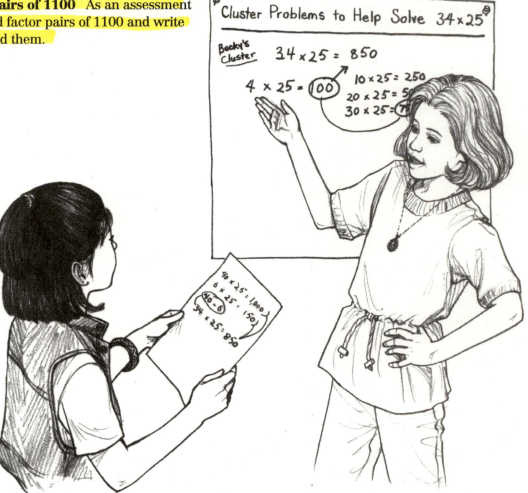

What to Plan Ahead of Time

Materials

- Chart paper (Sessions 1–4)
- Calculators (Session 1)
- Class lists from Investigation 2, Factor Pairs of 100 and Factor Pairs of 1000 (Sessions 2–5)
- Overhead projector (Sessions 2–5, optional)

Other Preparation

- Duplicate student sheets and teaching resources, located at the end of this unit, in the following quantities. If you have Student Activity Booklets, no copying is needed.

For Session 1

Student Sheet 11, What Could You Count By? (p. 123): 1 per student (homework)

For Sessions 2–4

Student Sheet 12, Multiplication Clusters (p. 124): 1 per student

Student Sheet 13, More Multiplication Clusters (p. 126): 1 per student (optional, for further practice)

Student Sheet 14, Challenging Multiplication Clusters (p. 127): 1 per student (optional, for added challenge)

Student Sheet 15, Division Clusters (p. 128): 1 per student

Student Sheet 16, More Division Clusters (p. 129): 1 per student (optional, for further practice)

Student Sheet 17, Challenging Division Clusters (p. 130): 1 per student (optional, for added challenge)

Student Sheet 18, Writing About Multiplication Clusters (p. 131): 1 per student (homework)

Student Sheet 19, Make Your Own Cluster (p. 132): 1 per student (homework)

For Session 5

Student Sheet 20, Factor Pairs of 950 (p. 133): 1 per student (homework)

Comparing Factors of 100, 1000, and 10,000

Materials

- Chart paper
- Calculators
- Student Sheet 11 (1 per student, homework)

What Happens

In small groups, students find numbers they can count by to land exactly on 100, 1000, and 10,000. They discuss how knowing factor pairs of 100 and 1000 can help them find factor pairs of 10,000. Their work focuses on:

- becoming familiar with skip-counting patterns (sequences of multiples such as 500, 1000, 1500, . . .) leading to 10,000
- using knowledge of landmarks up to 1000 (including factors of 1000 and multiples of those factors) to explore landmarks up to 10,000
- finding relationships among factors of 100, 1000, and 10,000

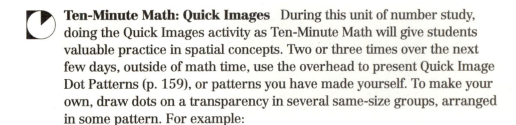 **Ten-Minute Math: Quick Images** During this unit of number study, doing the Quick Images activity as Ten-Minute Math will give students valuable practice in spatial concepts. Two or three times over the next few days, outside of math time, use the overhead to present Quick Image Dot Patterns (p. 159), or patterns you have made yourself. To make your own, draw dots on a transparency in several same-size groups, arranged in some pattern. For example:

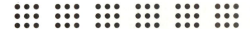

Flash the dot pattern for 3 seconds and then cover it. Ask:

Can you draw the dot pattern you saw?

Give students time to draw what they remember, then flash the pattern for another 3 seconds and let students revise their drawings. Ask:

Can you figure out how many dots you saw?

When most have finished drawing, show the pattern again and leave it visible for further revision and for checking the number of dots shown.

Ask students to describe how they saw and remembered the pattern. You may notice students using different strategies: some will see a multiplication problem (such as 6×9) and will not draw the dots until reminded to do so; others will draw the dots and then figure out how many there are.

For full directions and variations on this activity, see p. 98.

On a piece of chart paper, set up a three-column chart as follows:

Counting Around the Class		
Numbers to count by so someone will say . . .		
100	1000	10,000

Suppose we do some counting around the class. What are some numbers we could count by and be sure that somewhere in the count, someone would say 100?

Record one or two suggestions on the chart. Students will likely have many ideas, but gather only a couple of suggestions now since students will be working on their own to find other numbers.

What are some numbers we could count by and be sure that somewhere in the count, someone would say 1000? What about 10,000?

Again, record only one or two suggestions for each, since students will be finding more numbers in their groups.

How can you use what you already know to find some more numbers without actually doing the counting all the way to 1000 or 10,000?

Possible strategies include using what they know about factors of 1000 and about the dimensions of rectangles with 1000 squares. Some might multiply by 10 those numbers that work for 100, because if someone in the class will say 100 when you count by 4's, then someone will say 1000 when you count by 40's.

Extending the Chart Students work in groups of four to find additional numbers for the class chart. Each group will need calculators, and each student makes his or her own chart on notebook paper for recording the group's findings. Students first copy the numbers from the class chart, then find at least three other numbers for each column.

As students work on this activity, circulate to observe how they say the number names. For example, some students will express the number 7500 as "75 hundred" while others will say "7 thousand 5 hundred." Probe to find out if students recognize equivalent ways of saying the same number:

What's another way to say 7 thousand 5 hundred? How do you know?

If students have difficulty providing another way, encourage them to think about relationships between hundreds and thousands.

How many hundreds are in a thousand? in 2 thousand? in 7 thousand? How many hundreds are the same as half of 1 thousand?

Students who finish early with their work on the chart might try finding numbers that work for 1000 but not for 100, and numbers that work for 10,000 but not for 1000. They could also try to find *all* the numbers for each column of the chart. Or, students could pick a multiple of 1000 (such as 4000) and add a fourth column to the chart, filling in numbers that they could count by to say that number.

Pooling Our Counting Numbers   Bring students together to add their groups' findings to the class chart. Gather and record answers until students have given you all the different numbers they found. Encourage them to explain how they found their answers.

How did you use factors of 100 to find factors of 1000? Why does it work to multiply a factor of 100 by 10? What about doubling a factor of 100? How did you use factors of 1000 to find factors of 10,000?

Leave the chart posted so that students can continue to add other numbers as they find them over the next few days. If they think they have found them all, ask them to explain or write about how they can be sure.

As students begin exploring relationships among powers of 10, they are often surprised at just how much larger each successive power of 10 is than the one before. See the **Teacher Note**, Powers of 10: How Much Larger, and How Many Times as Large? (p. 54), for some ways to help students better understand the relative size of these numbers.

Session 1 Follow-Up

What Could You Count By?   Each student chooses a number that is a multiple of 100 (such as 300 or 500) or a multiple of 1000 (such as 2000 or 6000). On Student Sheet 11, What Could You Count By?, students find and record at least five numbers that they could count by, so that somewhere in the count they will reach the chosen number. They might count around a group.

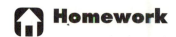
Homework

What Could We *Not* Count By?   Students might be interested in making another chart to record numbers they could *not* count by to get to 100. For example, if they started at 0 and counted by 3, they would not say 100. After recording the numbers they find, students might choose one and write about how they know for sure that they would not say 100. Students could also find numbers they could *not* count by to get to 1000 or 10,000.

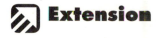
Extension

Powers of 10: How Much Larger, and How Many Times as Large?

Understanding relationships among powers of ten is an essential part of understanding the structure of our number system. When students first begin exploring powers of ten, they are often surprised at just how much larger each power of ten is than the one before. Even students who have memorized the place headings, and the fact that each is ten times more than the previous one, may not have a sense of the size of these numbers.

For example, some students may at first assume that it is just as far from 1 to 1000 as it is from 1000 to 1,000,000. They may be likely to respond "1 million" to questions such as: "What's 1 thousand more than 1 thousand?" or "What number is 10 times as large as 1 thousand?" In order to grasp relationships among powers of ten, students need a chance to develop their intuition about the magnitude of large numbers, and time to explore just how much larger each successive power of ten is.

Most upper elementary students are familiar with number patterns that grow according to an additive rule: You *add* 10 in order to go from one multiple of 10 to the next; you add 2 in order to go from one even number to the next. Each multiple of 10 is always 10 larger than the previous one; each even number is always 2 more than the one before.

Fewer students are familiar with number patterns that grow according to a multiplicative rule (or exponentially): you *multiply by 10* in order to go from one power of ten to the next; you *multiply by 2* in order to go from one power of two to the next. While each power of ten is 10 times as large as the previous one, each successive power of ten is increasingly larger than the one before.

Many of the activities in this unit are designed to help students develop their understanding of relationships among large numbers. You can provide additional ways for students to explore the distance between large numbers. For example:

- Use counting sequences to emphasize distance between large numbers.

  I listed the numbers we said when we counted around the class by 500's up to 10,000. How many people counted to get to 1000? How many counted to get to 10,000? If each person said only one number, how many people would we need to get to 100,000? How do you know?

- Provide opportunities for visualizing the distance between numbers. Some students will find it easiest to think about the distance between numbers visually. The 20 × 50 and 25 × 40 rectangles of 1000 squares and the Many Squares Poster in Investigation 4 can help them. For example, you might draw two or three horizontal lines across a Many Squares Poster to divide it into horizontal strips. The strips do not need to be equally spaced. Post the poster at the front of the room, and ask students to make a few quick estimates of which strip different numbers would be in.

  Which strip would 10 be in? Why do you think so? What about 100? 1000? 5000? 7500?

- Encourage students to make additive and multiplicative comparisons. When students are working with numbers of different sizes, they might compare *how much larger* and *how many times as large* one is than the other.

  We found that 100 is one of the factors of 10,000. How much larger is 10,000 than 100? How many times as large?

Multiples of 10	How much larger than previous multiple of 10?
10	—
20	10
30	10
40	10
50	10
60	10
70	10

Powers of 10	How many times as large as previous power of 10?	How much larger than previous power of 10?
1	—	—
10	10	9
100	10	90
1000	10	900
10,000	10	9000
100,000	10	90,000
1,000,000	10	900,000

Multiplication and Division Clusters

What Happens

Students work with clusters of multiplication and division problems that focus students on using their knowledge of factor pairs for 100 and 1000 and their multiples to solve problems. Student work focuses on:

- developing mental multiplication and division strategies that rely on land-marks up to 10,000

Materials

- Overhead projector (optional)
- Class lists, Factor Pairs of 100 and 1000
- Student Sheet 12 (1 per student)
- Student Sheets 13–14 (as needed)
- Chart paper (optional)
- Student Sheet 15 (1 per student)
- Student Sheets 16–17 (as needed)
- Student Sheet 18 (1 per student, homework)
- Student Sheet 19 (1 per student, homework)

Activity

Solving Multiplication Clusters

Write the following cluster of related problems on the board:

2×5	42×10
20×5	42×5
40×5	

Pair up students to work together on these. Partners may refer to the class lists of Factor Pairs of 100 and 1000, but *not* use standard algorithms or calculators. As students work, circulate to ask how they are solving the problems. Encourage them to use the factor pairs they know and the problems they have already solved to help them with the others.

How can knowing that $2 \times 5 = 10$ help you solve 20×5? How does the answer to 20×5 help you with 40×5? Which of the problems in this cluster helped you to figure out 42×5? Are there other problems that were *not* included in this cluster that might have helped you?

After students have been working for several minutes, call them together to share a few strategies. Then, add the following problem to the cluster:

18×5

Ask how the answers to 20×5 and 2×5 can help us with 18×5.

For more information on cluster problems, see the **Teacher Note**, About Cluster Problems (p. 62).

Teacher Checkpoint

Multiplication Clusters

Distribute a copy of Student Sheet 12, Multiplication Clusters, to each student. Explain that students will be working in pairs on these clusters of multiplication problems. They will use the factor pairs they know and other problems in the cluster to solve the final problem in the cluster.

Your job is to solve the last problem in each cluster. Use any of the other problems in the cluster to help you solve the last problem. If you think of a problem you can use to help you solve the last problem, you can add it to the cluster. You don't have to solve every problem in the cluster. Select the ones that help you figure out the final problem in each set.

Refer to any strategies used to solve 42 × 5 in the previous activity.

Observing the Students   While students are working, observe each pair at least once with the following questions in mind:

■ What strategies do they have for relating known factor pairs to new multiplication problems? For example, can they find an answer to a multiplication problem by *doubling* one of the factors in a known pair? by multiplying one of the factors in a known pair by 10?

■ Can students put together answers to two or more easier multiplication problems to solve a more difficult one?

■ What factor pairs do they know by heart?

If students have difficulty, encourage them to talk about how what they already know can help them solve more difficult problems. Some students may need help seeing how to put together the answers to two multiplication problems to find the answer to a third. For example, if a student can solve 3 × 50 and 20 × 50, but not 23 × 50, you might follow a line of questioning like this:

You wrote down 1000 for the answer to 20 × 50. How did you find that answer? If you have one more 50—that is, twenty-one 50's—how much would you have? How could you write a problem for that? What if you had two more 50's? Three more 50's? Is there a problem like that in the cluster?

If students easily find one solution, ask them to find a second solution that uses problems in the cluster they didn't use the first time. When pairs finish, they join with another pair to compare their answers and solution strategies. As they listen to one another, they see if they can learn a new way to solve the final problem in each cluster.

For More Practice or Extra Challenge   Make available Student Sheet 13, More Multiplication Clusters, to students who would benefit from more practice. Other students might be ready for Student Sheet 14, Challenging Multiplication Clusters, which includes problems with answers 10,000 and larger and some that use decimals. Students might also enjoy making up their own clusters and exchanging them with partners to solve.

Sharing Our Cluster Strategies

Which of the problems in this cluster were easy for you? How did you figure out the harder ones?

Encourage students to think about which multiplication pairs or relationships they "just knew," which they recognized as factor pairs of some landmark numbers, and which they determined by using skip counting or some other strategy.

4×25	10×25
40×25	50×25
6×25	46×25

Ask for explanations of how students solved 46 × 25. Here are some of the strategies they might have used:

- Breaking the problem into 40 × 25 and 6 × 25 and adding the two results
- Breaking the problem into 50 × 25 and 4 × 25 and subtracting one from the other
- Skip counting by 25's up from 40 × 25
- Skip counting down from 50 × 25
- Transforming the problem by halving one factor and doubling the other, twice, first making 23 × 50, then 11.5 × 100, which is easy to multiply mentally.

All of these are acceptable approaches. See the **Dialogue Box**, Ways to Solve 46 × 25 (p. 65), for the discussion that occurred in one class.

As students explain their strategies, listen for examples where students are multiplying by 10 or 100, putting together the results of two problems to find an answer to a third, and partitioning larger numbers into smaller components. For example, to solve 50 × 25, a student might explain:

> You can break it into two parts. There's 40 × 25. I know that's 1000 because of the rectangles we made. Then there's 10 × 25, and we figured out that's 250. You put them together, and you get 1250.

Many students will see a pattern when a number is multiplied by 10. They may notice that you always add a zero but be unable to explain why. Encourage students to double-check their work using other strategies, and to be able to estimate that their answer is a reasonable one.

For example, if a student solves 10 × 25 by saying that "It's like 1 × 25 and add a zero, so it's 250," you might ask, "And how do you know 250 is a reasonable answer? Is there another way you can prove it? How do you know it's not 2500?"

Now that students have spent some time exploring how "difficult" problems can become easier when we see them in terms of simpler related problems, they have a chance to form their own clusters of related problems.

Making Our Own Problem Clusters

Now that students have spent some time exploring how "difficult" problems can become easier when we see them in terms of simpler related problems, they have a chance to form their own clusters of related problems.

Put the multiplication problem 34×25 on the board or overhead. Working in pairs, students create a cluster of several problems that would help them solve 34×25.

If students are having difficulty getting started, ask two or three volunteers to suggest another problem that might help them think about how to solve 34×25 in their head. Record the suggested problems on the board or overhead, and ask how these problems could help. Explain that the clusters they create may include some or all of the problems on the board.

As students work, circulate to observe what strategies they are using. If some students continue to have difficulty, suggest that they think about factor pairs they know.

Could 4×25 help? How?

When pairs finish their clusters, they write them on the board or on a piece of chart paper. Set aside five or ten minutes for students to walk around and look at each other's sets of cluster problems. As students circulate, encourage them to look at each cluster and see if they can understand why the authors chose that particular set of problems. If there is time, students can share observations and ask questions about cluster problems they do not understand.

Solving Division Clusters

Note: Most of your students will have already had some experience with division. If your students did the fourth grade unit, *Packages and Groups,* they will have had opportunities to interpret and solve division problems. In the following activities students will solve clusters of division problems that emphasize using knowledge of familiar factor pairs (such as 4×8 and 4×25) to solve division problems. Students will explore division in more depth in the unit *Building on Numbers You Know,* as they solve a variety of numeric and story problems.

Introduce division cluster problems by encouraging students to share what they already know about division and what it means. Write the following problem on the board:

$16 \div 4$

We've been solving multiplication problems. This is a different kind of problem. Who has an idea about what this problem means? What is this problem asking?

Some students may want to give the answer. At this point, keep the focus on the meaning of the expression. Students might explain 16 ÷ 4 as "How many 4's in 16?" or "How many times does 4 go into 16?" Once students have had a chance to share their ideas, ask them what the answer is, and to explain their thinking. Students might say that 16 ÷ 4 is 4 because "4, 8, 12, 16—4 fours is 16" or "4 goes into 16 4 times because 4 times 4 is 16."

Many elementary students are more comfortable with multiplication than division, just as they are often more comfortable with addition than subtraction. Some do not recognize that multiplication and division are related operations. Both involve two factors and the multiple created by multiplying those two factors (4 × 4 = 16, and 16 ÷ 4 = 4). (See the **Teacher Note**, The Relationship Between Division and Multiplication, p. 63.)

While it is important that all students can recognize and interpret standard division notation, some may find it helpful to think of division as a missing factor problem. You might suggest that students think of 16 ÷ 4 as finding the missing factor for the factor pair 4 × _?_ = 16. (See the **Teacher Note**, What About Notation?, p. 64).

Now write the following cluster of related division problems on the board:

4 ÷ 4	100 ÷ 4
80 ÷ 4	16 ÷ 4

96 ÷ 4

After students have been working for several minutes, call the class together to share solution strategies. If students do not recognize the strategy of breaking a problem into two components, encourage them to think more about relationships among the problems.

How can knowing 80 ÷ 4 help you to solve 96 ÷ 4? Once you know there are twenty 4's in 80, what can you do to figure out how many 4's are in 96? Are there other problems that were not included in this cluster that might have helped you?

Distribute Student Sheet 15, Division Clusters, to each student. Students continue to work in pairs. If they have difficulty, encourage them to talk about how they can use what they know, such as familiar factor pairs, to solve more difficult problems. When pairs finish, they meet with another pair to compare answers and solution strategies.

For More Practice or Extra Challenge For students who need more practice, make available copies of Student Sheet 16, More Division Clusters. Others might be ready for Student Sheet 17, Challenging Division Clusters (with some numbers 10,000 and larger). Students could also continue working on multiplication clusters (Student Sheets 13–14).

Division Cluster Strategies

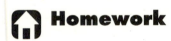

$$24 \div 4 \qquad 100 \div 4$$
$$200 \div 4 \qquad 224 \div 4$$
$$248 \div 4$$

Put on the board the second division cluster from Student Sheet 15. As you did with the multiplication clusters, ask students to share their strategies for mentally solving the final problem in the cluster. Do they recognize relationships between multiplication and division? Do they multiply or divide by 10? Do they combine the results of two problems to find an answer to a third? Do they partition larger numbers into smaller components? Do they recognize some of these division problems as related to factor pairs of 100, 1000, or other landmark numbers?

Sessions 2, 3, and 4 Follow-Up

Homework

Writing About Multiplication Clusters After Session 2, solve both clusters on Student Sheet 18, Writing About Multiplication Clusters, and write about how they found each answer. Remind them to add to the cluster any other problems they use to solve the last problem. Collect these papers so you can get a sense of how students are thinking about the cluster problems.

Robby

① 3 × 25 = 75
② 40 × 25 = 1,000
③ 80 × 25 = 2,000
④ 77 × 25 = 1,925

I knew what #2 was so 80 × 25 is twice as much as that so the answer is 2,000. And I knew that #1 is 75. To get the answer to #4 I said 77 is 3 × 25 less than 80 × 25 so just subtract the answer of 3 × 25 from 2,000.

❖ **Tip for the Linguistically Diverse Classroom** Encourage students who are not writing comfortably in English to indicate numerically and with arrows and diagrams how one or more problems helped them find the answer to another problem. For example:

$$3 \times 25 = 75$$
$$40 \times 25 = 1000$$
$$80 \times 25 = 2000$$
$$2000 - 75$$
$$(80-3) \quad 77 \times 25 = 1925$$

If you have difficulty following their strategies, ask them to explain orally what they did.

Make Your Own Cluster After Session 3 or 4, students make up a set of cluster problems for 47×40 or $336 \div 4$ on Student Sheet 19, Make Your Own Cluster. They write about how they used the problems in their cluster to solve the original problem.

About Cluster Problems

Cluster problems are sets of problems that help students think about using what they know to solve harder problems. For example, what do you know that would help you solve 12×25? If you know that $4 \times 25 = 100$, you might think of 12×25 as $(4 \times 25) + (4 \times 25) + (4 \times 25)$ or $100 + 100 + 100$. Or, you might start with 10×25. If you know that $10 \times 25 = 250$, then you can start with 250 and add two more 25's to get 300. As students work with clusters, they learn to think about all the number relationships they know that might help them solve the problem they are working on.

In this unit, the clusters focus particularly on using the factor pairs of 100, 1000, and their multiples. Students do not need to know by heart all the single-digit multiplication pairs or all the factor pairs of 100 and 1000 in order to do these cluster problems. As students work on the cluster problems, they will become more fluent with these factor pairs. They will also develop strategies for "using what they know" to find answers and will increase their understanding of relationships among factor pairs.

Students' work with cluster problems in this unit helps them make sense of multiplication and division with large numbers and provides a foundation for later work. In the *Investigations* grade 5 unit, *Building on Numbers Your Know,* they will build upon the strategy of pulling apart numbers into manageable pieces and then working with each piece as they solve more difficult problems, such as 37×26. They will also use the strategies they develop in this unit to find approximate answers to multiplication and division problems and to check that an answer obtained with a calculator or algorithm is "in the ballpark."

The Relationship Between Division and Multiplication

Teacher Note

Multiplication and division are related operations: Both involve two factors and the multiple created by multiplying those two factors. For example, here is a set of linked multiplication and division relationships:

$$24 \times 3 = 72 \qquad 3 \times 24 = 72$$
$$72 \div 24 = 3 \qquad 72 \div 3 = 24$$

Mathematics educators call all of these "multiplicative" situations because they all involve the relationship of factors and multiples. Many problem situations your students will encounter can be described by either multiplication or division. For example:

> I bought a package of 72 treats for my dog. If I give her 3 treats every day, how many days will this package last?

The elements in this problem are 24 treats, 3 treats per day, and a number of days to be determined. This problem could be written in standard notation as either division or multiplication:

$$72 \div 3 = \underline{\quad} \quad \text{or} \quad 3 \times \underline{\quad} = 72$$

Once the problem is solved, the relationships can still be expressed as either division or multiplication:

> 72 treats divided into 3 treats per day results in 24 days ($72 \div 3 = 24$)
>
> 3 treats per day for 24 days is equivalent to 72 treats ($3 \times 24 = 72$)

Many elementary students are more comfortable with multiplication than with division, just as they are often more comfortable with addition than with subtraction. We want students to recognize and interpret standard division and multiplication notation. However, we do not want to insist they use one or the other to record their work when both provide good descriptions of a problem situation. In the dog-treat problem, either notation is a perfectly good description of the results.

Similarly, the order of the factors doesn't matter when describing a multiplication situation. Both examples that follow provide good descriptions of the dog-treat problem:

> 3 treats per day for 24 days is equivalent to 72 treats ($3 \times 24 = 72$)
>
> (3 per group in 24 groups is 72 total)
>
> 24 days with 3 treats per day is equivalent to 72 treats ($24 \times 3 = 72$)
>
> (24 groups with 3 per group is 72 total)

While some people prefer one or the other way to write these factors, we do not feel that a standard order (putting either the number of groups first or the number in each group first) should be taught or insisted on. As long as students can explain their problem and their solution and can relate the notation clearly to the problem, the order of the factors in multiplication equations is not critical.

It is important that your students learn to recognize, interpret, and use the standard forms and symbols for multiplication and division, both on paper and on the calculator. These include:

$$42 \qquad 3 \times 42 \qquad 42 \div 3 \qquad 3\overline{)42} \qquad \frac{42}{3}$$
$$\underline{\times\ 3}$$

Your challenge is to introduce these symbols in a way that allows students to interpret them meaningfully. That is, students must understand what is being asked in a problem that is written in standard notation. They can then devise their own way to find an answer. Notation is also useful as an efficient way to record a problem and its solution. It is *not* a directive to carry out a particular procedure, or a signal to forget everything you ever knew about the relationships of the numbers in the problem.

Your students may come to you already believing that when they see a problem like $3\overline{)42}$, written in the familiar division format, they must carry out the traditional long-division procedure. Instead, we want them to use everything they know about these two numbers in order to solve the problem. They might skip count by 3's out loud or on the calculator. Or they might use reasoning based on their understanding of number relationships:

It takes ten 3's to make 30. Then there are three more 3's to get up to 39, that's thirteen 3's so far. Then 40, 41, 42—that's one more 3—it's 14.

Well, half of 42 is 21, and I can divide 21 into 7 groups of 3, so you can double that, and it's 14.

Similarly, when students see a multiplication problem like 4×55 written vertically, they are likely to forget everything they know about these numbers and try to carry out multiplication with carrying. Instead, we want students to use what they know about number composition and relationships. For example:

I know that two 50's make 100, and there's four 50's, so that's 200. Then I know that four 5's is 20, so it's 220.

Students need to get used to interpreting multiplication in both horizontal and vertical form as simply indicating a multiplication situation, not a particular way to carry out the problem. So, while you help students to read standard notation and to use it to record their work, keep the emphasis on understanding the problem context and using good number sense to solve the problem.

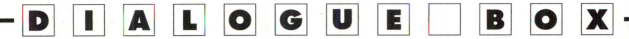

Ways to Solve 46 × 25

This class has been working on Student Sheet 12, Multiplication Clusters. Now, in a follow-up discussion (p. 57), they are sharing their strategies for thinking about one of the problems in the fifth cluster, 46 × 25.

4 × 25	10 × 25
40 × 25	50 × 25
6 × 25	**46 × 25**

Rachel: I didn't finish getting the answer yet, but I made a plan for how to find it. If you do the answer of 50 × 25, and you take away the answer of 4 × 25, you get 46 × 25. You can get 50 × 25 if you add 40 × 25 and 10 × 25. So you do that, and then you minus 4 × 25.

Maricel: I did it her way. I knew that 4 × 25 is 100. Then you think of 40 × 25 as ten times that. It's like ten 100's, so it's 1000. Then, ten 25's is 250. You go 10 × 25 plus 40 × 25 to get 50 × 25. 1000 plus 250 is 1250. Then you have to take away the 4 × 25 . . . 1250 minus 100 is 1150.

Antonio: I started with 40 × 25, because I knew that from the rectangles we made. Then you need another 6 × 25. It's like three 50's, because 25 is two 50's—so it's 50, 100, 150. So you put it together and the answer is 1150.

Cara: I got 50 × 25 the way Maricel did. I knew it would be 100 less than 1250, so 1250 take away 100 is 1150.

Robby: I noticed that 50 × 25 is the same as 5 × 10 × 25. So I started with 10 × 25—that's 250. You need five of those. I knew that's 1250 because 5 × 25 is 125, so 5 × 250 must be 1250. Then you just need to take away 4 × 25, or 100.

Marcus: I put together 40 × 25 and 4 × 25 and half of 4 × 25 to get 46 × 25. You put the 40 and the 4 together, that's 44, and then half again of the 4 to get 46 × 25. So it's 1000 plus 100 plus 50.

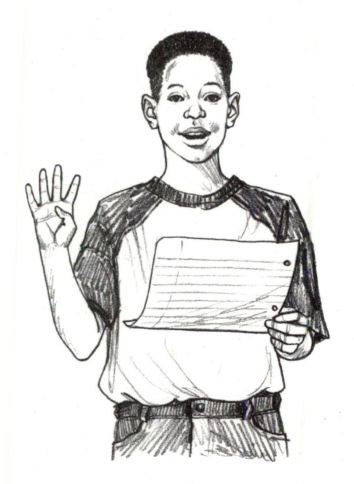

Factor Pairs of 1100

Materials

- Class lists, Factor Pairs of 100 and 1000
- Student Sheet 20 (1 per student, homework)
- Overhead projector (optional)

What Happens

As an assessment activity, students find factor pairs of 1100 and write about how they found them. Their work focuses on:

- finding factor pairs of one number by using knowledge of related factor pairs and number relationships
- explaining mathematical thinking and reasoning in writing

Activity

Assessment

Finding Factor Pairs of 1100

Write the following on the board or overhead:

1. Find some factor pairs of 1100.
2. Write about how you found each factor pair.

Explain that students will be working on these two tasks for most of the session, and that you will be walking around to observe their work. Emphasize that it is not necessary for students to find *all* the factor pairs of 1100. It is more important for them to find only a few and to write a clear explanation of how they found each one.

Students work individually. They may refer to the class lists of Factor Pairs of 100 and 1000. Encourage students to work without calculators (but allow their use if students feel it is necessary).

Circulate quickly to make sure students understand the task. If students are having difficulty beginning, encourage them to think of the different ways they have found factor pairs throughout the unit, such as skip counting, working cluster problems, and using what they know about factor pairs of some numbers to find others.

Most students will have time to find and write about several factor pairs. Some may tell you they could find more factor pairs of 1100, given more time. Remind these students that they are not expected to find all the factor pairs of 1100, and encourage them to find additional factor pairs outside of class time.

Be sure students understand that the two parts of this assessment carry equal weight: (1) finding the factor pairs, and (2) communicating clearly about their strategies. If students have difficulty with the writing, ask to them *tell* you how they found a particular factor pair, and then to put that same explanation in writing. Encourage students to add to their writing if it is not clear enough.

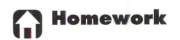

❖ **Tip for the Linguistically Diverse Classroom** Students who are not writing comfortably in English may indicate with numbers and symbols how they found each factor pair.

Observing the Students As you circulate to observe students' work and listen to what they say, consider how students are using what they know about factor pairs of 100, 1000, and other landmarks to find factor pairs of 1100. For example:

- Are they skip counting up from a known factor pair? ("I know that 20×50 is a factor pair of 1000. One more 50 gives you 1050, that's 21, and one more after that is 1100, that's 22, so 22×50 would work.")

- Are they combining answers to related problems? ("There are twenty 50's in 1000, and there are two 50's in 100, so there are twenty-two 50's in 1100.")

- Are they using what they know about factors of multiples of 100? ("There are eleven 100's in 1100, so you can multiply one part of a factor pair of 100 by 11; and 2×50 is a factor pair of 100, so 22×50 is a factor pair of 1100.")

- Do students have strategies for using one factor pair of 1100 to find others? ("I figured out that 22×50 is a factor pair of 1100, so 44×25 would also work, because it's twice 22 and half of 50.")

See the **Teacher Note**, Assessment: Finding Factor Pairs of 1100 (p. 68) for other examples of student work on this assessment.

Students who finish early might try to find *all* the factor pairs of 1100 and write about how they can be sure they found them all. Alternatively, they could begin working on the homework.

When everyone has finished, collect the work. Then invite students to share with the class the factor pairs they found and their strategies for finding them.

Session 5 Follow-Up

Factor Pairs of 950 Students find factor pairs of 950 and write about how they found each factor pair on Student Sheet 20, Factor Pairs of 950. If 950 feels like an unmanageable number for some of your students, assign a smaller number.

🏠 **Homework**

The following classroom examples demonstrate the range of responses you might expect on the assessment Finding Factor Pairs of 1100 (p. 66). The teacher is circulating to observe students working, to read what they are writing, and to ask questions to help them explain their thinking and reasoning more clearly.

Building up from 1000 to 1100 After students have been working for about 15 minutes, the teacher arrives at Tai's desk. Tai explains that he has been finding factor pairs of 1000 and then "building them up" to factor pairs of 1100. His written explanations show that he uses a variety of strategies for building up: skip counting, repeated addition, and using his knowledge of factor pairs of 100.

Tai

50 × 22 = 1100 —— I got this one by just adding 2 more 50s to 1000 and that equals 1100.

44 × 25 = 1100 —— I added 4 more 25s to 1000 and got 1100.

100 × 11 = 1100 —— I added just 1 more 100 to 100 and got 1100.

110 × 10 = 1100 —— I flipped the third problem around (100 × 11) and instead of adding 100 to 1000 I added 10 more 10s.

55 × 20 = 1100 —— I flipped the first problem around and instead of adding 2 50s to 1000 I added 5 20s to 1000.

550 × 2 = 1100 —— I did 2 × 500 = 1000 and tried to figure out how to get a 100 so I split 100 in half and got 50 than added that to 500.

4 × 275 = 1100 —— I did 4 × 250 = 1000 and I wanted to get another 100 so I added 25 4 times.

Continued on next page

Using Factors to Find Factor Pairs   Next, the teacher visits Natalie. She has written only 2, 5, and 10 on her paper.

Can you tell me something about what you have on your paper?

Natalie: I know 2 is a factor of 1100 because 1100 ends in 0, so it's even. 5 goes into 100 so it also goes into 1000 because it's 10 times it. Same with 10. You need to see how many times it goes in to find the other number. Like, how many times 2 goes into 1100.

Can you use what you know about factor pairs of 100 or 1000 to find out how many times it goes in?

Natalie [*hesitantly*]: 2 goes into 100 fifty times, and 2 goes into 1000 . . . [*she finds 2 × 500 on her list of factor pairs of 1000*] 500 times. So you need to put those together to find out how many times 2 goes in. 500 plus 50, that's 550. [*She writes "× 550" next to the "2" on her paper.*]

Natalie's explanation shows that she recognizes that if one number is a factor of another number, it is also a factor of 10 times that number; she knows that if a number is a factor of each of two numbers, it is also a factor of the sum of those numbers; and she understands that if you know one member of a factor pair of a number, you can divide it into the number to find the other member of the factor pair. However, since Natalie seems to have more difficulty retrieving factor pairs of 100 and 1000 than many of her classmates, the teacher decides to offer her the use of a calculator to help her to use what she does know. By the end of the session, she has found five factor pairs of 1000 and written explanations of how she found them.

Using Relationships Between 100 and 1100
Next the teacher visits Danny, who has just completed a list of all the factor pairs of 1100. He has not yet written an explanation of how he found them.

$$
\begin{aligned}
100 &\times 11 \\
50 &\times 22 \\
25 &\times 44 \\
4 &\times 275 \\
5 &\times 220 \\
2 &\times 550 \\
10 &\times 110 \\
1 &\times 1100 \\
20 &\times 55
\end{aligned}
$$

Can you tell me how you found these factor pairs?

Danny: First I listed the factors of 100 because all the factors of 100 go into 1100. The multiples of a number have the same factors as the number you began with, and 1100 is a multiple of 100. The factors of 100 are 100, 50, 25, 4, 5, 2, 10, 1 and 20. Then I took 1100 and divided it by the factors of 100 in my head, and then I matched them up.

Can you give me an example of what you did? How did you find this first one (100 × 11)?

Danny: I did 1100 divided by 100 and I got 11, so it's 100 × 11. Then I did the same thing with the next factor of 100 on my list, 50 . . . 1100 divided by 50 is 22, so it's 50 × 22.

Danny's explanation shows a strong understanding of number relationships and ability to express these relationships in general terms. The teacher asks Danny to put his explanation in writing and to illustrate his general procedure for finding factor pairs with two or three specific examples.

Continued on next page

Shakita

$50 \times 22 = 1100$

$550 \times 2 = 1100$ — I cut 1100 in half to get this number, and I knew if 550 is half of 1100 I just multiply by 2.

$225 \times 4 = 1100$ — This is the same as the last problem except I cut 550 in half and doubled $2 = 4$.

$25 \times 44 = 1100$ — Now I'm at the point where I can't split 225 in half so I'm splitting 50 in half from the first problem and doubling 22 to get 44.

$100 \times 11 = 1100$ — Now I can't split 25 in half so instead I'm doubling 50 and cutting 22 in half.

$220 \times 5 = 1100$

$110 \times 10 = 1100$ — I just cut 220 in half and doubled 5 to get 10.

$55 \times 20 = 1100$ — Again I cut 110 in half and I doubled 10.

$1100 \times 1 = 1100$ — I found this out because 1 X times anything is always that anything.

Halving and Doubling The teacher visits Shakita toward the end of the session. Her written explanations show that she approached the task by finding factor pairs of 1100, and then systematically halving one member of the factor pair and doubling the other to find more factor pairs.

The teacher asks Shakita to tell how she found the two factor pairs she began with: 50×22 and 220×5, and to add these explanations to her paper. Shakita thinks she has found all the factor pairs of 1100, and the teacher suggests that if Shakita has time, she should write about how she can be sure she found them all.

Reasoning About Landmarks up to 10,000

What Happens

Session 1: Close to 1000 and Close to 0   Students play a game that involves arranging digits to make two three-digit numbers that have a sum as close as possible to 1000. In a variation of the game, they arrange digits to make two three-digit numbers that have a *difference* as close as possible to 0.

Sessions 2, 3, and 4: Using Landmarks up to 10,000   Students are introduced to Choice Time, during which they choose from among four activities: finding and describing particular squares on the Many Squares Poster (a rectangle of 10,000 squares); solving number puzzles with clues related to the factors of 1000 and their multiples; and playing the two games Close to 1000 and Close to 0.

Sessions 5 and 6: Reasoning About 1000 and 10,000   As an assessment, students add a clue to a number puzzle that gives it only one answer, and they write about their reasoning. Students also record everything they know about 10,000. They find factor pairs of 10,000 and write about how they found them.

Mathematical Emphasis

- Using knowledge of landmarks up to 10,000 (including factors of 1000 and multiples of those factors) to solve a variety of puzzles and problems
- Developing mental and written strategies for finding sums and differences of three- and four-digit numbers
- Reading, writing, and ordering numbers to 10,000
- Developing a sense of the magnitude of 10,000

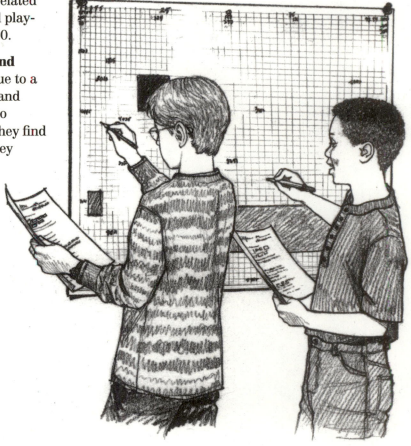

What to Plan Ahead of Time

Materials

- Numeral Cards: 2 decks and 1 transparent set (Sessions 1–4)

- Many Squares Posters: 2 per class (Sessions 2–4)

- Letter-size envelopes (to hold number puzzles): 16, plus 12 (optional) for the challenge puzzles (Sessions 2–4)

- Students' Number Puzzle Recording Sheets (p. 107) from Investigation 1 (Sessions 2–4)

- Square tiles: 200 to share (Sessions 2–4)

- Class lists of Factor Pairs of 100 and 1000 (Session 5)

- Overhead projector (Session 1)

- Calculators (Sessions 2–6)

Other Preparation

- Duplicate student sheets and teaching resources, located at the end of this unit, in the following quantities. If you have Student Activity Booklets, copy only the items marked with an asterisk.

For Session 1

Student Sheet 21, How to Play Close to 1000 (p. 134): 1 per student (homework)

Student Sheet 22, Close to 1000 Score Sheet (p. 135): 2 per student (1 for class, 1 for homework)

Student Sheet 23, How to Play Close to 0 (p. 136): 1 per student (homework)

Student Sheet 24, Close to 0 Score Sheet (p. 137): 2 per student (1 for class, 1 for homework)

Numeral Cards (p. 147): 1 deck per pair; 1 set per student (homework)

For Sessions 2–4

Student Sheet 25, Many Squares Poster Tasks, Groups A, B, C, D (p. 138): Refer to the activity (p. 82) to determine how many to copy for your classroom.

Student Sheet 26, Exploring the Many Squares Poster (p. 142): 1 per student

Student Sheet 27, Problems from Close to 1000 (p. 143): 1 per student (homework)

Student Sheet 28, Problems from Close to 0 (p. 144): 1 per student (homework)

Number Puzzles 15–22* (p. 150): 2 of each for the class, cut apart and placed in prepared envelopes. Challenge Number Puzzles 23☆–28☆* (p. 154) are optional.

300 charts (p. 158): 2–3 per student (or reusable 300 charts from Investigation 1)

For Sessions 5–6

Student Sheet 29, Add a Clue (p. 145): 1 per student

Student Sheet 30, Another Add a Clue (p. 146): 1 per student (homework)

300 Charts (p. 158): available as needed

- Prepare letter-size envelopes to hold the puzzle clues, two identical sets per class. Label each envelope with the puzzle number, using a star for the challenge puzzles.

- It will be easier to manage these sessions if you are able to laminate the Many Squares Posters. To laminate a poster, fold it in half and slide it through the laminating machine. Use a razor to cut the 3 open edges. Then fold it in half the other way, and repeat the process. (Sessions 2–4)

Close to 1000 and Close to 0

Materials

- Overhead projector
- Numeral Cards (1 deck per pair, 1 transparent set, and 1 set per student for homework)
- Student Sheet 21 (1 per student, homework)
- Student Sheet 22 (2 per student)
- Student Sheet 23 (1 per student, homework)
- Student Sheet 24 (2 per student)

What Happens

Students play a game that involves arranging digits to make two three-digit numbers that have a sum as close as possible to 1000. In a variation of the game, they arrange digits to make two three-digit numbers that have a *difference* as close as possible to 0. Their work focuses on:

- developing mental and written strategies for finding sums and differences of three- and four-digit numbers
- finding pairs of three-digit numbers that sum to 1000 or near 1000
- understanding relationships among place values up to the thousands place

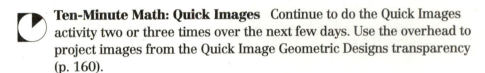 **Ten-Minute Math: Quick Images** Continue to do the Quick Images activity two or three times over the next few days. Use the overhead to project images from the Quick Image Geometric Designs transparency (p. 160).

Flash one design for 3 seconds, and give students time to try to draw what they remember.

Flash it for another 3 seconds, and let students revise their drawings. Then, leave the design visible for further revision.

After students finish an image, encourage them to talk about what they saw in successive flashes. You may hear comments such as "I saw two wheels of six triangles each." If students are having difficulty, suggest that students try to find the shapes that make up the figure:

Each design is made from familiar geometric shapes. Find these shapes and try to figure out how they are put together.

As students describe their figures, you might begin to introduce correct terminology for these shapes—*parallelograms, hexagons, equilateral triangles, trapezoids,* and so forth.

Close to 1000

Students who have worked with the *Investigations* grade 4 curriculum units may already be familiar with the game Close to 1000. Even so, plan to review the game directions with the class. You may want to enlist those who know the game to help you teach it to the rest of the class.

Reviewing the Game Rules In the game Close to 1000, each player is dealt eight Numeral Cards (the digits 0 to 9 and Wild Cards, which can be used as any digit). Players arrange six of their cards to make two numbers that have a sum as close as possible to 1000. Encourage students to play the game *without* calculators.

Student Sheet 21, How to Play Close to 1000 (p. 134), will be sent home for reference (for homework, students play the game with family members), but the sheet could be distributed during class if you feel the students would benefit from having written directions. The **Teacher Note**, Playing Close to 1000 and Close to 0 (p. 79), demonstrates the basic game and its variations.

For a practice round, display a hand of eight transparent cards on the overhead (or draw these cards on the board):

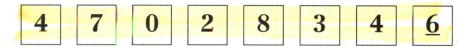

Ask students to suggest some numbers that could be made from three of these digits. Record their suggestions. Note that students are allowed to form 078, which is not considered a three-digit number but is a legitimate answer in this game. Then pose the problem:

We're going to play a game called Close to 1000. Some of you may remember this game from last year. Using these six of these eight numbers, make two three-digit numbers and add them together. Try to get a sum (a total) as close to 1000 as possible.

As students are working individually on this problem, circulate and talk to as many of them as you can about strategies they are using. After a few minutes, collect several answers on the board. Explain how to score the game.

Your score for each round is how far your answer is from 1000. Suppose you made the two numbers 734 and 264.

Write 734 + 264 = on the board. Write the equation horizontally; that is, do not put one number below the other.

What's 734 + 264 ? (998) How far is 998 from 1000? (2) Your score for this set of numbers would be 2.

Suppose you made 603 and 424. [*Write 603 + 424 = on the board.*] **What's 603 + 424?** (1027) **How far is 1027 from 1000?** (27) **Your goal is to get the lowest score, so the score of 2 is better than the score of 27.**

Playing the Game   Students arrange themselves in pairs. Each pair needs one deck of Numeral Cards, and each student needs a copy of Student Sheet 22, Close to 1000 Score Sheet.

Point out on the score sheet that each game consists of five rounds. For the first round, each player is dealt eight cards. After Round 1, players discard the six cards they used and retain the two unused cards. They are then dealt six new cards so they have eight for Round 2. After Round 2, they discard the six used cards and again receive six new ones, and so on for five rounds.

Note: Students sometimes limit themselves by using multiples of ten whenever possible. To avoid this, you might leave out the Wild Cards when students first play, or establish a rule that Wild Cards can't be made into zeros.

Many students will play Close to 1000 cooperatively, helping one another find the best combinations. Encourage this cooperation:

After you have dealt eight cards to each player, take turns and help each other. Work together to get the best answer you can for each person.

Circulate quickly to make sure everyone understands the game. If students seem stuck, choose three of their cards and make a three-digit number; then ask them to make a second number that will bring the sum close to 1000.

Students continue playing until everyone has completed at least one game (five rounds). Students who want to play more than two games may set up their score sheets on the back of Student Sheet 21 or on notebook paper.

Observe as students play to learn what strategies they are using for making combinations and for choosing the sum closest to 1000. Ask questions as needed to understand their thinking. Some students may at first play by trial and error, picking digits randomly to make numbers and then adding them with paper and pencil. Encourage these students to estimate mentally before they do written addition.

A more efficient approach involves trying to come as close as possible to 1000, one place at a time, starting with the hundreds place. For example, we might look for combinations of digits that make 9 (900) in the hundreds place, 9 (90) in the tens place, and 10 in the ones place. Or, we might try to pick digits that add to 10 (1000) for the hundreds place, and then aim for the smallest number possible in the tens place, and the next-smallest number possible in the ones place.

To determine how far various sums are from 1000, students might use strategies involving mental arithmetic. For example: "I made 1013 and 971. I know 1013 is closer because it's 13 away from 1000, and if you add 20 to 971, it still would be less than 1000." Or, students might draw upon their knowledge of number composition: "I made 1039 and 975. 1039 is 39 away from 1000. 975 is only 25 away, because when you count by 25's, you go 900, 925, 950, 975, 1000."

Close to 0

Introduce Close to 0, a variation of the game Close to 1000. Student Sheet 23, How to Play Close to 0 (p. 136), offers written directions that will be sent home; you can distribute this sheet during class if you feel it would be helpful.

You've been making two numbers that have a sum as close as possible to 1000. Now we're going to switch the game around—you will try to make two numbers that have a *difference* as close as possible to 0. That is, if you subtract one of the numbers from the other, you want to get a number close to 0.

Display this hand of eight transparent cards on the overhead (or draw the cards on the board):

| 3 | 7 | 2 | 1 | 5 | 8 | 1 | 0 |

Ask students to choose six of these eight digits to make two numbers that have a difference as close as possible to 0. Encourage students to work without calculators.

As students are working individually on this problem, circulate to make sure they understand the task. After a few minutes, collect several answers on the board.

As with the game Close to 1000, the goal is to get the lowest score. Ask students to decide which would be a better choice of numbers from this set of eight cards, 130 and 128, or 138 and 127. Ask them to explain their reasoning. ($130 - 128 = 2$, and $138 - 127 = 11$, so the first pair is a better choice, 2 being a lower score than 11.)

To start the game, each pair needs a deck of Numeral Cards, and each student needs a copy of Student Sheet 24, Close to 0 Score Sheet.

Students play until everyone has completed at least one game (five rounds).

As students play, observe the strategies they are using. One successful strategy involves trying to make two numbers that are nearly alike, working from the hundreds place, to the tens place, and then the ones place.

Some students may find it difficult to think about the difference between two numbers without writing them as a vertical subtraction problem. Encourage these students to think of other ways they might find how far apart the numbers are. For example:

Is there a different way you could think about how far apart 702 and 685 are? What if you tried counting up by 5's from 685?

Students will continue playing Close to 1000 and Close to 0 as part of Choice Time in Sessions 2–4. For additional games, students can easily set up their own score sheets on notebook paper, using Student Sheets 22 and 24 as models.

Session 1 Follow-Up

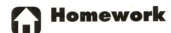 **Homework**

Close to 1000 and Close to 0   Students teach the games Close to 1000 and Close to 0 to someone at home. Each student needs a copy of the directions on Student Sheets 21 and 23, a clean copy of each score sheet (Student Sheets 22 and 24), and a set of Numeral Cards (pages 1–3) to cut out. If students are unlikely to have scissors at home, allow time during the school day for them to make the decks of Numeral Cards.

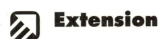 **Extension**

Close to 1000: Using Negative and Positive Integers   Students who seem to be having no difficulty with Close to 1000 might try playing it with the alternative scoring method described in the **Teacher Note**, Playing Close to 1000 and Close to 0 (p. 79).

Playing Close to 1000 and Close to 0

Here is a sample of two students playing Close to 1000, using the basic scoring.

Round 1

Sofia is dealt: 4 5 8 3 2 9 9 0

Zach is dealt: 9 1 3 8 4 7 1 5

Sofia makes 420 + 583 = 1003.
Zach makes 847 + 153 = 1000.

Round 2

Sofia has 9, 9 left from
Round 1 and is dealt: 2 8 5 1 5 0

Zach has 9, 1 left from
Round 1, and is dealt: 7 0 8 5 2 6

Sofia makes 915 + 085 = 1000.
Zach makes 296 + 701 = 997.

Note: Zach could have gotten closer to 1000 in Round 2. Do you see how?

Play continued for five rounds. Here are the score sheets for their complete games:

Name Sofia		Date
		Student Sheet 22

Close to 1000 Score Sheet

Game 1		Score
Round 1:	420 + 583 = 1003	3
Round 2:	915 + 085 = 1000	0
Round 3:	607 + 407 = 1014	14
Round 4:	364 + 634 = 998	2
Round 5:	785 + 215 = 1000	0
	TOTAL SCORE	19

Name Zach		Date
		Student Sheet 22

Close to 1000 Score Sheet

Game 1		Score
Round 1:	847 + 153 = 1000	0
Round 2:	296 + 701 = 997	3
Round 3:	714 + 303 = 1017	17
Round 4:	819 + 180 = 999	1
Round 5:	503 + 481 = 984	16
	TOTAL SCORE	37

Variation: Playing with Negative and Positive Integers

Note: Students should be very comfortable with the basic game before trying this variation.

In this variation, students score the game Close to 1000 using negative and positive integers. If a player's total is above 1000, the score is recorded as positive. If the total is below 1000, the score is negative. For example: A total of 1003 is scored as +3 (3 above 1000), while a total of 997 is scored as –3 (3 below 1000). If using this variation, the score sheets from Sofia's and Zach's game would look like this:

Name Sofia		Date
		Student Sheet 22

Close to 1000 Score Sheet

Game 1		Score
Round 1:	420 + 583 = 1003	3
Round 2:	915 + 085 = 1000	0
Round 3:	607 + 407 = 1014	14
Round 4:	364 + 634 = 998	–2
Round 5:	785 + 215 = 1000	0
	TOTAL SCORE	+15

Name Zach		Date
		Student Sheet 22

Close to 1000 Score Sheet

Game 1		Score
Round 1:	847 + 153 = 1000	0
Round 2:	296 + 701 = 997	–3
Round 3:	714 + 303 = 1017	17
Round 4:	819 + 180 = 999	1
Round 5:	503 + 481 = 984	–16
	TOTAL SCORE	–1

The player with the total score closest to zero wins. So in this case, Zach wins (Sofia's +15 is 15 away from 0, and Zach's –1 is only 1 away from 0).

Continued on next page

Scoring this way changes the strategy for the game. Even though Sofia got two perfect 1000's, she did not compensate for her positive scores with enough negative ones. Zach had some totals quite far away from 1000, but he balanced his negative and positive scores more evenly to come out with a total score closer to zero.

Close to 0

Close to 0 is played fundamentally the same way as Close to 1000, except that students find the *difference* between the two numbers they make. The strategy changes, as the best score now comes from two numbers that are as close to alike as possible.

There is only one scoring system for Close to 0. Just as in Close to 1000, the goal is to get the lowest total score. Shown here are sample games for two students playing Close to 0.

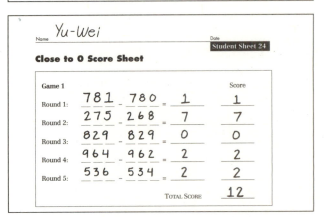

Name	Katrina			Date
				Student Sheet 24

Close to 0 Score Sheet

Game 1				Score
Round 1:	862	− 851	= 11	11
Round 2:	956	− 954	= 2	2
Round 3:	608	− 607	= 1	1
Round 4:	749	− 749	= 0	0
Round 5:	257	− 256	= 1	1
			TOTAL SCORE	15

Name	Yu-Wei			Date
				Student Sheet 24

Close to 0 Score Sheet

Game 1				Score
Round 1:	781	− 780	= 1	1
Round 2:	275	− 268	= 7	7
Round 3:	829	− 829	= 0	0
Round 4:	964	− 962	= 2	2
Round 5:	536	− 534	= 2	2
			TOTAL SCORE	12

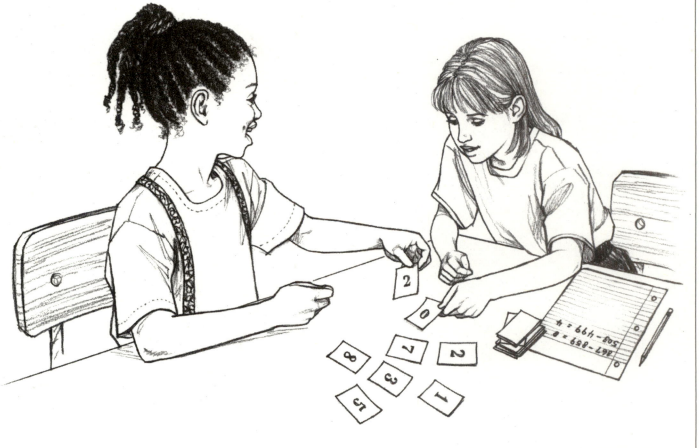

Using Landmarks up to 10,000

What Happens

Students are introduced to Choice Time, during which they choose from among four activities: finding and describing particular squares on the Many Squares Poster (a rectangle of 10,000 squares); solving number puzzles with clues related to the factors of 1000 and their multiples; and playing the two games Close to 1000 and Close to 0. Their work focuses on:

- using knowledge of landmarks up to 10,000 (including factors of 1000 and multiples of those factors) to solve a variety of puzzles and problems

- reading, writing, and ordering numbers to 10,000

- developing a sense of the magnitude of 10,000

Materials

- Many Squares Posters (2)
- Student Sheet 25 (1 Task Sheet per student)
- Student Sheet 26 (1 per student)
- Number Puzzles 15–22 (2 sets, in envelopes)
- Number Puzzles 23☆–28☆ (optional)
- Students' Number Puzzle Recording Sheets
- Square tiles (200 to share)
- 300 charts
- Numeral Cards (at least 2 decks available)
- Student Sheets 27–28 (1 each per student, homework)
- Calculators (available)

Introducing Choice Time Sessions 2–4 are set up as Choice Time. Pairs and small groups of students will choose from four activities designed to give them experience in working with important landmarks up to 10,000.

Choice Time is a format that recurs throughout the *Investigations* units, so this is a good time for students to become familiar with its structure. The **Teacher Note**, About Choice Time (p. 87), offers some guidelines and describes how students might use a Choice List to keep track of their work.

Introduce your rules and students' responsibilities for Choice Time. Suggest that they set up a Choice List for keeping track of what they have done. Students should try each choice at least once during the three sessions. They may repeat any activity except Filling in the Many Squares Poster.

Activity

Choice Time: Numbers to 10,000

How to Set Up the Choices Set up centers in the classroom where students will either work or obtain materials for each of the activities, as follows:

Choice 1: Filling in the Many Squares Poster—two Many Squares Posters, displayed where students can easily write on them (wall, floor, table, hallway); copies of Student Sheets 25 and 26 (plan to distribute these to small groups as they come to work at their poster); calculators

Choice 2: Number Puzzles—labeled envelopes containing number puzzle clues, gathered in a "puzzle pool"; 300 charts; calculators; square tiles; students' own Number Puzzle Recording Sheets

Choice 3: Close to 1000—decks of Numeral Cards, paper and pencil for score sheets

Choice 4: Close to 0—decks of Numeral Cards, paper and pencil for score sheets

The most structured of the four choices is Filling in the Many Squares Poster. Divide the class in half for work on the two posters. Then divide each half into four groups, designated group A, group B, group C, and group D. Depending on your class size, each poster group will have 2–5 members. One group at a time works at each poster, in sequence (group A first, group D last). Be sure that each group understands which of the two posters they will be working on.

Student Sheet 25 provides four different sets of tasks, one set each for groups A–D. How many copies of each task you will need depends on how you group your students for this activity. Each student needs a copy of the appropriate task for his or her group. For example, in a class of 33 students, the poster groups might be set up as shown in the following diagram.

The groups who are not working on the posters will be busy with the other three choices—they may solve number puzzles, or they may break into pairs to play the "Close to" games at their seats. You or an aide will need to keep the eight poster groups moving in sequence through the poster activity. If some members of a group are playing a game when it is their turn for the poster tasks, suggest that they finish their game later.

Introduce the Four Choices   At the beginning of Session 2, spend a few minutes introducing the procedure for Choice 1, Filling in the Many Squares Poster. As necessary, review how to solve the number puzzles (introduced in Investigation 1) and how to play the two "Close to" games.

Choice 1: Filling in the Many Squares Poster

The Many Squares Poster is a rectangle of 10,000 squares. A few of the squares are numbered as reference points, following a left-to-right, top-to-bottom numbering system. Avoid telling students the total number of squares, as they will discover this number through their poster tasks.

Working at the poster, groups of students find squares specified on their task sheet and write in the numbers. Individually, students write about their strategies for finding the size of rectangular areas on the poster.

As Choice Time begins, the group A students will be working at their poster. While at the poster, they do everything on their task sheet (Student Sheet 25, group A tasks) and individually answer the questions on Student Sheet 26. When the group A students have completed their poster work, group B gathers at each poster, and so on until all four groups for each poster have had their turn.

Students write on the posters in *pencil* only (unless you have laminated posters, in which case they will use fine-tipped markers). They write only the numbers they are asked to find on the poster. Otherwise, they may end up putting in numbers that other groups are asked to find, or they may label so many "landmark" numbers that subsequent groups do not have the chance to develop their own strategies for finding numbers.

Observe students to see how they are finding the numbers. Are they skip counting? Can they use numbers already on the poster to help them find others? Do they understand that the right edge of the poster shows multiples of 100? If you can't tell how some students are finding numbers, point to a random square on the poster and ask how we could find the number for that square. Or, you might choose two or three of the numbers the group has written on the poster and ask individuals to explain how they know these numbers are correctly placed.

If students seem to be having difficulty tracking across rows or down columns, suggest using a ruler, meterstick, or other straightedge.

Choice 2: Number Puzzles

Students work in groups of four to solve Number Puzzles 15 through 22, which include clues about the factors of 1000 and their multiples. Decide whether you want to make available the more challenging puzzles 23☆–28☆, which require more sophisticated reasoning about factors of 1000 and their multiples.

Number Puzzles 1 through 8 in Investigation 1 are *not* prerequisite to these puzzles; in fact, you might want to include the envelopes for puzzles 1–8 and 9☆–14☆ in this Choice Time for students who did not do them earlier.

Groups who are working on puzzles 15 and 16 may want to take square tiles to work with. Some of the puzzles have more than one answer, and some are impossible. When a group finishes a puzzle, each member writes the answer on his or her own recording sheet. They put the clues back in the envelope, return the puzzle to the pool, and take another one.

Following are the answers for number puzzles 15–22 and 23☆–28☆. As with the first set of puzzles, we urge you to try the problems yourself to better understand the mathematical thinking students are doing. Use these answers for confirmation of your solutions:

Puzzle 15—2, 8	Puzzle 23☆—40
Puzzle 16—25, 100	Puzzle 24☆—875
Puzzle 17—1000, 2000	Puzzle 25☆—2500, 1250
Puzzle 18—25, 100	Puzzle 26☆—900
Puzzle 19—20	Puzzle 27☆—16
Puzzle 20—impossible	Puzzle 28☆—impossible
Puzzle 21—250	
Puzzle 22—750	

Choice 3: Close to 1000

Student pairs play Close to 1000, the game introduced in Session 1. Players are dealt eight Numeral Cards each and work simultaneously, each choosing six of their cards to make two numbers that have a sum as close as possible to 1000. Encourage students to play the game without calculators. Students record their scores on notebook paper (using the Student Sheet 22 score sheet as a model, if necessary). The goal is to get the lowest possible score.

For an added challenge, students might try the alternative scoring method, using both negative and positive integers, as described in the **Teacher Note**, Playing Close to 1000 and Close to 0 (p. 79).

Choice 4: Close to 0

Student pairs play Close to 0, the variation on Close to 1000 introduced in Session 1. In this game, players are trying to make two numbers that have a difference as close as possible to 0. Encourage students to play the game without calculators. Students record their scores on notebook paper (using the Student Sheet 24 score sheet as a model, if necessary). Again, the goal is to get the lowest possible score.

Observing the Students

Throughout Choice Time, meet with groups who need help or with those you have not had much chance to observe. As you circulate, introduce the more challenging variations or more challenging puzzles to particular groups or students who seem ready. Encourage students to get help from other groups while you are busy.

Once you are settled into working, I will visit with different groups to learn about your thinking. If you have a question while I am meeting with someone else, you may ask another group for help.

You might also enlist the help of particular students as helpers for their peers who have questions.

During this Choice Time, look for the following:

- How are students handling making decisions about how to organize their time and activity?

- Are there too many (or not enough) activities going on at once?

- Are students keeping track of the choices they have completed?

- Are students becoming fluent in finding factors of 1000 and in skip counting by factors of 1000?

- Are students able to use their answers to one of the problems to help them find an answer to another?

- Are students using calculators appropriately?

- Which activities give students the most difficulty? What mathematics in that activity needs more discussion and practice?

At the end of Session 2, you may want to hold a 5-minute class discussion about the activity choices. Ask students to share what they have particularly enjoyed and what has challenged them. Do some planning for Choice Time during Sessions 3 and 4. Do students need any help with the activities? Are any groups ready for the more challenging variations? You may decide to adjust the number of choices offered in Session 3, to regroup students, or spend time on some related work you feel is needed, such as sharing strategies for some of the activities.

Sessions 2, 3, and 4 Follow-Up

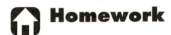 **Homework**

Problems from Close to 1000   Students complete Student Sheet 27, Problems from Close to 1000, using the given sets of eight digits as if they were playing Close to 1000. Students may want to use their home sets of Numeral Cards to duplicate the given digits so that they can physically move around the digits.

Problems from Close to 0   Students complete Student Sheet 28, Problems from Close to 0.

Extensions

Different Paths to 1000   As an addition to Choice Time or as a separate activity, small groups might play a game of Different Paths to 1000. To start, each person in the group enters the same number on his or her calculator. Each student in the group needs to find a different path to 1000 on the calculator display. They may use as many operations as they want for each path, but at least one path should include multiplication, and another path division. Students may use any keys except those that clear the calculator display.

Provide a few starting numbers, such as 17; 775; 996; 3048; and (for practice with decimals) 60.25. Students may also choose their own starting numbers. As they work, observe and talk with them to discover how they are using their knowledge of number composition to find ways to get to 1000. Take some whole-group time for students to explain how they found one of their paths. You could start the discussion with some of the explanations you heard.

Kevin got to 1000 from 17 by adding 8 to get 25, and then multiplying by 40. Did anyone else use factor pairs to get to 1000? What did you do?

Shakita said she got to 1000 from 725 by adding 75 to get 800, then counting by 100's to get to 1000. Did anyone else count by some number to get to 1000? What did you count by?

Further Exploration of the Many Squares Poster   Students can challenge each other by pointing to blank squares on the poster and asking partners to find what number goes there. Students can also find and label "favorite" numbers on the poster, such as their birth year or the last four digits of their telephone number.

About Choice Time

Choice Time is an opportunity for students to work on a variety of activities that focus on similar content. The activities are not sequential; as students move among them, they continually revisit some of the important concepts and ideas from earlier sessions. For the Choice Time activities in this unit, students work in pairs and small groups. In other units, some Choice Time activities may be done individually. Most activities involve some type of recording or writing; these records will help you assess students' growth.

Students can create a Choice List on a piece of notebook paper, for keeping track of which activities they have done. As students finish a choice, they write it on their list along with the names of classmates they worked with. They attach to the list any individual written work they have done. Some teachers list the choices for each day on the board or overhead and have students copy the list at the beginning of class, leaving room to add specifics about their work on that choice. Students are then responsible for checking off completed activities.

In any classroom there will be a range of how much work students can complete. For each choice there may be extensions or additional problems for students who have completed the required work. Choice Time encourages students to return to choices they have done before, doing another puzzle or playing a game again. Students benefit from such repeated experiences. You may also want to make the choices available at other times of the day.

If you and your students have not used a structure like Choice Time before, establish some clear guidelines when you introduce it. Discuss what students' responsibilities are during Choice Time:

- Try every choice at some time.
- Be productively engaged during Choice Time.
- Work quietly with your group or partner.
- Keep track, on paper, of the choices you have worked on.
- Keep all your work in your math folder.
- Ask other students when you don't understand or feel stuck.

Some teachers establish the rule, "Ask two other students before me," requiring students to check with two peers before coming to the teacher for help.

Noah

Choice List
1. Many Squares Poster Group C   10/5
2. Number Puzzles #15, 18, 19, 20 23★, 25★   10/4
3. Close to 1000   —
4. Close to 0 with Marcus   10/4
5. Different Paths to 1000   —

Although the activities in this unit can be done with two posters, extra copies would give each student more practice with numbers to 10,000. Therefore, you may want to purchase or make additional copies of the Many Squares Poster.

To make additional posters of the same size, you might start with rolls of centimeter graph paper, which run 75 centimeters wide. Cut off two 100-centimeter lengths and tape these together, overlapping or trimming to create a square 100 centimeters on a side. (Alternatively, any smaller sheets of graph paper can be taped together to make a poster 100 by 100 squares.)

Once your 100-by-100 grid is prepared, copy the given reference numbers and highlighted rectangles from the Many Squares Poster. If each grid square is one centimeter, a meterstick can help you locate the squares to be numbered or marked. Students should *not* be enlisted to help, as they will then be unlikely to develop their own approaches to finding numbers on the poster.

The following key will help you locate the three rectangular areas marked on the poster, but note that these areas are to have no reference numbers written inside:

> The area marked with stars is 10 by 10 squares; its upper left corner square would be 2625.

> The area marked with triangles is 2 squares wide by 4 squares high; its upper left corner square would be 6803.

> The large rectangle marked with dots is 50 squares wide by 20 squares high; its upper left corner square would be 6536.

You can make these rectangular areas more prominent by marking their borders or coloring them in with a highlighter or a light-colored marker that students can write over.

If you can laminate your posters, student work (in fine-tipped marker) can be erased and the posters can be reused in subsequent years.

With more than two posters, you might want to structure the students' poster work in a different way. For example:

- Students might work alone or in pairs at posters set up in different parts of the classroom or hallway. The fewer students working on a poster, the more opportunities each student has to find numbers on it.

- If you can provide one poster to each group of four students, each group could complete all four task sheets. Since in this case they will not be interfering with other groups' work, they might be allowed to label or mark additional squares to help them locate numbers on the poster. For example, some will find it helpful to label every multiple of 1000 or to draw a vertical guide line through the numbers that end with 25, 50 and 75.

Reasoning About 1000 and 10,000

What Happens

As an assessment, students add a clue to a number puzzle that gives it only one answer, and they write about their reasoning. Students also record everything they know about 10,000. They find factor pairs of 10,000 and write about how they found them. Their work focuses on:

- reasoning about factors of 1000 and 10,000 and multiples of those factors
- explaining mathematical thinking and reasoning in writing

Materials

- Student Sheet 29 (1 per student)
- Class lists, Factor Pairs of 100 and 1000
- Student Sheet 30 (1 per student, homework)
- Calculators (available)
- 300 charts (available)

What Can You Say About 10,000?

Today you are going to write, on a sheet of notebook paper, everything you know about 10,000. For example, think about questions like these:

How much larger is 10,000 than 10? than 100? than 1000?

How much smaller is 10,000 than 100,000? than 1,000,000?

What are some of the factors of 10,000? some of its multiples?

What are some dimensions of rectangles that would contain exactly 10,000 squares? How large is a rectangle made of 10,000 centimeter squares?

Is 10,000 a square number? a prime number? How do you know?

....

❖ **Tip for the Linguistically Diverse Classroom** Students who are not writing comfortably in English can be encouraged to use mathematical signs and simple drawings to convey their ideas about 10,000. For example:

$1000 \times 10 = 10,000$

$1,000,000 = 990,000 + 10,000$

$10,000 =$

Allow about 20 minutes for work on this activity in class. Then introduce the assessment activity, Add a Clue (p. 91). After they have completed the assessment, students may continue recording what they know about 10,000. They may also continue working on this activity for homework.

Plan to take some whole-group time in Session 6 to share the students' ideas about 10,000, perhaps making a class list or poster.

1. 10,000 is 9000 more than 1000. It is 9900 more than 100.
2. 10,000 is 1000 times as big as 10, because if you count ten times by 1000 you get 10,000.
3. It's 100 times as big as 100 because you can divide the 1000 by 10 and get 100 and put the extra 10 times on the 10 to get 100. I also know it's 100 times as big as 100 because the poster was 100 across and 100 down.
4. A poster with 10,000 squares fills most of the board in our room.
5. It is 10 times smaller than 100,000.
6. These are some of the factor pairs of 10,000
    1,000 × 10   50 × 200   100 × 100

✷ You can divide 10,000 by lots of numbers. 2 goes into it and 25 and 50 and 5 because they are also factors of 100. 8 and 125 are factors of 10,000 because a factor pair of 100 is 8 and 12.5. For 10,000 it's 8 and 1250. You multiply 12.5 × 100 because 10,000 is 100 times more than 100.

✷ 10,000 meters is 10 Kilometers.

✷ It is a composite number because it has other factors besides 1 and 10,000.

✷ It is a square number because you can make a square from 10,000 squares like on the poster.

✷ 10,000 is even because if you keep going 2+2+2 etc. you get to 10,000.

Each student completes Student Sheet 29, Add a Clue, which presents a number puzzle like the others students have solved in groups during this unit. In their work, students may use calculators, 300 charts, and the class lists of Factor Pairs of 100 and 1000.

Note: It is *not* necessary for students to have finished all the number puzzles from Investigations 1 and 4 in order to do this assessment.

Allow at least 30 minutes for the assessment activity, although some students will not need the entire time. Those who finish early continue recording what they know about 10,000.

As students work, circulate and ask individuals to explain how they are thinking about the puzzle. If some students are having difficulty with the writing, ask them to tell you what they did, and then simply put these explanations in writing. As you review the writing, make sure their explanations are clear and complete. Encourage them to add to or clarify their writing as needed.

❖ **Tip for the Linguistically Diverse Classroom** Do this assessment sheet orally with students who have limited English proficiency.

When everyone has finished, collect students' work and then invite students to share with the class the clues they added and their reasoning.

As you assess students' work (both written and discussion), consider the following questions:

- Does the student understand what factors and multiples are? What strategies does he or she use for finding them?
- Can the student explain how he or she used each clue to eliminate possible answers?
- Can the student devise a fourth clue that involves a number relationship such as factor, multiple, odd, or square?

Examples of student work for this assessment are discussed in the **Teacher Note**, Assessment: Add a Clue (p. 94).

Write the following challenge on the board or overhead:

Find some factor pairs of 10,000. Write about how you found each factor pair.

Emphasize that it is not necessary for students to find all the factor pairs of 10,000. It is more important for them to find only a few and to write a clear explanation of how they found each one.

Allow about 30 minutes for this activity. Most students will have time to find and write about several factor pairs. Some students may tell you they could find more factor pairs of 10,000, given more time. Acknowledge this and encourage them to find additional factor pairs outside of class time.

Students work individually. They may refer to the class lists of Factor Pairs of 100 and 1000. Encourage them to work without calculators (but allow their use if students feel it is necessary).

Observing the Students Circulate as students work. If students are having difficulty getting started, encourage them to think of the different things that have helped them find factor pairs throughout the unit, such as skip counting, working cluster problems, and using what they know about factor pairs of some numbers to find others. As you look at students' work and listen to what they say, consider the following questions:

■ How are students using what they know about factor pairs of 100, 1000, and other landmarks to find factor pairs of 10,000? For example:

Are they using relationships between 1000 and 10,000 to find factor pairs? ("I know that 25 is a factor of 1000, so it also goes into 10,000. 10,000 is ten times more than 1000, so instead of 25×40, it's 25×400.")

Are they using what they know about factors of multiples of 1000? ("There are forty 25's in 1000, and 10,000 is ten 1000's. So you need four hundred 25's to get to 10,000.")

■ Do students have strategies for using one factor pair of 10,000 to find others? ("I figured out that 400×25 is a factor pair of 10,000. 200×50 would also work because it's half 400 and twice 25.")

Students who finish early might try to find all the factor pairs of 10,000 and write about how they can be sure they found them all.

When everyone has finished, collect students' work. Invite students to share the factor pairs they found and their strategies for finding them.

Choosing Student Work to Save

As the unit ends, encourage students to spend 20–30 minutes revisiting their work for the last few weeks. You may want to use one of the following options for creating a record of students' work on this unit:

■ Students look back through their folders or notebooks and write about what they learned in the unit, what they remember most, and what was hard or easy for them. You might have students complete this work during their writing time.

■ Students select one or two pieces of their work as their best, and you also choose one or two pieces of their work to be saved. This work is saved in a portfolio for the year. You might include students' written responses to the assessments Finding Factor Pairs of 1100 (p. 66) and Add a Clue (p. 91). Students can create a separate page with brief comments describing each piece of work.

■ You may want to send a selection of work home for families to see. Students write cover letters, describing their work in this unit. This work should be returned if you are keeping a year-long portfolio of mathematics work for each student.

Sessions 5 and 6 Follow-Up

Another Add a Clue   Students solve another Add a Clue problem on Student Sheet 30, Another Add a Clue.

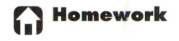 **Homework**

Two different approaches to the assessment tasks on Student Sheet 29, Add a Clue (p. 145), are illustrated by the work of Manuel and Lindsay. Manuel responded this way:

1. What numbers fit these three clues?

25, 50, 100

2. How did you find the numbers that fit the clues?

I found the factors of 1000 and 300. I know some of the factor pairs of 1000 by heart. I started with those and did twice one and half the other to find more. I know the factors of 100 by heart and I multiplied them by 3 to get the factors of 300. I counted by 25 and I checked to see if each number I counted is a factor of 300 and 1000. I circled those ones.

Factors were listed in the margins of his page, as follows:

3. Write a fourth clue that gives the puzzle just one answer.

My number is a factor of 75.

4. What is the answer to your puzzle? How do you know?

The answer is 25 because it is the only one that is a factor of 75. 25 × 3 = 75.

50 is not a factor of 75 because the smallest thing you can do is 50 × 2 and that's 100.

100 is not a factor of 75 because it is more than 75.

Manuel's responses to questions 1 and 2 demonstrate a strong grasp of factors and multiples. He recognizes that if a number is a factor of 100, then 3 times that number is a factor of 300; he has strategies for using one factor pair of a number to find others; and he uses repeated addition to find multiples.

For question 3, Manuel's clue eliminates two of the three answers he found. His explanation in question 4 demonstrates solid reasoning about factor and multiple relationships.

This was Lindsay's response:

1. What numbers fit these three clues?

50, 100

2. How did you find the numbers that fit the clues?

I started with the middle clue because that gets rid of the most numbers. I counted by 25 and found all the multiples of 25 up to 150 because 150 is half of 300. That's 50, 75, 100, 125, 150. With each of these numbers I counted to see if it would hit 300 and if it did I divided to see if it goes into 1000.

3. Write a fourth clue that gives the puzzle just one answer.

This number of tiles will make a square.

4. What is the answer to your puzzle? How do you know?

The answer is 100 because 10 × 10 = 100 so you can make a square that is 10 wide and 10 long and has 100 tiles in it. You can't make a square from 50 tiles because there isn't a number you can times by itself to get 50.

Lindsay sought an efficient approach to the initial problem. She began with the clue that she thought would eliminate the most numbers, and she recognized that she need only find numbers up to 150. She used repeated addition to find multiples of 25 and to determine whether these numbers are factors of 300. She also used division to find factors.

Continued on next page

However, she failed to include 25 as a multiple of 25. It is not clear from her explanation if this was an oversight, or if she actually thinks that 25 is not a multiple of 25.

Lindsay's added clue in question 3 eliminates one of the two answers she found. Her explanation in question 4 demonstrates that she has developed geometric and numeric meaning for square numbers.

When Lindsay handed in her paper, the teacher looked it over and then asked if she could say what a multiple is. Lindsay began her explanation:

"Multiples are the numbers you get when you keep adding a number to itself—25, that's one 25, then 50, that's two 25's . . ." then suddenly realized that she had not included 25 as a multiple of 25 when listing numbers that match all three clues. She wrote in 25 as one of her answers to question 1. That meant her added clue no longer worked, as both 25 and 100 tiles will make a square.

She then changed her fourth clue to read, "This number of tiles will *not* make a square." She explained that the answer is now 50, since of 25, 50, and 100, 50 is the only number that is not square.

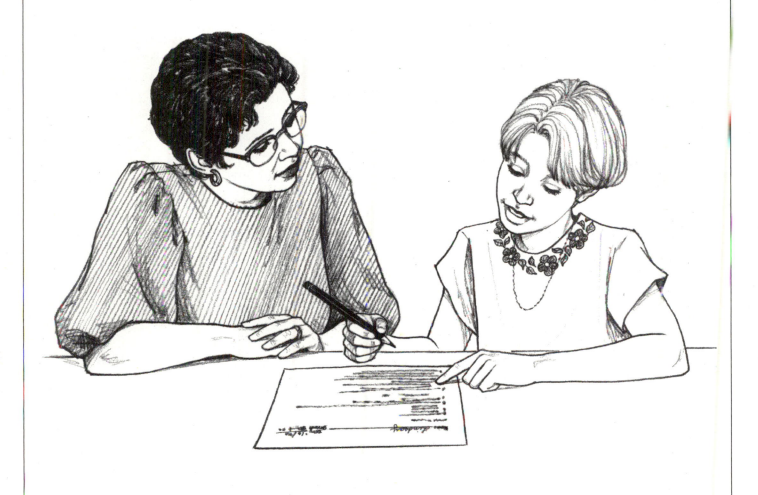

Exploring Data

Basic Activity

You or the students decide on something to observe about themselves. Because this is a Ten-Minute Math activity, the data they collect must be something they already know or can observe easily around them. Once the question is determined, quickly organize the data as students give individual answers to the question. The data can be organized as a line plot, a list, a table, or a bar graph. Then students describe what they can tell from the data, generate some new questions, and, if appropriate, make predictions about what will happen the next time they collect the same data.

Exploring Data is designed to give students many quick opportunities to collect, graph, describe, and interpret data about themselves and the world around them. Students focus on:

- describing important features of the data
- interpreting and posing questions about the data

Procedure

Step 1. Choose a question. Make sure the question involves data that students know or can observe: How many buttons are you wearing today? What month is your birthday? What is the best thing you ate yesterday? Are you wearing shoes or sneakers or sandals? How did you get to school today?

Step 2. Quickly collect and display the data. Use a list, a table, a line plot, or a bar graph. For example, a line plot for data about how many buttons students are wearing could look something like this:

```
              X
    X         X         X
    X         X         X
    X         X  X  X   X
    X         X  X  X   X
    X  X  X   X  X  X   X
   ─────────────────────────
    0  1  2   3  4  5   6
```

Number of Buttons

Step 3. Ask students to describe the data. What do they notice about their data? For data that have a numerical order (How many buttons do you have today? How many people live in your house? How many months until your birthday?), ask questions like these:

"Are the data spread out or close together? What is the highest and lowest value? Where do most of the data seem to fall? What seems typical or usual for this class?"

For data in categories (What is your favorite book? How do you get to school? What month is your birthday?), ask questions like these: "Which categories have a lot of data? few data? none? Is there a way to categorize the data differently to get other information?"

Step 4. Ask students to interpret and predict. "Why do you think that the data came out this way? Does anything about the data surprise you? Do you think we'd get similar data if we collected it tomorrow? next week? in another class? with adults?"

Step 5. List any new questions. Keep a running list of questions you can use for further data collection and analysis. You may want to ask some of these questions again.

Variations

Data from Home For homework, have students collect data that involves asking questions or making observations at home: What time do your brothers and sisters go to bed? What do you usually eat for breakfast?

Data from Another Class or Other Teachers Depending on your school situation, you may be able to assign students to collect data from other classrooms or other teachers. Students are always interested in surveying others about questions that interest them, such as this one: When you were little, did you like school?

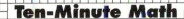

Categories If students take surveys about "favorites"—flavor of ice cream, breakfast cereal, book, color—or other data that falls into categories, the graphs are often flat and uninteresting. There is not too much to say, for example, about a graph like this:

```
X
X        X                    X        X
X        X        X           X        X        X
X        X        X           X        X        X
vanilla  chocolate straw-    chocolate Rocky    vanilla
                   berry     chip      Road     fudge
```

It is more interesting for students to group their results into fewer, more descriptive categories, so that they can see other things about the data. In this case, even though vanilla seems to be the favorite in the graph above, another way of grouping the data seems to show that flavors with some chocolate in them are really the favorites.

Chocolate flavors   //// //// /

Flavors without chocolate   //// /

Familiar Fractions Once data is grouped into two or three categories, students express the data as fractions and then find familiar fractions and percents to describe the amounts. For example, in the ice cream choices survey, $6/17$ prefer flavors without chocolate. This is less than half. It is about a third since $6/18$ is a third. Seventeenths are larger than eighteenths, so it's more than $33\frac{1}{3}\%$, maybe about 35%. Students can check by dividing 6 by 17 on the calculator.

Quick Images

Basic Activity

Students are briefly shown a picture of a figure. Depending on the kind of figure, they either draw it or build it.

For each type of figure—dot patterns, geometric shapes, cube images, or pattern block arrangements—students must find meaningful ways to see and develop a mental image. They might see the figure as a whole ("It looks like a window, three cubes high and five cubes wide"), or decompose it into memorable parts ("It looks like a flower with a square center and four diamond petals"), or use their knowledge of number relationships to remember a pattern ("There were 6 groups of 5 dots, so it's 30"). Their work focuses on:

- organizing and analyzing visual images
- developing concepts and language needed to reflect on and communicate about spatial relationships
- using geometric vocabulary to describe shapes and patterns
- using number relationships to describe patterns

Materials

- Overhead projector
- Overhead transparencies of the dot patterns or geometric figures you will use as images for the session. To use the images, first make a transparency, then cut out the separate figures and keep them in an envelope. Include the numbers beside the figures; they will help you properly orient the figures on the overhead.
- Pencil and paper
- Interlocking cubes, pattern blocks, or other shapes for the variations

Procedure

Step 1. Flash an image for 3 seconds. It's important to keep the picture up for as close to 3 seconds as possible. If you show the picture too long, students will draw or build from the picture rather than their image of it; if you show it too briefly, they will not have time to form a mental image. Suggest to students that they study the figure carefully while it is visible, then try to draw or build it from their mental image.

Step 2. Students draw or build what they saw. Give students a few minutes with their pencil and paper or the manipulatives to try to draw or construct a figure based on the mental image they have formed. After you see that most students' activity has stopped, go on to step 3.

Step 3. Flash the image again, for revision. After you show the image for another 3 seconds, students revise their building or drawing, based on this second view.

It is essential to provide enough time between the first and second flashes for most students to complete their attempts at drawing or building. While they may not have completed their figure, they should have done all they can until they see the picture on the screen again.

Step 4. Show the image a final time. When student activity subsides again, show the picture a third time. This time leave it visible so that all students can complete or revise their solutions.

Step 5. Students describe how they saw the drawing as they looked at it on successive "flashes."

Variations

In this unit you will find transparency masters for two types of Quick Images: dot patterns and geometric designs. You can supplement any of these with your own examples or make up other types. Following are some options.

Quick Image Geometric Designs. Use the Quick Image Geometric Designs transparency. When students talk about what they saw in successive flashes, many students will say things like "I saw four circles in a row, overlapping." You might suggest this strategy for students having difficulty: "Each design is made from familiar geometric shapes. Find these shapes and try to figure out how they are put together."

As students describe their figures, you can introduce correct terms for the shapes: *parallelogram, rhombus, trapezoid, equilateral triangle,* and so forth. As you use these terms naturally as part of the discussion, students will begin to use and recognize them.

Quick Image Dot Patterns Use the Quick Image Dot Patterns transparency. The procedure is the same, except that now students are asked two questions: "Can you draw the dot patterns you see? Can you figure out how many dots you saw?"

When students answer only one question, ask them the other again. You will see different students using different strategies. For instance, some will see a multiplication problem, 9 × 3, and will not draw the dots unless asked. Others will draw the dots, then figure out how many there are.

Quick Image Cubes Each student should have a supply of 15–20 cubes. Flash a drawing of a three-dimensional cube figure, like this:

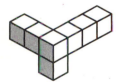

Follow the same procedure, giving students time to build what they saw.

Quick Image Pattern Blocks or Other Shapes
Use a set of transparent overhead pattern blocks or other shapes if you have them, or use a regular set and leave small spaces between the pieces. Arrange three or four shapes on the overhead to form a larger shape or design. Follow the usual procedure. Students create the shapes they see using their own set of shapes or by drawing the figure.

Using the Calculator You can integrate the calculator into the Quick Image Dot Patterns. As you draw larger or more complex dot patterns, students may begin to count the groups and the number of groups. They should use a variety of strategies to find the total number of dots, including mental calculation and the calculator.

Related Homework Options

- **Creating Quick Images** Students can make up their own Quick Images to challenge the rest of the class. Talk with students about keeping these reasonable—challenging, but not overwhelming. If they are too complex and difficult, other students will just become frustrated.

- **Family Quick Images** You can also send images home for students to try with their families. Instead of using the overhead projector, they can simply show a picture for a few seconds; cover it up while members of the family try to draw it; then show it again, and so forth. Other members of the family may also be interested in creating images.

The following activities will help ensure that this unit is comprehensible to students who are acquiring English as a second language. The suggested approach is based on *The Natural Approach: Language Acquisition in the Classroom* by Stephen D. Krashen and Tracy D. Terrell (Alemany Press, 1983). The intent is for second-language learners to acquire new vocabulary in an active, meaningful context.

Note that *acquiring* a word is different from *learning* a word. Depending on their level of proficiency, students may be able to comprehend a word upon hearing it during an investigation without being able to say it. Other students may be able to use the word orally, but not read or write it. The goal is to help students naturally acquire targeted vocabulary at their present level of proficiency.

We suggest using these activities just before the related investigations. The activities can also be led by English-proficient students.

Investigations 1–4

possible, impossible

1. Ask students if they can wiggle their ears without touching them. Group students who can and cannot do this.

2. Ask students in the "possible" group to demonstrate their skill. Nod your head as you confirm that it is *possible* for these students to wiggle their ears without touching them.

3. Now ask students in the "impossible" group to try to wiggle. Shake your head as you note that the task is *impossible* for these students.

4. Next, challenge students to raise one eyebrow and to curl their tongue. For each challenge, repeat the format above, with emphasis on the words *possible* and *impossible*.

row, in order, rearrange, even, odd

1. Verbalize what you are doing as you write the numbers 1 to 10 on the board.

   I'm going to write 1 to 10 *in order*. First I'll write the number 1, followed by the number 2 . . .

   1 2 3 4 5 6 7 8 9 10

2. Now tell students that you are going to *rearrange* these numbers. Below the first row, write the numbers 1–10 with all the evens first.

   2 4 6 8 10 1 3 5 7 9

3. Once again tell students you will *rearrange* the numbers. In a third row, write the numbers 1–10 with the *odd* numbers first.

   1 3 5 7 9 2 4 6 8 10

4. Separate the three rows with long horizontal lines and number the rows from 1 to 3. Ask questions about each row.

1. 1	2	3	4	5	6	7	8	9	10
2. 2	4	6	8	10	1	3	5	7	9
3. 1	3	5	7	9	2	4	6	8	10

   Which row has the numbers in order?
   Which row has the even numbers first?
   Which row has the odd numbers first?
   Which rows end with the number 10?
   Which rows begin with the number 1?
   Which rows did I rearrange?
   Which row is in order?

Blackline Masters

Investigation 4

General Resources for the Unit

Dear Family,

We are starting a unit called *Mathematical Thinking at Grade 5*. In this unit your child will learn about the number system and about the "landmark" numbers—like 100, 1000, 10,000, and their factors and multiples—that help us find our way around that system.

During this unit, your child will explore questions like these:

What factors do the numbers 100, 250, and 1000 have in common? What multiples?

How many 25's are there in 1000? How many 25's in 10,000?

What numbers could we count by and land exactly on 10,000?

If we count by 50's, and there are 26 of us, what number will the last person say? What if we count by 100's? by 250's?

How much larger is 10,000 than 1000? How many 1000's are in 10,000?

What else do you know about 10,000?

Your child will be solving problems that take considerable time, thought, and discussion. Children are expected to think about the problems in their own ways, and to be able to talk and write about their solutions. Throughout the year, you can help in several ways:

■ Sometimes your child's homework will ask for your participation. For example, in this unit your child will bring home some mathematical games. Play them together, and see what your child is learning.

■ Any time you need to estimate amounts at home, try to involve your child. Look for ways to count or estimate large numbers of things, like floor tiles, or windowpanes, or the number of cookies you'll need to make for the big picnic. Encourage your child to think of different ways to figure out about how many.

■ Look with your child for large numbers in newspapers, on packages, on signs, and around your home and neighborhood. Talk together about what the numbers mean.

We are looking forward to an exciting few weeks as we create a mathematical community in our classroom.

Sincerely,

Mr. Porter

Number Shape Clues

Find and record a number that fits each clue.

Draw one or more rectangles to show that your number fits the clue.

Record the factor pair that your rectangle shows.

Clues

1. You can make this number of tiles into a rectangle 2 tiles wide.

2. You can make this number of tiles into a rectangle 5 tiles wide.

3. You can make this number of tiles into *only* 1 rectangle.

4. You can make this number of tiles into a square.

5. You can make this number of tiles into *only* 2 rectangles.

6. You can make this number of tiles into at least 4 different rectangles.

Factor Pairs from 1 to 25

On the graph paper provided, draw rectangles to show the factor pairs for each number from 1 to 25. Label the dimensions of each rectangle and list the factor pair that each rectangle shows.

Below, record any observations or discoveries about the rectangles and factors for these numbers. (For example, which numbers have the most factors? The fewest? How many numbers have 2 as a factor?)

_____

_____

_____

_____

_____

_____

_____

_____

_____

Skip Counting

In the space below, record the first 20 numbers you would say if you counted by a large one-digit number, such as 7 or 9, or a small two-digit number, such as 11 or 12. Try this task without a calculator.

The number I chose to count by is _____.

The numbers I said were:

Number Puzzle Recording Sheet

Check off each puzzle you solve. Record your answer.

Investigation 1 Number Puzzles

Puzzle	Answer
1	
2	
3	
4	
5	
6	
7	
8	

Puzzle	Answer
9☆	
10☆	
11☆	
12☆	
13☆	
14☆	

Save this recording sheet for use in Investigation 4.

Investigation 4 Number Puzzles

Puzzle	Answer
15	
16	
17	
18	
19	
20	
21	
22	

Puzzle	Answer
23☆	
24☆	
25☆	
26☆	
27☆	
28☆	

Make Your Own Puzzle

Here are three clues of a number puzzle:

My number is a multiple of 9.
My number is odd.
My number has two digits.

1. What numbers fit these three clues?

2. How did you find all the numbers that fit the clues?

3. Write a fourth clue that gives the puzzle just one answer.

4. What is the answer to your new puzzle?

What's the Number?

Three of these puzzles have more than one answer.
Try to find all the possible answers for each puzzle.
One of these puzzles is impossible.

1. My number is a factor of 20. It's also a factor of 30.

2. My number is a multiple of 10. It's a factor of 45.

3. My number is between 40 and 50. It is prime.

4. My number is a multiple of 4. It's a square number.
It's less than 50.

Make an Impossible Puzzle

Here are three clues of a number puzzle:

My number is less than 100.
My number is a multiple of 7.
My number is a multiple of 3.

1. What numbers fit these three clues?

2. How did you find all the numbers that fit the clues?

3. Write a fourth clue that makes the puzzle impossible.

4. Explain how you know your new puzzle is impossible.

Sample Puzzle

My number is a multiple of 15.

Sample Puzzle

My number is odd.

Sample Puzzle

My number is greater than 50.

Sample Puzzle

My number is less than 100.

This page presents two identical copies of the sample puzzle clues. Duplicate enough so that each small group of four students can have one set of the clues, cut apart and clipped together.

Sample Puzzle

My number is a multiple of 15.

Sample Puzzle

My number is odd.

Sample Puzzle

My number is greater than 50.

Sample Puzzle

My number is less than 100.

Puzzle 1

My number is less than 30.

Puzzle 1

My number of tiles will make
a square.

Puzzle 1

My number of tiles will make
a rectangle 2 tiles wide.

Puzzle 1

My number is greater than 5.

Puzzle 2

My number of tiles will make
a rectangle 3 tiles wide.

Puzzle 2

My number of tiles will make
a rectangle 4 tiles wide.

Puzzle 2

My number is greater than 20.

Puzzle 2

My number is less than 30.

Investigation 1 • Resource
Mathematical Thinking at Grade 5

Puzzle 3

My number of tiles will make a rectangle 4 tiles wide.

Puzzle 3

My number of tiles will make a rectangle 2 tiles wide.

Puzzle 3

My number of tiles will make a rectangle 5 tiles wide.

Puzzle 3

My number is less than 50.

Puzzle 4

My number is less than 25.

Puzzle 4

My number of tiles will make only one rectangle.

Puzzle 4

My number is odd.

Puzzle 4

My number is a factor of 36.

Puzzle 5

You say my number when you start at 0 and count by 15's.

Puzzle 5

You say my number when you start at 0 and count by 25's.

Puzzle 5

My number is less than 200.

Puzzle 5

My number is even.

Puzzle 6

My number has three digits.

Puzzle 6

My number is less than 300.

Puzzle 6

My number is a multiple of 40.

Puzzle 6

My number is a multiple of 60.

Puzzle 7

My number is a square number.

Puzzle 7

My number has two digits.

Puzzle 7

My number is a multiple of 9.

Puzzle 7

My number is even.

Puzzle 8

My number is prime.

Puzzle 8

My number is a factor of 42.

Puzzle 8

My number is less than 10.

Puzzle 8

My number is a factor of 70.

☆☆☆☆☆ ☆ **Puzzle 9**☆

My number is a factor of 60.

☆☆☆☆☆ ☆ **Puzzle 9**☆

My number has two digits.

☆☆☆☆☆ **Puzzle 9**☆

The sum of the digits in my number is 3.

☆☆☆☆☆ **Puzzle 9**☆

One factor of my number is 4.

☆☆☆☆☆ **Puzzle 10**☆

My number is not a factor of 20.

☆☆☆☆☆ **Puzzle 10**☆

My number is a factor of 42.

☆☆☆☆☆ **Puzzle 10**☆

My number is less than 30.

☆☆☆☆☆ **Puzzle 10**☆

My number is even.

☆☆☆☆☆   **Puzzle 11**☆

My number is a square number.

☆☆☆☆☆   **Puzzle 11**☆

My number is even.

☆☆☆☆☆   **Puzzle 11**☆

My number is less than 100.

☆☆☆☆☆   **Puzzle 11**☆

My number is prime.

☆☆☆☆☆   **Puzzle 12**☆

My number is a multiple of 35.

☆☆☆☆☆   **Puzzle 12**☆

My number is a multiple of 25.

☆☆☆☆☆   **Puzzle 12**☆

My number is a multiple of 2.

☆☆☆☆☆   **Puzzle 12**☆

My number is less than 400.

☆☆☆☆☆   **Puzzle 13☆**

My number is odd.

☆☆☆☆☆   **Puzzle 13☆**

My number has two digits.

☆☆☆☆☆   **Puzzle 13☆**

My number is a multiple of 3.

☆☆☆☆☆   **Puzzle 13☆**

The sum of the digits in my number is greater than 15.

☆☆☆☆☆   **Puzzle 14☆**

My number is less than 200.

☆☆☆☆☆   **Puzzle 14☆**

My number is a multiple of 11.

☆☆☆☆☆   **Puzzle 14☆**

My number has three digits.

☆☆☆☆☆   **Puzzle 14☆**

The sum of the digits in my number is 10.

Find the Counting Numbers

Find *all* the counting numbers that fit each clue.

1. If you count by this number, you will say 100, but you will *not* say 10.

2. If you count by this number, you will say 200, but you will *not* say 40.

3. If you count by this number, you will say 300, but you will *not* say 75.

More Factor Pairs

The multiple of 100 I have chosen is _____.

Find several factor pairs for the multiple of 100 you chose
and list them below.

_____

_____

_____

_____

_____

Write about the strategies you used to find the factor pairs.

Counting Backward

Choose a multiple of 100 and count backward by one of the factors on our class list of factor pairs.

The multiple I chose is _____.

The factor I am counting by is _____.

The numbers I said when I counted backward:

What Could You Count By?

Choose a multiple of 100 (such as 300 or 500) or a multiple of 1000 (such as 2000 or 6000).

The multiple I chose is _____.

Find and record at least 5 different numbers you could count by so that somewhere in the count you would reach your chosen number.

How did you decide what numbers to try?

Number I tried that did not reach my multiple:

Multiplication Clusters (page 1 of 2)

Use problems in the cluster to help you solve the last problem.
Add any other problems you use to help solve the last problem.

20 × 4	25 × 4
2 × 4	**23 × 4**

4 × 25	10 × 25
12 × 25	**13 × 25**

3 × 50	20 × 50
7 × 50	**17 × 50**

Multiplication Clusters (page 2 of 2)

Use problems in the cluster to help you solve the last problem.
Add any other problems you use to help solve the last problem.

30×5 200×5

233×10 **233×5**

4×25 10×25

40×25 50×25

6×25 **46×25**

500×4 1000×4

2500×4 **2507×4**

More Multiplication Clusters

Use problems in the cluster to help you solve the last problem.
Add any other problems you use to help solve the last problem.

8×25	30×25
40×25	**38×25**

25×40	70×10
75×40	**74×40**

25×4	200×4
250×4	275×4
	277×4

25×5	200×5
2000×5	**2025×5**

Challenging Multiplication Clusters

Use problems in the cluster to help you solve the last problem.
Add any other problems you use to help solve the last problem.

7×40	25×40
250×40	275×40
	282×40

3×50	20×50
200×50	**197×50**

0.5×50	2.5×5 2×5 $2.$
25×5	**2.5×50**

12×24	25×12
$.5 \times 24$	**12.5×24**

Division Clusters

Use problems in the cluster to help you solve the last problem.
Add any other problems you use to help solve the last problem.

5 ÷ 5   100 ÷ 5

30 ÷ 5   **135 ÷ 5**

24 ÷ 4   100 ÷ 4

200 ÷ 4   224 ÷ 4

248 ÷ 4

100 ÷ 20   1000 ÷ 20

800 ÷ 20   **900 ÷ 20**

More Division Clusters

Use problems in the cluster to help you solve the last problem.
Add any other problems you use to help solve the last problem.

$100 \div 4$ $16 \div 4$

$116 \div 4$ **$232 \div 4$**

$100 \div 2$ $200 \div 2$

$90 \div 2$ $10 \div 2$

$190 \div 2$

$100 \div 25$ $1000 \div 25$

$2000 \div 25$ $300 \div 25$

$2300 \div 25$

Challenging Division Clusters

Use problems in the cluster to help you solve the last problem.
Add any other problems you use to help solve the last problem.

100 ÷ 50	1000 ÷ 5
10,000 ÷ 50	**10,100 ÷ 50**

NCAS
P. 131
※ 1

100 ÷	1000 ÷ 25
500 ÷	10,000 ÷ 25
10,500 ÷ 25	

500 ÷ 50	1000 ÷ 50
2000 ÷ 50	**2500 ÷ 50**

2000 ÷ 400	8000 ÷ 400
4,000 ÷ 400	**20,000 ÷ 400**

Writing About Multiplication Clusters

Solve each cluster. Add to the cluster any other problem(s)
you used to solve the last problem. Write about how you
used the problems in the cluster to solve the final problem.

5×20 10×20

50×20 60×20

$$65 \times 20$$

3×25 40×25

80×25 **77×25**

Make Your Own Cluster

Write a cluster of problems to help you solve one of the
following problems.

$$47 \times 40 \qquad\qquad\qquad 336 \div 4$$

Record your cluster below. Write about how the problems
in the cluster helped you solve the original problem.

Factor Pairs of 950

Find factor pairs of 950 and write about how you found
each pair.

How to Play Close to 1000

Materials

- One deck of Numeral Cards
- Close to 1000 Score Sheet for each player

Players: 1, 2, or 3

How to Play

1. Deal out eight Numeral Cards to each player.

2. Use any six cards to make two numbers. For example, a 6, a 5, and a 2 could make 652, 625, 526, 562, 256, or 265. Wild Cards can be used as any numeral. Try to make two numbers that, when added, give you a total that is close to 1000.

3. Write these numbers and their total on the Close to 1000 Score Sheet. For example: 652 + 347 = 999.

4. Find your score. Your score is the difference between your total and 1000.

5. Put the cards you used in a discard pile. Keep the two cards you didn't use for the next round.

6. For the next round, deal six new cards to each player. Make more numbers that come close to 1000. When you run out of cards, mix up the discard pile and use them again.

7. After five rounds, total your scores. Lowest score wins.

Scoring Variation   Write the score with plus and minus signs to show the direction of your total away from 1000. For example: If your total is 999, your score is −1. If your total is 1005, your score is +5. The total of these two scores would be +4. Your goal is to get a total score for five rounds that is close to 0.

Close to 1000 Score Sheet

Game 1   Score

Round 1: ___ ___ ___ + ___ ___ ___ = _____   _____

Round 2: ___ ___ ___ + ___ ___ ___ = _____   _____

Round 3: ___ ___ ___ + ___ ___ ___ = _____   _____

Round 4: ___ ___ ___ + ___ ___ ___ = _____   _____

Round 5: ___ ___ ___ + ___ ___ ___ = _____   _____

                                                      TOTAL SCORE   _____

Game 2   Score

Round 1: ___ ___ ___ + ___ ___ ___ = _____   _____

Round 2: ___ ___ ___ + ___ ___ ___ = _____   _____

Round 3: ___ ___ ___ + ___ ___ ___ = _____   _____

Round 4: ___ ___ ___ + ___ ___ ___ = _____   _____

Round 5: ___ ___ ___ + ___ ___ ___ = _____   _____

                                                      TOTAL SCORE   _____

How to Play Close to 0

Materials

- One deck of Numeral Cards
- Close to 0 Score Sheet for each player

Players: 1, 2, or 3

How to Play

1. Deal out eight Numeral Cards to each player.

2. Use any six cards to make two numbers. For example, a 6, a 5, and a 2 could make 652, 625, 526, 562, 256, or 265. Wild Cards can be used as any numeral. Try to make two numbers that, when subtracted, give you a difference that is close to 0.

3. Write these numbers and their difference on the Close to 0 Score Sheet. For example: 652 − 647 = 5. The difference is your score.

4. Put the cards you used in a discard pile. Keep the two cards you didn't use for the next round.

5. For the next round, deal six new cards to each player. Make two more numbers with a difference close to 0. When you run out of cards, mix up the discard pile and use them again.

6. After five rounds, total your scores. Lowest score wins.

Close to 0 Score Sheet

Game 1   Score

Round 1:   __ __ __ – __ __ __ = _____   _____

Round 2:   __ __ __ – __ __ __ = _____   _____

Round 3:   __ __ __ – __ __ __ = _____   _____

Round 4:   __ __ __ – __ __ __ = _____   _____

Round 5:   __ __ __ – __ __ __ = _____   _____

TOTAL SCORE   _____

Game 2   Score

Round 1:   __ __ __ – __ __ __ = _____   _____

Round 2:   __ __ __ – __ __ __ = _____   _____

Round 3:   __ __ __ – __ __ __ = _____   _____

Round 4:   __ __ __ – __ __ __ = _____   _____

Round 5:   __ __ __ – __ __ __ = _____   _____

TOTAL SCORE   _____

Many Squares Poster Tasks (Group A)

1. Label these squares on the poster:

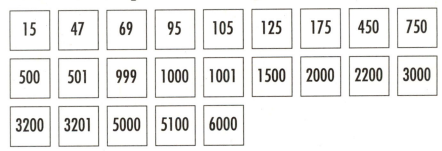

15	47	69	95	105	125	175	450	750
500	501	999	1000	1001	1500	2000	2200	3000
3200	3201	5000	5100	6000				

2. Find each number described below. Label the square on the poster, and record the number on this sheet.

What number is . . .

1 row below 750? _____

2 rows below 750? _____

5 rows below 750? _____

10 rows below 750? _____

20 rows below 750? _____

3. Find each number described below. Label the square on the poster, and record the number on this sheet.

What number is . . .

25 more than 5725? _____

50 more than 5725? _____

53 more than 5725? _____

100 more than 5725? _____

1000 more than 5725? _____

100 less than 5725? _____

150 less than 5725? _____

Many Squares Poster Tasks (Group B)

1. Label these squares on the poster:

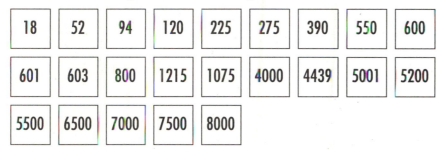

| 18 | 52 | 94 | 120 | 225 | 275 | 390 | 550 | 600 |

| 601 | 603 | 800 | 1215 | 1075 | 4000 | 4439 | 5001 | 5200 |

| 5500 | 6500 | 7000 | 7500 | 8000 |

2. Find each number described below. Label the square on the poster, and record the number on this sheet.

What number is . . .

1 row below 1075? _____

2 rows below 1075? _____

5 rows below 1075? _____

10 rows below 1075? _____

20 rows below 1075? _____

3. Find each number described below. Label the square on the poster, and record the number on this sheet.

What number is . . .

25 more than 6050? _____

50 more than 6050? _____

53 more than 6050? _____

100 more than 6050? _____

1000 more than 6050? _____

100 less than 6050? _____

150 less than 6050? _____

Many Squares Poster Tasks (Group C)

1. Label these squares on the poster:

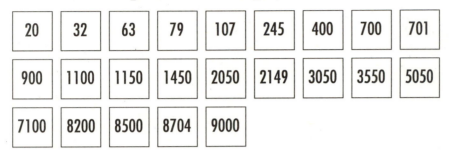

20	32	63	79	107	245	400	700	701
900	1100	1150	1450	2050	2149	3050	3550	5050
7100	8200	8500	8704	9000				

2. Find each number described below. Label the square on the poster, and record the number on this sheet.

What number is . . .

2 rows below 1150? _____

4 rows below 1150? _____

5 rows below 1150? _____

10 rows below 1150? _____

20 rows below 1150? _____

3. Find each number described below. Label the square on the poster, and record the number on this sheet.

What number is . . .

25 more than 9525? _____

50 more than 9525? _____

53 more than 9525? _____

100 more than 9525? _____

100 less than 9525? _____

150 less than 9525? _____

1000 less than 9525? _____

Many Squares Poster Tasks (Group D)

1. Label these squares on the poster:

| 11 | 30 | 55 | 80 | 109 | 129 | 350 | 425 | 725 |

| 801 | 1025 | 1050 | 2025 | 2275 | 3500 | 4050 | 7203 | 7750 |

| 8215 | 9100 | 9500 | 9900 | 10,000 |

2. Find each number described below. Label the square on the poster, and record the number on this sheet.

What number is . . .

2 rows above 10,000? _____

3 rows above 10,000? _____

4 rows above 10,000? _____

11 rows above 10,000? _____

5500 less than 10,000? _____

3. Find each number described below. Label the square on the poster, and record the number on this sheet.

What number is . . .

25 more than 3250? _____

50 more than 3250? _____

53 more than 3250? _____

100 more than 3250? _____

2000 more than 3250? _____

25 less than 3250? _____

75 less than 3250? _____

Exploring the Many Squares Poster

1. What are the numbers of the squares in the box marked with triangles? (Write the numbers here. Do *not* label these squares on your poster.)

2. How many squares are in the box marked with stars? _____

   How many squares on the poster are *not* in the box marked with stars? _____

   How do you know?

3. How many squares are in the box marked with dots? _____

   How many squares on the poster are *not* in the box marked with dots? _____

   How do you know?

4. What advice would you give someone who wanted to find 8250 on the poster?

Problems from Close to 1000

Suppose you are dealt these hands in Close to 1000.
What numbers would you make for the best score?
(Best score = sum as close to 1000 as possible)

Score

Round 1 | 4 | 6 | 0 | 5 | 3 | 2 | 7 | 9 |

_____ + _____ = _____   _____

Round 2 | 2 | 8 | 4 | 4 | 7 | 2 | 1 | 4 |

_____ + _____ = _____   _____

Round 3 | 3 | 7 | 1 | 9 | 6 | 0 | 5 | 3 |

_____ + _____ = _____   _____

Round 4 | 8 | 5 | 0 | 3 | 0 | 1 | 4 | 2 |

_____ + _____ = _____   _____

Round 5 | 0 | 5 | 6 | 3 | 7 | 4 | 2 | 1 |

_____ + _____ = _____   _____

TOTAL SCORE _____

Problems from Close to 0

Suppose you are dealt these hands in a game of Close to 0.
What numbers would you make for the best score?
(Best score = difference as close to 0 as possible)

Score

Round 1   5   3   <u>6</u>   <u>9</u>   0   <u>6</u>   2   1

_____ − _____ = _____   _____

Round 2   4   8   1   5   7   2   8   <u>6</u>

_____ − _____ = _____   _____

Round 3   1   0   1   5   <u>9</u>   0   2   <u>6</u>

_____ − _____ = _____   _____

Round 4   <u>6</u>   2   3   2   4   8   5   0

_____ − _____ = _____   _____

Round 5   8   4   0   2   7   3   <u>9</u>   1

_____ − _____ = _____   _____

TOTAL SCORE _____

Add a Clue

Here are three clues of a number puzzle:

My number is a factor of 1000.
My number is a multiple of 25.
My number is a factor of 300.

1. What numbers fit these three clues?

2. How did you find the numbers that fit the clues?

3. Write a fourth clue that gives the puzzle just one answer. Do *not* use a clue about what the number is greater than, and do *not* use a clue about what the number is less than.

4. What is the answer to your new puzzle? How do you know?

Another Add a Clue

Here are three clues of a number puzzle:

My number is a factor of 3000.
My number is a factor of 50.
My number is a factor of 900.

1. What numbers fit these three clues?

2. How did you find the numbers that fit the clues?

3. Write a fourth clue that gives the puzzle just one answer. *Do not* use a clue about what the number is greater than, and *do not* use a clue about what the number is less than.

4. What is the answer to your new puzzle? How do you know?

0	0	1	1
0	0	1	1
2	2	3	3
2	2	3	3

4	4	5	5
4	4	5	5
6	6	7	7
6	6	7	7

Investigation 4 • Resource
Mathematical Thinking at Grade 5

8	8	9	9
8	8	9	9
WILD CARD	WILD CARD		
WILD CARD	WILD CARD		

NUMBER PUZZLES 15-16

Puzzle 15

My number is a factor of 200.

Puzzle 15

My number has one digit.

Puzzle 15

My number of tiles cannot be made into a square.

Puzzle 15

My number of tiles will make a rectangle 2 tiles wide.

Puzzle 16

My number is a factor of 100.

Puzzle 16

My number of tiles will make a rectangle 5 tiles wide.

Puzzle 16

My number is greater than 10.

Puzzle 16

My number of tiles can be made into a square.

Puzzle 17 My number is a factor of 10,000.	**Puzzle 17** My number is less than 3000.
Puzzle 17 My number has four digits.	**Puzzle 17** Three of the digits in my number are 0.

Puzzle 18 My number is a factor of 1000.	**Puzzle 18** My number is a multiple of 25.
Puzzle 18 My number is a factor of 600.	**Puzzle 18** My number is a square number.

Puzzle 19

My number is a factor of 1000.

Puzzle 19

My number is a multiple of 10.

Puzzle 19

My number is a factor of 500.

Puzzle 19

My number is less than 45.

Puzzle 20

My number is prime.

Puzzle 20

My number is a factor of 100.

Puzzle 20

My number has two digits.

Puzzle 20

My number is a factor of 1000.

Investigation 4 • Resource
Mathematical Thinking at Grade 5

Puzzle 21

My number is a factor of 1000.

Puzzle 21

My number is a multiple of 50.

Puzzle 21

My number is not a multiple of 100.

Puzzle 21

My number has three digits.

Puzzle 22

You say my number when you start at 0 and count by 75's.

Puzzle 22

You say my number when you start at 0 and count by 125's.

Puzzle 22

My number is even.

Puzzle 22

My number has three digits.

☆☆☆☆☆   **Puzzle 23**☆

My number is a factor of 1000.

☆☆☆☆☆   **Puzzle 23**☆

My number has fewer than three digits.

☆☆☆☆☆   **Puzzle 23**☆

My number is not a factor of 100.

☆☆☆☆☆   **Puzzle 23**☆

My number is a multiple of 5.

☆☆☆☆☆   **Puzzle 24**☆

My number is a multiple of 25.

☆☆☆☆☆   **Puzzle 24**☆

My number has three digits.

☆☆☆☆☆   **Puzzle 24**☆

My number is greater than 500.

☆☆☆☆☆   **Puzzle 24**☆

The sum of the digits in my number is 20.

☆☆☆☆☆   **Puzzle 25☆**

My number is a factor
of 10,000.

☆☆☆☆☆   **Puzzle 25☆**

My number has four digits.

☆☆☆☆☆   **Puzzle 25☆**

My number is not a multiple
of 1000.

☆☆☆☆☆   **Puzzle 25☆**

My number is a multiple
of 250.

☆☆☆☆☆   **Puzzle 26☆**

My number is a multiple of 50.

☆☆☆☆☆   **Puzzle 26☆**

My number is a multiple of 90.

☆☆☆☆☆   **Puzzle 26☆**

My number has three digits.

☆☆☆☆☆   **Puzzle 26☆**

My number is greater
than 500.

☆☆☆☆☆   **Puzzle 27**☆

My number is a square
number.

☆☆☆☆☆   **Puzzle 27**☆

My number is a factor
of 10,000.

☆☆☆☆☆   **Puzzle 27**☆

My number is even.

☆☆☆☆☆   **Puzzle 27**☆

My number has two digits.

☆☆☆☆☆   **Puzzle 28**☆

My number is a factor of 1000.

☆☆☆☆☆   **Puzzle 28**☆

My number is not a factor
of 10,000.

☆☆☆☆☆   **Puzzle 28**☆

My number is a multiple of 50.

☆☆☆☆☆   **Puzzle 28**☆

My number is a multiple of 8.

© Dale Seymour Publications®

Investigation 4 • Resource
Mathematical Thinking at Grade 5

300 CHART

1	2	3	4	5	6	7	8	9	10
11	12	13	14	15	16	17	18	19	20
21	22	23	24	25	26	27	28	29	30
31	32	33	34	35	36	37	38	39	40
41	42	43	44	45	46	47	48	49	50
51	52	53	54	55	56	57	58	59	60
61	62	63	64	65	66	67	68	69	70
71	72	73	74	75	76	77	78	79	80
81	82	83	84	85	86	87	88	89	90
91	92	93	94	95	96	97	98	99	100
101	102	103	104	105	106	107	108	109	110
111	112	113	114	115	116	117	118	119	120
121	122	123	124	125	126	127	128	129	130
131	132	133	134	135	136	137	138	139	140
141	142	143	144	145	146	147	148	149	150
151	152	153	154	155	156	157	158	159	160
161	162	163	164	165	166	167	168	169	170
171	172	173	174	175	176	177	178	179	180
181	182	183	184	185	186	187	188	189	190
191	192	193	194	195	196	197	198	199	200
201	202	203	204	205	206	207	208	209	210
211	212	213	214	215	216	217	218	219	220
221	222	223	224	225	226	227	228	229	230
231	232	233	234	235	236	237	238	239	240
241	242	243	244	245	246	247	248	249	250
251	252	253	254	255	256	257	258	259	260
261	262	263	264	265	266	267	268	269	270
271	272	273	274	275	276	277	278	279	280
281	282	283	284	285	286	287	288	289	290
291	292	293	294	295	296	297	298	299	300

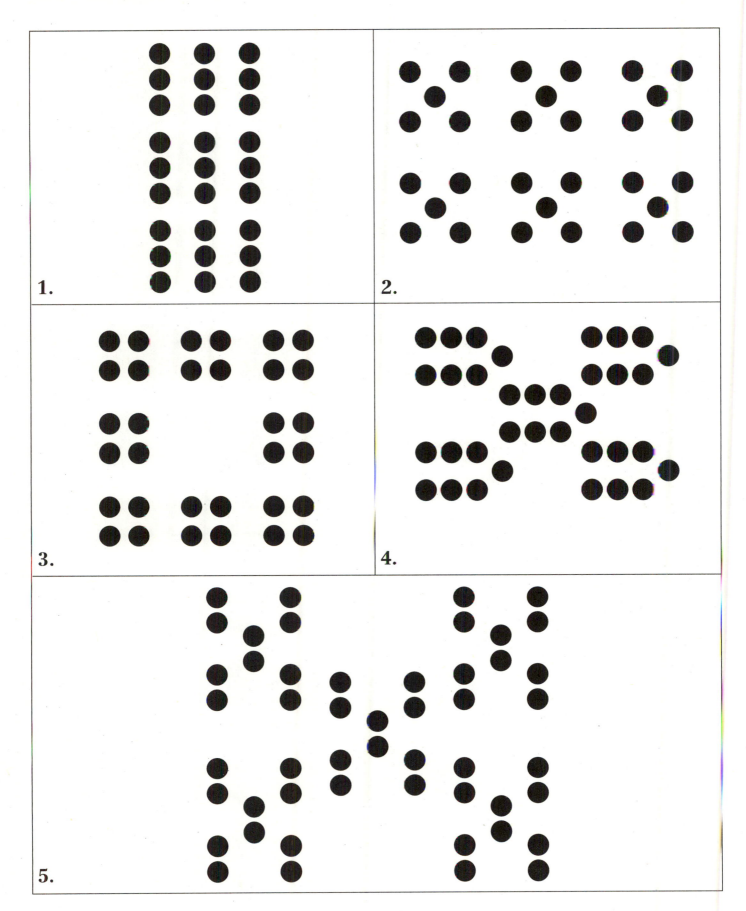

Ten-Minute Math
Mathematical Thinking at Grade 5

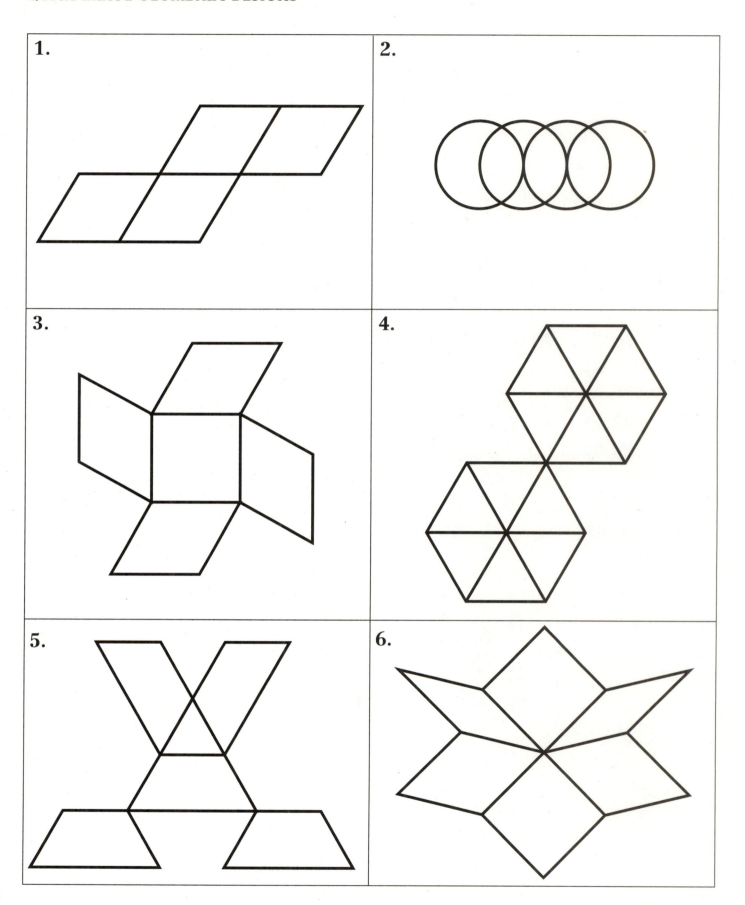

1.

2.

3.

4.

5.

6.

Practice Pages

This optional section provides homework ideas for teachers who want or need to give more homework than is assigned to accompany the activities in this unit. The problems included here provide additional practice in learning about number relationships and in solving computation and number problems. For number units, you may want to use some of these if your students need more work in these areas or if you want to assign daily homework. For other units, you can use these problems so that students can continue to work on developing number and computation sense while they are focusing on other mathematical content in class. We recommend that you introduce activities in class before assigning related problems for homework.

Solving Problems in Two Ways   Students explore different ways to solve computation problems in the units *Mathematical Thinking at Grade 5* and *Building on Numbers You Know*. Here, we provide five sheets of problems that students solve in two different ways. Problems may include addition, subtraction, multiplication, or division. Students record each way they solved the problem.

Story Problems   Story problems at various levels of difficulty are used throughout the *Investigations* curriculum. The three story problem sheets provided here help students review and maintain skills that have already been taught. You can make up other problems in this format, using numbers and contexts that are appropriate for your students. Students solve the problems and then record their strategies.

Practice Page A

Solve this problem in two different ways, and write about how you solved it:

$$307 - 289 =$$

Here is the first way I solved it:

Here is the second way I solved it:

Practice Page B

Solve this problem in two different ways, and write about
how you solved it:

$$354 + 534 =$$

Here is the first way I solved it:

Here is the second way I solved it:

Practice Page C

Solve this problem in two different ways, and write about how you solved it:

$$42 \times 19 =$$

Here is the first way I solved it:

Here is the second way I solved it:

Practice Page D

Solve this problem in two different ways, and write about
how you solved it:

789 + 1038 =

Here is the first way I solved it:

Here is the second way I solved it:

Practice Page E

Solve this problem in two different ways, and write about
how you solved it:

104 ÷ 8 =

Here is the first way I solved it:

Here is the second way I solved it:

Practice Page F

In our classroom we have 4 bookcases. Each bookcase has 4 shelves. On each shelf there are 10 books. How many books do we have in our classroom?

Show how you solved this problem. You can use numbers, words, or pictures.

Practice Page G

We have 140 music cassettes that we want to sell at the flea market. We will put 14 cassettes in each bag to sell. How many bags of cassettes will we have?

Show how you solved this problem. You can use numbers, words, or pictures.

Practice Page H

My friend has 24 pencils in a box. She wants to divide them equally among herself, her sister, and me. How many pencils will we each get?

Show how you solved this problem. You can use numbers, words, or pictures.